insulin (regular)	isoproterenol	lactated Ringer's	lidocaine	methylprednisolone sodium succinate	mezlocillin	midazolam	morphine sulfate	nafcillin	norepinephrine	normal saline solution	ondansetron	oxacillin	oxytocin	penicillin G potassium	phenylephrine	phenytoin	phytonadione	piperacillin	potassium chloride	procainamide	ranitidine	sodium bicarbonate	ticarcillin	tobramycin	vancomycin	verapamil
acyclovir			4		4			4	4			4		4					4	4		4	4	4	4	4	4
albumin																											
amikacin			24				24	4		24	24	4	8		8			24		4		24	24			24	24
aminophylline			24	24	?			24		24							4	24		24	24					4	4
amiodarone	24	24		24			24	24	24		24	4						4	24		24	24			4	4	24
ampicillin	2				4				8						3		4		?	?				?			
calcium gluconate			24	24		24			24			24						4			?			1			48
cefazolin	2		24			24			24	4		24	4					?						?		2	24
cefoxitin	24		24				4		24	4								24		24							
ceftazidime					4				24	4							?	6									
cimetidine	24	24		24	24		24		48	4			24		24		24									24	24
ciprofloxacin		48	24		24							24	24		24				24							24	24
clindamycin		24		24		24	4		24	4			4				48	24		?	24		48				24
dexamethasone sodium phosphate										4										24	4	4					24
dextrose 5% in water (D₅W)		24		24	?	24			24	24		48	6	6	24			24	24	24	48	24	24	24	24	24	24
D₅W in lactated Ringer's		24		24					24			24			24				24								
D₅W in normal saline solution		24		24	?			24				48	?		24				24	24		24		48			24
diazepam																				?							24
diphenhydramine					4	1/4			4			4			24				4	1							
dobutamine		24	24	24		4	4		4	24	24				24				?	24	48						24
dopamine		48	24	18		4	4		48		24							24	48								24
epinephrine		24			4	4		4	24						3		4		24								24
erythromycin lactobionate		18			24	4			22										24	24							24
esmolol		24			24	8	24	24	24			24		24		24	24		24				24	24	24	24	
gentamicin	2		24			24	1		24	4					1				24								24
heparin sodium	2	24		24		24	1			4	4	4	?		4	6	24	4	24	24	6						24
hydrocortisone sodium succinate	4	4	24		?		4			24	4	4		4	24		4		24								24
insulin (regular)			24			24	1			4			2				4		24	3	2	2	2	48			
isoproterenol			24							24									24								24
lactated Ringer's		24		24	?	72			24				24						24	24			24	24			48
lidocaine	24		24					4	48		24										24	24	24				48
methylprednisolone sodium succinate		?				24	4					?			24					?		48	2				24
mezlocillin		72									48																
midazolam	24			24				24		24		24							24	24					24	24	
morphine sulfate	1		4	4		24		4	4		4	4	4		4	1			4	4		1	3	4	1	4	24
nafcillin			24	48			4						24						24		24						
norepinephrine			24	4					24		4										4						
normal saline solution		24		24	?	48			24	24		48	24		24				24	24	24	48	24	24	48	24	24
ondansetron					24	4			48				4						4		4		4		4		
oxacillin			24					4			4								24								
oxytocin	2							1											4			24					24
penicillin G potassium		24		24				4			24								24			24					24
phenylephrine																			24			24					24
phenytoin																				24			24				48
phytonadione																			4			24					
piperacillin		24			24	4			24										24		4						24
potassium chloride	4		24		?		24	4	24		24	4		4			24		4	24		4	48	24			24
procainamide			24							24										24							48
ranitidine	24	24		24	48			1		4	48	4			24				4	48	24			24	24	24	
sodium bicarbonate	3		24	2					3	24		24			24		24	24	24								
ticarcillin	2		24							4		1		48						24							24
tobramycin	2		24						24	1			48						24	4				24			24
vancomycin	2		24						24	4			24	4					24	4				24			24
verapamil	48	24	24	48	24			24		24	24			24	24			48		24	24	48			24	24	24

8th Edition

Nursing

I.V. DRUG HANDBOOK

LIPPINCOTT WILLIAMS & WILKINS
A **Wolters Kluwer** Company

Philadelphia • Baltimore • New York • London
Buenos Aires • Hong Kong • Sydney • Tokyo

Staff

Publisher
Judith A. Schilling McCann, RN, MSN

Editorial Director
William J. Kelly

Clinical Director
Joan M. Robinson, RN, MSN

Senior Art Director
Arlene Putterman

Art Director
Elaine Kasmer

Clinical Manager
Eileen Cassin Gallen, RN, BSN

Drug Information Editor
Melissa M. Devlin, PharmD

Senior Editor
Ann E. Houska

Editors
Rita Doyle, Patricia Nale, Carol Turkington

Clinical Editors
Lisa M. Bonsall, RN, MSN, CRNP;
Christine M. Damico, RN, MSN, CPNP;
Kimberly A. Zalewski, RN, MSN

Copy Editors
Louise Quinn, Patricia Turkington

Digital Composition Services
Diane Paluba (manager),
Donald G. Knauss (project manager),
Joyce Rossi Biletz (senior desktop assistant)

Manufacturing
Patricia K. Dorshaw (manager),
Beth Janae Orr (book production manager)

Editorial Assistants
Carol A. Caputo, Tara Carter-Bell,
Arlene P. Claffee

Indexer
Deborah K. Tourtlotte

Visit our Web site at NDHnow.com

IVDH8–D N
05 04 03 10 9 8 7 6 5 4 3 2 1
ISSN 1040-2373
ISBN 1-58255-265-7

CONTENTS

Pharmacologic Classes

I.V. Drugs, Solutions, and Blood Products

Appendices and Index

Appendices

Drug Updates on the Internet .... NDHnow.com

CONTRIBUTORS AND CONSULTANTS

Lauren D. Blough, RN, BSN, CRNI
Clinical Specialist and Educator,
    Infusion Therapy
Florida Hospital
Orlando, Fla.

James Caldwell, PharmD
Clinical Pharmacy Coordinator
Anne Arundel Medical Center
Annapolis, Md.

Lawrence P. Carey, PharmD
Assistant Professor, Physician
    Assistant Studies
Philadelphia University
Philadelphia, Pa.

Lisa Colodny, PharmD, BCNSP
Regional Pharmacy Manager
Coral Springs Medical Center
Coral Springs, Fla.

Noreen Coyne, RN, MSN, CRNI, OCN
National Director of Clinical Standards
    & Development
Tender Loving Care, Staff Builders
    Home Health Care
Lake Success, N.Y.

Tracy Farnese, PharmD
Medical Information Specialist
McNeil Consumer & Specialty
    Pharmaceuticals
Fort Washington, Pa.

Christopher A. Fausel, PharmD, BCPS,
BCOP
Clinical Pharmacist
Indiana University Hospital
Indianapolis, Ind.

Tatyana Gurvich, PharmD
Clinical Pharmacologist
Glendale Adventist FPRP
Glendale, Calif.

AnhThu Hoang, PharmD
North York, Ontario

Kristy H. Lucas, PharmD
Assistant Professor
West Virginia University–Charleston
Charleston, W. Va.

Randall A. Lynch, PharmD
Assistant Director, Pharmacy
Presbyterian Medical Center
University of Pennsylvania Health
    System
Philadelphia, Pa.

Nicole M. Maisch, RPh, PharmD
Assistant Clinical Professor of
    Pharmacy Practice
St. John's University College of
    Pharmacy and Allied Health
    Professions
Jamaica, N.Y.

Marie Maloney, PharmD
Clinical Pharmacist
University Medical Center
Tucson, Ariz.

George Melko, RPh, PharmD
Independent Consultant
West Chester, Pa.

William O'Hara, PharmD
Clinical Coordinator
Thomas Jefferson Hospital
Philadelphia, Pa.

David Pipher, RPh, PharmD
Director of Pharmacy
Forbes Regional Hospital
Monroeville, Pa.

Christine Price, PharmD
Clinical Coordinator
Morton Plant Mease Health Care
Dunedin, Fla.

Jeffrey B. Purcell, PharmD
Clinical Lead Pharmacist
Harborview Medical Center
Seattle, Wash.

Barbara Reville, CRNP, MS, BC, AOCN
Clinical Instructor
University of Pennsylvania School of
    Nursing
Philadelphia, Pa.

Susan W. Sard, PharmD
Clinical Pharmacist
Anne Arundel Medical Center
Annapolis, Md.

Michele F. Shepherd, PharmD, MS, BCPS,
FASHP
Clinical Specialist
Abbott Northwestern Hospital
Minneapolis, Minn.

Wendy J. Smith, RN, MSN, ACNP, AOCN
Nurse Practitioner
The West Clinic
Memphis, Tenn.

Joseph F. Steiner, RPh, PharmD
Dean and Professor of Pharmacy
    Practice
Idaho State University College of
    Pharmacy
Pocatello, Idaho

Joanne Whitney, RPh, PharmD, PhD
Director, Drug Products Laboratory
Associate Clinical Professor
University of California
San Francisco, Calif.

Barbara S. Wiggins, PharmD
Pharmacy Clinical Specialist
University of Virginia Health System
Charlottesville, Va.

Every year, as the pharmacopoeia of I.V. drugs expands, the body of knowledge increases. For each drug you encounter, you need precise information on indications, dosages, preparation and incompatibilities, administration techniques, and interactions. You also need clear guidelines on how to prevent complications such as extravasation, infection, hypersensitivity, phlebitis, and occluded catheters. Should complications develop during or after therapy, you need immediate guidelines on how to respond.

Nursing I.V. Drug Handbook, Eighth Edition, provides quick access to the crucial details that make safe and effective administration of I.V. drugs possible. This edition contains new features to enhance nursing knowledge and skills. New in this edition are a section describing pharmacologic classes; an updated table showing drug compatibilities; a special symbol to alert you to drugs containing benzyl alcohol; a special symbol for off-label uses; expanded information about availability and mixing, compatibility, and storage; a new section showing effects on laboratory test results; and several new appendices on topics including chemotherapeutic drugs, drug errors, dialysis, and therapeutic monitoring.

PHARMACOLOGIC CLASSES

Listed alphabetically at the front of the book are synopses of 25 major pharmacologic classes of I.V. drugs. This section lets you compare the effects and uses of drugs within their classes. Each entry describes the pharmacology, clinical indications and actions, adverse reactions, and special considerations for drugs that belong to a pharmacologic group, along with tips for use in pregnant, breast-feeding, pediatric, and geriatric patients and pointers for patient education. You'll also find tables throughout this section that allow you to compare drugs within and between pharmacologic classes.

COMPREHENSIVE ENTRIES

The heart of the book contains complete, easy-to-use entries on I.V. drugs as well as blood products, amino acid solutions, dextrose solutions, colloid and crystalloid solutions, and fat emulsions. Entries are listed alphabetically by generic name. Trade names appear under generic names.

Generic and trade names are followed by pharmacologic class, therapeutic class, pregnancy risk category and, when appropriate, controlled substance schedule and pH. Normal pH is 7.35 to 7.45. Drugs with a pH below 7.35 are acidic; those with a pH above 7.45, basic. Drugs that are highly acidic or basic are more likely to contribute to phlebitis.

Indications & dosages gives you the indications for I.V. use of the drug and dosages for adults and children. Dosage adjustments, such as those needed for patients with renal impairment, are highlighted with the **Adjust-a-dose** logo. *Administration* gives you specific instructions for delivering the drug by the appropriate methods: direct injection, intermittent infusion, and continuous infusion. Rates are provided when available. *Incompatibilities* tells you which other drugs and solutions shouldn't be mixed with the drug.

Contraindications & cautions explains when the drug is contraindicated and when you should be especially careful giving it. Classified by body system, *Adverse reactions* lists potential common, uncommon, life-threatening, and common and life-threatening reactions.

Interactions details the effects of using the drug with other drugs, herbs, or food as well as the effects resulting from lifestyle practices such as using tobacco or alcohol.

Effects on lab test results lists altered levels, counts, and other values in laboratory test results that a drug may cause.

Action describes how the drug achieves its therapeutic effects. *Pharmacokinetics* provides information on the drug's distribution, metabolism, and excretion. For solutions and blood products that don't have these characteristics, *Composition* appears in place of these two headings, offering a breakdown of the product's components.

Clinical considerations covers key nursing concerns not included elsewhere—including osmolarity, osmolality, tips on drug administration, therapy modification for certain patients, and treatment for overdose. Osmolarity is the measure of a solute concentration in terms of liters of solution, whereas osmolality is measured in terms of kilograms of water. This information, like a drug's pH, is helpful in determining a drug's or a fluid's potential for causing phlebitis.

Finally, *Patient teaching* includes topics to teach patients, such as the purpose of the drug and the importance of reporting burning at the I.V. site and other adverse reactions.

APPENDICES AND INDEX

New appendices include acronyms and protocols used in chemotherapy regimens, drug names that look or sound alike, the most common drug errors, therapeutic monitoring guidelines, and drugs removed by dialysis.

Other appendices cover major electrolyte components for I.V. solutions, preventing and treating drug extravasation, guidelines for handling chemotherapeutic drugs, and selected drugs for conscious sedation. Also included

are flow rates for dobutamine, dopamine, epinephrine, isoproterenol, nitroglycerin, and nitroprusside infusions.

The inside front cover contains a compatibility table for 60 commonly used I.V. drugs. The inside back cover features a blood-type compatibility table, helpful information about calculating I.V. drug dosages, and definitions of osmolality, osmolarity, and pH.

The index lets you look up drug information by generic name, trade name, and indication.

NDHnow.com

As an added benefit, you can access **NDHnow.com**, the Web site that keeps your handbook current by providing drug updates and important drug news.

ACE	angiotensin-converting enzyme	**g**	gram
ADH	antidiuretic hormone	**G**	gauge
AIDS	acquired immunodeficiency syndrome	**GFR**	glomerular filtration rate
		GGT	gamma-glutamyltransferase
ALT	serum alanine aminotransferase	**GI**	gastrointestinal
		gtt	drops
aPTT	activated partial thromboplastin time	**G6PD**	glucose-6-phosphate dehydrogenase
AST	serum aspartate aminotransferase	**GU**	genitourinary
		H_1	histamine$_1$
AV	atrioventricular	H_2	histamine$_2$
b.i.d.	twice daily	**HIV**	human immunodeficiency virus
BPH	benign prostatic hyperplasia		
BUN	blood urea nitrogen	**hr**	hour
cAMP	cyclic 3′,5′ adenosine monophosphate	**h.s.**	at bedtime
		ICU	intensive care unit
CBC	complete blood count	**I.D.**	intradermal
CK	creatine kinase	**I.M.**	intramuscular
CMV	cytomegalovirus	**INR**	international normalized ratio
CNS	central nervous system		
COPD	chronic obstructive pulmonary disease	**IPPB**	intermittent positive-pressure breathing
CPR	cardiopulmonary resuscitation	**IU**	International Unit
		I.V.	intravenous
CSF	cerebrospinal fluid	**kg**	kilogram
CV	cardiovascular	**L**	liter
CVA	cerebrovascular accident	**lb**	pound
D_5W	dextrose 5% in water	**LDH**	lactate dehydrogenase
DIC	disseminated intravascular coagulation	**M**	molar
		m^2	square meter
DNA	deoxyribonucleic acid	**MAO**	monoamine oxidase
ECG	electrocardiogram	**mcg**	microgram
EEG	electroencephalogram	**mEq**	milliequivalent
EENT	eyes, ears, nose, throat	**mg**	milligram
FDA	Food and Drug Administration	**MI**	myocardial infarction
		min	minute

ml	milliliter
mm^3	cubic millimeter
mOsm	milliosmol
ng	nanogram (millimicrogram)
NG	nasogastric
NSAID	nonsteroidal anti-inflammatory drug
OTC	over-the-counter
PABA	para-aminobenzoic acid
PCA	patient-controlled analgesia
P.O.	by mouth
P.R.	by rectum
p.r.n.	as needed
PT	prothrombin time
PTT	partial thromboplastin time
PVC	premature ventricular contraction
q	every
q.i.d.	four times daily
RBC	red blood cell
RDA	recommended daily allowance
REM	rapid eye movement
RNA	ribonucleic acid
RSV	respiratory syncytial virus
SA	sinoatrial
S.C.	subcutaneous
SIADH	syndrome of inappropriate antidiuretic hormone
S.L.	sublingual
SSRI	selective serotonin reuptake inhibitor
T$_3$	triiodothyronine
T$_4$	thyroxine
t.i.d.	three times daily
TPN	total parenteral nutrition
UTI	urinary tract infection
WBC	white blood cell

Pharmacologic classes

adrenergics

albuterol sulfate, arbutamine
hydrochloride, bitolterol mesylate,
brimonidine tartrate, dobutamine
hydrochloride, dopamine
hydrochloride, ephedrine,
epinephrine, epinephryl borate,
isoetharine hydrochloride,
isoproterenol, levalbuterol,
metaproterenol sulfate,
naphazoline hydrochloride,
norepinephrine bitartrate,
phenylephrine hydrochloride,
pirbuterol acetate,
pseudoephedrine, salmeterol
xinafoate, terbutaline sulfate,
tetrahydrozoline hydrochloride,
xylometazoline hydrochloride

The cellular causes of alpha-receptor activation aren't fully understood. Adenylate cyclase activation and cAMP accumulation cause beta-receptor activation.

Alpha$_1$ receptors are located on smooth muscle and glands and are excitatory; alpha$_2$ receptors are prejunctional regulatory receptors in the CNS and postjunctional receptors in many peripheral tissues. Beta$_1$ receptors are located in cardiac tissues and are excitatory; beta$_2$ receptors are located primarily on smooth muscle and glands and are inhibitory.

Adrenergic drugs may mimic the naturally occurring catecholamines norepinephrine, epinephrine, and dopamine. They also may stimulate the release of norepinephrine.

PHARMACOLOGY
Most adrenergics affect peripheral excitatory actions on glands and vascular smooth muscle; cardiac and CNS excitatory actions; peripheral inhibitory actions on smooth muscle of the bronchial tree and blood vessels supplying skeletal muscles and gut; and metabolic and endocrine effects. Because tissues respond differently to adrenergic agonists, catecholamine actions vary according to which receptor type—alpha or beta—is found in the tissues.

INDICATIONS & ACTIONS
Most adrenergics affect alpha and beta activity. Dopaminergic and serotonergic activity may occur, possibly stimulating receptors in the CNS to release histamine.

Appetite suppression is a temporary drug effect, which often causes weight gain after the patient develops tolerance or the drug is discontinued. Drug is used also to treat hypotension, control urinary incontinence and enuresis, and relieve pain of dysmenorrhea.

➤**Hypotension**—
Alpha agonists, such as norepinephrine, phenylephrine, and pseudoephedrine, constrict arteries and veins, which increases blood pressure. This helps treat hypotension and manage serious allergic conditions. Topical alpha agonists induce local vasoconstriction (decongestion), stop superficial hemorrhage (styptic), stimulate radial smooth muscle of the iris (mydriasis), and, with local anesthetics, localize anesthesia and prolong duration of action. Ophthalmic preparations reduce aqueous humor production and increase uveoscleral outflow.

➤**Cardiac stimulation**—
Beta$_1$ agonists, such as dobutamine, act primarily in the heart, producing a positive inotropic effect. Because they increase heart rate, enhance AV conduction, and increase the strength of the heartbeat, beta$_1$ agonists may be used

---

♦ Off-label use

to restore heartbeat in cardiac arrest, to relieve heart block in syncopal seizures (not a treatment of choice), or to treat acute heart failure and cardiogenic or other types of shock. The use of beta$_1$ agonists in shock is controversial because these drugs increase free fatty acids, leading to metabolic acidosis, and because they may cause arrhythmias, which pose a special threat in cardiogenic shock.

➤**Bronchodilation—**
Beta$_2$ agonists, such as albuterol, bitolterol, isoetharine, isoproterenol, metaproterenol, salmeterol, pirbuterol, and terbutaline, act primarily on smooth muscle of the bronchial tree, vasculature, intestines, and uterus. They also induce hepatic and muscle glycogenolysis, which results in hyperglycemia (sometimes useful in insulin overdose) and hyperlactic acidemia.

Some beta$_2$ agonists are used as bronchodilators, others as vasodilators. They're also used to relax the uterus, delay delivery in premature labor, and relieve symptoms of dysmenorrhea. Some degree of cardiac stimulation may occur because all beta$_2$ agonists (especially isoproterenol) have some degree of beta$_1$ activity.

➤**Renal vasodilation—**
Dopamine is the only commercially available sympathomimetic with significant dopaminergic activity, although some other sympathomimetics seem to act on dopamine receptors in the CNS. Dopamine receptors are prominent in the splanchnic and renal vasculature, where they mediate vasodilation. This helps induce diuresis in patients with acute renal failure, heart failure, and shock.

ADVERSE REACTIONS
Geriatric patients, infants, and patients with thyrotoxicosis or CV disease are more sensitive to the effects of these drugs.

Alpha agonists usually produce CV reactions. Extreme hypertension is a major adverse effect of systemic alpha agonists. Hypertensive or geriatric patients may develop an exaggerated pressor response, which may cause vagal reflex responses leading to bradycardia and AV block. Alpha agonists also interfere with breast-feeding and may cause nausea, vomiting, sweating, piloerection, rebound congestion or miosis, difficulty urinating, and headache. Ophthalmic use may cause mydriasis, photophobia, burning or stinging eyes, and blurred vision.

Beta agonists often cause tachycardia, tachyarrhythmias, palpitations, premature atrial and ventricular contractions, and myocardial necrosis. Reflex tachycardia and palpitations result from hypotension.

Metabolic reactions to beta agonists include hyperglycemia, increased metabolic rate, hyperlactic acidosis, and local and systemic acidosis (decreased bronchodilator response). Respiratory reactions include COPD and mucus plugs from increased mucus secretion. Other reactions include tremors, vertigo, insomnia, and anxiety.

Centrally acting adrenergics have similar effects and may also cause dry mouth, flushing, diarrhea, impotence, hyperthermia (in excessive doses), agitation, anorexia, dizziness, dyskinesia, and changes in libido. Long-term use of adrenergics in children may cause arrested growth; however, growth usually recovers after drug is stopped.

LIFESPAN CONSIDERATIONS
● Pregnancy risk categories range from B to D in this group.
● Avoid using adrenergics in breast-feeding patients.
● Lower doses of adrenergics are recommended in children.
● Geriatric patients usually need lower doses because they may be more sensitive to therapeutic and adverse effects of some adrenergics.

adrenocorticoids

Glucocorticoids: betamethasone, cortisone acetate, dexamethasone, hydrocortisone, methylprednisolone, prednisolone, prednisone, triamcinolone

Mineralocorticoid: fludrocortisone acetate

Adrenocorticoids (also known as corticosteroids) are classified according to their activity into two groups: glucocorticoids and mineralocorticoids. *Glucocorticoids* regulate carbohydrate, lipid, and protein metabolism, inflammation, and the body's immune responses to diverse stimuli. *Mineralocorticoids* regulate electrolyte homeostasis. Many adrenocorticoids exert both kinds of activity. (See *Comparing systemic glucocorticoids,* page 4.)

PHARMACOLOGY

Adrenocorticoids dramatically affect almost all body systems. They control the rate of protein synthesis, reacting with receptor proteins in the cytoplasm of sensitive cells to form a steroid-receptor complex. The steroid-receptor complex migrates into the nucleus of the cell, where it binds to chromatin. Information carried by the steroid of the receptor protein directs the genetic apparatus to transcribe RNA, resulting in the synthesis of specific proteins that serve as enzymes in various biochemical pathways. Because the maximum pharmacologic activity lags behind peak blood levels, the effects of adrenocorticoids may result from modification of enzyme activity rather than from direct action by the drugs.

Glucocorticoids stimulate transcription of messenger RNA in individual cell nuclei to synthesize enzymes that decrease inflammation. These enzymes stimulate biochemical pathways that decrease the inflammatory response by stabilizing leukocyte lysosomal membranes, which prevent the release of destructive acid hydrolases from leukocytes; inhibiting macrophage accumulation in inflamed areas; reducing leukocyte adhesion to the capillary endothelium; reducing capillary wall permeability and edema formation; decreasing complement components; antagonizing histamine activity and release of kinin from substrates; reducing fibroblast proliferation, collagen deposition, and scar tissue formation; and by other unknown mechanisms.

Mineralocorticoids act renally at the distal tubules to enhance the reabsorption of sodium ions—and water—from the tubular fluid into the plasma, and the urinary excretion of both potassium and hydrogen ions.

INDICATIONS & ACTIONS
➤**Asthma**—
Systemic glucocorticoids treat status asthmaticus and acute asthma episodes, when combined with sympathomimetics and aminophylline.
➤**Sarcoidosis**—
Systemic glucocorticoids treat ocular, CNS, glandular, myocardial, and severe pulmonary involvement; they're also used for hypercalcemia and severe skin lesions.
➤**Advanced pulmonary or extrapulmonary tuberculosis**—
Systemic glucocorticoids help decrease inflammation caused by *Mycobacterium tuberculosis.*
➤**Pericarditis ♦**—
An unlabeled use for systemic glucocorticoids is to treat pain, fever, and inflammation of pericarditis.
➤**Inflammation**—
A major use of these drugs is to treat inflammation. The anti-inflammatory effects depend on the direct local action of the steroids. Glucocorticoids decrease the inflammatory response by stabilizing leukocyte lysosomal mem-

Comparing systemic glucocorticoids

Drug	Equivalent dose (mg)	Relative glucocorticoid (anti-inflammatory) potency	Relative mineralo-corticoid potency	Plasma half-life (hr)	Biological half-life (hr)
betamethasone, oral	0.6-0.75	20-30	0	> 5	36-54
betamethasone acetate	0.6-0.75	20-30	0	> 5	36-54
betamethasone sodium phosphate	0.6-0.75	20-30	0	> 5	36-54
cortisone acetate	25	0.8	2	$\frac{1}{2}$	8-12
dexamethasone, oral	0.5-0.75	20-30	0	$2-3\frac{1}{2}$	36-54
dexamethasone acetate	0.5-0.75	20-30	0	$2-3\frac{1}{2}$	36-54
dexamethasone sodium phosphate	0.5-0.75	20-30	0	$2-3\frac{1}{2}$	36-54
hydrocortisone, oral	20	1	2	$1\frac{1}{2}-2$	8-12
hydrocortisone acetate	20	1	2	$1\frac{1}{2}-2$	8-12
hydrocortisone cypionate	20	1	2	$1\frac{1}{2}-2$	8-12
hydrocortisone sodium phosphate	20	1	2	$1\frac{1}{2}-2$	8-12
hydrocortisone sodium succinate	20	1	2	$1\frac{1}{2}-2$	8-12
methylprednisolone, oral	4	5	0	1-3	18-36
methylprednisolone acetate	4	5	0	1-3	18-36
methylprednisolone sodium succinate	4	5	0	1-3	18-36
prednisolone, oral	5	4	1	$2\frac{1}{4}-3\frac{1}{2}$	18-36
prednisolone acetate	5	4	1	$2\frac{1}{4}-3\frac{1}{2}$	18-36
prednisolone sodium phosphate	5	4	1	$2\frac{1}{4}-3\frac{1}{2}$	18-36
prednisolone tebutate	5	4	1	$2\frac{1}{4}-3\frac{1}{2}$	18-36
prednisone	5	4	1	1	18-36
triamcinolone, oral	4	5	0	$> 3\frac{1}{3}$	18-36
triamcinolone acetonide	4	5	0	$> 3\frac{1}{3}$	18-36
triamcinolone diacetate	4	5	0	$> 3\frac{1}{3}$	18-36
triamcinolone hexacetonide	4	5	0	$> 3\frac{1}{3}$	18-36

branes, which prevent the release of destructive acid hydrolases from leukocytes; inhibiting macrophage accumulation in inflamed areas; reducing leukocyte adhesion to the capillary endothelium; reducing capillary wall permeability and edema formation; decreasing complement components; antagonizing histamine activity and release of kinin from substrates; reducing fibroblast proliferation, collagen deposition, and subsequent scar tissue formation; and by other unknown mechanisms.

➤Immunosuppression—
All the mechanisms of immunosuppressive action are unknown. Glucocorticoids reduce activity and volume of the lymphatic system, producing lymphocytopenia, decreasing immunoglobulin and complement levels, decreasing passage of immune complexes through basement membranes, and possibly depressing reactivity of tissue to antigen-antibody interaction.

➤Adrenal insufficiency—
Combined mineralocorticoid and glucocorticoid therapy is used to treat adrenal insufficiency and salt-losing forms of congenital adrenogenital syndrome.

➤Rheumatic and collagen diseases and other severe diseases—
Glucocorticoids are used to treat rheumatic and collagen diseases, such as arthritis, polyarteritis nodosa, and systemic lupus erythematosus; thyroiditis; severe dermatologic diseases, such as pemphigus, exfoliative dermatitis, lichen planus, and psoriasis; allergic reactions; ocular disorders; respiratory diseases, such as asthma, sarcoidosis, and lipid pneumonitis; hematologic diseases, such as autoimmune hemolytic anemia and idiopathic thrombocytopenia; neoplastic diseases, such as leukemias and lymphomas; and GI diseases, such as ulcerative colitis, regional enteritis, and celiac disease. Other indications include myasthenia

gravis, organ transplantation, nephrotic syndrome, and septic shock.

➤Antenatal use in preterm labor—
Dexamethasone and betamethasone may be used as short-course I.M. therapy in women with preterm labor to hasten fetal maturation of lungs and cerebral blood vessels.

➤Hypercalcemia—
Glucocorticoids are used to treat hypercalcemia resulting from sarcoidosis, vitamin D intoxication, multiple myeloma, and breast cancer in postmenopausal women.

➤Cerebral edema—
High-dose parenteral glucocorticoid administration may decrease cerebral edema in brain tumors and during neurosurgery.

➤Acute spinal cord injury—
Large I.V. doses of glucocorticoids, when given shortly after injury, may improve motor and sensory function in patients with acute spinal cord injury.

ADVERSE REACTIONS
Suppression of the hypothalamic-pituitary-adrenal (HPA) axis is the major effect of systemic therapy with adrenocorticoids. When given in high doses or for long term, glucocorticoids suppress release of corticotropin from the pituitary gland. Subsequently, the adrenal cortex stops secreting endogenous corticosteroids. The degree and duration of HPA axis suppression are highly variable among patients and depend on the dose, frequency and time of administration, and duration of therapy.

Patients with a suppressed HPA axis caused by exogenous glucocorticoid administration who stop therapy abruptly may experience severe withdrawal symptoms, such as fever, myalgia, arthralgia, malaise, anorexia, nausea, desquamation of skin, orthostatic hypotension, dizziness, fainting, dyspnea, and hypoglycemia. Therefore,

♦ Off-label use

long-term adrenocorticoid therapy should always be withdrawn gradually.

Adrenal suppression may persist for as long as 12 months in patients who have received large doses for prolonged periods. Until he completely recovers, a patient subjected to stress may show signs and symptoms of adrenal insufficiency and may need glucocorticoid and mineralocorticoid replacement therapy.

Patients receiving large doses of glucocorticoids over a long term may develop cushingoid symptoms, including moon face, central obesity, striae, hirsutism, acne, ecchymoses, hypertension, osteoporosis, muscle atrophy, sexual dysfunction, diabetes, cataracts, hyperlipidemia, peptic ulcer, increased susceptibility to infection, and fluid and electrolyte imbalances.

Other adverse reactions may include CNS effects, such as euphoria, insomnia, psychotic behavior, pseudotumor cerebri, mental changes, nervousness, and restlessness; CV effects, such as heart failure, hypertension, and edema; GI effects, including peptic ulcer, irritation, and increased appetite; metabolic effects, such as hypokalemia, sodium and fluid retention, weight gain, hyperglycemia, and osteoporosis; musculoskeletal effects, including acute tendon rupture, muscle wasting and pain, and myopathy; skin effects, such as delayed wound healing, acne, skin eruptions, muscle atrophy, striae, and Kaposi's sarcoma; and immunosuppression, including increased susceptibility to infection, activation of latent infection, and exacerbation of other infections.

LIFESPAN CONSIDERATIONS
• Pregnancy risk category is C for drugs that are rated.
• Glucocorticoids and mineralocorticoids may cause fetal abnormalities. Avoid using in pregnant patients, if possible.

• Drugs of this class appear in breast milk and can suppress growth or cause other unwanted effects in the nursing infant. Mothers who need to take a corticosteroid should consider another form of feeding the baby. Some studies suggest the amount of drug appearing in the milk is negligible at certain doses and an alternative to consider would include waiting 3 to 4 hours after the dose before breast-feeding and selecting prednisolone rather than prednisone which would result in a lower corticosteroid dose to the infant.
• Long-term administration of pharmacologic doses of glucocorticoids in children may retard bone growth. Signs and symptoms of adrenal suppression include retardation of linear growth, delayed weight gain, low plasma cortisol levels, and lack of response to corticotropin stimulation. Alternate-day therapy is recommended to minimize growth suppression. Benefits of therapy should strongly outweigh adverse effects.
• Consider using lower dose in elderly patients because of body changes caused by aging such as decreased muscle mass and plasma volume. Monitor blood pressure, blood glucose and electrolytes at least every 6 months. Because of their reduced ability to metabolize and eliminate drugs, monitor elderly patients closely.

alpha-adrenergic blockers
dihydroergotamine mesylate, doxazosin mesylate, ergotamine tartrate, phentolamine mesylate, prazosin hydrochloride, tamsulosin hydrochloride, terazosin hydrochloride

Adrenergic blockers obstruct the effects of peripheral neurohormonal transmitters, such as norepinephrine and epinephrine, on adrenergic receptors. Alpha and beta adrenoreceptors and blockers may be divided according to whether they are selective or nonselective for a particular receptor. Alpha blockers antagonize mydriasis, vasoconstriction, nonvascular smooth-muscle excitation, and other adrenergic responses caused by alpha-receptor stimulation.

PHARMACOLOGY

Nonselective alpha blockers—dihydroergotamine, ergotamine, and phentolamine—antagonize both alpha$_1$ and alpha$_2$ receptors. Alpha blockade causes tachycardia, palpitations, and increased renin secretion because adrenergic nerve endings release excessive norepinephrine. Norepinephrine counteracts nonselective alpha blockers, which may be used to treat peripheral vascular disorders such as Raynaud's disease, acrocyanosis, frostbite, acute atrial occlusion, phlebitis, phlebothrombosis, diabetic gangrene, shock, and pheochromocytoma.

Selective alpha$_1$ receptor blockers decrease vascular resistance and increase venous capacitance, which lowers blood pressure; causes pink warm skin, nasal and scleroconjunctival congestion, ptosis, orthostatic and exercise hypotension, and mild to moderate miosis; and interferes with ejaculation. They also relax nonvascular smooth muscle, notably in the prostate capsule, reducing urinary symptoms in men with BPH. Doxazosin, prazosin, and terazosin are used to treat hypertension and terazosin, tamsulosin, and doxazosin to treat prostatic outflow obstruction caused by BPH.

INDICATIONS & ACTIONS

➤**Peripheral vascular disorders**—
Alpha-adrenergic blockers are used to treat peripheral vascular disorders, including Raynaud's disease, acrocyanosis, frostbite, acute atrial occlusion, phlebitis, and diabetic gangrene. Dihydroergotamine and ergotamine have been used to treat vascular headaches. Prazosin has been used to treat Raynaud's disease. Phentolamine is used to treat dermal necrosis caused by extravasation of norepinephrine, dopamine, or phenylephrine (alpha agonists).

➤**Hypertension**—
Prazosin, doxazosin, and terazosin are used in managing essential hypertension. Phentolamine is used to control hypertension and is a useful adjunct in surgical treatment of pheochromocytoma.

➤**BPH**—
Terazosin, tamsulosin, and doxazosin are used to control mild to moderate urinary obstructive symptoms in men with BPH. As an off-label use, prazosin is also used to treat BPH.

ADVERSE REACTIONS

Nonselective alpha-adrenergic blockers cause orthostatic hypotension, tachycardia, palpitations, fluid retention (from excess renin secretion), nasal and ocular congestion, and aggravation of respiratory infection. These drugs are contraindicated in patients with severe cerebral and coronary atherosclerosis and in those with renal insufficiency.

Selective alpha blockers may cause severe orthostatic hypotension and syncope, especially with the first dose. The most common adverse effects of alpha blockade are dizziness, headache, and malaise.

LIFESPAN CONSIDERATIONS

● Pregnancy risk category ranges from B to X. Avoid using in pregnant women.
● These agents should be used with caution in breast-feeding women.
● Safety and efficacy of many of these drugs haven't been established for children. Refer to specific drug monograph for more information.
● In elderly patients, the hypotensive effects may be more pronounced.

aminoglycosides

amikacin sulfate, gentamicin sulfate, kanamycin sulfate, neomycin sulfate, netilmicin sulfate, paromomycin sulfate, streptomycin sulfate, tobramycin sulfate

Aminoglycoside antibiotics were discovered during the search for drugs to treat serious, penicillin-resistant, gram-negative infections. Streptomycin, derived from soil actinomycetes, was the first therapeutically useful aminoglycoside. Bacterial resistance to this prototype and adverse reactions soon led to the development of kanamycin, gentamicin, neomycin, netilmicin, tobramycin, and amikacin.

The basic structure of aminoglycosides is an aminocyclitol nucleus joined with one to two amino sugars by glycosidic linkage; hence the name aminoglycosides.

Aminoglycosides share some pharmacokinetic properties, such as poor oral absorption, poor CNS penetration, and poor renal excretion, as well as serious adverse reactions and toxicity. Their clinical use may require close monitoring of serum levels.

PHARMACOLOGY

Aminoglycosides are bactericidal. The drugs appear to bind directly and irreversibly to 30S ribosomal subunits, inhibiting bacterial protein synthesis. Bacterial resistance to aminoglycosides may be from decreased bacterial cell wall permeability, low affinity of the drug for ribosomal binding sites, or enzymatic degradation by microbial enzymes.

Aminoglycosides are active against many aerobic gram-negative organisms and some aerobic gram-positive organisms. They don't kill fungi, viruses, or anaerobic bacteria.

Gram-negative organisms susceptible to aminoglycosides include *Acinetobacter, Citrobacter, Enterobacter, Escherichia coli, Klebsiella,* indole-positive and indole-negative *Proteus, Providencia, Pseudomonas aeruginosa, Salmonella, Serratia,* and *Shigella* species. Streptomycin is active against *Brucella* species, *Calymmatobacterium granulomatis, Francisella tularensis, Haemophilus influenzae, H. ducreyi, Pasteurella multocida,* and *Yersinia pestis.*

Susceptible aerobic gram-positive organisms include *Staphylococcus aureus* and *S. aureus epidermidis.* Streptomycin is active against *Nocardia, Erysipelothrix, Enterococcus faecalis,* and some mycobacteria, including *Mycobacterium tuberculosis, M. marinum,* and certain strains of *M. kansasii* and *M. leprae.*

Paromomycin is active against protozoa, especially *Entamoeba histolytica* and is somewhat effective against *Taenia saginata, Hymenolepis nana, Diphyllobothrium latum,* and *T. solium.* Neomycin and paromomycin have some activity against *Acanthamoeba.*

Aminoglycosides are poorly absorbed after oral administration in patients with intact GI mucosa and usually are used parenterally for systemic infections. Intraventricular or intrathecal administration is necessary for CNS infections. Kanamycin and neomycin are given orally for bowel sterilization.

Aminoglycosides are distributed widely throughout the body after parenteral administration. CSF levels are minimal, even in patients with inflamed meninges. Over time, aminoglycosides accumulate in body tissue, especially in the kidney and inner ear, causing drug saturation. The drug is released slowly from these tissues. Most aminoglycosides are minimally protein-bound and aren't metabolized. They don't penetrate abscesses well.

Aminoglycosides: Renal function and half-life

Aminoglycosides, which are excreted by the kidneys, have significantly prolonged half-lives in patients with end-stage renal disease. Knowing this can help you assess a patient's potential for drug accumulation and toxicity. Nephrotoxicity, a major hazard of therapy with aminoglycosides, is linked to serum levels that exceed the therapeutic levels listed below. Therefore, monitoring peak and trough levels is essential for safe use of these drugs.

	Half-life (hr)		Therapeutic levels (mcg/ml)	
Drug and route	**Normal renal function**	**End-stage renal disease**	**Peak**	**Trough**
amikacin I.M., I.V.	2-3	24-60	16-32	< 10
gentamicin I.M., I.V., topical	2	24-60	4-8	< 2
kanamycin I.M., I.V., topical	2-3	24-60	15-40	< 10
neomycin oral, topical	2-3	12-24	Not applicable	Not applicable
netilmicin I.M., I.V.	2-2½	< 10	6-10	< 2
streptomycin I.M., I.V.	2½	100	20-30	Not applicable
tobramycin I.M., I.V., topical	2-2½	24-60	4-8	< 2

Aminoglycosides are excreted primarily in urine, chiefly by glomerular filtration. Neomycin is chiefly excreted unchanged in feces when taken orally. Elimination half-life ranges from 2 to 4 hours and is prolonged in patients with decreased renal function. (See *Aminoglycosides: Renal function and half-life.*)

INDICATIONS & ACTIONS

➤ **Infection caused by susceptible organisms—**
Aminoglycosides are used alone for the following conditions:

• Infections caused by susceptible aerobic gram-negative bacilli, including septicemia; postoperative, pulmonary, intra-abdominal, and serious, recurrent urinary tract infections; and infections of skin, soft tissue, bones, and joints

• Infections from aerobic gram-negative bacillary meningitis (not susceptible to other antibiotics); in ventriculitis, drugs are given intrathecally or intraventricularly because of poor CNS penetration

• Ammonia-forming bacteria in the GI tract of patients with hepatic encephalopathy (kanamycin or paromomycin used orally and neomycin used orally or as a retention enema as an adjunct therapy)

• Disseminated *M. avium* complex infections (gentamicin encapsulated in liposomes is being evaluated for this use)

Aminoglycosides are combined with other antibacterials for the following conditions:

• Serious staphylococcal infections (with an antistaphylococcal penicillin)

• Serious *P. aeruginosa* infections (with an antipseudomonal penicillin or cephalosporin)

♦ Off-label use

- Enterococcal infections, including endocarditis (with penicillin G, ampicillin, or vancomycin)
- Febrile, leukopenic compromised host (as initial empiric therapy with an antipseudomonal penicillin or cephalosporin)
- Serious *Klebsiella* species infections (with a cephalosporin)
- Nosocomial pneumonia (with a cephalosporin)
- Anaerobic infections involving *Bacteroides fragilis* (with clindamycin, metronidazole, cefoxitin, doxycycline, chloramphenicol, or ticarcillin)
- Tuberculosis (use of parenteral streptomycin with other antituberculotics)
- Pelvic inflammatory disease (gentamicin with clindamycin)

ADVERSE REACTIONS

Adverse reactions may be systemic or local. Ototoxicity and nephrotoxicity are the most serious systemic complications of aminoglycoside therapy. Ototoxicity involves both vestibular and auditory functions and usually is related to persistently high drug levels. Damage is reversible only if detected early and if drug is discontinued promptly.

Any aminoglycoside may cause usually reversible nephrotoxicity. The damage results in tubular necrosis. Mild proteinuria and casts are early signs of declining renal function. An elevated creatinine level follows several days after the decline has begun. Nephrotoxicity usually begins on day 4 to 7 of therapy and appears to be dose-related.

Neuromuscular blockade results in skeletal weakness and respiratory distress similar to that seen with the use of neuromuscular blockers, such as tubocurarine and succinylcholine.

Oral aminoglycoside therapy most often causes nausea, vomiting, and diarrhea. Less common adverse reactions include hypersensitivity reactions (ranging from mild rashes, fever, and eosinophilia to fatal anaphylaxis) and hematologic reactions (hemolytic anemia, transient neutropenia, leukopenia, and thrombocytopenia). Transient elevations of liver function values also occur.

Parenteral aminoglycosides may cause local adverse reactions such as vein irritation, phlebitis, and sterile abscess.

LIFESPAN CONSIDERATIONS

- Pregnancy risk category is D. Drugs cross the placenta, creating the potential for fetal toxicity and possibly causing congenital deafness.
- Small amounts of drugs appear in breast milk. Recommend an alternative to breast-feeding during therapy.
- The half-life of aminoglycosides is prolonged in neonates and premature infants because of their immature renal systems. Dosage changes may be needed.
- Geriatric patients have decreased renal function and are at greater risk for nephrotoxicity. They may require a lower drug dose and longer dosing intervals. A creatinine clearance determination may be more useful than routine screening tests such as BUN and creatinine levels, to determine in assessing renal function. Geriatric patients are also susceptible to ototoxicity and superinfection.

---

angiotensin-converting enzyme inhibitors

benazepril hydrochloride, captopril, enalapril maleate, enalaprilat, fosinopril sodium, lisinopril, moexipril hydrochloride, perindopril erbumine, quinapril hydrochloride, ramipril, trandolapril

---

Angiotensin-converting enzyme (ACE) inhibitors may be used to manage hypertension and to treat heart failure. Captopril is indicated to prevent diabet-

Comparing doses of ACE inhibitors for hypertension

Drug	Target adult daily dose	Dosage adjustments
benazepril	10-40 mg in single or divided doses	Creatinine clearance < 30 ml/min or patient taking diuretic: initially, 5 mg/day
captopril	25-150 mg 2-3 times daily	Renal impairment, hyponatremia, or hypovolemia: reduce dosage and titrate slowly.
enalapril	P.O.: 10-40 mg in single or divided doses I.V.: 1.25 mg (≥ 5 min) q 6 hr	Creatinine clearance ≤ 30 ml/min or patient taking diuretic: initially, 2.5 mg/day
fosinopril	20-40 mg in single or divided doses	None
lisinopril	20-40 mg in a single dose	Creatinine clearance ≤ 10-30 ml/min or patient taking diuretic: initially, 5 mg/day Creatinine clearance < 10 ml/min: initially, 2.5 mg/day
moexipril	7.5-30 mg in single or divided doses	Creatinine clearance < 40 ml/min: initially, 3.75 mg/day
perindopril	4-8 mg in single or divided doses	Creatinine clearance 30-60 ml/min: initially, 2 mg/day
quinapril	20-80 mg in single or divided doses	Creatinine clearance 30-60 ml/min or patient taking diuretic: initially, 5 mg/day Creatinine clearance 10-30 ml/min: initially, 2.5 mg/day
ramipril	2.5-20 mg in single or divided doses	Creatinine clearance < 40 ml/min or creatinine > 2.5 mg/dl: initially, 1.25 mg/day
trandolapril	1-4 mg in single dose	Creatinine clearance < 30 ml/min, concurrent diuretic therapy, or hepatic cirrhosis: initially, 0.5 mg/day

ic nephropathy, and captopril and lisinopril are useful in improving survival rates in patients after an MI.

PHARMACOLOGY

ACE inhibitors prevent the conversion of angiotensin I to angiotensin II, a potent vasoconstrictor. Besides decreasing vasoconstriction, and thus reducing peripheral arterial resistance, inhibition of angiotensin II decreases adrenocortical secretion of aldosterone. This results in decreased sodium and water retention and extracellular fluid volume.

INDICATIONS & ACTIONS

➤Hypertension, heart failure— Decreased peripheral resistance and sodium and water retention cause the antihypertensive effects of ACE inhibitors.

ACE inhibitors manage heart failure by decreasing systemic vascular resistance (afterload) and pulmonary capillary wedge pressure (preload). They're also used after MI to reduce the risk of death. (See *Comparing doses of ACE inhibitors for hypertension.*)

Ramipril, in combination with other antihypertensive, antiplatelet, and antilipemic drugs, may decrease the risk of CV events in high-risk patients age 55 and older. Captopril, enalapril, and trandolapril manage patients with left ventricular dysfunction after an MI and help reduce incidence of post-MI heart failure in these patients.

♦ Off-label use

➤**Diabetic nephropathy—**
Captopril slows the progression of renal insufficiency in patients with type 1 diabetes mellitus.

ADVERSE REACTIONS
The most common adverse effects of therapeutic doses of ACE inhibitors are headache, fatigue, hypotension, tachycardia, dysgeusia, proteinuria, hyperkalemia, rash, cough, and angioedema of the face and limbs. Severe hypotension may occur at toxic drug levels. ACE inhibitors should be used cautiously in patients with impaired renal function or serious autoimmune disease, and in patients taking other drugs known to depress WBC count or immune response.

LIFESPAN CONSIDERATIONS
● Stop ACE inhibitors if patient becomes pregnant. Pregnancy risk category is C during the first trimester. Drug may harm or kill fetus during the second and third trimesters (pregnancy risk category is D).
● Captopril and enalapril appear in breast milk. Tell patient not to breast-feed during therapy.
● Safety and efficacy of ACE inhibitors in children haven't been established.
● Elderly patients may need lower doses because of impaired drug clearance and because they may be more sensitive to hypotensive effects.

anticholinergics
Antiparkinsonians: benztropine mesylate, biperiden, trihexyphenidyl hydrochloride

Belladonna alkaloids: atropine sulfate, hyoscyamine sulfate, scopolamine hydrobromide

Synthetic quaternary anticholinergics: glycopyrrolate, ipratropium bromide, mepenzolate bromide, methscopolamine bromide, propantheline bromide

Tertiary synthetic and semisynthetic (antispasmodic) derivatives: dicyclomine hydrochloride, homatropine, oxybutynin chloride, tolterodine tartrate

Anticholinergics are used to treat various spastic conditions, including acute dystonic reactions, muscle rigidity, parkinsonism, and extrapyramidal disorders. They're also used to reverse neuromuscular blockade, prevent nausea and vomiting resulting from motion sickness, as adjunctive treatment for peptic ulcer disease and other GI disorders, and preoperatively to decrease secretions and block cardiac reflexes. Belladonna alkaloids are naturally occurring anticholinergics that have been used for centuries. Many semisynthetic alkaloids and synthetic anticholinergic compounds are available, but most offer few advantages over naturally occurring alkaloids.

PHARMACOLOGY
Anticholinergics competitively antagonize the actions of acetylcholine and other cholinergic agonists at muscarinic and nicotinic receptors within the parasympathetic nervous system and smooth muscles that lack cholinergic innervation. Lack of specificity for site of action increases the hazard of adverse effects in association with therapeutic effects.

Antispasmodics are structurally similar to anticholinergics, but their anticholinergic activity usually occurs only at high doses. Their mechanism of action is unknown, but they're thought to directly relax smooth muscle.

INDICATIONS & ACTIONS
➤**Hypersecretory conditions—**
Many anticholinergics, such as atropine, belladonna leaf, glycopyrrolate,

hyoscyamine, levorotatory alkaloids of belladonna, and mepenzolate, are used therapeutically for their antisecretory properties. These properties derive from competitive blockade of cholinergic receptor sites, causing decreased gastric acid secretion, salivation, bronchial secretions, and sweating.

➤**GI tract disorders—**
Some anticholinergics, as well as the antispasmodics such as dicyclomine, are used to treat spasms and other GI tract disorders. These drugs competitively block the actions of acetylcholine at cholinergic receptor sites. Antispasmodics presumably act by a nonspecific, direct spasmolytic action on smooth muscle. These drugs are used to treat pylorospasm, ileitis, and irritable bowel syndrome. Transdermal scopolamine prevents nausea and vomiting that may occur during recovery from anesthesia and surgery. Atropine may be used to relieve nausea and vomiting caused by morphine used to treat an MI.

➤**Sinus bradycardia—**
Atropine is used to treat sinus bradycardia caused by drugs, poisons, or sinus node dysfunction. It blocks normal vagal inhibition of the SA node and increases heart rate. Atropine may be given to rectify sustained bradycardia and hypotension caused by nitroglycerin used to treat an MI.

➤**Dystonia and parkinsonism—**
Biperiden, benztropine, and trihexyphenidyl hydrochloride are used to treat acute dystonic reactions and drug-induced extrapyramidal adverse effects. They act centrally by blocking cholinergic receptor sites, balancing cholinergic activity with dopamine.

➤**Perioperative use—**
Atropine, glycopyrrolate, and hyoscyamine are used postoperatively with anticholinesterases to reverse nondepolarizing neuromuscular blockade. These drugs block muscarinic effects of anticholinesterases by competitively blocking muscarinic receptor sites.

Atropine, glycopyrrolate, and scopolamine are used preoperatively to decrease secretions and block cardiac vagal reflexes. They diminish secretions by competitively inhibiting muscarinic receptor sites and block cardiac vagal reflexes by preventing normal vagal inhibition of the SA node.

➤**Bronchospasm—**
Atropine and ipratropium are potent bronchodilators used to treat antigen-, methacholine-, histamine-, or exercise-induced bronchospasm (oral inhalation and I.M. atropine). Oral inhalation of atropine or ipratropium is used to treat chronic bronchitis and asthma. Oral inhalation of atropine sulfate has been used for the short-term treatment and prevention of bronchospasm caused by chronic bronchial asthma, bronchitis, and COPD.

➤**Genitourinary tract disorders—**
Atropine, oxybutynin, propantheline, and tolterodine are used to treat reflex neurogenic bladder.

➤**Poisoning—**
Atropine is used to reverse the cholinergic effects of toxic exposure to organophosphate and carbamate anticholinesterase pesticides, and to treat ingestion of cholinomimetic plants and fungi.

➤**Motion sickness—**
Scopolamine prevents nausea and vomiting caused by motion sickness. Its exact mechanism of action is unknown, but it's thought to affect neural pathways originating in the ear.

ADVERSE REACTIONS
Dry mouth, decreased sweating or anhidrosis, headache, mydriasis, blurred vision, cycloplegia, xerophthalmia, dry skin, urinary hesitancy and urine retention, constipation, palpitations, and tachycardia most commonly occur with therapeutic doses and usually disappear once the drug is discontinued. Signs and symptoms of drug toxicity include CNS signs resembling psychosis (dis-

orientation, confusion, hallucinations, delusions, anxiety, agitation, and restlessness) and such peripheral effects as dilated, nonreactive pupils; blurred vision; hot, dry, flushed skin; dry mucous membranes; dysphagia; stupor, seizures, decreased or absent bowel sounds; urine retention; hyperthermia; tachycardia; hypertension; and increased respiration.

LIFESPAN CONSIDERATIONS
● The safety of anticholinergic therapy during pregnancy hasn't been determined.
● Some anticholinergics may appear in breast milk. Breast-feeding women should avoid these drugs. Anticholinergics may decrease milk production.
● Safety and efficacy in children haven't been established.
● Give cautiously to elderly patients. Even patients older than age 40 may be more sensitive to the effects of these drugs.

---

antihistamines
azelastine hydrochloride,
brompheniramine maleate,
cetirizine hydrochloride,
chlorpheniramine maleate,
clemastine fumarate, cyclizine
hydrochloride, cyclizine lactate,
cyproheptadine hydrochloride,
desloratadine, dimenhydrinate,
diphenhydramine hydrochloride,
fexofenadine hydrochloride,
hydroxyzine hydrochloride,
loratadine, meclizine hydrochloride,
promethazine hydrochloride,
tripelennamine hydrochloride,
triprolidine hydrochloride

Antihistamines, synthetically produced H_1-receptor antagonists have many applications related specifically to chemical structure. Some antihistamines are used primarily to treat rhinitis or pruritus, whereas others are used for their antiemetic and antivertigo effects. Still others are used as sedative-hypnotics, antitussives and to treat dyskinesias.

PHARMACOLOGY
Antihistamines are structurally related chemicals that compete with histamine for H_1-receptor sites on the smooth muscle of the bronchi, GI tract, uterus, and large blood vessels, binding to the cellular receptors and preventing access and subsequent activity of histamine. They don't directly alter histamine or prevent its release. Also, antihistamines antagonize the action of histamine that causes increased capillary permeability and resultant edema. They also suppress flare and pruritus caused by the endogenous release of histamine.

INDICATIONS & ACTIONS
➤ Allergy—
Most antihistamines (azelastine, brompheniramine, cetirizine, chlorpheniramine, clemastine, cyproheptadine, desloratadine, diphenhydramine, fexofenadine, hydroxyzine, loratadine, promethazine, and triprolidine) are used to treat allergic signs and symptoms, such as rhinitis, sneezing, itchy nose, and itchy, watery, red eyes.
➤ Urticaria—
Cetirizine, clemastine, cyproheptadine, desloratadine, fexofenadine, hydroxyzine, loratadine, and triprolidine are used systemically. It's believed that these drugs counteract histamine-induced pruritus by a combination of peripheral effects on nerve endings and local anesthetic and sedative activity.
    Tripelennamine and diphenhydramine are used topically to relieve itching caused by minor skin irritation. Structurally related to local anesthetics, these compounds prevent initiation and transmission of nerve impulses.

➤**Vertigo, nausea, and vomiting—**
Cyclizine, dimenhydrinate, and
meclizine are used only as antivertigo
drugs and antiemetics. Their antihistaminic activity hasn't been evaluated.
Diphenhydramine and promethazine
are used as antiallergic and antivertigo
drugs and as antiemetics and antinause-
ants. Although the mechanisms aren't
fully understood, antiemetic and antivertigo effects probably result from
central antimuscarinic activity.
➤**Sedation—**
Diphenhydramine and promethazine
are used for their sedative action. The
mechanism of antihistamine-induced
CNS depression is unknown.
➤**Suppression of cough—**
Diphenhydramine syrup is used as an
antitussive. The cough reflex is suppressed by a direct effect on the
medullary cough center.
➤**Dyskinesia—**
The central antimuscarinic action of
diphenhydramine reduces drug-induced
dyskinesias and parkinsonism through
inhibition of acetylcholine (anticholinergic effect).

ADVERSE REACTIONS
At therapeutic dosage levels, all antihistamines, except loratadine, are likely
to cause drowsiness and impaired motor function during initial therapy. Also,
their anticholinergic action usually
causes dry mouth and throat, blurred
vision, and constipation. Antihistamines that are also phenothiazines,
such as promethazine, may cause other
adverse effects, including cholestatic
jaundice (thought to be a hypersensitivity reaction), and may predispose patients to photosensitivity. Patients taking such drugs should avoid prolonged
exposure to sunlight.
  Toxic doses elicit a combination of
CNS depression and excitation as well
as atropine-like symptoms, including
sedation, reduced mental alertness,
apnea, CV collapse, hallucinations,

tremors, seizures, dry mouth, flushed
skin, and fixed, dilated pupils. Toxic
effects reverse when drug is discontinued. Used appropriately, in correct doses, antihistamines are safe for prolonged use.

LIFESPAN CONSIDERATIONS
● Pregnancy risk category ranges from
B to C, depending on agent. Safe use of
antihistamines during pregnancy hasn't
been established. Some manufacturers
recommend avoiding these drugs during the third trimester of pregnancy because of the risk of severe reactions in
neonates and premature infants.
● Antihistamines shouldn't be used during breast-feeding.
● Children, especially those younger
than age 6, may experience paradoxical
hyperexcitability with restlessness, insomnia, nervousness, euphoria,
tremors, and seizures.
● Elderly patients are usually more sensitive to the effects of antihistamines
and are especially likely to experience
a greater degree of dizziness, sedation,
hypotension, and urine retention.

barbiturates
amobarbital, mephobarbital,
methohexital sodium,
pentobarbital sodium,
phenobarbital, primidone,
secobarbital sodium, thiopental
sodium

Although barbiturates have been used
extensively as sedative-hypnotics and
anxiolytics, benzodiazepines are the
current drugs of choice for sedative-
hypnotic effects. Phenobarbital, mephobarbital, and primidone remain effective for anticonvulsant therapy. A
few short-acting barbiturates are used
as general anesthetics.

PHARMACOLOGY

Barbiturates are structurally related compounds that act throughout the CNS. They induce an imbalance in central inhibitory and facilitatory mechanisms and decrease both presynaptic and postsynaptic membrane excitability.

The exact mechanisms of action of barbiturates aren't known, and it's unclear which cellular and synaptic actions result in sedative-hypnotic effects. Barbiturates can produce all levels of CNS depression, from mild sedation to coma to death. Barbiturates exert their effects by facilitating the actions of gamma-aminobutyric acid (GABA). They also exert a central effect, which depresses respiration and GI motility. Barbiturates have no analgesic action and may increase the reaction to painful stimuli at subanesthetic doses. The principal anticonvulsant mechanism of action is reduction of nerve transmission and decreased excitability of the nerve cell. Barbiturates also raise the seizure threshold.

INDICATIONS & ACTIONS

➤**Seizure disorders**—
Phenobarbital and mephobarbital are used to treat and manage seizure disorders. They're used mainly in tonic-clonic (grand mal) and partial seizures. At anesthetic doses, all barbiturates have anticonvulsant activity. Phenobarbital is an effective parenteral agent for status epilepticus (with airway support).

Barbiturates suppress the spread of seizure activity produced by epileptogenic foci in the cortex, thalamus, and limbic systems by enhancing the effects of GABA.

➤**Sedation, hypnosis**—
Most currently available barbiturates are used as sedative-hypnotics for short-term (up to 2 weeks) treatment of insomnia because of their nonspecific CNS effects.

Barbiturates aren't used routinely as sedatives. Barbiturate-induced sleep differs from physiologic sleep in that REM sleep cycles are reduced.

➤**Preanesthesia sedation**—
Barbiturates are also used as preanesthetic sedatives and for relief of anxiety.

➤**Psychiatric use**—
Barbiturates (especially amobarbital) have been used parenterally in narcoanalysis and narcotherapy and in identifying schizophrenia.

ADVERSE REACTIONS

Drowsiness, lethargy, vertigo, headache, and CNS depression are common with barbiturates. After hypnotic doses, a hangover effect, subtle distortion of mood, and impaired judgment or motor skills may continue for many hours. After a decrease in dose or discontinuation of barbiturates used for hypnosis, patients may experience rebound insomnia, increased dreaming or nightmares, and hyperalgesia. Hypersensitivity reactions (rash, angioedema, Stevens-Johnson syndrome) are rare. Acquired hypersensitivity reactions are more likely to occur in patients with a history of asthma or allergies to other drugs. Barbiturates can cause paradoxical excitement at low doses, confusion in geriatric patients, and hyperactivity in children. High fever, severe headache, stomatitis, conjunctivitis, or rhinitis may precede skin eruptions. Because of the potential for fatal consequences, discontinue barbiturates if dermatologic reactions occur.

Withdrawal symptoms may occur after as few as 2 weeks of uninterrupted therapy. Symptoms usually occur within 8 to 12 hours after the last dose but may be delayed up to 5 days. They may include weakness, anxiety, nausea, vomiting, insomnia, hallucinations, and seizures.

LIFESPAN CONSIDERATIONS
● Pregnancy risk category is D. Barbiturates may harm the fetus in pregnant women. These drugs may cause postpartum hemorrhage and hemorrhagic disease of the newborn, reversible with vitamin K. If a woman takes barbiturates in the last trimester of pregnancy, her neonate may exhibit withdrawal symptoms.
● Barbiturates appear in breast milk and may cause infant CNS depression. Use cautiously in these patients.
● Premature infants are more susceptible to the depressant effects of barbiturates because of immature hepatic metabolism. Children receiving barbiturates may experience hyperactivity, excitement, or hyperalgesia.
● Geriatric patients and patients receiving subhypnotic doses may experience hyperactivity, excitement, confusion, depression, or hyperalgesia. Use cautiously in these patients.

---

benzodiazepines

alprazolam, chlordiazepoxide hydrochloride, clonazepam, clorazepate dipotassium, diazepam, estazolam, flurazepam hydrochloride, lorazepam, midazolam hydrochloride, oxazepam, quazepam, temazepam, triazolam

---

Benzodiazepines have replaced barbiturates as the treatment of choice for anxiety, seizure disorders, and sedation. They are preferred because therapeutic doses produce less drowsiness, respiratory depression, and impairment of motor function, and toxic doses are less likely to be fatal.

PHARMACOLOGY
Benzodiazepines are a group of structurally related chemicals that act on polysynaptic neuronal pathways in the CNS. Although their action isn't completely understood, they enhance or facilitate the action of gamma-aminobutyric acid (GABA), an inhibitory CNS neurotransmitter, and may act at the limbic, thalamic, and hypothalamic levels of the CNS. They produce anxiolytic, sedative, hypnotic, skeletal muscle relaxant, and anticonvulsant effects. Although all benzodiazepines are CNS depressants, certain kinds act more selectively at specific sites, allowing them to be divided into several categories based on their predominant clinical use.

INDICATIONS & ACTIONS
➤Seizure disorders—
Five of the benzodiazepines (diazepam, clonazepam, clorazepate, midazolam, and parenteral lorazepam) are used as anticonvulsants. They suppress the spread of seizure activity produced by epileptogenic foci in the cortex, thalamus, and limbic systems by enhancing presynaptic inhibition. Clonazepam is a useful adjunct to treat petit mal variant (Lennox-Gastaut syndrome), myoclonic, or akinetic seizures. Benzodiazepines are also useful adjuncts to help prevent partial seizures with elementary symptoms (jacksonian seizures), psychomotor seizures, and petit mal seizures. The parenteral form of diazepam, midazolam, and lorazepam is indicated to treat status epilepticus.
➤Anxiety, tension, and insomnia—
Most benzodiazepines work as anxiolytics or sedative-hypnotics. They're thought to facilitate the effects of GABA in the ascending reticular activating system, increasing inhibition and blocking both cortical and limbic arousal.

Benzodiazepines are used to treat anxiety and tension that occur alone or as an adverse effect of a primary disorder. They aren't recommended for tension caused by everyday stress. Which benzodiazepine is chosen depends on its metabolic characteristics. For instance, in patients with depressed renal or hepatic function, alprazolam, lorazepam, or oxazepam may be selected because they have a relatively short duration of action and no active metabolites.

The sedative-hypnotic properties of chlordiazepoxide, clorazepate, diazepam, lorazepam, and oxazepam make these the drugs of choice as preoperative medication and as an adjunct in the rehabilitation of alcoholics.

➤**Surgical adjuncts for conscious sedation or amnesia—**
Diazepam, midazolam, and lorazepam have amnestic effects. The mechanism of such action isn't known. Parenteral administration before procedures such as endoscopy or elective cardioversion impairs recent memory and interferes with the establishment of memory trace, producing anterograde amnesia.

➤**Skeletal muscle spasm or tremor—**
Because oral forms of diazepam and chlordiazepoxide have skeletal muscle relaxant properties, they're often used to treat neurologic conditions involving muscle spasms and tetanus. The mechanism of such action is unknown, but these drugs are believed to inhibit spinal polysynaptic and monosynaptic afferent pathways.

➤**Delirium—**
Benzodiazepines may be used alone or with antipsychotic drugs to treat delirium, but caution should be used because benzodiazepines may also exacerbate delirium.

➤**Schizophrenia—**
Benzodiazepines may be used as an adjunct to antipsychotic drugs to manage schizophrenia.

➤**Chemotherapy-induced nausea and vomiting—**
Benzodiazepines may be used as an adjunct to control nausea and vomiting caused by emetogenic cancer chemotherapy.

➤**Neonatal opiate withdrawal—**
Parenteral diazepam relieves agitation caused by neonatal opiate withdrawal.

ADVERSE REACTIONS

Therapeutic dosage of the benzodiazepines usually causes drowsiness and impaired motor function, which should be monitored early in treatment. These drugs also cause GI discomfort, such as constipation, diarrhea, vomiting, appetite changes, and urinary changes. Visual disturbances and CV irregularities are common. Continuing problems with short-term memory, confusion, severe depression, shakiness, vertigo, slurred speech, staggering, bradycardia, shortness of breath or difficulty breathing, and severe weakness usually indicate a toxic dose level. Prolonged or frequent use of benzodiazepines can cause physical dependency and withdrawal when use is discontinued.

LIFESPAN CONSIDERATIONS

● Pregnancy risk category for some agents ranges from D to X. Other agents, such as clonazepam, are unknown. Benzodiazepines can cause fetal harm if administered during pregnancy. There's an increased risk of congenital malformation if given during the first trimester. Use of benzodiazepines during labor may cause neonatal flaccidity.

● Breast-fed infants may show sedation, feeding difficulties, and weight loss. Safe use in breast-feeding hasn't been established.

● Because children, particularly very young ones, are sensitive to the CNS depressant effects of benzodiazepines, use caution. Neonates exposed to the drug in utero may exhibit withdrawal symptoms.

● Geriatric patients receiving benzodiazepines require lower doses. Use cautiously. Parenteral administration of these drugs in elderly patients is more likely to cause apnea, hypotension, bradycardia, and cardiac arrest. Geriatric patients may show prolonged elimination of benzodiazepines, except possibly oxazepam, lorazepam, temazepam, and triazolam.

beta blockers

Beta₁ blockers: acebutolol, atenolol, betaxolol hydrochloride, bisoprolol, esmolol, metoprolol

Beta₁ and beta₂ blockers: carteolol hydrochloride, carvedilol, labetalol, levobunolol hydrochloride, metipranolol hydrochloride, nadolol, penbutolol sulfate, pindolol, propranolol, sotalol, timolol maleate

Beta blockers are used to treat hypertension, angina pectoris, and arrhythmias. These drugs are well tolerated by most patients.

PHARMACOLOGY
Beta blockers compete with beta agonists for available beta-receptor sites. Individual drugs differ in their ability to affect beta receptors. Some available drugs are considered nonselective, that is, they block both beta₁ receptors in cardiac muscle and beta₂ receptors in bronchial and vascular smooth muscle. Several drugs are cardioselective and, in lower doses, primarily inhibit beta₁ receptors. Some beta blockers have intrinsic sympathomimetic activity and simultaneously stimulate and block beta receptors, decreasing cardiac output. Still others also have membrane-stabilizing activity, which affects cardiac action potential. (See *Comparing beta blockers,* page 20.)

INDICATIONS & ACTIONS
➤**Hypertension**—
Most beta blockers are used to treat hypertension. Although the exact mechanism of their antihypertensive effect is

unknown, the action is thought to result from decreased cardiac output, decreased sympathetic outflow from the CNS, and suppression of renin release.
➤**Angina**—
Propranolol, atenolol, nadolol, and metoprolol are used to treat angina pectoris. They decrease myocardial oxygen requirements through the blockade of catecholamine-induced increases in heart rate, blood pressure, and the extent of myocardial contraction.
➤**Heart failure**—
Carvedilol increases survival rates and decreases the risk of hospitalization in patients.
➤**Arrhythmias**—
Propranolol, acebutolol, sotalol, and esmolol are used to treat arrhythmias. They prolong the refractory period of the AV node and slow AV conduction.
➤**Glaucoma**—
The mechanism by which betaxolol, levobunolol, metipranolol, and timolol reduce intraocular pressure is unknown, but the drug effect is at least partially caused by decreased production of aqueous humor.
➤**Myocardial infarction**—
Timolol, propranolol, atenolol, and metoprolol are used to reduce cardiovascular mortality and risk of reinfarction post-MI.
➤**Migraine prevention**—
Atenolol, metoprolol, nadolol, propranolol, and timolol are used to prevent recurrent attacks of migraine and other vascular headaches. It's unknown exactly how these drugs decrease migraine headache attacks, but it's probably because they inhibit vasodilation of cerebral vessels.
➤**Other uses**—
Some beta blockers have been used as anxiolytics, for managing subaortic stenosis, as adjunctive therapy of bleeding esophageal varices or pheochromocytomas, and to treat portal hypertension or essential tremors. Carvedilol and metoprolol are used to treat heart

Comparing beta blockers

Drug	Half-life (hr)	Lipid solubility	Membrane-stabilizing activity	Intrinsic sympathomimetic activity
Nonselective				
carteolol	6	low	0	++
carvedilol	7-10	high	not known	0
labetalol	6-8	moderate	0	0
metipranolol	4	low to moderate	0	0
nadolol	20	low	0	0
penbutolol	5	high	0	+
pindolol	3-4	moderate	+	+++
propranolol	4	high	++	0
timolol	4	low to moderate	0	0
Beta₁-selective				
acebutolol	3-4	low	+	+
atenolol	6-7	low	0	0
betaxolol	14-22	low	+	0
bisoprolol	9-12	low	0	0
esmolol	0.15	low	0	0
metoprolol	3-7	moderate	*	0

* Only in higher-than-usual doses.
+ Activity that drug possesses in comparison to other beta blockers.

failure with cardiac glycosides, diuretics, or ACE inhibitors.

ADVERSE REACTIONS

Therapeutic doses may cause bradycardia, fatigue, and dizziness. Adverse reactions include other CNS disturbances, such as nightmares, depression, memory loss, or hallucinations. Impotence, cold limbs, and elevated cholesterol levels may also occur. Severe hypotension, bradycardia, heart failure, or bronchospasm usually indicates toxic dose levels.

LIFESPAN CONSIDERATIONS

● Pregnancy risk category is C or D. Avoid beta blocker therapy in pregnant women. Atenolol may cause intrauterine growth retardation.
● Beta blockers appear in breast milk and can possibly cause cyanosis or bradycardia in the nursing infant. Women taking beta-blockers shouldn't breast-feed.
● Safety and efficacy of beta blockers in children haven't been established. Use only if benefit outweighs risk.
● Geriatric patients may need lower maintenance dosages of beta blockers.

They also may experience enhanced adverse effects.

calcium channel blockers

amlodipine besylate, bepridil hydrochloride, diltiazem hydrochloride, felodipine, isradipine, nicardipine hydrochloride, nifedipine, nimodipine, nisoldipine, verapamil hydrochloride

Calcium channel blockers have become increasingly popular as a treatment for angina and have come to be the preferred drugs for Prinzmetal's variant angina (vasospastic angina). They have been used as antihypertensives. Verapamil and diltiazem have proved effective in treating supraventricular tachycardias (SVTs).

PHARMACOLOGY
The main physiologic action of calcium channel blockers is to inhibit calcium influx across the slow channels of myocardial and vascular smooth-muscle cells. By inhibiting calcium influx into these cells, calcium channel blockers reduce intracellular calcium concentrations. This, in turn, dilates coronary arteries, peripheral arteries, and arterioles, and slows cardiac conduction.

When used to treat Prinzmetal's variant angina, calcium channel blockers inhibit coronary spasm, increasing oxygen delivery to the heart. Peripheral artery dilation leads to decreased total peripheral resistance. This reduces afterload, which, in turn, decreases myocardial oxygen consumption. Inhibition of calcium influx into the specialized cardiac conduction cells (specifically, those in the SA and AV nodes) slows conduction through the heart. This effect is most pronounced with verapamil and diltiazem.

INDICATIONS & ACTIONS
➤**Angina**—
Calcium channel blockers are useful in managing Prinzmetal's variant angina, chronic stable angina, and unstable angina. In Prinzmetal's variant angina, these drugs inhibit spontaneous and ergonovine-induced coronary spasm, thereby increasing coronary blood flow and maintaining myocardial oxygen delivery. In unstable and chronic stable angina, their effectiveness presumably stems from their ability to reduce afterload.
➤**Arrhythmias**—
Of the calcium channel blockers, verapamil and diltiazem have the greatest effect on the AV node, slowing the ventricular rate in atrial fibrillation or flutter and converting SVT to normal sinus rhythm.
➤**Hypertension**—
Because they dilate systemic arteries, most of these drugs are useful in mild to moderate hypertension.
➤**Other uses**—
Calcium channel blockers, especially verapamil, may also be effective as adjunctive management of hypertrophic cardiomyopathy by improving the filling of the heart and reducing symptoms such as chest pain, breathlessness, and palpitations. They've been used to treat migraine headaches, peripheral vascular disorders, and subarachnoid hemorrhage (nimodipine) and as adjunctive therapy to treat esophageal spasm.

ADVERSE REACTIONS
Verapamil may cause adverse effects on the conduction system, including bradycardia and various degrees of heart block. It may exacerbate heart failure and cause hypotension after rapid I.V. administration. Prolonged oral verapamil therapy may cause constipation.

Nifedipine can cause hypotension, reflex tachycardia, peripheral edema, flushing, light-headedness, and headache.

◆ Off-label use

Diltiazem most commonly causes anorexia, nausea, various degrees of heart block, bradycardia, heart failure, and peripheral edema.

LIFESPAN CONSIDERATIONS

● Pregnancy risk category is C. Use in pregnant women only when clearly needed and the potential benefits outweigh the potential for harm to the fetus.

● Calcium channel blockers (verapamil and diltiazem) may appear in breast milk. To avoid possible adverse effects in infants, women should discontinue breast-feeding during therapy.

● Adverse hemodynamic effects of parenteral verapamil may occur in neonates and infants. Safety and effectiveness of diltiazem and nifedipine haven't been established.

● Use cautiously because decreased clearance may increase the half-life of calcium channel blockers.

---

cephalosporins

First-generation cephalosporins: cefadroxil, cefazolin sodium, cephalexin monohydrate, cephapirin, cephradine

Second-generation cephalosporins: cefaclor, cefotetan disodium, cefoxitin sodium, cefprozil, cefuroxime axetil, cefuroxime sodium, loracarbef

Third-generation cephalosporins: cefdinir, cefditoren pivoxil, cefoperazone sodium, cefotaxime sodium, cefpodoxime proxetil, ceftazidime, ceftibuten, ceftizoxime sodium, ceftriaxone sodium

Fourth-generation cephalosporin: cefepime hydrochloride

Cephalosporins are beta-lactam antibiotics first isolated from the fungus

Cephalosporium acremonium. Their mechanism of action is similar to that of penicillins, but their antibacterial effects differ.

PHARMACOLOGY

Cephalosporins are chemically and pharmacologically similar to penicillin. Their structure contains a beta-lactam ring, a dihydrothiazine ring, and side chains. They act by inhibiting bacterial cell wall synthesis, causing rapid cell lysis. (See *Comparing cephalosporins.*)

The sites of action for cephalosporins are enzymes known as penicillin-binding proteins (PBP). The affinity of certain cephalosporins for PBP in various microorganisms helps explain the differing activity in this class of antibiotics.

Cephalosporins are bactericidal. They act against many gram-positive and gram-negative bacteria and some anaerobic bacteria. They don't kill fungi or viruses.

First-generation cephalosporins act against many gram-positive cocci, including penicillinase-producing *Staphylococcus aureus* and *S. epidermidis; Streptococcus pneumoniae, Str. agalactiae* (group B streptococci), and *Str. pyogenes* (group A beta-hemolytic streptococci); susceptible gram-negative organisms include *Escherichia coli, Klebsiella pneumoniae, Proteus mirabilis,* and *Shigella* species.

Second-generation cephalosporins are effective against all organisms attacked by first-generation drugs and have additional activity against *Acinetobacter, Moraxella catarrhalis, Citrobacter, Enterobacter, Haemophilus influenzae, Neisseria, Providencia,* and *Serratia* species; *Bacteroides fragilis* is susceptible to cefotetan and cefoxitin.

Third-generation cephalosporins are less active than first- and second-generation drugs against gram-positive bacteria but more active against gram-

Comparing cephalosporins

Drug and route	Elimination half-life (hr)		Sodium (mEq/g)	CSF penetration
	Normal renal function	End-stage renal disease		
cefaclor oral	$1/2$-1	3-$5^1/_2$	Unknown	No
cefadroxil oral	1-2	20-25	Unknown	No
cefazolin I.M., I.V.	1-2	3-7	2-2.1	No
cefdinir P.O.	$1^1/_2$	16	Unknown	Unknown
cefepime I.M., I.V.	2	17-21	Unknown	Yes
cefoperazone I.M., I.V.	$1^1/_2$-$2^1/_2$	$1^1/_2$-3	1.5	Sometimes
cefotaxime I.M., I.V.	1-$1^1/_2$	3-11	2.2	Yes
cefotetan I.M., I.V.	3-5	13-35	3.5	No
cefoxitin I.M., I.V.	$1/2$-1	$6^1/_2$-$21^1/_2$	2.3	No
cefpodoxime oral	2-3	10	Unknown	Unknown
cefprozil oral	1-$1^1/_2$	5-6	Unknown	Unknown
ceftazidime I.M., I.V.	$1^1/_2$-2	35	2.3	Yes
ceftibuten oral	$2^1/_2$	$13^1/_2$-$22^1/_2$	Unknown	Unknown
ceftizoxime I.M., I.V.	$1^1/_2$-2	30	2.6	Yes
ceftriaxone I.M., I.V.	$5^1/_2$-11	$15^3/_4$	3.6	Yes
cefuroxime I.M., I.V.	1-2	15-22	2.4	Yes
cephalexin oral	$1/2$-1	19-22	Unknown	No
cephapirin I.M., I.V.	$1/2$-1	1-$1^1/_2$	2.4	No
cephradine oral, I.M., I.V.	$1/2$-2	8-15	6	No

♦ Off-label use

negative organisms, including those resistant to first- and second-generation drugs. Third-generation cephalosporins have the greatest stability against beta-lactamases produced by gram-negative bacteria. Susceptible gram-negative organisms include *Acinetobacter, Enterobacter, E. coli, Klebsiella, Morganella, Neisseria, Proteus, Providencia,* and *Serratia* species. Some third-generation drugs are active against *B. fragilis* and *Pseudomonas* species.

The fourth-generation cephalosporin cefepime is active against a wide range of gram-positive and gram-negative bacteria. Susceptible gram-negative organisms include *Enterobacter* species, *E. coli, K. pneumoniae, P. mirabilis,* and *Pseudomonas aeruginosa.* Susceptible gram-positive organisms include *S. aureus* (methicillin-susceptible strains only), *S. pneumoniae,* and *S. pyogenes* (Lancefield's group A streptococci).

Oral absorption of cephalosporins varies widely. Many must be given parenterally. Most are distributed widely into the body, the actual amount varying with individual drugs. CSF penetration by first- and second-generation drugs is minimal. Third-generation drugs achieve much greater penetration, and although the fourth-generation drug cefepime is known to cross the blood-brain barrier, to what degree isn't known. Cephalosporins cross the placental barrier. Degree of metabolism varies with individual drugs. Some aren't metabolized at all, whereas others are extensively metabolized.

Cephalosporins are excreted primarily in urine, chiefly by renal tubular effects. Elimination half-life ranges from 30 minutes to 10 hours in patients with normal renal function. Some drug appears in breast milk. Most cephalosporins can be removed by hemodialysis or peritoneal dialysis. Patients on dialysis may require dosage adjustment.

INDICATIONS & ACTIONS

➤ **Infection caused by susceptible organisms—**
Parenteral cephalosporins are used to treat serious infections of the lungs, skin, soft tissue, bones, joints, urinary tract, blood (septicemia), abdomen, and heart (endocarditis).

Third-generation cephalosporins (except cefoperazone) and the second-generation drug cefuroxime are used to treat CNS infections caused by susceptible strains of *H. influenzae, N. meningitidis,* and *S. pneumoniae;* meningitis caused by *E. coli* or *Klebsiella* species can be treated with ceftriaxone, cefotaxime, or ceftizoxime.

First-generation and some second-generation cephalosporins also can be given prophylactically to reduce postoperative infection after some surgical procedures. Third-generation drugs aren't usually indicated in those cases.

Penicillinase-producing *N. gonorrhoeae* can be treated with cefoxitin, cefotaxime, ceftriaxone, ceftizoxime, cefpodoxime, cefoperazone, or cefuroxime.

Cefepime, ceftazidime, and ceftriaxone have been used parenterally for empiric anti-infective therapy of probable bacterial infections in febrile neutropenic patients. Ceftriaxone may also be used to treat Lyme disease.

ADVERSE REACTIONS

Hypersensitivity reactions range from mild rash, fever, and eosinophilia to fatal anaphylaxis and are more common in patients with penicillin allergy. Hematologic reactions include positive direct and indirect antiglobulin (Coombs' test), thrombocytopenia or thrombocythemia, transient neutropenia, and reversible leukopenia. Adverse renal effects, nausea, vomiting, diarrhea, abdominal pain, glossitis, dyspepsia, tenesmus, and minimal elevation of liver function test values have occurred. Hemolytic anemia with extravascular hemolysis and some fatalities have occurred in patients receiving cefotaxime, ceftizoxime, ceftriaxone, or cefotetan.

Local venous pain and irritation are common after I.M. injection. Such reactions occur more often with higher doses and long-term therapy.

Disulfiram-type reactions occur when cefoperazone or cefotetan is given within 48 to 72 hours of alcohol ingestion.

Bacterial and fungal superinfection results from suppression of normal flora.

LIFESPAN CONSIDERATIONS
• Pregnancy risk category is B. Safety in pregnancy hasn't been established because relatively few controlled studies exist. Use only when clearly needed.
• Cephalosporins appear in breast milk. Use cautiously in breast-feeding women, taking into consideration the effects of the drug on the infants normal bowel flora or interference of culture results if the infant needs a fever or infection work-up.
• Drug half-life is prolonged in neonates and in infants up to age 1.
• Geriatric patients are susceptible to superinfection and to coagulopathies. Lower doses of cephalosporins may be needed.

diuretics, loop
bumetanide, ethacrynate sodium, ethacrynic acid, furosemide, torsemide

Loop diuretics are sometimes referred to as high-ceiling diuretics because they produce a peak diuresis greater than that produced by other drugs. Loop diuretics are particularly useful in edema caused by heart failure, hepatic cirrhosis, and renal disease. Ethacrynic acid may cause ototoxicity and a higher risk of GI reactions and is used less frequently. Structurally similar to furosemide, bumetanide is about 40 times more potent. Torsemide is the newest loop diuretic. (See *Comparing loop diuretics,* page 26.)

PHARMACOLOGY
Loop diuretics inhibit sodium and chloride reabsorption in the ascending loop of Henle, thus increasing renal excretion of sodium, chloride, and water. Like thiazide diuretics, loop diuretics increase excretion of potassium. They produce greater maximum diuresis and electrolyte loss than thiazide diuretics.

INDICATIONS & ACTIONS
➤Edema—
Loop diuretics effectively relieve edema caused by heart failure and may be useful in patients refractory to other diuretics. Because furosemide and bumetanide may increase glomerular filtration rate, they're useful in patients with renal impairment. I.V. loop diuretics are used adjunctively in patients with acute pulmonary edema to decrease peripheral vascular resistance. Loop diuretics also are used to treat edema caused by hepatic cirrhosis and nephrotic syndrome.
➤Hypertension—
Loop diuretics are used in patients with mild to moderate hypertension, although thiazides are the initial diuretics of choice in most patients. Loop diuretics are preferred in patients with heart failure or renal impairment. Used I.V., they're a helpful adjunct in managing hypertensive crises.

Loop diuretics have been used to increase excretion of calcium in patients with hypercalcemia.

Loop diuretics have been used to enhance the elimination of drugs and toxic substances after intoxication.

ADVERSE REACTIONS
The most common adverse effects of loop diuretics are metabolic and elec-

Comparing loop diuretics

Drug and route	Usual dosage	Onset (min)	Peak (hr)	Duration (hr)
bumetanide				
I.V.	0.5-1 mg ≤ t.i.d.	≤ 5	$^1/_4$-$^3/_4$	4-6
P.O.	0.5-2 mg/day	30-60	1-2	$^1/_2$-1
ethacrynic acid				
I.V.	50 mg/day	≤ 5	$^1/_4$-$^1/_2$	2
P.O.	50-100 mg/day	≤ 30	2	6-8
furosemide				
I.V.	20-40 mg q 2 hr, p.r.n.	≤ 5	$^1/_3$-1	2
P.O.	20-80 mg ≤ b.i.d.	30-60	1-2	6-8
torsemide				
I.V.	5-20 mg/day	≤ 10	≤ 1	6-8
P.O.	5-20 mg/day	≤ 60	1-2	6-8

trolyte disturbances (particularly potassium depletion), hypochloremic alkalosis, hyperglycemia, hyperuricemia, and hypomagnesemia. Rapid parenteral administration may cause hearing loss (including deafness) and tinnitus. High doses may produce profound diuresis, leading to hypovolemia and CV collapse.

LIFESPAN CONSIDERATIONS
• Pregnancy risk category ranges from B to C. There are no adequately controlled studies for use of loop diuretics in pregnant women. Avoid use if possible.
• Don't use loop diuretics in breast-feeding women.
• Use loop diuretics cautiously in neonates. Don't use ethacrynic acid and ethacrynate sodium in infants. The usual pediatric dose can be used, but extend dose intervals.
• Elderly and debilitated patients are more susceptible to drug-induced diuresis. Monitor carefully. Excessive diuresis can quickly lead to dehydration, hypovolemia, hypokalemia, and hyponatremia and may cause circulatory collapse. Reduced doses may be indicated.

diuretics, thiazide
bendroflumethiazide, chlorothiazide, chlorothiazide sodium, hydrochlorothiazide, hydroflumethiazide, methyclothiazide, polythiazide, trichlormethiazide

diuretics, thiazide-like
chlorthalidone, indapamide, metolazone

Thiazide diuretics were discovered and synthesized as an outgrowth of studies on carbonic anhydrase inhibitors. Thiazides proved a major advance because they were the first potent, and safe, diuretic.

PHARMACOLOGY
Thiazide diuretics interfere with sodium transport across tubules of the cortical diluting segment of the nephron, thereby increasing renal excretion of sodium, chloride, water, potassium, and calcium. Bicarbonate, magnesium, phosphate, bromide, and iodide excretion are also increased. These drugs may also decrease excretion of ammo-

Comparing thiazide diuretics

Drug	Equivalent dose (mg)	Onset (hr)	Peak (hr)	Duration (hr)
bendroflumethiazide	5	within 2	4	6-12
chlorothiazide	500	within 2	4	6-12
hydrochlorothiazide	50	within 2	4-6	6-12
methyclothiazide	5	within 2	4-6	24

nia, causing increased serum ammonia level. Long-term thiazide therapy can cause mild metabolic alkalosis caused by hypokalemia and hypochloremia.

The exact mechanism of thiazides' antihypertensive effect is unknown, but it's thought to be partially caused by direct dilation of the arteries. Thiazides initially decrease extracellular fluid volume, plasma volume, and cardiac output. Extracellular fluid volume and plasma volume revert to near baseline levels in several weeks but remain slightly below normal. Cardiac output returns to normal or slightly above. Total body sodium level remains slightly below pretreatment level. Peripheral vascular resistance is initially elevated but falls below pretreatment level with long-term diuretic therapy. (See *Comparing thiazide diuretics*.)

In patients with diabetes insipidus, thiazides cause a decrease in urine volume and increase in renal concentration of urine, possibly because of sodium depletion and decreased plasma volume. This leads to an increase in renal water and sodium reabsorption. In addition, thiazides can cause hyperglycemia, exacerbation of diabetes mellitus, or precipitation of diabetes mellitus.

INDICATIONS & ACTIONS
➤**Edema**—
Thiazide diuretics are used to treat edema caused by heart failure and nephrotic syndrome and, with spironolactone,

to treat edema and ascites caused by hepatic cirrhosis. Thiazides may also be used to control edema during pregnancy except if caused by renal disease. This treatment isn't indicated for mild edema.

Efficacy and toxicity profiles of thiazide and thiazide-like diuretics are equivalent at comparable doses. The single exception is metolazone, which may be more effective in patients with impaired renal function. Usually, thiazide diuretics are less effective than loop diuretics in patients with renal insufficiency.

➤**Hypertension**—
Thiazide diuretics are commonly used for initial management of all degrees of hypertension. Used alone, they reduce mean blood pressure by only 10 to 15 mm Hg. In mild hypertension, thiazide diuresis alone will usually reduce blood pressure to desired levels. However, in moderate to severe hypertension that doesn't respond to thiazides alone, combination therapy with another antihypertensive is needed.

➤**Diabetes insipidus**—
In diabetes insipidus, thiazides cause a decrease in urine volume. Urine becomes more concentrated, possibly because of sodium depletion and decreased plasma volume. Thiazides are particularly effective in nephrogenic diabetes insipidus.

➤**Other uses**—
Thiazides are used for prophylaxis of renal calculi formation from hypercal-

ciuria and to treat electrolyte disturbances caused by renal tubular necrosis.

ADVERSE REACTIONS

Thiazide diuretics cause electrolyte and metabolic disturbances, the most common being potassium depletion. Patients may require dietary supplementation.

Other abnormalities include hypochloremic alkalosis, hypomagnesemia, hyponatremia, hypercalcemia, hyperuricemia, elevated cholesterol levels, and hyperglycemia. Overdose of thiazides may produce lethargy that can progress to coma within a few hours.

LIFESPAN CONSIDERATIONS

• Pregnancy risk category ranges from B to C. Thiazides cross the placental barrier and appear in cord blood. Risks and benefits must be evaluated. Results are inconclusive, but teratogenic effects have been reported. Some prescribers recommend avoiding use in the first trimester. Routine use isn't recommended with mild edema.
• Thiazides appear in breast milk. Safety and effectiveness in breast-feeding women haven't been established.
• Safety and effectiveness in children haven't been established for all thiazide diuretics. Indapamide and metolazone aren't recommended for use in children.
• Elderly and debilitated patients require close observation and may need reduced doses. In elderly patients, excess diuresis can quickly lead to dehydration, hypovolemia, hyponatremia, hypomagnesemia, and hypokalemia.

estrogens

esterified estrogens, estradiol, estradiol acetate, estradiol cypionate, estradiol hemihydrate, estradiol valerate, estrogen and progestin, estrogenic substances (conjugated), estropipate, ethinyl estradiol

Estrogens have several uses: treatment of the symptoms of menopause, atrophic vaginitis, breast cancer, vulva and vaginal atrophy, treatment of hypoestrogenism, and other diseases; prophylaxis of osteoporosis; and contraception, when in combination with progestins.

PHARMACOLOGY

Estrogens are hormones secreted by ovarian follicles, the adrenals, corpus luteum, placenta, and testes. Conjugated estrogens and estrogenic substances are normally obtained from the urine of pregnant mares. Other estrogens are manufactured synthetically or from plant sources.

Estrogens promote the development and maintenance of the female reproductive system and secondary sexual characteristics. They inhibit the release of pituitary gonadotropins and have various metabolic effects, including retention of fluid and electrolytes, retention and deposition in bone of calcium and phosphorus, and mild anabolic activity. They increase high-density lipoproteins and decrease low-density lipoproteins.

Estrogens and estrogenic substances administered as drugs have effects related to endogenous estrogen's mechanism of action. They can mimic the action of endogenous estrogen when used as replacement therapy or produce such useful effects as inhibiting ovulation or growth of certain hormone-sensitive cancers.

Use of estrogens isn't risk-free. Long-term use is linked to an increased risk of endometrial cancer, gallbladder disease, and thromboembolic disease. Elevations in blood pressure often occur as well.

INDICATIONS & ACTIONS
➤**Moderate to severe vasomotor symptoms of menopause—**
Endogenous estrogens are significantly reduced after menopause. This usually results in vasomotor symptoms, such as hot flashes and dizziness. Estradiol, estradiol acetate, estradiol valerate, and estradiol cypionate mimic the action of endogenous estrogens in preventing these symptoms.
➤**Breast cancer—**
Conjugated estrogens, esterified estrogens, and estradiol inhibit the growth of hormone-sensitive cancers in certain carefully selected men and postmenopausal women.
➤**Prostate cancer—**
Conjugated estrogens, esterified estrogens, estradiol, and estradiol valerate inhibit growth of hormone-sensitive cancer tissue in men with advanced disease.
➤**To prevent postmenopausal osteoporosis—**
Estradiol and conjugated estrogens replace or augment activity of endogenous estrogen in causing calcium and phosphate retention and preventing bone decalcification.
➤**Hypoestrogenism—**
Estradiol and estradiol valerate supplement depleted hormones which cause hypogonadism, castration, or primary ovarian failure. Estradiol cypionate is indicated for the treatment of female hypogonadism only.
➤**Vulva and vaginal atrophy—**
Estradiol, estradiol acetate, and estradiol valerate decrease the destruction of these areas in women.

➤**Contraception—**
Ethinyl estradiol is used with progestins for ovulation control to prevent conception.

ADVERSE REACTIONS
Acute reactions include changes in menstrual bleeding patterns (spotting, prolonged or absent bleeding), abdominal cramps, swollen feet or ankles, bloated sensation (fluid and electrolyte retention), breast swelling and tenderness, weight gain, nausea, loss of appetite, headache, photosensitivity, and loss of libido.

With long-term administration, adverse reactions include increased blood pressure (sometimes into the hypertensive range), thromboembolic disease, cholestatic jaundice, benign hepatomas and endometrial carcinoma (rare). Risk of thromboembolic disease increases significantly with cigarette smoking, especially in women older than age 35. Increased risk of thromboembolic events also may occur in postmenopausal women, women undergoing surgery, and those who have fractures or are immobilized.

LIFESPAN CONSIDERATIONS
● Estrogens are contraindicated in pregnant women.
● Estrogens are contraindicated in breast-feeding women.
● Because of the effects of estrogen on epiphyseal closure, use estrogens cautiously in adolescents whose bone growth isn't complete. Estrogens aren't used in children.
● Postmenopausal women with a uterus who are on long-term estrogen therapy have an increased risk of endometrial cancer. This risk can be reduced by adding a progestin to the regimen.

♦ Off-label use

Comparing fluoroquinolones

Drug	Oral bioavailability (%)	Plasma protein–binding (%)	Half-life (hr)
ciprofloxacin	70-80 (with food)	20-40	Normal renal function: 4-6 Severe renal failure: 6-8
gatifloxacin	96 (without regard to food)	20	Normal renal function: 7-14 Severe renal failure: 36
gemifloxacin	60-84 (without regard to food)	60-70	Normal renal function: 7
levofloxacin	100 (without regard to food)	50	Normal renal function: 6 Severe renal failure: 76
lomefloxacin	78-86 (without regard to food)	10	Normal renal function: not stated Severe renal failure: 21-45
moxifloxacin	90 (without regard to food)	50	Normal renal function: 10-14
norfloxacin	30-40 (without regard to food)	10-15	Normal renal function: 3-4 Severe renal failure: 9-10
ofloxacin	98 (without regard to food)	20-25	Normal renal function: $4^{1}/_{2}$-7 Severe renal failure: 28-37
sparfloxacin	92 (without regard to food)	45	Normal renal function: 16-30 Severe renal failure: 38.5

fluoroquinolones

ciprofloxacin, gatifloxacin, gemifloxacin, levofloxacin, lomefloxacin, moxifloxacin, norfloxacin, ofloxacin

Fluoroquinolones are broad-spectrum, systemic antibacterial drugs active against a wide range of aerobic gram-positive and gram-negative organisms. Gram-positive aerobic bacteria include *Staphylococcus aureus, Staphylococcus epidermis, Staphylococcus hemolyticus, Staphylococcus saprophyticus;* penicillinase- and non–penicillinase-producing staphylococci and some methicillin-resistant strains; *Strepto-coccus pneumoniae;* group A (beta) he-molytic streptococci *(S. pyogenes);* group B streptococci *(S. agalactiae); viridans streptococci;* groups C, F, and G streptococci and nonenterococcal group D streptococci; *Enterococcus faecalis.* These drugs are active against gram-positive aerobic bacilli including *Corynebacterium* species, *Listeria monocytogenes,* and *Nocardia aster-oides.*

Fluoroquinolones are effective against gram-negative aerobic bacteria including, but not limited to, *Neisseria meningitidis* and most strains of penicillinase- and non–penicillinase-producing *Haemophilus ducreyi, H. influenzae, H. parainfluenzae, Moraxel-la catarrhalis, N. gonorrhoeae,* and most clinically important *Enterobacte-riaceae, Pseudomonas aeruginosa, Vibrio cholerae,* and *V. parahaemolyti-cus.* Certain fluoroquinolones are active against *Chlamydia trachomatis, Le-gionella pneumophila, Mycobacterium avium-intracellulare, Mycoplasma ho-minis,* and *M. pneumoniae.*

Peak concentration (hr)	Elimination	Dialyzability
1-2	40%-70% of drug is cleared unchanged by the kidneys in 24 hr	< 10% removed by hemodialysis
1-2	70% unchanged by the kidneys	Not defined
1/2-2	36% of drug is cleared unchanged by the kidneys	20-30% removed by hemodialysis
1	Almost entirely eliminated unchanged in the urine	Not defined
1 1/2	60%-80% of drug is cleared unchanged by the kidneys in 48 hr	< 3% removed by hemodialysis
1-3	45% unchanged (20% in urine, 25% in feces)	Not defined
1-2	26% of drug is cleared unchanged by the kidneys in 24 hr	< 10% removed by hemodialysis
1-2	70%-90% of drug is cleared unchanged by the kidneys in 36 hr	< 10%-30% removed by hemodialysis
3-6	10% is excreted unchanged in the urine	Not defined

PHARMACOLOGY
Fluoroquinolones produce a bactericidal effect by inhibiting intracellular DNA topoisomerase II (DNA gyrase) or topoisomerase IV. These enzymes are essential catalysts in the duplication, transcription, and repair of bacterial DNA. (See *Comparing fluoroquinolones.*)

INDICATIONS & ACTIONS
➤Bone and joint infections, bacterial bronchitis, endocervical and urethral chlamydial infections, bacterial gastroenteritis, endocervical and urethral gonorrhea, intra-abdominal infections, febrile neutropenia, pelvic inflammatory disease, bacterial pneumonia, bacterial prostatitis, acute sinusitis, skin and soft tissue infections, typhoid fever, bacterial UTIs, chancroid, meningococcal carriers, and bacterial septicemia—
Fluoroquinolones are used to treat infections caused by many aerobic gram-positive and gram-negative organisms.
➤To prevent bacterial UTIs—
Fluoroquinolones are used to prevent infections caused by susceptible organisms.

ADVERSE REACTIONS
The following adverse effects are observed rarely with fluoroquinolones but require medical attention: CNS stimulation (acute psychosis, agitation, hallucinations, tremors), hepatotoxicity, hypersensitivity reactions, interstitial nephritis, phlebitis, pseudomembranous colitis, and tendinitis or tendon rupture. The following adverse effects require no medical attention unless they persist or become intolerable: CNS effects (dizziness, headache, ner-

◆ Off-label use

vousness, drowsiness, insomnia), GI reactions, and photosensitivity.

LIFESPAN CONSIDERATIONS
● Pregnancy risk category is C. Adequate, well-controlled trials haven't been completed, but these drugs cross the placental barrier and may cause arthropathies.
● It's unknown if a fluoroquinolone appears in breast milk. Breast-feeding patients should avoid therapy with this drug because it may cause arthropathies in newborns and infants.
● Fluoroquinolones aren't recommended in children because they can cause joint problems.
● Geriatric patients may require a reduction in their daily dose because of slower renal function.

histamine₂-receptor antagonists
cimetidine, famotidine, nizatidine, ranitidine

The introduction of H₂-receptor antagonists had revolutionized the treatment of peptic ulcer disease. These drugs structurally resemble histamine and competitively inhibit the action of histamine on gastric H₂-receptor. (See *Comparing adult dosages of histamine₂-receptor antagonists.*)

PHARMACOLOGY
All H₂-receptor antagonists inhibit the action of histamine at H₂-receptors, reducing gastric acid output and concentration.

INDICATIONS & ACTIONS
➤**Duodenal ulcer**—
Cimetidine, famotidine, nizatidine, and ranitidine are used to treat acute duodenal ulcer and to prevent ulcer recurrence.

➤**Gastric ulcer**—
Cimetidine, famotidine, nizatidine, and ranitidine are indicated for acute gastric ulcer. However, the benefits of long-term therapy (over 8 weeks) have not been proven.
➤**Hypersecretory states**—
Cimetidine, famotidine, nizatidine, and ranitidine are used to treat hypersecretory states such as Zollinger-Ellison syndrome. Because patients with these conditions need much higher doses than those with peptic ulcer disease, they may experience more pronounced adverse effects.
➤**Reflux esophagitis**—
Cimetidine, famotidine, nizatidine, and ranitidine are used to provide short-term relief from gastroesophageal reflux in patients who don't respond to conventional therapy (lifestyle changes, antacids, diet modification). These drugs raise the stomach pH. Some prescribers prefer to combine the H₂-receptor antagonist with metoclopramide, but further study is needed to confirm effectiveness of the combination.
➤**Stress ulcer prevention ♦** —
In unlabeled use, cimetidine, famotidine, nizatidine, and ranitidine help prevent stress ulcers in critically ill patients, particularly those in ICU. Some prescribers prefer intensive antacid therapy for such patients.
➤**Unlabeled uses ♦** —
H₂-receptor antagonists are used for many unlabeled indications, including short-bowel syndrome, prevention of allergic reactions to I.V. contrast medium, and to eradicate *H. pylori* in treatment of peptic ulcers. Other uses include relief of occasional heartburn, acid indigestion, or sour stomach.

ADVERSE REACTIONS
Although H₂-receptor antagonists rarely cause adverse reactions, patients may develop mild transient diarrhea, dizziness, fatigue, headache, muscle

Comparing adult dosages of histamine$_2$-receptor antagonists

Indication	cimetidine	famotidine	nizatidine	ranitidine
Duodenal ulcer	I.M., I.V. 300 mg q 6-8 hr P.O. 800 mg h.s. or 300 mg q.i.d. with meals and h.s. or 400 mg b.i.d.	I.V. 20 mg q 12 hr P.O. 40 mg h.s. or 20 mg b.i.d.	P.O. 300 mg h.s. or 150 mg b.i.d.	I.M., I.V. 50 mg q 6-8 hr P.O. 150 mg b.i.d. or 300 mg once per day after evening meal or h.s.
Duodenal ulcer maintenance	P.O. 400 mg h.s.	P.O. 20 mg h.s.	P.O. 150 mg h.s.	P.O. 150 mg h.s.
Gastric ulcer	I.M., I.V. 300 mg q 6-8 hr P.O. 800 mg h.s. or 300 mg q.i.d. with meals and h.s.	I.V. 20 mg q 12 hr P.O. 40 mg h.s.	P.O. 300 mg h.s. or 150 mg b.i.d.	P.O. 150 mg b.i.d.
Gastric ulcer maintenance	No approved dosage	No approved dosage	No approved dosage	P.O. 150 mg h.s.
Gastroesophageal reflux disease	P.O. 400 mg q.i.d. or 800 mg b.i.d.	P.O. 20 mg b.i.d.	P.O. 150 mg b.i.d.	P.O. 150 mg b.i.d.
Erosive esophagitis	P.O. 400 mg q.i.d. or 800 mg b.i.d.	P.O. 20-40 mg b.i.d.	P.O. 150 mg b.i.d.	P.O. 150 mg q.i.d.
Erosive esophagitis healing maintenance	No approved dosage	No approved dosage	No approved dosage	P.O. 150 mg b.i.d.
Pathological hypersecretory conditions	I.M., I.V. 300 mg q 6-8 hr P.O. 300 mg q.i.d. with meals and h.s.	I.V. 20 mg q 12 hr P.O. 20 mg q 6 hr	No approved dosage	I.M., I.V. 50 mg q 6-8 hr P.O. 150 mg b.i.d.
Prevention of upper GI bleeding	I.V.: 50 mg/hr continuous infusion	No approved dosage	No approved dosage	No approved dosage
Heartburn, acid indigestion, sour stomach	P.O. 200 mg, p.r.n., up to 400 mg daily.	P.O. 10 mg, p.r.n., up to 10 mg b.i.d.	P.O. 75 mg, p.r.n., up to 75 mg b.i.d.	P.O. 75 mg p.r.n., up to 75 mg b.i.d.

pain, and irritation at I.V. site. Cimetidine may also cause impotence and mild gynecomastia.

Cimetidine may inhibit hepatic enzymes, thereby impairing the metabolism of certain drugs. Ranitidine may also produce this effect but to a lesser extent. Famotidine and nizatidine don't inhibit hepatic enzymes or drug clearance.

LIFESPAN CONSIDERATIONS
• Pregnancy risk category B. No adequate controlled studies have been done in pregnant women.
• H$_2$-receptor antagonists may appear in breast milk. Use cautiously.
• Safety and efficacy in children haven't been established.
• Use cautiously when giving these drugs to geriatric patients because of the increased risk of adverse reactions, particularly those affecting the CNS.

♦ Off-label use

Dosage adjustment is required in patients with impaired renal function.

---

nitrates
amyl nitrite, isosorbide, nitroglycerin

Nitroglycerin is the therapeutic mainstay for classic and variant angina. A commercial I.V. nitroglycerin form is used to reduce afterload and preload in various cardiac disorders.

PHARMACOLOGY
The major pharmacologic property of nitrates is vascular smooth-muscle relaxation, resulting in generalized vasodilation. Venous effects predominate; however, nitroglycerin produces dose-dependent dilatation of both arterial and venous beds.

Nitrates are metabolized to a free radical nitric oxide thought to be an endothelium-derived relaxing factor, which is usually impaired in patients with coronary artery disease.

Decreased peripheral venous resistance results in venous pooling of blood and decreased venous return to the heart (preload); decreased arteriolar resistance reduces systemic vascular resistance and arterial pressure (afterload). These vascular effects reduce myocardial oxygen consumption, promoting a more favorable oxygen supply to demand ratio.

Although nitrates reflexively increase heart rate and myocardial contractility, reduced ventricular wall tension results in a net decrease in myocardial oxygen consumption. In the coronary circulation, nitrates redistribute circulating blood flow along collateral channels and preferentially increase subendocardial blood flow, improving perfusion to the ischemic myocardium.

Nitrates relax all smooth muscle, not just vascular smooth muscle, regardless of autonomic innervation, including bronchial, biliary, GI, ureteral, and uterine smooth muscle.

INDICATIONS & ACTIONS
➤ **Angina pectoris—**
By relaxing vascular smooth muscle in both the venous and arterial beds, nitrates decrease myocardial oxygen consumption. By dilating coronary vessels, they redistribute blood flow to ischemic tissue. Although systemic and coronary vascular effects vary slightly, depending on which nitrate is used, both smooth-muscle relaxation and vasodilation probably account for the value of nitrates in treating angina. Because individual nitrates have similar pharmacologic and therapeutic properties, the best nitrate to use in a specific situation depends mainly on the onset of action and duration of effect required.

S.L. nitroglycerin is the drug of choice for acute angina pectoris because of its rapid onset of action, low cost, and effectiveness. Lingual or buccal nitroglycerin and other rapidly acting nitrates, such as amyl nitrite and S.L. or chewable isosorbide dinitrate, also may be useful for this indication. Amyl nitrite is rarely used because it's expensive, inconvenient, and carries a high risk of adverse effects. S.L., lingual, or buccal nitroglycerin or S.L. or chewable isosorbide dinitrate typically are effective in circumstances likely to provoke an angina attack.

Beta blockers usually are considered the drug of choice in the prophylactic management of angina pectoris. Nitrates with a relatively long duration of effect include oral preparations of isosorbide mononitrate and isosorbide dinitrate, and oral or topical nitroglycerin. Combination treatment of beta blockers and nitrates appears to be the therapy of choice.

The effectiveness of oral nitrates is debatable, although isosorbide dinitrate, isosorbide mononitrate, and nitroglycerin generally are considered effective. However, the effectiveness of topical nitroglycerin preparations hasn't been fully determined. Some experts believe oral nitrates are ineffective or less effective than rapidly acting I.V. nitrates in reducing frequency of angina and increasing exercise tolerance. Also, prolonged use of oral nitrates may cause cross-tolerance to S.L. nitrates.

I.V. nitroglycerin may be used to treat unstable angina pectoris, Prinzmetal's angina, and angina pectoris in patients who haven't responded to recommended doses of nitrates or a beta blocker.

Sedatives may be useful in the adjunctive management of angina pectoris caused by psychogenic factors. However, if combination therapy is required, each drug should be adjusted individually. Fixed combinations of oral nitrates and sedatives should be avoided.

➤ Acute MI—
The hemodynamic effects of I.V., S.L., or topical nitroglycerin may prove beneficial in treating left-sided heart failure and pulmonary congestion caused by acute MI. However, the effect of the drug on morbidity and mortality in patients with these conditions is controversial.

I.V., S.L., and topical nitroglycerin and isosorbide dinitrate are effective in managing acute and chronic heart failure. S.L. administration can quickly reverse the signs and symptoms of pulmonary congestion in acute pulmonary edema. The I.V. form may control hemodynamic status more accurately.

➤ Other uses—
I.V. nitroglycerin is used to control perioperative hypertension, hypertensive emergencies, heart failure, and pulmonary edema caused by MI.

I.V. nitroglycerin has been used to treat severe hypertension and hypertensive crises. Other forms have been used to treat refractory heart failure. Nitroglycerin also has been used to relieve pain, dysphagia, and spasm in patients with diffuse esophageal spasm without gastroesophageal reflux.

ADVERSE REACTIONS
Headache is most common early in therapy. It may be severe but usually diminishes rapidly. Orthostatic hypotension, dizziness, weakness, and transient flushing may occur. Patients sensitive to hypotensive effects may experience nausea, vomiting, weakness, restlessness, pallor, cold sweats, tachycardia, syncope, or CV collapse. Dosage reduction may control GI upset. Therapy should be discontinued if patient develops blurred vision, dry mouth, or rash. Dependence can occur with repeated, prolonged use.

Tolerance, caused by a high or sustained drug level, occurs usually with oral, I.V., and topical therapy and rarely with intermittent S.L. use. Patients taking oral isosorbide dinitrate or topical nitroglycerin haven't exhibited cross-tolerance to S.L. nitroglycerin. Patients may become tolerant of the vascular and antianginal effects of the drugs, and cross-tolerance between the nitrates and nitrites may occur. To prevent tolerance, the lowest effective dose and an intermittent dosing schedule should be used. A nitrate-free interval of 10 to 12 hours daily may also be helpful.

LIFESPAN CONSIDERATIONS
• Pregnancy risk category is C. No adequate controlled studies have been done in pregnant women. Use only if clearly indicated.
• It's unknown if drugs appear in breast milk. Use cautiously.
• Safety and effectiveness of nitrates in children haven't been established.

opioids

alfentanil hydrochloride, codeine,
difenoxin hydrochloride,
diphenoxylate hydrochloride,
fentanyl citrate, hydromorphone
hydrochloride, levomethadyl
acetate hydrochloride, meperidine
hydrochloride, methadone
hydrochloride, morphine sulfate,
oxycodone hydrochloride,
oxymorphone hydrochloride,
propoxyphene, remifentanil
hydrochloride, sufentanil citrate

Opioids, previously called narcotic
agonists, usually include natural and
semisynthetic alkaloid derivatives from
opium and their synthetic surrogates,
whose actions mimic those of morphine. Most of these drugs are classified as Schedule II by the Federal Drug
Enforcement Agency because they
have a high potential for addiction and
abuse. In the past, opioids were used
indiscriminately for analgesia and sedation and to control diarrhea and
cough. (See *Comparing opioids*.)

PHARMACOLOGY

Opioids act as agonists at specific opiate receptor binding sites in the CNS
and other tissues. These are the same
receptors occupied by endogenous opioid peptides (enkephalins and endor-
phins) to alter CNS response to painful
stimuli. Opiate agonists don't alter the
cause of pain, only the patient's perception of it. They relieve pain without affecting other sensory functions. Opiate
receptors are present in highest concentrations in the limbic system, thalamus,
striatum, hypothalamus, midbrain, and
spinal cord.

Opioids produce respiratory depression by a direct effect on the respiratory centers in the brain stem, resulting
in decreased sensitivity and responsiveness to increases in carbon dioxide tension. These drugs offer direct suppression of the cough reflex center. They
also cause nausea.

Opioids cause drowsiness, sedation,
euphoria, dysphoria, mental clouding,
and EEG changes. Higher than usual
analgesic doses cause anesthesia. Most
opioids cause miosis, although meperidine and its derivatives may also cause
mydriasis or no pupillary change.

Because opioids decrease gastric,
biliary, and pancreatic secretions and
delay digestion, constipation is a common adverse effect. At the same time,
these drugs increase tone in the biliary
tract and may cause biliary spasms.
Some patients may have no biliary effects, whereas others may have biliary
spasms that increase plasma amylase
and lipase levels up to 15 times normal
values.

Opioids increase smooth-muscle
tone in the urinary tract and induce
spasms, causing the urge to urinate.
These drugs may cause orthostatic hypotension. They are linked to signs and
symptoms of histamine release or peripheral vasodilation, including pruritus, flushing, red eyes, and sweating—
effects often mistakenly attributed to
allergy, which should be evaluated
carefully.

Opiates can be divided chemically
into three groups: phenanthrenes
(codeine, hydrocodone, hydromorphone, morphine, oxycodone, and
oxymorphone); diphenylheptanes
(levomethadyl, methadone, and propoxyphene); and phenylpiperidines
(alfentanil, diphenoxylate, fentanyl,
meperidine, remifentanil, and sufentanil). If a patient is hypersensitive to
an opioid, agonist-antagonist, or antagonist of a given chemical group, use
extreme caution when considering the
use of another agent from the same
chemical group. However, a drug from
the other groups might be well tolerated.

Comparing opioids

Drug	Route	Onset (min)	Peak	Duration (hr)
alfentanil	I.V.	Immediate	Not available	Not available
codeine	I.M., P.O., S.C.	15-30	30-60 min	4-6
fentanyl	I.M., I.V.	7-8	Not available	1-2
hydrocodone	P.O.	30	60 min	4-6
hydromorphone	I.M., I.V., S.C.	15	30 min	4-5
	P.O., rectal	30	60 min	4-5
meperidine	I.M.	10-15	30-50 min	2-4
	P.O.	15-30	60 min	2-4
	S.C.	10-15	40-60 min	2-4
methadone	I.M., P.O., S.C.	30-60	30-60 min	4-6†
morphine	I.M.	≤ 20	30-60 min	3-7
	P.O., rectal	≤ 20	≤ 60 min	3-7
	S.C.	≤ 20	50-90 min	3-7
oxycodone	P.O.	15-30	30-60 min	4-6
oxymorphone	I.M., S.C.	10-15	30-60 min	3-6
	I.V.	5-10	30-60 min	3-6
	rectal	15-30	30-60 min	3-6
propoxyphene	P.O.	20-60	2-2½ hr	4-6
remifentanil	I.V.	Immediate	Not available	Not available
sufentanil	I.V.	1.3-3	Not available	Not available

† Because of cumulative effects, duration of action increases with repeated doses.

Some opioids are well absorbed after oral or rectal administration, whereas others must be given parenterally. I.V. dosing is the most rapidly effective and reliable method. Absorption after I.M. or S.C. dosing may be erratic. Opioids vary in onset and duration of action. They are removed rapidly from the bloodstream and distributed, in decreasing order of concentration, into skeletal muscle, kidneys, liver, intestinal tract, lungs, spleen, and brain. They readily cross the placental barrier.

Opioids are metabolized mainly in the endoplasmic reticulum of the liver (first-pass effect) and also in the CNS, kidneys, lungs, and placenta. They undergo conjugation with glucuronic acid, hydrolysis, oxidation, or N-dealkylation.

They are excreted primarily in the urine, but small amounts are excreted in the feces.

INDICATIONS & ACTIONS

The opioids produce varying degrees of analgesia and have antitussive, antidiarrheal, and sedative effects. Clinical response is dose-related and varies with each patient.

➤Analgesia—

Opioids may be used in the symptomatic management of moderate to severe pain caused by acute and some chronic disorders, including renal or biliary colic, MI, acute trauma, postoperative pain, or terminal cancer. They also may be used to provide analgesia during diagnostic and orthopedic procedures and during labor. Drug selection, route of administration, and dose depend on a variety of factors. For example, in mild pain, oral therapy with codeine or oxycodone is usually sufficient. In acute pain of short duration, such as that caused by diagnostic procedures or orthopedic manipulation, a short-acting drug, such as meperidine or fentanyl, is effective.

These drugs are often given to alleviate postoperative pain, but because they influence CNS function, carefully monitor the course of recovery to detect early signs of complications. Opioids are used to manage severe, chronic pain caused by terminal cancer, which requires careful evaluation and adjustment of drug, dose, and route of administration.

➤**Pulmonary edema**—
Morphine, meperidine, oxymorphone, hydromorphone, and similar drugs have been used to relieve anxiety in patients with dyspnea caused by acute pulmonary edema and acute left-sided heart failure. These drugs shouldn't be used to treat pulmonary edema resulting from a chemical respiratory stimulant. Opioids decrease peripheral resistance, causing pooling of blood in the limbs and decreased venous return, cardiac workload, and pulmonary venous pressure. Blood is shifted from the central to the peripheral circulation.

➤**Preoperative sedation**—
Routine use of opioids for preoperative sedation in patients without pain isn't recommended because it may cause complications during and after surgery. To ease preoperative anxiety, a barbiturate or benzodiazepine is equally effective, with a lower risk of postoperative vomiting.

➤**Anesthesia**—
Certain opioids, including alfentanil, fentanyl, remifentanil, and sufentanil, may be used for induction of anesthesia, as an adjunct in the maintenance of

general and regional anesthesia, or as a primary anesthetic agent in surgery.

➤**Cough suppression**—
Some opioids, most commonly codeine and its derivative, hydrocodone, are used as antitussives to relieve dry, nonproductive cough.

➤**Diarrhea**—
Diphenoxylate and other opioids are used as antidiarrheals. All opioids cause constipation to some degree, but only a few are indicated for this use. Usually, opiate antidiarrheals are empirically combined with antacids, absorbing drugs, and belladonna alkaloids in commercial preparations.

ADVERSE REACTIONS

Respiratory depression and circulatory depression, including orthostatic hypotension, are the major hazards of treatment with opioids. Rapid I.V. administration increases the risk of these serious adverse effects. Respiratory arrest, shock, and cardiac arrest have occurred. It's likely that equianalgesic doses of individual opiates produce a comparable degree of respiratory depression, but its duration may vary.

Other adverse CNS effects include dizziness, visual disturbances, mental clouding or depression, sedation, coma, euphoria, dysphoria, weakness, faintness, agitation, restlessness, nervousness, seizures, and, rarely, delirium and insomnia.

Adverse effects seem to be more common in ambulatory patients and those not experiencing severe pain. Adverse GI effects include nausea, vomiting, and constipation, as well as increased biliary tract pressure that may result in biliary spasm or colic. Tolerance, psychological dependence, and physical dependence may follow prolonged, high-dose therapy (more than 100 mg of morphine daily for longer than 1 month).

Use opiate agonists extremely cautiously during pregnancy and labor be-

cause they readily cross the placental barrier. Premature infants are especially sensitive to their respiratory and CNS depressant effects.

Opiate agonists have a high potential for addiction and should always be administered cautiously in patients susceptible to physical or psychological dependence. The agonist-antagonists have a lower potential for addiction and abuse, but the possibility still exists.

LIFESPAN CONSIDERATIONS
● Meperidine and oxymorphone hydrochloride are classified as pregnancy risk category B, but D if used for a long time or for high doses used at term. Most opioids are listed as pregnancy risk category C.
● Administration of an opiate to a woman shortly before delivery may cause respiratory depression in the neonate. Watch neonate closely and be prepared to resuscitate.
● Codeine, meperidine, methadone, morphine, and propoxyphene appear in breast milk and should be used cautiously in breast-feeding women. Methadone may cause physical dependence in breast-feeding infants of women on maintenance therapy.
● Safety and efficacy in children haven't been established. Give cautiously to children.
● Elderly patients usually need lower doses because they may be more sensitive to the therapeutic and adverse effects of drug.

opioid agonist-antagonists
buprenorphine hydrochloride, butorphanol tartrate, nalbuphine hydrochloride, pentazocine hydrochloride

These drugs have varying degrees of agonist and antagonist activity. They are potent analgesics, with less addiction potential than the pure opioid agonists.

PHARMACOLOGY
Each drug in this class is believed to act differently on the various opiate receptors in the CNS, thus yielding slightly different effects. Like the opioid agonists, these drugs can be divided into related chemical groups. Buprenorphine, butorphanol, and nalbuphine are phenanthrenes, like morphine, whereas pentazocine is a benzomorphan.

INDICATIONS & ACTIONS
➤Pain—
Opioid agonist-antagonists are primarily used as analgesics, particularly in patients at high risk for drug dependence or abuse. Some are used as preoperative or preanesthetic medication, to supplement balanced anesthesia, or to relieve prepartum pain.
➤Other uses—
Buprenorphine reverses fentanyl-induced anesthesia. Buprenorphine and naloxone reduce opiate consumption in patients who are physically dependent on opiates.

ADVERSE REACTIONS
Major hazards of agonist-antagonists are respiratory depression, apnea, shock, and cardiopulmonary arrest, possibly causing death. All opioid agonist-antagonists can cause respiratory depression, but the severity of depression each drug can cause has a "ceiling"; for example, each drug depresses respiration to a certain point, but increased doses don't depress it further. All opioid agonist-antagonists have been reported to cause withdrawal symptoms after abrupt discontinuation of long-term use. They have some addiction potential, but less than the pure opioid agonists.

CNS effects are the most common adverse reactions and may include drowsiness, sedation, light-headedness, dizziness, hallucinations, disorientation, agitation, euphoria, dysphoria, insomnia, confusion, headache, tremor, miosis, seizures, and psychological dependence. CV reactions may include tachycardia, bradycardia, palpitations, chest wall rigidity, hypertension, hypotension, syncope, and edema. GI reactions may include nausea, vomiting, and constipation (most common), dry mouth, anorexia, and biliary spasms. Other effects include urine retention or hesitancy, decreased libido, flushing, rash, pruritus, and pain at the injection site.

Opioid agonist-antagonists can produce morphinelike dependence and thus have abuse potential. Psychological and physiologic drug dependence and tolerance can develop after prolonged repeated administration. Patients with dependence or tolerance to opioid agonist-antagonists usually demonstrate an acute abstinence syndrome or withdrawal signs and symptoms, of which the severity is related to the degree of dependence, abruptness of withdrawal, and the drug used.

Common signs and symptoms of withdrawal are yawning, lacrimation, and sweating (early); mydriasis, piloerection, facial flushing, tachycardia, tremor, irritability, and anorexia (intermediate); and muscle spasms, fever, nausea, vomiting, and diarrhea (late).

LIFESPAN CONSIDERATIONS
• Most drugs in this class are pregnancy risk category C. Giving an opiate agonist-antagonist to a woman shortly before delivery may cause respiratory depression in the neonate. The infant must be closely monitored. Be prepared to resuscitate.
• These drugs aren't recommended for breast-feeding women.
• Neonates may be more susceptible to the respiratory depressant effects of opiate agonist-antagonists.

• Elderly patients usually need lower doses because they may be more sensitive to the therapeutic and adverse effects of drug.

penicillins

Natural penicillins: penicillin G benzathine, penicillin G potassium, penicillin G procaine, penicillin G sodium, penicillin V potassium

Aminopenicillins: amoxicillin trihydrate, amoxicillin trihydrate with clavulanate potassium, ampicillin sodium, ampicillin sodium with sulbactam sodium, ampicillin trihydrate

Penicillinase-resistant penicillins: dicloxacillin sodium, nafcillin sodium, oxacillin sodium

Extended-spectrum penicillins: carbenicillin indanyl sodium, piperacillin sodium, piperacillin sodium with tazobactam sodium, ticarcillin disodium, ticarcillin with clavulanate potassium

Penicillins are effective antibiotics with low toxicity. Penicillin is naturally derived from a mold, *Penicillium chrysogenum.* Synthetic derivatives are created by chemical reactions that modify their structure, resulting in increased GI absorption, resistance to destruction by beta-lactamase (penicillinase), and a broader spectrum of susceptible organisms.

PHARMACOLOGY
The basic structure of penicillin is a thiazolidine ring connected to a beta-lactam ring that contains a side chain. This nucleus is the main structural requirement for antibacterial activity. Modifications of the side chain alter the antibacterial and pharmacologic effects of penicillin.

Comparing penicillins

Drug	Route	Adult dosage	Penicillinase-resistant
amoxicillin	P.O.	250-500 mg q 8 hr 3 g with 1 g probenecid for gonorrhea as single dose	No
amoxicillin and clavulanate potassium	P.O.	250-500 mg q 8 hr 500-875 mg q 12 hr	Yes
ampicillin	I.M., I.V. P.O.	2-14 g daily in divided doses given q 4-6 hr 250-500 mg q 6 hr 2.5 g with 1 g probenecid (for gonorrhea) as single dose	No
ampicillin sodium and sulbactam sodium	I.M., I.V.	1.5-3 g q 6-8 hr	Yes
dicloxacillin	P.O.	125-500 mg q 6 hr	Yes
nafcillin	I.V.	250 mg-2 g q 4-6 hr	Yes
penicillin G benzathine	I.M.	1.2-2.4 million units as single dose	No
penicillin G potassium	I.M., I.V.	200,000-4 million units q 4 hr	No
penicillin G procaine	I.M.	600,000-1.2 million units q 1-3 days 4.8 million units with 1 g probenecid as single dose for primary, secondary, and early latent syphilis; weekly for 3 weeks for late latent syphilis	No
penicillin G sodium	I.M., I.V.	200,000-4 million units q 4 hr	No
penicillin V potassium	P.O.	250-500 mg q 6-8 hr	No
piperacillin	I.M., I.V.	100- 300 mg/kg daily as divided doses given q 4-6 hr	No
piperacillin sodium and tazobactam sodium	I.V.	3.375 g q 6 hr	Yes
ticarcillin	I.M., I.V.	150-300 mg/kg daily as divided doses given q 3-6 hr	No
ticarcillin and clavulanate potassium	I.V.	3.1 g q 4-6 hr	Yes

Penicillins are generally bactericidal. They inhibit synthesis of the bacterial cell wall, causing rapid cell lysis, and are most effective against fast-growing susceptible bacteria.

Oral absorption of penicillin varies widely. The most variable in gastric acid is penicillin G. Side-chain changes in penicillin V, ampicillin, amoxicillin, and other P.O. penicillins are more stable in gastric acid and permit better absorption from the GI tract. (See *Comparing penicillins*.)

Penicillins are distributed widely throughout the body. CSF penetration is minimal but is enhanced in patients with inflamed meninges. Most penicillins are only partially metabolized. With the exception of nafcillin, penicillins are excreted primarily in urine, chiefly through renal tubular effects. Nafcillin undergoes enterohepatic circulation and is excreted chiefly through the biliary tract.

INDICATIONS & ACTIONS
➤**Infection caused by susceptible organisms—**
These infections may be treated with natural penicillins, aminopenicillins, penicillinase-resistant penicillins, or extended-spectrum penicillins.

Penicillin G is the prototype of the natural penicillins. Derivatives such as penicillin V are more acid stable and thus better absorbed orally. All natural penicillins may be inactivated by beta-lactamase–producing bacteria. Natural penicillins act primarily against gram-positive organisms.

Clinical indications for natural penicillins include streptococcal pneumonia, enterococcal and nonenterococcal group D endocarditis, diphtheria, anthrax, meningitis, tetanus, botulism, actinomycosis, syphilis, relapsing fever, Lyme disease, rat-bite fever, Whipple's disease, and others. Natural penicillins are used prophylactically against pneumococcal infections, rheumatic fever, bacterial endocarditis, and neonatal group B streptococcal disease.

Susceptible aerobic gram-positive cocci include enterococcus (usually with an aminoglycoside), non–penicillinase-producing *Staphylococcus aureus* and *S. epidermis,* nonenterococcal group D streptococci, *Streptococcus viridans,* and groups A, B, C, D, G, H, K, L, and M streptococci. Susceptible aerobic gram-negative cocci include *Neisseria meningitidis* and non–penicillinase-producing *N. gonorrhoeae.*

Susceptible aerobic gram-positive bacilli include *Bacillus anthracis, Corynebacterium* (both diphtheria and opportunistic species), and *Listeria* species. Susceptible anaerobes include

Actinomyces, Clostridium, Fusobacterium, Peptococcus, Peptostreptococcus, Veillonella, and non–beta-lactamase-producing strains of *Streptococcus pneumoniae.* The drugs are also active against some gram-negative aerobic bacilli, including some strains of *Haemophilus influenzae, Pasteurella multocida, Streptococcus moniliformis,* and *Spirillum minus.*

Susceptible spirochetes include *Borrelia* recurrentis, *Leptospira* species, *Treponema pallidum, T. pertenue,* and possibly *Borrelia burgdorferi.*

Aminopenicillins (amoxicillin and ampicillin) offer a broader spectrum of activity including many gram-negative organisms. Like natural penicillins, aminopenicillins are vulnerable to inactivation by penicillinase. They are primarily used to treat septicemia, gynecologic infections, and infections of the urinary, respiratory, and GI tracts, and skin, soft tissue, bones, and joints. Their activity spectrum includes *Escherichia coli, H. influenzae, Listeria monocytogenes, N. gonorrhoeae, Proteus mirabilis, Salmonella, Shigella, S. aureus, S. epidermidis* (non–penicillinase-producing *Staphylococcus*), and *S. pneumoniae.*

Penicillinase-resistant penicillins (dicloxacillin, nafcillin, and oxacillin) are semisynthetic penicillins designed to remain stable against hydrolysis by most staphylococcal penicillinases and thus are the drugs of choice against susceptible penicillinase-producing staphylococci. They also retain activity against most organisms susceptible to natural penicillins. Clinical indications are much the same as for aminopenicillins.

Extended-spectrum penicillins (carbenicillin, piperacillin, and ticarcillin) offer a wider range of bactericidal action than the other three classes. They are used in hard-to-treat gram-negative infections and are usually combined with aminoglycosides. They are used most often against susceptible strains of *Bacteroides fragilis, Citrobacter, Enterobacter, Klebsiella, Pseudomonas aeruginosa,* and *Serratia* species. Their gram-negative spectrum also includes *Morganella morganii, Proteus mirabilis, P. vulgaris, Providencia rettgeri, Salmonella,* and *Shigella* species. These penicillins are also vulnerable to destruction by beta-lactamase or penicillinases.

ADVERSE REACTIONS
Systemic hypersensitivity reactions range from mild rash, fever, and eosinophilia to fatal anaphylaxis. Hematologic reactions include hemolytic anemia, transient neutropenia, leukopenia, and thrombocytopenia.

Certain adverse reactions are more common with specific classes of penicillin: bleeding episodes are usually seen at high-dose levels of extended-spectrum penicillins; acute interstitial nephritis is reported most often with methicillin; GI adverse effects are most common with ampicillin. High doses, especially of penicillin G, irritate the CNS in patients with renal disease, causing confusion, twitching, lethargy, dysphagia, seizures, and coma. Hepatotoxicity is most common with penicillinase-resistant penicillins; hyperkalemia and hypernatremia occur with extended-spectrum penicillins.

Jarisch-Herxheimer reaction can occur when penicillin G is used to treat secondary syphilis. Signs and symptoms are chills, fever, headache, myalgia, tachycardia, malaise, sweating, hypotension, and sore throat.

Local irritation from parenteral therapy may be severe enough to require discontinuation of the drug or administration by subclavian catheter if drug therapy is to continue.

LIFESPAN CONSIDERATIONS
• Pregnancy risk category is B. Safe use of penicillins in pregnancy hasn't been established, but the level of safety is considered acceptable based on standards of care. Penicillin G is used to treat syphilis and amoxicillin and ampicillin are used to treat urinary tract infections during pregnancy without adverse effects.
• See drug monographs for specific recommendations for breast-feeding patients.
• Specific dosage recommendations for pediatric patients have been established for most penicillins.
• Use cautiously. Elderly patients are susceptible to superinfection. Lower the dose in elderly patients with diminished creatinine clearance.

phenothiazines
Aliphatic derivatives:
chlorpromazine hydrochloride,
promethazine hydrochloride,
triflupromazine
Piperazine derivatives:
fluphenazine hydrochloride,
perphenazine, prochlorperazine,
trifluoperazine hydrochloride
Piperidine derivatives:
mesoridazine besylate,
thioridazine
Thioxanthene: thiothixene

This group of drugs has many effects, including strong antipsychotic activity.

PHARMACOLOGY
Phenothiazines are classified in terms of chemical structure: the aliphatic agent (chlorpromazine) has a greater sedative, hypotensive, and allergic activity. Piperazines (perphenazine, prochlorperazine, fluphenazine, and trifluoperazine) are more likely to produce extrapyramidal symptoms. Piperidines (thioridazine and mesoridazine) have intermediate effects. Thioxanthenes are chemically similar to phenothiazines

and are pharmacologically similar to piperazine phenothiazines. Promethazine is a derivative that has antihistaminic qualities.

All antipsychotic drugs have similar mechanisms of action. They're believed to function as dopamine antagonists, blocking postsynaptic dopamine receptors in various parts of the CNS. Their antiemetic effects result from blockage of the chemoreceptor trigger zone. They also produce varying degrees of anticholinergic and alpha-adrenergic receptor blocking actions. They are structurally similar to tricyclic antidepressants (TCAs) and share many adverse reactions.

All antipsychotic drugs have equal clinical efficacy when given in equivalent doses. Choice of specific therapy is determined primarily by the individual patient's response and adverse reaction profile. A patient who doesn't respond to one drug may respond to another.

Onset of full therapeutic effects requires 6 weeks to 6 months. Therefore, dosage adjustment is recommended at not less than weekly intervals.

INDICATIONS & ACTIONS
➤**Psychoses**—
Phenothiazines (except promethazine) and thiothixene are indicated to treat agitated psychotic states. They're especially effective in controlling hallucinations in schizophrenic patients, the manic phase of manic-depressive illness, and excessive motor and autonomic activity.
➤**Nausea and vomiting**—
Chlorpromazine, perphenazine, promethazine, and prochlorperazine are effective in controlling severe nausea and vomiting induced by CNS disturbances. They don't prevent motion sickness or vertigo.
➤**Anxiety**—
Chlorpromazine, mesoridazine, promethazine, prochlorperazine, and trifluoperazine also may be used for short-term treatment of moderate anxiety in selected nonpsychotic patients, for example, to control anxiety before surgery.
➤**Severe behavior problems**—
Chlorpromazine and thioridazine are indicated to control combativeness and hyperexcitability in children with severe behavior problems. They're also used in hyperactive children for short-term treatment of excessive motor activity with labile moods, impulsive behavior, aggressiveness, attention deficit, and poor tolerance of frustration. Mesoridazine is used to manage hypersensitivity and to promote cooperative behavior in patients with mental deficiency and chronic brain syndrome.
➤**Tetanus**—
Chlorpromazine is an effective adjunct in treating tetanus.
➤**Porphyria**—
Because of its effects on the autonomic nervous system, chlorpromazine is effective in controlling abdominal pain in patients with acute intermittent porphyria.
➤**Delirium**—
Phenothiazines may be used to treat delirium. Antipsychotic drugs remain first-line therapy.
➤**Intractable hiccups**—
Chlorpromazine may be used to treat patients with intractable hiccups.
➤**Neurogenic pain**—
Fluphenazine is a useful adjunct to manage selected chronic pain states.
➤**Allergies and pruritus**—
Because of their potent antihistaminic effects, many of these drugs are used to relieve itching.

ADVERSE REACTIONS
Phenothiazines may produce extrapyramidal symptoms (dystonic movements, torticollis, oculogyric crises, parkinsonian symptoms) from akathisia during early treatment, to tardive dyskinesia after long-term use.

In rare cases, a syndrome resembling severe parkinsonism may occur. It consists of rapid onset of hyperthermia, muscular hyperreflexia, marked extrapyramidal and autonomic dysfunction, arrhythmias, and sweating.

Other adverse reactions are similar to those seen with TCAs, including sedative and anticholinergic effects, orthostatic hypotension, reflex tachycardia, fainting, dizziness, arrhythmias, anorexia, nausea, vomiting, abdominal pain, local gastric irritation, seizures, endocrine effects, hematologic disorders, ocular changes, skin eruptions, and photosensitivity. Allergic manifestations are usually marked by elevation of liver enzyme levels progressing to obstructive jaundice.

Piperidine derivatives have the most pronounced CV effects, whereas piperazine derivatives have the least. Parenteral administration is often caused by CV effects because of more rapid absorption. Seizures are more common with aliphatic derivatives.

LIFESPAN CONSIDERATIONS
• Safety of phenothiazine use during pregnancy hasn't been established.
• If possible, patient shouldn't breast-feed while taking antipsychotic drugs. Most phenothiazines appear in breast milk and have a direct effect on prolactin levels.
• Unless otherwise specified, antipsychotic drugs aren't recommended for children younger than age 12. Use phenothiazines carefully for nausea and vomiting because children suffering from chickenpox, measles, CNS infections, or dehydration are at greatly increased risk for dystonic reactions.
• Elderly patients are more sensitive to therapeutic and adverse effects, especially cardiac toxicity, tardive dyskinesia, and other extrapyramidal effects. Adjust dosage to patient response.

tetracyclines
demeclocycline hydrochloride, doxycycline, minocycline hydrochloride, oxytetracycline hydrochloride, tetracycline hydrochloride

Usually well tolerated with few serious adverse effects, tetracyclines have an unusually broad spectrum of antibacterial activity, including gram-negative and gram-positive anaerobic and aerobic bacteria, *Chlamydia* species, and protozoa. Longer-acting tetracyclines have enhanced activity against *Chlamydia* and *Legionella* species.

Demeclocycline has a higher risk of severe photosensitivity reactions. Because of its renal effects, it's rarely prescribed for clinical use, although it's used investigationally to treat SIADH secretion.

PHARMACOLOGY
Tetracyclines are bacteriostatic but may be bactericidal against certain organisms. They bind reversibly to 30S and 50S ribosomal subunits, inhibiting bacterial protein synthesis. Bacterial resistance to tetracyclines is usually mediated by plasmids (R-factor resistance), which decrease bacterial cell wall permeability. This is the most important cause of resistance by staphylococci, streptococci, most aerobic gram-negative organisms, and *Pseudomonas aeruginosa.* With two exceptions, cross-resistance occurs with all tetracyclines: doxycycline is active against *Bacteroides fragilis,* and minocycline is active against *Acinetobacter* species, *Enterobacteriaceae* species, and *Staphylococcus aureus.*

Tetracyclines attack many pathogens but aren't antifungal or antiviral.

Susceptible gram-positive organisms include *Actinomyces israelii, Bacillus anthracis, Clostridium perfringens,*

♦ Off-label use

Clostridium tetani, Listeria monocytogenes, and *Nocardia* species. Initial but transient activity exists against staphylococci and streptococci. Infections caused by these organisms are usually treated with other drugs.

Susceptible gram-negative organisms include *Bartonella bacilliformis, Bordetella pertussis, Brucella* species, *Calymmatobacterium granulomatis,* Campylobacter *fetus, Francisella tularensis, Haemophilus ducreyi, H. influenzae, Legionella pneumophila, Leptotrichia buccalis, Neisseria gonorrhoeae, N. meningitidis, Pasteurella multocida, Shigella* species, *Spirillum minus, Streptobacillus moniliformis, Vibrio cholerae, V. parahaemolyticus, Yersinia enterocolitica, Y. pestis,* and many other common pathogens.

Other susceptible organisms include *Borrelia recurrentis, Chlamydia psittaci, C. trachomatis, Coxiella burnetii, Leptospira* species, *Mycoplasma hominis, M. pneumoniae, Rickettsia akari, R. prowazekii, R. tsutsugamushi, R. typhi, Treponema pallidum,* and *T. pertenue.*

Tetracyclines are absorbed systemically after oral administration, chiefly from the duodenum. Except for doxycycline and minocycline, absorption is decreased by food, milk, and divalent and trivalent cations. Oral absorption of tetracyclines is affected by chelation with certain minerals such as calcium (doxycycline is least involved); chelation causes tetracyclines to localize in bones and teeth. Because of hepatotoxicity and thrombophlebitis, only doxycycline and, to a lesser extent, minocycline, are used I.V.

Tetracyclines distribute widely into body tissues and fluid, but CSF penetration is minimal. Lipid-soluble minocycline and doxycycline penetrate fluids and tissues better. All tetracyclines cross the placental barrier.

Tetracyclines are excreted primarily in urine, chiefly by glomerular filtration. Some drug appears in breast milk, and some inactivated drug is excreted in feces. Unlike other tetracyclines, minocycline undergoes enterohepatic circulation and is excreted in feces.

Oxytetracycline is moderately hemodialyzable. Other tetracyclines are removed only minimally by hemodialysis or peritoneal dialysis.

INDICATIONS & ACTIONS
➤**Bacterial, antiprotozoal, rickettsial, and fungal infections—**
Tetracyclines are used as first-line therapy for chlamydial infections and are the drugs of choice for lymphogranuloma venereum, non–lymphogranuloma venereum strains of *C. trachomatis* in sexually transmitted diseases, psittacosis, and nongonococcal urethritis if the primary pathogen is *M. hominis* or *C. trachomatis.* They're also the drugs of choice for rickettsial infections (Rocky Mountain spotted fever, scrub and endemic typhus, rickettsial pox, and Q fever) and brucellosis. Tetracyclines also are used to treat infections caused by *Campylobacter,* mycoplasma pneumonia (after Legionnaire's disease is ruled out), anthrax, pertussis, cholera (in United States only), leprosy, and gonorrhea.

Tetracyclines are used as second-line therapy for syphilis, actinomycosis, listeriosis, chancroid, and infections caused by *P. multocida* and *Y. pestis.* They also provide affordable protection in chronic pulmonary disease.

Tetracyclines are used orally to treat inflammatory acne vulgaris, topically for mild to moderate inflammatory acne, and as eyedrops for superficial eye infections, for inclusion conjunctivitis, and to prevent ophthalmia neonatorum.

Individual tetracyclines are more effective against certain species or strains of a particular organism.
➤**Diuretic in SIADH—**
Demeclocycline causes diuresis by blocking antidiuretic hormone-induced

reabsorption of water in the distal tubules and collecting ducts of the kidney.

➤**Pleural or pericardial effusion**— Parenteral tetracycline hydrochloride may be given by intracavitary injection as a sclerosing agent in pleural or pericardial effusion. Parenteral doxycycline hyclate may be used as a sclerosing agent to control pleural effusions caused by metastatic tumors.

➤**Other uses**—

Tetracycline is used as an adjunct to treat *H. pylori* infection.

Doxycycline is used to suppress or prevent malaria caused by chloroquine-resistant or sulfadoxine- and pyrimethamine-resistant *Plasmodium falciparum* in individuals traveling to endemic areas for fewer than 4 months.

Oral doxycycline and oral tetracycline are used to treat Lyme disease.

Tetracycline is used to treat various GI infections including balantidiasis caused by *Balantidium coli,* Whipple's disease, blind-loop syndrome, and tropical sprue.

Oral doxycycline can also be used as an alternative agent to treat anthrax. It has also been used as an anti-inflammatory drug to treat adult periodontitis, acne, and rosacea.

ADVERSE REACTIONS

The most common adverse effects of tetracyclines are dose-related. Among them are anorexia, flatulence, nausea, vomiting, bulky and loose stools, epigastric burning, and abdominal discomfort.

Hypersensitivity reactions are infrequent and include urticaria, rash, pruritus, eosinophilia, and exfoliative dermatitis.

Photosensitivity reactions may be severe. They commonly occur with demeclocycline, rarely with minocycline.

Renal effects are minor and include occasional elevations in BUN level (without increase in creatinine level) and a reversible diabetes insipidus syndrome (only with demeclocycline). Renal failure has been attributed to Fanconi's syndrome after use of outdated tetracycline.

Rare adverse effects include hepatotoxicity—often in pregnant women receiving more than 2 g I.V. daily—leukocytosis, thrombocytopenia, hemolytic anemia, leukopenia, neutropenia, and atypical lymphocytes. There have also been reports of vaginal candidiasis, microscopic thyroid discoloration after long-term use, dizziness, light-headedness, drowsiness, vein irritation after I.V. use, and permanent discoloration of teeth in children younger than age 8.

Use of these drugs with hormonal contraceptives can decrease the effectiveness of the contraceptive.

LIFESPAN CONSIDERATIONS

● Pregnancy risk category is D. Tetracyclines may cause fetal toxicity in pregnant women.

● Don't use tetracyclines in breast-feeding women.

● Don't use in children younger than age 8 unless there's no alternative. Tetracyclines can cause permanent discoloration of teeth, enamel hypoplasia, and a reversible decrease in bone calcification.

● Some elderly patients have decreased esophageal motility. Use tetracyclines cautiously, and watch for local irritation from slowly passing oral dosage forms. Elderly patients are more susceptible to superinfection.

thrombolytic enzymes

alteplase, reteplase (recombinant), streptokinase, tenecteplase, urokinase

When a thrombus obstructs a blood vessel, permanent damage to the is-

Comparing thrombolytic enzymes

Thrombolytic enzymes dissolve clots by accelerating the formation of plasmin by activated plasminogen. Plasminogen activators, found in most tissues and body fluids, help plasminogen (an inactive enzyme) convert to plasmin (an active enzyme), which dissolves the clot. Doses of the enzymes listed below may vary according to the patient's condition.

Drug	Action	Initial dose	Maintenance therapy
alteplase	Directly converts plasminogen to plasmin	I.V. bolus: 6-10 mg over 1 to 2 min	I.V. infusion: 60 mg/hr in the 1st hr; then 20 mg/hr for the next 2 hr for a total of 100 mg
reteplase	Enhances the cleavage of plasminogen to generate plasmin	Double I.V. bolus injection of 10 + 10 units	Not necessary
streptokinase	Indirectly activates plasminogen, which converts to plasmin	Intracoronary bolus: 15,000 to 20,000 units I.V. bolus: none needed	Intracoronary infusion: 2,000 to 4,000 units/min over 1 hr; total dose 140,000 units I.V. infusion: 1,500,000 units over 1 hr
tenecteplase	Directly converts plasminogen to plasmin	I.V. bolus over 5 seconds. If patient weighs less than 60 kg, give 30 mg; if 60-69 kg, give 35 mg; if 70-79 kg, give 40 mg; if 80-89 kg, give 45 mg; if 90 kg or more, give 50 mg.	Not necessary
urokinase	Directly converts plasminogen to plasmin	Intracoronary bolus: none needed	Intracoronary infusion: 2,000 IU/lb/hr (4,400 IU/kg/hr); rate of 15 ml of solution/hr for total of 12 hr (total volume shouldn't exceed 200 ml)

chemic area may occur before the body can dissolve the clot. Thrombolytics were developed to speed lysis of the clot and prevent permanent ischemic damage. It isn't clear whether these drugs significantly reduce thrombosis-induced ischemic damage in all situations for which they are currently used. (See *Comparing thrombolytic enzymes.*)

PHARMACOLOGY

Streptokinase is a proteinlike substance produced by group C beta-hemolytic streptococci. Urokinase is an enzyme isolated from human kidney tissue cultures. Alteplase and tenecteplase are tissue-type plasminogen activators synthesized by recombinant DNA tech-

nology. Reteplase is a recombinant-plasminogen activator. Thrombolytic enzymes act to lyse clots mainly by converting plasminogen to plasmin. In contrast, anticoagulants act by preventing thrombi from developing. Thrombolytics are more likely to produce bleeding than are oral anticoagulants.

INDICATIONS & ACTIONS
➤**Thrombosis and thromboembolism—**
Alteplase, streptokinase, and urokinase are used to treat acute pulmonary thromboembolism. Streptokinase and urokinase are used to treat deep vein thrombosis, acute arterial thromboembolism, or acute coronary arterial

thrombosis, and to clear arteriovenous cannula occlusion and venous catheter obstruction. Alteplase, reteplase, streptokinase, tenecteplase, and urokinase are indicated in acute MI. These drugs are given to lyse coronary artery thrombi, which may cause improved ventricular function and decreased risk of heart failure. Alteplase is used to manage acute ischemic CVA.

ADVERSE REACTIONS
Adverse reactions to these drugs are essentially an extension of their actions, with hemorrhage being the most common adverse effect. These drugs cause bleeding twice as often as does heparin. Streptokinase is more likely to cause an allergic reaction than urokinase. Information regarding hypersensitivity to alteplase is limited.

LIFESPAN CONSIDERATIONS
• All thrombolytics are rated pregnancy risk category C, except urokinase, which is rated B. Thrombolytics should be used in pregnancy only if clearly indicated.
• Safety in breast-feeding women hasn't been established.
• Safety in children hasn't been established.
• Patients age 75 and older are at greater risk for cerebral hemorrhage because they're more apt to have cerebrovascular disease.

abciximab
ReoPro

Pharmacologic class: glycoprotein IIb/IIIa inhibitor
Therapeutic class: platelet aggregation inhibitor
Pregnancy risk category: C

INDICATIONS & DOSAGES
➤ **Adjunct to percutaneous transluminal coronary angioplasty (PTCA) or atherectomy to prevent acute cardiac ischemic complications in patients at high risk for abrupt closure of the treated coronary vessel—**
Adults: 0.25 mg/kg as an I.V. bolus given 10 to 60 minutes before start of PTCA or atherectomy, followed by a continuous I.V. infusion of 0.125 mcg/kg/minute, up to a maximum of 10 mcg/minute for 12 hours.
➤ **Unstable angina unresponsive to conventional medical therapy when percutaneous coronary intervention (PCI) is planned within 24 hours—**
Adults: 0.25 mg/kg as an I.V. bolus, followed by an 18- to 24-hour infusion at 10 mcg/minute, concluding 1 hour after PCI.

Use abciximab with heparin and aspirin.

ADMINISTRATION
Direct injection: Administer 10 to 60 minutes before procedure.
Intermittent infusion: Not recommended.
Continuous infusion: Infuse at a maximum rate of 10 mcg/minute for the du-

ration of the infusion through a continuous infusion pump equipped with an in-line filter. After infusion, discard unused portion.

PREPARATION & STORAGE
Available in 5-ml vials at a concentration of 2 mg/ml. Withdraw the needed amount of abciximab through a sterile, nonpyrogenic, low protein-binding 0.2-micron or 0.22-micron filter. For continuous infusion, mix with appropriate amount of sterile normal saline solution or D_5W. Inspect solution before giving it, and discard if you see any opaque particles. Don't freeze or shake it. Store at 36° to 46° F (2° to 8° C).

Incompatibilities
None reported. Give drug in a separate I.V. line. Don't add other drugs to the infusion solution.

CONTRAINDICATIONS & CAUTIONS
• Contraindicated in patients hypersensitive to any component of the drug or to murine proteins.
• Contraindicated in those who have active internal bleeding, intracranial neoplasm, arteriovenous malformation or aneurysm, severe uncontrolled hypertension, bleeding diathesis, platelet count less than 100,000/mm³, or a history of vasculitis.
• Contraindicated in those who have had significant GI or GU bleeding within the past 6 weeks; CVA within the past 2 years or one with significant residual neurologic deficit; major surgery or trauma within the past 6 weeks. Also contraindicated in those who have received oral anticoagulants within the

---

past 7 days, unless PT is 1.2 times control or less.
• Contraindicated with use of I.V. dextran before or during PTCA.
• Use cautiously in patients at increased risk for bleeding, including those who weigh less than 165 lb (75 kg), are older than age 65, have a history of GI disease, or are receiving thrombolytics. Other conditions that increase a patient's risk of bleeding include PTCA within 12 hours of onset of symptoms for an acute MI, PTCA lasting longer than 70 minutes, or failed PTCA. Using heparin with abciximab also may contribute to the risk of bleeding.

ADVERSE REACTIONS
CNS: hyperesthesia, hypesthesia, confusion, pain, headache.
CV: *hypotension,* **bradycardia,** peripheral edema, *chest pain.*
EENT: abnormal vision.
GI: *nausea,* vomiting, abdominal pain.
Hematologic: *bleeding, thrombocytopenia,* anemia, leukocytosis.
Musculoskeletal: *back pain.*
Respiratory: pleural effusion, pleurisy, pneumonia.

INTERACTIONS
Drug-drug. *Anticoagulants, antiplatelet drugs, heparin, NSAIDs, thrombolytics:* Increases risk of bleeding. Monitor hematologic and coagulation studies.

EFFECTS ON LAB TEST RESULTS
• May increase WBC count. May decrease hemoglobin, hematocrit, and platelet count.

ACTION
Binds to the glycoprotein IIb/IIIa (GP IIb/IIIa) receptor of platelets and inhibits platelet aggregation.

PHARMACOKINETICS
Onset and peak occur almost immediately after I.V. infusion. Effects on platelet aggregation persist for about 48 hours. Low levels of GP IIb/IIIa receptor blockade occur for up to 10 days after infusion ends.
Distribution: Occurs in free plasma after I.V. bolus.
Metabolism: Unknown.
Excretion: Initial half-life, less than 10 minutes; second-phase half-life, about 30 minutes.

CLINICAL CONSIDERATIONS
• Before treatment, measure platelet count, PT, INR, and PTT. During and after treatment, monitor platelet count, activated clotting time, and PTT.
• Monitor patient closely for bleeding. Bleeding caused by therapy falls into two broad categories: that observed at the arterial access site used for cardiac catheterization, and internal bleeding involving the GI or GU tract or retroperitoneal sites.
• Avoid noncompressible I.V. sites.
• Take steps to prevent bleeding. Keep patient on bed rest for 6 to 8 hours after sheath is removed or drug infusion is stopped, whichever is later. Minimize or avoid, if possible, arterial and venous punctures; I.M. injections; use of urinary catheters, NG tubes, or automatic blood pressure cuffs; and nasotracheal intubation.
• Consider saline or heparin locks when drawing blood.
• Remove dressings gently.

PATIENT TEACHING
• Explain to patient and family need for drug and how it's given.
• Instruct patient to report adverse reactions, especially bleeding, immediately.

acetazolamide sodium
Diamox

Pharmacologic class: carbonic anhydrase inhibitor
Therapeutic class: antiglaucoma drug, anticonvulsant, diuretic
Pregnancy risk category: C
pH: 9.2

INDICATIONS & DOSAGES
➤ **To rapidly lower intraocular pressure or to treat a patient unable to take the drug orally—**
Adults: 500 mg I.V. May repeat I.V. dose in 2 to 4 hours, if needed. Therapy is usually continued with 125 to 250 mg P.O. q 4 to 6 hours, depending on patient's response.
➤ **Acute glaucoma—**
Children: 5 to 10 mg/kg I.V. q 6 hours.
➤ **Diuresis—**
Adults: 5 mg/kg I.V. p.r.n.
Children: 5 mg/kg or 150 mg/m² I.V. once daily in morning.
➤ **Petit mal, unlocalized seizures—**
Adults and children: 8 to 30 mg/kg I.V. daily in up to four divided doses. Usual dosage range is 375 mg to 1,000 mg. If drug is given in combination therapy, give 250 mg daily initially, and titrate dosage further.

ADMINISTRATION
Direct injection: Using a 21G or 23G needle, inject 100 to 500 mg/minute into a large vein.
Intermittent infusion: Not recommended.
Continuous infusion: Not recommended.

PREPARATION & STORAGE
Available as a powder in a 500-mg vial. Reconstitute with 5 ml of sterile water for injection to provide a solution containing no more than 100 mg/ml. Refrigerate reconstituted drug and use within 24 hours because it contains no preservatives.

Incompatibilities
Multivitamins.

CONTRAINDICATIONS & CAUTIONS
• Contraindicated in those with hepatic or renal disease or dysfunction because of increased risk of hepatotoxicity or nephrotoxicity; in those with hyponatremia, hypokalemia, or hyperchloremic acidosis because of increased risk of further electrolyte imbalances; in those with adrenal gland failure; and in those undergoing long-term therapy for chronic noncongestive angle-closure glaucoma.
• Use cautiously in those sensitive to sulfonamides because of increased risk of hypersensitivity and in those with respiratory acidosis, emphysema, or chronic pulmonary disease because of increased risk of respiratory acidosis. Use cautiously in those with diabetes mellitus because drug may raise glucose levels and in those with gout or renal calculi because drug may exacerbate these conditions.

ADVERSE REACTIONS
CNS: drowsiness, paresthesia, depression, headache, dizziness, confusion, stimulation, fatigue, fever, *seizures.*
CV: flushing.
EENT: transient myopia, tinnitus.
GI: anorexia, *altered taste,* nausea, vomiting, diarrhea.
GU: crystalluria, *decreased uric acid excretion,* polyuria, hematuria, *renal failure.*
Hematologic: *aplastic anemia, agranulocytosis, leukopenia, thrombocytopenia, thrombocytopenia purpura.*
Metabolic: hyperchloremic acidosis, hypokalemia, growth retardation in children, hyponatremia, *hypoglycemia,* hyperglycemia.

Skin: pain at injection site, urticaria, photosensitivity.
Other: *anaphylaxis.*

INTERACTIONS

Drug-drug. *Amphetamines, procainamide, quinidine:* Enhances or prolongs effects of these drugs because their excretion may be decreased. Monitor patient closely.
Amphotericin B, corticosteroids, corticotropin, diuretics: Increases risk of hypokalemia. Monitor potassium level.
Cardiac glycosides: Increases risk of toxic reaction in hypokalemic patients. Monitor potassium and cardiac glycoside levels.
Cyclosporine: May cause nephrotoxicity and cause elevated cyclosporine levels. Monitor renal function and cyclosporine levels closely.
Lithium, methenamine: Reduces effects of these drugs. Monitor patient closely.
Phenytoin: May increase phenytoin levels, speed up bone demineralization, and adversely affect calcium metabolism. Monitor patient closely.

EFFECTS ON LAB TEST RESULTS

• May increase uric acid, chloride, and liver function enzyme levels. May decrease potassium, sodium, and bicarbonate levels. May increase or decrease glucose level.
• May decrease hemoglobin, hematocrit, WBC, granulocyte, and platelet counts, and thyroid iodine uptake.

ACTION

Decreases production of aqueous humor, thus reducing intraocular pressure 50% to 60%. By inhibiting renal tubular secretion of hydrogen ions, it increases excretion of sodium, potassium, bicarbonate, and water, thus producing an alkaline diuresis.

PHARMACOKINETICS

Onset, 2 minutes; peak effect, 15 minutes; duration, 4 to 5 hours.
Distribution: Throughout body tissues and, in unknown quantities, across the placental barrier. It's unknown if drug appears in breast milk. Highest levels found in erythrocytes, plasma, and kidneys; lower levels appear in liver, muscle, eyes, and CNS. Drug doesn't accumulate in tissues.
Metabolism: None.
Excretion: By renal tubular secretion and passive reabsorption, with 70% to 100% excreted unchanged in urine in 24 hours.

CLINICAL CONSIDERATIONS

• Continuously supervise any patient receiving the drug because I.V. administration reduces intraocular pressure rapidly.
• When used in diuretic therapy, consult with prescriber and dietitian to provide high-potassium diet.
• Carefully monitor intake and output and electrolyte levels, especially potassium level.
• Weigh patient daily. Rapid or excessive fluid loss causes weight loss and hypotension. Geriatric patients are especially susceptible to excessive diuresis.
• Monitor arterial blood gas levels of patients with COPD for respiratory acidosis.
• Monitor diabetic patients carefully for hyperglycemia and glycosuria.
• *Alert:* Don't confuse acetazolamide sodium (Diamox) with acyclovir sodium (Zovirax) vials, which may look alike.

PATIENT TEACHING

• Instruct patient to report adverse reactions.
• Caution patient not to perform hazardous activities if adverse CNS reactions occur.

acyclovir sodium (acycloguanosine)
Avirax ◇, Zovirax

Pharmacologic class: synthetic purine nucleoside
Therapeutic class: antiviral
Pregnancy risk category: C
pH: 10.5 to 11.6

INDICATIONS & DOSAGES
➤ **Mucocutaneous herpes simplex virus I (HSV-I) and HSV-II infections in immunocompromised patients with normal renal function—**
Adults and children age 12 and older: 5 mg/kg I.V. q 8 hours for 7 days.
Infants and children younger than age 12: 10 mg/kg I.V. q 8 hours for 7 days.
➤ **Initial genital herpes infection in immunocompetent patients—**
Adults and children age 12 and older: 5 mg/kg I.V. q 8 hours for 5 days.
➤ **Herpes simplex encephalitis—**
Adults and children age 12 and older: 10 mg/kg I.V. q 8 hours for 10 days.
Children ages 3 months to 12 years: 20 mg/kg I.V. q 8 hours for 10 days.
Children from birth to 3 months: 10 mg/kg to 20 mg/kg I.V. q 8 hr for 10 days.
➤ **Varicella zoster in immunocompromised patients—**
Adults and children age 12 and older: 10 mg/kg I.V. q 8 hours for 7 days.
Children younger than age 12: 20 mg/kg I.V. q 8 hours for 7 days.
Adjust-a-dose: For adults with a creatinine clearance of 25 to 50 ml/minute, give 100% of dose q 12 hours; if clearance is 10 to 25 ml/minute, give 100% of dose q 24 hours; if clearance is less than 10 ml/minute, give 50% of dose q 24 hours. For patients on hemodialysis, 60% of drug is removed after a 6-hour dialysis session. Give supplemental dose after each session.

ADMINISTRATION
Direct injection: Not recommended.
Intermittent infusion: Give over at least 1 hour using an intermittent infusion device or an I.V. line containing a free-flowing, compatible solution. Shorter infusion time increases the risk of nephrotoxicity.
Continuous infusion: Not recommended.

PREPARATION & STORAGE
Available as a powder supplied in 10-ml and 20-ml sterile vials, which are equivalent to 500 and 1,000 mg of acyclovir, respectively.
  Store unopened vials at 59° to 77° F (15° to 25° C).
  To reconstitute, add 10 ml of sterile water for injection to the 10-ml vial and 20 ml to the 20-ml vial to yield a concentration of 50 mg/ml. Don't reconstitute with bacteriostatic water because a precipitate may form.
  If refrigerated, the reconstituted solution may form a precipitate, which dissolves when warmed to room temperature. Once you reconstitute the drug, use it within 12 hours.
  For intermittent infusion, dilute reconstituted drug with commercially available electrolyte and glucose solutions and use within 24 hours. Dilute with at least 70 ml for a concentration of 7 mg/ml or less. Greater concentrations can cause phlebitis.

Incompatibilities
Biological or colloidal solutions, idarubicin hydrochloride, parabens.

CONTRAINDICATIONS & CAUTIONS
• Contraindicated in patients hypersensitive to the drug.
• Use cautiously in those with previous CNS reaction to cytotoxic drugs or neurologic abnormalities because of increased risk of adverse neurologic effects; in those with renal impairment or dehydration because of increased risk

of nephrotoxicity; and in those with serious hepatic impairment, electrolyte imbalances, or significant hypoxia.

ADVERSE REACTIONS
CNS: lethargy, confusion, agitation, *coma, seizures,* delirium, hallucinations, obtundation, psychosis, headache, malaise, pain, fever.
GI: nausea, vomiting, diarrhea, constipation.
GU: *renal failure.*
Hematologic: *leukopenia,* blood dyscrasia.
Skin: rash, *inflammation or phlebitis at injection site,* diaphoresis.

INTERACTIONS
Drug-drug. *Interferon, intrathecal methotrexate:* May cause neurologic abnormalities. Monitor patient.
Nephrotoxic drugs: Increases risk of nephrotoxicity. Monitor patient closely.
Probenecid: Prolongs half-life of acyclovir. Avoid using together.
Zidovudine: May cause neurotoxicity due to increased acyclovir level. Monitor patient.

EFFECTS ON LAB TEST RESULTS
• May increase BUN and creatinine levels.
• May decrease WBC count. May increase or decrease platelet count.

ACTION
Cells infected with HSV take up acyclovir and convert it to its active form, acyclovir triphosphate, which slows viral DNA replication. Acyclovir is active against *Herpesviridae,* including HSV-I and HSV-II, varicella-zoster virus, Epstein-Barr virus, and CMV.

PHARMACOKINETICS
Levels peak at end of standard 1-hour infusion.
Distribution: Extensive, in tissues and body fluids, including brain, kidney, liver, lung, muscle, spleen, uterus, vaginal mucosa and secretions, CSF, saliva, semen, and herpetic vesicular fluid. Drug crosses the placental barrier. Drug may appear in breast milk.
Metabolism: Partly in liver.
Excretion: In urine by glomerular filtration and renal tubular secretion, with 60% to 90% excreted unchanged in 24 hours. Plasma levels follow a biphasic decline: initial phase half-life averages 20 minutes; terminal phase, 2 to $3\frac{1}{2}$ hours.

CLINICAL CONSIDERATIONS
• Use drug for infusion only. Avoid rapid infusion or bolus I.V. injection.
• Solutions with 10 mg/ml or more of drug may increase the risk of phlebitis.
• Carefully monitor intake and output. Drug level peaks in the kidneys during the first 2 hours of infusion, so keep the patient adequately hydrated and maintain urine output during this period.
• Monitor creatinine level. Be prepared to increase hydration, adjust dose, or stop drug if level doesn't return to normal after a few days.
• If overdose occurs, maintain enough urine flow to prevent precipitation in renal tubules. Recommended urine output is 500 ml/g of drug infused or more. Hemodialysis removes the drug.
• *Alert:* Don't confuse acyclovir sodium (Zovirax) with acetazolamide sodium (Diamox) vials, which may look alike.

PATIENT TEACHING
• Inform patient that drug helps manage disease but it doesn't eliminate or cure it. Drug won't prevent spread of infection to others.
• Teach patient to recognize tingling, itching, or pain—early symptoms of herpes infection—and to seek treatment before the infection fully develops.
• Instruct patient to avoid sexual contact during active infections.

adenosine
Adenocard

Pharmacologic class: nucleoside
Therapeutic class: antiarrhythmic
Pregnancy risk category: C
pH: 4.5 to 7.5

INDICATIONS & DOSAGES
➤ **To convert paroxysmal supraventricular tachycardia (PSVT) to sinus rhythm—**
Adults: 6 mg I.V. by bolus injection over 1 to 2 seconds. If PSVT isn't eliminated in 1 to 2 minutes, give 12 mg by rapid I.V. push. Repeat 12-mg dose once, if needed.

ADMINISTRATION
Direct injection: Rapid I.V. injection is needed for drug action. Give over 1 to 2 seconds directly into a peripheral vein if possible; if using an I.V. line, use the most proximal port and follow the injection with a rapid saline flush to hasten drug delivery to systemic circulation.
Intermittent infusion: Not recommended.
Continuous infusion: Not recommended.

PREPARATION & STORAGE
Supplied in vials containing 6 mg/2 ml or syringes containing 6 mg/2 ml, 12 mg/4 ml, or 15 mg/5 ml. Store at controlled room temperature (59° to 86° F [15° to 30° C]). Don't refrigerate.
Observe solution for crystals, which may appear if solution has been refrigerated. If you see crystals, gently warm solution to room temperature. Don't use cloudy solutions. Discard any drug that you don't use because drug lacks preservatives.

Incompatibilities
Other I.V. drugs.

CONTRAINDICATIONS & CAUTIONS
• Contraindicated in patients hypersensitive to adenosine.
• Contraindicated in those with atrial flutter, atrial fibrillation, or ventricular tachycardia because drug is ineffective in treating these arrhythmias.
• Contraindicated in those with second- or third-degree heart block or sick sinus syndrome unless they have an artificial pacemaker because drug decreases conduction through the AV node and may induce a first-, second-, or third-degree heart block. Because the drug has a short half-life, these effects are usually transient; however, patients who develop significant block after a dose of adenosine shouldn't receive additional doses.
• Contraindicated in those who may have bronchoconstrictive, bronchospastic, or obstructive lung disease, such as asthma or emphysema.
• Drug may cause new arrhythmias when used to convert to normal sinus rhythm. These effects are usually transient and include sinus bradycardia or tachycardia, atrial premature contractions, various degrees of AV block, PVCs, and skipped beats.

ADVERSE REACTIONS
CNS: headache, light-headedness, dizziness.
CV: *asystole;* *chest, throat, neck, or jaw discomfort;* **arrhythmias; first-, second-, or third-degree heart block;** hypotension, *flushing.*
EENT: blurred vision.
GI: metallic taste, nausea.
GU: groin pressure.
Musculoskeletal: heaviness in arms, back pain, lower-extremity discomfort.
Respiratory: *dyspnea,* cough.

INTERACTIONS
Drug-drug. *Carbamazepine:* May cause higher-degree heart block. Monitor ECG.

Reactions may be *common,* uncommon, ***life-threatening,*** or COMMON AND LIFE-THREATENING.

Dipyridamole: May potentiate drug's effects, requiring smaller doses. Monitor patient closely.

Methylxanthines: May antagonize drug's effects. Patients receiving theophylline or caffeine may require higher doses or may not respond to adenosine.

Drug-herb. *Guarana:* May decrease response. Monitor patient.

Drug-food. *Caffeine:* May antagonize drug's effects. Patient may require higher doses or may not respond to adenosine.

EFFECTS ON LAB TESTS
None reported.

ACTION
Acts on the AV node to slow conduction and inhibit reentry pathways.

PHARMACOKINETICS
Effect is immediate.
Distribution: Rapidly removed from the systemic circulation, presumably by erythrocytes and vascular endothelial cells.
Metabolism: Once taken up into the body pool of nucleosides, drug is used in several ways. May be converted to inosine and adenosine monophosphate. Estimated plasma half-life, under 10 seconds.
Excretion: Unknown.

CLINICAL CONSIDERATIONS
• Give drug only with continuous ECG monitoring. Watch for arrhythmias.
• Don't give single doses over 12 mg.
• Boluses of 6 or 12 mg usually don't cause systemic hemodynamic effects.
• To provide adequate therapeutic effect, rapid I.V. bolus injection is needed so that enough drug may reach the systemic circulation.
• **Alert:** Some patients with bronchial asthma may experience no adverse reactions to I.V. adenosine, but the potential for bronchoconstriction exists. Inhaled drug causes bronchoconstriction in patients with asthma.

• Because half-life is only 10 seconds, adverse effects usually resolve quickly when injection is stopped.
• Drug is useful for treating Wolff-Parkinson-White syndrome and PSVT caused by accessory bypass tracts.

PATIENT TEACHING
• Explain procedure to patient, and warn him that he may experience facial flushing.
• If appropriate, before giving adenosine, ask patient to attempt vagal maneuvers, such as Valsalva's maneuver.
• Instruct patient to report adverse reactions promptly, such as discomfort at the I.V. site.

albumin (normal human-serum albumin)
Albuminar 5% and 25%, Albutein 5% and 25%, Buminate 5% and 25%, Plasbumin 5% and 25%

Pharmacologic class: blood derivative
Therapeutic class: plasma protein
Pregnancy risk category: C
pH: 6.4 to 7.4

INDICATIONS & DOSAGES
➤ **Shock—**
Adults: 25 g I.V. over 15 to 30 minutes. If patient shows no response after 30 minutes, repeat dose. Thereafter, adjust dosage based on patient's condition. Maximum dosage is 125 g/day for up to 2 days (5 L of 5% solution or 1 L of 25% solution).
Children: 25 g I.V. over 15 to 30 minutes.
Premature infants: 1 g/kg I.V.
Adults with nephrosis: 25 to 50 gI.V. repeated q 1 to 2 days.
➤ **Hypoproteinemia—**
Adults: 50 to 75 g I.V. of 25% solution daily.

Children: 25 g/day I.V.
➤ **Burns—**
Adults: Enough dosage to keep albumin level at 2 to 3 g/dl.
   Note: Dosage reflects extent of burn, protein loss, denuded skin areas, and decreased albumin synthesis, which may persist for up to 60 days.
➤ **Preoperative adjunct in cardiopulmonary bypass procedures—**
Adults: Enough dosage to keep albumin level at 2 to 3 g/dl.
➤ **Hyperbilirubinemia—**
Premature infants: 4 ml (1 g)/kg or 120 ml (30 g)/m² I.V. of 25% solution given 1 to 2 hours before transfusion.
Premature infants with low protein levels: 1.4 to 1.8 ml/kg I.V. of 25% solution.

ADMINISTRATION
Direct injection: Not recommended.
Intermittent infusion: Infuse at rate appropriate to patient's condition, usually over 15 to 30 minutes. When albumin is used for plasma volume expansion, don't exceed rate of 2 to 4 ml/minute with 5% solution and 1 ml/minute with 25% solution. For patients with hypoproteinemia, don't exceed 5 to 10 ml/minute of 5% solution or 2 to 3 ml/minute of 25% solution. For patients with hypertension or mild to moderate heart failure, infuse 10% solution slowly.
Continuous infusion: Infuse diluted solution slowly; adjust according to patient response and changes in blood pressure.

PREPARATION & STORAGE
Available in sterile, nonpyrogenic vials packed with infusion kits; 5% solution supplied in 50-, 250-, 500-, and 1,000-ml vials and 25% solution in 20-, 50-, and 100-ml vials.
   Store below 99° F (37° C), but don't freeze. Discard unused portion after 4 hours.

For continuous infusion, add 25% solution to 500 to 1,000 ml of D₅W or normal saline. To obtain a 10% solution, dilute one part 25% solution in 1½ parts dextrose 10% in water.

Incompatibilities
Verapamil hydrochloride.

CONTRAINDICATIONS & CAUTIONS
• Contraindicated in patients hypersensitive to albumin.
• Contraindicated in those with severe anemia because volume expansion may worsen disorder.
• Contraindicated in those with severe cardiac failure because of risk of circulatory overload and in those with normal or increased intravascular volume because of risk of hypertension.
• Use cautiously in those with low cardiac reserve without albumin deficiency because circulatory overload and pulmonary edema may occur.

ADVERSE REACTIONS
CNS: chills, fever.
CV: *fluid overload,* hypotension, tachycardia.
GI: nausea, vomiting, increased saliva.
Skin: rash, urticaria.
Other: *anaphylaxis.*

INTERACTIONS
None reported.

EFFECTS ON LAB TEST RESULTS
• May increase albumin level.

COMPOSITION
Consisting of at least 96% protein, normal albumin is a solution made from pooled blood, plasma, serum, or placentas obtained from healthy donors. Clear to yellow-brown, odorless, and moderately viscous, albumin solutions have a pH between 6.4 and 7.4, adjusted with sodium carbonate, sodium bicarbonate, or acetic acid. Solutions contain sodium caprylate and sodium

acetyltryptophanate as stabilizers but have no preservatives or antimicrobials.

Both 5% and 25% solutions contain 130 to 160 mEq/L of sodium; 5% albumin is isotonic and 25% albumin is hypertonic, equivalent to five times the normal oncotic pressure.

Albumin includes no clotting factors, is nonreactive to hepatitis B surface antigen, and contains no significant isoagglutinins or other antibodies. It may be given regardless of blood type or Rhesus factor. Albumin is pasteurized at 140° F (60° C) for 10 hours.

CLINICAL CONSIDERATIONS
• Minimize allergic reactions by giving antihistamines before infusion and by slowing infusion rate.
• One volume of 25% albumin is equivalent to five volumes of 5% albumin in producing hemodilution and relative anemia.
• Albumin's sodium content ranges between 130 and 160 mEq/L, so dosage may need to be reduced for patients on sodium-restricted diets.
• Monitor vital signs before, during, and after infusion. Also monitor hemoglobin, hematocrit, and albumin, total protein, and electrolyte levels.
• Watch closely for signs of circulatory overload or pulmonary edema. If signs occur, stop infusion, keep vein open with ordered solution, and notify prescriber.
• Check intake and output, and report changes in output. Increases colloid pressure mobilizes extracellular fluid, causing diuresis for 3 to 20 hours.
• Monitor patient with cerebral edema. Withhold fluids for 8 hours after infusion to avoid fluid overload.
• In surgical or trauma patients, watch for possible bleeding points undetected at lower blood pressures.

PATIENT TEACHING
• Explain to patient and family the use and administration of albumin.

• Tell patient to report adverse reactions promptly.

aldesleukin (interleukin-2, IL-2)
Proleukin

Pharmacologic class: lymphokine
Therapeutic class: immunoregulatory protein
Pregnancy risk category: C
pH: 7.2 to 7.8

INDICATIONS & DOSAGES
➤ **Metastatic renal cell carcinoma; metastatic melanoma—**
Adults age 18 and older: 600,000 IU/kg (0.037 mg/kg) I.V. over 15 minutes q 8 hours for 5 days, for a total of 14 doses. After a 9-day rest, repeat the sequence for another 14 doses. Repeat courses may be given after a rest period of at least 7 weeks from hospital discharge.
➤ **Metastatic renal cell carcinoma ♦—**
Adults: 18 million IU/m² by continuous I.V. infusion for 5 days; repeat in 1 week.
Adjust-a-dose: Withhold dose if patient develops atrial fibrillation, sustained ventricular tachycardia, or bradycardia that requires treatment; systolic blood pressure below 90 mm Hg with increasing need for pressors; ECG change indicating MI or ischemia with or without chest pain; suspected cardiac ischemia; oxygen saturation less than 94% on room air or less than 90% on 2 liters oxygen by nasal cannula; mental status changes; sepsis syndrome; creatinine level of 4.5 mg/dl or higher or of 4 mg/dl with symptoms of severe volume overload, acidosis, hyperkalemia, or persistent oliguria (urine output of 10 ml/hour or less for 16 to 24 hours with increasing creatinine levels); signs and symptoms of hepatic failure including encephalopathy, increasing ascites, pain, hypoglycemia;

repeated positive stool guaiac (3 to 4+); bullous dermatitis or marked worsening of existing skin condition. Subsequent doses may be given if situation resolves. See specific dosing instructions.

ADMINISTRATION

Direct injection: Not recommended.
Intermittent infusion: Infuse diluted dose over 15 minutes. Avoid using an in-line filter.
Continuous infusion: Give diluted solution over 24 hours.

PREPARATION & STORAGE

Available as a powder for injection containing 22 million IU (1.3 mg)/vial.

Reconstitute by adding 1.2 ml of sterile water for injection; the resultant solution contains 18 million IU (1.1 mg)/ml. To avoid excessive foaming, direct water diluent toward side of vial and swirl gently; don't shake. The reconstituted drug should be particle-free and colorless to slightly yellow.

To dilute, add the ordered dose of reconstituted drug to 50 ml of 5% dextrose injection, preferably in a plastic container for more consistent drug delivery.

Store powder for injection and reconstituted solutions in the refrigerator. After reconstitution and dilution, drug must be given within 48 hours. Discard unused drug. Return solution to room temperature before administration.

Incompatibilities

Albumin, bacteriostatic water for injection, normal saline solution, other I.V. drugs.

CONTRAINDICATIONS & CAUTIONS

• Contraindicated in patients hypersensitive to drug or any of its components.
• Contraindicated in those with abnormal results from a thallium stress test or pulmonary function test and in those with organ allografts.
• Retreatment is contraindicated in those who experience pericardial tamponade, disturbances in cardiac rhythm that are uncontrolled or unresponsive to intervention; sustained ventricular tachycardia of five consecutive beats or more; recurrent chest pain accompanied by ECG changes consistent with an MI or angina; renal dysfunction requiring dialysis for longer than 72 hours or intubation for longer than 72 hours; coma or toxic psychosis lasting longer than 48 hours; seizures that are repetitive or difficult to control; ischemia or perforation of the bowel; or GI bleeding requiring surgery.
• Don't use drug unless patient has had definitive test results documenting normal cardiac, pulmonary, hepatic, and CNS function. Use extremely cautiously in patients with normal results if they have had cardiac or pulmonary disease and in patients with history of seizure disorders because the drug may cause seizures.
• Use cautiously in all patients and monitor closely because severe adverse effects generally accompany therapy at the recommended dosage. Only use in a hospital setting under the direction of a prescriber experienced in the use of chemotherapeutic drugs. An ICU and intensive care or cardiopulmonary specialists must be available.
• Use cautiously in those who need large volumes of fluid, such as those who are hypercalcemic, because fluid management or administration of pressors may be needed to treat capillary leak syndrome.

ADVERSE REACTIONS

CNS: *mental status changes, dizziness, sensory dysfunction,* special senses disorders, syncope, motor dysfunction, *seizures, coma,* fatigue, weakness, *malaise,* headache, *fever, CVA.*
CV: *hypotension, arrhythmias, sinus tachycardia, bradycardia,* PVCs, premature atrial contractions, myocardial

ischemia, *MI, cardiac arrest, heart failure, thrombosis,* pericardial effusion, endocarditis, gangrene, *edema, chest pain.*
EENT: conjunctivitis.
GI: *nausea, vomiting, diarrhea, stomatitis, anorexia,* GI bleeding, dyspepsia, constipation, intestinal perforation or ileus, *abdominal pain.*
GU: *oliguria, anuria,* proteinuria, hematuria, dysuria, renal impairment requiring dialysis, urine retention, urinary frequency.
Hematologic: *anemia, thrombocytopenia, leukopenia,* coagulation disorders, *capillary leak syndrome resulting in substantial fluid retention,* leukocytosis, eosinophilia.
Hepatic: jaundice, ascites, hepatomegaly.
Metabolic: *weight gain,* weight loss.
Musculoskeletal: arthralgia, myalgia, arthritis, muscle spasm, *back pain.*
Respiratory: *pulmonary congestion,* pulmonary edema, *respiratory failure, dyspnea,* tachypnea, pleural effusion, wheezing, *apnea, pneumothorax,* hemoptysis.
Skin: *pruritus,* erythema, *rash,* dry skin, *exfoliative dermatitis,* purpura, petechiae, urticaria, alopecia, phlebitis, injection site reactions.
Other: *chills, infection,* allergic reactions.

INTERACTIONS
Drug-drug. *Antihypertensives, beta blockers:* Increases risk of hypotension. Monitor blood pressure.
Bone marrow depressants: Causes additive bone marrow depression. Monitor hematologic study results.
Cardiotoxic drugs, including daunorubicin, doxorubicin: Increases cardiotoxicity. Avoid using together.
Hepatotoxic drugs, nephrotoxic drugs: Causes additive toxicity. Monitor renal and hepatic function study results.

Psychotropics: Increases CNS depression, altered CNS function. Monitor mental status.
Systemic corticosteroids, glucocorticoids: Reduces antitumorigenic effect. Avoid using together.

EFFECTS ON LAB TEST RESULTS
• May increase bilirubin, creatinine, AST, and alkaline phosphatase levels. May decrease magnesium and calcium levels.
• May increase eosinophil count. May decrease hemoglobin, hematocrit, and RBC, platelet, neutrophil, and lymphocyte counts. May increase or decrease WBC count.

ACTION
Highly purified immunoregulatory protein synthesized using recombinant DNA technology. Its biologic activity is similar to human interleukin-2 (IL-2): it enhances lymphocyte mitogenesis, stimulates long-term growth of IL-2–dependent cell lines, enhances lymphocyte cytotoxicity, induces both lymphokine-activated and natural killer cell activity, and initiates interferon gamma production. Immunologic effects include activation of cellular immunity, production of cytokines, including tumor necrosis factor, interleukin-1 (IL-1), and gamma interferon, and inhibition of tumor growth. Its specific antitumorigenic action is unknown.

PHARMACOKINETICS
Onset, peak, and duration of drug are unknown.
Distribution: Rapidly distributed after I.V. infusion into extravascular and extracellular space. Preferential uptake into liver, kidneys, and lungs.
Metabolism: In the kidneys.
Excretion: Glomerular filtration and peritubular extraction remove aldesleukin from the blood, then proximal convoluted tubule cells metabolize it.

CLINICAL CONSIDERATIONS

• Because of drug's short half-life of 85 minutes, adverse effects usually reverse when therapy is complete.

• Use drug in patients with normal cardiac and pulmonary functions, as determined by thallium stress testing and formal pulmonary function tests.

• Before therapy, obtain a chest X-ray and perform standard hematologic measurements, including, electrolyte levels, renal and hepatic function tests, and CBC, differential, and platelet counts. Repeat daily during therapy.

• *Alert:* Drug is linked to capillary leak syndrome, a condition caused by the loss of vascular tone, in which plasma proteins and fluids escape into the extravascular space. Mean arterial blood pressure begins to drop within 2 to 12 hours of treatment; edema and effusions may be severe, and death can result from hypoperfusion of major organs. Other conditions that can accompany capillary leak syndrome include arrhythmia, MI, angina, mental status changes, renal insufficiency, respiratory distress or failure, and GI bleeding, ischemia, and perforation.

• When treating capillary leak syndrome, carefully monitor fluid status, pulse rate, mental status, urine output, organ perfusion, and central venous pressure.

• If patient develops moderate to severe lethargy or somnolence, withhold dose and notify prescriber because continued administration can cause coma.

• Adjust dosage of concomitant drugs to compensate for aldesleukin-induced renal and hepatic impairment.

• Patients should be neurologically stable, with a computed tomography scan negative for CNS metastases. Drug may exacerbate symptoms in patients with unrecognized or undiagnosed CNS metastases.

• Toxic reactions are commonly related to dosage. If patient develops such a reaction, expect to withhold a dose or interrupt therapy rather than reducing the dose.

• Drug has been used investigationally for several cancers, including Kaposi's sarcoma, colorectal cancer, and malignant lymphoma.

• Severe anemia or thrombocytopenia may occur. Give packed RBCs or platelets.

• Tumor may continue to regress for up to 12 months after therapy.

• In case of overdose, treat symptoms supportively and life-threatening toxic reactions with I.V. dexamethasone, which may decrease aldesleukin's therapeutic effect.

PATIENT TEACHING

• Encourage patient to discuss risks and benefits of therapy with prescriber.

• Explain administration schedule to patient and caregivers, and stress importance of compliance.

• Instruct patient to report adverse reactions promptly.

alefacept
Amevive

Pharmacologic class:
immunosuppressive
Therapeutic class: antipsoriatic
Pregnancy risk category: B

INDICATIONS & DOSAGES

➤ **Moderate to severe chronic plaque psoriasis in patients who are candidates for systemic therapy or phototherapy—**
Adults: 7.5 mg I.V. push over 5 seconds once weekly for 12 weeks. An additional 12-week course of therapy may be given if CD4+ T lymphocyte count is normal and at least 12 weeks have passed since the previous treatment.
Adjust-a-dose: Withhold dose if CD4+ T lymphocyte count is below 250 cells/

mm³. Stop drug if CD4+ count remains below 250 cells/mm³ for 1 month.

ADMINISTRATION
Direct injection: Prime infusion set provided in the kit with 3 ml normal saline before giving the drug. Flush infusion set with 3 ml normal saline after drug is given. Give as I.V. bolus over 5 seconds.
Intermittent infusion: Not recommended.
Continuous infusion: Not recommended.

PREPARATION & STORAGE
Available as 7.5 mg single-dose vial for I.V. use. Reconstitute 7.5-mg vial with 0.6 ml of supplied diluent to yield a final concentration of 7.5 mg/0.5 ml. Don't filter the reconstituted solution. Slowly inject diluent toward the side of the vial. Swirl vial gently; don't shake. Make sure reconstituted solution is clear and colorless to slightly yellow; discard solution if it's discolored or cloudy. After reconstitution, use immediately or store in the refrigerator and use within 4 hours. Store powder at room temperature, protected from light.

Incompatibilities
Diluents other than the one provided, other I.V. drugs.

CONTRAINDICATIONS & CAUTIONS
Contraindicated in patients hypersensitive to the drug or any of its components, in breast-feeding women, and in patients with a history of systemic malignancy or infection.

Use cautiously in patients at high risk for malignancy, in patients with chronic or recurrent infections, and in pregnant patients.

ADVERSE REACTIONS
CNS: dizziness.
CV: *coronary artery disorder, MI.*
EENT: pharyngitis.

GI: nausea.
Hematologic: LYMPHOPENIA.
Musculoskeletal: myalgia.
Respiratory: cough.
Skin: pruritus; injection site pain, inflammation, bleeding, edema, or mass.
Other: *infection,* chills, *malignancy, hypersensitivity reaction,* accidental injury, antibody formation.

INTERACTIONS
Drug-drug. *Immunosuppressants, phototherapy:* Increases risk of excessive immunosuppression. Avoid using together.

EFFECTS ON LAB TEST RESULTS
● May decrease CD4+ and CD8+ T lymphocyte counts.

ACTION
An immunosuppressive protein that interferes with lymphocyte activation and reduces subsets of CD2+ T lymphocytes, which reduces circulating total CD4+ and CD8+ T lymphocyte counts.

PHARMACOKINETICS
Onset, peak and duration of drug are unknown.
Distribution: Unknown.
Metabolism: Unknown.
Excretion: After I.V. administration, the elimination half-life is 270 hours.

CLINICAL CONSIDERATIONS
● Monitor CD4+ T lymphocyte count weekly for 12 weeks of treatment. Patient should have normal CD4+ T lymphocyte count before starting therapy.
● Monitor patient carefully for signs of infection and malignancy. Stop drug if malignancy or serious infection occurs.
● Enroll pregnant women using alefacept into the Biogen Pregnancy Registry, by phoning 1-866-263-8483, so that the drug's effects can be studied.
● Signs and symptoms of overdose may include chills, headache, arthralgia, and sinusitis. In case of overdose, monitor

patient closely for effects on total lymphocyte count and CD4+ T lymphocyte count.

PATIENT TEACHING
• Inform patient of potential adverse reactions.
• Advise patient to immediately report signs of infection or malignancy.
• Tell patient that blood tests will be done regularly to monitor WBC counts.
• Tell patient to notify prescriber if she is or may be pregnant within 8 weeks of taking drug.

alemtuzumab
Campath

Pharmacologic class: monoclonal antibody
Therapeutic class: antineoplastic
Pregnancy risk category: C
pH: 6.8 to 7.4

INDICATIONS & DOSAGES
➤ **B-cell chronic lymphocytic leukemia in patients treated with alkylating drugs and in whom fludarabine therapy has failed—**
Adults: Initially, 3 mg I.V. infusion over 2 hours daily; if tolerated, increase dose to 10 mg daily. Once the 10-mg dose is tolerated, increase to 30 mg daily, usually within 3 to 7 days. For maintenance, give 30 mg I.V. three times weekly on nonconsecutive days (such as Monday, Wednesday, Friday) for up to 12 weeks. Don't give single doses of more than 30 mg or weekly doses of more than 90 mg.
Adjust-a-dose: For patients with hematologic toxicity, see *Adjusting dosages for hematologic toxicity,* page 65.

ADMINISTRATION
Direct injection: Not recommended.

Intermittent infusion: Not recommended.
Continuous injection: Premedicate patient with 50 mg diphenhydramine and 650 mg acetaminophen 30 minutes before first dose, at dose increases, and as indicated. Infuse diluted 100-ml solution over 2 hours.

PREPARATION & STORAGE
Available in 3-ml glass ampules of clear solution containing 10 mg/ml.
Discard solution if it's discolored or if it develops precipitate. Don't shake ampule before use. Withdraw the necessary amount of drug from the ampule and filter with a sterile, low–protein-binding, non–fiber-releasing 5-micron filter before dilution. Dilute with 100 ml normal saline or D_5W. Gently invert the bag to mix the solution.
Diluted solutions must be used within 8 hours of preparation. Protect ampules from direct sunlight. Store at 36° to 46° F (2° to 8° C). Don't freeze solution, and discard if the ampule has been frozen.

Incompatibilities
Other I.V. drugs.

CONTRAINDICATIONS & CAUTIONS
• Contraindicated in patients with active systemic infections, underlying immunodeficiency (such as HIV), or type I hypersensitivity or anaphylactic reactions to alemtuzumab or its components.
• Patient who has recently received alemtuzumab shouldn't be immunized with live viral vaccines due to his suppressed immune system.
• Breast-feeding women should stop breast-feeding during treatment and for at least 3 months after the last dose of alemtuzumab.

ADVERSE REACTIONS
CNS: *insomnia,* depression, somnolence, *asthenia, headache, dysthesia,*

Adjusting dosages for hematologic toxicity

Hematologic toxicity	Dosage adjustment
First occurrence of absolute neutrophil count (ANC) < 250/mm³ or platelets ≤ 25,000/mm³	Withhold therapy; resume at same dose when ANC ≥ 500/mm³ or platelets ≥ 50,000/mm³. If delay between doses is ≥ 7 days, start therapy at 3 mg; escalate to 10 mg; then 30 mg as tolerated.
Second occurrence of ANC < 250/mm³ or platelets ≤ 25,000/mm³	Withhold therapy; when ANC ≥ 500/mm³ or platelets ≥ 50,000/mm³, resume at 10 mg. If delay between doses is ≥ 7 days, start therapy at 3 mg; escalate to 10 mg only.
Third occurrence of ANC < 250/mm³ or platelets ≤ 25,000/mm³	Discontinue therapy.
For a decrease of ANC or platelet count ≤ 50% of the baseline value in patients starting therapy with ANC ≤ 500/mm³ or platelet count ≤ 25,000/ mm³	Withhold therapy; when ANC or platelet count returns to baseline, resume therapy. If delay between dosing is ≥ 7 days, start therapy at 3 mg and escalate to 10 mg; then 30 mg as tolerated.

dizziness, fatigue, fever, malaise, tremor.
CV: *edema, peripheral edema, chest pain, hypotension, hypertension, tachycardia,* **supraventricular tachycardia.**
EENT: epistaxis, rhinitis, *pharyngitis.*
GI: *anorexia, nausea, vomiting, diarrhea, stomatitis, ulcerative stomatitis, mucositis, abdominal pain, dyspepsia, constipation.*
Hematologic: NEUTROPENIA, *anemia,* **pancytopenia,** THROMBOCYTOPENIA, *purpura,* **leukopenia.**
Musculoskeletal: *pain, skeletal pain, back pain, myalgia.*
Respiratory: *dyspnea, cough, bronchitis, pneumonitis,* **bronchospasm.**
Skin: *rash, urticaria, pruritus, increased sweating.*
Other: INFECTION, SEPSIS, *herpes simplex, rigors,* temperature change sensation, candidiasis.

INTERACTIONS
None reported.

EFFECTS ON LAB TEST RESULTS
• May decrease hemoglobin, hematocrit, and CD4+, RBC, WBC, platelet, neutrophil, and lymphocyte counts.

ACTION
Binds to CD52 antigen, which is present on the surface of most immune modulators, and causes antibody-dependent lysis of leukemic cells after cell-surface binding.

PHARMACOKINETICS
Drug peak and trough levels rise during the first few weeks of treatment. Steady state is reached at 6 weeks but may vary among individuals. Increase in concentration corresponds with reduction of malignant lymphocytosis.
Distribution: Binds to various tissues.
Metabolism: Unknown.
Excretion: Half-life, 12 days.

CLINICAL CONSIDERATIONS
• Give 200 mg hydrocortisone to decrease severity of any severe infusion-related events. Give anti-infective prophylaxis while patient is receiving therapy; TMP-sulfa DS b.i.d. three times a week and 250 mg famciclovir (or equivalent) b.i.d. have been used at the beginning of alemtuzumab therapy. Continue for 2 months after last dose of alemtuzumab or until CD4+ count is 200 cells/mm³ or higher.

• *Alert:* If patient has systemic infection at scheduled dose time, withhold drug.

• Monitor blood pressure and hypotensive symptoms during administration.

• Monitor hematologic studies carefully.

• Check CBC and platelet counts weekly during therapy and more frequently if anemia, neutropenia, or thrombocytopenia worsens.

• Don't immunize with live viral vaccines.

• If therapy is interrupted for 7 days or longer, restart with gradual dose increase.

• Irradiate blood if transfusions are needed to protect against graft-versus-host disease.

PATIENT TEACHING

• Tell patient to report immediately any infusion-related reactions, such as rigors, chills, fever, nausea, or vomiting.

• Advise patient that blood tests will be done frequently during therapy to monitor for adverse effects.

• Advise patient to report immediately any signs or symptoms of infection.

• Instruct women of childbearing age and men to use effective contraceptive methods during therapy and for at least 6 months after completion of therapy.

alfentanil hydrochloride
Alfenta

Pharmacologic class: opioid
Therapeutic class: analgesic, anesthetic
Pregnancy risk category: C
Controlled substance schedule: II
pH: 4 to 6

INDICATIONS & DOSAGES

➤ **Adjunct to general anesthesia—**
Adults: Initially, 8 to 50 mcg/kg I.V., then in increments of 3 to 15 mcg/kg.

➤ **As a primary anesthetic—**
Adults: Initially, 130 to 245 mcg/kg I.V., then 0.5 to 1.5 mcg/kg/minute.

➤ **In monitored anesthesia care—**
Adults: Initially, 3 to 8 mcg/kg I.V., then in increments of 3 to 5 mcg/kg q 5 to 20 minutes. Total dose is 3 to 40 mcg/kg.

Adjust-a-dose: For debilitated patients, reduce dosage. For obese patients, base dosage on lean body weight.

ADMINISTRATION

Only staff trained in giving I.V. anesthetics and managing their potential adverse effects should give this drug.

Direct injection: Over 90 seconds to 3 minutes, inject undiluted drug into I.V. tubing of a free-flowing, compatible solution.

Intermittent infusion: Not recommended.

Continuous infusion: Using an I.V. piggyback, infuse diluted drug at ordered rate through tubing containing a free-flowing, compatible solution.

PREPARATION & STORAGE

Available in ampules containing 2, 5, 10, or 20 ml at a concentration of 500 mcg/ml.

Drug may be injected full strength using a tuberculin or 1-ml syringe. For continuous infusion, dilute in normal saline solution, D_5W, dextrose 5% in normal saline, or lactated Ringer's solution.

Store undiluted drug between 59° and 86° F (15° and 30° C); avoid freezing. Protect from light.

Incompatibilities
None reported.

CONTRAINDICATIONS & CAUTIONS

• Contraindicated in patients hypersensitive to fentanyl derivatives.

• Use cautiously in those with head injury, pulmonary disease, decreased

---

Reactions may be *common*, uncommon, *life-threatening*, or COMMON AND LIFE-THREATENING.

respiratory reserve, or hepatic or renal dysfunction.
• Use cautiously in obese, geriatric, or pediatric patients because decreased metabolism prolongs drug effect.

ADVERSE REACTIONS
CNS: dizziness, sleepiness, postoperative sedation.
CV: *arrhythmias, cardiac arrest, bradycardia,* hypotension, hypertension, tachycardia.
EENT: blurred vision.
GI: *nausea, vomiting.*
Musculoskeletal: muscle rigidity.
Respiratory: *apnea, respiratory depression.*

INTERACTIONS
Drug-drug. *Antihypertensives, diuretics:* Increases hypotension. Monitor blood pressure.
Benzodiazepines, CNS depressants: Enhances CNS depression. Use together cautiously.
Buprenorphine, nalbuphine, pentazocine: Antagonizes or enhances effects, depending on dose. Monitor patient closely.
Hepatic enzyme inducers such as cimetidine: Decreases clearance and prolongs action of alfentanil. Monitor patient for prolonged drug effects.
Naloxone, naltrexone: Antagonizes effects of alfentanil. Monitor patient for reversal of alfentanil effects.

EFFECTS ON LAB TEST RESULTS
• May increase amylase and lipase levels.

ACTION
Acts as an agonist at stereospecific opioid receptor sites in the CNS. As a result, drug alters the perception of pain and the emotional response to it.

PHARMACOKINETICS
Onset, within 1 minute for analgesia and 1 to 2 minutes for loss of consciousness; duration, 5 to 10 minutes for analgesia and 10 minutes to regain consciousness.
Distribution: Rapidly dispersed into body tissues and across blood-brain barrier, with 92% bound to plasma proteins. Drug readily crosses placental barrier. Drug appears in breast milk.
Metabolism: In liver.
Excretion: Primarily by liver. Inactive metabolites and less than 1% of unchanged drug are excreted in urine.

CLINICAL CONSIDERATIONS
• As a primary anesthetic, alfentanil may be prescribed to induce anesthesia for general surgery requiring endotracheal intubation and medical ventilation.
• Discontinue drug 10 to 15 minutes before surgery ends.
• Closely monitor respiratory, CV, and neurologic systems during and after surgery.
• Periodically monitor postoperative vital signs and bladder function. Monitoring arterial oxygen saturation may help you assess respiratory depression.
• Patient may need analgesics shortly after surgery.
• If overdose occurs, reverse effects with naloxone and then give symptomatic care. For apnea, give oxygen, provide mechanical ventilation, and use positive-pressure ventilation by bag or mask. For hypotension, give I.V. fluids and vasopressors; for muscle rigidity, a neuromuscular blocker.

PATIENT TEACHING
• Explain to patient and family the anesthetic effect of alfentanil as well as preoperative and postoperative care measures.

• Inform patient that another analgesic will be available to relieve pain after effects of the drug have worn off.

---

allopurinol sodium
Aloprim

Pharmacologic class: xanthine oxidase inhibitor
Therapeutic class: antigout drug
Pregnancy risk category: C
pH: 11.1 to 11.8

INDICATIONS & DOSAGES
➤ **Prevention or acute, short-term treatment of transient hyperuricemia resulting from rapid cell destruction during antineoplastic therapy—tumor lysis syndrome—in patients unable to take oral allopurinol—**
Adults: 200 to 400 mg/m² I.V. daily as a single infusion or given in divided doses at 6-, 8-, or 12-hour intervals. Don't exceed 600 mg daily.
Children: 200 mg/m² I.V. daily in four divided doses. Don't exceed 600 mg/day.
Adjust-a-dose: For patients with creatinine clearance between 10 and 20 ml/minute, give 200 mg/day I.V. If clearance is 3 to 10 ml/minute, give 100 mg/day; if clearance is less than 3 ml/minute, give 100 mg/day at extended intervals.

ADMINISTRATION
Direct injection: Not recommended.
Intermittent infusion: Give diluted drug in four to six intermittent doses; rate depends on volume.
Continuous infusion: Infuse diluted drug over 24 hours.

PREPARATION & STORAGE
Available as a 30-ml vial of lyophilized powder containing 500 mg of allopuri-nol. Store powder at 59° to 77° F (15° to 25° C).
To reconstitute, add 25 ml of sterile water for injection to the vial. Further dilute to desired concentration with sterile normal saline or D_5W injection. Final concentration shouldn't exceed 1.2 mg/ml. Store reconstituted solution at room temperature. Infusion should begin within 10 hours of preparation. Use within 24 hours because the drug contains no preservatives.

Incompatibilities
Amikacin, amphotericin B, carmustine, cefotaxime, chlorpromazine, cimetidine, clindamycin phosphate, cytarabine, dacarbazine, daunorubicin, diphenhydramine, doxorubicin, doxycycline hyclate, droperidol, floxuridine, gentamicin, haloperidol lactate, hydroxyzine, idarubicin, imipenem and cilastatin sodium, mechlorethamine, meperidine, methylprednisolone sodium succinate, metoclopramide, minocycline, nalbuphine, netilmicin, ondansetron, prochlorperazine edisylate, promethazine, sodium bicarbonate, streptozocin, tobramycin sulfate, vinorelbine.

CONTRAINDICATIONS & CAUTIONS
• Stop therapy at first sign of rash or hypersensitivity reaction; severe reactions may be fatal.
• Use cautiously in patients with impaired renal or hepatic function or with concurrent illnesses that may affect renal function, such as hypertension or diabetes. Dosage may need to be adjusted.

ADVERSE REACTIONS
CNS: *seizures.*
CV: *allergic vasculitis, arterial nephrosclerosis.*
GI: nausea, vomiting.
GU: *renal failure.*
Hematologic: *leukopenia, neutropenia, thrombocytopenia, pancytopenia.*

Reactions may be *common*, uncommon, *life-threatening*, or COMMON AND LIFE-THREATENING.

Respiratory: *pulmonary embolism, respiratory failure or insufficiency.*
Skin: *severe exfoliative dermatitis, toxic epidermal necrolysis,* rash.
Other: *hypersensitivity reactions, sepsis.*

INTERACTIONS

Drug-drug. *Amoxicillin, ampicillin:* Increases incidence of rash. Avoid using together.
Azathioprine, mercaptopurine: Inhibits metabolism of azathioprine and mercaptopurine, increasing the risk of toxic reaction from both. Monitor for signs and symptoms of toxicity.
Chlorpropamide: Increases risk of hypoglycemia. Avoid using together.
Cyclophosphamide, other cytotoxic drugs: May enhance bone marrow depression. Monitor hematologic studies.
Dicumarol: Increases anticoagulant effects. Monitor coagulation values.
Diuretics: Causes more frequent hypersensitivity reactions. Monitor patient closely.
Uricosurics: Increases urine excretion of oxypurinol. May enhance therapy.

EFFECTS ON LAB TEST RESULTS

• May increase alkaline phosphatase, BUN, creatinine, glucose, phosphate, bilirubin, AST, and ALT levels. May decrease magnesium and uric acid levels. May increase or decrease calcium, potassium, and sodium levels.
• May increase eosinophil count. May decrease hemoglobin, hematocrit, and WBC, neutrophil, and platelet counts.

ACTION

Reduces uric acid production by inhibiting the enzyme xanthine oxidase.

PHARMACOKINETICS

Half-life, 1 to 3 hours; for oxypurinol, 18 to 30 hours.
Distribution: Uniformly in total tissue water, except in the brain; small

amounts found in muscles. Drug and its active metabolite, oxypurinol, appear in breast milk.
Metabolism: Rapidly oxidized to oxypurinol.
Excretion: 70% in urine, 20% in feces.

CLINICAL CONSIDERATIONS

• Monitor hemoglobin, WBC and platelet counts, and alkaline phosphatase, ALT, BUN, creatinine, electrolyte, and uric acid levels before starting therapy and daily during therapy.
• To prevent xanthine calculi from forming and to prevent renal precipitation of urates when used with other uricosurics, make sure patient takes in enough fluids so that urine output is at least 2 L daily and urine remains neutral or slightly alkaline.
• Dialysis removes allopurinol and oxypurinol.

PATIENT TEACHING

• Explain to patient and family the use and administration of allopurinol.
• Tell patient to report adverse reactions or discomfort at I.V. site promptly.
• Warn patient to avoid performing hazardous activities until the adverse CNS reactions are known.

alpha₁-proteinase inhibitor (human)
Prolastin

Pharmacologic class: enzyme inhibitor
Therapeutic class: replacement protein
Pregnancy risk category: C

INDICATIONS & DOSAGES

➤ **Replacement therapy for patients with congenital alpha₁-antitrypsin**

deficiency and signs of panacinar emphysema—
Adults: 60 mg/kg I.V. once weekly. Infusion rate of 0.08 ml/kg/minute or more.

ADMINISTRATION
Direct injection: Inject directly into vein at a rate of 0.08 ml/kg/minute or more. Drug takes about 30 minutes to administer.
Intermittent infusion: Not recommended.
Continuous infusion: Not recommended.

PREPARATION & STORAGE
Available in single-dose vials containing 500 or 1,000 mg of alpha₁-proteinase inhibitor. The package includes a vial of sterile water for injection (20 ml for 500 mg and 40 ml for 1,000 mg), a double-ended transfer needle, and a filter needle. Refrigerate package before use.

To reconstitute, bring vials to room temperature and follow manufacturer's directions. Use within 3 hours. Dilute with normal saline solution, if needed.

Incompatibilities
Other I.V. drugs or solutions.

CONTRAINDICATIONS & CAUTIONS
• Use cautiously in those with circulatory overload because the colloidal solution increases plasma volume.

ADVERSE REACTIONS
CNS: dizziness, light-headedness, fever.
Hematologic: transient leukocytosis, dilution anemia.
Other: viral transmission.

INTERACTIONS
None reported.

EFFECTS ON LAB TEST RESULTS
• May increase WBC count. May decrease hemoglobin and hematocrit.

COMPOSITION
Prepared from pooled human plasma that has tested negative for hepatitis and HIV, this drug contains alpha₁-proteinase inhibitor, the deficient protein in alpha₁-antitrypsin deficiency. It also contains small amounts of other plasma proteins.

ACTION
Increases alpha₁-antitrypsin levels in plasma and the epithelial lining of the lungs, thus preventing panacinar emphysema from worsening.

PHARMACOKINETICS
Distribution: Unknown.
Metabolism: Unknown.
Excretion: Half-life is about 4½ days.

CLINICAL CONSIDERATIONS
• In patients who haven't been previously immunized against hepatitis B, give 0.06 ml/kg body weight of hepatitis B immune globulin (human) I.M. when you give the first dose of hepatitis B vaccine.
• Many commercial assays for alpha₁-proteinase inhibitor measure immunoreactivity of the protein and not inhibitor activity. Monitoring drug level may not accurately reflect clinical response.

PATIENT TEACHING
• Teach patient about AIDS. If he tests negative for the hepatitis B surface antigen, encourage him to get immunized for hepatitis B.
• Tell patient to report adverse reactions to prescriber promptly.
• Instruct patient not to smoke during therapy.

Reactions may be *common*, uncommon, ***life-threatening**,* or COMMON AND LIFE-THREATENING.

alprostadil (prostaglandin E₁)

Prostin VR ◇, Prostin VR Pediatric

Pharmacologic class: prostaglandin

Therapeutic class: prostaglandin derivative

Pregnancy risk category: NR

INDICATIONS & DOSAGES

➤ **To keep the arterial duct patent until surgery can be performed—**
Neonates: 0.05 to 0.1 mcg/kg/minute I.V., not to exceed 0.4 mcg/kg/minute. When therapeutic response is achieved, reduce dosage to lowest level that maintains it.

Patients with low partial pressure of oxygen values will have best response and require lowest dose.

ADMINISTRATION

Only staff trained in pediatric intensive care should give drug.

Direct injection: Not recommended.

Intermittent infusion: Not recommended.

Continuous infusion: Using a continuous-rate pump, infuse drug through large peripheral or central vein or through umbilical artery catheter placed at level of the arterial duct.

PREPARATION & STORAGE

Available in 500 mcg/ml ampules.

Dilute 1 ml (500 mcg/ml) in 25 to 250 ml of normal saline solution or D_5W to yield a concentration of 2 to 20 mcg/ml. Don't use diluents that contain benzyl alcohol because they can cause fatal toxic syndrome.

Store solution at 36° to 46° F (2° to 8°C). Don't freeze. Use prepared solution within 24 hours.

Incompatibilities

None reported.

CONTRAINDICATIONS & CAUTIONS

• Contraindicated in neonates with respiratory distress syndrome because a patent duct can cause circulatory overload.

• Use cautiously in neonates with bleeding disorders because drug inhibits platelet aggregation.

ADVERSE REACTIONS

CNS: *seizures, fever.*

CV: *bradycardia,* hypotension, tachycardia, *flushing,* edema.

GI: diarrhea.

Hematologic: *DIC.*

Metabolic: *hypokalemia.*

Respiratory: APNEA, *respiratory distress.*

Other: *sepsis.*

INTERACTIONS

Drug-drug. *Anticoagulants, antiplatelet drugs, thrombolytics:* Increases risk of bleeding. Monitor hematologic and coagulation values.

EFFECTS ON LAB TEST RESULTS

• May decrease potassium level.

ACTION

Inhibits platelet aggregation and produces vasodilation by acting directly on vascular smooth muscle. By relaxing the smooth muscle of the arterial duct, drug prevents the closure that normally occurs 24 to 96 hours after birth.

PHARMACOKINETICS

Onset, 1½ to 3 hours in acyanotic congenital heart disease and 15 to 30 minutes in cyanotic heart disease; effect peaks at 3 hours in coarctation of aorta, 1½ hours in interruption of aortic arch, 30 minutes in cyanotic heart disease; duration, length of infusion. Duct usually begins to close 1 to 2 hours after end of infusion.

Distribution: In plasma.

Metabolism: Pulmonary, with up to 80% metabolized by oxidation on first pass through lungs.

Excretion: Primarily by the kidneys, as metabolites, within 24 hours. Half-life ranges from 5 to 10 minutes.

CLINICAL CONSIDERATIONS

• To maintain patency, give drug before duct closes.

• If flushing occurs from peripheral vasodilation, reposition catheter.

• Infusion may continue during cardiac catheterization.

• Drug may be given by intra-aortic or intra-arterial infusion.

• *Alert:* Monitor respiratory status during treatment and keep resuscitation equipment readily available. Apnea usually occurs in first hour of infusion in 10% to 12% of neonates weighing less than 2 kg (4 lb) at birth.

• Use an umbilical artery catheter, auscultation, or a Doppler transducer to monitor arterial pressure. Expect to reduce infusion rate if hypotension or fever develops and to stop drug if apnea or bradycardia develops.

• In infants with restricted pulmonary blood flow, measure drug's effectiveness by monitoring blood oxygenation. In infants with restricted systemic blood flow, measure drug's effectiveness by monitoring systemic blood pressure and blood pH.

PATIENT TEACHING

• Explain to family the use and administration of drug.

• Encourage parents to ask questions and express concerns.

alteplase, recombinant alteplase, tissue plasminogen activator (t-PA)

Activase, Activase rt-PA ◊ , Cathflo Activase

Pharmacologic class: tissue plasminogen activator
Therapeutic class: thrombolytic enzyme
Pregnancy risk category: C
pH: 7.3

INDICATIONS & DOSAGES

➤ **To destroy coronary artery thrombi in an acute MI—**

Adults weighing 65 kg (143 lb) or more: 100 mg I.V. over 3 hours, with 60 mg given in first hour. Give 6 to 10 mg in first 1 to 2 minutes, 20 mg in second hour, and 20 mg in third hour. Don't exceed dosage; doses above 100 mg have been linked with intracranial bleeding.

Adults weighing less than 65 kg: 1.25 mg/kg I.V. over 3 hours, with 60% of dose given in first hour. Give 10% in first 1 to 2 minutes and remainder over next 2 hours.

➤ **Accelerated dosing for an acute MI—**

Adults weighing more than 67 kg (148 lb): Total dose of 100 mg I.V. given as follows: 15 mg by rapid I.V. bolus over 1 to 2 minutes, then 50 mg I.V. over the next 30 minutes, followed by remaining 35 mg I.V. over the next hour.

Adults weighing 67 kg or less: Initially, 15 mg I.V. bolus over 1 to 2 minutes; followed by 0.75 mg/kg, not to exceed 50 mg, over the next 30 minutes; then 0.5 mg/kg, not to exceed 35 mg, over the next hour.

Reactions may be *common,* uncommon, *life-threatening,* or COMMON AND LIFE-THREATENING.

➤ **Acute ischemic stroke within 3 hours of symptom onset—**
Adults: 0.9 mg/kg I.V., to a maximum of 90 mg, I.V. infusion over 1 hour, with 10% of the dose given initially as an I.V. bolus over 1 minute.

➤ **Lysis of acute pulmonary emboli—**
Adults: 100 mg I.V. over 2 hours.

➤ **To restore function to central venous access devices as assessed by the ability to withdraw blood—**
Adults and children older than age 2: For patients weighing 30 kg (66 lb) or more, instill 2 mg I.V. Cathflo Activase in 2 ml sterile water into catheter. For patients weighing 10 kg (22 lb) to less than 30 kg (66 lb), instill 110% of the internal lumen volume of the catheter, not to exceed 2 mg in 2 ml. After 30 minutes of dwell time, assess catheter function by aspirating blood. If function is restored, aspirate 4 to 5 ml of blood to remove Cathflo Activase and residual clot, and gently irrigate the catheter with normal saline solution. If catheter function not restored after 120 minutes, instill a second dose.

ADMINISTRATION
Direct injection: Bolus doses of Activase can be given over 1 to 2 minutes. Don't use excessive pressure while instilling Cathflo Activase into the catheter, which could cause catheter rupture or expulsion of the clot into the circulation.
Intermittent infusion: Not recommended.
Continuous infusion: Infuse diluted solution at recommended rate.

PREPARATION & STORAGE
Available as lyophilized powder in 50-mg and 100-mg vials (Activase) and 2-mg single-patient vials for intra-catheter instillation (Cathflo Activase). Store Activase vials at room temperature or refrigerate; store Cathflo Activase vials in the refrigerator.

Activase
Reconstitute just before injection. Using an 18G needle, reconstitute to 1 mg/ml by adding 50 ml or 100 ml of the preservative-free, sterile water for injection that the manufacturer provided. Don't use bacteriostatic water for injection. Aim diluent at lyophilized cake and expect slight foaming. Let vial stand for several minutes.

If needed, dilute drug to 0.5 mg/ml in glass bottles or polyvinyl chloride bag. For 50-ml vial, add 50 ml of normal saline solution or D_5W; for 100-ml vial, add 100 ml. Avoid undue agitation. Diluted solution remains stable for 8 hours at room temperature.

Cathflo Activase
Reconstitute with 2.2 ml sterile water; dissolve completely into a colorless to pale yellow solution that yields a concentration of 1 mg/ml. Solutions are stable for up to 8 hours at room temperature.

Incompatibilities
None reported, but don't mix with other drugs.

CONTRAINDICATIONS & CAUTIONS
● Contraindicated in those with evidence of intracranial hemorrhage, suspicion of subarachnoid hemorrhage, seizure at onset of stroke, internal bleeding, aneurysm, arteriovenous malformation, bleeding diathesis, history of CVA, brain tumor, CNS surgery or trauma in previous 2 months, or systolic blood pressure above 179 mm Hg or diastolic blood pressure above 109 mm Hg.
● Use cautiously in those with acute pericarditis, cerebrovascular disease, diabetic hemorrhagic retinopathy, significant hepatic disease, or risk of left-sided heart thrombus, as in mitral stenosis with atrial fibrillation, marked hypertension, subacute bacterial endocarditis, septic thrombophlebitis, or an

occluded arteriovenous cannula at an infected site.

• Use cautiously in those older than age 75; in those who within the past 10 days have had GI or GU bleeding, major surgery, or trauma; and in those receiving oral anticoagulant therapy.

• In pregnant patients and in those who have had obstetric delivery within the past 10 days, the risk of therapy should be weighed against the possible benefits.

ADVERSE REACTIONS

CNS: fever.
CV: *accelerated idioventricular rhythm, PVCs, ventricular tachycardia, cardiogenic shock, heart failure, cardiac arrest, myocardial rupture, reinfarction, cardiac tamponade, venous thrombosis and embolism, electromechanical dissociation,* recurrent ischemia, mitral insufficiency, pericardial effusion, pericarditis, hypotension, *sinus bradycardia.*
GI: nausea, vomiting.
Hematologic: *bleeding.*
Respiratory: *pulmonary edema.*
Skin: urticaria.

INTERACTIONS

Drug-drug. *Aspirin, dipyridamole, heparin, oral anticoagulants:* Increases risk of bleeding. Monitor hematologic and coagulation values closely.

EFFECTS ON LAB TEST RESULTS

• May alter coagulation and fibrinolytic test results.

ACTION

Binds to fibrin in thrombi and converts plasminogen to plasmin, thus initiating local fibrinolysis and limited systemic proteolysis.

PHARMACOKINETICS

Onset, rapid; duration, short.
Distribution: In plasma. Not known if drug appears in breast milk.

Metabolism: In liver.
Excretion: 86% in urine, 5% in feces. Half-life ranges from 3 to 5 minutes.

CLINICAL CONSIDERATIONS

• Recanalization of occluded coronary arteries and improvement of heart function are time-dependent and require that treatment be started within 6 to 12 hours after onset of symptoms.

• Before starting therapy, obtain results from coagulation studies (such as PT, PTT, INR, and fibrin split products), if possible.

• To prevent new clot formation, give heparin during or after alteplase infusion, if ordered. Don't give heparin when treating acute ischemic stroke with t-PA.

• Coronary thrombolysis is linked to arrhythmias induced by reperfusion of ischemic myocardium. Such arrhythmias don't differ from those commonly caused by MI. Keep antiarrhythmics available, and carefully monitor ECG.

• Start to treat acute ischemic stroke within 3 hours of symptom onset.

• Rule out intracranial hemorrhage by computed tomography or another diagnostic imaging method sensitive to hemorrhage.

• Blood pressure should be monitored frequently and controlled during and after administration in management of acute ischemic stroke.

• *Alert:* Avoid I.M. injections because of high risk of bleeding into muscle. Also avoid turning and moving the patient excessively during infusion.

• Avoid venipuncture and arterial puncture during therapy because of increased risk of bleeding. If arterial puncture is needed, select a site on an arm and apply pressure for 30 minutes afterward. Also, prevent bleeding by using pressure dressings, sandbags, or ice packs on recent puncture sites.

Reactions may be *common,* uncommon, *life-threatening,* or **COMMON AND LIFE-THREATENING.**

• If unable to stop severe bleeding with local pressure, stop alteplase and heparin infusions.

• *Alert:* Assess the cause of catheter dysfunction before using Cathflo Activase. Some conditions that occlude the catheter include: catheter malposition, mechanical failure, constriction by a suture, and lipid deposits or drug precipitates within the catheter lumen. Don't suction because of the risk of damage to the vascular wall or collapse of soft-walled catheters.

PATIENT TEACHING
• Explain to patient and family the use and administration of alteplase.
• Tell patient to report adverse reactions promptly.

amifostine
Ethyol

Pharmacologic class: organic thiophosphate
Therapeutic class: cytoprotective drug
Pregnancy risk category: C
pH: 7

INDICATIONS & DOSAGES
➤ **To reduce the cumulative renal toxicity caused by repeated administration of cisplatin in patients with advanced ovarian cancer or non–small-cell lung cancer—**
Adults: 910 mg/m^2/day as a 15-minute I.V. infusion, starting 30 minutes before chemotherapy. If hypotension occurs and blood pressure doesn't return to normal within 5 minutes after treatment is stopped, subsequent cycles should use a dose of 740 mg/m^2.
➤ **To reduce the incidence of moderate to severe xerostomia in patients undergoing radiation therapy for head and neck cancers—**
Adults: 200 mg/m^2/day I.V. infusion over 3 minutes, initiated 15 to 30 minutes before radiation.

ADMINISTRATION
Direct injection: Not recommended.
Intermittent infusion: Infuse over 15 minutes to prevent renal toxicity; infuse over 3 minutes to prevent xerostomia.
Continuous infusion: Not recommended.

PREPARATION & STORAGE
Supplied as a sterile lyophilized powder mixture in 10-ml single-use vials requiring reconstitution for I.V. infusion. Each single-use vial contains 500 mg of amifostine (anhydrous basis) and 500 mg of mannitol. Reconstitute with 9.7 ml of normal saline solution; reconstituted solution and diluted solution in normal saline solution at concentrations of 5 mg/ml to 40 mg/ml are stable for up to 5 hours at room temperature (about 77° F [25° C]) or up to 24 hours if refrigerated (35° to 46° F [2° to 8° C]).
    Don't use solution if it's cloudy or develops a precipitate.

Incompatibilities
Solutions other than normal saline for injection.

CONTRAINDICATIONS & CAUTIONS
• Contraindicated in patients hypersensitive to aminothiol compounds or mannitol.
• Contraindicated in hypotensive or dehydrated patients and in those receiving chemotherapy for potentially curable malignancies, including certain malignancies of germ cell origin, except for those involved in clinical studies.
• Contraindicated in those receiving antihypertensives that can't be stopped

during the 24 hours preceding amifostine administration.

● Use cautiously in geriatric patients with preexisting CV or cerebrovascular conditions and in those for whom nausea, vomiting, or hypotension may be more likely to have serious consequences.

ADVERSE REACTIONS

CNS: dizziness, somnolence.
CV: *hypotension,* flushing or feeling of warmth.
GI: *nausea, vomiting.*
Metabolic: hypocalcemia.
Respiratory: hiccups.
Other: chills or feeling of coldness, sneezing, allergic reactions ranging from rash to rigors.

INTERACTIONS

Drug-drug. *Antihypertensives, other drugs that could potentiate hypotension:* May cause profound hypotension. Monitor blood pressure closely.

EFFECTS ON LAB TEST RESULTS

● May decrease calcium level.

ACTION

Alkaline phosphatase removes the phosphate group from amifostine, producing a pharmacologically active, free thiol metabolite. Free thiol in normal tissues binds and detoxifies reactive metabolites of cisplatin, reducing the toxic effects of cisplatin on renal tissue. Free thiol can also act as a scavenger of free radicals that may be generated in tissues exposed to cisplatin.

PHARMACOKINETICS

Rapid; found in bone marrow cells 5 to 8 minutes after administration. Rapidly cleared from plasma; distribution half-life, less than 1 minute; elimination half-life, about 8 minutes.
Distribution: Throughout body tissues.
Metabolism: Unknown.

Excretion: Renal excretion of parent drug and its two metabolites was low during the first hour after administration.

CLINICAL CONSIDERATIONS

● *Alert:* Don't infuse for longer than designated time; a longer infusion can increase the risk of adverse reactions.
● Make sure the patient is adequately hydrated before administration.
● Keep patient supine during infusion.
● Give an antiemetic, such as 20 mg of dexamethasone I.V. or a serotonin 5-hydroxytryptamine-3 receptor antagonist, before and in conjunction with amifostine. Additional antiemetics may be needed, based on the chemotherapeutic drugs given.
● Monitor blood pressure every 5 minutes during infusion. If hypotension occurs and therapy must be interrupted, notify prescriber and place patient in the Trendelenburg position. Then give an infusion of normal saline solution, using a separate I.V. line. If blood pressure returns to normal within 5 minutes and patient is asymptomatic, you may restart the infusion so the patient receives the full dose of the drug. If you can't give the full dose, limit subsequent doses to 740 mg/m^2.
● Monitor calcium levels in patients at risk for hypocalcemia such as those with nephrotic syndrome. Give calcium supplements, if needed.

PATIENT TEACHING

● Instruct patient to remain supine throughout infusion.
● Advise patient not to breast-feed; it's unknown if drug or its metabolites appear in breast milk.

amikacin sulfate
Amikin

Pharmacologic class: semi-synthetic aminoglycoside
Therapeutic class: antibiotic
Pregnancy risk category: D
pH: 3.5 to 5.5

INDICATIONS & DOSAGES
➤ **Septicemia, peritonitis, and severe burn, bone, joint, respiratory tract, skin, and soft-tissue infections caused by susceptible organisms—**
Adults and children: 15 mg/kg/day I.V. in equally divided doses at 8-hour or 12-hour intervals for 7 to 10 days, not to exceed 1.5 g/day.
Neonates: Initially, 10 mg/kg, then 7.5 mg/kg q 12 hours.
Adjust-a-dose: In adults and children with renal impairment, loading dose is 7.5 mg/kg. Subsequent doses are based on levels and degree of impairment. In patients undergoing hemodialysis, give supplemental doses of about 50% to 70% of initial loading dose after each dialysis session.
➤ **Uncomplicated UTI—**
Adults: 250 mg I.V. twice daily.

ADMINISTRATION
Direct injection: Not recommended.
Intermittent infusion: Using a 21G to 23G needle, infuse diluted drug over 30 to 60 minutes in children and adults and over 1 to 2 hours in infants.
Continuous infusion: Not recommended.

PREPARATION & STORAGE
Supplied as a 50 mg/ml concentration in 2- and 4-ml vials or as a 250 mg/ml concentration in 2-ml and 4-ml vials.
  For infusion, add 500 mg of amikacin to 100 to 200 ml of normal saline solution, D_5W, 5% dextrose and half-normal saline solution, 5% dextrose and 0.2% saline solution, lactated Ringer's, Normosol M in 5% dextrose, and Normosol R in 5% dextrose. All solutions remain stable for 24 hours at room temperature. Yellowing of solution doesn't indicate loss of potency.

Incompatibilities
Amphotericin B, bacitracin, cephapirin, cisplatin, heparin sodium, other I.V. drugs, phenytoin, thiopental, vancomycin, vitamin B complex with C.

CONTRAINDICATIONS & CAUTIONS
• Contraindicated in patients hypersensitive to aminoglycosides.
• Use cautiously in premature infants, neonates, and geriatric patients; in those who are dehydrated or have renal impairment because of increased risk of toxic reaction; and in those who have eighth cranial nerve damage because of risk of ototoxicity.
• Use cautiously in those with myasthenia gravis or Parkinson's disease because drug can cause neuromuscular blockade.

ADVERSE REACTIONS
CNS: neuromuscular blockade, peripheral neuritis, *encephalopathy.*
EENT: *auditory and vestibular ototoxicity.*
GU: *nephrotoxicity.*
Other: *hypersensitivity reactions.*

INTERACTIONS
Drug-drug. *Dimenhydrinate:* May mask symptoms of ototoxicity. Use together with caution.
General anesthetics, neuromuscular blockers: May potentiate neuromuscular blockade. Monitor patient closely.
Indomethacin: May increase trough and peak amikacin levels. Monitor amikacin level closely.

I.V. loop diuretics, such as furosemide: Increases ototoxicity. Monitor hearing function test results.

Other aminoglycosides, acyclovir, amphotericin B, cephalosporins, cisplatin, methoxyflurane, vancomycin: May increase nephrotoxicity. Use together cautiously and monitor renal function test results.

Parenteral penicillins, such as ticarcillin: Inactivates amikacin in vitro. Don't mix together.

EFFECTS ON LAB TEST RESULTS

• May increase BUN, creatinine, nonprotein nitrogen, and urine urea levels.

ACTION

Appears to inhibit protein synthesis by binding to the 30S ribosomal subunit. As a result, DNA is misread, resulting in nonfunctional protein.

Acts against such aerobic bacteria as gram-negative *Acinetobacter, Citrobacter, Enterobacter, Escherichia coli, Klebsiella, Proteus, Providencia, Pseudomonas aeruginosa, Salmonella, Serratia,* and *Shigella.* Susceptible gram-positive bacteria include *Staphylococcus aureus* and *S. epidermidis.*

PHARMACOKINETICS

Drug level peaks from 30 minutes to 2 hours.

Distribution: In most extracellular fluids, including serum, ascitic, pericardial, pleural, synovial, lymphatic, peritoneal, and abscess. Crosses the placental barrier. Low levels appear in breast milk and in CSF.

Metabolism: Not metabolized.

Excretion: By glomerular filtration, with 94% to 98% recovered in urine in 24 hours. Half-life is 2 to 3 hours in adults with normal renal function. It can extend up to 100 hours in patients with renal impairment.

CLINICAL CONSIDERATIONS

• To calculate the correct dose, obtain patient's pretreatment body weight.

• Obtain specimens for culture and sensitivity tests before giving first dose; therapy may begin before results are available.

• Evaluate patient's hearing before and during treatment.

• *Alert:* Obtain periodic peak and trough levels, and adjust dosage. Normal peak level is 20 to 30 mcg/ml; normal trough level, 5 to 10 mcg/ml. Higher levels accompany toxic reaction. Draw trough level before next dosage and peak level 30 minutes after end of infusion.

• If therapy is prolonged for longer than 2 weeks, check ambulatory patients for loss of balance.

• To assess renal function, obtain periodic BUN and creatinine levels.

• To reduce risk of nephrotoxicity, keep patient well hydrated; measure intake and output. Monitor urine for decreased specific gravity.

• *Alert:* Drug may contain sulfites.

• If overdose occurs, use hemodialysis or peritoneal dialysis to remove drug, if ordered. Exchange transfusions may be considered for neonates.

• *Alert:* Don't confuse amikacin (Amikin) with anakinra (Kineret).

PATIENT TEACHING

• Explain to patient and family the use and administration of amikacin.

• Tell patient to report adverse reactions promptly.

• Encourage patient to maintain adequate fluid intake.

---

amino acid solution

Aminosyn, Aminosyn II, Aminosyn-PF, Aminosyn-RF, FreAmine, FreAmine HBC, HepatAmine, NephrAmine, ProcalAmine, Travasol, TrophAmine

Pharmacologic class: protein substrates
Therapeutic class: parenteral nutritional therapy and caloric drug
Pregnancy risk category: C
pH: 5 to 6.8

INDICATIONS & DOSAGES

➤ **Total parenteral nutrition in patients who can't or won't eat—**
Adults: 1 to 1.5 g/kg I.V. daily.
Children weighing more than 10 kg (22 lb): 20 to 25 g/kg I.V. daily for the first 10 kg, then 1 to 1.25 g/kg daily for each kilogram over 10 kg.
Children weighing less than 10 kg: 2 to 4 g/kg I.V. daily.
➤ **Nutritional support in patients with cirrhosis, hepatitis, or hepatic encephalopathy—**
Adults: 80 to 120 g I.V. of amino acids (12 to 18 g of nitrogen) daily of Hepat-Amine.
➤ **Nutritional support in patients with high metabolic stress—**
Adults: 1.5 g/kg I.V. daily of FreAmine HBC.
➤ **Nutritional support in patients with renal failure—**
Adults: 0.3 to 0.5 g/kg I.V. daily (up to total of 26 g daily). Patients on dialysis may require 1 to 1.2 g/kg daily.
Adjust-a-dose: Dosage adjustment must be based on nitrogen balance and body weight corrected for fluid balance.

ADMINISTRATION

Direct injection: Not recommended.
Intermittent infusion: Not recommended.

Continuous infusion: Infuse solution based on patient tolerance, usually over 8 hours. In severely debilitated patients or those requiring long-term parenteral nutrition, give hypertonic solutions containing more than 12.5% dextrose via subclavian catheter into the superior vena cava. In moderately debilitated patients, give solutions mixed with D_5W or dextrose 10% in water via peripheral route.

PREPARATION & STORAGE

Available in bottles containing 250 to 1,000 ml.
   Add dextrose 5% to 70% in water, electrolytes, trace elements, and vitamins, as needed. When modifying solutions, use strict aseptic technique, follow manufacturer's instructions, and give within 24 hours. Discard remaining solution.
   Use only clear solution; hold up to light to find precipitate or evidence of damaged container.

Incompatibilities

Bleomycin, ganciclovir, and indomethacin. Because of the high risk of incompatibility with other substances, add only needed nutritional products.

CONTRAINDICATIONS & CAUTIONS

• Contraindicated in patients hypersensitive to any solution component and in those with inborn error of amino acid metabolism.
• Contraindicated in those with severe uncorrected electrolyte or acid-base imbalance, which could be exacerbated; hyperammonemia, which could worsen; or reduced blood volume, which could lead to acid-base imbalance.
• General amino acid solutions are contraindicated in those with renal failure, severe hepatic disease, hepatic coma, or encephalopathy.
• Special solutions for hepatic failure, encephalopathy, and metabolic stress

---

◆ Off-label use   *May contain benzyl alcohol   ◇ Canada

are contraindicated in those with anuria.

• Hyperosmolar solutions are contraindicated in those with intracranial or intraspinal hemorrhage because fluid overload can exacerbate the condition.

• Use cautiously in those with cardiac disease because of possible fluid overload or diabetes because of increased insulin requirements and in children, especially those with renal failure.

ADVERSE REACTIONS
CNS: *seizures,* fever.
CV: *heart failure,* flushing, edema.
GI: nausea, vomiting, abdominal pain.
GU: glycosuria, osmotic diuresis.
Hepatic: fatty liver.
Metabolic: *hyperosmolar hyperglycemic nonketotic syndrome,* dehydration, electrolyte imbalance, hyperammonemia, hyperglycemia, *rebound hypoglycemia,* metabolic acidosis or alkalosis.
Respiratory: pulmonary edema.
Skin: *edema at injection site,* tissue sloughing.
Other: *anaphylaxis, septicemia from contaminated solution,* chills.

INTERACTIONS
Drug-drug. *Tetracyclines:* May reduce protein-sparing effect. Monitor patient closely.

EFFECTS ON LAB TEST RESULTS
• May increase ammonia and liver enzyme levels. May decrease phosphate, magnesium, and potassium levels. May increase or decrease glucose level.

COMPOSITION
Amino acid injection and solution provide various concentrations of parenteral nutrients, including essential and nonessential amino acids, nitrogen, electrolytes, and calories. They supply nitrogen in a form that's assimilated easily. Solutions vary in amount of protein and nitrogen, osmolarity, and elec-

trolyte level. Nonprotein calories are usually provided as dextrose and, to a lesser extent, as glycerin, fructose, alcohol, or fat.

The pharmacy can prepare special solutions for patients with specific nutrient requirements or intolerance to the components of conventional solutions. For example, solutions are available for patients with renal or hepatic impairment.

CLINICAL CONSIDERATIONS
• Osmolarity is 316 to 1,300 mOsm/L.
• Add electrolytes, vitamins, and trace elements, using strict aseptic technique.
• Begin with a 5% to 10% dextrose concentration and gradually increase to hypertonicity greater than 12.5% dextrose, if needed.
• If flow rate lags behind ordered rate, don't try to catch up by increasing rate beyond original order.
• Monitor electrolyte, glucose, and BUN levels and renal and liver function test results. Check calcium level frequently. If glycosuria occurs, expect to give insulin.
• Monitor for extraordinary electrolyte losses that may occur during NG suction, vomiting, or drainage from GI fistula.
• Monitor patient for signs of fluid overload.
• Check infusion site frequently. Change peripheral I.V. site every 48 hours or per facility policy to prevent irritation and infection.
• To guide dosage of dextrose and insulin, if needed, check blood glucose level every 6 hours.
• Replace all I.V. equipment (I.V. lines, filter, and bottle) every 24 hours.
• Observe infusion site for signs of infection, drainage, edema, and extravasation. Check for fever or other possible signs of infection or hypersensitivity.
• Use TPN line solely for providing nutrition, not for collecting blood samples, transfusing blood, or giving drugs.

Reactions may be *common,* uncommon, **life-threatening,** or COMMON AND LIFE-THREATENING.

- Essential fatty acid deficiency may result from long-term fat-free I.V. feedings. Fat emulsion (500 ml) weekly may be needed.
- If TPN must be interrupted, give D_5W or $D_{10}W$ by peripheral vein to prevent rebound hypoglycemia.
- Provide frequent, meticulous mouth care to prevent parotitis.
- Give 10 mg of phytonadione weekly to prevent vitamin K deficiency.
- Monitor intake, output, weight, and pattern as well as caloric intake for significant changes.

PATIENT TEACHING
- Explain to patient and family the use and administration of amino acids. Encourage them to ask questions.
- Tell patient to report adverse reactions promptly.
- Tell patient receiving TPN that he may imagine taste or smell of food. Explain that these sensations are common, and suggest some distracting activity during mealtimes.
- Encourage patient to take special care with oral hygiene. Advise him to use a soft toothbrush and fluoride toothpaste and floss teeth daily.
- Inform patient that fewer bowel movements occur while receiving TPN.

aminocaproic acid
Amicar*

Pharmacologic class: carboxylic acid derivative
Therapeutic class: fibrinolysis inhibitor
Pregnancy risk category: C
pH: 6 to 7.6

INDICATIONS & DOSAGES
➤ **Life-threatening hemorrhage caused by systemic hyperfibrinolysis linked to complications of cardiac** surgery and portacaval shunt; lung, prostate, cervical, or stomach cancer; abruptio placentae; hematologic disorders such as aplastic anemia; and urinary fibrinolysis caused by severe trauma, shock, or anoxia—
Adults: Initially, 4 to 5 g I.V., then 1 to 1.25 g hourly. Or, initially, 4 to 5 g, then continuous infusion of 1 g/hour for about 8 hours to maintain drug level of 130 mcg/ml. Maximum dose, 30 g/day.
Children ◆: 100 mg/kg or 3 g/m² body surface area I.V. during first hour, then continuous infusion of 33 mg/kg/hour or 1 g/m²/hour. Maximum dose is 18 g/m²/day.

ADMINISTRATION
Direct injection: Not recommended.
Intermittent infusion: Not recommended.
Continuous infusion: Slowly infuse 4 to 5 g of diluted drug during first hour. Then infuse 1 g/hour to maintain level of 130 mcg/ml.

PREPARATION & STORAGE
Available in 250 mg/ml solutions containing 5 g (20 ml) with benzyl alcohol. Place 4 to 5 g in 250 ml of diluent and 1 to 1.25 g in 50 ml of diluent. Acceptable diluents include normal saline solution, D_5W, Ringer's solution, or sterile water for injection; sterile water for injection produces a hypo-osmolar solution. Don't use sterile water for injection when patient has subarachnoid hemorrhage. Store at 59° to 86° F (15° to 30° C); avoid freezing.

Incompatibilities
Fructose solution.

CONTRAINDICATIONS & CAUTIONS
- Contraindicated in patients with active intravascular clotting linked to possible fibrinolysis and bleeding as a primary disorder.

• Contraindicated in those with DIC, unless it's used with heparin. Otherwise, drug could cause potentially fatal thrombi.

• Use cautiously in those with upper urinary tract bleeding because glomerular capillary thrombosis or clots in the renal pelvis and ureter could cause intrarenal obstruction; in those with renal disorders because drug may accumulate and cause renal damage; and in those with hepatic disease because the cause of bleeding may be more difficult to diagnose.

• Use cautiously in those with cardiac disorders because of possible hypotension and bradycardia and in those predisposed to thrombosis.

ADVERSE REACTIONS

CNS: confusion, *seizures,* delirium, dizziness, *CVA,* syncope, headache, malaise, fever.
CV: *arrhythmias with rapid I.V. infusion, bradycardia,* hypotension, ischemia, thrombosis, thrombophlebitis, edema.
EENT: conjunctival injection, nasal congestion, tinnitus, watery eyes.
GI: abdominal pain, diarrhea, nausea, vomiting.
GU: *reversible acute renal failure,* prolonged menstruation with cramping.
Metabolic: hyperkalemia.
Musculoskeletal: muscle weakness, myalgia, myopathy, *rhabdomyolysis.*
Respiratory: dyspnea, *pulmonary embolism.*
Skin: pruritus, rash.

INTERACTIONS

Drug-drug. *Estrogens, hormonal contraceptives containing estrogen:* Causes hypercoagulability, resulting from increased clotting factors. Monitor patient for signs and symptoms of blood clots, and monitor coagulation study results.

EFFECTS ON LAB TEST RESULTS

• May increase BUN, creatinine, potassium, CK, AST, and ALT levels.

ACTION

Inhibits fibrinolysis—and thus clot dissolution—by inhibiting plasminogen activator substances and, to a lesser degree, by blocking antiplasmin activity.

PHARMACOKINETICS

Drug peak levels vary.
Distribution: Throughout intravascular and extravascular compartments. Drug readily penetrates RBCs and tissues and probably crosses the placental barrier. Drug isn't bound to plasma proteins. It's unknown if drug appears in breast milk.
Metabolism: Mechanism unknown; major portion not metabolized.
Excretion: In urine by glomerular filtration and reabsorption within 12 hours, largely unchanged with 11% excreted as the metabolite adipic acid.

CLINICAL CONSIDERATIONS

• *Alert:* Don't confuse Amikin (amikacin) with Amicar.
• *Alert:* Rapid infusion may induce hypotension and bradycardia.
• Monitor patient for muscle weakness. Rhabdomyolysis has occurred with prolonged use.
• Drug is sometimes helpful as an adjunct in treating hemophilia.
• Drug is also used as antidote for alteplase, streptokinase, or urokinase, but it isn't beneficial in treating thrombocytopenia.
• Monitor coagulation study results, heart rhythm, and blood pressure. Tell prescriber immediately if any change occurs.
• Guard against thrombophlebitis by using proper technique for needle insertion and positioning.

PATIENT TEACHING
• Explain to patient and family the use and administration of drug.
• Tell patient to report adverse reactions promptly.

aminophylline*

Pharmacologic class: xanthine derivative
Therapeutic class: bronchodilator
Pregnancy risk category: C
pH: 8.6 to 9

INDICATIONS & DOSAGES
➤ **Acute bronchial asthma and reversible bronchospasm caused by chronic bronchitis and emphysema—**
Adults not receiving theophylline: Initially, 6 mg/kg I.V., followed by maintenance doses; for nonsmoking adults, 0.7 mg/kg/hour for first 12 hours, then 0.5 mg/kg/hour for next 12 hours; for geriatric patients and those with cor pulmonale, 0.6 mg/kg/hour for first 12 hours, then 0.3 mg/kg/hour for next 12 hours; for patients with heart failure or liver failure, 0.5 mg/kg/hour for first 12 hours, then 0.1 to 0.2 mg/kg/hour for next 12 hours.
Children not receiving theophylline: Initially, 6 mg/kg I.V., followed by maintenance doses; for children ages 6 months to 9 years, 1.2 mg/kg/hour for first 12 hours, then 1 mg/kg/hour for next 12 hours; for children ages 9 to 16, 1 mg/kg/hour for first 12 hours, then 0.8 mg/kg/hour for next 12 hours.
Adults and children receiving theophylline: Dosage form, amount, time, and administration rate of last theophylline dose determine first dose. Ideally, first dose should be postponed until theophylline level is obtained. For patients with sufficient respiratory distress, you may give a loading dose of 2.5 mg/kg I.V.

Adjust-a-dose: Expect to reduce dosage in neonates, geriatric patients, and those with COPD, active influenza, or cardiac, renal, or hepatic dysfunction because of decreased theophylline clearance.
➤ **Cystic fibrosis ♦ —**
Infants: 10 to 12 mg/kg I.V. daily for maintenance dosing.

ADMINISTRATION
• *Alert: Direct injection:* Not commonly used. Give undiluted loading dose (25 mg/ml) very slowly, not exceeding 25 mg/minute. Don't give through a central venous catheter. Rapid injection can be fatal.
Intermittent infusion: Not recommended.
Continuous infusion: For maintenance therapy, give desired dose in a large volume (500 to 1,000 ml) of compatible solution. Adjust infusion rate to deliver prescribed amount each hour.

PREPARATION & STORAGE
Available as a 25-mg/ml solution in 10-ml (250-mg) and 20-ml (500-mg) ampules, vials, and syringes. Syringes may contain benzyl alcohol.
    Drug is compatible with most common I.V. solutions such as D_5W in normal saline solution.
    Store containers at room temperature and protect from freezing and light. Inspect for precipitate and discoloration before use.

Incompatibilities
Amikacin, amiodarone, ascorbic acid, bleomycin, cephapirin, chlorpromazine, ciprofloxacin, clindamycin phosphate, codeine phosphate, corticotropin, dimenhydrinate, dobutamine, doxapram, doxorubicin, epinephrine hydrochloride, fat emulsion 10%, fructose 10% in normal saline, hydralazine, hydroxyzine hydrochloride, invert sugar 10% in normal saline injection, invert sugar 10% in water,

levorphanol, meperidine, methadone, methylprednisolone sodium succinate, morphine, nafcillin, norepinephrine, ondansetron, papaverine, penicillin G potassium, pentazocine lactate, phenobarbital sodium, phenytoin sodium, procaine, prochlorperazine edisylate, promazine, promethazine hydrochloride, regular insulin, vancomycin, verapamil hydrochloride, vitamin B complex with C.

CONTRAINDICATIONS & CAUTIONS
• Contraindicated in patients hypersensitive to theophylline, caffeine, theobromine, and other xanthine compounds.
• Use cautiously in patients with severe cardiac disease, severe hypoxemia, hypertension, hyperthyroidism, peptic ulcer, diabetes mellitus, acute MI, or heart failure because drug may exacerbate symptoms; also use cautiously in those with cor pulmonale, prolonged fever, or febrile viral respiratory infections because these conditions prolong theophylline's half-life.
• Use cautiously in neonates, geriatric patients, and those with liver disease because of increased risk of toxic reaction; also use cautiously in those with enlarged prostate because of increased risk of urine retention.

ADVERSE REACTIONS
CNS: dizziness, *generalized tonic-clonic seizures,* irritability, reflex hyperexcitability, restlessness, syncope, light-headedness.
CV: *cardiac arrest, circulatory collapse,* hypotension, *ventricular fibrillation, arrhythmias, bradycardia,* palpitations, precordial pain, *tachycardia,* flushing.
EENT: tinnitus.
GI: *nausea, vomiting,* diarrhea, epigastric pain, hematemesis.
Metabolic: hyperglycemia, SIADH, severe dehydration.

Musculoskeletal: muscle twitching.
Respiratory: *tachypnea.*

INTERACTIONS
Drug-drug. *High-dose allopurinol, cimetidine, corticosteroids, diltiazem, erythromycin or other macrolides, felodipine, fluoroquinolones, hormonal contraceptives, mexiletine, propranolol, thiabendazole, verapamil:* Increases aminophylline concentrations. Monitor patient for toxicity.
Barbiturates, ketoconazole, phenytoin, rifampin: Decreases effectiveness of aminophylline. Monitor patient for therapeutic effect.
Beta blockers: Increases aminophylline level and risk of arrhythmias. Monitor patient for clinical effect and monitor ECG.
CNS stimulants, ephedrine: Increases risk of CNS adverse effects. Monitor patient closely.
Lithium: Increases lithium excretion. Adjust lithium dosage.
Warfarin: Increases risk of bleeding. Monitor PT and INR.
Drug-food. *Caffeine:* Increases risk of CNS adverse effects. Discourage use together.
Drug-lifestyle. *Smoking:* Increases elimination of drug, increasing dose requirements. Monitor drug levels and therapeutic response.

EFFECTS ON LAB TEST RESULTS
• May increase glucose and free fatty acid levels.

ACTION
Either acts as an adenosine receptor antagonist or inhibits phosphodiesterase, the enzyme that degrades cAMP. This action alters intracellular calcium levels, relaxing bronchial smooth muscles and pulmonary vessels. Theophylline and aminophylline also cause coronary vasodilation, diuresis, and cardiac, cerebral, and skeletal muscle stimula-

---

Reactions may be *common,* uncommon, *life-threatening,* or **COMMON AND LIFE-THREATENING.**

tion; theophylline also increases medullary sensitivity to carbon dioxide.

PHARMACOKINETICS
Onset, upon completion of infusion; duration, varies with age, sex, and activities.

Distribution: Rapidly dispersed throughout extracellular fluids and body tissues. Drug crosses the placenta and partially penetrates RBCs. Drug also appears in breast milk in levels about 70% of normal levels.

Metabolism: In liver.

Excretion: Drug and metabolites are mainly excreted in the urine with small amounts removed unchanged in the feces. Renal clearance only contributes 8% to 12% of the overall plasma clearance of drug; rest is caused by hepatic metabolism. Half-life, 3 to 12 hours in nonsmoking asthmatic adults; 1½ to 9½ hours in children.

CLINICAL CONSIDERATIONS
• Base dosage on lean body weight and theophylline level. Monitor trough level to manage regimen; monitor peak levels to assess for toxic reaction. Optimum therapeutic levels are 10 to 20 mcg/ml.
• I.V. administration can cause vein irritation and burning. Dilute drug with compatible solution, if needed.
• *Alert:* When interpreting orders, don't confuse aminophylline with theophylline. Aminophylline is about 79% theophylline.

PATIENT TEACHING
• Explain to patient and family the use and administration of drug.
• Tell patient to report adverse reactions promptly.
• Warn geriatric patient that dizziness, a common adverse reaction, may occur at the start of therapy.

amiodarone hydrochloride
Cordarone*

Pharmacologic class: benzofuran derivative
Therapeutic class: ventricular and supraventricular antiarrhythmic, group III antiarrhythmic
Pregnancy risk category: D
pH: 4.1

INDICATIONS & DOSAGES
➤ **To treat and prevent frequently recurring ventricular fibrillation VF) and hemodynamically unstable ventricular tachycardia (VT) in patients unresponsive to other therapy; in patients with VF or VT who can't take oral amiodarone—**
Adults: Initially, rapid loading infusion of 150 mg I.V. given over first 10 minutes (15 mg/minute), then a slow loading phase of 1 mg/minute over 6 hours for a total of 360 mg, followed by a maintenance phase of 0.5 mg/minute for 18 hours for a total of 540 mg. After the first 24 hours, continue the maintenance infusion of 0.5 mg/minute; may be increased to control arrhythmia. Experience using I.V. amiodarone for longer than 3 weeks is limited.

ADMINISTRATION
Direct injection: Give initial bolus of 15 mg/kg over 10 minutes; must be diluted in 100 ml of D_5W.
Intermittent infusion: Not recommended.
Continuous infusion: Must give by volumetric infusion pump. Use central venous catheter when possible. Use an in-line filter.

PREPARATION & STORAGE

Available in 3-ml ampules at a concentration of 50 mg/ml. Store at room temperature and protect from light.

I.V. amiodarone must be diluted before use. When possible, give amiodarone via a central venous catheter. For rapid loading dose, dilute 150 mg of drug in 100 ml D_5W; for maintenance infusion, final concentrations can range from 1 to 6 mg/ml. However, for infusions longer than 1 hour in duration, don't exceed a 2 mg/ml concentration unless a central venous catheter is used. Infusions exceeding 2 hours must be given in glass or polyolefin bottles containing D_5W.

Incompatibilities

Aminophylline, cefazolin sodium, heparin sodium, sodium bicarbonate.

CONTRAINDICATIONS & CAUTIONS

• Contraindicated in patients hypersensitive to drug or severe sinus bradycardia or second- or third-degree AV block.

• Use cautiously in those with preexisting pulmonary disease and in geriatric patients because the cardiopulmonary effects of drug can be fatal.

• To minimize risk, use lowest effective dose. Pediatric dosage isn't established.

• Closely monitor patient during loading phase.

• Drug may leach out plasticizers such as DEHP, adversely affecting male reproductive tract development in fetuses, infants, and toddlers.

• Drug contains benzyl alcohol, which has caused "gasping syndrome" in neonates (younger than 1 month old). Symptoms include sudden onset of gasping respiration, hypotension, bradycardia, and cardiovascular collapse.

ADVERSE REACTIONS

CNS: fever.

CV: HYPOTENSION, *bradycardia, heart failure, cardiac arrest, ventricular tachycardia, AV block, cardiogenic shock,* edema.
GI: nausea, vomiting, diarrhea.
Hematologic: *thrombocytopenia.*
Hepatic: *hepatic dysfunction.*

INTERACTIONS

Drug-drug. *Amphotericin B in systemic form, corticosteroids:* Enhances toxic reactions in patients with hypokalemia caused by these drugs. Monitor potassium level, and monitor patient for toxicity.
Anticoagulants: Increases PT and INR, which may last for months. Monitor PT and INR.
Beta blockers, calcium channel blockers: Potentiates AV block, bradycardia, sinus arrest. Monitor ECG and vital signs.
Cimetidine, indinavir: Increases amiodarone levels. Monitor patient for toxicity.
Digoxin, flecainide, phenytoin, procainamide, quinidine: Increases levels of these drugs. Monitor patient closely. Decrease dosages of these drugs.
Disopyramide: Prolongs QT interval and, rarely, causes torsades de pointes. Monitor ECG.
Potassium-wasting diuretics: Increases risk of arrhythmias linked to hypokalemia. Monitor potassium level and ECG.
Drug-herb. *Pennyroyal:* May change the rate at which toxic metabolites of pennyroyal form. Discourage use together.
St. John's wort: May decrease amiodarone levels. Discourage use together.

EFFECTS ON LAB TEST RESULTS

• May increase ALT, AST, alkaline phosphatase, and GGT levels.
• May increase PT, INR, and QT interval. May decrease platelet count and uptake of sodium iodide ^{131}I and sodi-

um pertechnetate ^{99m}Tc in thyroid imaging tests.

ACTION
Prolongs the refractory period and repolarization. Also antagonizes alpha and beta responses to catecholamine stimulation.

PHARMACOKINETICS
Onset, minutes to hours; duration, about 6 hours when given over 30 to 60 minutes.
Distribution: Rapid and widespread throughout body tissues, with 96% bound to plasma proteins. Crosses blood-brain and placental barriers. Appears in breast milk.
Metabolism: Extensively metabolized, probably in liver and possibly in intestinal lumen.
Excretion: Mainly unchanged in feces. The metabolite N-desethylamiodarone is eliminated through bile. Half-life averages 25 days after single dose, longer after multiple doses.

CLINICAL CONSIDERATIONS
• Obtain baseline ophthalmologic data. Monitor patient for dry eyes, halo vision, and photophobia. Recommend use of sunscreen or sunglasses.
• Obtain baseline pulmonary function tests. Assess respiratory system for pulmonary toxicity.
• Monitor ECG status continuously for AV block, bradycardia, paradoxical arrhythmias, and prolonged QT intervals.
• Monitor thyroid and liver enzyme levels.
• If overdose occurs, provide symptomatic and supportive care. Monitor ECG and blood pressure. To treat bradycardia, give an I.V. beta blocker such as isoproterenol or assist with transvenous pacemaker insertion. To correct hypotension, infuse I.V. fluids and place patient in Trendelenburg's position. To improve tissue perfusion, give an I.V. vasopressor or an inotropic

drug such as norepinephrine or dopamine. Hemodialysis and peritoneal dialysis don't help remove drug.

PATIENT TEACHING
• Explain to patient and family the use and administration of drug.
• Tell patient to report adverse reactions promptly.
• Inform patient that drug's adverse effects are more prevalent at high doses but are generally reversible when therapy is stopped.

ammonium chloride

Pharmacologic class: acid-forming salt
Therapeutic class: systemic acidifier, expectorant
Pregnancy risk category: C
pH: 4 to 6

INDICATIONS & DOSAGES
➤ **Metabolic alkalosis caused by chloride loss from vomiting, gastric suction, pyloric stenosis, or gastric fistula drainage; diuretic-induced chloride depletion—**
Adults: Estimated in milliequivalents, I.V. dosage reflects severity of alkalosis, amount of chloride deficit, and patient tolerance. Estimate the patient's fluid volume by multiplying 20% of his body weight in kg by his chloride level. For example, if the patient weighs 70 kg (154 lb) and has a chloride level of 94 mEq/ml, the equation is as follows: 14 kg $\times$ 94 mEq/ml = 1,316 mEq. (1 L of 2.14% solution provides 400 mEq of ammonium and chloride ions.)

ADMINISTRATION
Direct injection: Not recommended.
Intermittent infusion: Not recommended.

Continuous infusion: To avoid pain, toxic effects, and local irritation, infuse diluted solution at no more than 5 ml/minute. Infuse the 2.14% solution at 0.9 to 1.3 ml/minute, but always less than 2 ml/minute. Start infusion at half the calculated rate to determine patient tolerance.

PREPARATION & STORAGE
Available as 26.75% (5 mEq/ml) in 20 ml (100 mEq) vials.

Prepare diluted solution by adding one or two vials equaling 100 or 200 mEq of aqueous ammonium chloride to 500 or 1,000 ml of normal saline for injection.

Ammonium chloride for injection concentrate should be stored at 40° C or less; avoid freezing. Solution may crystallize if stored at low temperature. Crystals dissolve when solution is placed in warm water.

Incompatibilities
Alkalies and their carbonates, strong oxidizing drugs such as potassium chloride, and dimenhydrinate, levorphanol, and methadone.

CONTRAINDICATIONS & CAUTIONS
• Contraindicated in patients hypersensitive to drug, severe hepatic disease, hepatic coma, or renal impairment.
• Contraindicated in those with primary respiratory acidosis because of risk of developing systemic acidosis.
• Use cautiously in those with pulmonary insufficiency and edema because of possible changes in arterial blood gas levels.

ADVERSE REACTIONS
CNS: *coma, tonic seizures,* excitement, headache, confusion, drowsiness.
CV: *arrhythmias, bradycardia.*
GI: nausea, thirst, anorexia.
GU: glycosuria.

Metabolic: hypokalemia, hyponatremia, hyperglycemia.
Musculoskeletal: muscle twitching.
Respiratory: Kussmaul's respirations, hyperventilation.
Skin: pain and irritation at injection site (with rapid administration), rash.

INTERACTIONS
Drug-drug. *Antidepressants, ephedrine, methadone, salicylates:* Increases urine excretion. Monitor patient for clinical effects.
Spironolactone: Decreases urine excretion. Monitor patient for toxicity.

EFFECTS ON LAB TEST RESULTS
• May increase chloride level. May decrease potassium and sodium levels.

ACTION
Increases free hydrogen ions, which then react with bicarbonate ions to form water and carbon dioxide. Chloride anions then combine with bases in extracellular fluid, displacing bicarbonate and causing acidosis. After 1 to 3 days, the kidneys increase ammonium production and chloride ion excretion to compensate for sodium loss.

PHARMACOKINETICS
Onset, 15 to 60 minutes; duration, 1 to 3 days.
Distribution: Throughout body in circulating plasma. Unknown if drug crosses placental barrier or appears in breast milk.
Metabolism: In liver, where ammonium ions are metabolized to urea and hydrochloric acid.
Excretion: In urine.

CLINICAL CONSIDERATIONS
• Osmolarity is 10 mOsm/ml.
• Check for pain at infusion site and adjust rate of infusion, if needed.
• To prevent acidosis, check electrolyte levels during therapy.

Reactions may be *common*, uncommon, *life-threatening*, or COMMON AND LIFE-THREATENING.

• Monitor input and output, edema, weight, and urine pH during therapy. Expect diuresis for the first 2 days.
• Assess respiratory pattern frequently.
• If overdose occurs, stop the drug and give potassium chloride I.V. or sodium bicarbonate I.V. for acidosis. Signs and symptoms of overdose include arrhythmias, asterixis, bradycardia, coma, irregular breathing, local or generalized twitching, pallor, sweating, tonic seizures, and vomiting.

PATIENT TEACHING
• Explain to patient and family the use and administration of drug.
• Tell patient to report adverse reactions, including discomfort at I.V. site, promptly.

amobarbital sodium
Amytal

Pharmacologic class: barbiturate
Therapeutic class: sedative-hypnotic, anticonvulsant
Pregnancy risk category: D
Controlled substance schedule: II
pH: 9.6 to 10.4

INDICATIONS & DOSAGES
➤ **Agitation in psychoses, insomnia, seizures, and status epilepticus—**
Adults and children older than age 6: 65 to 500 mg, not to exceed 1 g. I.V. route typically used only in emergencies; dosage varies by patient.

ADMINISTRATION
Direct injection: Don't exceed rate of 100 mg/minute. Extravasation can cause necrosis.
Intermittent infusion: Not recommended.
Continuous infusion: Not recommended.

PREPARATION & STORAGE
To prepare the standard 100-mg/ml (10%) injection, dissolve 250 or 500 mg of sterile powder in 2.5 or 5 ml, respectively, of sterile water for injection. Rotate the ampule to facilitate mixing; don't shake it. If solution becomes cloudy after 5 minutes, discard; drug breaks down in solution or on exposure to air. Drug also precipitates if diluent pH is 9.2 or less. Give within 30 minutes of reconstitution.

Incompatibilities
Cefazolin, chlorpromazine, cimetidine, clindamycin phosphate, droperidol, isoproterenol hydrochloride, methyldopate, norepinephrine, penicillin G, pentazocine lactate, succinylcholine, thiamine.

CONTRAINDICATIONS & CAUTIONS
• Contraindicated in those with liver impairment from cirrhosis, drug or alcohol abuse, or lengthy exposure to hepatic carcinogens.
• Contraindicated in those with history of acute intermittent or variegate porphyria because of possible aggravation of symptoms.
• Use cautiously in those with history of drug abuse.
• Use cautiously in geriatric or debilitated patients because of possible excitement, depression, or confusion; in those with renal impairment, uremia, or shock because of prolonged or intensified hypnotic effects; in those with cardiac disease because of adverse circulatory effects, especially with overly rapid administration; in those with pulmonary disease because of possible ventilatory depression; and in those with acute or chronic pain because of induced paradoxical reaction.
• Use cautiously in asthmatic patients because risk of hypersensitivity reaction is increased; in those with hyperthyroidism or hyperkinesis because symptoms may be exacerbated; in

those with borderline hyperadrenalism because the effect of exogenous hydrocortisone and endogenous cortisol may be reduced; and in those with hypertension because drug may cause hypotension.

ADVERSE REACTIONS

CNS: *drowsiness, lethargy, CNS depression,* agitation, ataxia, confusion, nightmares, physical dependence, syncope.
CV: *cardiac arrest, circulatory collapse,* hypotension, edema.
GI: nausea, vomiting, diarrhea, constipation, epigastric pain.
Musculoskeletal: hyperkinesia.
Respiratory: *bronchospasm, respiratory arrest, apnea,* hypoventilation.
Skin: rash, *severe subcutaneous tissue necrosis;* urticaria; pain, irritation, and sterile abscess at injection site.

INTERACTIONS

Drug-drug. *Anticonvulsants:* Worsens lethargy and motor disturbances. Monitor patient for these effects.
Corticosteroids, doxycycline, estrogens, hormonal contraceptives, metronidazole, mexiletine, oral anticoagulants, tricyclic antidepressants: Reduces effectiveness of these drugs. Monitor therapeutic response.
Haloperidol, maprotiline, primidone: May change frequency or pattern of epileptiform seizures. Monitor patient closely. Avoid using together.
Hypnotics, MAO inhibitors, tranquilizers, other CNS depressants: Potentiates hypnotic and sedative effects. Monitor patient for increased CNS depression.
Ketamine: Increases risk of hypotension and respiratory depression. Monitor respiratory rate and vital signs.
Drug-lifestyle. *Alcohol use:* Causes CNS depression. Discourage use together.

EFFECTS ON LAB TEST RESULTS

● May cause false-positive phentolamine test results.

ACTION

Depresses sensory cortex, motor activity, and cerebellar function to produce drowsiness, sedation, and hypnosis.

PHARMACOKINETICS

Onset, 1 to 5 minutes; duration, 3 to 6 hours, depending on dose and distribution rate.
Distribution: Rapidly dispersed throughout body tissues, with highest level in liver and brain. Drug crosses the placental barrier and appears in breast milk.
Metabolism: Hepatic microsomal enzymes slowly metabolize drug to an inactive metabolite.
Excretion: In urine and, less commonly, in feces. Inactive metabolites are excreted as conjugates of glucuronic acid. After I.V. bolus, plasma level follows biphasic decline: first phase of half-life, about 40 minutes; second phase, 20 to 25 hours.

CLINICAL CONSIDERATIONS

● *Alert:* Give drug only to hospitalized patients under close observation and respiratory monitoring. Keep resuscitation equipment available.
● Barbiturates potentiate opioid effect. If given during labor, reduce opioid dose to lessen risk of neonatal respiratory depression.
● Don't give drug within 24 hours of liver function tests because it may cause elevated readings.
● Monitor PT and INR carefully when patient starts or ends anticoagulant therapy. Anticoagulant dose may need to be adjusted.
● When patient is receiving hypnotic dose, remove cigarettes, help him walk, and raise bed rails, especially if he's elderly.

• Signs and symptoms of drug overdose include clammy skin, coma, cyanosis, hypotension, and pupillary constriction.
• If overdose occurs, maintain airway and, if needed, provide ventilatory support. Monitor vital signs and fluid balance. For shock, give fluids and follow standard care measures; for hypotension, give vasopressors. In patients with normal renal function, forced diuresis may help remove drug; hemodialysis or hemoperfusion may enhance removal.

PATIENT TEACHING
• Dependence and severe withdrawal symptoms may follow long-term therapy. When stopping drug after prolonged use, withdraw over 5 to 6 days to prevent withdrawal symptoms and rebound rapid eye movement (REM) sleep.
• Morning hangover commonly occurs with hypnotic dose because of disrupted REM sleep.

amphotericin B
Amphocin, Fungizone

Pharmacologic class: polyene macrolide
Therapeutic class: antifungal
Pregnancy risk category: B
pH: 5.7

INDICATIONS & DOSAGES
➤ **Systemic fungal infections, such as aspergillosis, blastomycosis, candidiasis, coccidioidomycosis, cryptococcosis, histoplasmosis, and phycomycosis**—
Adults and children: Initially, 0.25 mg/kg I.V. over 6 hours; if tolerated, may be infused over 3 to 4 hours. A test dose of 1 mg in 20 ml of D_5W is infused over 20 to 30 minutes. Monitor

patient's vital signs q 30 minutes for 4 hours. Dosage is increased gradually, depending on patient tolerance and infection severity, to a maximum of 1 mg/kg/day. Dosage must never exceed 1.5 mg/kg/day. If stopped for 1 week or more, therapy resumes with first dose and gradually increases, as described. Therapy may last for months.
➤ **To prevent fungal infection in neutropenic cancer patients or patients undergoing bone marrow transplantation ◆**—
Adults: 0.1 mg/kg/day I.V. infusion.
➤ **Paracoccidioidomycosis ◆**—
Adults: 0.4 to 0.5 mg/kg/day slow I.V. infusion for 4 to 12 weeks.
➤ **Mucocutaneous leishmaniasis caused by *L. braziliensis;* American cutaneous leishmaniasis caused by *Leishmania braziliensis* or *L. mexicana* ◆**—
Adults, children: Initially, 0.25 to 0.5 mg/kg/day I.V. infusion; gradually increase to 0.5 to 1 mg/kg/day, and then give on alternate days. Continue therapy for 3 to 12 weeks with a total dose of 1 to 3 g.

ADMINISTRATION
Direct injection: Not recommended.
Intermittent infusion: Not recommended.
Continuous infusion: Give 500 ml of diluted solution over 3 to 6 hours. Inline filter should have a pore diameter exceeding 1 micron. Flush line with D_5W rather than normal saline.

PREPARATION & STORAGE
For 50-mg vial, reconstitute with 10 ml of sterile, not bacteriostatic, water for injection. Shake until solution clears. Further dilute in 500 ml of D_5W with a pH above 4.2. Final concentration will be 0.1 mg/ml.
    Store concentrate at room temperature for 24 hours or refrigerate for 1

week. When diluted, use drug promptly. Protect from light until ready to hang.

Incompatibilities
Amikacin, calcium chloride, chlorpromazine, cimetidine, diphenhydramine, edetate calcium disodium, gentamicin, kanamycin, lactated Ringer's injection, melphalan, methyldopa, normal saline solution, paclitaxel, penicillin G potassium, penicillin G sodium, polymyxin B, potassium chloride, prochlorperazine mesylate, streptomycin, verapamil.

CONTRAINDICATIONS & CAUTIONS
• Contraindicated in patients hypersensitive to drug, unless infection is life threatening and susceptible only to this drug.
• Use only in those with confirmed diagnosis of potentially fatal fungal infection.
• Use cautiously in patients with renal impairment.
• Closely supervise any patient receiving the drug.

ADVERSE REACTIONS
CNS: neurologic toxicity, *headache, malaise, fever, pain.*
CV: hypotension, thrombophlebitis at injection site, *cardiac arrest after rapid injection, ventricular fibrillation, shock.*
EENT: hearing loss.
GI: anorexia, nausea, vomiting, diarrhea, dyspepsia, cramping epigastric pain.
GU: *reduced renal function,* azotemia, hypokalemia, urine with low specific gravity, *renal tubular acidosis.*
Hematologic: normochromic normocytic anemia, *agranulocytosis, thrombocytopenia, leukopenia,* coagulation defects.
Hepatic: *acute liver failure.*
Metabolic: *hypomagnesemia,* hypokalemia, weight loss.

Musculoskeletal: muscle and joint pain.
Skin: rash, *pain at injection site.*
Other: shaking chills, *anaphylactic reaction.*

INTERACTIONS
Drug-drug. *Amiodarone, cardiac glycosides:* Increases toxicity in patients with amphotericin-induced hypokalemia. Monitor potassium and drug levels.
Antineoplastics, cyclosporine, nephrotoxic antibiotics, potassium-wasting diuretics: Increases risk of nephrotoxicity. Monitor renal function test results.
Carbonic anhydrase inhibitors, corticosteroids, corticotropin, potassium-wasting diuretics: Causes severe hypokalemia. Monitor potassium level.
Flucytosine: May increase antifungal effects. Monitor therapeutic response.
Nondepolarizing neuromuscular blockers: Enhances effects of these drugs. Monitor patient closely.
Drug-herb. *Gossypol:* Increases risk of renal toxicity. Discourage use together.

EFFECTS ON LAB TEST RESULTS
• May increase urine urea, uric acid, BUN, creatinine, alkaline phosphatase, ALT, AST, GGT, LDH, and bilirubin levels. May decrease potassium and magnesium levels. May increase or decrease glucose level.
• May decrease hemoglobin, hematocrit, and platelet and granulocyte counts. May increase or decrease WBC and eosinophil counts.

ACTION
Binds to sterols in fungal cell walls, changing cell permeability and allowing leakage of potassium and other cellular constituents.

PHARMACOKINETICS
Onset, rapid; peak, end of infusion.
Distribution: Penetrates well into inflamed pleural cavities, peritoneum, and joints; 90% to 95% bound to plasma proteins. Poorly distributed to aqueous humor, bone, brain, and pancreas; may cross the placental barrier.
Metabolism: Mechanism unknown.
Excretion: Eliminated slowly in urine, with 40% removed in 7 days; 2% to 5% of dose is excreted in a biologically active form. Initial phase half-life, 24 to 48 hours; second phase half-life, 15 days.

CLINICAL CONSIDERATIONS
• Adding 1,200 to 1,600 units of heparin to solution may reduce risk of thrombophlebitis.
• Assess I.V. site for signs of thrombophlebitis. Rotate I.V. sites regularly.
• Monitor vital signs every 30 minutes for 4 hours during initial therapy. Fever may appear 1 to 2 hours after start of infusion; it should subside within 4 hours after stopping drug.
• Antiemetics, antihistamines, antipyretics, and corticosteroids may be ordered to prevent adverse reactions.
• Giving meperidine before infusion of amphotericin B may decrease rigors.
• Don't use any diluent that contains a bacteriostatic agent, which can cause drug to precipitate.
• Monitor intake and output, reporting change in urine appearance or volume. If therapy is stopped at first sign of renal dysfunction, damage is usually reversible.
• Monitor potassium and magnesium levels and expect to give supplements if levels are low. Monitor hemoglobin and hematocrit for anemia.
• Obtain liver and kidney function studies two to three times weekly. If BUN level exceeds 40 mg/dl or creatinine level exceeds 3 mg/dl, drug may be stopped until kidney function improves.

Drug also may be stopped if alkaline phosphatase levels or bilirubin levels rise.
• Before sending the patient home with an I.V. line, fully evaluate him for reactions and make sure his condition is stable on the drug.

PATIENT TEACHING
• Explain to patient and family the use and administration of drug.
• Warn patient of possible discomfort at I.V. site and of other potential adverse reactions.
• Tell patient to report adverse reactions promptly, especially hypersensitivity reactions.
• Inform patient that therapy requires compliance and monitoring of his condition.

amphotericin B cholesteryl sulfate
Amphotec

Pharmacologic class: polyene macrolide
Therapeutic class: antifungal
Pregnancy risk category: B

INDICATIONS & DOSAGES
➤ **Invasive aspergillosis in patients whose renal impairment or toxicity precludes use of effective doses of amphotericin B deoxycholate or whose previous amphotericin B deoxycholate therapy has failed—**
Adults and children: 3 to 4 mg/kg/day I.V.; can increase to 6 mg/kg/day if patient shows no improvement or if fungal infection progresses.

Dilute in D_5W and give by continuous infusion at 1 mg/kg/hour. A test dose is advised when a new course of treatment is started; infuse a small amount of drug—10 ml of final preparation containing 1.6 to 8.3 mg of drug—over 15 to 30 minutes and monitor for next 30 minutes. Infusion time may be shortened to 2 hours or lengthened based on tolerance.

➤ **Invasive fungal infections caused by** *Candida* **or** *Cryptococcus* **in patients who can't tolerate or fail to respond to conventional amphotericin B** ♦ —
Adults: 3 to 6 mg/kg/day I.V infusion.
➤ **Visceral leishmaniasis** ♦ —
Adults: 2 mg/kg I.V. infusion once daily for 7 to 10 days.

ADMINISTRATION
Direct injection: Not recommended.
Intermittent infusion: Infuse over at least 2 hours. Don't mix with other drugs. If given through an existing I.V. line, flush line with D_5W before infusion or use a separate line.
Continuous infusion: Not recommended.

PREPARATION & STORAGE
Available in preservative-free 50-mg and 100-mg lyophilized powder vials. Store vials at room temperature. Reconstitute 50-mg vial with rapid addition of 10 ml of sterile water for injection and 100-mg vial with rapid addition of 20 ml of sterile water with a sterile syringe and 20G needle. Shake vial gently. Use only sterile water for injection as a diluent.

Reconstituted drug is clear or opalescent liquid and is stable for 24 hours if refrigerated. Discard partially used vials.

Dilute to a final concentration of about 0.6 mg/ml (range, 0.16 to 0.83 mg/ml) with D_5W only. Final product is stable for 24 hours refrigerated when diluted with D_5W. Don't give undiluted. Don't filter or use an in-line filter; don't freeze.

Incompatibilities
Bacteriostatic agents, electrolyte solutions, saline solutions.

CONTRAINDICATIONS & CAUTIONS
• Contraindicated in patients hypersensitive to any component of the drug, unless the benefits outweigh the risks.
• It's unknown if drug appears in breast milk. Because of the potential for serious adverse reactions in breast-feeding infants, prescriber should consider importance of drug to the mother and determine whether she should stop breast-feeding or stop drug treatment. Use in pregnant women only if anticipated benefits outweigh potential risks to the fetus.

ADVERSE REACTIONS
CNS: headache, confusion, abnormal thoughts, anxiety, agitation, somnolence, stupor, depression, hallucinations, dizziness, paresthesia, neuropathy, hypertonia, *seizures,* syncope, asthenia, *fever.*
CV: *hypotension, tachycardia,* chest pain, hypertension, *arrhythmias, heart failure, cardiac arrest, supraventricular tachycardia, hemorrhage, shock,* atrial fibrillation, *bradycardia,* phlebitis, ventricular extrasystoles, orthostatic hypotension, edema, peripheral edema.
EENT: eye hemorrhage, tinnitus, mucous membrane disorder.
GI: *nausea, vomiting,* melena, stomatitis, abdominal pain, anorexia, GI disorder, GI hemorrhage, hematemesis.
GU: *kidney failure,* hematuria, abnormal kidney function.
Hematologic: coagulation disorders, anemia, hypochromic anemia, leukocytosis, *thrombocytopenia, leukopenia.*
Hepatic: jaundice, *hepatic failure, bilirubinemia.*
Metabolic: *hypokalemia,* hypomagnesemia, hypocalcemia, hyperglycemia, hypophosphatemia, hyponatremia, hyperkalemia, hypervolemia.
Musculoskeletal: arthralgia, myalgia, back pain.

Respiratory: dyspnea, hypoxia, epistaxis, increased cough, lung or respiratory disorders, hemoptysis, hyperventilation, asthma, *apnea, pulmonary edema.*
Skin: sweating, skin disorder, reaction and pain at injection site, rash, pruritus.
Other: *chills,* facial edema, *sepsis,* infection, *allergic reaction, anaphylaxis.*

INTERACTIONS
No formal drug interaction studies have been done with amphotericin B cholesteryl sulfate. However, the following drugs are known to interact with amphotericin B:
Drug-drug. *Antineoplastics:* Enhances renal toxicity, bronchospasm, hypotension. Avoid using together.
Corticosteroids: Enhances potassium depletion. Monitor potassium level.
Cardiac glycosides: Enhances potassium excretion; increases risk of digitalis toxicity. Monitor potassium and digoxin levels.
Cyclosporine, tacrolimus: May increase creatinine level. Monitor renal function tests.
Flucytosine: Has synergistic effect, may increase toxicity of flucytosine. Monitor for drug toxicity.
Imidazoles, such as clotrimazole, ketoconazole, miconazole: Has antagonistic effects; significance undetermined. Monitor patient closely.
Nephrotoxic drugs, such as aminoglycosides, pentamidine: May enhance renal toxicity. Monitor renal function tests.
Skeletal muscle relaxants: Amphotericin B–induced hypokalemia may enhance curariform effects of skeletal muscle relaxants, such as tubocurarine. Monitor potassium level.

EFFECTS ON LAB TEST RESULTS
• May increase BUN, creatinine, alkaline phosphatase, ALT, AST, bilirubin, GGT, and LDH levels. May decrease calcium, phosphate, magnesium, and protein levels. May increase or decrease glucose, sodium, and potassium levels.
• May decrease hemoglobin, platelet count, and INR. May increase or decrease WBC count and PT.

ACTION
Binds to sterols in cell membranes to sensitive fungi, resulting in leakage of intracellular contents and causing cell death caused by changes in membrane permeability. Also binds to mammalian cell membranes, which is believed to account for human toxicity.

PHARMACOKINETICS
Onset, rapid; peak, end of infusion.
Distribution: Multicompartmental; steady-state volume increases with higher doses, possibly from uptake by tissues.
Metabolism: Unclear.
Excretion: Unclear; elimination half-life, 27 to 29 hours; increasing doses increase the elimination half-life. Dialysis doesn't remove drug.

CLINICAL CONSIDERATIONS
• To decrease the risk of acute infusion-related reactions, consider pretreating the patient with an antihistamine or a corticosteroid. If such a reaction occurs, reduce the rate of infusion and promptly give an antihistamine or a corticosteroid, as needed.
• Monitor vital signs every 30 minutes during initial therapy. Acute infusion-related reactions, such as fever, chills, hypotension, nausea, and tachycardia usually occur 1 to 3 hours after starting I.V. infusion. These reactions are usually most severe after the first dose and diminish with subsequent doses. If severe respiratory distress occurs, stop infusion immediately and don't treat further with drug.
• Monitor intake and output; report change in urine appearance or volume.

• Monitor renal and hepatic function test results and CBC, PT, and electrolyte—especially potassium, magnesium, and calcium—levels.

PATIENT TEACHING
• Instruct patient to report signs and symptoms of hypersensitivity immediately.
• Warn patient of possible discomfort at I.V. site and of adverse effects.

amphotericin B lipid complex
Abelcet

Pharmacologic class: polyene antibiotic
Therapeutic class: antifungal
Pregnancy risk category: B
pH: 5 to 7

INDICATIONS & DOSAGES
➤ **Invasive fungal infections including** *Aspergillus fumigatus, Candida albicans, C. guillermondii, C. stellatoideae,* **and** *C. tropicalis, Cryptococcus* **species,** *Coccidioidomycosis* **species,** *Histoplasma* **species, and** *Blastomyces* **species in patients refractory to or intolerant of conventional amphotericin B therapy—**
Adults and children: 5 mg/kg daily as a single I.V. infusion. Give by continuous I.V. infusion at a rate of 2.5 mg/kg/hour.
➤ **Visceral leishmaniasis that failed to respond to or relapsed after treatment with an antimony compound** ◆ —
Adults: 1 to 3 mg/kg I.V. infusion once daily for 5 days.

ADMINISTRATION
Direct injection: Not recommended.
Intermittent infusion: Not recommended.

Continuous infusion: Don't use an inline filter. If infusing through an existing I.V. line, flush first with D_5W. Give at a rate of 2.5 mg/kg/hour. If infusion time exceeds 2 hours, shake bag every 2 hours to ensure that the contents are mixed.

PREPARATION & STORAGE
To prepare, shake the vial gently until yellow sediment is gone. Using aseptic technique, draw the calculated dose into one or more 20-ml syringes, using an 18G needle. More than one vial is needed. Attach a 5-micron filter needle to the syringe and inject the dose into an I.V. bag of D_5W. One filter needle can be used for up to four vials of drug. The volume of D_5W should be enough to yield a final concentration of 1 mg/ml. For pediatric patients and those with CV disease, the recommended final concentration is 2 mg/ml.

Shake the bag and check the contents for any foreign material. Discard any unused drug because it doesn't contain a preservative.

Infusions are stable for up to 48 hours if refrigerated at 36° to 46° F (2° to 8° C) and up to 6 hours if kept at room temperature. Don't freeze.

Incompatibilities
Eectrolytes, other I.V. drugs, saline solutions.

CONTRAINDICATIONS & CAUTIONS
• Contraindicated in patients hypersensitive to amphotericin B or any of its components.
• Use cautiously in those with renal impairment.

ADVERSE REACTIONS
CNS: headache, pain, *fever.*
CV: chest pain, *cardiac arrest,* hypertension, hypotension.
GI: abdominal pain, diarrhea, *GI hemorrhage,* nausea, vomiting.
GU: *kidney failure.*

Hematologic: anemia, *leukopenia, thrombocytopenia.*
Hepatic: bilirubinemia.
Metabolic: hypokalemia.
Respiratory: dyspnea, respiratory disorder, *respiratory failure.*
Skin: rash.
Other: *chills,* infection, MULTIPLE ORGAN FAILURE, *sepsis.*

INTERACTIONS

Drug-drug. *Antineoplastics:* Increases risk of renal toxicity, bronchospasm, and hypotension. Monitor renal function, respiratory status, and vital signs closely.
Cardiac glycosides: Increases risk of digitalis toxicity caused by amphotericin B–induced hypokalemia. Monitor potassium and digoxin levels closely.
Corticosteroids, corticotropin: Enhances hypokalemia, which may lead to cardiac toxicity. Monitor electrolyte levels and cardiac function.
Cyclosporine: Increases renal toxicity. Monitor renal function test results.
Flucytosine: Increases risk of flucytosine toxicity caused by increased cellular uptake or impaired renal excretion. Use together cautiously and monitor patient for toxicity.
Imidazoles, such as clotrimazole, itraconazole, ketoconazole, miconazole: Decreases efficacy of amphotericin B because ergosterol synthesis is inhibited. Significance is unknown. Monitor patient closely.
Leukocyte transfusions: Causes acute pulmonary toxicity. Avoid using together.
Nephrotoxic drugs, such as aminoglycosides and pentamidine: Increases risk of renal toxicity. Use together cautiously. Monitor renal function closely.
Skeletal muscle relaxants: Enhances effects of skeletal muscle relaxants caused by amphotericin B–induced hypokalemia. Monitor potassium level closely.

Zidovudine: Increases myelotoxicity and nephrotoxicity. Monitor renal and hematologic function.

EFFECTS ON LAB TEST RESULTS
● May increase BUN, creatinine, alkaline phosphatase, ALT, AST, bilirubin, GGT, and LDH levels. May decrease potassium level.
● May decrease hemoglobin, hematocrit, and WBC and platelet counts.

ACTION
Active component, amphotericin B, binds to sterols in fungal cell membranes, resulting in enhanced cellular permeability and cell damage. Has fungistatic or fungicidal effects depending on fungal susceptibility.

PHARMACOKINETICS
Onset, unknown; peak, unknown; duration, unknown.
Distribution: Well distributed. The distribution volume increases with increasing dose. Amphotericin B lipid complex yields measurable amphotericin B levels in spleen, lung, liver, lymph nodes, kidney, heart, and brain.
Metabolism: Unknown.
Excretion: Although rapidly cleared from blood, drug has a terminal half-life of 173 hours, probably caused by slow elimination from tissues.

CLINICAL CONSIDERATIONS
● Premedication with acetaminophen, an antihistamine, and a corticosteroid may prevent or lessen the severity of infusion-related reactions, such as fever, chills, nausea, and vomiting, which occur 1 to 2 hours after the start of the infusion.
● Slowing the infusion rate may also decrease the incidence of infusion-related reactions. For infusions lasting longer than 2 hours, shake the I.V. bag every 2 hours to ensure an even suspension.

• If severe respiratory distress occurs, stop infusion. Drug shouldn't be reinstituted in this situation.

• During therapy, monitor liver function, CBC, and creatinine and electrolyte levels, especially magnesium and potassium levels.

• Base the need for dosage adjustment on the patient's overall status.

• Renal toxicity is more common at higher doses.

PATIENT TEACHING

• Inform patient that fever, chills, nausea, and vomiting may occur during the infusion but usually subside with subsequent doses.

• Instruct patient to report any redness or pain at the infusion site.

• Teach patient to recognize and report any symptoms of acute hypersensitivity, such as respiratory distress.

• Warn patient that therapy may take several months.

• Tell patient to expect frequent laboratory testing to monitor kidney and liver function.

amphotericin B liposomal
AmBisome

Pharmacologic class: polyene antibiotic
Therapeutic class: antifungal
Pregnancy risk category: B
pH: 5 to 6

INDICATIONS & DOSAGES

➤ **Empirical therapy for presumed fungal infection in febrile, neutropenic patients—**
Adults and children: 3 mg/kg I.V. infusion daily.

➤ **Systemic fungal infections caused by *Aspergillus, Candida,* or *Cryptococcus* species in patients unresponsive to amphotericin B deoxycholate** or in those for whom renal impairment or unacceptable toxicity precludes the use of amphotericin B deoxycholate—
Adults and children: 3 to 5 mg/kg I.V. infusion daily.

➤ **Visceral leishmaniasis in immunocompetent patients—**
Adults and children: 3 mg/kg I.V. infusion daily on days 1 to 5, 14, and 21. A repeat course of therapy may be beneficial if initial treatment fails.

➤ **Visceral leishmaniasis in immunocompromised patients—**
Adults and children: 4 mg/kg I.V. infusion daily on days 1 to 5, 10, 17, 24, 31, and 38. Further treatment is recommended if initial therapy fails or patient experiences a relapse.

➤ **Cryptococcal meningitis in HIV-infected patients—**
Adults and children: 6 mg/kg/day I.V. infusion over 2 hours. Infusion time may be reduced to 1 hour if well tolerated. Infusion time may be increased if discomfort occurs.

ADMINISTRATION

Direct injection: Not recommended.
Intermittent infusion: An existing I.V. line must be flushed with D_5W before drug is infused. If this isn't feasible, give drug through a separate line. Also, give drug using a controlled infusion device. Give over 120 minutes; may be reduced to 60 minutes if drug is well tolerated.
Continuous infusion: Not recommended.

PREPARATION & STORAGE

Reconstitute with 12 ml of sterile water for injection.

Don't reconstitute with bacteriostatic water for injection, and don't allow any bacteriostatic agent to get into the solution. Shake vial vigorously for 30 seconds or until particulate matter is dispersed after reconstitution.

The reconstituted solution is withdrawn into a sterile syringe, injected through a 5-micron filter into the appropriate amount of D_5W to a final concentration of 1 to 2 mg/ml. Lower concentrations (0.2 to 0.5 mg/ml) may be appropriate for infants and small children. Infusion should be completed within 6 hours of reconstitution.

After reconstitution with sterile water, drug may be stored for up to 24 hours at 36° to 46° F (2° to 8° C).

Incompatibilities
Other I.V. drugs, saline solutions.

CONTRAINDICATIONS & CAUTIONS
• Contraindicated in patients hypersensitive to drug or any of its components.
• Use cautiously in those with impaired renal function, those receiving chemotherapy or bone marrow transplantation, geriatric patients, and pregnant women.

ADVERSE REACTIONS
CNS: *anxiety, confusion, headache, insomnia, asthenia,* fever, *pain.*
CV: *chest pain, hypotension, tachycardia,* hypertension, *edema,* vasodilation, *peripheral edema.*
EENT: *epistaxis, rhinitis.*
GI: *nausea, vomiting, abdominal pain, diarrhea,* **GI hemorrhage.**
GU: *hematuria.*
Hepatic: ***hepatocellular damage,*** *hepatomegaly, bilirubinemia.*
Metabolic: *hyperglycemia,* hypernatremia, *hypocalcemia, hypokalemia, hypomagnesemia.*
Musculoskeletal: *back pain.*
Respiratory: *increased cough, dyspnea,* hypoxia, *pleural effusion, lung disorder,* hyperventilation.
Skin: *pruritus, rash,* sweating.
Other: *chills, infection,* ***anaphylaxis,*** SEPSIS, *blood product infusion reaction.*

INTERACTIONS
Drug-drug. *Antibiotics, nephrotoxic drugs:* May cause additive nephrotoxicity. Give cautiously, and monitor renal function closely.
Antineoplastics: May enhance potential for renal toxicity, bronchospasm, and hypotension. Monitor renal function, respiratory status, and vital signs.
Cardiac glycosides: Increases risk of digitalis toxicity in potassium-depleted patients. Monitor digoxin and potassium levels closely.
Clotrimazole, ketoconazole, miconazole: May induce fungal resistance to amphotericin B. Use together with caution.
Corticosteroids, corticotropin: May result in cardiac dysfunction. Monitor potassium level and cardiac function.
Flucytosine: May increase flucytosine toxicity. Monitor patient for toxicity.
Leukocyte transfusions: May cause acute pulmonary toxicity. Avoid using together.
Skeletal muscle relaxants: Enhances effects of skeletal muscle relaxants caused by amphotericin-induced hypokalemia. Monitor potassium levels.

EFFECTS ON LAB TEST RESULTS
• May increase BUN, creatinine, glucose, sodium, alkaline phosphatase, ALT, AST, bilirubin, GGT, and LDH levels. May decrease potassium, calcium, and magnesium levels.

ACTION
Active component, amphotericin B, binds to the sterol component of a fungal cell membrane leading to alterations in cell permeability and cell death.

PHARMACOKINETICS
Onset, unknown; peak, unknown; duration, unknown.
Distribution: Unknown.
Metabolism: Unknown.

Excretion: Initial half-life is 7 to 10 hours with once daily, 24-hour dosing; terminal elimination half-life is 100 to 153 hours.

CLINICAL CONSIDERATIONS

• Patients also receiving chemotherapy or bone marrow transplantation are at greater risk for additional adverse reactions including seizures, arrhythmias, thrombocytopenia, and respiratory failure.

• To lessen the risk or severity of adverse reactions, premedicate patient with antipyretics, antihistamines, antiemetics, or corticosteroids.

• Therapy may take several weeks to months.

• Patients treated with AmBisome had a lower incidence of chills, elevated BUN, hypokalemia, and vomiting than patients treated with regular amphotericin B.

• Use a controlled infusion device and an in-line filter with a mean pore diameter larger than 1 micron. Initially, infuse drug over at least 2 hours. If the treatment is well-tolerated, infusion time may be reduced to 1 hour. If the patient experiences discomfort during infusion, infusion time may be increased.

• Observe the patient closely for adverse reactions during the infusion. If anaphylaxis occurs, stop the infusion immediately, provide supportive therapy, and notify prescriber.

• Monitor liver function studies, CBC, creatinine, BUN, and electrolyte levels, particularly magnesium and potassium.

• Monitor for signs of hypokalemia, such as ECG changes, muscle weakness, cramping, and drowsiness.

PATIENT TEACHING

• Teach patient signs and symptoms of hypersensitivity, and stress importance of reporting them immediately.

• Warn patient that therapy may take several months; teach personal hygiene and other measures to prevent spread and recurrence of lesions.

• Instruct the patient to report any adverse reactions that occur while receiving the drug.

• Instruct the patient to watch for and report any signs or symptoms of hypokalemia, such as muscle weakness, cramping, drowsiness.

ampicillin sodium

Pharmacologic class: aminopenicillin
Therapeutic class: antibiotic
Pregnancy risk category: B
pH: 8 to 10.4

INDICATIONS & DOSAGES

➤ **Systemic, respiratory tract, skin, and GI infections and acute UTIs—**
Adults: 250 to 500 mg I.V. q 6 hours; in more severe infections, 500 mg q 6 hours, to a maximum of 12 g/day.
Children: 25 to 50 mg/kg I.V. q 6 hours.
➤ **Bacterial meningitis; septicemia—**
Adults: 1 to 2.5 g I.V. q 3 to 4 hours.
Children: 12.5 to 50 mg/kg I.V. q 3 to 4 hours.
➤ **Enterococcal endocarditis—**
Adults: 12 g daily I.V. continuously or in equally divided doses q 4 hours along with gentamicin.
➤ **Urethritis caused by** *Neisseria gonorrhoeae—*
Men: 500 mg I.V. q 8 to 12 hours for two doses.
➤ **To prevent bacterial endocarditis ◆ —**
Adults: 2 g I.V. 30 minutes before procedure.
Children: 50 mg/kg I.V. 30 minutes before procedure.
Adjust-a-dose: For patients with renal impairment, adjust dosage based on degree of renal impairment, severity of the infection, and susceptibility of the causative organism. Increase dosing interval to 6 to 12 hours if creatinine

---

clearance is 10 to 50 ml/minute; 12 to 24 hours if clearance is less than 10 ml/minute. Hemodialysis patients should receive a supplemental dose after each dialysis session.

ADMINISTRATION
Direct injection: Inject reconstituted drug into a large vein or cannula over 10 to 15 minutes. After injection, flush cannula with normal saline.
Intermittent infusion: Give diluted solution through I.V. piggyback or cannula over 30 to 60 minutes.
Continuous infusion: Not recommended.

PREPARATION & STORAGE
Supplied in vials containing 125 mg, 250 mg, 500 mg, 1 g, and 2 g. Reconstitute by adding 5 ml of sterile water for injection to the 125-, 250-, or 500-mg vial; 7.5 ml to 1-g vial; or 10 ml to 2-g vial. Dilute for infusion with 50 or 100 ml of normal saline solution, D_5W, 1/6 M sodium lactate, lactated Ringer's solution, 10% invert sugar, or sterile water for injection. Concentration of the drug shouldn't exceed 30 mg/ml.

At room temperature (77° F [25° C]), solutions containing 30 mg/ml or less remain stable for 8 hours in sterile water for injection, normal saline solution; solutions containing 2 mg/ml or less remain stable for 4 hours in D_5W; solutions containing 10 to 20 mg/ml remain stable for 2 hours in D_5W.

When refrigerated at 39° F (4° C), ampicillin solutions containing 30 mg/ml are stable for 48 hours in sterile water for injection or normal saline solution; solutions containing 20 mg/ml or less are stable for 72 hours in sterile water for injection or normal saline solution, 4 hours in D_5W.

Incompatibilities
Amikacin, amino acid solutions, chlorpromazine, dextran solutions, dopamine, erythromycin lactobionate, 10% fat emulsions, fructose, gentamicin, heparin sodium, hetastarch, hydrocortisone sodium succinate, hydromorphone, kanamycin, lidocaine, lincomycin, polymyxin B, prochlorperazine edisylate, sodium bicarbonate, streptomycin, tobramycin.

CONTRAINDICATIONS & CAUTIONS
● Contraindicated in patients hypersensitive to penicillin.
● Contraindicated in those with infectious mononucleosis because of high risk of maculopapular rash.
● Use cautiously in patients hypersensitive to cephalosporins, geriatric patients, and those with renal impairment. Dosage may need to be reduced.

ADVERSE REACTIONS
CNS: lethargy, *seizures,* anxiety, confusion, dizziness, fatigue.
CV: vein irritation, thrombophlebitis.
GI: *nausea,* vomiting, *diarrhea, pseudomembranous colitis,* glossitis, stomatitis.
GU: *acute interstitial nephritis.*
Hematologic: *bone marrow depression.*
Skin: pain at injection site.
Other: *anaphylaxis,* bacterial or fungal superinfection, hypersensitivity reactions (rash, urticaria).

INTERACTIONS
Drug-drug. *Allopurinol:* Increases risk of rash. Monitor patient closely.
Hormonal contraceptives: Reduces contraceptive effectiveness. Recommend use of second contraceptive method.
Methotrexate: Decreases methotrexate excretion. Monitor patient for toxicity.
Probenecid: Decreases ampicillin excretion. Avoid using together.

EFFECTS ON LAB TEST RESULTS
● May increase eosinophil count. May decrease hemoglobin, hematocrit, and platelet, WBC, and granulocyte counts.
● May falsely increase uric acid level with the copper chelate method. May

cause false-positive results in urine glucose when tested with copper sulfate, such as Benedict's solution and Clinitest.

ACTION

Joins with penicillin-binding proteins in susceptible bacteria, inhibiting cell wall synthesis. Acts against non–penicillinase-producing strains of *Staphylococcus aureus, S. epidermidis, Streptococcus pneumoniae, S. viridans,* some strains of enterococci, and groups A, B, C, and G streptococci.

Susceptible gram-negative bacteria include *Bordetella pertussis, Branhamella catarrhalis, Eikenella corrodens, Escherichia coli, Gardnerella vaginalis, Haemophilus influenzae, Legionella, Pasteurella multocida, Neisseria gonorrhoeae, N. meningitidis, Proteus mirabilis, Salmonella,* and *Shigella.* Susceptible anaerobic bacteria include *Actinomyces, Arachnia, Bifidobacterium, Campylobacter fetus, Clostridium perfringens, C. tetani, Eubacterium, Fusobacterium, Lactobacillus, Peptococcus, Peptostreptococcus,* and *Propionibacterium.*

PHARMACOKINETICS

Drug level peaks immediately after 15-minute infusion.
Distribution: Readily distributed to most body tissues and bone. Normally poor distribution to eye, brain, and CSF; improves when inflammation is present. Drug crosses the placental barrier and appears in cord blood and amniotic fluid. Small amounts appear in bile and breast milk.
Metabolism: Partially, in liver.
Excretion: Largely by glomerular filtration and renal tubular secretion. Elimination half-life averages about 1 hour; in neonates and patients with renal impairment, 10 to 24 hours.

CLINICAL CONSIDERATIONS

• Obtain specimens for culture and sensitivity testing before giving first dose.

Therapy may start before results are available.
• Check for previous penicillin or cephalosporin hypersensitivity before first dose. Normal history doesn't rule out future allergic reaction.
• Intermittent infusion reduces risk of vein irritation. Change I.V. site every 48 hours or per facility policy.
• If acute interstitial nephritis, bone marrow depression, or pseudomembranous colitis develops, stop drug.
• Monitor for signs of bacterial or fungal superinfection.
• If diarrhea persists during therapy, collect stool specimens to rule out possible pseudomembranous colitis.
• To prevent false results, use Clinistix or glucose enzymatic test strip to determine urine glucose levels.

PATIENT TEACHING

• Explain to patient and family the use and administration of drug.
• Tell patient to report adverse reactions promptly, including rash, fever, and chills.
• Tell patient to report discomfort at I.V. site promptly.

ampicillin sodium and sulbactam sodium
Unasyn

Pharmacologic class: aminopenicillin and beta-lactamase inhibitor combination
Therapeutic class: antibiotic
Pregnancy risk category: B
pH: 8 to 10

INDICATIONS & DOSAGES

➤ **Peritonitis and gynecologic, skin, and skin structure infections caused by susceptible organisms—**
Adults and children weighing 40 kg or more: 1.5 (1 g ampicillin, 0.5 g sulbac-

tam) to 3 g (2 g ampicillin, 1 g sulbactam) I.V. q 6 hours, not to exceed 4 g/ day of sulbactam.

➤ **Skin and skin structure infections—**
Children age 1 and older: 300 mg/kg daily (200 mg ampicillin, 100 mg sulbactam) I.V. in equally divided doses given q 6 hours. Don't exceed 14 days of therapy.
Adjust-a-dose: In an adult, if creatinine clearance is 30 ml/minute or more, give 1.5 to 3 g q 6 to 8 hours; if clearance is 15 to 29 ml/minute, give 1.5 to 3 g q 12 hours; and if clearance is 5 to 14 ml/ minute, give 1.5 to 3 g q 24 hours.

ADMINISTRATION
Direct injection: Inject reconstituted drug into large vein or cannula over at least 10 to 15 minutes. Then flush with normal saline solution.
Intermittent infusion: After diluting reconstituted drug (usually in 100 ml of solution), infuse over 15 to 30 minutes.
Continuous infusion: Not used.

PREPARATION & STORAGE
Available in 1.5-g and 3-g vials and in piggyback vials. Reconstitute with sterile water for injection to yield a concentration of 375 mg/ml. For infusion, immediately dilute reconstituted solution with compatible diluent to yield 3 to 45 mg/ml.

Storage times depend on diluent and concentration. Using sterile water for injection or normal saline injection, a 45 mg/ml solution remains stable for 8 hours at 77° F (25° C) and for 48 hours at 39° F (4° C); a 30 mg/ml solution remains stable for 72 hours at 39° F.

Using D₅W, a 30 mg/ml solution is stable for 2 hours at 77° F and for 4 hours at 39° F.

Using lactated Ringer's solution, a 45 mg/ml solution remains stable for 8 hours at 77° F and for 24 hours at 39° F.

Other compatible diluents include dextrose 5% and half-normal saline solution or 10% invert sugar.

Incompatibilities
Amikacin, amino acid solutions, chlorpromazine, dextran solutions, dopamine, erythromycin lactobionate, 10% fat emulsions, fructose, gentamicin, heparin sodium, hetastarch, hydrocortisone sodium succinate, kanamycin, lidocaine, lincomycin, netilmicin, polymyxin B, prochlorperazine edisylate, sodium bicarbonate, streptomycin, tobramycin.

CONTRAINDICATIONS & CAUTIONS
● Contraindicated in patients hypersensitive to penicillin or sulbactam.
● Contraindicated in those with mononucleosis because of increased risk of maculopapular rash.
● Use cautiously in patients hypersensitive to cephalosporins, geriatric patients, and those with renal impairment. Dosage may need to be reduced.

ADVERSE REACTIONS
CV: thrombophlebitis.
GI: diarrhea, *pseudomembranous colitis.*
Skin: rash, pain at injection site.
Other: bacterial or fungal superinfections, *anaphylaxis.*

INTERACTIONS
Drug-drug. *Allopurinol:* Increases risk of rash. Monitor patient closely.
Hormonal contraceptives: Reduces effectiveness. Recommend second method of birth control.
Methotrexate: Diminishes excretion. Monitor patient for toxicity.
Probenecid: Decreases ampicillin and sulbactam excretion. Monitor levels, and watch for signs of toxic reaction.

EFFECTS ON LAB TEST RESULTS
● May increase BUN, creatinine, ALT, AST, alkaline phosphatase, bilirubin, LDH, CK, and GGT levels.
● May increase eosinophil count. May decrease hemoglobin and platelet, WBC, and granulocyte counts.
● May cause false elevations with copper chelate method in uric acid levels. May cause false-positive results in urine glucose when tested with copper sulfate, such as Benedict's solution and Clinitest.

ACTION
Inhibits bacterial cell wall synthesis by joining with penicillin-binding proteins. Addition of sulbactam, a beta-lactamase inhibitor, makes the compound effective against many beta-lactamase–producing bacteria that are normally resistant to ampicillin alone. Susceptible aerobic bacteria include *Acinetobacter calcoaceticus, Bacteroides fragilis, Enterobacter, Escherichia coli, Klebsiella, Neisseria gonorrhoeae, Proteus mirabilis, Staphylococcus aureus, S. epidermidis, S. saprophyticus, Streptococcus pneumoniae, S. pyogenes,* and *S. viridans.*

PHARMACOKINETICS
Drug level peaks immediately after 15-minute infusion; half-life, about 1 hour.
Distribution: Widely distributed in body fluids and tissues. Brain and CSF penetration increases with meningeal inflammation. Drug crosses the placental barrier. Drug appears in breast milk.
Metabolism: Ampicillin partly metabolized in liver; sulbactam metabolism unknown.
Excretion: In patients with normal renal function, 75% to 85% excreted unchanged in urine, primarily by glomerular filtration and renal tubular secretion.

CLINICAL CONSIDERATIONS
● Obtain specimens for culture and sensitivity testing before giving first dose. Therapy may start before results of tests are known.
● Check patient's history for previous hypersensitivity to penicillin or cephalosporins before giving first dose. Normal history doesn't rule out the possibility of future allergic reaction.
● If anaphylaxis or pseudomembranous colitis develops, stop drug.
● Give ampicillin sulbactam at least 1 hour before bacteriostatic antibiotics.
● If diarrhea persists during therapy, collect stool specimens to rule out possible pseudomembranous colitis.
● Observe patient for fungal and bacterial superinfection with large doses or prolonged use.
● Patients with renal impairment must be monitored frequently for signs of toxic reaction resulting from high drug levels.
● If overdose occurs, hemodialysis may be used to remove ampicillin and probably sulbactam.
● Use Clinistix or Tes-Tape to test for urine glucose levels.

PATIENT TEACHING
● Explain to patient and family how drug works and is given.
● Tell patient to report adverse reactions promptly, especially rash, fever, or chills. Rash is the most common allergic reaction.
● Tell patient to report discomfort at I.V. site promptly.

Reactions may be *common,* uncommon, ***life-threatening,*** or COMMON AND LIFE-THREATENING.

antihemophilic factor (AHF, factor VIII)

Helixate FS, Hemofil M, Hyate:C, Koate-DVI, Kogenate, Kogenate FS, Monoclate-P, Recombinate, ReFacto

Pharmacologic class: blood derivative
Therapeutic class: antihemophilic
Pregnancy risk category: C

INDICATIONS & DOSAGES

Drug provides hemostasis in factor VIII deficiency, hemophilia A. The specific dosage depends on the patient's weight, severity of hemorrhage, and presence of inhibitors. Mild bleeding episodes require a circulating factor VIII level of 20% to 40% or more of normal; moderate to major bleeding episodes and minor surgery, a level of 30% to 60% of normal; severe bleeding or major surgery, a level of 80% to 100% of normal. The following dosages provide guidelines. Refer to specific brand for actual dosing.
➤ **Mild bleeding—**
Adults and children: 10 to 20 IU/kg I.V. daily.
➤ **Moderate to major bleeding and minor surgery—**
Adults and children: Initially, 15 to 30 IU/kg I.V. Repeat one dose at 12 to 24 hours, if needed.
➤ **Severe bleeding and bleeding near vital organs—**
Adults and children: Initially, 40 to 50 IU/kg I.V., then 20 to 25 IU/kg q 8 to 12 hours, p.r.n.
➤ **Major surgery—**
Adults and children: 50 IU/kg I.V. 1 hour before surgery, then repeat 6 to 12 hours after first dose p.r.n. Maintain circulating factor levels at 30% of normal for 10 to 14 days after surgery.

ADMINISTRATION

Direct injection: Using a plastic syringe, because concentrate may adhere to glass, and the winged infusion set, inject into vein at 2 ml/minute. Consult specific product information; some can be given at a rate of 10 ml/minute.
Intermittent infusion: Not recommended.
Continuous infusion: Not recommended.

PREPARATION & STORAGE

Available in a kit, including single-dose vial with diluent, sterile needles for reconstitution and withdrawal, winged infusion set with microbore tubing, and alcohol swabs. Refrigerate drug that hasn't been reconstituted, freeze Hyate:C, and avoid freezing all others.

Before reconstitution, vials of lyophilized powder and diluents should be warmed to room temperature.

Reconstitute by using the double-ended needle to transfer diluent into vial, which is drawn in by vacuum. Gently swirl vial until contents dissolve. Use within 3 hours. Hemofil M should be used within 1 hour.

• *Alert:* Kogenate FS and Helixate FS should be kept refrigerated at all times at temperatures of 36° F to 46° F (2° C to 8° C) (*not* room temperature) to ensure the drugs' potency through the expiration date. Previously, the manufacturers of these agents allowed for storage at room temperature for up to 2 months as an alternative to refrigeration.

Incompatibilities

Protein precipitants.

CONTRAINDICATIONS & CAUTIONS

• Contraindicated in patients hypersensitive to mouse protein.

ADVERSE REACTIONS
CNS: fever.
CV: chest tightness, hypotension.
GI: nausea, vomiting.
Hematologic: *hemolytic anemia, thrombocytopenia.*
Hepatic: *viral hepatitis.*
Respiratory: wheezing.
Skin: *stinging at infusion site,* urticaria.
Other: *anaphylaxis,* mild chills, *thrombosis, hepatitis B, HIV.*

INTERACTIONS
None reported.

EFFECTS ON LAB TEST RESULTS
• May increase fibrinogen level.
• May decrease hemoglobin, hematocrit, and platelet count.

COMPOSITION
Factor VIII is a sterile, lyophilized concentrate of factor VIII:C, a coagulant portion of factor VIII complex, and small amounts of factor VIII:R, the protein responsible for von Willebrand's factor activity.

This highly purified concentrate of pooled human plasma is tested for hepatitis and HIV. Preparations are either heat- or detergent-treated to inactivate potential viruses. These treatments sharply lower the risk of hepatitis and AIDS.

CLINICAL CONSIDERATIONS
• I.V. administration of 1 IU/kg increases circulating antihemophilic factor by about 2%.
• Monitor coagulation studies before therapy and at regular intervals during treatment.
• Monitor hematocrit and Coombs' test result in patients with type A, B, or AB blood because trace amounts of type A and B isohemagglutinins are present in antihemophilic factor, and large or frequent dosing may cause

progressive anemia or intravascular hemolysis.

PATIENT TEACHING
• Explain to patient and family the use and administration of antihemophilic factor.
• Tell patient to report adverse reactions promptly.
• Instruct patient to wear medical identification tag.
• Tell patient to notify prescriber if drug seems less effective; a change may signal development of antibodies.

anti-inhibitor coagulant complex
Autoplex T, Feiba VH Immuno

Pharmacologic class: activated prothrombin complex
Therapeutic class: hemostatic
Pregnancy risk category: C

INDICATIONS & DOSAGES
➤ **Patients with factor VIII inhibitors who are about to have surgery or are bleeding—**
Adults and children: 25 to 100 factor VIII correctional units/kg I.V. Autoplex T, depending on severity of hemorrhage. May repeat q 6 hours p.r.n.
➤ **Joint hemorrhage in patients with factor VIII inhibitors—**
Adults and children: 50 units/kg I.V. Feiba VH Immuno q 12 hours, increasing to 100 units/kg q 12 hours until patient's condition improves.
➤ **Mucous membrane hemorrhage in patients with factor VIII inhibitors—**
Adults and children: 50 units/kg I.V. Feiba VH Immuno q 6 hours, increasing to 100 units/kg q 6 hours if hemorrhage continues. Maximum daily dose, 200 units/kg.

Reactions may be *common,* uncommon, *life-threatening,* or COMMON AND LIFE-THREATENING.

➤ **Soft-tissue hemorrhage in patients with factor VIII inhibitors—**
Adults and children: 100 units/kg I.V. Feiba VH Immuno q 12 hours. Maximum daily dose, 200 units/kg.
➤ **Other severe hemorrhages in patients with factor VIII inhibitors—**
Adults and children: 100 units/kg I.V. Feiba VH Immuno q 12 hours (occasionally, q 6 hours).

ADMINISTRATION

Direct injection: Inject Autoplex T directly into vein of 2 ml/minute, increasing to 10 ml/minute based on patient tolerance. Stop if patient develops a headache, flushing, or change in pulse or blood pressure. Resume at a slower rate when symptoms disappear.

Inject Feiba VH Immuno no faster than 2 units/kg/minute.
Intermittent infusion: Not recommended for Autoplex T. For Feiba VH Immuno, follow manufacturer's directions for using the administration set. Make sure to use a standard blood filter. Infuse no faster than 2 units/kg/minute.
Continuous infusion: Not recommended.

PREPARATION & STORAGE

Available in a package containing a vial of dry concentrate, a vial of sterile water for injection, a double-ended transfer needle, and a filter needle. Refrigerate vials before use.

To reconstitute, bring vials to room temperature and follow manufacturer's instructions. If drawing more than 1 vial into a syringe, use a new filter needle for each vial.

Don't refrigerate after reconstitution. Use Autoplex T within 1 hour and Feiba VH Immuno within 3 hours; otherwise, the patien will become hypotensive because of increased prekallikrein activator.

Incompatibilities

Other I.V. drugs or solutions.

CONTRAINDICATIONS & CAUTIONS

• Contraindicated in those with fibrinolysis or DIC because drug increases risk of intravascular clotting.
• Use cautiously in infants because hepatitis, if contracted, causes higher mortality in them than in adults.
• Use cautiously in those with hepatic disease because risk of hepatotoxicity increases if hepatitis is contracted.

ADVERSE REACTIONS

CNS: headache, lethargy, fever.
CV: *pulse and blood pressure changes,* chest pain, ***acute MI, thromboembolic events,*** flushing.
Hematologic: *DIC.*
Respiratory: cough, dyspnea.
Other: ***anaphylaxis, hepatitis B and HIV,*** chills.

INTERACTIONS

Drug-drug. *Antifibrinolytics:* May alter effects of anti-inhibitor coagulant complex. Avoid using together.

EFFECTS ON LAB TEST RESULTS

• May alter coagulation test results.

COMPOSITION

Prepared from pooled human plasma that has tested negative for hepatitis and HIV, drug contains varying amounts of clotting factor precursors, activated clotting factors, and factors of the kinin-generating system.

CLINICAL CONSIDERATIONS

• Drug controls hemorrhage in hemophilia A patients who have a factor VIII inhibitor level above 10 Bethesda units. Patients with a level of 2 to 10 Bethesda units may receive the drug if they have severe hemorrhage or respond poorly to factor VIII infusion.
• Before therapy, verify that patient has a diagnosed clotting deficiency caused by factor VIII inhibitors.
• Stop infusion and monitor for DIC if signs and symptoms of intravascular co-

agulation develop, such as dyspnea, chest pain, cough, and pulse and blood pressure changes. Laboratory indicators of DIC include prolonged thrombin time, PT, INR, and PTT; reduced fibrinogen levels and platelet count; and the presence of fibrin split products.

PATIENT TEACHING
● Teach patient about AIDS, and encourage immunization against hepatitis B in patients who have tested negative for hepatitis B surface antigen.
● Explain to patient and family how drug works and is given.
● Tell patient to report adverse reactions promptly.

antithrombin III, human
Thrombate III

Pharmacologic class: glycoprotein
Therapeutic class: anticoagulant, antithrombotic
Pregnancy risk category: B

INDICATIONS & DOSAGES
➤ Patients with hereditary antithrombin III deficiency who are having surgical or obstetric procedures or those with thromboembolism—
Adults and children: First dose is individualized to the quantity needed to increase antithrombin III activity to 120% of normal activity as determined 30 minutes after administration. Usual dose is 50 to 100 IU/minute I.V., not to exceed 100 IU/minute. Dose is calculated based on anticipated 1.4% increase in antithrombin III activity produced by 1 IU/kg of body weight using the following formula:

$$\text{Dose} = \frac{\left[\begin{array}{c}\text{desired} \\ \text{AT-III} \\ \text{level (\%)}\end{array} - \begin{array}{c}\text{baseline} \\ \text{AT-III} \\ \text{level (\%)}\end{array}\right] \times \begin{array}{c}\text{weight} \\ \text{(kg)}\end{array}}{1.4\% \text{ (IU/kg)}}$$

The denominator in this formula is the expected increase in antithrombin III activity, in percent, produced by 1 IU/kg, as determined 20 minutes after administration of first dose. Maintenance dose is individualized to quantity needed to increase antithrombin III activity to 80% of prior normal activity and is given at 24-hour intervals.

To calculate the dose, multiply the desired antithrombin III activity, as percent of normal, minus the baseline antithrombin III activity as percent of normal by body weight in kilograms. Divide by actual increase in antithrombin III activity in percent produced by 1 IU/kg as determined 30 minutes after administration of first dose.

Treatment usually continues for 2 to 8 days but may be prolonged when given to pregnant, postsurgical, or immobilized patients.

ADMINISTRATION
Direct injection: Not recommended.
Intermittent infusion: Infuse over 10 to 20 minutes at rate of 50 IU/minute (1 ml/minute), not to exceed 100 IU/minute (2 ml/minute).
Continuous infusion: Not recommended.

PREPARATION & STORAGE
Available as a lyophilized powder in 50-ml infusion bottles containing 500 or 1,000 IU of antithrombin III. Store at 36° to 46° F (2° to 8° C).

Warm diluent to room temperature before reconstitution. Reconstitute using 10 or 20 ml sterile water for injection that is provided. Gently swirl the vial to dissolve the powder. Don't shake. Bring solution to room temperature and give within 3 hours of reconstitution. Further dilute in same diluent solution if needed. Inspect for precipitate and discoloration before use.

Incompatibilities
None reported.

Reactions may be *common,* uncommon, *life-threatening,* or COMMON AND LIFE-THREATENING.

CONTRAINDICATIONS & CAUTIONS
• Use extremely cautiously in children and neonates because safety and efficacy haven't been established.
• Use cautiously. Drug is prepared from pooled plasma from human donors. It carries a minimal risk of viral transmission. Plasma used in the manufacturing process is screened for hepatitis B surface antigen and HIV, and the product is heat-treated for 10 hours at 140° F (60° C) to further reduce the risk of viral transmission.

ADVERSE REACTIONS
CNS: dizziness.
CV: chest tightness, lowered blood pressure, vasodilation, diuresis.
GI: foul taste in mouth, nausea.
Other: chills, cramps.

INTERACTIONS
Drug-drug. *Heparin:* Increases anticoagulant effects of both drugs. May need to reduce heparin dosage.

EFFECTS ON LAB TEST RESULTS
None reported.

ACTION
Replaces deficient antithrombin III in patients with hereditary antithrombin III deficiency, normalizing coagulation-inhibiting capability and inhibiting formation of thromboemboli. It inactivates thrombin and activated forms of factors IX, X, XI, and XII.

PHARMACOKINETICS
Special receptors on hepatocytes bind antithrombin III clotting factor complexes, rapidly removing them from circulation.
Distribution: Binds to epithelium and is redistributed into the extravascular compartment; distribution into breast milk is highly unlikely because of large molecular size.
Metabolism: Unknown.

Excretion: Biologic half-life, 2 to 3 days.

CLINICAL CONSIDERATIONS
• Drug isn't recommended for long-term prevention of thrombotic episodes.
• Because of risk of neonatal thromboembolism in children of parents with hereditary antithrombin III deficiency, measure antithrombin III levels immediately after birth. Fatal neonatal thromboembolism has occurred.
• Diagnosis of hereditary antithrombin III deficiency should be based on a clear family history of venous thrombosis, decreased antithrombin III levels, and the exclusion of acquired deficiency. Antithrombin III levels may be measured with amidolytic assays using synthetic chromogenic substrates or with clotting assays or immunoassays.
• One IU is equivalent to the quantity of endogenous antithrombin III present in 1 ml of normal plasma.
• Heparin binds to antithrombin III lysine binding sites in a 1:1 M ratio, which results in increased efficacy of heparin.
• Measure antithrombin III levels before and 20 minutes after treatment, and calculate the anticipated recovery. If the recovery differs from the anticipated rise of 1.4% for each IU/kg given, modify the formula.
• *Alert:* Dyspnea and increased blood pressure may occur if administration rate is too rapid, about 1,500 IU in 5 minutes.
• *Alert:* Because product is made from human plasma, there is a risk of infection. If infection is thought to be caused by this product, notify the Bayer Corporation at 888-765-3203.

PATIENT TEACHING
• Explain to patient and parents the use and administration of drug. Encourage them to ask questions and express concerns.

• Tell patient to report adverse reactions promptly.

aprotinin
Trasylol

Pharmacologic class: naturally occurring protease inhibitor
Therapeutic class: system hemostatic
Pregnancy risk category: B

INDICATIONS & DOSAGES
➤ **To reduce excessive blood loss and blood transfusions during cardiopulmonary bypass—**
Adults: 1 ml (1.4 mg or 10,000 kallikrein-inhibiting units [KIUs]) I.V. test dose 10 minutes before scheduled administration time, followed by a loading dose of 200-ml (280 mg or 2 million KIU) given over 20 to 30 minutes after induction of anesthesia. Patient should be in a supine position. A 200-ml pump-priming dose is provided for the bypass machine before the bypass is begun. During surgery, a constant infusion of 50 ml/hour (70 mg/ hour or 500,000 KIU/hour) of aprotinin is given until the incision is closed. Once closed, the infusion is stopped. Alternative dose is 1 million KIU as a loading dose, pump prime of 1 million KIU, then a constant infusion of 250,000 KIU/hour.

ADMINISTRATION
Direct injection: By slow I.V. injection over at least 4 minutes.
Intermittent infusion: By slow I.V. infusion at a rate of 200 ml over 20 to 30 minutes.
Continuous infusion: During surgery at a rate of 50 ml/hour until incision is closed.

PREPARATION & STORAGE
Available as 100-ml and 200-ml vials containing 1.4 mg/ml (10,000 KIU) aprotinin. Store at room temperature. May dilute with D₅W or normal saline solution before infusion.

Incompatibilities
Corticosteroids, heparin, nutrient solutions containing amino acids or fat emulsions, other I.V. drugs, tetracycline.

CONTRAINDICATIONS & CAUTIONS
• Contraindicated in patients hypersensitive to the drug or its components or to bovine products.
• Contraindicated in those with thromboembolic disease requiring anticoagulant therapy.
• Use cautiously in those with renal impairment because renal toxicity may occur.
• Use cautiously in those receiving aprotinin for the second, third, or fourth time because such use may cause significant adverse reactions. Safety and efficacy haven't been established in children.

ADVERSE REACTIONS
CNS: confusion, *fever,* asthenia, insomnia.
CV: ATRIAL FIBRILLATION, *cardiac failure, MI, arrhythmias, shock,* hypotension, chest pain, tachycardia, peripheral edema, hypertension, *thrombosis.*
GI: *nausea,* vomiting, diarrhea, constipation.
GU: *kidney failure,* UTI, urine retention.
Hematologic: leukocytosis, *thrombocytopenia,* anemia.
Metabolic: hyperglycemia.
Respiratory: *apnea,* respiratory tract disorder, pleural effusion, pneumonia, dyspnea, asthma, pneumothorax, atelectasis, hypoxia.
Skin: rash.
Other: infection, *sepsis, anaphylaxis.*

Reactions may be *common,* uncommon, *life-threatening,* or COMMON AND LIFE-THREATENING.

INTERACTIONS

Drug-drug. *ACE inhibitors:* May block antihypertensive effect of ACE inhibitors. Monitor blood pressure closely.
Fibrinolytics: May inhibit effects of fibrinolytics. Monitor patient closely.
Heparin: Prolonged activated clotting time. Monitor coagulation study results.

EFFECTS ON LAB TEST RESULTS

• May increase AST, ALT, creatinine, and glucose levels. May decrease potassium level.
• May increase WBC count. May decrease platelet count. May alter liver function test values.

ACTION

A natural proteinase inhibitor from bovine lungs with a complex mechanism of action. By inhibiting chymotrypsin, kallikrein, plasmin, plasmin-streptokinase, and trypsin through the formation of reversible enzyme-inhibitor complexes, aprotinin inhibits both fibrinolysis and turnover of coagulation factors. It also protects blood platelets from becoming dysfunctional when exposed to the bypass machine.

PHARMACOKINETICS

With recommended dosing at induction of anesthesia, therapeutic levels are achieved at the beginning of cardiopulmonary bypass.
Distribution: Rapidly distributed into total extracellular space; followed by active accumulation in proximal renal tubules after glomerular filtration.
Metabolism: In kidneys to small peptides or amino acids.
Excretion: Mostly excreted as peptides and amino acids within 6 days of administration.

CLINICAL CONSIDERATIONS

• A test dose is recommended before infusion because aprotinin may cause allergic reactions, including anaphylaxis.
• Give drug through a central line.

• To avoid hypotension, make sure patient is supine when giving test dose.
• Watch for increased creatinine level, which signals nephrotoxicity. If nephrotoxicity occurs, it's usually mild and reversible.

PATIENT TEACHING

• Explain to patient and family the use and administration of drug.
• Tell patient to report adverse reactions promptly.
• Reassure patient and family that patient will be monitored continuously throughout therapy for adverse reactions. arbutamine hydrochloride

arbutamine hydrochloride
GenESA

Pharmacologic class: adrenergic agonist
Therapeutic class: sympathomimetic diagnostic aid
Pregnancy risk category: B
pH: 3.8

INDICATIONS & DOSAGES

➤ **Single-dose diagnostic aid in patients with suspected coronary artery disease (CAD) who can't exercise adequately. Stress induction with arbutamine is indicated as an aid in diagnosing the presence or absence of CAD—**
Adults: 0.1 mcg/kg/minute for 1 minute via GenESA I.V. infusion system. The device adjusts dose until the maximum heart rate limit set by user is achieved or a maximum infusion rate of 0.8 mcg/kg/minute. Maximum total dose, 10 mcg/kg.

ADMINISTRATION

Direct injection: Give drug by direct I.V. infusion only with the GenESA device.

Intermittent infusion: Not recommended.
Continuous infusion: Not recommended.

PREPARATION & STORAGE
Drug is manufactured in a 20-ml prefilled glass syringe and plunger rod containing 0.05 mg/ml. Don't dilute before administration. Should only be given via the prefilled syringe using the GenESA system, which is a closed-loop, computer-controlled, I.V. infusion device. Inspect syringe for evidence of particulate matter or discoloration before administering.

Before using the GenESA system, read and understand the manufacturer's directions for use.

Store drug at 36° to 46° F (2° to 8° C), and make sure it's protected from light.

Incompatibilities
None reported.

CONTRAINDICATIONS & CAUTIONS
• Contraindicated in patients hypersensitive to drug, idiopathic hypertrophic subaortic stenosis, a history of recurrent sustained ventricular tachycardia, or New York Heart Association class III or IV heart failure.
• Contraindicated in those who have an implanted cardiac pacemaker or automated cardioverter or defibrillator and in those who are receiving atropine, digoxin, other anticholinergics, or tricyclic antidepressants.
• Avoid use in patients with unstable angina, mechanical left ventricular outflow obstruction such as severe valvular aortic stenosis, uncontrolled systemic hypertension, cardiac transplant, history of cerebrovascular disease, peripheral vascular disorder resulting in cerebral or aortic aneurysm, angle-closure glaucoma, supraventricular tachyarrhythmias or ventricular arrhythmias, or uncontrolled hyperthyroidism and in patients

receiving class I antiarrhythmics, such as flecainide, lidocaine, or quinidine.
• Safety and efficacy of drug in patients who have had an MI within the past 30 days haven't been evaluated; don't use in these patients.
• Use cautiously in patients with a known sulfite allergy. Drug contains sodium metabisulfite, which may produce an allergic response in susceptible patients.

ADVERSE REACTIONS
CNS: anxiety, dizziness, fatigue, headache, hypoesthesia, pain, paresthesia, *tremor.*
CV: *angina pectoris,* ARRHYTHMIAS, chest pain, flushing, hypotension, hot flashes, palpitation, vasodilation.
GI: nausea, dry mouth, taste perversion.
Respiratory: dyspnea.
Skin: increased sweating.

INTERACTIONS
Drug-drug. *Atropine, digoxin, tricyclic antidepressants:* Arbutamine dosing is based on heart rate. These drugs increase the heart rate and will interfere with dosing. Avoid using together.
Beta blockers: May attenuate arbutamine's effects. Stop beta blocker at least 48 hours before giving arbutamine.

EFFECTS ON LAB TEST RESULTS
None reported.

ACTION
Increases cardiac workload through both positive inotropic and chronotropic actions.

PHARMACOKINETICS
Onset, 1 minute; peak, unknown; duration, variable.
Distribution: 58% bound to plasma proteins.
Metabolism: Metabolized in the liver to methoxyarbutamine.
Excretion: After I.V. administration, 84% is excreted in the urine and 9% in

the feces within 48 hours. Elimination half-life, about 8 minutes.

CLINICAL CONSIDERATIONS

• *Alert:* Don't give atropine to enhance drug-induced chronotropic response; coadministration may lead to tachyarrhythmias.
• Monitor blood pressure, heart rate, and a diagnostic quality ECG continuously throughout drug infusion.
• Emergency resuscitative equipment should be at the bedside during drug administration.
• Transient prolongation of the corrected QT interval, as measured from a surface ECG, occurs with administration.
• Transient reductions in potassium levels may occur, but rarely to hypokalemic levels.

PATIENT TEACHING

• Instruct patient on need to stop beta blockers at least 48 hours before undergoing cardiac stress testing with arbutamine, as ordered by prescriber.
• Inform patient that drug temporarily increases heart rate but that he'll be closely monitored.
• Inform patient of potential adverse events.

argatroban

Pharmacologic class: direct thrombin inhibitor
Therapeutic class: anticoagulant
Pregnancy risk category: B
pH: 3.2 to 7.5

INDICATIONS & DOSAGES

➤ **To treat or prevent thrombosis in patients with heparin-induced thrombocytopenia (HIT)—**
Adults: 2 mcg/kg/minute, given as a continuous I.V. infusion; adjust dose

until the steady state aPTT is 1.5 to 3 times the initial baseline value, not to exceed 100 seconds; maximum dose is 10 mcg/kg/minute.

Before giving argatroban, stop heparin therapy and obtain a baseline aPTT. Allow aPTT to decrease from the effects of heparin therapy.
Adjust-a-dose: For patients with moderate hepatic impairment, the first dose should be reduced to 0.5 mcg/kg/min, given as a continuous infusion. The aPTT should be monitored closely and the dosage adjusted if indicated.
➤ **Anticoagulation in patients with or at risk for HIT during percutaneous coronary intervention (PCI)—**
Adults: 350 mcg/kg I.V. bolus over 3 to 5 minutes. Start a continuous I.V. infusion at a rate of 25 mcg/kg/minute. Check activated clotting time (ACT) 5 to 10 minutes after the bolus dose is given.
Adjust-a-dose: Follow the table below to adjust the dose:

ACT	Additional I.V. bolus	Continuous I.V. infusion
< 300 sec	150 mcg/kg	30 mcg/kg/min***
300-450 sec	None needed	25 mcg/kg/min
> 450 sec	None needed	15 mcg/kg/min***

***Check ACT again after 5 to 10 min.

In case of dissection, impending abrupt closure, thrombus formation during the procedure, or inability to achieve or maintain an ACT for longer than 300 seconds, give an additional bolus of 150 mcg/kg and increase infusion rate to 40 mcg/kg/minute. Check ACT again after 5 to 10 minutes.

ADMINISTRATION
Direct injection: Give bolus doses over 3 to 5 minutes when indicated.
Intermittent infusion: Not recommended.
Continuous injection: Give drug at specified rates.

PREPARATION & STORAGE
Available as 250-mg/2.5-ml clear, colorless to pale yellow, slightly viscous solution in single-use vials at a concentration of 100 mg/ml. Store at room temperature. Keep the vials in their original cartons to protect drug from light.

Dilute drug in 250 ml of normal saline solution, D_5W, or lactated Ringer's injection to a final concentration of 1 mg/ml. Mix the constituted solution by repeatedly inverting the diluent bag for 1 minute. During preparation, the solution may show a slight haziness because of microprecipitates, which will dissolve rapidly upon mixing. Prepared solutions are stable for up to 24 hours at 77° F (25° C).

Incompatibilities
Other I.V. drugs.

CONTRAINDICATIONS & CAUTIONS
• Contraindicated in patients hypersensitive to the drug or any of its components and in those with overt major bleeding
• Use cautiously in patients with hepatic disease or conditions that increase the risk of hemorrhage, such as severe hypertension.
• Use cautiously in patients who have just had lumbar puncture, spinal anesthesia, or major surgery, especially of the brain, spinal cord, or eye; patients with hematologic conditions caused by increased bleeding tendencies, such as congenital or acquired bleeding disorders; and those with GI ulcers or other lesions.

• It's unknown whether argatroban appears in breast milk. A decision should be made to stop either breast-feeding or the drug, taking into account the importance of the drug to the mother.

ADVERSE REACTIONS
CNS: fever, pain, *CVA.*
CV: *atrial fibrillation, cardiac arrest,* hypotension, *ventricular tachycardia.*
GI: abdominal pain, diarrhea, GI bleeding, nausea, vomiting.
GU: abnormal renal function, *hematuria,* urinary tract infection.
Hematologic: *anemia.*
Respiratory: cough, dyspnea, pneumonia, hemoptysis.
Other: groin bleeding, *allergic reactions,* brachial bleeding, infection, *sepsis.*

INTERACTIONS
Drug-drug. *Oral anticoagulants:* May prolong PT and INR and may increase the risk of bleeding. Monitor patient closely.
Thrombolytic agents: Increases risk of intracranial bleeding. Avoid using together.

EFFECTS ON LAB TESTS RESULTS
• May increase aPTT, ACT, PT, INR, and thrombin time. May decrease hemoglobin and hematocrit.

ACTION
Argatroban reversibly binds to the thrombin-active site and inhibits thrombin-catalyzed or -induced reactions, including fibrin formation, coagulation factor V, VIII, and XIII activation, protein C activation, and platelet aggregation. Argatroban can inhibit the action of free and clot-associated thrombin and doesn't need the cofactor antithrombin III for antithrombotic activity.

Reactions may be *common,* uncommon, ***life-threatening,*** or **COMMON AND LIFE-THREATENING.**

PHARMACOKINETICS
Onset, rapid; peak, 1 to 3 hours; duration, until the end of the infusion.
Distribution: Distributed mainly in the extracellular fluid with a steady-state volume of 174 ml/kg. Argatroban is 54% bound to human proteins, of which 34% is bound to a_1-acid glycoprotein and 20% to albumin.
Metabolism: Metabolized mainly in the liver by hydroxylation. The formation of four metabolites is catalyzed in the liver by the cytochrome P-450 enzymes CYP 3A4/5. The primary metabolite (M1) is 20% weaker than that of the parent drug. The other metabolites are detected in low concentrations in the urine.
Excretion: Primary excretion of argatroban is in the feces, presumably through the biliary tract. Half-life, 39 to 51 minutes.

CLINICAL CONSIDERATIONS
• *Alert:* Discontinue all parenteral anticoagulants before giving argatroban. Giving argatroban together with antiplatelets, thrombolytics, and other anticoagulants may increase the risk of bleeding.
• Obtain baseline coagulation tests, platelets, hemoglobin, and hematocrit before starting therapy.
• *Alert:* To treat or prevent HIT, monitor aPTT. Check aPTT 2 hours after giving drug; dose adjustments may be required to get a targeted aPTT of 1.5 to 3 times the baseline, no longer than 100 seconds. Steady state is achieved 1 to 3 hours after starting argatroban.
• *Alert:* Hemorrhage in patient receiving argatroban can occur at any site in the body. Any unexplained fall in hematocrit or blood pressure or any other unexplained symptoms may signal a hemorrhage.
• To convert to oral anticoagulant therapy, give warfarin P.O. with argatroban at up to 2 mcg/kg/minute until the INR exceeds 4. After argatroban is stopped,

check the INR in 4 to 6 hours. If the repeat INR is below the desired therapeutic range, resume the I.V. argatroban infusion. Repeat the procedure daily until the desired therapeutic range of warfarin alone is reached.
• Additional ACT should be drawn about every 20 to 30 minutes during a prolonged PCI procedure.
• *Alert:* Don't confuse argatroban with Aggrastat (tirofiban).
• Ask patient if she is pregnant, breastfeeding, or recently had a baby.

PATIENT TEACHING
• Tell patient to report immediately to prescriber any unusual bruising or bleeding (nosebleeds, bleeding gums, ecchymosis, or hematuria) or tarry or bloody stools.
• Advise patient to avoid activities that carry a risk of injury and to use a soft toothbrush and an electric razor while undergoing drug therapy.
• Instruct patient to tell prescriber if he experiences wheezing, trouble breathing, or skin rash.
• Tell patient to notify prescriber if he has GI ulcers, hepatic disease, recent surgery, radiation treatment, falling episodes, or injury.

arsenic trioxide
Trisenox

Pharmacologic class: arsenic trioxide
Therapeutic class: antineoplastic
Pregnancy risk category: D
pH: 7 to 9

INDICATIONS & DOSAGES
➤ **Acute promyelocytic leukemia (APL) in patients who have relapsed from, or are refractory to, retinoid and anthracycline chemotherapy, and whose APL is characterized by**

the t(15;17) translocation or PML/RAR-alpha gene expression—
Adults and children older than age 5: For induction phase, 0.15 mg/kg I.V. daily until bone marrow remission. Maximum 60 doses. For consolidation phase, 0.15 mg/kg I.V. daily for 25 doses over a period up to 5 weeks, beginning 3 to 6 weeks after completion of induction therapy.

ADMINISTRATION
Direct injection: Not recommended.
Intermittent infusion: Not recommended.
Continuous infusion: Infuse over 1 to 2 hours. If vasomotor reactions occur, infusion time may be extended up to 4 hours

PREPARATION & STORAGE
Available as a 10-mg single-use ampule containing a clear, colorless solution with a concentration of 1 mg/ml. Dilute with 100 to 250 ml of D_5W or normal saline injection. Discard any unused portions. Use the diluted drug within 24 hours if the solution is stored at room temperature and within 48 hours if the solution is refrigerated. Follow facility policy regarding preparation, handling, and disposal of antineoplastic drugs. The active ingredient is a carcinogen.

Incompatibilities
Other I.V. drugs.

CONTRAINDICATIONS & CAUTIONS
• Contraindicated in patients hypersensitive to arsenic.
• Use extreme caution in patients with renal impairment because arsenic is excreted renally.
• Use cautiously in patients with heart failure, prolonged QT interval, conditions that result in hypokalemia or hypomagnesemia, or a history of torsades de pointes.

• Caution woman of childbearing age to avoid becoming pregnant during therapy or to notify prescriber before becoming pregnant.

ADVERSE REACTIONS
CNS: *fever, headache, insomnia, paresthesia, dizziness,* tremor, **seizures,** somnolence, **coma,** *anxiety, depression, agitation, confusion, fatigue, weakness, pain.*
CV: tachycardia, PROLONGED QT INTERVAL, COMPLETE AV BLOCK, *palpitations, edema, chest pain,* ECG abnormalities, *hypotension, flushing, hypertension.*
EENT: *eye irritation, epistaxis, blurred vision,* dry eye, earache, tinnitus, *sore throat, postnasal drip,* eyelid edema, *sinusitis,* nasopharyngitis, painful red eye, oral blistering, oral candidiasis.
GI: *nausea, vomiting, diarrhea, anorexia, abdominal pain, constipation, loose stools, dyspepsia,* fecal incontinence, **GI hemorrhage,** dry mouth, abdominal tenderness or distention, bloody diarrhea.
GU: *renal failure,* renal impairment, oliguria, incontinence, **vaginal hemorrhage,** intermenstrual bleeding.
Hematologic: *hyperleukocytosis, anemia,* THROMBOCYTOPENIA, NEUTROPENIA, **APL differentiation syndrome, DIC, hemorrhage,** lymphadenopathy.
Metabolic: *hypokalemia, hypomagnesemia, hyperglycemia, hypocalcemia,* **hypoglycemia,** acidosis, *weight gain,* weight loss, HYPERKALEMIA.
Musculoskeletal: *arthralgia, myalgia, bone pain, back pain, neck pain, limb pain.*
Respiratory: *cough, dyspnea, hypoxia, pleural effusion, wheezing, decreased breath sounds, crepitations, rales,* hemoptysis, tachypnea, rhonchi, *upper respiratory tract infection.*
Skin: *dermatitis, pruritus, ecchymosis, dry skin, erythema, increased sweating,* night sweats, petechiae, hyperpigmen-

tation, urticaria, skin lesions, local exfoliation, *pallor, pain at injection site.*
Other: *drug hypersensitivity, rigors,* lymphadenopathy, facial edema, *herpes simplex infection,* bacterial infection, herpes zoster, **sepsis.**

INTERACTIONS

Drug-drug. *Drugs that can lead to electrolyte abnormalities, such as diuretics and amphotericin B:* Increases risk of electrolyte abnormalities. Use together cautiously.
Drugs that can prolong the QT interval, such as antiarrhythmics or thioridazine: May further prolong QT interval. Use together cautiously and monitor ECG closely.

EFFECTS ON LAB TEST RESULTS

• May increase ALT and AST levels. May decrease magnesium and calcium levels. May increase or decrease glucose and potassium levels.
• May increase WBC count. May decrease hemoglobin, hematocrit, and neutrophil and platelet counts.

ACTION

Although the mechanism of action for arsenic trioxide isn't completely understood, it's thought to cause morphologic changes and DNA fragmentation, and it may damage or degrade the fusion protein PML-RAR alpha, thereby killing promyelocytic leukemic cells.

PHARMACOKINETICS

Onset, peak, and duration of action are unknown.
Distribution: Unknown.
Metabolism: Metabolized in the liver by arsenate reductase to trivalent arsenic. Trivalent arsenic undergoes methylation reactions to dimethylarsinic acid. Stored mainly in the liver, kidney, heart, lung, hair, and nails.
Excretion: Excreted in the urine.

CLINICAL CONSIDERATIONS

• *Alert:* Arsenic trioxide can cause fatal arrhythmias and complete AV block.
• *Alert:* Arsenic trioxide has been linked to APL differentiation syndrome, characterized by fever, dyspnea, weight gain, pulmonary infiltrates, and pleural or pericardial effusions, with or without leukocytosis. This syndrome can be fatal and requires treatment with high-dose corticosteroids.
• Before starting drug, perform baseline ECG, obtain potassium, calcium, magnesium, and creatinine levels, and correct electrolyte abnormalities.
• Arsenic trioxide may increase or decrease blood pressure. Monitor blood pressure closely.
• Monitor electrolytes and hematologic and coagulation profiles at least twice weekly during treatment. Keep potassium levels above 4 mEq/dl and magnesium levels above 1.8 mg/dl.
• Monitor patient for syncope and rapid or irregular heart rate. If these occur, stop drug, hospitalize patient, and monitor electrolytes and QT interval. Drug may be restarted when electrolyte abnormalities are corrected and QTc interval falls below 460 msec.
• *Alert:* Monitor patient closely for any adverse reactions or signs or symptoms of acute toxicity. Symptoms of acute toxicity include confusion, muscle weakness, and seizures. If overdose occurs, immediately stop arsenic trioxide. Consider treatment with 3 mg/kg dimercaprol I.M. every 4 hours until life-threatening toxicity has subsided, followed by penicillamine 250 mg P.O. up to q.i.d. (up to 1 g daily).
• Monitor ECG at least weekly during therapy. Prolonged QTc interval commonly occurs between 1 and 5 weeks after infusion, and returns to baseline about 8 weeks after infusion. If QTc interval is higher than 500 msec at any time during therapy, assess patient closely and consider stopping drug.

PATIENT TEACHING

● Tell patient to report fever, shortness of breath, or weight gain immediately.
● Instruct patient to tell prescriber about all drugs he currently takes and to check with prescriber before starting any new drug.
● Inform diabetic patient that drug may cause hyperglycemia or hypoglycemia, and instruct him to monitor glucose level closely.
● Because of the potential for serious adverse reactions in breast-feeding infants, instruct patient to stop breast-feeding during therapy.

ascorbic acid (vitamin C)

Pharmacologic class: water-soluble vitamin
Therapeutic class: vitamin
Pregnancy risk category: A; C if recommended allowance exceeded
pH: 5.5 to 7

INDICATIONS & DOSAGES

➤ **Vitamin C deficiency—**
Adults: 100 to 250 mg I.V. once daily, b.i.d., or t.i.d.
Pregnant or breast-feeding women: 60 to 80 mg daily, not to exceed 1 g/day.
Children: 100 to 300 mg I.V. once daily, b.i.d., or t.i.d.
Infants: 50 to 100 mg I.V. daily.
➤ **Scurvy—**
Adults: 100 to 250 mg I.V. once or twice daily.
Infants and children: 100 to 300 mg I.V. daily in divided doses.

ADMINISTRATION

Direct injection: Slowly inject into vein over 2 to 3 minutes. Alternately, inject into I.V. tubing containing a compatible solution. Avoid rapid injection, which may cause transient dizziness or faintness.
Intermittent infusion: Infuse diluted drug over 20 to 30 minutes.
Continuous infusion: Add drug to compatible I.V. solution.

PREPARATION & STORAGE

Available in 500-mg/ml parenteral formulations. If the manufacturer recommends refrigerating it, do so.
    If needed, dilute drug in 50 to 100 ml of compatible solution.
    Solution remains stable at room temperature for 96 hours. Light exposure darkens drug but doesn't reduce its effectiveness.

Incompatibilities

Aminophylline, bleomycin, cefazolin, cephapirin, chloramphenicol, chlorothiazide, conjugated estrogens, erythromycin lactobionate, hydrocortisone, nafcillin, sodium bicarbonate.

CONTRAINDICATIONS & CAUTIONS

● Use cautiously in those with G6PD deficiency or renal failure.
● Avoid high doses in pregnant patients because of risk of scurvy in neonates. A neonate dependent on high doses of the drug may develop scurvy when doses of ascorbic acid are reduced or withdrawn.
● Avoid high doses in patients with hyperoxaluria because of risk of calculi.

ADVERSE REACTIONS

CNS: headache, fatigue, insomnia dizziness, faintness.
CV: leg swelling, flushing.
GI: nausea, diarrhea, abdominal cramps, heartburn, vomiting.
Skin: necrotic skin lesion, urticaria with doses exceeding 1 g/day, discomfort at injection site.

INTERACTIONS

Drug-drug. *Salicylates:* Inhibits ascorbic acid uptake by leukocytes and

---

platelets. Watch for symptoms of ascorbic acid deficiency.

Warfarin: May decrease warfarin activity. Monitor PT and INR.

Drug-herb. *Bearberry:* Inactivation of bearberry in urine. Discourage use together.

EFFECTS ON LAB TEST RESULTS
• May increase levels of urine calcium.
• May cause false-negative occult blood test results. May cause false-positive urine glucose results using Benedict's solution and false-negative results using glucose oxidase method.

ACTION
Vitamin is needed for collagen formation and tissue repair. It's involved in oxidation-reduction reactions throughout the body.

PHARMACOKINETICS
Onset, 15 to 60 minutes; duration, until deficiency resolves, usually in about 3 days.

Distribution: Throughout body tissues, especially liver, leukocytes, glandular tissue, and ocular lenses, with about 25% bound to proteins. Vitamin crosses placental barrier. Fetal levels are two to four times higher than maternal levels. Vitamin appears in breast milk.

Metabolism: Mainly in liver.

Excretion: Unchanged, in urine.

CLINICAL CONSIDERATIONS
• Therapeutic value of ascorbic acid is controversial when used for acne, anemia, burns, cancer, common cold, depression, fractures, hemorrhage, infections, infertility, and pressure sores.
• Prolonged use of high doses may increase metabolism.
• Infiltration may cause local tissue irritation and damage. Frequently assess I.V. site.
• Monitor patient for kidney stones (1 to 3 g); excessive oxalate secretion

is the result of ascorbic acid metabolism.
• Hemodialysis can remove vitamin.
• *Alert:* Drug may contain sulfites.

PATIENT TEACHING
• Explain to patient and family the use and administration of ascorbic acid.
• Tell patient to report adverse reactions promptly.
• Stress proper nutritional habits to prevent recurrence of deficiency.

asparaginase (colaspase, B-asparaginase)
Elspar, Kidrolase ◇

Pharmacologic class: enzyme (L-asparagine amidohydrolase, G_1–phase specific)
Therapeutic class: antineoplastic
Pregnancy risk category: C
pH: 7.4

INDICATIONS & DOSAGES
➤ **Induction phase of acute lymphocytic leukemia, combined with prednisone and vincristine—**
Children: 1,000 IU/kg I.V. daily for 10 days, starting on day 22 of the treatment period.
➤ **Induction phase of acute lymphocytic leukemia (as sole drug)—**
Adults and children: 200 IU/kg I.V. daily for 28 days. Dosage varies with protocol.

ADMINISTRATION
Direct injection: Not recommended.
Intermittent infusion: Start new I.V. site in distal vein to allow for successive venipunctures, if needed, using a 23G or 25G butterfly needle. Give drug through side port of rapidly infusing D_5W or normal saline solution and give over at least 30 minutes.

Continuous infusion: Not recommended.

PREPARATION & STORAGE
Available in 10,000-IU vials, which are stable for 2 years if kept at room temperature and 4 years if refrigerated. Reconstitute drug with 5 ml of normal saline solution without a preservative or sterile water for injection. Drug may be clear or slightly cloudy. Dilute in D_5W or normal saline solution within 8 hours after reconstitution.

Use extreme caution when preparing or giving drug to avoid mutagenic, teratogenic, and carcinogenic risks. Use a biological containment cabinet and avoid contact with skin. Wear mask and gloves. If solution comes in contact with skin or mucosa, immediately wash thoroughly with soap and water. Correctly dispose of needles, syringes, vials, and unused drug.

Incompatibilities
None reported.

CONTRAINDICATIONS & CAUTIONS
• Contraindicated in patients hypersensitive to the drug.
• Contraindicated in those with chickenpox, herpes, or recent exposure to these viral illnesses because of risk of severe, generalized disease and in those with pancreatitis or a history of it.
• Use cautiously in those with diabetes mellitus because of elevated glucose levels; in those with gout or history of urate stones because of increased uric acid levels; in patients with hepatic impairment because of heightened risk of hepatotoxicity; or in patients with infection because of increased risk of generalized disease.

ADVERSE REACTIONS
CNS: headache, irritability, *intracranial hemorrhage,* CNS toxicity, depression, somnolence, fatigue, *coma,* confusion, hallucinations, malaise.

CV: thrombophlebitis.
GI: anorexia, nausea, vomiting, abdominal cramps, *pancreatitis.*
GU: glycosuria, polyuria, *renal failure.*
Hematologic: *hypofibrinogenemia, bone marrow suppression, thrombocytopenia, neutropenia.*
Hepatic: *hepatotoxicity.*
Metabolic: hyperglycemia, weight loss, hypocholesterolemia, hyperuricemia.
Other: *anaphylaxis,* allergic reactions, *death, fatal hyperthermia.*

INTERACTIONS
Drug-drug. *Methotrexate:* Decreases methotrexate effectiveness. Avoid using together.
Prednisone, vincristine: Increases toxicity. Monitor patient for signs of toxicity.

EFFECTS ON LAB TEST RESULTS
• May increase creatinine, BUN, AST, ALT, alkaline phosphatase, bilirubin, glucose, uric acid, and ammonia levels. May decrease cholesterol, fibrinogen, and albumin levels.
• May decrease hemoglobin, hematocrit, and thyroid-binding globulin, platelet, and WBC counts.

ACTION
Derived from *Escherichia coli,* this enzyme depletes neoplastic cells of exogenous asparagine, thus inhibiting the DNA and protein synthesis essential for neoplastic cell survival.

PHARMACOKINETICS
Onset, immediate in plasma; duration, 23 to 33 days; active enzyme can be detected in plasma.
Distribution: Minimal outside vascular compartment. Drug doesn't cross blood-brain barrier.
Metabolism: Unknown.

Reactions may be *common,* uncommon, *life-threatening,* or COMMON AND LIFE-THREATENING.

Excretion: Unknown. Drug isn't excreted in urine. Initial half-life, 4 to 9 hours; terminal half-life, 1 to 5 days.

CLINICAL CONSIDERATIONS

• *Alert:* Skin testing and desensitization are mandatory before first dose or if longer than 1 week has elapsed between treatments. Life-threatening hypersensitivity occurs in 20% to 35% of patients. For skin test, inject 2 IU intradermally at least 1 week before first asparaginase dose, and observe injection site for at least 1 hour for flare or wheal. If skin test results are abnormal or if patient was previously treated with asparaginase, desensitize by gradually increasing I.V. doses until reaching ordered daily dose, provided no allergic reaction occurs. Normal skin test results don't rule out future allergic reactions. Keep emergency equipment nearby during therapy.

• Risk of hypersensitivity is lower with daily dose schedule than with weekly one and rises with repeated courses of therapy. Give drug in a hospital under direction of an experienced prescriber.

• Adequate hydration, alkalization of urine, and allopurinol administration may reduce the risk of uric acid nephropathy.

• Patients taking an antidiabetic or an antigout drug may require increased dosages because asparaginase raises glucose and uric acid levels.

• Loss of potency has been observed with use of 0.2-micron filter.

• Drug has low therapeutic index; therapeutic effects are unlikely without some signs of toxic reaction.

• Resistance to cytotoxic effects of drug develops rapidly.

• Monitor CBC, serum amylase, blood and urine glucose, hepatic and renal function test results.

• Keep epinephrine, diphenhydramine, and I.V. corticosteroids available for treatment of anaphylaxis.

• Observe patient for signs of CNS toxicity or thromboembolism. Be especially alert for dyspnea and chest pain, which may indicate pulmonary embolism.

PATIENT TEACHING

• Tell women not to breast-feed during therapy because of potential adverse effects on infant.

• Teach patient to recognize signs of hepatic impairment—jaundice, dark orange urine, and clay-colored stools.

• Tell patient to watch for signs and symptoms of infection, such as fever, sore throat, and fatigue, and of bleeding, such as easy bruising, nosebleeds, bleeding gums, and melena, and to take his temperature daily.

• Stress the importance of maintaining an adequate fluid intake to help prevent hyperuricemia. If adverse GI reactions prevent patient from drinking fluids, tell him to notify prescriber.

---

atenolol
Tenormin

Pharmacologic class: beta blocker
Therapeutic class: antianginal
Pregnancy risk category: D
pH: 5.5 to 6.5

INDICATIONS & DOSAGES

➤ **Reduce CV mortality and risk of reinfarction in hemodynamically stable patients who have survived the acute phase of an MI—**
Adults: 5 mg I.V., followed in 10 minutes by another 5 mg I.V. Start oral therapy 10 minutes after the final I.V. dose in patient who can tolerate the full I.V. dose. Give 50 mg P.O., followed 12 hours later by another 50 mg dose. Then give 50 mg b.i.d. or 100 mg once daily P.O. for at least 6 to 9 days, or until patient is discharged from the hospi-

---

tal. If not contraindicated, therapy may be continued for 1 to 3 years.
➤ **To slow rapid ventricular response to atrial fibrillation following acute MI without left ventricular dysfunction and AV block** ◆ —
Adults: 2.5 to 5 mg I.V. over 2 to 5 minutes p.r.n., to control rate. Don't exceed 10 mg over a 10- to 15-minute period.

ADMINISTRATION
Direct injection: Give over at least 5 minutes into a large vein.
Intermittent infusion: Not recommended.
Continuous infusion: Not recommended.

PREPARATION & STORAGE
Available in 10-ml ampules containing 5 mg atenolol. Store the drug at room temperature (59° to 86° F [15° to 30° C]) and protect it from light. Dilute with normal saline solution, D_5W, or saline and dextrose injection. Dilutions are stable for 48 hours.

Incompatibilities
Other I.V. drugs.

CONTRAINDICATIONS & CAUTIONS
• Contraindicated in those with sinus bradycardia, heart block greater than first degree, cardiogenic shock, or overt cardiac failure.
• Contraindicated in those with an acute MI accompanied by cardiac failure that isn't effectively and promptly controlled and in hypotensive patients.
• Use cautiously in patients with history of bronchospastic disease. The relative selectivity of atenolol for beta$_1$ receptors may allow drug to be used in this condition. Have a bronchodilator available, preferably a beta$_2$ stimulant.
• Use cautiously in diabetic patients. Beta blockers may block some symptoms of hypoglycemia.
• Use cautiously in those with heart failure controlled by cardiac glycosides

or diuretics. Intrinsic sympathetic stimulation is needed to support circulatory function in heart failure, and excessive beta blockade may exacerbate heart failure.

ADVERSE REACTIONS
CNS: dizziness, light-headedness, depression, fatigue, fever.
CV: *heart failure,* hypotension, cold extremities, *bradycardia,* peripheral vascular disease.
GI: nausea, vomiting, diarrhea.
Respiratory: dyspnea, *bronchospasm.*
Skin: rash.

INTERACTIONS
Drug-drug. *Antihypertensives:* Enhances hypotensive effect. Monitor blood pressure.
Cardiac glycosides, diltiazem, verapamil: Causes excessive bradycardia and increases depressant effect on myocardium. Use together cautiously and monitor ECG closely.
Insulin, oral antidiabetics: May alter dosage requirements in diabetic patients whose condition was previously stabilized. Monitor glucose level.
Reserpine: May cause hypotension. Monitor blood pressure.

EFFECTS ON LAB TEST RESULTS
• May increase BUN, creatinine, potassium, uric acid, glucose, transaminase, alkaline phosphatase, and LDH levels. May decrease glucose level.
• May increase platelet count.

ACTION
The mechanism whereby atenolol, a cardioselective beta$_1$ blocker, improves survival in patients with an MI is unknown. It reduces the frequency of ventricular premature beats, reduces chest pain, reduces myocardial oxygen consumption, and inhibits cardiac muscle enzyme level elevation after MI.

PHARMACOKINETICS
Levels peak within 5 minutes after I.V. administration; elimination half-life, 6 to 7 hours.
Distribution: Into most tissues. Drug crosses the placental barrier and is 5% to 15% bound to plasma proteins. Drug appears in breast milk.
Metabolism: Not metabolized.
Excretion: Primarily renal. Over 85% of an I.V. dose is excreted in the urine within 24 hours.

CLINICAL CONSIDERATIONS
• *Alert:* Administration of I.V. atenolol should be restricted to a critical care area such as the cardiac care unit.
• During the acute phase of an MI, beta blocker therapy should supplement standard cardiac care unit treatment.
• I.V. atenolol affords a rapid onset of the protective effects of beta blockade against reinfarction. I.V. route is preferred immediately after MI because gastric absorption may be delayed in the early phase of an MI. This may be a result of physiologic changes linked to the MI or of decreased GI motility caused by morphine administration. Oral therapy alone may still provide benefits.
• Give drug as soon as patient's eligibility is established and his hemodynamic condition has stabilized. A reduction in mortality appears to be most significant during the first 24 hours after infarct.
• Patients with renal failure may need their dosage adjusted.
• During administration, monitor patient's blood pressure, heart rate, and ECG readings. Stop drug if significant hypotension or bradycardia occurs.
• If patient can't tolerate I.V. atenolol, he may still be a candidate for oral therapy. Give 100 mg of atenolol daily P.O., either as 50 mg b.i.d. or 100 mg once daily, for at least 7 days.
• Closely monitor I.V. administration of atenolol in patients who may have thyroid disease. Beta blockade may mask certain signs of hyperthyroidism.
• If overdose occurs, provide symptomatic treatment for drug overdose. Hemodialysis removes atenolol from general circulation.

PATIENT TEACHING
• Explain to patient and family the use and administration of atenolol. Encourage them to ask questions and express concerns.
• Teach patient about drug's adverse reactions and tell him to report them promptly.

atracurium besylate
Tracrium*

Pharmacologic class: competitive, nondepolarizing neuromuscular blocker
Therapeutic class: skeletal muscle relaxant
Pregnancy risk category: C
pH: 3.25 to 3.65

INDICATIONS & DOSAGES
➤ **To facilitate endotracheal intubation and muscle relaxation during surgery or mechanical ventilation—**
Adults: Initially, 0.4 to 0.5 mg/kg I.V., which is double the dose needed for nearly complete neuromuscular blockade. Maintenance dose of 0.08 to 0.1 mg/kg, p.r.n., depending on patient response.
Children ages 1 month to 2 years: Initially, 0.3 to 0.4 mg/kg I.V. Frequent maintenance doses may be needed.
  Dosage must be individualized.

ADMINISTRATION
Only staff trained in giving I.V. anesthetics and managing adverse reactions should give drug.

Direct injection: Inject rapidly into an I.V. line containing a free-flowing, compatible solution.

Intermittent infusion: Infuse diluted drug into I.V. line containing a compatible solution, as needed, during procedure.

Continuous infusion: After direct injection, give at 5 to 10 mcg/kg/minute during procedure.

PREPARATION & STORAGE

Available in 5-ml and 10-ml ampules with 0.9 % benzyl alcohol. Each milliliter contains 10 mg of drug. Refrigerate at 36° to 46° F (2° to 8° C). Don't freeze. Dilute the drug with D_5W or normal saline solution for intermittent or continuous infusion.

Concentrations of 0.2 or 0.5 mg/ml are stable for 24 hours at room temperature or refrigerated.

Incompatibilities

Alkaline solutions because of drug's acid pH, lactated Ringer's solution.

CONTRAINDICATIONS & CAUTIONS

• Contraindicated in patients hypersensitive to the drug.

• Use cautiously in those with a history of severe anaphylactic reaction, asthma, or disorders exacerbated by substantial histamine release.

• Use cautiously in those with bronchogenic cancer and such neuromuscular diseases as myasthenia gravis and Eaton-Lambert syndrome because drug potentiates neuromuscular blockade, in those with hypotension because drug may exacerbate the condition, and in those with pulmonary impairment because drug deepens respiratory depression.

• Use cautiously in those with hyperthermia because drug's duration of action may be intensified or prolonged.

• Use cautiously in patients with electrolyte imbalance or dehydration, which may alter drug action.

ADVERSE REACTIONS

CV: *bradycardia,* tachycardia, hypotension, flushing.

Respiratory: increased bronchial secretions, *prolonged dose-related apnea, bronchospasm, laryngospasm,* wheezing.

Skin: erythema, pruritus, urticaria, rash.

Other: *anaphylaxis.*

INTERACTIONS

Drug-drug. *Aminoglycoside antibiotics, corticosteroids, lithium, magnesium, procainamide, quinidine, succinylcholine, thiazide diuretics, verapamil:* Potentiates neuromuscular blockade. Use cautiously during and after surgery.

Edrophonium, neostigmine, pyridostigmine: Reverses neuromuscular blockade. Monitor patient closely.

Lithium, magnesium salts, opioid analgesics: Increases skeletal muscle relaxation and may cause respiratory paralysis. Reduce dose of atracurium.

Phenytoin, theophylline: Resistance to or reversal of neuromuscular blockade. Monitor patient closely.

Succinylcholine: Quickens onset and may increase depth of neuromuscular blockade. Monitor patient.

EFFECTS ON LAB TEST RESULTS

None reported.

ACTION

Produces muscle relaxation by blocking acetylcholine's effect at the myoneural junction. This action prevents muscle depolarization and leads to short-term paralysis.

PHARMACOKINETICS

Onset is dose-related; 0.4 to 0.5 mg/kg produces maximum neuromuscular blockade in 3 to 5 minutes; duration, 20 to 35 minutes for effects to start subsiding and 60 to 70 minutes for them to end.

Reactions may be *common,* uncommon, *life-threatening,* or COMMON AND LIFE-THREATENING.

Distribution: Into extracellular space. Drug crosses placental barrier and is 82% bound to plasma proteins. It's unknown if drug appears in breast milk.
Metabolism: Rapid, by enzymatic pathways—nonoxidative ester hydrolysis catalyzed by nonspecific esterase—and nonenzymatic pathways via Hofmann elimination, a chemical degradation.
Excretion: In urine and bile, with a small fraction unchanged. About 90% of drug is eliminated in 7 hours.

CLINICAL CONSIDERATIONS
• Osmolality: 22 mOsm/kg (10 mg/ml atracurium).
• Size of first dose depends on degree of muscle relaxation needed and whether drug will be combined with inhalation anesthetics or narcotics. When possible, use a peripheral nerve stimulator to assess depth of blockade and to determine subsequent doses.
• Ensure adequate sedation during therapy.
• Maintenance doses have no cumulative effect on duration of neuromuscular blockade if recovery is allowed to begin before their administration.
• *Alert:* Keep emergency resuscitation equipment available at all times.
• Maintain a patent airway.
• Make sure corneas are protected because patient will be unable to blink.
• Patient won't have usual reflexes, such as cough and gag reflexes, while under effects of drug, except for pupillary constriction to light.
• If overdose occurs, maintain a patent airway and assist breathing, as needed. Give fluids and vasopressors for hypotension and edrophonium, neostigmine, or pyridostigmine for neuromuscular blockade. Usually reverses in 8 to 10 minutes.
• Reduce dose and administration rate in patients in whom histamine release may be hazardous.
• Previous administration of succinylcholine doesn't prolong duration of action of atracurium, but it quickens onset and may deepen neuromuscular blockade.
• Atracurium has a longer duration of action than succinylcholine and a shorter duration than tubocurarine or pancuronium.
• Drug has little or no effect on heart rate and doesn't counteract or reverse the bradycardia caused by anesthetics or vagal stimulation. Thus, bradycardia is seen more frequently with atracurium than with other neuromuscular blocking agents. Pretreatment with anticholinergics (atropine or glycopyrrolate) is advised.
• *Alert:* Use drug only if endotracheal intubation, administration of oxygen under positive pressure, artificial respiration, and assisted or controlled ventilation are immediately available.
• Until head and neck muscles recover from blockade effects, patient may find speech difficult.
• Assess need for pain medication or sedation. Drug doesn't affect consciousness or relieve pain.
• Recommend monitoring for bradycardia during administration; patient may require I.V. atropine.
• Use a peripheral nerve stimulator to monitor responses during ICU administration; it may be used to detect residual paralysis during recovery and to avoid atracurium overdose.

PATIENT TEACHING
• Explain to patient and family how drug works and is given. Tell them patient will be closely monitored during therapy and his needs anticipated because he'll be unable to move or communicate.
• Explain all procedures to patient during therapy because he can still hear.

atropine sulfate

Pharmacologic class: anticholinergic, belladonna alkaloid
Therapeutic class: antiarrhythmic, vagolytic
Pregnancy risk category: C
pH: 3 to 6.5

INDICATIONS & DOSAGES
➤ **Symptomatic bradycardia—**
Adults: 0.5 to 1 mg I.V. q 5 minutes until desired heart rate, usually 60 beats/minute, is reached. Maximum total dose, 3 mg; minimum dose, 0.5 mg. Lower dose could cause paradoxical bradycardia by vagal stimulation.
➤ **Ventricular asystole in advanced life support—**
Adults: 1 mg I.V. q 5 minutes.
Adolescents and children: 0.02 mg/kg I.V. in children, minimum 0.1 mg; maximum 1 mg q 5 minutes, if needed. In adolescents, maximum total dose is 2 mg.
➤ **Blocked muscarinic effects of anticholinesterases—**
Adults: 0.6 to 1.2 mg I.V. for each 0.5 to 2.5 mg of neostigmine methylsulfate or each 10 to 20 mg of pyridostigmine bromide.
➤ **Antidote for anticholinesterase toxicity—**
Adults: Initially, 1 to 2 mg I.V., then 2 mg q 5 to 60 minutes until symptoms subside. In severe cases, first dose may be as much as 6 mg q 5 to 60 minutes, p.r.n.

ADMINISTRATION
Direct injection: Inject prescribed amount of undiluted drug into vein or I.V. tubing over 1 to 2 minutes.
Intermittent infusion: Not recommended.
Continuous infusion: Not recommended.

PREPARATION & STORAGE
Available in single-dose ampules or vials of 0.3 mg/ml, 0.4 mg/ml, 0.5 mg/ml, 0.8 mg/ml, and 1 mg/ml; in multidose 20-ml vials of 0.4 mg/ml; in multidose 30-ml vials of 0.3 mg/ml and 0.4 mg/ml; and in prefilled syringes containing 0.5, 0.8, and 1 mg of drug. Store at room temperature.

Incompatibilities
Alkalies, bromides, iodides, isoproterenol, methohexital, norepinephrine, pentobarbital sodium, sodium bicarbonate.

CONTRAINDICATIONS & CAUTIONS
● Contraindicated in those with glaucoma, except those with open-angle glaucoma who are being treated with miotics, because drug may raise intraocular pressure.
● Contraindicated in those with myasthenia gravis, obstructive uropathy, or unstable CV status caused by acute hemorrhage.
● Use cautiously in those with autonomic neuropathy, benign prostatic hyperplasia, or other obstructive uropathy because drug may cause urine retention; in children with brain damage because drug may exacerbate CNS effects; in those with hypertension or pregnancy-induced hypertension because drug may aggravate the condition; and in those with xerostomia because drug may further decrease salivary flow.
● Use cautiously in those with Down syndrome because of abnormal pupillary dilation and tachycardia; in those with reflux esophagitis because of increased reflux; in those with fever because of possible suppressed sweat gland secretions; in those with hepatic or renal impairment because of decreased drug metabolism or excretion; in those with hyperthyroidism because of risk of severe tachycardia; and in those with obstructive GI disease, in-

testinal atony, paralytic ileus, or ulcerative colitis because of impaired motility.
• Use cautiously in patients with tachycardia that threatens to cause cardiac decompensation.

ADVERSE REACTIONS
CNS: dizziness, headache, ataxia, confusion, delirium, drowsiness, insomnia, light-headedness, nervousness, restlessness, *coma.*
CV: tachycardia, *aggravated AV block, ventricular fibrillation, ventricular tachycardia,* flushing.
EENT: *blurred vision,* increased intraocular pressure, *mydriasis,* photophobia.
GI: nausea, *dry mouth,* vomiting, bloating, constipation.
GU: urinary hesitancy, urine retention.
Skin: *local irritation at injection site,* rash, urticaria, decreased sweating.
Other: *anaphylaxis.*

INTERACTIONS
Drug-drug. *Anticholinergics:* Causes additive effects. Monitor patient closely.
Digoxin: May elevate digoxin levels. Monitor digoxin levels.
Levodopa, ketoconazole: Reduces absorption. Avoid using together.
Potassium chloride supplements (extended-release oral preparations): Increases risk of GI lesions. Avoid using together.
Drug-herb. *Jaborandi tree, pill-bearing spurge:* Decreases effectiveness of drug. Discourage use together.
Jimsonweed: May adversely affect CV function. Discourage use together.
Squaw vine: May decrease metabolic breakdown. Discourage use together.

EFFECTS ON LAB TEST RESULTS
None reported.

ACTION
Binds to postganglionic receptors and blocks acetylcholine, thereby obstruct-

ing vagal effects on the SA node and increasing heart rate. Increases conduction through the AV node. Has antimuscarinic effects on bronchial and intestinal smooth muscle.

PHARMACOKINETICS
Onset, 2 to 4 minutes; duration, 4 to 6 hours.
Distribution: Throughout body tissues and across the blood-brain and placental barriers; 18% of drug binds to albumin. Trace amounts appear in breast milk.
Metabolism: In liver, into several metabolites, including tropine acids and esters.
Excretion: Mainly in urine, with small amounts in feces and expired air. Half-life, 2 to 3 hours.

CLINICAL CONSIDERATIONS
• *Alert:* Watch for tachycardia in cardiac patients because the drug may precipitate ventricular fibrillation.
• Monitor blood pressure closely to evaluate drug tolerance.
• Initial drug bolus may cause bradycardia, which usually resolves in 1 to 2 minutes.
• Monitor ECG for patients receiving drug for bradycardia or heart block. Watch for heart rate exceeding 100 beats/minute, increased PVCs, and ventricular tachycardia. Notify prescriber if any of these occur.
• Encourage patient to drink fluids and provide mouth care when appropriate.
• Patients sensitive to other belladonna alkaloids or salicylates may show atropine intolerance.
• Assess for urine retention by monitoring intake and output. Palpate patient's bladder every 4 hours.
• When assessing patient with CNS injury who has received atropine, realize that his pupil size isn't a reliable diagnostic sign.
• If overdose occurs, give fluids for shock, diazepam for CNS irritability,

pilocarpine for mydriasis, and cooling blanket for hyperthermia. Catheterize patient to prevent urine retention. Provide respiratory support and possibly give physostigmine to treat delirium, hallucinations, coma, or supraventricular tachycardia.

PATIENT TEACHING
● Explain to patient and family the drug's use, administration, and adverse effects.
● Tell patient to report adverse reactions promptly.
● Tell patient to report discomfort at I.V. site promptly.

azithromycin
Zithromax

Pharmacologic class: azalide macrolide
Therapeutic class: antibiotic
Pregnancy risk category: B
pH: 6.4 to 6.8

INDICATIONS & DOSAGES
➤ **Community-acquired pneumonia caused by** *Chlamydia pneumoniae, H. influenzae, Mycoplasma pneumonia, Streptococcus pneumoniae; Legionella pneumophila, M. catarrhalis,* **and** *Staphylococcus aureus*—
Adults and adolescents ages 16 and older: 500 mg I.V. as a single daily dose for 2 days, followed by 500 mg P.O. as a single daily dose to complete a 7- to 10-day course of therapy.
➤ **Pelvic inflammatory disease caused by** *C. trachomatis, Neisseria gonorrhoeae,* **or** *M. hominis*—
Adults and adolescents age 16 and older: 500 mg I.V. as a single daily dose for 1 to 2 days, followed by 250 mg P.O. daily to complete a 7-day course of therapy.

ADMINISTRATION
Direct injection: Not recommended.
Intermittent infusion: Infuse a 500-mg dose over 1 hour or more.
Continuous infusion: Not recommended.

PREPARATION & STORAGE
Reconstitute 500 mg vial with 4.8 ml of sterile water for injection and shake well until dissolved to yield a concentration of 100 mg/ml. Dilute solution further in at least 250 ml of normal saline solution, half-normal saline solution, D_5W, or lactated Ringer's solution to yield a final concentration between 1 and 2 mg/ml.

Reconstituted solution is stable for 24 hours when stored below 86° F (30° C).

Incompatibilities
None reported.

CONTRAINDICATIONS & CAUTIONS
● Contraindicated in patients hypersensitive to erythromycin or other macrolides.

ADVERSE REACTIONS
CNS: dizziness, vertigo, headache, fatigue, somnolence.
CV: palpitations, chest pain.
GI: nausea, vomiting, diarrhea, abdominal pain, dyspepsia, flatulence, melena, *pseudomembranous colitis.*
GU: candidiasis, vaginitis, nephritis.
Hepatic: cholestatic jaundice.
Skin: rash, photosensitivity.
Other: *angioedema.*

INTERACTIONS
Drug-drug. *Carbamazepine, cyclosporine, phenytoin:* May increase levels of these drugs. Monitor drug levels.
Digoxin: May increase digoxin level. Monitor digoxin level.
Ergotamine: Causes acute ergotamine toxicity. Monitor patient closely.

Reactions may be *common*, uncommon, *life-threatening*, or COMMON AND LIFE-THREATENING.

Pimozide: Prolongs QT interval and ventricular tachycardia. Monitor ECG closely.

Theophylline: May increase theophylline level. Monitor theophylline level.

Triazolam: May decrease clearance of triazolam. Monitor patient for increased adverse effects.

Warfarin: May increase INR. Monitor INR closely.

Drug-lifestyle. *Sun exposure:* May cause photosensitivity reactions. Advise patient to avoid excessive sunlight exposure.

EFFECTS ON LAB TEST RESULTS
None reported.

ACTION
Binds to the 50S subunit of bacterial ribosomes, blocking protein synthesis; bacteriostatic or bactericidal, depending on concentration.

PHARMACOKINETICS
Onset, unknown; peak, unknown; duration, unknown.

Distribution: Unknown.
Metabolism: Unknown.
Excretion: Unknown.

CLINICAL CONSIDERATIONS
● Obtain specimen for culture and sensitivity tests before giving first dose. Therapy may begin pending results.
● The move from I.V. to P.O. therapy should be at the prescriber's discretion and should be based on patient response.
● Monitor for superinfection. May cause overgrowth of nonsusceptible bacteria or fungi.

PATIENT TEACHING
● Tell patient to take drug as prescribed, even after he feels better.
● Advise patient to report signs of a rash or itching to his prescriber.

aztreonam
Azactam

Pharmacologic class: monobactam
Therapeutic class: antibiotic
Pregnancy risk category: B
pH: 4.5 to 7.5

INDICATIONS & DOSAGES
➤ **Infections of the respiratory or GU tract, bone, skin, and soft tissues caused by susceptible organisms—**
Adults: 500 mg to 2 g I.V. q 8 to 12 hours. For severe systemic or life-threatening infections, give 2 g q 6 to 8 hours. Maximum daily dose is 8 g.

Adjust-a-dose: If estimated creatinine clearance is 10 to 30 ml/minute, decrease dosage by 50% after an initial 1 to 2 g loading dose; if clearance is less than 10 ml/minute or patient is on hemodialysis, give the first dose of 500 mg to 2 g, then give 25% of the usual dose at the usual fixed intervals of 6, 8, or 12 hours. For serious or life-threatening infections, give ⅛ of the first dose after each hemodialysis session in addition to the maintenance doses.

Children age 9 months and older: For mild to moderate infections, 30 mg/kg I.V. q 8 hours; for moderate to severe infections, 30 mg/kg q 6 or 8 hours. Maximum dose of 120 mg/kg/day.

ADMINISTRATION
Direct injection: Using a 21G to 23G needle, inject reconstituted drug over 3 to 5 minutes into vein or I.V. line containing a free-flowing, compatible solution.

Intermittent infusion: Over 20 to 60 minutes, infuse into I.V. tubing of a free-flowing, compatible solution, or give using a volume-control device. If you're using a volume-control device,

final dilution shouldn't exceed 2%, or 20 mg/ml.
Continuous infusion: Not recommended.

PREPARATION & STORAGE

Available in 15-ml vials or 100-ml piggyback infusion bottles containing 500 mg, 1 g, or 2 g of drug; and 30-ml vial containing 2 g. For direct injection, add 6 to 10 ml of sterile water for injection to vial and shake well. For infusion, add at least 3 ml sterile water for each g of drug. Dilute with 50 to 100 ml of normal saline solution, D_5W, dextrose 5% in normal saline injection, or lactated Ringer's solution. Solutions reconstituted with normal saline solution or sterile water remain potent for 48 hours if kept at room temperature and for 7 days if refrigerated. Slight pink tint doesn't affect potency.

Before reconstitution, store drug at room temperature. After reconstitution, promptly use any solution over 2% concentration and discard the unused amount.

Incompatibilities

Ampicillin sodium, cephradine, metronidazole, nafcillin, other I.V. drugs, vancomycin.

CONTRAINDICATIONS & CAUTIONS

• Contraindicated in patients hypersensitive to the drug.
• Use cautiously in patients hypersensitive to penicillins or cephalosporins, in geriatric patients, and in those with renal impairment.

ADVERSE REACTIONS

CV: phlebitis, thrombophlebitis.
GI: altered taste, nausea, vomiting, diarrhea.
Hematologic: *neutropenia,* anemia, *pancytopenia, thrombocytopenia,* leukocytosis, thrombocytosis.
Skin: discomfort or swelling at injection site, rash.

Other: bacterial or fungal superinfections, *anaphylaxis.*

INTERACTIONS

Drug-drug. *Aminoglycosides, beta-lactam antibiotics, other anti-infectives:* Causes synergistic effectiveness; may be used together for this effect. Monitor patient closely.
Cefoxitin, imipenem and cilastatin: May cause antagonistic effect. Avoid using together.
Furosemide, probenecid: Increases aztreonam level. Avoid using together.

EFFECTS ON LAB TEST RESULTS

• May increase BUN, creatinine, ALT, AST, and LDH levels.
• May increase PT, PTT, and INR. May decrease hemoglobin, hematocrit, and neutrophil and RBC counts. May increase or decrease WBC and platelet counts.
• May cause false-positive results in Coombs' test and in urine glucose test when copper sulfate (Benedict's solution, Clinitest) is used.

ACTION

A narrow-spectrum, bactericidal monobactam antibiotic, aztreonam inhibits bacterial cell wall synthesis, causing cell wall destruction. It's effective against many gram-negative aerobic bacteria, including *Neisseria meningitidis, N. gonorrhoeae, Haemophilus influenzae, Moraxella catarrhalis, Citrobacter diversus, Enterobacter agglomerans, Escherichia coli, Hafnia alvei, Klebsiella pneumoniae, Morganella morganii, Proteus mirabilis, P. vulgaris, Providencia, Serratia marcescens, Salmonella, Shigella, Pasteurella multocida,* and *Pseudomonas aeruginosa.*

Aztreonam exerts little or no effect against gram-positive aerobic bacteria, anaerobic bacteria, *Chlamydia,* fungi, *Mycoplasma,* or viruses. It's usually

---

Reactions may be *common,* uncommon, *life-threatening,* or COMMON AND LIFE-THREATENING.

combined with other antibiotics for life-threatening infections.

PHARMACOKINETICS

Level peaks 2 to 3 minutes after a single dose by I.V. injection; duration, 6 to 8 hours.

Distribution: Widely distributed in fluids and tissues, with 40% to 60% bound to proteins. CSF level is higher when meninges are inflamed. Drug crosses placental barrier and appears in breast milk.

Metabolism: Hydrolysis of the beta-lactam ring metabolizes 6% to 16% of drug to inactive metabolites.

Excretion: In urine, primarily as unchanged drug, by glomerular filtration and renal tubular secretion. In patients with normal renal function, half-life averages about 90 minutes.

CLINICAL CONSIDERATIONS

● Obtain specimens for culture and sensitivity testing before giving first dose. Therapy may start before results are available.

● Aztreonam's effectiveness against gram-negative organisms is comparable to that of the aminoglycosides but without their ototoxic or nephrotoxic adverse effects.

● Check for previous antibiotic hypersensitivity. Normal history doesn't rule out future allergic reaction.

● Monitor for phlebitis at infusion site.

● Monitor BUN and creatinine levels during therapy. Patients with renal dysfunction or geriatric patients may need their dosage adjusted.

● Observe patient for fungal and bacterial superinfection with prolonged use.

● If overdose occurs, hemodialysis, peritoneal dialysis, or both may be used to clear aztreonam from serum.

PATIENT TEACHING

● Explain to patient and family the use and administration of aztreonam.

● Tell patient to report adverse reactions promptly.

● Tell patient to alert nurse if discomfort occurs at I.V. site.

basiliximab
Simulect

Pharmacologic class: chimeric (murine or human) monoclonal antibody (IgG1k)
Therapeutic class: interleukin-2 (IL-2) receptor antagonist
Pregnancy risk category: B

INDICATIONS & DOSAGES
➤ **To prevent acute organ rejection in patients receiving renal transplantation when used as part of an immunosuppressive regimen that includes cyclosporine and corticosteroids—**
Adults and children weighing 35 kg (77 lb) or more: 20 mg I.V. given within 2 hours before transplant surgery and 20 mg I.V. given 4 days after transplantation.
Children weighing less than 35 kg: 10 mg I.V. given within 2 hours before transplant surgery and 10 mg I.V. given 4 days after transplantation.

ADMINISTRATION
Direct injection: Not recommended.
Intermittent infusion: Infuse drug over 20 to 30 minutes via a central or peripheral vein.
Continuous infusion: Not recommended.

PREPARATION & STORAGE
Supplied as 20 mg powder for injection in single-use vials.

When mixing solution, gently invert bag to avoid foaming. Don't shake. Reconstitute with 5 ml of sterile water for injection. Shake vial gently to dissolve powder. Dilute reconstituted solution to a volume of 50 ml with normal saline or dextrose 5% for infusion.

Use reconstituted solution immediately, or refrigerate it at 36° to 46° F (2° to 8° C) for up to 24 hours, or keep it at room temperature for up to 4 hours.

Incompatibilities
Other I.V. drugs.

CONTRAINDICATIONS & CAUTIONS
• Contraindicated in those hypersensitive to the drug or its components.
• Use cautiously in geriatric patients.

ADVERSE REACTIONS
CNS: agitation, anxiety, asthenia, depression, *dizziness, headache,* hypoesthesia, *insomnia,* neuropathy, paresthesia, *tremor,* fatigue, *fever.*
CV: abnormal heart sounds, angina pectoris, **arrhythmias,** atrial fibrillation, **heart failure,** chest pain, *general edema, hypertension,* hypotension, *leg or peripheral edema,* tachycardia.
EENT: abnormal vision, cataract, conjunctivitis, *pharyngitis, rhinitis,* sinusitis.
GI: *abdominal pain, candidiasis, constipation, diarrhea, dyspepsia,* esophagitis, enlarged abdomen, flatulence, gastroenteritis, GI disorder, **GI hemorrhage,** gum hyperplasia, melena, *nausea,* ulcerative stomatitis, *vomiting.*
GU: abnormal renal function, albuminuria, bladder disorder, *dysuria,* frequent micturition, genital edema in men, hematuria, impotence, *increased nonprotein nitrogen levels,* oliguria, renal tubular necrosis, ureteral disorder, *UTI,* urine retention.

Hematologic: *anemia,* hematoma, ***hemorrhage,*** polycythemia, purpura, ***thrombocytopenia,*** thrombosis.
Metabolic: *acidosis,* dehydration, diabetes mellitus, fluid overload, hypercalcemia, *hypercholesterolemia, hyperglycemia, hyperkalemia,* hyperlipidemia, *hyperuricemia, hypocalcemia, hypokalemia,* hypomagnesemia, *hypophosphatemia,* hypoproteinemia, *weight increase.*
Musculoskeletal: arthralgia, arthropathy, *back pain,* bone fracture, cramps, *leg pain,* myalgia.
Respiratory: abnormal breath sounds, bronchitis, ***bronchospasm,*** *cough, dyspnea,* pharyngitis, pneumonia, pulmonary disorder, pulmonary edema, *upper respiratory tract infection.*
Skin: *acne,* cyst, hypertrichosis, pruritus, rash, skin disorder or ulceration, *surgical wound complications.*
Other: herpes simplex, herpes zoster, accidental trauma, *CMV infection,* hernia, infection, ***sepsis,*** *viral infection.*

INTERACTIONS
None reported.

EFFECTS ON LAB TEST RESULTS
• May increase calcium, cholesterol, glucose, lipid, and uric acid levels. May decrease magnesium, phosphorus, and protein levels. May increase or decrease potassium level.
• May increase RBC count. May decrease hemoglobin and platelet count.

ACTION
Binds specifically to and blocks the IL-2 receptor alpha-chain on the surface of activated T-lymphocytes. This inhibits IL-2–mediated activation of lymphocytes, a critical pathway in the cellular immune response involved in allograft rejection.

PHARMACOKINETICS
Onset, unknown; peak, immediate; duration, unknown.

Distribution: Unknown.
Metabolism: Unknown.
Excretion: Elimination half-life is about 7 days in adults and about 11 days in pediatric patients.

CLINICAL CONSIDERATIONS
• *Alert:* Use only under the supervision of a prescriber qualified and experienced in immunosuppression therapy and management of organ transplantation.
• Use basiliximab as adjunct to cyclosporine and corticosteroids.
• It's unknown whether the response to vaccines will be altered with drug administered.
• *Alert:* Anaphylactoid reactions may result after administration of proteins. If this occurs, have drugs for treating severe hypersensitivity reactions available for immediate use and withhold further basiliximab treatments.
• Monitor patient for electrolyte imbalances and acidosis during drug therapy.
• Monitor patient's intake and output, vital signs, hemoglobin level, and hematocrit during therapy.
• Watch for signs of opportunistic infections during drug therapy.

PATIENT TEACHING
• Inform patient of potential benefits of therapy and risks linked to immunosuppressive therapy, including a decreased incidence of graft loss or acute rejection.
• Inform women of childbearing age to use effective contraception before beginning therapy and up to 2 months after completing therapy.
• Instruct patient to report adverse reactions and signs of infection immediately.
• Explain that drug is used with cyclosporine and corticosteroids.
• Advise patient that immunosuppressive therapy increases the risk of developing lymphoproliferative disorders and opportunistic infections.

benztropine mesylate
Cogentin

Pharmacologic class: anticholinergic
Therapeutic class: antiparkinsonian
Pregnancy risk category: C
pH: 5 to 8

INDICATIONS & DOSAGES
➤ **Arteriosclerotic, idiopathic, or
postencephalitic parkinsonian syndrome—**
Adults: Usual daily dose is 1 to 2 mg
I.V.; range, 0.5 to 6 mg I.V. daily. Initiated at low dose and gradually increased by 0.5-mg increments over 5-
to 6-day intervals until symptomatic relief occurs or maximum dose of 6 mg
I.V. daily is reached.
➤ **Drug-induced extrapyramidal
symptoms—**
Adults: 1 to 4 mg I.V. once daily or
b.i.d. Dosage adjusted as needed and
tolerated.
➤ **Drug-induced extrapyramidal
symptoms that develop shortly after
antipsychotic therapy begins—**
Adults: 1 to 2 mg I.V. b.i.d. or t.i.d.
Reevaluate after 1 to 2 weeks of therapy.
➤ **Acute dystonic reactions—**
Adults: Initially, 1 to 2 mg I.V. daily,
then 1 to 2 mg P.O. b.i.d. Dosage adjusted as needed and tolerated.

ADMINISTRATION
Direct injection: Aspirate solution from
ampule. Over 3 to 5 minutes, inject
into vein or into I.V. tubing containing
a free-flowing, compatible solution.
Intermittent infusion: Not recommended.
Continuous infusion: Not recommended.

PREPARATION & STORAGE
Supplied in 1-mg/ml concentration.
    Store in light-resistant container at
room temperature.

Incompatibilities
None reported.

CONTRAINDICATIONS & CAUTIONS
• Contraindicated in those hypersensitive to the drug.
• Contraindicated in those with tardive
dyskinesia because symptoms may
worsen.
• Use cautiously in older children and
geriatric patients because of anticholinergic effects.
• Individualize dosage in children age 3
and older.
• Use cautiously in those with alcoholism or CNS disorders because of
possible anhidrosis leading to hyperthermia and in those with hypertension
or myasthenia gravis because of possible aggravation.
• Use cautiously in those with a history
of extrapyramidal reactions because of
possible intensified symptoms and in
those with hepatorenal impairment because of possible toxic reactions.
• Use cautiously in those with cardiac
instability or arrhythmias because of
increased risk of arrhythmias, in those
with dementia because of increased
risk of confusion and psychosis and
possible impaired memory, and in
those with angle-closure glaucoma
because of increased intraocular pressure.
• Use cautiously in those with intestinal
obstruction because of decreased GI
tone and motility.
• Use cautiously in those with prostatic
hyperplasia or urine retention because
urine retention may worsen.

ADVERSE REACTIONS
CNS: confusion.
CV: tachycardia.

EENT: dry mouth, blurred vision, mydriasis.
GI: paralytic ileus, constipation, vomiting, nausea.
GU: urine retention.
Skin: decreased sweating.

INTERACTIONS

Drug-drug. *Amantadine, antihistamines, haloperidol, MAO inhibitors, phenothiazines, procainamide, quinidine, tricyclic antidepressants:* Causes additive anticholinergic effects. Reduce dosage before giving.
Other CNS depressants: Deepens CNS depression. Avoid using together.
Drug-herb. *Jimson weed:* May adversely affect CV function. Avoid using together.
Drug-lifestyle. *Alcohol use:* Increases CNS depression. Discourage use together.

EFFECTS ON LAB TEST RESULTS
None reported.

ACTION
Drug probably decreases acetylcholine activity in the basal ganglia.

PHARMACOKINETICS
Onset, within a few minutes; duration, 24 hours.
Distribution: Throughout the body, especially in CNS, CV system, GI tract, and urinary tract smooth muscle. Drug crosses the placental barrier, and small amounts appear in breast milk.
Metabolism: Minimal in liver.
Excretion: Most excreted unchanged or as metabolites in urine.

CLINICAL CONSIDERATIONS
• Use I.V. or I.M. route for patients unable to tolerate the oral drug or for emergencies when rapid response is desired. I.V. route is rarely used because of small difference in onset time compared with I.M. route.

• Individualize dosage according to age, weight, and type of parkinsonism being treated.
• Dosage may be given as a single daily dose, usually h.s. or divided into separate doses up to four times daily, depending on patient response.
• Drug's full effects may not be apparent for 2 to 3 days.
• Monitor heart rate and ECG for tachycardia, input and output for anhidrosis and urine retention, and temperature.
• Watch for signs and symptoms of paralytic ileus, such as abdominal distention and pain; decreased or absent bowel sounds; and constipation.
• Closely monitor patients with a history of mental illness because symptoms may intensify.
• *Alert:* Never stop drug abruptly. Reduce dosage gradually.
• If overdose occurs, give 1 to 2 mg of physostigmine salicylate S.C. or I.V. Repeat dose in 2 hours, if needed.

PATIENT TEACHING
• Encourage patient to perform good mouth care to prevent oral lesions caused by dry mouth.
• Tell patient that drug may impair mental or physical ability needed for operating machinery or driving a car.
• Stress the importance of reporting GI symptoms, fever, or heat intolerance if patient is also receiving a phenothiazide, haloperidol, or another anticholinergic, because of risk of paralytic ileus, hyperthermia, and heat stroke.
• Caution patient about the risk of anhidrosis, especially if he performs manual labor or if the weather is hot.
• Advise breast-feeding patient before use that drug may inhibit lactation.

betamethasone sodium phosphate
Celestone Phosphate

Pharmacologic class: glucocorticoid
Therapeutic class: anti-inflammatory
Pregnancy risk category: C
pH: 8.5

INDICATIONS & DOSAGES
➤ **Severe inflammation or immunosuppression—**
Adults: 0.5 to 9 mg I.V. daily. After achieving satisfactory response, reduce dosage gradually and maintain at lowest level that produces therapeutic response.

ADMINISTRATION
Direct injection: Use only in severe or life-threatening conditions.
Intermittent infusion: Not recommended.
Continuous infusion: Not recommended.

PREPARATION & STORAGE
Available in 5-ml multidose vials containing 3 mg/ml.
    Store between 59° and 86° F (15° and 30° C); don't freeze. Protect from light.

Incompatibilities
Parenteral local diluents or anesthetics containing preservatives, such as parabens or phenols.

CONTRAINDICATIONS & CAUTIONS
• Contraindicated in those hypersensitive to corticosteroids or with systemic fungal infections.
• Use cautiously in those with hypothyroidism or cirrhosis because drug response may be exaggerated, in those with hyperthyroidism because drug metabolism may be accelerated, and in those with cardiac disease or renal impairment because fluid retention may be hazardous.
• Use cautiously in those with uncontrolled viral, fungal, or bacterial infection because drug increases susceptibility to infection and masks symptoms.
• Use cautiously in those with heart failure, diverticulitis, hypertension, nonspecific ulcerative colitis, peptic ulcer, or psychosis because drug may aggravate these conditions.
• Use cautiously in those with a history of tuberculosis because drug may reactivate disease and in those with hyperlipidemia because drug may raise fatty acid and cholesterol levels.
• Use cautiously in those with diabetes mellitus or osteoporosis because of possible exacerbation, in those with Strongyloides infestation because of risk of hyperinfection, and in those with myasthenia gravis because of worsened weakness.
• Use cautiously in those with glaucoma because of elevated intraocular pressure and in those with hypoalbuminemia because of an increased risk of toxic reaction.
• Use cautiously in children because safe and effective dosages haven't been established. Intracranial pressure may rise, leading to headache, oculomotor or abducens nerve paralysis, papilledema, and vision loss. Long-term use may retard bone growth, whereas high doses may cause pancreatic inflammation or destruction.

ADVERSE REACTIONS
CNS: headache, vertigo, *euphoria, insomnia, seizures, increased intracranial pressure.*
CV: *heart failure,* hypertension, edema.
EENT: cataracts, increased intraocular pressure, glaucoma.
GU: menstrual irregularities.

Reactions may be *common*, uncommon, *life-threatening*, or COMMON AND LIFE-THREATENING.

Metabolic: sodium retention, fluid retention, hypocalcemia, hypercholesterolemia, hyperglycemia, hypokalemia.
Musculoskeletal: muscle weakness, osteoporosis.
Skin: impaired wound healing, acne, hirsutism.
Other: cushingoid state, *acute adrenal insufficiency.*

INTERACTIONS

Drug-drug. *Amiodarone, cardiac glycosides:* Betamethasone-induced hypokalemia may worsen toxic effects of the drugs. Dosage may need to be adjusted.
Amphotericin B (parenteral), carbonic anhydrase inhibitors, diuretics: May worsen hypokalemia. Monitor patient closely.
Antidiabetics: Reduces effectiveness caused by betamethasone-induced hyperglycemia. Dosage may need to be adjusted.
Drugs that induce cytochrome P-450 (barbiturates, phenytoin, rifampin, and ephedrine), phenobarbital: Decreases effectiveness because of enhanced metabolism of betamethasone. Dosage may need to be adjusted.
Estrogens: Decreases steroid clearance. Monitor patient for toxicity.
Ketoconazole, other drugs that inhibit cytochrome P-450, troleandomycin: Decreases clearance of betamethasone and increases adverse effects. Consider decreasing betamethasone dosage.
Vaccines with killed virus: Decreases antibody response. Avoid using together.
Vaccines with live virus: Increases risk of neurologic toxicity. Avoid using together.

EFFECTS ON LAB TEST RESULTS

• May increase potassium, glucose, calcium, and cholesterol levels. May decrease protein-bound iodine levels in thyroid function tests.
• May cause false-negative results in the nitroblue tetrazolium tests for systemic bacterial infections. Suppresses skin test reactions. Alters gonadorelin test results and decreases ^{131}I uptake during radionuclide brain and bone imaging.

ACTION

A synthetic glucocorticoid that reduces inflammation mainly by stabilizing leukocyte lysosomal membranes. Drug also suppresses pituitary release of corticotropin, which stops adrenocortical production of corticosteroids.

PHARMACOKINETICS

Onset, 1 to 5 minutes; duration varies, depending on dose and time of administration.
Distribution: Rapidly distributed to intestines, kidneys, liver, muscles, and skin. Drug crosses placental barrier and appears in breast milk.
Metabolism: Primarily in liver. Lesser amounts metabolized in kidneys and other tissues.
Excretion: By kidneys. Small amount of unmetabolized drug is excreted in urine, negligible amount in bile.

CLINICAL CONSIDERATIONS

• *Alert:* Use I.V. administration only in emergencies or when oral therapy is impossible.
• *Alert:* Don't confuse Celestone Phosphate with Celestone Soluspan, a suspension that can't be given I.V.
• *Alert:* Drug may contain sulfites.
• Adrenal function recovery may take 1 week after high-dose therapy lasting 1 to 5 days and up to 1 year after prolonged therapy.
• Before and during long-term therapy, monitor ECG, blood pressure, chest and spinal X-rays, glucose tolerance test results, potassium levels, and hypothalamic and pituitary function test results. Also, periodically check electrolyte levels, CBC, height, weight, and intraocular pressure.
• Watch for signs of infection.

• Because drug increases catabolism, patient may need more protein.
• Patient may need a potassium supplement.
• Stop drug gradually and as soon as possible.

PATIENT TEACHING
• Instruct patient to stay on a low-sodium diet if needed.
• Warn patient of increased risk of infection.
• Instruct patient on long-term corticosteroid therapy to wear or carry medical identification indicating need for supplemental steroid therapy during stress.
• Tell patient to report adverse reactions.

biperiden lactate
Akineton

Pharmacologic class: anticholinergic
Therapeutic class: antiparkinsonian
Pregnancy risk category: C

INDICATIONS & DOSAGES
➤ **Drug-induced extrapyramidal disorders—**
Adults: Initially, 2 mg (0.4 ml) I.V., repeated q 30 minutes until symptoms subside. Maximum of four doses (8 mg) over 24 hours.

ADMINISTRATION
Direct injection: Using a 21G to 23G needle, inject drug over at least 1 minute into vein or into I.V. tubing containing a free-flowing, compatible solution.
Intermittent infusion: Not recommended.
Continuous infusion: Not recommended.

PREPARATION & STORAGE
Available in 1-ml ampules containing 5 mg/ml. Drug is stable at room temperature. Protect from light.

Incompatibilities
None reported.

CONTRAINDICATIONS & CAUTIONS
• Contraindicated in those hypersensitive to biperiden and in those with acute angle-closure glaucoma, bowel obstruction, or megacolon.
• Use cautiously in febrile patients or those exposed to heat because drug decreases the ability to sweat.
• Use cautiously in those with angle-closure glaucoma because drug may raise intraocular pressure and in debilitated patients or those with tachycardia because drug may cause thyrotoxicosis or decreased cardiac output.
• Use cautiously in those with a prostate disorder because of possible urine retention and in confused or geriatric patients because of possible euphoria, confusion, and agitation.
• Use cautiously in those with hypertension or tardive dyskinesia because of possible aggravation and in those with a history of extrapyramidal reactions because of possible worsening of symptoms.
• Use cautiously in those with cardiac instability or arrhythmias because of increased risk of arrhythmias and in those with hepatic or renal impairment because of increased risk of toxic reaction.
• Use cautiously in those with intestinal obstruction because of decreased GI motility and tone and in those with myasthenia gravis because of worsened weakness.

ADVERSE REACTIONS
CNS: drowsiness, euphoria, disorientation, agitation.
CV: *bradycardia,* hypotension.
EENT: dry mouth, blurred vision.

GI: *constipation.*
GU: urine retention.

INTERACTIONS
Drug-drug. *Anticholinesterases:* Reduces effects. Monitor patient closely.
Amantadine, antihistamines, meperidine, phenothiazines, quinidine, tricyclic antidepressants: Enhances anticholinergic effects. Monitor patient closely.
CNS depressants: Deepens sedation. Avoid using together.
Digoxin: May elevate plasma digoxin levels if slow-dissolving oral digoxin is administered. Monitor digoxin levels.
Haloperidol, phenothiazines: May decrease antipsychotic actions of these drugs, possibly by direct CNS antagonism. Monitor patient for clinical effect.
Drug-lifestyle. *Alcohol use:* Increases sedative effects. Discourage use together.

EFFECTS ON LAB TEST RESULTS
None reported.

ACTION
Exerts a central anticholinergic effect similar to that of atropine by inhibiting acetylcholine's muscarinic effects. Relaxes smooth muscle diminishes GI, bronchial, and sweat gland secretions, and dilates pupils.

PHARMACOKINETICS
Onset and duration, unknown.
Distribution: Probably throughout most body tissues. Unknown if drug appears in breast milk.
Metabolism: Probably in the liver.
Excretion: Mainly in urine as unchanged drug or metabolites.

CLINICAL CONSIDERATIONS
• Expect prescriber to switch patient to oral form of drug as soon as possible.

• **Alert:** Bradycardia and hypotension can be minimized or avoided by slow I.V. administration.
• Obtain baseline blood pressure and heart rate. Monitor patient for hypotension and tachycardia during and after drug administration. Keep patient in bed during injection and until blood pressure stabilizes.
• If photophobia occurs, keep patient's room dark.
• If patient becomes confused or disoriented, institute safety precautions.
• Provide frequent mouth care to relieve dry mouth. Monitor bladder and bowel functions for urine retention and constipation.
• To treat drug overdose, give vasopressors for persistent hypotension. Provide respiratory support, antipyretics, and fluid replacement. Don't give phenothiazines because they could cause coma.
• For a life-threatening overdose, give physostigmine.

PATIENT TEACHING
• Tell patient he may become drowsy.
• Instruct patient to change positions slowly after administration.
• Instruct patient to use caution when driving a car or operating machinery.

bivalirudin
Angiomax

Pharmacologic class: direct thrombin inhibitor
Therapeutic class: anticoagulant
Pregnancy risk category: B
pH: 5 to 6

INDICATIONS & DOSAGES
➤ **Unstable angina in patients undergoing percutaneous transluminal coronary angioplasty (PTCA)—**
Adults: 1 mg/kg I.V. bolus just before PTCA; then begin 4-hour I.V. infusion

at 2.5 mg/kg/hour. After initial 4-hour infusion, an additional I.V. infusion at a rate of 0.2 mg/kg/hour for up to 20 hours may be given p.r.n. Used in conjunction with 300 to 325 mg aspirin.

Adjust-a-dose: For patients with creatinine clearance 30 to 59 ml/minute, reduce dose by 20%. For clearance 10 to 29 ml/minute, reduce dose by 60%. For dialysis-dependent patients (off dialysis), reduce dose by 90%.

ADMINISTRATION
Direct injection: Not recommended.
Intermittent infusion: Give 1 mg/kg I.V. bolus, followed by continuous infusion.
Continuous infusion: After bolus dose is given, infuse at rate of 2.5 mg/kg/hour over 4 hours. At the end of the infusion, an additional 0.2 mg/kg/hour for fewer than 20 hours may be given.

PREPARATION & STORAGE
Available as a powder contained in a 250-mg single-use vial. Reconstitute each 250-mg vial with 5 ml of sterile water for injection. Gently swirl the vial until all material is dissolved. Further dilute each reconstituted vial in 50 ml D_5W or normal saline solution to yield a final concentration of 5 mg/ml.

To prepare a low-rate infusion to be given after the initial infusion, further dilute each reconstituted vial in 500 ml D_5W or normal saline solution to yield a final concentration of 0.5 mg/ml.

Store vials at room temperature. The reconstituted solution is stable for 24 hours at 36° to 46° F (2° to 8° C). The diluted drug is stable at room temperature for up to 24 hours. Discard any unused portion of reconstituted solution.

Incompatibilities
Other I.V. drugs.

CONTRAINDICATIONS & CAUTIONS
● Contraindicated in patients hypersensitive to drug or its components and in those with active major bleeding.

● Avoid use in patients with unstable angina who aren't undergoing PTCA and in patients with other acute coronary syndromes.
● Use cautiously in patients with heparin-induced thrombocytopenia or heparin-induced thrombocytopenia-thrombosis syndrome, and in patients with diseases linked to increased risk of bleeding.
● Use cautiously in pregnant, breast-feeding, and elderly patients. Puncture-site hemorrhage and catheterization-site hematoma may occur more often in patients age 65 and older than in younger patients.

ADVERSE REACTIONS
CNS: fever, anxiety, *headache,* insomnia, nervousness, cerebral ischemia, confusion, *pain.*
CV: *bradycardia,* hypertension, syncope, vascular anomaly, *ventricular fibrillation, hypotension.*
GI: abdominal pain, dyspepsia, *nausea,* vomiting.
GU: urine retention, *kidney failure.*
Hematologic: *severe, spontaneous bleeding* (cerebral, retroperitoneal, GU, GI).
Musculoskeletal: *back pain,* pelvic pain.
Skin: pain at injection site.
Other: *sepsis.*

INTERACTIONS
Drug-drug. *Glycoprotein IIb/IIIa inhibitors:* Safety and efficacy not established. Avoid using together.
Heparin, warfarin, other oral anticoagulants: May increase risk of bleeding. Use together cautiously. Stop heparin at least 8 hours before giving bivalirudin.

EFFECTS ON LAB TEST RESULTS
None reported.

ACTION
Drug binds specifically and rapidly to thrombin and directly inhibits both

clot-bound and circulating thrombin. By inhibiting thrombin, bivalirudin prevents the generation of fibrin and any further activation of the clotting cascade by inhibiting thrombin-induced platelet activation, granule release, and aggregation to produce an anticoagulant effect.

PHARMACOKINETICS
Onset, rapid; peak, immediate; duration, until end of infusion.
Distribution: Drug binds rapidly to thrombin.
Metabolism: Cleared from plasma by a combination of renal mechanisms and proteolytic cleavage.
Excretion: Eliminated renally. Clearance is reduced about 20% in patients with moderate-to-severe renal impairment and about 80% in those receiving dialysis. Half-life is 25 minutes in patients with normal renal function.

CLINICAL CONSIDERATIONS
• *Alert:* Stop low–molecular-weight heparin 8 hours before giving drug.
• Give bolus dose immediately before PTCA.
• Monitor baseline coagulation tests, hemoglobin, and hematocrit before and during therapy.
• *Alert:* Hemorrhage can occur at any body site in patients receiving bivalirudin. Suspect a hemorrhage if unexplained drop in hematocrit, fall in blood pressure, or another unexplained symptom occurs.
• If overdose occurs, stop drug infusion and monitor patient closely for bleeding.
• About 25% of bivalirudin dose is removed by dialysis.

PATIENT TEACHING
• Tell patient drug can cause bleeding and to report unusual bruising or bleeding (nosebleeds, bleeding gums) or tarry or bloody stools to prescriber immediately.

• Tell patient that drug is given with aspirin, and caution him to avoid other aspirin-containing drugs during treatment.
• Advise patient to avoid activities that carry a risk of injury, cuts, or bruises, and instruct him to use a soft toothbrush and electric razor during treatment.

bleomycin sulfate
Blenoxane

Pharmacologic class: antibiotic antineoplastic (G_2- and M-phase specific)
Therapeutic class: antineoplastic
Pregnancy risk category: D
pH: 4.5 to 6 when reconstituted, depending on diluent

INDICATIONS & DOSAGES
➤ **Hodgkin's and non-Hodgkin's malignant lymphomas, testicular cancer, and squamous cell carcinomas of the buccal mucosa, cervix, epiglottis, gingivae, head, larynx, lips, mouth, nasopharynx, neck, oropharynx, palate, paralarynx, penis, sinuses, skin, tongue, tonsils, and vulva—** *Adults:* 0.25 to 0.5 unit/kg I.V. or 10 to 20 units/m² once or twice weekly. Because of risk of anaphylactoid reactions, treat patient with lymphoma with 2 units or fewer for the first two doses. If tolerated, follow above dosage schedule. In Hodgkin's disease, after tumor is reduced by 50%, give 1 unit daily or 5 units weekly as maintenance therapy.

ADMINISTRATION
Direct injection: Using a 23G or 25G butterfly needle, inject reconstituted drug over 10 minutes at a new I.V. site.
Intermittent infusion: Using a secondary line, infuse dose into an estab-

lished line containing a free-flowing, compatible solution.
Continuous infusion: Not recommended.

PREPARATION & STORAGE
Preparation is linked to carcinogenic, mutagenic, and teratogenic risks. Follow facility policy to reduce risks.

Vials contain 15 units or 30 units of drug.

For I.V. use, dilute the 15-unit or 30-unit vial with at least 5 ml or 10 ml, respectively, of normal saline solution.

Refrigerate powdered drug. Diluted solution is stable for 24 hours at room temperature. Because preparation doesn't contain preservatives, use within 24 hours. Discard unused portion.

Incompatibilities
Amino acids; aminophylline; ascorbic acid injection; cefazolin; diazepam; drugs containing sulfhydryl groups; fluids containing dextrose; furosemide; hydrocortisone; methotrexate; mitomycin; nafcillin; penicillin G; riboflavin; solutions containing divalent and trivalent cations, especially calcium salts and copper; terbutaline sulfate.

CONTRAINDICATIONS & CAUTIONS
• Contraindicated in those hypersensitive to drug.
• Use cautiously in those with pulmonary impairment because 10% of patients develop pulmonary toxicity and 1% die of pulmonary fibrosis. Geriatric patients are also at risk for pulmonary toxicity.
• Use cautiously in those with hepatic or renal impairment because of increased risk of toxic reaction.
• After receiving the drug, patient may experience lung damage from reduced oxygen levels.

ADVERSE REACTIONS
CNS: fever.
EENT: ulcerations of lips and tongue.

GI: vomiting, anorexia, stomatitis.
Hematologic: anemia, *thrombocytopenia, leukopenia.*
Metabolic: weight loss.
Respiratory: *pneumonitis, pulmonary fibrosis,* wheezing.
Skin: *erythema, rash, striae, vesiculation, tenderness of skin,* pruritus, urticaria, *hyperpigmentation,* hyperkeratosis, alopecia, nail changes.
Other: chills, *anaphylactoid reaction.*

INTERACTIONS
Drug-drug. *Antineoplastics:* Increases bleomycin toxicity. Monitor patient closely.
Digoxin: Decreases level and renal excretion of digoxin. Monitor digoxin level closely.
Phenytoin: Decreases phenytoin level. Monitor patient closely.

EFFECTS ON LAB TEST RESULTS
• May increase uric acid level.

ACTION
May inhibit synthesis of DNA, RNA, and proteins by binding directly with DNA.

PHARMACOKINETICS
Onset, immediate; serum level peaks, 30 to 60 minutes.
Distribution: Mainly to kidneys, lungs, lymphatic system, peritoneum, and skin. Studies suggest higher level occurs in squamous cell carcinoma than in sarcoma. Low level in bone marrow probably results from high level of bleomycin enzymes.
Metabolism: Unknown; however, extensive tissue inactivation occurs in the liver and kidneys and less in the skin and lungs.
Excretion: In patients with normal renal function, 60% to 70% is excreted unchanged in urine within 24 hours; terminal half-life is about 2 hours. In patients with renal impairment, less

than 20% is excreted in urine as active drug.

CLINICAL CONSIDERATIONS
• Because risk of bone marrow toxicity is low, drug is commonly used in patients with bone marrow suppression, as a supplement to other chemotherapeutic drugs, or as a temporary treatment until bone marrow suppression has improved.
• Follow procedures for proper handling and disposal of chemotherapeutic drugs.
• *Alert:* Toxic reaction may occur at lower dosages when used with other antineoplastics.
• *Alert:* Assess respiratory function carefully before each treatment, especially if patient is at high risk for pulmonary toxicity. Signs include dyspnea, bibasilar crackles, and a nonproductive cough. Patients older than age 70 or those receiving a total dose over 400 units are at increased risk for toxic reaction.
• Monitor patient closely during infusion and for 1 hour after.
• Obtain BUN and creatinine clearance levels, liver and pulmonary function tests, ECGs, and chest X-rays before and during treatment. Expect drug to be stopped if tests show marked deterioration.
• In patients prone to posttreatment fever, give acetaminophen before treatment and for 24 hours after.
• After treatment, give supplemental oxygen at a fraction of inspired oxygen, not exceeding 25% to avoid potential lung damage.
• Monitor patient's blood pressure.
• Hodgkin's disease and testicular tumors usually improve within 2 weeks. If no improvement is noted during this time, it's unlikely to occur.
• Improvement of squamous cell carcinoma commonly takes 3 weeks or longer.

• Monitor lymphoma patients for idiosyncratic reactions such as hypotension, confusion, fever, chills, wheezing occurring after the first 2 doses.

PATIENT TEACHING
• Warn patient about possible hair loss, which is usually temporary.
• Tell patient to report adverse reactions promptly and to take infection control and bleeding precautions.

bretylium tosylate
Bretylate ◇ , Bretylol

Pharmacologic class: adrenergic blocker
Therapeutic class: class III ventricular antiarrhythmic
Pregnancy risk category: C
pH: 4.5 to 7

INDICATIONS & DOSAGES
➤ **Ventricular fibrillation or hemodynamically unstable ventricular tachycardia—**
Adults: 5 mg/kg I.V. given undiluted over 1 minute. If persistent, follow with 10 mg/kg q 5 to 30 minutes, p.r.n. Maximum dose, 30 to 35 mg/kg/day.
Children ◆ : For acute ventricular fibrillation, initially 5 mg/kg I.V., followed by 10 mg/kg q 15 to 30 minutes, with a maximum total dose of 30 mg/kg; maintenance dosage, 5 to 10 mg/kg q 6 hours.
➤ **Persistent ventricular tachycardia—**
Adults: 5 to 10 mg/kg I.V. infused over 8 to 10 minutes. Maintenance dosage, 5 to 10 mg/kg over 8 minutes or more, repeated q 6 to 8 hours; or continuous infusion at rate of 1 to 2 mg/minute.
➤ **Other life-threatening arrhythmias—**
Adults: 5 to 10 mg/kg I.V. over at least 8 minutes, repeated at 1- to 2-hour in-

tervals if persistent. Maintenance dosage, 5 to 10 mg/kg q 6 hours, or continuous infusion at a rate of 1 to 2 mg/minute.

Children ♦ *:* 5 to 10 mg/kg I.V. q 6 hours.

Adjust-a-dose: For patients with renal impairment, increase dosage interval.

ADMINISTRATION

Direct injection: Using a 20G to 22G needle, inject undiluted over about 8 to 10 minutes into I.V. line.

Intermittent infusion: Dilute to at least 50 ml with D_5W or normal saline injection and infuse ordered dose over 8 minutes or more.

Continuous infusion: Give diluted drug at rate of 1 to 2 mg/minute.

PREPARATION & STORAGE

Supplied as single-dose, 10-ml ampule containing 500 mg drug.

For infusion, dilute with at least 50 ml of D_5W or normal saline solution.

Store at 59° to 86° F (15° to 30° C). Diluted drug remains stable for 48 hours at room temperature, 7 days if refrigerated.

Prediluted, commercially prepared solutions are also available.

Incompatibilities

None reported.

CONTRAINDICATIONS & CAUTIONS

• Contraindicated in those receiving cardiac glycoside therapy unless they have a life-threatening arrhythmia that isn't caused by that therapy. Avoid starting bretylium and cardiac glycoside therapies at the same time.

• Use cautiously in those with impaired cardiac output, aortic stenosis, or pulmonary hypertension because of the risk of severe hypotension.

• Reduce dosage in those with renal impairment because of high risk of toxic reaction.

ADVERSE REACTIONS

CNS: vertigo, dizziness, faintness, light-headedness, syncope.

CV: SEVERE HYPOTENSION, ESPECIALLY ORTHOSTATIC, *transient arrhythmias,* transient hypertension.

GI: nausea and vomiting with rapid administration.

INTERACTIONS

Drug-drug. *Antiarrhythmics (such as lidocaine, quinidine, procainamide, and propranolol), cardiac glycosides:* Causes additive or antagonistic antiarrhythmic effects and risk of toxic reaction. Monitor patient for additive toxic effects.

Antihypertensives: May potentiate hypotension. Monitor blood pressure.

Pressor catecholamines (dopamine, norepinephrine): Potentiates effects of these drugs. Monitor blood pressure closely.

EFFECTS ON LAB TEST RESULTS

None reported.

ACTION

May increase the threshold for ventricular fibrillation by prolonging repolarization, perhaps by blocking postganglionic sympathetic neurons or depleting catecholamines. This causes an adrenergic-blocking action, prolonging repolarization. The drug also may have vasodilating, cardiostimulating, and weak local anesthetic effects.

PHARMACOKINETICS

In ventricular fibrillation, onset is a few minutes; duration average, 6 to 24 hours. In ventricular tachycardia, onset is 20 minutes to 2 hours; peak, 6 to 9 hours; duration average, 6 to 24 hours. Onset is occasionally delayed 30 minutes to several hours.

Distribution: Appears in tissues of high adrenergic innervation, including sympathetic ganglia, heart, and spleen. Traces concentrate in adrenals. Drug doesn't cross blood-brain barrier; about 1% to 10% is protein-bound. Unknown if drug crosses placental barrier or appears in breast milk.

Metabolism: Not metabolized.
Excretion: By kidneys, unchanged. Half-life averages 5 to 10 hours but can extend up to 4 days in patients with creatinine clearance less than 30 ml/minute.

CLINICAL CONSIDERATIONS
• Osmolarity: 174 mOsm/L. For premixed solution: 2 mg/ml is 260 to 264 mOsm/L and 4 mg/ml is 270 to 278 mOsm/L.
• *Alert:* Bretylium is used as a second-line agent when other therapy, such as lidocaine, has failed.
• Subtherapeutic doses of less than 5 mg/kg may cause hypotension.
• Stop therapy as soon as possible after arrhythmias are under control.
• Rapid administration may cause severe nausea and vomiting.
• Closely monitor ECG, heart rate, pulse, and blood pressure. Notify prescriber of significant change.
• Keep patient in supine position until tolerant of hypotension, which may be after several days of therapy. Notify prescriber of significant change. He may order norepinephrine, dopamine, or volume expanders to raise blood pressure.
• Watch for increased angina in susceptible patients.
• Monitor temperature because of risk of hyperthermia, which may develop within 1 hour of administration and peak within 1 to 3 days.
• To manage overdose, give nitroprusside or another short-acting antihypertensive to treat initial hypertensive effects. Don't use long-acting drugs that may potentiate the subsequent hypotensive effects. Treat hypotension with fluids and dopamine or norepinephrine. Dialysis doesn't remove drug.

PATIENT TEACHING
• Instruct patient to remain in supine position until tolerant of hypotension.
• Tell patient to report adverse reactions immediately and to alert nurse if he experiences discomfort at the I.V. site.

bumetanide*

Pharmacologic class: sulfonamide-type loop diuretic
Therapeutic class: diuretic
Pregnancy risk category: C
pH: 6.8 to 7.8

INDICATIONS & DOSAGES
➤ **Edema linked to heart failure and hepatic or renal disease—**
Adults: Initially, 0.5 to 1 mg I.V. daily. Repeat q 2 to 3 hours, if needed, up to maximum of 10 mg daily.
Adjust-a-dose: For patients with impaired renal function, maximum dosages of 20 mg I.V. daily may be given. For patients with creatinine clearance less than 5 ml/minute, doses greater than 2 mg I.V. are needed to achieve diuresis. For patients with chronic renal insufficiency, a continuous infusion of 12 mg I.V. over 12 hours may be more effective and less toxic than I.V. bolus therapy.

ADMINISTRATION
Direct injection: Using a 21G or 23G needle, inject desired dose of 0.25 mg/ml solution over 1 to 2 minutes.
Intermittent infusion: Give diluted drug through an intermittent infusion device or piggyback into an I.V. line containing a free-flowing, compatible solution. Infuse at ordered rate.
Continuous infusion: Patients with renal insufficiency may benefit from 12 mg I.V. over 12 hours, instead of bolus dosing.

PREPARATION & STORAGE
Available with premixed preservative in 2-ml (0.25-mg/ml) ampules and 2-ml, 4-ml, and 10-ml (0.25-mg/ml) vials.

Drug can be further diluted for I.V. infusion using D_5W, normal saline solution, or lactated Ringer's solution in either a glass or a plastic container. Prepare solution for I.V. infusion within 24 hours of use. Protect drug from light to avoid discoloration. Store at room temperature.

When large doses are needed, use vials to prevent glass particles from broken ampules from entering the solution. If ampules must be used, add a filter to I.V. tubing.

Incompatibilities
Dobutamine, midazolam.

CONTRAINDICATIONS & CAUTIONS
● Contraindicated in those hypersensitive to the drug and in those with anuria.
● Contraindicated in those hypersensitive to sulfonylureas.
● Contraindicated in those with hepatic impairment or severe electrolyte depletion because of increased risk of dehydration and electrolyte imbalance, which could lead to hepatic coma and death, and in those with severe renal impairment because of increased risk of toxic reaction.
● Use cautiously in those with sulfonamide sensitivity because of possible enhanced bumetanide sensitivity.
● Use cautiously in those with increased risk of hypokalemia, such as those with potassium-losing nephropathy or diarrhea-causing conditions; in those receiving a cardiac glycoside and diuretic for heart failure; in those with hepatic cirrhosis and ascites; and in those in a state of aldosterone excess with normal renal function.
● Use cautiously in those with a history of ventricular arrhythmias because drug-induced hypokalemia increases their risk, and in those with an acute MI because excessive diuresis can precipitate shock.
● Use cautiously in those with gout or hyperuricemia because drug raises uric acid levels.
● Too-vigorous diuresis may result in profound water loss and dehydration, especially in geriatric patients.

ADVERSE REACTIONS
CNS: dizziness.
CV: hypotension.
GU: *renal failure,* azotemia.
Hematologic: *thrombocytopenia.*
Metabolic: *hyperuricemia, hypochloremia, hypokalemia, hyponatremia,* hypophosphatemia, hypocalcemia, hypercholesterolemia, hyperglycemia.
Musculoskeletal: muscle cramps.

INTERACTIONS
Drug-drug. *Aminoglycosides, other nephrotoxic and ototoxic drugs:* Increases risk of nephrotoxicity and ototoxicity. Use together cautiously.
Amphotericin B, corticosteroids, corticotropin: Increases risk of hypokalemia. Use together cautiously.
Antihypertensives: Potentiates hypotensive effects. Use together cautiously.
Cardiac glycosides: Enhances risk of toxicity in patients with drug-induced hypokalemia. Monitor potassium and cardiac glycoside levels.
Indomethacin, probenecid: Reduces diuresis. Use together cautiously.
Lithium: Toxicity from reduced renal clearance. Monitor lithium level.
Drug-herb. *Dandelion:* May interfere with diuretic activity. Discourage use together.

EFFECTS ON LAB TEST RESULTS
● May increase AST, ALT, LDH, alkaline phosphatase, bilirubin, creatinine, glucose, uric acid, and cholesterol levels. May decrease potassium, sodium chloride, phosphorus, and calcium levels.
● May decrease platelet count. May increase or decrease WBC count.

Reactions may be *common,* uncommon, *life-threatening,* or COMMON AND LIFE-THREATENING.

ACTION
Inhibits sodium and chloride reabsorption primarily in the ascending loop of Henle. Precise mechanism of action is unknown, but drug may affect phosphate reabsorption in the proximal tubule. It doesn't act on the distal tubule.

PHARMACOKINETICS
Onset, a few minutes; peak, 15 to 30 minutes; duration, 2 to 4 hours.
Distribution: Highest levels found in kidneys, liver, and plasma; lowest levels found in heart, lung, muscle, and adipose tissue. Unknown if drug crosses the placental barrier or appears in breast milk.
Metabolism: Partly in liver to at least five inactive metabolites.
Excretion: 80% excreted in urine by glomerular filtration and possibly by renal tubular secretion, with 45% to 50% as unchanged drug or metabolites; 10% to 20% excreted in feces and bile almost entirely as metabolites. Elimination half-life, 60 to 90 minutes.

CLINICAL CONSIDERATIONS
• Osmolality: 453 mOsm/kg.
• I.V. route is used when rapid onset is needed, GI absorption is impaired, or P.O. route is impractical. I.V. route should be changed to oral as soon as the patient can safely tolerate it.
• Because drug causes potassium loss, give potassium replacements, as needed.
• If excessive diuresis or electrolyte imbalance occurs, expect the drug to be stopped or the dosage to be reduced until imbalance returns to normal.
• Monitor blood pressure and pulse rate during rapid diuresis. Use cautiously with other potassium-wasting drugs.
• Monitor electrolyte, BUN, creatinine, and carbon dioxide levels frequently.
• If BUN or creatinine level markedly increases or if oliguria develops during treatment, stop the drug.

• Observe for signs of hypokalemia, such as weakness, dizziness, confusion, anorexia, vomiting, and cramps.
• Monitor glucose levels in patients with diabetes and uric acid levels in patients with gout.
• Periodically monitor patient's weight to monitor fluid status.
• If overdose occurs, monitor urine output and serum and urine electrolyte levels to determine appropriate treatment. Provide replacement fluids and electrolytes, as needed.

PATIENT TEACHING
• Instruct patient to inform prescriber if signs or symptoms of electrolyte imbalance occur, such as weakness, dizziness, fatigue, faintness, mental confusion, lassitude, muscle cramps, headache, paresthesia, thirst, anorexia, nausea, or vomiting.
• Advise patient to stand up slowly to prevent dizziness, and to limit alcohol intake and strenuous exercise in hot weather to avoid exacerbating orthostatic hypertension.

buprenorphine hydrochloride
Buprenex

Pharmacologic class: narcotic agonist-antagonist, opioid partial agonist
Therapeutic class: analgesic
Pregnancy risk category: C
Controlled substance schedule: V
pH: 3.5 to 5.5

INDICATIONS & DOSAGES
➤ **Moderate to severe postoperative pain or pain from cancer, trigeminal neuralgia, trauma—**
Adults and children age 13 or older: 0.3 mg I.V q 6 hours, p.r.n. Initial dose may be repeated once in 30 to 60 minutes, if needed.

Continuous infusion of 25 to 250 mcg/hour has been used experimentally for postoperative pain in adults. ♦

Children ages 2 to 12: 2 to 6 mcg/kg I.V. q 4 to 6 hours. Dosage shouldn't exceed 6 mcg/kg.

➤ **Reversal of fentanyl-induced anesthesia and to provide subsequent analgesia ♦ —**

Adults: 0.3 to 0.8 mg I.V. 1 to 4 hours after anesthesia induction and about 30 minutes before the end of surgery.

Adjust-a-dose: In geriatric patients, give lower doses because of increased sensitivity to the drug and delayed clearance.

For patients at risk for respiratory depression, reduce dosage by 50%.

ADMINISTRATION

Direct injection: Inject over at least 2 minutes into an I.V. line containing a free-flowing, compatible solution. Avoid rapid injection to prevent possibly fatal anaphylactoid reaction or cardiopulmonary problems.

Intermittent infusion: Not recommended.

Continuous infusion: Used experimentally. Using a controller, infuse diluted drug at prescribed rate through an I.V. line containing a free-flowing, compatible solution.

PREPARATION & STORAGE

Supplied as 0.324 mg, equivalent to 0.3 mg, buprenorphine in 1-ml preservative-free ampules.

Drug can be diluted in D_5W, dextrose 5% and normal saline solution, or lactated Ringer's and normal saline solution. For continuous infusion, dilute with normal saline solution to a concentration of 15 mcg/ml.

Prevent prolonged exposure to light and exposure to temperatures above 104° F (40° C) or below 32° F (0° C).

Incompatibilities

Diazepam, furosemide, lorazepam.

CONTRAINDICATIONS & CAUTIONS

● Contraindicated in those hypersensitive to the drug.

● Avoid use in children younger than age 2 because safety and effectiveness haven't been established.

● Use extremely cautiously in those with respiratory disorders because of possible decreased respiratory drive and increased airway resistance, and in those with prostatic hyperplasia, urethral stricture, or recent urinary tract surgery because of possible urine retention.

● Use cautiously in those with hypothyroidism, myxedema, or adrenocortical insufficiency because of increased risk of respiratory depression, and in those with a history of drug abuse or emotional instability because of increased risk of drug dependence.

● Use cautiously in those with head injury, coma, CNS depression, or increased intracranial pressure because drug may increase CSF pressure and decrease level of consciousness, and in those with narcotic dependence because drug may induce withdrawal symptoms.

● Use cautiously in those with hepatic disease because drug metabolism and excretion are impaired and in geriatric or debilitated patients and those with severe renal impairment because renal clearance is reduced.

● Use cautiously in those with gallbladder disease because increased intracholedochal pressure stimulates contraction of the sphincter of Oddi.

ADVERSE REACTIONS

CNS: *dizziness, sedation,* headache, confusion, nervousness, euphoria, *vertigo,* **increased intracranial pressure,** fatigue, weakness, depression, dreaming, psychosis, slurred speech, paresthesia.

Reactions may be *common*, uncommon, *life-threatening*, or COMMON AND LIFE-THREATENING.

CV: hypotension, *bradycardia,* tachycardia, hypertension, Wenckebach block, cyanosis, flushing.

EENT: miosis, blurred vision, diplopia, visual abnormalities, tinnitus, conjunctivitis.

GI: *nausea,* vomiting, constipation, dry mouth.

GU: urine retention.

Respiratory: *respiratory depression,* hypoventilation, dyspnea.

Skin: *pruritus, diaphoresis, injection site reactions.*

Other: chills, withdrawal syndrome.

INTERACTIONS

Drug-drug. *Antihistamines, barbiturate anesthetics, CNS depressants, MAO inhibitors, narcotics, sedatives, tranquilizers:* Deepens CNS and respiratory depression, hypotension. Use together cautiously.

Naloxone, naltrexone: Reduces buprenorphine effects. Avoid using together.

Opioid analgesics: May decrease analgesic effect. Avoid using together.

Drug-lifestyle. *Alcohol use:* Causes additive effects. Use together cautiously.

EFFECTS ON LAB TEST RESULTS

• May increase amylase and lipase levels.

• May cause delayed emptying during gastric studies. May increase CSF pressure during lumbar puncture.

• May cause misleading hepatobiliary imaging results.

ACTION

Effects may result from binding with opiate receptors at many CNS sites. Drug also possesses opioid antagonist activity, which alters the perception of pain and emotional response to it. Long duration of action may result from drug's slow dissociation from receptor sites.

PHARMACOKINETICS

Onset, immediately after administration; peak level, after 2 minutes; duration, 6 to 10 hours.

Distribution: 96% protein bound, with levels found in liver, brain, and GI tract. Drug crosses the blood-brain barrier, but it's unclear if it crosses the placental barrier or appears in the breast milk.

Metabolism: Hepatic; undergoes N-dealkylation to form norbuprenorphine and then conjugates with glucuronic acid.

Excretion: Primarily in feces as free buprenorphine and metabolites and secondarily in urine as conjugated buprenorphine and metabolites. Elimination half-life for first phase, 2 minutes; for second phase, 11 minutes; and for last phase, 132 minutes.

CLINICAL CONSIDERATIONS

• Osmolality: 297 mOsm/kg.

• Monitor blood pressure and respiratory status frequently for at least 1 hour after administration. Keep resuscitation equipment and naloxone readily available. If respiratory rate drops below 8 breaths/minute, wake patient to stimulate breathing and notify prescriber.

• Patients who become physically dependent on this drug may have acute withdrawal syndrome if given an antagonist. Use cautiously and monitor patient closely.

• Assess bowel function. Patient may need stool softener.

• To treat overdose, maintain airway and provide respiratory support. Naloxone may be used to reverse respiratory depression; however, it may antagonize respiratory depression or potentiate other adverse reactions. If ineffective, give 1 to 2 mg/kg of doxapram by I.V. push to stimulate respiration. Give I.V. fluids, oxygen, and vasopressors as needed to maintain blood pressure.

PATIENT TEACHING
• When used postoperatively, encourage patient to turn, cough, and breathe deeply to prevent atelectasis.
• Notify patient that drug may interfere with ability to operate machinery or drive a car.
• Instruct patient to avoid alcohol and other CNS depressants.
• Advise ambulatory patient to get out of bed or walk cautiously because of risk of orthostatic hypotension.

butorphanol tartrate
Stadol

Pharmacologic class: opioid agonist-antagonist, opioid partial agonist
Therapeutic class: analgesic, adjunct to anesthesia
Pregnancy risk category: C
Controlled substance schedule: IV
pH: 3 to 5.5

INDICATIONS & DOSAGES
➤ **Moderate to severe pain from acute and chronic disorders—**
Adults: 1 mg I.V. q 3 to 4 hours; range, 0.5 to 2 mg q 3 to 4 hours, p.r.n.
➤ **Preoperative anesthesia—**
Adults: 2 mg I.V. shortly before induction. During maintenance anesthesia, 0.5 to 1 mg I.V. Total dose varies; patients rarely require less than 4 mg or more than 12.5 mg.
➤ **Pain during labor—**
Adults: 1 to 2 mg I.V. q 4 hours in mother with fetus of at least 37 weeks' gestation and without signs of fetal distress.
Adjust-a-dose: Dose should be reduced to 0.5 mg q 6 hours in patients with hepatic or renal impairment and in geriatric patients.

ADMINISTRATION
Direct injection: Inject drug directly into the vein or an established I.V. line over several minutes.
Intermittent infusion: Not recommended.
Continuous infusion: Not recommended.

PREPARATION & STORAGE
Available in single- and multiple-dose vials and disposable syringes with concentrations of 1 and 2 mg/ml. No dilution needed. Store at room temperature away from light.

Incompatibilities
Dimenhydrinate, pentobarbital sodium.

CONTRAINDICATIONS & CAUTIONS
• Contraindicated in those hypersensitive to the drug.
• Contraindicated in those with acute respiratory depression or diarrhea caused by poisoning or pseudomembranous colitis because of delayed toxin removal.
• Avoid use in patients younger than age 18 because pediatric safety and effectiveness haven't been established.
• Use cautiously in opioid-dependent patients. Detoxification should precede butorphanol administration.
• Use cautiously in those with a history of drug abuse or emotional instability because of the risk of dependence and in those with hypothyroidism because of deepened respiratory and prolonged CNS depression.
• Use cautiously in those with hepatic or renal disease and in geriatric patients because of increased risk of toxic reaction and in those with an MI or coronary artery disease because of increased cardiac workload.
• Use cautiously in those with hypertension, arrhythmias, or seizures to avoid exacerbation; in those with head trauma or increased intracranial pressure to avoid increasing the pressure

---

Reactions may be *common*, uncommon, *life-threatening*, or COMMON AND LIFE-THREATENING.

further and masking key symptoms; and in those with respiratory compromise to reduce the risk of respiratory depression.
• Use cautiously in those with inflammatory bowel disease because of possible toxic megacolon and in those with prostatic hyperplasia, urethral stricture, or recent urinary tract surgery because of possible urine retention.
• Use cautiously in those with acute abdominal conditions because significant symptoms can be obscured.

ADVERSE REACTIONS
CNS: *sedation, dizziness,* headache, vertigo, confusion, light-headedness, paresthesia, lethargy, asthenia, anxiety, euphoria, nervousness, floating feeling.
CV: vasodilation, palpitations.
EENT: dry mouth, blurred vision.
GI: *nausea, vomiting,* anorexia.
Respiratory: *respiratory depression.*
Skin: clamminess, sweatiness, pruritus.

INTERACTIONS
Drug-drug. *CNS depressants:* Increases CNS and respiratory depression. Avoid using together.
Antihypertensives: May cause hypotension. Monitor blood pressure closely.
Buprenorphine, naloxone, naltrexone: Reduces therapeutic effects of butorphanol. Avoid using together.
Pancuronium: May cause conjunctival changes. Monitor patient closely.
Drug-lifestyle. *Alcohol use:* Causes additive effects. Discourage use together.

EFFECTS ON LAB TEST RESULTS
None reported.

ACTION
Thought to bind with opiate receptors at many CNS sites, altering the perception of pain and the emotional response to it.

PHARMACOKINETICS
Onset, 1 minute; peak, almost immediately; duration, 2 to 4 hours.
Distribution: Throughout body tissues, with highest levels in lungs, spleen, heart, endocrine tissue, blood cells, and fat tissue. Drug crosses placental barrier; fetal levels are ½ to 1½ times maternal levels. Drug also appears in breast milk. Cerebral levels are lower than serum levels.
Metabolism: Extensively by the liver.
Excretion: Mostly in urine; rest appears in bile and feces and undergoes enterohepatic recycling. Elimination half-life, 3 to 4 hours.

CLINICAL CONSIDERATIONS
• Osmolality: 284 mOsm/kg.
• Drug may cause delayed emptying during gastric studies and may increase CSF pressure during lumbar puncture.
• Drug can cause physical and psychological dependence. Abrupt withdrawal after long-term use produces intense withdrawal symptoms.
• To minimize hypotension and dizziness, give drug with patient in recumbent position.
• *Alert:* Rapid I.V. injection can cause severe respiratory depression, hypotension, circulatory collapse, and cardiac arrest.
• *Alert:* Keep emergency resuscitation equipment available when giving drug.
• Individualize preoperative dose based on age, body weight, physical status, underlying condition, use of other drugs, type of anesthesia, and surgical procedure being performed.
• Individualize dose used in labor based on initial response, other analgesics or sedatives used, and expected time of delivery. Don't repeat dose in less than 4 hours and don't give within 4 hours of anticipated delivery.
• Assess bowel function. Patient may need a stool softener.
• Periodically monitor postoperative vital signs and bladder function. Because

drug decreases both rate and depth of respirations, monitoring of arterial oxygen saturation may aid in assessing respiratory depression.
• If overdose occurs, give naloxone and monitor cardiopulmonary status. Provide oxygen, respiratory support, I.V. fluids, and vasopressors.

PATIENT TEACHING
• Caution patient against performing hazardous tasks, such as operating machinery or driving a car.
• Notify patient of potential for dependence.

C

calcitriol
Calcijex

Pharmacologic class: vitamin D
analogue
Therapeutic class: antihypocal-
cemic
Pregnancy risk category: C
pH: 6.5 to 8

INDICATIONS & DOSAGES
➤ **To manage hypocalcemia in patients undergoing long-term renal
dialysis—**
Adults: 1 to 2 mcg I.V. three times
weekly, about every other day. Dosage
may be increased by 0.25 to 0.5 mcg at
2- to 4-week intervals. Maintenance
dose, 0.5 to 4 mcg three times weekly.

ADMINISTRATION
Direct injection: Aspirate solution from
ampule and inject directly into vein or
into I.V. tubing containing a free-
flowing, compatible solution.
Intermittent infusion: Not recommended.
Continuous infusion: Not recommended.

PREPARATION & STORAGE
Available in ampules containing 1 or
2 mcg/ml.
  Compatible with D_5W, normal saline
solution, or water for injection.
  Store at room temperature. Avoid
freezing.
  Discard unused portions immediately, because calcitriol injection doesn't
contain a preservative.

Incompatibilities
None reported.

CONTRAINDICATIONS & CAUTIONS
● Contraindicated in those with hypercalcemia or vitamin D toxicity. Don't
use with preparations containing vitamin D.
● Use cautiously in those taking a cardiac glycoside because hypercalcemia
may precipitate cardiac arrhythmias.

ADVERSE REACTIONS
CNS: headache, somnolence, weak-
ness.
CV: hypertension, *arrhythmias.*
EENT: conjunctivitis, rhinorrhea, dry
mouth, metallic taste, photophobia.
GI: nausea, vomiting, constipation,
anorexia.
GU: polyuria, nocturia.
Metabolic: weight loss; increased
magnesium, phosphorus, and calcium
levels.
Musculoskeletal: bone pain, muscle
pain.
Skin: pruritus.
Other: hyperthermia, decreased libido.

INTERACTIONS
Drug-drug. *Barbiturates, phenytoin:*
Increases metabolism of calcitriol and
decreases activity. May need to increase calcitriol dose.
Cardiac glycosides: Hypercalcemia
may precipitate cardiac arrhythmias.
Avoid using together.
Corticosteroids: Decreases effectiveness of vitamin D analogues. Avoid using together.
Verapamil: Causes atrial fibrillations
with hypercalcemia. Avoid using together.

EFFECTS ON LAB TEST RESULTS
• May increase calcium, magnesium, and phosphorus levels.
• May falsely increase cholesterol level with Zlatkis-Zak test.

ACTION
Promotes absorption of calcium from the intestine by forming a calcium-binding protein, increases tubular reabsorption of calcium, and suppresses secretion and synthesis of parathyroid hormone.

PHARMACOKINETICS
Onset, shortly after injection.
Distribution: Widely distributed, with known sites of action in intestine, bone, kidney, and parathyroid gland. Metabolites are transported in blood and bound to proteins. It's unknown if drug appears in breast milk.
Metabolism: In liver and kidney.
Excretion: Primarily in feces.

CLINICAL CONSIDERATIONS
• Tonicity: isotonic.
• Maintain calcium level at 9 to 10 mg/dl. Give an oral calcium supplement, as needed.
• Monitor calcium and phosphorus levels at least twice weekly early in treatment and during dosage adjustment. Stop drug and notify prescriber if calcium level × phosphorus level exceeds 70 mg/dl.
• Monitor magnesium, alkaline phosphatase, and 24-hour urine calcium and phosphorus levels periodically during treatment.
• If overdose occurs, provide supportive care. Calcitonin administration may help to reverse hypercalcemia. Peritoneal dialysis using a calcium-free dialysate may remove drug.

PATIENT TEACHING
• Inform patient of symptoms of hypercalcemia, and tell him to report adverse reactions to prescriber immediately.
• Tell patient about diet and calcium supplementation. Tell patient to take in a consistent amount of dietary calcium and to take a calcium supplement if his prescriber has instructed him to do so.

calcium chloride
calcium gluceptate
calcium gluconate

Pharmacologic class: calcium supplement
Therapeutic class: therapeutic drug for electrolyte balance, cardiotonic
Pregnancy risk category: C
pH: calcium chloride, 5.5 to 7.5; calcium gluceptate, 5.6 to 7; calcium gluconate, 6 to 8.2

INDICATIONS & DOSAGES
➤ **Emergency treatment of hypocalcemia—**
Adults: 7 to 14 mEq I.V.
Children: 1 to 7 mEq I.V.
Infants: Less than 1 mEq I.V.; repeat q 1 to 3 days p.r.n.
➤ **Hypocalcemic tetany—**
Adults: 4.5 to 16 mEq I.V.
Children: 0.5 to 0.7 mEq/kg I.V. t.i.d. or q.i.d. or until tetany is controlled.
Infants: 2.4 mEq/kg I.V. daily in divided doses.
➤ **Hyperkalemia with secondary cardiac toxicity—**
Adults: 2.25 to 14 mEq I.V. given while monitoring ECG; repeat in 1 to 2 minutes p.r.n.
➤ **Advanced cardiac life support—**
Adults: 0.027 to 0.054 mEq/kg calcium chloride, 4.5 to 6.3 mEq calcium glu-

ceptate, or 2.3 to 3.7 mEq calcium gluconate I.V.; repeated p.r.n.
Children: 0.25 to 0.35 mEq/kg calcium chloride I.V.; repeat in 10 minutes p.r.n.
➤ **Magnesium toxicity—**
Adults: 7 mEq I.V.; subsequent doses based on response.
➤ **Transfusion of citrated blood—**
Adults: 1.35 mEq/100 ml of citrated blood I.V.
Neonates: 0.45 mEq/100 ml of citrated blood I.V.

ADMINISTRATION

Direct injection: Give slowly through a small needle into a large vein or through an I.V. line containing a free-flowing, compatible solution at a rate not exceeding 1 ml/minute (1.5 mEq/minute) for calcium chloride, 1.5 to 5 ml/minute for calcium gluconate, and 2 ml/minute for calcium gluceptate. Don't use scalp veins in children.
Intermittent infusion: Infuse diluted solution through an I.V. line containing a compatible solution. Maximum rate of 100 mg/minute for calcium chloride or 200 mg/minute suggested for calcium gluceptate and calcium gluconate.
Continuous infusion: Infuse after addition of large volume of fluid at a maximum rate of 100 mg/minute for calcium chloride or 200 mg/minute for calcium gluceptate and calcium gluconate.

PREPARATION & STORAGE

Calcium chloride comes in a 10-ml ampule, vial, and syringe of 10% solution containing 1.36 mEq calcium/ml. Calcium gluceptate comes in a 5-ml ampule and in 50-ml and 100-ml bulk containers of a 22% solution containing 0.9 mEq calcium/ml. Calcium gluconate is available in 10-ml ampules and vials and 20-ml vials as a 10% solution containing 0.45 to 0.48 mEq calcium/ml. Calcium salts may be diluted with compatible solutions, including most I.V. and total parenteral nutrition solutions, before infusion.

Warm injection to body temperature before giving in nonemergencies.

Store from 59° to 86° F (15° to 30° C), unless the manufacturer specifies otherwise. Use only clear solutions. If crystals are present in calcium gluceptate, discard solution. If crystals are present in calcium gluconate, warm solution to 86° to 104° F (30° to 40° C) to dissolve them.

Incompatibilities

Calcium chloride: amphotericin B, chlorpheniramine, dobutamine, magnesium sulfate.
Calcium gluceptate: magnesium sulfate, prednisolone sodium phosphate, prochlorperazine edisylate.
Calcium gluconate: amphotericin B, dobutamine, indomethacin sodium trihydrate, magnesium sulfate, methylprednisolone sodium succinate, prochlorperazine edisylate.

CONTRAINDICATIONS & CAUTIONS

• Contraindicated in those with digitalis toxicity or ventricular fibrillation because of an increased risk of arrhythmias and in those with hypercalciuria, calcium renal calculi, or hypercalcemia because of possible exacerbation.
• Contraindicated in those with sarcoidosis because this condition may potentiate hypercalcemia.
• Use cautiously in those with renal impairment, dehydration, or electrolyte imbalance because of an increased risk of hypercalcemia and in those with cardiac disease because of an increased risk of arrhythmias.
• Use calcium chloride cautiously in those with cor pulmonale, respiratory acidosis, renal disease, or respiratory failure because of its acidifying effects.

ADVERSE REACTIONS

CNS: tingling sensations, weakness, syncope (especially with rapid I.V. injection).
CV: vasodilation, hypotension, ***bradycardia, cardiac arrhythmias, cardiac arrest, vein irritation.***
Other: sense of oppression or heat waves.

INTERACTIONS

Drug-drug. *Calcium channel blockers:* Antagonizes effects. Avoid using together.
Cardiac glycosides: Causes arrhythmias from potentiated inotropic and toxic glycoside effects. Use together cautiously, if at all.
Parenteral magnesium sulfate, nondepolarizing neuromuscular blockers: Reduces muscle paralysis. Avoid using together.
Potassium supplements: May cause arrhythmias. Avoid using together.
Thiazide diuretics: Reduces calcium excretion, possibly resulting in hypercalcemia. Avoid using together.

EFFECTS ON LAB TEST RESULTS

• May increase calcium level.
• May cause false-negative serum and urine magnesium test results using Titan yellow method.

ACTION

Maintains nervous system integrity, muscular and skeletal function, and cell membrane and capillary permeability. Essential for coagulation, release and storage of neurotransmitters and hormones, amino acid uptake and binding, vitamin B_{12} absorption, gastrin secretion, and contraction of cardiac and smooth muscle.

PHARMACOKINETICS

Onset, immediately after infusion; duration, 30 minutes to 2 hours.
Distribution: Into extracellular fluid; then 99% is rapidly incorporated into bone and 1% is divided between intracellular and extracellular fluid; 45% of calcium binds to protein. Calcium crosses placental barrier, reaching higher level in fetal blood than in maternal blood, and appears in breast milk and sweat.
Metabolism: Not metabolized.
Excretion: Mainly removed in feces as unabsorbed calcium or part of bile and pancreatic juices. Also filtered by renal glomeruli but reabsorbed in loop of Henle and convoluted tubules. Small amounts of calcium appear in urine.

CLINICAL CONSIDERATIONS

• Osmolality: calcium chloride, 1,765 mOsm/kg measured for 10% solution; calcium gluconate, 276 mOsm/kg.
• Osmolarity: calcium chloride, 2,040 mOsm/L for 10% solution; calcium glucepate, 555 mOsm/L; calcium gluconate, 680 mOsm/L for American Regent product and 270 mOsm/L for Abbott product.
• Review results of renal function tests before giving calcium.
• *Alert:* Never give drug S.C. or I.M., only I.V.
• After I.V. injection, briefly keep patient in a recumbent position.
• Monitor blood pressure and watch for a moderate drop. In hypertensive or geriatric patients, blood pressure may rise briefly.
• Closely monitor calcium level and possibly ECG. Check urine calcium level to help avoid hypercalciuria.
• Hypocalcemia may cause muscle twitching and spasms. Hypercalcemia may cause bradycardia, depressed nervous and neuromuscular function, arrhythmias, and impaired renal function.
• If calcium level exceeds 12 mg/dl, give normal saline, I.V. fluids, and furosemide or ethacrynic acid to promote calcium excretion. Closely monitor potassium and magnesium levels and ECG to detect complications. As-

sist with hemodialysis and give calcitonin and adrenocorticosteroids, if ordered.

PATIENT TEACHING
• Tell patient he may experience tingling sensations, heat waves, and weakness after drug administration.
• Instruct patient to report discomfort at I.V. site immediately.

carboplatin
Paraplatin

Pharmacologic class: alkylating drug (cell cycle phase–nonspecific)
Therapeutic class: antineoplastic
Pregnancy risk category: D
pH: 5 to 7 for a 1% solution

INDICATIONS & DOSAGES
➤ Ovarian cancer—
Adults: 360 mg/m² I.V. on day 1 q 4 weeks, as single agent therapy. For combination chemotherapy regimen with cyclophosphamide, initial carboplatin dose is 300 mg/m² I.V.
Adjust-a-dose: If creatinine clearance is between 41 and 59 ml/minute, adjust dose to 250 mg/m²; if clearance is between 16 and 40 ml/minute, adjust dose to 200 mg/m².

Reduce dose 25% if platelet count is below 50,000/mm³ or neutrophil count is below 500/mm³. Dose may be increased by 25% if platelet count is over 100,000/mm³ and neutrophil count is over 2,000/mm³. Don't repeat dose unless neutrophil count is at least 2,000/mm³ and platelet count is at least 100,000/mm³.

ADMINISTRATION
Direct injection: Not recommended.
Intermittent infusion: Usually infused over 15 minutes or longer into vein or with a free-flowing, compatible I.V. solution.
Continuous infusion: Not recommended.

PREPARATION & STORAGE
To avoid mutagenic, teratogenic, and carcinogenic risks, use extreme caution when preparing or giving carboplatin. Use a biological containment cabinet, wear gloves and mask, and use syringes with luer-lock fittings to prevent leakage of drug solution. Also, correctly dispose of needles, vials, and unused drug, and avoid contaminating work surfaces. Avoid inhalation of dust or vapors and contact with skin or mucous membranes.

Available in vials containing 50, 150, and 450 mg. Immediately before use, reconstitute with D_5W, normal saline solution, or sterile water for injection to a concentration of 10 mg/ml.

Dilute reconstituted carboplatin with normal saline injection or D_5W to a concentration as low as 0.5 mg/ml.

Store unopened vials at room temperature and protect from light. Once reconstituted and diluted, solution remains stable at room temperature for 8 hours. Because the drug doesn't contain antibacterial preservatives, discard unused drug after 8 hours.

Don't use needles or I.V. administration sets containing aluminum because carboplatin may precipitate and lose potency.

Incompatibilities
Fluorouracil, mesna, sodium bicarbonate.

CONTRAINDICATIONS & CAUTIONS
• Contraindicated in those hypersensitive to cisplatin, platinum-containing compounds, or mannitol.
• Contraindicated in those with severe bone marrow depression or bleeding.
• Use cautiously in those with creatinine clearance below 60 ml/minute be-

cause they may experience more severe bone marrow depression, and in those older than age 65 because they're at greater risk for neurotoxicity. Dosage may need to be adjusted in these patients.

ADVERSE REACTIONS
CNS: *CVA, peripheral neuropathies, asthenia, pain.*
CV: *heart failure, embolism.*
EENT: *ototoxicity,* visual disturbances, change in taste, oral ulceration.
GI: *vomiting, nausea,* abdominal pain, diarrhea, constipation.
Hematologic: THROMBOCYTOPENIA, NEUTROPENIA, LEUKOPENIA, bleeding, infections, *anemia.*
Metabolic: *hyponatremia, hypokalemia, hypocalcemia, hypomagnesemia.*
Skin: rash, urticaria, erythema, pruritus, *alopecia.*
Other: *allergic reactions, infection.*

INTERACTIONS
Drug-drug. *Aminoglycosides, other nephrotoxic or ototoxic drugs:* Increases risk of nephrotoxicity or ototoxicity. Use together cautiously.
Aspirin: Increases risk of bleeding. Avoid using together.
Myelosuppressants: Causes additive bone marrow suppression. Monitor patient.

EFFECTS ON LAB TEST RESULTS
• May increase BUN, creatinine, AST, and alkaline phosphatase levels. May decrease electrolyte levels.
• May decrease hemoglobin, hematocrit, and neutrophil, WBC, RBC, and platelet counts.

ACTION
Has properties similar to alkylating drugs. It cross-links strands of DNA material, inhibiting DNA synthesis and leading to cell death. It also has immunosuppressive, radiosensitizing, and antimicrobial properties.

PHARMACOKINETICS
Drug level peaks immediately.
Distribution: Widely distributed into body tissues and fluids with highest levels in kidneys, liver, skin, and tumor tissue. No significant protein binding of the parent compound occurs, but free platinum may irreversibly bind to protein. Unknown if drug appears in breast milk.
Metabolism: Carboplatin compounds are believed to be displaced by water to form complexes that bind with DNA.
Excretion: 65% eliminated by kidneys within 12 hours and 71% within 24 hours. Half-life is 2 to 5 hours with possible enterohepatic recirculation. However, platinum from carboplatin is slowly excreted, with a minimum half-life of 5 days.

CLINICAL CONSIDERATIONS
• Osmolality: 10 mg/ml solution in sterile water, 94 mOsm/kg.
• Only one increase in dosage is recommended. Subsequent doses shouldn't exceed 125% of starting dose.
• Determine electrolytes, creatinine, BUN, CBC, and creatinine clearance levels before the first infusion and before each course.
• Drug can produce severe vomiting. Begin antiemetic therapy before carboplatin therapy.
• *Alert:* Because aluminum adversely reacts with carboplatin, don't use aluminum-containing I.V. sets or needles in preparing or giving the drug.
• *Alert:* Have epinephrine, corticosteroids, and antihistamines available for use in hypersensitivity reactions.
• Patients with anemia resulting from cumulative doses may require a transfusion.
• Observe closely for hypersensitivity reactions, which may occur within minutes of administration.
• Monitor vital signs during infusion.
• Monitor CBC and platelet count frequently during therapy and, when indi-

cated, until recovery. Leukocyte and platelet nadirs usually occur by day 21. Levels usually return to baseline by day 28. Don't repeat dose unless platelet count exceeds 100,000/mm³ and neutrophil count is above 2,000/mm³.
• Patient may require periodic audiometric testing.

PATIENT TEACHING
• Advise women of childbearing age to avoid becoming pregnant during therapy.
• Because drug may cause toxic reaction in infants, advise patients not to breast-feed during therapy.
• Advise patient to watch for signs and symptoms of infection, such as fever, sore throat, or fatigue, or of bleeding, such as easy bruising, melena, bleeding gums, or nosebleeds. Tell patient to take his temperature daily.

carmustine (BCNU)
BiCNU

Pharmacologic class: alkylating drug, cell cycle phase–nonspecific nitrosourea
Therapeutic class: antineoplastic
Pregnancy risk category: D
pH: 5.6 to 6

INDICATIONS & DOSAGES
➤ **Brain tumors, Hodgkin's disease, lymphomas, malignant melanoma ◆, multiple myeloma—**
Adults and children: 150 to 200 mg/m² I.V. given as a single dose or divided into daily injections, such as 75 to 100 mg/m² on two successive days. Repeat full dose q 6 to 8 weeks.
Adjust-a-dose: Give 70% of dose if WBC count is between 2,000/mm³ and 3,000/mm³ and platelet count is between 25,000/mm³ and 75,000/mm³. Give 50% of previous dose for WBC

counts below 2,000/mm³ and platelet counts below 25,000/mm³.

ADMINISTRATION
Direct injection: Not recommended.
Intermittent infusion: Infuse 250 to 500 ml of diluted solution over 1 to 2 hours. If patient reports pain, dilute drug further or slow infusion.
Continuous infusion: Not recommended.

PREPARATION & STORAGE
Take special precautions when preparing drug because of its mutagenic, teratogenic, and carcinogenic effects: Wear gloves and mask, use a biological containment cabinet, and prevent work surface contamination. Avoid contact with skin because drug causes burning and a brown stain. If contact occurs, wash the area immediately and thoroughly. Correctly dispose of all equipment and unused drug.
    Drug comes as a powder in 100-mg vials. Before preparation, check for oily film at bottom of vial, which is a sign of decomposition, and discard if present.
    Dilute 100 mg with 3 ml of sterile, dehydrated ethyl alcohol that the manufacturer has supplied. After dissolving, add 27 ml of sterile water for injection to produce clear, colorless to yellow solution with a concentration of 3.3 mg of carmustine/ml of 10% alcohol. Preparation remains stable for 8 hours if kept at room temperature and 24 hours if refrigerated. Protect from light. Reconstituted solution may be further diluted with 250 to 500 ml of D₅W or normal saline solution for infusion. If refrigerated and protected from light, this solution remains stable for 48 hours if prepared in a glass container; solution becomes unstable in plastic I.V. bag.
    Store in original container, protected from light, at 36° to 46° F (2° to 8° C).

Incompatibilities
Sodium bicarbonate.

CONTRAINDICATIONS & CAUTIONS
• Contraindicated in those hypersensitive to the drug.
• Contraindicated in those with chickenpox or recent exposure to it or herpes zoster because of risk of severe generalized disease.
• Dosage may need to be reduced in those receiving drug along with other myelosuppressives.
• Use cautiously in those with myelosuppression, existing infection, or renal, hepatic, or pulmonary impairment because of the increased risk of toxic or adverse reactions.
• Use cautiously in smokers and in those who have received radiation therapy (especially to the mediastinum) or cytotoxic drug therapy because of an increased risk of pulmonary toxicity.

ADVERSE REACTIONS
GI: nausea, vomiting.
GU: decreased kidney size, azotemia, *renal failure.*
Hematologic: *thrombocytopenia, leukopenia,* anemia.
Hepatic: *hepatotoxicity,* jaundice.
Respiratory: pulmonary infiltrates, *pulmonary fibrosis.*
Skin: local irritation, facial flushing.

INTERACTIONS
Drug-drug. *Anticoagulants, aspirin:* Increases risk of bleeding. Avoid using together.
Cimetidine, myelosuppressives: Enhances toxicity. Avoid using together.
Digoxin, phenytoin: Reduces drug level. Monitor level closely.
Mitomycin: Causes damage to corneal and conjunctival epithelium. Monitor patient closely.
Toxoids, vaccines with killed virus: Reduces effectiveness. Avoid using together.

Vaccines with live virus: Increases risk of neurotoxicity. Avoid using together.

EFFECTS ON LAB TEST RESULTS
• May increase urine urea, AST, bilirubin, and alkaline phosphatase levels.
• May decrease hemoglobin and WBC and platelet counts.

ACTION
Interferes with DNA and RNA synthesis by acting as an alkylating drug.

PHARMACOKINETICS
Onset, rapid; drug level peaks at end of infusion.
Distribution: Throughout body tissues. Drug crosses the blood-brain and placental barriers and appears in breast milk.
Metabolism: By the liver within 15 minutes of administration. Some metabolites are active.
Excretion: Primarily by the kidneys; up to 10% by lungs as carbon dioxide; 1% in feces.

CLINICAL CONSIDERATIONS
• Osmolality: 3.3 mg/ml solution, reconstituted as directed in ethanol and water, exceeds 2,000 mOsm/kg.
• **Alert:** Give an antiemetic before carmustine. Monitor patient for nausea and vomiting, which may last up to 6 hours after administration.
• **Alert:** Obtain baseline pulmonary function tests, then monitor function during therapy. Risk of pulmonary toxicity increases with cumulative doses exceeding 1,400 mg/m^2.
• Avoid all I.M. injections when platelet count is less than 100,000/mm^3.
• Intense flushing of the skin may occur during I.V. infusion but usually disappears in 2 to 4 hours.
• At first sign of extravasation, stop infusion and infiltrate area with liberal injections of 0.5 mEq/ml sodium bicarbonate solution.

Reactions may be *common,* uncommon, *life-threatening,* or COMMON AND LIFE-THREATENING.

- *Alert:* Don't exceed frequency of every 6 weeks.
- Administration over less than 1 to 2 hours may produce severe pain and burning at the injection site and along the vein.
- Check CBC weekly for at least 6 weeks after dose to monitor extent of myelosuppression. Thrombocytopenia usually occurs 4 to 6 weeks after dose and lasts 1 to 2 weeks. Leukopenia occurs 5 to 6 weeks after dose and lasts for 1 to 2 weeks.
- Avoid immunizing patient or exposing him to patients who have received a live vaccine.
- Periodically monitor hepatic and renal function.

PATIENT TEACHING
- Advise any woman of childbearing age to avoid becoming pregnant during treatment because drug may harm the fetus.
- Because drug may cause toxic reaction in infants, advise patients not to breast-feed while receiving drug.
- Advise patient to watch for signs and symptoms of infection, such as fever, sore throat, and fatigue, or of bleeding, such as easy bruising, melena, bleeding gums, and nosebleeds. Tell patient to take his temperature daily.

caspofungin acetate
Cancidas

Pharmacologic class: glucan synthesis inhibitor, echinocandin
Therapeutic class: antifungal
Pregnancy risk category: C
pH: 6.6

INDICATIONS & DOSAGESS
➤ **Invasive aspergillosis in patients refractory to or intolerant of other therapies (amphotericin B, lipid formulations of amphotericin B, or itraconazole)—**
Adults: 70-mg I.V. loading dose on day 1, followed by 50 mg daily thereafter. Duration of treatment should be based on severity of patient's underlying disease, recovery from immunosuppression, and clinical response.
Adjust-a-dose: For patients with Child-Pugh score 7 to 9, after initial 70-mg loading dose, give 35 mg daily.

ADMINISTRATION
Direct injection: Not recommended.
Intermittent infusion: Not recommended.
Continuous infusion: Give drug by slow I.V. infusion over 1 hour.

PREPARATION & STORAGE
Available as a lyophilized powder for injection in 50-mg and 70-mg single-use vials.

To prepare, allow refrigerated vial to warm to room temperature. Reconstitute vial with 10.5 ml of normal saline solution and gently mix. Transfer 10 ml of the reconstituted solution (for all 70-mg, 50-mg, 35-mg doses) to 250 ml normal saline solution. For patients on fluid restriction, the 50-mg and 35-mg doses may be diluted in 100 ml normal saline solution.

Use reconstituted vials within 1 hour or discard. Refrigerate vials at 36° to 46° F (2 ° to 8° C). Store reconstituted and diluted solution at less than 77° F (25° C).

Incompatibilities
Dextrose solutions, other I.V. drugs.

CONTRAINDICATIONS & CAUTIONS
- Contraindicated in patients hypersensitive to drug or its components.
- Use cautiously in breast-feeding women.

ADVERSE REACTIONS
CNS: *fever,* headache, *paresthesia.*
CV: *tachycardia, phlebitis, thrombo-phlebitis,* infused vein complications.
GI: nausea, vomiting, diarrhea, abdominal pain, *anorexia.*
GU: proteinuria, hematuria.
Hematologic: eosinophilia, *anemia.*
Metabolic: hypokalemia.
Musculoskeletal: *pain, myalgia.*
Respiratory: *tachypnea.*
Skin: histamine-mediated symptoms including rash, facial swelling, pruritus, warm sensation; *sweating.*
Other: *chills.*

INTERACTIONS
Drug-drug. *Cyclosporine:* May significantly increase caspofungin and ALT levels. Don't use together unless potential benefit outweighs potential risk.
Inducers of drug clearance or mixed inducer-inhibitors (carbamazepine, dexamethasone, efavirenz, nelfinavir, nevirapine, phenytoin, rifampin): May reduce caspofungin level. May need to adjust dosage.
Tacrolimus: May reduce tacrolimus level. Monitor tacrolimus level. May need to adjust dosage.

EFFECTS ON LAB TEST RESULTS
• May increase alkaline phosphatase level. May decrease potassium and urinary protein levels.
• May increase eosinophil and WBC counts, urine RBC count, and urine pH. May decrease hemoglobin.

ACTION
Inhibits the synthesis of an integral component of the fungal cell wall in susceptible *Aspergillus* species.

PHARMACOKINETICS
Onset, immediate.
Distribution: Extensively distributed and has a prolonged plasma half-life. About 97% bound to albumin with minimal distribution into RBCs.

Metabolism: Slowly metabolized in the liver.
Excretion: 35% in feces, 41% in urine.

CLINICAL CONSIDERATIONS
• The efficacy of a 70-mg dose regimen in patients who aren't clinically responding to the 50-mg daily dose isn't known. Limited safety data suggest that an increase in dosage to 70 mg daily is well-tolerated. Safety and efficacy of doses above 70 mg haven't been adequately studied.
• Monitor I.V. site carefully for phlebitis.
• Observe patients for histamine-mediated reactions, including rash, facial swelling, pruritus, and a sensation of warmth.
• Obtain baseline liver function test before beginning drug therapy. Assess lab values periodically during drug therapy to monitor patient's hepatic function.

PATIENT TEACHING
• Instruct patient to report to prescriber any signs and symptoms of phlebitis.
• Tell patient to report to prescriber immediately any adverse reactions during drug therapy.

cefazolin sodium
Ancef

Pharmacologic class: semi-synthetic first-generation cephalosporin
Therapeutic class: antibiotic
Pregnancy risk category: B
pH: 4.5 to 6 for reconstituted product from vial, 4.5 to 7 for frozen premixed solution

INDICATIONS & DOSAGES
➤ **Septicemia, endocarditis, and infections of the respiratory tract, GU tract, skin, soft tissue, biliary tract,**

bones, and joints caused by susceptible organisms—
Adults: In mild infection, 250 to 500 mg
I.V. q 8 hours; in moderate to severe infection, 500 mg to 1 g q 6 to 8 hours; in
life-threatening infection, 1 to 1.5 g q
6 hours. Maximum daily dose, 12 g.
Children older than age 1 month: 25
to 50 mg/kg I.V. daily in three or
four equally divided doses; in life-
threatening infection. 100 mg/kg daily
may be needed.
➤ **Surgical prophylaxis**—
Adults: 1 g I.V. 30 to 60 minutes before
surgery; during surgery, 0.5 to 1 g q
2 hours; after surgery, 0.5 to 1 g q 6 to
8 hours for 24 hours.
Adjust-a-dose: Dosage for patients
with renal impairment depends on creatinine clearance.
Adults: If creatinine clearance is 10 ml/
minute or less, give half usual dose q
18 to 24 hours; if clearance is 11 to
34 ml/minute, give half usual dose q
12 hours; if clearance is 35 to 54 ml/
minute, give full dose q 8 hours or less
frequently; and if it exceeds 55 ml/
minute, give usual adult dose.
Children: If creatinine clearance is 5 to
20 ml/minute, give 10% of the usual
daily dose q 24 hours; if clearance is
20 to 40 ml/minute, give 25% of the
usual daily dose divided equally q 12
hours; if clearance is 40 to 70 ml/
minute, give 60% of the usual daily
dose divided equally q 12 hours; and if
it exceeds 70 ml/minute, give usual pediatric dose.

ADMINISTRATION
Direct injection: Inject the solution into
a vein over 3 to 5 minutes or into I.V.
tubing containing a free-flowing, compatible solution.
Intermittent infusion: Insert a 21G or
23G needle into port of primary tubing,
and infuse 50 to 100 ml of solution
over 30 minutes.
Continuous infusion: Not recommended.

PREPARATION & STORAGE
Available in 500-mg and 1-g vials.
   To reconstitute, add 2 ml of normal
saline solution or sterile or bacteriostatic water to the 500-mg vial or 2.5 ml to
the 1-g vial. Shake well. This dilution
yields a concentration of 225 mg/ml
and 330 mg/ml, respectively. Further
dilute reconstituted drug with 5 ml of
sterile water for injection.
   For intermittent infusion, add reconstituted drug to 50 to 100 ml of compatible solution, such as D_5W; dextrose 5%
in lactated Ringer's; dextrose 5% in
0.2%, half-normal or normal saline solution; dextrose 5% and Normosol-M;
or dextrose 5% and Ionosol B or
Plasma-Lyte.
   Reconstituted and diluted drug remains stable for 24 hours if kept at
room temperature or 10 days if refrigerated.
   Solutions reconstituted with sterile
water or bacteriostatic water or normal
saline injection are stable for 12 weeks
when stored at -4° F (-20° C). Don't
use a cloudy or precipitated solution.
Don't refreeze thawed solutions.
   Also available in 500 mg and 1 g in
50 ml of D_5W frozen piggybacks.

Incompatibilities
Aminoglycosides, amiodarone, amobarbital, ascorbic acid injection, bleomycin, calcium glucceptate, calcium
gluconate, cimetidine, colistimethate,
erythromycin glucceptate, hydrocortisone, idarubicin, lidocaine, norepinephrine, oxytetracycline, pentobarbital sodium, polymyxin B, ranitidine,
tetracycline, theophylline, vitamin B
complex with C.

CONTRAINDICATIONS & CAUTIONS
• Contraindicated in those hypersensitive to cephalosporins, penicillins, or
penicillin-like products.
• Use cautiously in those with renal
disease to prevent toxic reaction.

• Use cautiously in those with a history of ulcerative colitis, regional enteritis, or antibiotic-associated colitis because of an increased risk of pseudomembranous colitis.

ADVERSE REACTIONS
CV: phlebitis at injection site.
GI: diarrhea, oral candidiasis, vomiting, nausea, pseudomembranous colitis.
GU: genital and anal pruritus, vaginitis, vaginal candidiasis.
Hematologic: *neutropenia, leukopenia, thrombocytopenia.*
Other: *hypersensitivity reactions.*

INTERACTIONS
Drug-drug. *Nephrotoxic drugs:* Additive nephrotoxicity. Avoid using together.
Probenecid: Reduces renal excretion of cefazolin. Use together cautiously.

EFFECTS ON LAB TEST RESULTS
• May increase ALT, AST, alkaline phosphatase, bilirubin, GGT, and LDH levels.
• May increase eosinophil count. May decrease neutrophil, WBC, and platelet counts.
• May falsely elevate serum or urine creatinine levels in tests using Jaffe reaction. May cause false-positive Coombs' test results and false-positive results in urine glucose tests using cupric sulfate (Benedict's reagent or Clinitest).

ACTION
Inhibits mucopeptide synthesis in the bacterial cell wall, promoting osmotic instability. Its spectrum of activity includes many gram-positive aerobic cocci, including *Staphylococcus aureus, S. epidermidis, Streptococcus pneumoniae,* group A beta-hemolytic streptococci, and group B streptococci.

PHARMACOKINETICS
Drug level peaks at 1 to 2 hours.
Distribution: Widely distributed into body tissues and fluids, including pleural and synovial fluid, bile, and bone. Not readily distributed into CSF, even when meninges are inflamed. Drug crosses the placental barrier and appears in breast milk in low levels.
Metabolism: Not metabolized.
Excretion: In urine by glomerular filtration and tubular secretion; 60% excreted in 6 hours, 80% to 100% in 24 hours. Half-life is about 1 to 2 hours.

CLINICAL CONSIDERATIONS
• Osmolality: 325 mOsm/kg for 20 mg/ml in D_5W; 347 mOsm/ml for 20 mg/ml in normal saline solution; 412 mOsm/kg for 50 mg/ml in D_5W; 426 mOsm/kg for 50 mg/ml in normal saline solution; 260 to 320 mOsm/kg for 500 mg/5 ml frozen premixed solution; 310 to 380 mOsm/kg for 1 g/50 ml frozen premixed solution.
• Check for previous penicillin or cephalosporin hypersensitivity. Negative history doesn't rule out future allergic reaction. Expect to treat anaphylaxis with epinephrine.
• Obtain specimens for culture and sensitivity testing before giving first dose. Therapy may start before results are available.
• Monitor renal and liver function.
• For patients on sodium restriction, note that drug contains 2 mEq of sodium per gram of drug.
• To avoid inaccurate results when checking urine for glucose, use glucose oxidase methods, such as Clinistix or glucose enzymatic test strip.
• If patient is undergoing long-term therapy, observe him for fungal and bacterial superinfection.
• *Alert:* Names of some cephalosporins are similar. Use caution when giving.
• *Alert:* If seizures occur, promptly stop drug; give anticonvulsants.
• Dialysis may help to remove drug.

PATIENT TEACHING

• Advise patient to report adverse reactions promptly.
• Instruct patient to report discomfort at I.V. site immediately.

cefepime hydrochloride
Maxipime

Pharmacologic class: semi-synthetic fourth-generation cephalosporin
Therapeutic class: antibiotic
Pregnancy risk category: B
pH: 4 to 6 for reconstituted product

INDICATIONS & DOSAGES

➤ **Mild to moderate uncomplicated or complicated UTI, including pyelonephritis—**
Adults and children ages 12 and older: 0.5 to 1 g I.V. q 12 hours for 7 to 10 days.
➤ **Severe uncomplicated or complicated UTI, including pyelonephritis—**
Adults and children ages 12 and older: 2 g I.V. q 12 hours for 10 days.
➤ **Moderate to severe pneumonia—**
Adults and children ages 12 and older: 1 to 2 g I.V. q 12 hours for 10 days.
➤ **Moderate to severe uncomplicated skin and skin structure infection—**
Adults and children ages 12 and older: 2 g I.V. q 12 hours for 10 days.
➤ **Empiric therapy in febrile neutropenia—**
Adults: 2 g I.V. q 8 hours for 7 days or until neutropenia resolves.
Children weighing less than 88 lb (40 kg): 50 mg/kg I.V. q 8 hours.
➤ **Complicated intra-abdominal infections in combination with metronidazole—**
Adults: 2 g I.V. q 12 hours for 7 to 10 days.

Adjust-a-dose: For patients with renal impairment, initial dose should be the same as in normal renal function; maintenance dose depends on creatinine clearance. No data are available for children with renal impairment, but dosage adjustments similar to those for adults are recommended. (See table on page 166.)

For patients on hemodialysis, about 68% of drug is removed after a 3-hour dialysis session. Give a repeat dose, equivalent to the initial dose, at the completion of dialysis.

For patients on continuous ambulatory peritoneal dialysis, give normal dose every 48 hours.

ADMINISTRATION

Direct injection: Not recommended.
Intermittent infusion: Infuse reconstituted solution over 30 minutes.
Continuous infusion: Not recommended.

PREPARATION & STORAGE

Available in 500-mg, 1-g, and 2-g vials, 1-g ADD-Vantage vials, and 1-g and 2-g piggyback bottles. For intermittent infusion, reconstitute the 1-g or 2-g piggyback bottle with 50 or 100 ml of normal saline injection, dextrose 5% and 10% injection, 1/6 M sodium lactate injection, dextrose 5% and normal saline injection, lactated Ringer's and dextrose 5% injection, or Normosol-R and Normosol-M in dextrose 5% injection. Alternatively, reconstitute 500-mg vial with 5 ml, 1-g vial with 10 ml, or 2-g vial with 10 ml and add an appropriate quantity of the resulting solution to an I.V. container with one of the compatible fluids.

Reconstitute ADD-Vantage only with 50 or 100 ml of dextrose 5% injection or normal saline injection in ADD-Vantage flexible diluent containers.

Reconstituted solution is stable for 24 hours if kept between 68° and 77° F

Dosage adjustments for renal impairment

| Creatinine clearance (ml/min) | 500 mg q 12 hr | If normal dosage would be | | |
		1 g q 12 hr	2 g q 12 hr	2 g q 8 hr
30-60	500 mg q 24 hr	1 g q 24 hr	2 g q 24 hr	2 g q 12 hr
11-29	500 mg q 24 hr	500 mg q 24 hr	1 g q 24 hr	2 g q 24 hr
< 11	250 mg q 24 hr	250 mg q 24 hr	500 mg q 24 hr	1 g q 24 hr

(20° and 25° C) or 7 days if refrigerated between 36° and 46° F (2° and 8° C).

Incompatibilities
Aminophylline, gentamicin, metronidazole, netilmicin, tobramycin, vancomycin.

CONTRAINDICATIONS & CAUTIONS
• Contraindicated in those who have shown immediate hypersensitivity reactions to the drug or to cephalosporin antibiotics, penicillins, or other beta-lactam antibiotics.
• Use cautiously in those with renal or hepatic impairment or poor nutritional state and in those receiving a protracted course of antimicrobial therapy because of potential alteration of PT and INR.
• Use cautiously in those with a history of GI disease, especially colitis, because of increased risk of pseudomembranous colitis.

ADVERSE REACTIONS
CNS: headache, pain, fever.
CV: phlebitis.
GI: diarrhea, colitis, nausea, vomiting, oral candidiasis.
GU: vaginitis.
Hematologic: eosinophilia.
Skin: rash, pruritus, urticaria; pain or inflammation at injection site.

INTERACTIONS
Drug-drug. *Aminoglycosides:* Increases risk of nephrotoxicity, ototoxicity. Monitor patient closely.
Furosemide: Increases risk of nephrotoxicity. Monitor patient closely.
Probenecid: May inhibit excretion of cefepime. Monitor patient closely.

EFFECTS ON LAB TEST RESULTS
• May falsely elevate serum or urine creatinine level in tests using Jaffe reaction. May cause false-positive Coombs' test results and false-positive results in urine glucose tests using cupric sulfate (Benedict's reagent or Clinitest).

ACTION
Broad-spectrum antibiotic that inhibits cell-wall synthesis, promoting osmotic instability.

PHARMACOKINETICS
Onset, within 30 minutes; drug peak level, 1 to 2 hours; duration unknown.
Distribution: Throughout body, including bronchial mucosa, sputum, urine, and blister fluid. Drug may cross the blood-brain barrier and appears in breast milk; about 20% is bound to protein.
Metabolism: Metabolized to N-methylpyrrolidine, which is rapidly converted to N-oxide.
Excretion: Primarily in urine.

Reactions may be *common*, uncommon, *life-threatening*, or COMMON AND LIFE-THREATENING.

CLINICAL CONSIDERATIONS

• Check for previous penicillin or cephalosporin hypersensitivity. Negative history doesn't rule out future allergic reaction.

• Obtain specimens for culture and sensitivity before giving first dose. Therapy may start before results are available.

• If diarrhea persists during therapy, collect stool specimens to rule out pseudomembranous colitis.

• If patient is undergoing high-dose or long-term therapy, monitor patient for superinfection.

• Monitor PT and INR in patients at risk for altered prothrombin activity.

• *Alert:* Names of some cephalosporins are similar. Use caution when giving.

• Monitor BUN and liver enzyme levels and creatinine clearance in patients with potential renal or hepatic impairment.

• To avoid inaccurate results when checking urine for glucose, use glucose oxidase methods, such as Clinistix or glucose enzymatic test strip.

• *Alert:* In patients with renal impairment, serious adverse events including encephalopathy, myoclonus, seizures, and renal failure have been reported when doses weren't adjusted.

• If overdose occurs, provide supportive treatment. Hemodialysis may remove drug.

PATIENT TEACHING

• Advise patient to report unusual bleeding or bruising.

• Advise patient to report any diarrhea.

• Warn patients with renal insufficiency of serious adverse reactions, including encephalopathy, myoclonus, seizures, and renal failure, when taking unadjusted doses of drug.

cefoperazone sodium
Cefobid

Pharmacologic class: semisynthetic third-generation cephalosporin
Therapeutic class: antibiotic
Pregnancy risk category: B
pH: 4.5 to 6.5

INDICATIONS & DOSAGES

➤ **Septicemia, peritonitis, and gynecologic, skin, and urinary and respiratory tract infections caused by susceptible organisms—**
Adults: 2 to 4 g I.V. daily in divided doses q 12 hours. For severe infections, 6 to 12 g/day in divided doses b.i.d, t.i.d., or q.i.d., ranging from 1.5 to 4 g/dose.
Children ages 1 month to 12 years ♦ : 100 to 150 mg/kg I.V. daily in two or three divided doses.
Adjust-a-dose: For adults with hepatic impairment, dosage shouldn't exceed 4 g I.V. daily. Monitor drug level if higher doses are used. Patients with both hepatic and renal impairment shouldn't receive more than 1 to 2 g (base) daily without having their drug levels checked.

ADMINISTRATION
Direct injection: Not recommended.
Intermittent infusion: Infuse solution over 15 to 30 minutes into I.V. tubing containing a compatible solution.
Continuous infusion: Infuse solution containing 2 to 25 mg/ml at ordered rate.

PREPARATION & STORAGE
Available in 1-g and 2-g vials. Reconstitute 1 g of drug with 5 ml of compatible diluent. Shake vial vigorously until drug dissolves. Let vial stand to allow foam to dissipate before drawing up.

After reconstitution, dilute further by adding 20 to 40 ml of compatible diluent for intermittent infusion and enough diluent to make a solution of 2 to 25 mg/ml for a continuous infusion. Compatible solutions include D_5W or dextrose 10% in water, lactated Ringer's, dextrose 5% in lactated Ringer's, dextrose 5% in 0.2% or normal saline solution, Normosol-R, dextrose 5% and Normosol-M, and normal saline solution.

Solutions are stable for 24 hours if kept at room temperature and 72 hours if refrigerated.

Incompatibilities
Amifostine, aminoglycosides, diltiazem, doxapram hydrochloride, filgrastim, hetastarch, labetalol hydrochloride, meperidine hydrochloride, ondansetron hydrochloride, pentamidine isethionate, perphenazine, promethazine hydrochloride, sargramostim, vinorelbine tartrate.

CONTRAINDICATIONS & CAUTIONS
• Contraindicated in those hypersensitive to cephalosporins.
• Use cautiously in those allergic to penicillin because of risk of cross-reactivity.
• Use cautiously in those with a history of allergies, especially to drugs, because of increased risk of allergic reaction.
• Use cautiously in those with hypoprothrombinemia or a bleeding disorder because of possible exacerbation.
• Use cautiously in those with ulcerative colitis, regional enteritis, or antibiotic-associated colitis because of an increased risk of pseudomembranous colitis and in those with hepatic or biliary disease because of increased risk of toxic reaction.
• Use cautiously during prolonged parenteral or enteral nutrition and in those with poor nutritional status, malabsorption, or alcohol dependence because of an increased risk of vitamin K deficiency.

ADVERSE REACTIONS
CNS: fever.
GI: diarrhea, anorexia, nausea, vomiting, abdominal pain, colitis.
Hematologic: *eosinophilia, neutropenia,* anemia.
Skin: rash, urticaria, pruritus, inflammation, phlebitis, thrombophlebitis at infusion site.
Other: *hypersensitivity reactions.*

INTERACTIONS
Drug-drug. *Anticoagulants, platelet aggregation inhibitors, thrombolytics:* Increases risk of bleeding. Monitor patient closely.
Nephrotoxic drugs: Additive nephrotoxicity. Monitor patient closely.
Probenecid: Reduces renal excretion of cefoperazone. Use together cautiously.
Drug-lifestyle. *Alcohol use:* Disulfiram-like reaction. Warn patient not to drink alcohol for several days after stopping cefoperazone.

EFFECTS ON LAB TEST RESULTS
• May increase ALT, AST, alkaline phosphatase, bilirubin, GGT, and LDH levels.
• May increase INR and eosinophil count. May decrease hemoglobin and neutrophil count. May increase or decrease PT.
• May falsely elevate serum or urine creatinine levels in tests using Jaffe reaction. May cause false-positive Coombs' test results and false-positive results in urine glucose tests using cupric sulfate (Benedict's reagent or Clinitest).

ACTION
Inhibits mucopeptide synthesis in the bacterial cell wall, promoting osmotic instability. Its broad spectrum of activity includes gram-positive aerobic cocci, such as most strains of *Staphylococ-*

cus aureus, S. epidermidis, groups A and B streptococci, *Streptococcus durans, S. faecalis, S. faecium, S. pneumoniae,* and *S. viridans,* and some strains of *Listeria monocytogenes.*

Susceptible gram-negative aerobic bacteria include *Citrobacter diversus, C. freundii, Enterobacter aerogenes, E. cloacae, Escherichia coli, Haemophilus influenzae, H. parainfluenzae, Klebsiella oxytoca, Morganella morganii, Neisseria gonorrhoeae, N. meningitidis, Proteus mirabilis, P. vulgaris, Providencia, Pseudomonas, Salmonella, Shigella,* and *Yersinia enterocolitica.*

Susceptible anaerobes include *Bifidobacterium, Clostridium,* including some strains of *C. difficile, Eubacterium, Fusobacterium, Peptococcus, Peptostreptococcus, Propionibacterium,* and *Veillonella.*

PHARMACOKINETICS
Drug level peaks when infusion is completed.
Distribution: Throughout body tissues and fluids, including aqueous humor, bile, sputum, tonsils, sinus membranes, endometrium, myometrium, lungs, prostate, bone, and ascitic, pleural, and middle-ear fluid. Slight amounts appear in CSF with uninflamed meninges, higher amounts with inflammation. Drug crosses the placental barrier and appears in breast milk in small amounts; 82% to 93% is bound to protein.
Metabolism: None.
Excretion: Primarily in bile, with 15% to 30% excreted unchanged in urine within 24 hours. In patients with severe hepatic disease or biliary obstruction, 90% is excreted in urine. Mean half-life is about 2 hours.

CLINICAL CONSIDERATIONS
• Osmolality: 1 g in 50 ml D_5W is 302 mOsm/kg; 1 g in 50 ml normal saline solution is 328 mOsm/kg; 2 g in D_5W is 343 mOsm/kg; 2 g in 50 ml normal saline solution is 370 mOsm/kg.
• Check for cephalosporin or penicillin hypersensitivity before giving first dose. Negative history doesn't rule out future allergic reaction.
• Obtain specimens for culture and sensitivity testing before giving first dose. Therapy may start before results are available.
• Monitor BUN and creatinine levels to assess renal function.
• Monitor patient with hepatic disease or biliary obstruction often for signs and symptoms of toxic reaction.
• Monitor CBC, PT, and INR to assess bleeding disturbances.
• *Alert:* Names of some cephalosporins are similar. Use caution when giving.
• For patients on sodium restriction, note that drug contains 1.5 mEq of sodium per gram of drug.
• To avoid inaccurate results when checking urine for glucose, use Clinistix or glucose enzymatic test strips.
• If patient is undergoing long-term therapy, monitor him for fungal and bacterial superinfection.
• If diarrhea persists, culture stool to rule out *C. difficile* infection.
• If high doses are used in patients with hepatic disease, biliary obstruction, or renal impairment, monitor level of drug.
• Vitamin K may be given to patients receiving high doses, to debilitated patients, and to those with hepatic or renal impairment.
• Give prescribed dose after hemodialysis treatment.
• Treat overdose symptomatically. Hemodialysis enhances drug removal.

PATIENT TEACHING
• Advise patient to report diarrhea and other adverse reactions promptly.
• Instruct patient to report discomfort at I.V. site immediately.

cefotaxime sodium
Claforan

Pharmacologic class: third-generation cephalosporin
Therapeutic class: antibiotic
Pregnancy risk category: B
pH: 5 to 7.5

INDICATIONS & DOSAGES
➤ **Severe life-threatening infections caused by susceptible organisms**—
Adults: 2 g I.V. q 4 hours; maximum dosage, 12 g daily.
➤ **Moderate to severe infections caused by susceptible organisms**—
Adults and children weighing 50 kg (110 lb) or more: 1 to 2 g I.V. q 6 to 8 hours.
Children ages 1 month to 12 years (weighing less than 50 g): 50 to 180 mg/kg I.V. daily in four to six equally divided doses.
Neonates ages 1 to 4 weeks: 50 mg/kg I.V. q 8 hours.
Neonates younger than age 1 week: 50 mg/kg I.V. q 12 hours.
➤ **Uncomplicated infections caused by susceptible organisms**—
Adults: 1 g I.V. q 12 hours.
➤ **Disseminated gonorrhea ♦**—
Adults: 1 g I.V. q 8 hours for 7 days.
Neonates and children: 25 to 50 mg/kg I.V. q 8 to 12 hours for 7 days.
➤ **Gonococcal meningitis ♦**—
Neonates: 25 to 50 mg/kg I.V. q 8 to 12 hours for 10 to 14 days.
➤ **Surgical prophylaxis**—
Adults: 1 g I.V. 30 to 90 minutes before surgery.
➤ **Prophylaxis for cesarean section**—
Adults: 1 g I.V. once umbilical cord is clamped, then 1 g 6 and 12 hours later.
Adjust-a-dose: Adult patients with creatinine clearance below 20 ml/minute should receive half the usual dose at the usual time interval.

ADMINISTRATION
Direct injection: Give over 3 to 5 minutes directly into an intermittent infusion device or through an I.V. line containing a free-flowing, compatible solution.
Intermittent infusion: Infuse diluted solution over 20 to 30 minutes into a butterfly or scalp vein needle or through an I.V. line containing a compatible solution. If piggyback method is used, interrupt flow of primary I.V.
Continuous infusion: Give ordered infusion over 24 hours.

PREPARATION & STORAGE
Available in vials containing 500 mg, 1 g, or 2 g and in infusion bottles containing 1 g or 2 g. Reconstitute vials with 10 ml of sterile water for injection. Shake well to dissolve. I.V. infusion bottles can be further diluted in 50 to 100 ml of D_5W or normal saline solution.

Reconstituted drug can be diluted in 50 to 1,000 ml of compatible solution for continuous infusion. These solutions include D_5W or dextrose 10% in water; normal saline solution; dextrose 5% in 0.2% or half-normal or normal saline solution; invert sugar 10% in water; lactated Ringer's; or 1/6 M sodium lactate.

Reconstituted solution remains stable for 24 hours at 77° F (25° C) and for 10 days at below 41° F (5° C).

Incompatibilities
Allopurinol, aminoglycosides, aminophylline, doxapram, filgrastim, fluconazole, hetastarch, pentamidine isethionate, sodium bicarbonate injection, vancomycin.

CONTRAINDICATIONS & CAUTIONS
• Contraindicated in those hypersensitive to cephalosporins.
• Use cautiously in those hypersensitive to penicillin because of possible allergic reaction and in those with renal im-

---

pairment because of prolonged excretion.
• Use cautiously in those with a history of GI disease, especially colitis, because of an increased risk of pseudomembranous colitis.

ADVERSE REACTIONS

CNS: fever.
GI: *pseudomembranous colitis,* diarrhea, nausea, vomiting.
Hematologic: eosinophilia.
Skin: rash, pruritus, urticaria, injection site inflammation.
Other: *anaphylaxis.*

INTERACTIONS

Drug-drug. *Aminoglycosides, nephrotoxic drugs:* Additive nephrotoxicity. Monitor patient closely.
Probenecid: Reduces renal excretion of cefotaxime. Use together cautiously.

EFFECTS ON LAB TEST RESULTS

• May increase BUN, creatinine, ALT, AST, alkaline phosphatase, bilirubin, GGT, and LDH levels.
• May increase eosinophil count. May decrease hemoglobin and neutrophil, platelet, and granulocyte counts.
• May cause positive Coombs' test results.

ACTION

Inhibits mucopeptide synthesis in the bacterial cell wall, promoting osmotic instability. Its broad spectrum of activity includes most gram-negative aerobic bacteria, such as *Citrobacter diversus, C. freundii, Enterobacter aerogenes, E. cloacae, Escherichia coli, Haemophilus influenzae, Klebsiella oxytoca, K. pneumoniae, Morganella morganii, Proteus mirabilis, P. vulgaris, Providencia rettgeri, Salmonella, Serratia marcescens, Shigella,* and *Yersinia;* some strains of *Pseudomonas;* and ampicillin-resistant, penicillinase-resistant, and nonpenicillinase-resistant

strains of *Neisseria gonorrhoeae* and *N. meningitidis.*
   Drug is effective against some gram-positive aerobic bacteria, including most strains of *Staphylococcus aureus,* group A and group B streptococci, and *Streptococcus pneumoniae* and some strains of *S. viridans.*
   Susceptible anaerobic bacteria include *Bacteroides, Eubacterium, Fusobacterium, Peptococcus, Peptostreptococcus, Propionibacterium, Veillonella,* and some strains of *Clostridium.*

PHARMACOKINETICS

Drug level peaks when infusion is completed.
Distribution: Throughout most body tissues and fluids. Therapeutic levels reach middle ear and CSF, especially if meninges are inflamed. Drug readily crosses the placental barrier and appears in breast milk; 13% to 38% is bound to protein.
Metabolism: Partly metabolized in liver and kidneys.
Excretion: Excreted rapidly by glomerular filtration and renal tubular secretion. Half-life, about 60 to 90 minutes.

CLINICAL CONSIDERATIONS

• Osmolality: 1 g in 50 ml D_5W is 350 mOsm/kg; 1 g in 50 ml normal saline solution is 375 mOsm/kg; 2 g in 50 ml D_5W is 343 mOsm/kg; 2 g in 50 ml normal saline solution is 406 mOsm/kg.
• Check for previous penicillin or cephalosporin hypersensitivity. Negative history doesn't rule out future allergic reaction.
• Obtain specimens for culture and sensitivity testing before giving first dose. Therapy may start before test results are available.
• Assess I.V. site for inflammation or phlebitis and change site as needed.
• *Alert:* Names of some cephalosporins are similar. Use caution when giving.

• If diarrhea persists during therapy, collect stool specimens to rule out pseudomembranous colitis.

• If patient is undergoing long-term therapy, monitor him for fungal and bacterial superinfection.

• Monitor renally impaired patient often for signs and symptoms of toxic reaction. Dosage may need to be reduced.

• If course of treatment exceeds 10 days, monitor CBC because of risk of agranulocytosis and granulocytopenia.

• Treat patients with overdose symptomatically. Hemodialysis or peritoneal dialysis removes drug.

PATIENT TEACHING

• Instruct patient to report diarrhea and other adverse reactions promptly.

• Instruct patient to report discomfort at I.V. site immediately.

cefotetan disodium
Cefotan

Pharmacologic class: semi-synthetic second-generation cephalosporin, cephamycin
Therapeutic class: antibiotic
Pregnancy risk category: B
pH: 4.5 to 6.5 for reconstituted solutions

INDICATIONS & DOSAGES
➤ **Infections, except for UTI, caused by susceptible organisms—**
Adults: 1 to 2 g I.V. q 12 hours; in life-threatening infections, 3 g q 12 hours.
➤ **Skin and skin structure infections—**
Adults: 2 g I.V. daily or 1 g q 12 hours.
➤ **UTI—**
Adults: 500 mg I.V. q 12 hours or 1 to 2 g once daily or b.i.d.

➤ **Surgical prophylaxis—**
Adults: 1 to 2 g I.V. 30 to 60 minutes before surgery. For cesarean section, give dose as soon as umbilical cord is clamped. Maximum daily dose, 6 g.
Adjust-a-dose: For patients with renal impairment, adjust dosage based on the degree of renal impairment, severity of infection, and susceptibility of organisms. For adults with creatinine clearance under 10 ml/minute, give usual adult dose q 48 hours or one-fourth the usual dose q 12 hours; 10 to 30 ml/minute, usual dose q 24 hours or half usual dose q 12 hours; or 30 ml/minute or more, usual adult dose.

Give hemodialysis patients one-fourth the usual adult dose q 24 hours on days between treatments, and half the usual dose on the day of hemodialysis.

ADMINISTRATION
Direct injection: Inject reconstituted drug directly into vein over 3 to 5 minutes.
Intermittent infusion: Over 20 to 60 minutes, infuse solution through a butterfly or scalp vein needle or into the tubing of a free-flowing, compatible solution. Interrupt flow of primary I.V. solution during drug administration.
Continuous infusion: Not recommended.

PREPARATION & STORAGE
Available as a white to pale yellow powder in 1-g and 2-g vials and infusion vials.

Reconstitute drug with 10 to 20 ml of sterile water for injection. Reconstitute drug in infusion vials with 50 to 100 ml of D_5W or normal saline solution.

After reconstitution, solution remains stable for 24 hours if kept at room temperature, 96 hours if refrigerated, and 1 week if frozen.

Incompatibilities
Aminoglycosides, doxapram, heparin sodium, promethazine hydrochloride, vinorelbine tartrate.

CONTRAINDICATIONS & CAUTIONS
• Contraindicated in those hypersensitive to cephalosporins.
• Use cautiously in those hypersensitive to penicillin.
• Use cautiously in those with a history of GI disease, especially colitis, because of an increased risk of pseudomembranous colitis and in those with bleeding disorders because of increased risk of hypoprothrombinemia and hemorrhage.
• Use cautiously in patients with renal impairment because of prolonged excretion.

ADVERSE REACTIONS
GI: diarrhea, *pseudomembranous colitis.*
Hematologic: eosinophilia, thrombocytosis, *agranulocytosis,* hemolytic anemia, *leukopenia, thrombocytopenia.*
Skin: rash, itching, urticaria.
Other: *anaphylaxis.*

INTERACTIONS
Drug-drug. *Aminoglycosides, nephrotoxic drugs:* Causes additive nephrotoxicity. Monitor patient closely.
Probenecid: May inhibit excretion and increase cefotetan level. May be used for this effect.
Drug-lifestyle. *Alcohol use:* Causes disulfiram-like reaction. Urge patient to avoid alcohol within 72 hours of administration.

EFFECTS ON LAB TEST RESULTS
• May increase BUN, creatinine, ALT, AST, alkaline phosphatase, bilirubin, and LDH levels.
• May increase PT and INR and eosinophil count. May decrease hemoglobin and neutrophil and granulocyte counts.

May increase or decrease platelet count.
• May falsely elevate serum or urine creatinine level in tests using Jaffe reaction. May cause false-positive Coombs' test result and false-positive result in urine glucose test using cupric sulfate (Benedict's reagent or Clinitest).

ACTION
Inhibits mucopeptide synthesis in the bacterial cell wall, promoting osmotic instability. Its spectrum of activity includes gram-positive aerobic bacteria, including *Staphylococcus aureus;* most strains of group A beta-hemolytic streptococci and groups B, C, and G streptococci; and some strains of *Streptococcus pneumoniae* and *Staphylococcus epidermidis.*

Susceptible gram-negative aerobic bacteria include *Neisseria meningitidis;* most strains of *N. gonorrhoeae, Citrobacter diversus, C. freundii, Enterobacter aerogenes, E. agglomerans, E. cloacae, Escherichia coli, Haemophilus influenzae, Hafnia alvei, Klebsiella oxytoca, K. ozaenae, K. pneumoniae, Morganella morganii, Proteus mirabilis, P. vulgaris, Providencia rettgeri, P. stuartii, Salmonella, Serratia marcescens, Shigella,* and *Yersinia enterocolitica;* and some strains of *Alcaligenes odorans* and *Moraxella.*

Susceptible gram-positive anaerobic bacteria include *Actinomyces, Clostridium, Peptococcus, Peptostreptococcus,* and *Propionibacterium.* Susceptible gram-negative anaerobic bacteria include *Bacteroides, Fusobacterium,* and *Veillonella.*

PHARMACOKINETICS
Drug level peaks when infusion is completed.
Distribution: Throughout body tissues and fluids, but with limited distribution into CSF. Drug crosses the placental

barrier and appears in breast milk; 76% to 91% is bound to protein.
Metabolism: None.
Excretion: Unchanged by kidneys, primarily by glomerular filtration, with 50% to 80% removed in 24 hours. About 20% is excreted in bile. Half-life averages 4 hours.

CLINICAL CONSIDERATIONS

• Osmolarity: 100 mg in sterile water is 400 mOsm/L; 200 mg/ml in sterile water is 800 mOsm/L; 1 and 2 g infusion bottles reconstituted with D_5W or normal saline solution have osmolarity ranges of 340 to 480 mOsm/L.
• Check for previous penicillin or cephalosporin hypersensitivity. Negative history doesn't rule out future allergic reaction.
• Obtain specimens for culture and sensitivity testing before giving first dose. Therapy may start before results are available.
• If diarrhea persists during therapy, collect stool specimens to rule out pseudomembranous colitis.
• To avoid inaccurate results when checking urine for glucose, use Clinistix or glucose enzymatic test strip.
• If patient is undergoing high-dose or long-term therapy, monitor him for superinfection.
• Monitor PT and INR in patients with renal or hepatic impairment, malnutrition, or cancer and in geriatric patients.
• *Alert:* Names of some cephalosporins are similar. Use caution when giving.
• Treat overdose symptomatically. Hemodialysis or peritoneal dialysis may promote drug removal.

PATIENT TEACHING

• Instruct patient to report diarrhea and other adverse reactions promptly.
• Instruct patient to report discomfort at I.V. site immediately.

cefoxitin sodium
Mefoxin

Pharmacologic class: second-generation cephalosporin, cephamycin
Therapeutic class: antibiotic
Pregnancy risk category: B
pH: 4.2 to 7 for reconstituted solutions, about 6.5 for frozen premixed product

INDICATIONS & DOSAGES

➤ **Severe infections caused by susceptible organisms—**
Adults: 1 to 2 g I.V. q 6 to 8 hours; in life-threatening infections, up to 12 g.
Children age 3 months and older: 80 to 160 mg/kg/day I.V. divided into three to six equal doses.
➤ **To prevent infection after surgery—**
Adults: 2 g I.V. 30 to 60 minutes before surgery, then 2 g q 6 hours for 1 day after surgery.
Children ages 3 months and older: 30 to 40 mg/kg I.V. 30 to 60 minutes before surgery, then 30 to 40 mg/kg q 6 hours for up to 24 hours after surgery.
➤ **To prevent infection in patients having cesarean section—**
Adults: 2 g I.V. as a single dose after cord is clamped, or 2 g after cord is clamped and 2 g 4 and 8 hours later.
Adjust-a-dose: For adults with creatinine clearance under 5 ml/minute, give 500 mg to 1 g q 24 to 48 hours; 5 to 9 ml/minute, 500 mg to 1 g q 12 to 24 hours; 10 to 29 ml/minute, 1 to 2 g q 12 to 24 hours; 30 to 50 ml/minute, 1 to 2 g q 8 to 12 hours.

ADMINISTRATION

Direct injection: Inject diluted drug over 3 to 5 minutes directly into vein, through an intermittent infusion device,

---

or into an I.V. line containing a free-flowing, compatible solution.
Intermittent infusion: Give 50 to 100 ml solution through a butterfly or scalp vein needle, an intermittent infusion device, or a patent I.V. line at the ordered flow rate. Interrupt primary solution during cefoxitin infusion. Give over 15 to 30 minutes.
Continuous infusion: Infuse up to 1 L of solution over the prescribed duration.

PREPARATION & STORAGE
Available in 1-g and 2-g vials, PVC bags, and infusion bottles.

Reconstitute drug in 1-g and 2-g vials with 10 ml of sterile water for injection. For intermittent infusion, reconstitute drug in 1-g and 2-g infusion bags or bottles with 50 to 100 ml of a compatible solution. For continuous infusion, reconstitute and add up to 1 L of a compatible solution, such as D5W or dextrose 10% in water; dextrose 5% in 0.2% or half-normal or normal saline solution; Ringer's injection; lactated Ringer's; normal saline solution; 1/6 M sodium lactate; invert sugar 5% or 10% in water; and dextrose 5% and Ionosol B.

Solutions remain stable for 24 hours if kept at room temperature and 48 hours if refrigerated. Both powder and solutions may turn amber, but this doesn't indicate significant change in potency.

Store vials at 86° F (30° C).

Incompatibilities
Aminoglycosides, filgrastim, hetastarch, pentamidine isethionate, ranitidine.

CONTRAINDICATIONS & CAUTIONS
• Contraindicated in those hypersensitive to cephalosporins.
• Use cautiously in patients hypersensitive to penicillin or with other allergies.
• Use cautiously in those with a history of GI disease, especially colitis, because of increased risk of pseudomem-branous colitis and in those with renal impairment because of increased risk of toxic reaction.

ADVERSE REACTIONS
CV: thrombophlebitis.
GI: diarrhea, *pseudomembranous colitis.*
GU: *acute renal failure.*
Skin: rash.

INTERACTIONS
Drug-drug. *Nephrotoxic drugs:* Causes additive nephrotoxicity. Monitor patient closely.
Probenecid: Reduces renal excretion of cefoxitin. May be used for this effect.

EFFECTS ON LAB TEST RESULTS
• May increase ALT, AST, alkaline phosphatase, bilirubin, and LDH levels.
• May increase eosinophil count. May decrease hemoglobin and neutrophil and platelet counts.
• May falsely elevate serum or urine creatinine level in tests using Jaffe reaction. May cause false-positive Coombs' test results and false-positive results in urine glucose tests using cupric sulfate (Benedict's reagent or Clinitest).

ACTION
Inhibits mucopeptide synthesis in the bacterial cell wall. Its spectrum of activity includes gram-positive aerobic bacteria, including most strains of alpha- and beta-hemolytic streptococci, *Streptococcus pneumoniae,* and staphylococci, especially most strains of penicillin G-resistant *Staphylococcus aureus.*

Susceptible gram-negative aerobic bacteria include *Escherichia coli, Klebsiella, Morganella morganii, Proteus mirabilis, P. vulgaris, Providencia rettgeri, Salmonella, Shigella, Neisseria gonorrhoeae,* and most strains of *Haemophilus influenzae.* Susceptible anaerobic bacteria include *Bacteroides,*

Clostridium, Fusobacterium, Peptococcus, and *Peptostreptococcus.*

PHARMACOKINETICS
Level peaks immediately after infusion. *Distribution:* Widely distributed into most body tissues and fluids, including ascitic, pleural, and synovial fluid. Present in bile if no obstruction is present. Poor diffusion into CSF, even with inflamed meninges. Drug readily crosses the placental barrier and appears in breast milk in small amounts.
Metabolism: About 2% metabolized in liver.
Excretion: About 85% removed in urine by glomerular filtration and tubular secretion within 6 hours. Half-life after I.V administration, 41 to 59 minutes.

CLINICAL CONSIDERATIONS
• Osmolality: 1 g in 50 ml D_5W is 326 mOsm/kg; 1 g in 50 ml of normal saline solution is 352 mOsm/kg; 2 g in 50 ml D_5W is 388 mOsm/kg; 2 g in 50 ml normal saline solution is 415 mOsm/kg; 100 mg/ml reconstituted solution in sterile water is 468 mOsm/kg.
• Check for previous penicillin or cephalosporin hypersensitivity. Negative history doesn't rule out future allergic reaction.
• Obtain specimens for culture and sensitivity testing before giving first dose. Therapy may start before test results are available.
• *Alert:* Names of some cephalosporins are similar. Use caution when giving.
• If diarrhea persists during therapy, collect stool specimens to rule out pseudomembranous colitis.
• Monitor intake and output and creatinine and BUN levels to help detect nephrotoxicity.
• To avoid inaccurate results when checking urine for glucose, use Clinistix or glucose enzymatic test strip.

• If patient is undergoing high-dose or long-term therapy, monitor him for fungal and bacterial superinfection.
• Risk of thrombophlebitis decreases when butterfly or scalp vein needle is used.
• Loading dose of 1 to 2 g should be given after hemodialysis session. Maintenance doses should reflect patient's creatinine clearance.
• Treat overdose symptomatically. Hemodialysis helps remove drug.

PATIENT TEACHING
• Instruct patient to promptly report to prescriber diarrhea and other adverse reactions.
• Instruct patient to report discomfort at I.V. site immediately.

ceftazidime
Ceptaz, Fortaz, Tazicef, Tazidime

Pharmacologic class: semisynthetic third-generation cephalosporin
Therapeutic class: antibiotic
Pregnancy risk category: B
pH: 5 to 8 for reconstituted solutions

INDICATIONS & DOSAGES
➤ **Uncomplicated infections, except for UTI, caused by susceptible organisms—**
Adults and children older than age 12: 1 g I.V. q 8 to 12 hours; maximum daily dose, 6 g. Dosage depends on susceptibility of organism and severity of infection.
Children ages 1 month to 12 years: 25 to 50 mg/kg I.V. q 8 hours; maximum daily dose, 6 g.
Neonates: 30 mg/kg I.V. q 12 hours.
➤ **UTI—**
Adults and children older than age 12: In uncomplicated infection, 250 mg

I.V. q 12 hours; in severe infection, 500 mg q 8 to 12 hours.
➤ **Bone and joint infection—**
Adults and children older than age 12: 2 g I.V. q 12 hours.
➤ **Uncomplicated pneumonia, mild skin and skin-structure infections—**
Adults and children older than age 12: 500 mg to 1 g I.V. q 8 hours.
➤ **Peritonitis, meningitis, severe gynecologic infections, other life-threatening infections—**
Adults and children older than age 12: 2 g I.V. q 8 hours.
➤ **Pseudomonal lung infection in patients with cystic fibrosis who have normal renal function—**
Adults and children older than age 12: 30 to 50 mg/kg I.V. q 8 hours; maximum daily dose, 6 g.
Adjust-a-dose: For adults with renal impairment, give a 1-g loading dose. If creatinine clearance is between 31 and 50 ml/minute, give 1 g q 12 hours; between 16 and 30 ml/minute, 1 g q 24 hours; between 6 and 15 ml/minute, 500 mg q 24 hours; and below 6 ml/minute, give 500 mg q 48 hours.

For hemodialysis patients, give a loading dose of 1 g, then 1 g after each session. For peritoneal dialysis patients, give a loading dose of 1 g, then 500 mg q 24 hours.

ADMINISTRATION
Direct injection: First remove any carbon dioxide bubbles. Then inject reconstituted drug directly into vein over 3 to 5 minutes. Alternatively, give through an I.V. line containing a free-flowing, compatible solution.
Intermittent infusion: Using a Y-type administration set, infuse solution over 15 to 30 minutes. Stop primary solution during ceftazidime infusion.
Continuous infusion: Infuse prescribed volume over 24 hours. Don't use thawed solutions.

PREPARATION & STORAGE
Available as a white to off-white sterile powder in 500-mg, 1-g, and 2-g vials; also available in 1-g and 2-g piggyback vials for infusion. Powder and solution may darken, but potency isn't generally changed. Store powder at 59° to 86° F (15° to 30° C). Protect from light.

Piggyback vials may need venting because positive pressure develops when the drug is reconstituted. Follow each brand's reconstitution instructions.

To reconstitute drug in a 500-mg vial, add 5 ml of sterile water for injection, yielding a concentration of 100 mg/ml. To reconstitute drug in a 1-g vial, add 3 ml of sterile water for injection to yield a concentration of 280 mg/ml, or 10 ml to yield 95 to 100 mg/ml. To reconstitute drug in a 2-g vial, add 10 ml of sterile water for injection to yield a concentration of 180 mg/ml.

For the 1-g or 2-g piggyback vial, reconstitute with 10 ml of sterile water for injection and dilute with 90 ml of a compatible I.V. solution. The resultant solution will contain 10 mg/ml for the 1-g vial and 20 mg/ml for the 2-g vial.

If kept at room temperature, solutions usually remain potent for 18 to 24 hours; if refrigerated, 7 to 10 days; and if stored at -4° F (-20° C) immediately after reconstitution, 3 to 6 months. Avoid heating after thawing or refreezing. Thawed solutions usually retain potency for 8 to 24 hours at room temperature and for 4 to 7 days under refrigeration. Don't use if solution is cloudy or contains a precipitate.

For infusions at concentrations between 1 and 40 mg/ml, use these solutions: normal saline injection; 1/6 M sodium lactate injection; dextrose 5% in 0.2% or half-normal or normal saline solution; or D_5W or dextrose 10% in water. For concentrations between 1 and 20 mg/ml, use Ringer's injection, lactated Ringer's injection, invert sugar 10% in sterile water for injection, or dextrose

5% and Normosol-M. These solutions may be stored for 24 hours at room temperature or for 7 days if refrigerated. Solutions in D_5W or normal saline solution remain stable for at least 6 hours at room temperature in plastic tubing, drip chambers, or volume-control devices of infusion sets.

Incompatibilities
Aminoglycosides, aminophylline, fluconazole, idarubicin, midazolam, pentamidine isethionate, ranitidine hydrochloride, sargramostim, sodium bicarbonate solutions, vancomycin.

CONTRAINDICATIONS & CAUTIONS
• Contraindicated in those hypersensitive to cephalosporins.
• Use cautiously in those hypersensitive to penicillin or with other allergies.
• Use cautiously in those with history of GI disease, especially colitis, because of increased risk of pseudomembranous colitis.
• Use cautiously in those with hepatic or renal impairment or poor nutritional status and in those receiving protracted course of therapy because of increased risk of hypothrombinemia.
• Use cautiously in those with renal impairment because of higher and more prolonged drug levels.

ADVERSE REACTIONS
CNS: fever.
EENT: metallic taste.
GI: abdominal cramps, diarrhea, nausea, *pseudomembranous colitis,* vomiting.
GU: decreased glomerular filtration rate.
Hematologic: eosinophilia, thrombocytosis.
Skin: pruritus, rash, urticaria, photosensitivity, injection site inflammation or pain.
Other: *angioedema.*

INTERACTIONS
Drug-drug. *Aminoglycosides:* Causes additive or synergistic effect against some strains of *Pseudomonas aeruginosa* and *Enterobacteriaceae.* Monitor patient for effects.
Furosemide, nephrotoxic drugs: Increases nephrotoxicity. Monitor patient closely.

EFFECTS ON LAB TEST RESULTS
• May increase ALT, AST, alkaline phosphatase, bilirubin, and LDH levels.
• May increase eosinophil count. May decrease hemoglobin and WBC and granulocyte counts. May increase or decrease platelet count.
• May falsely elevate serum or urine creatinine level in test using Jaffe reaction. May cause false-positive result in Coombs' test and in urine glucose test using cupric sulfate (Benedict's reagent or Clinitest).

ACTION
Inhibits mucopeptide synthesis in the bacterial cell wall, promoting osmotic instability. Its broad spectrum of activity includes most gram-positive aerobic cocci, including *Staphylococcus aureus, S. epidermidis, Streptococcus pneumoniae,* group A beta-hemolytic streptococci, group B streptococci, and *Steptococcus viridans.*

Susceptible gram-negative aerobic bacteria include *Acinetobacter, Branhamella catarrhalis, Citrobacter diversus, C. freundii, Eikenella corrodens, Enterobacter aerogenes, E. agglomerans, E. cloacae, Escherichia coli, Haemophilus ducreyi, H. influenzae, H. parainfluenzae, Klebsiella oxytoca, K. pneumoniae, Morganella morganii, Neisseria gonorrhoeae, N. meningitidis, Pasteurella multocida, Proteus mirabilis, P. vulgaris, Providencia rettgeri, P. stuartii,* many *Pseudomonas* species, *Salmonella, Serratia marcescens, Shigella,* and *Yersinia enterocolitica.* Susceptible anaerobic organisms include *Bifidobacterium, Clostridium, Eubacterium, Lactobacillus, Peptococcus, Peptostreptococcus,* and *Propionibacterium.*

PHARMACOKINETICS

Onset, immediate; level peaks immediately after infusion.
Distribution: Widespread; therapeutic levels appear in bone, heart, skin, skeletal muscle, gallbladder, sputum, bile, urine, aqueous humor, CSF, and synovial, peritoneal, and lymphatic fluid. Average distribution half-life, 20 minutes; 5% to 24% is bound to protein. Drug crosses the placental barrier and appears in amniotic fluid and breast milk.
Metabolism: None.
Excretion: In urine by glomerular filtration as unchanged drug; about half is removed in 2 hours and 80% to 90% in 24 hours. Elimination half-life, 85 to 120 minutes.

CLINICAL CONSIDERATIONS

● Osmolality: 50 mg/ml in D_5W is 321 mOsm/kg; 50 mg/ml in normal saline solution is 333 mOsm/kg.
● Check for previous penicillin or cephalosporin hypersensitivity before giving first dose. Negative history doesn't rule out future allergic reaction.
● Obtain specimens for culture and sensitivity testing before giving first dose. Therapy may start before results are available.
● *Alert:* Names of some cephalosporins are similar. Use caution when giving.
● If diarrhea persists during therapy, collect stool specimens to rule out pseudomembranous colitis.
● If patient has renal impairment or is receiving aminoglycoside antibiotics or potent diuretics, closely monitor renal function because of potential for nephrotoxicity.
● If patient is undergoing long-term therapy, monitor him for superinfection.
● Monitor PT and INR.

● For patients who must restrict their sodium intake, include 54 mg of sodium per gram of drug in daily count.
● Because the safety of the arginine component of Ceptaz hasn't been established in children, sodium bicarbonate formulations, such as Fortaz, Tazicef, and Tazidime, should be used in children younger than age 12.
● Assess I.V. site for signs and symptoms of inflammation and change site as needed.
● Treat overdose and anaphylactic reaction symptomatically. Hemodialysis removes drug.

PATIENT TEACHING

● If patient is on a sodium-restricted diet, advise him of the sodium content of the drug.
● Instruct patient to report diarrhea and other adverse reactions promptly.
● Instruct patient to report discomfort at I.V. site immediately.

ceftizoxime sodium
Cefizox

Pharmacologic class: third-generation cephalosporin
Therapeutic class: antibiotic
Pregnancy risk category: B
pH: 6 to 8 for reconstituted product, 5.5 to 8 for frozen premixed solutions

INDICATIONS & DOSAGES

➤ **Life-threatening infections caused by susceptible organisms—**
Adults: 3 to 4 g I.V. q 8 hours; maximum dose, 12 g/day.
Children older than age 6 months: Up to 200 mg/kg I.V. daily in divided doses. Maximum dose, 12 g daily.
Adjust-a-dose: For patients with renal impairment, give a loading dose of 500 mg to 1 g I.V. If creatinine clear-

ance is 50 to 79 ml/minute, give 750 mg to 1.5 g q 8 hours; if clearance is 5 to 49 ml/minute, give 500 mg to 1 g q 12 hours; and if clearance is below 5 ml/minute, give 500 mg to 1 g q 48 hours or 500 mg q 24 hours.

➤ **Uncomplicated infections, except UTI, and severe infections caused by susceptible organisms—**
Adults: 1 to 2 g I.V. q 8 to 12 hours; maximum dosage, 12 g/day.
Children older than age 6 months: 50 mg/kg I.V. q 6 to 8 hours.

➤ **Uncomplicated UTI caused by susceptible organisms—**
Adults: 500 mg I.V. q 12 hours. Give higher dosage in patients with *P. aeruginosa* infection.

Adjust-a-dose: For patients with renal impairment, give a loading dose of 500 mg to 1 g I.V. If creatinine clearance is 50 to 79 ml/minute, 500 mg q 8 hours; 5 to 49 ml/minute, 250 to 500 mg q 12 hours; and below 5 ml/minute, 500 mg q 48 hours or 250 mg q 24 hours.

ADMINISTRATION

Direct injection: Inject reconstituted drug over 3 to 5 minutes directly into a vein or an I.V. line containing a compatible solution. Don't inject commercially available frozen solutions intended for infusion.
Intermittent infusion: Infuse 50 to 100 ml of diluted drug into established I.V. line over 15 to 30 minutes.
Continuous infusion: Using an infusion pump, give solution over 24 hours.

PREPARATION & STORAGE

Available as a white to pale yellow crystalline powder in 500-mg, 1-g, and 2-g vials. Also supplied as a frozen solution in 50-ml single-dose plastic containers, equivalent to 1 g or 2 g in D_5W.

When reconstituting powder, add 5 ml of sterile water for injection to the 500-mg vial, 10 ml to the 1-g vial, and

20 ml to the 2-g vial. This yields a concentration of 95 mg/ml.

Reconstitute drug in piggyback vials with 50 to 100 ml of normal saline injection. Alternatively, use D_5W or dextrose 10% in water; dextrose 5% in 0.2% or half-normal or normal saline solution; Ringer's injection; lactated Ringer's; invert sugar 10% in sterile water for injection; or 5% sodium bicarbonate in sterile water for injection. Shake well. For continuous infusion, add to compatible solution an amount appropriate for the patient's condition. Solution remains stable for 24 hours if kept at room temperature or for 96 hours if refrigerated. Although it may turn yellow to amber, this color change doesn't affect potency. However, don't use if solution is cloudy or contains precipitate.

Protect vials from light and store at 59° to 86° F (15° to 30° C). For solution, store frozen but not below -4° F (-20° C). Thaw frozen solution at room temperature. Discard if you detect leaks, cloudiness, precipitation, or a broken seal. After thawing, the solution remains stable for 24 hours at room temperature or for 10 days if refrigerated. Don't refreeze.

Incompatibilities
Aminoglycosides.

CONTRAINDICATIONS & CAUTIONS
● Contraindicated in those hypersensitive to cephalosporins.
● Use cautiously in those hypersensitive to penicillin or with other allergies.
● Use cautiously in those with a history of GI disease, especially colitis, because of increased risk of pseudomembranous colitis and in those with renal impairment because of risk of toxic reaction from increased clearance time.

ADVERSE REACTIONS
CNS: paresthesia, pain, fever.
CV: phlebitis.

Reactions may be *common*, uncommon, *life-threatening*, or COMMON AND LIFE-THREATENING.

Hematologic: eosinophilia, thrombocytosis, ***thrombocytopenia.***
Skin: pruritus, rash; burning, cellulitis, induration, or tenderness at injection site.

INTERACTIONS

Drug-drug. *Aminoglycosides, nephrotoxic drugs:* Causes additive nephrotoxicity. Monitor patient closely.
Probenecid: Reduces renal excretion of ceftizoxime. May be used for this effect.

EFFECTS ON LAB TEST RESULTS

• May increase BUN, creatinine, ALT, AST, alkaline phosphatase, bilirubin, GGT, and LDH levels. May decrease albumin and protein levels.
• May decrease hemoglobin and PT and RBC, WBC, granulocyte, and neutrophil counts. May increase or decrease platelet count.
• May falsely elevate serum or urine creatinine level in tests using Jaffe reaction. May cause false-positive results in Coombs' test and in urine glucose tests using cupric sulfate (Benedict's reagent or Clinitest).

ACTION

Inhibits mucopeptide synthesis in the bacterial cell wall, promoting osmotic instability. Drug's spectrum of activity includes such gram-positive aerobic bacteria as *Staphylococcus aureus,* many strains of *S. epidermidis,* group A and group B streptococci, *Streptococcus pneumoniae,* and *Corynebacterium diphtheriae.*

Susceptible gram-negative aerobic bacteria include *Citrobacter freundii, Enterobacter aerogenes, E. cloacae, Escherichia coli, Haemophilus influenzae,* including ampicillin-resistant strains, *Klebsiella pneumoniae, Morganella morganii, Neisseria gonorrhoeae,* including penicillin-resistant strains, *N. meningitidis, Proteus mirabilis, P. vulgaris, Providencia, Sal-*

monella, Serratia marcescens, Shigella, and some strains of *Acinetobacter, Aeromonas hydrophila, Moraxella, Pasteurella multocida, Pseudomonas aeruginosa,* and *Yersinia enterocolitica.*

Susceptible anaerobic bacteria include *Actinomyces, Bacteroides, Bifidobacterium, Eubacterium, Fusobacterium, Peptococcus, Peptostreptococcus, Propionibacterium, Veillonella,* and some strains of *Clostridium.*

PHARMACOKINETICS

Onset and peak levels immediately after administration.
Distribution: Widespread, appearing in gallbladder, bone, heart, prostate, uterus, saliva, aqueous humor, bile, surgical wounds, and pleural, ascitic, and peritoneal fluids. Drug crosses the placental barrier and appears in breast milk. Also appears in CSF when meninges are inflamed.
Metabolism: None.
Excretion: Primarily in urine; with 58% to 92% eliminated in 24 hours. Half-life, 85 to 115 minutes.

CLINICAL CONSIDERATIONS

• Osmolality: 1 g/50 ml premixed frozen solutions range from 330 to 405 mOsm/kg; 2 g/50 ml premixed frozen solutions range from 410 to 505 mOsm/kg; isotonic in a concentration of 1 g/13 ml sterile water.
• Frozen solution contains dextrose 5%.
• Check for previous penicillin or cephalosporin hypersensitivity before giving first dose. Negative history doesn't rule out future allergic reaction.
• Obtain specimens for culture and sensitivity testing before giving first dose. Therapy may start before results are available.
• For patients on sodium restriction, note that ceftizoxime contains 2.6 mEq of sodium per gram of drug.
• *Alert:* Names of some cephalosporins are similar. Use caution when giving.

- If diarrhea persists during therapy, collect stool specimens to rule out pseudomembranous colitis.
- If patient receives high doses, takes other antibiotics, especially aminoglycosides, or has renal impairment, monitor renal function and intake and output because of the risk of nephrotoxicity.
- For patients who must restrict their sodium intake, include 60 mg of sodium per gram of drug in daily count.
- If patient is undergoing high-dose or long-term therapy, monitor him for fungal and bacterial superinfection.
- If patient is undergoing hemodialysis, give dose after dialysis session. Supplemental doses are unnecessary.
- Treat overdose and anaphylactic reaction symptomatically and supportively. Hemodialysis may help to remove drug.

PATIENT TEACHING
- If patient is on a sodium-restricted diet, advise him of the sodium content of the drug.
- Instruct patient to report diarrhea and other adverse reactions promptly.
- Instruct patient to report discomfort at I.V. site immediately.

ceftriaxone sodium
Rocephin

Pharmacologic class: semisynthetic third-generation cephalosporin
Therapeutic class: antibiotic
Pregnancy risk category: B
pH: about 6.7 for reconstituted product, about 6.6 for frozen premixed solutions

INDICATIONS & DOSAGES
➤ **Severe infections caused by susceptible organisms—**
Adults: 1 to 2 g I.V. once daily or in divided doses q 12 hours; maximum, 4 g

daily. Dosage depends on infection type and severity.
Children younger than age 12: 50 to 75 mg/kg I.V. daily in divided doses q 12 hours; maximum, 2 g daily.
➤ **Meningitis—**
Adults and children: 100 mg/kg/day I.V. once daily or in equally divided doses q 12 hours. May give 100-mg/kg loading dose. Maximum, 4 g daily.
➤ **Disseminated gonococcal infections** ◆ **—**
Adults: 1 g I.V. daily, until 1 or 2 days after improvement begins.
➤ **Empiric therapy in febrile neutropenic patients (adjunct to amikacin)** ◆ **—**
Adults: 30 mg/kg I.V. once daily.
➤ **Surgical prophylaxis—**
Adults: 1 g I.V. 30 minutes to 2 hours before surgery.
Adjust-a-dose: For patients with both hepatic impairment and severe renal impairment, maximum dose is 2 g daily unless drug level is monitored closely.

ADMINISTRATION
Direct injection: Inject reconstituted drug over 2 to 4 minutes directly into a vein, through an intermittent infusion device, or into an I.V. line containing a compatible solution.
Intermittent infusion: Give diluted drug over 15 to 30 minutes, using an intermittent infusion device or an I.V. line containing a compatible solution. Give over 10 to 30 minutes in neonates or children.
Continuous infusion: Not recommended.

PREPARATION & STORAGE
Available as a white to yellowish orange crystalline powder in vials containing 250 mg, 500 mg, 1 g, or 2 g. Also available in 1-g and 2-g piggyback vials. When reconstituted, solution turns light yellow to amber, depending on the dilu-

ent, drug concentration, and storage duration.

Reconstitute with sterile water for injection, normal saline injection, D₅W or dextrose 10% injection, or a combination of saline and dextrose injection and other compatible solutions. These include sodium lactate, invert sugar 10%, sodium bicarbonate 5%, FreAmine III, dextrose 5% and Normosol-M, dextrose 5% and Ionosol B, and mannitol 5% or 10%.

Reconstitute by adding 2.4 ml diluent to the 250-mg vial, 4.8 ml to the 500-mg vial, 9.6 ml to the 1-g vial, or 19.2 ml to the 2-g vial. Reconstitute drug in 1-g piggyback vial with 10 ml diluent and the 2-g vial with 20 ml diluent. All reconstituted solutions yield a concentration that averages 100 mg/ml. After reconstitution, dilute further for intermittent infusion to desired concentration. Concentrations of 10 to 40 mg/ml are recommended, but lesser ones can be used. If kept at room temperature, I.V. dilutions are stable for 1 to 3 days; if refrigerated, 3 to 10 days.

Incompatibilities
Aminoglycosides, aminophylline, clindamycin phosphate, filgrastim, fluconazole, labetalol, lidocaine hydrochloride, pentamidine isethionate, theophylline, vancomycin, vinorelbine tartrate.

CONTRAINDICATIONS & CAUTIONS
• Contraindicated in patients hypersensitive to cephalosporins.
• Use cautiously in patients hypersensitive to penicillin, in those with history of allergies, and in those with renal or hepatic impairment. For most patients with renal or hepatic impairment, dosage doesn't need to be adjusted.
• Use cautiously in those with history of GI disease, especially colitis, because of increased risk of pseudomembranous colitis.

• Use cautiously in those with preexisting disease of the gallbladder, biliary tract, liver, or pancreas.

ADVERSE REACTIONS
GI: diarrhea, *pseudomembranous colitis.*
Hematologic: eosinophilia, thrombocytosis, *leukopenia.*
Skin: rash; induration, pain, ecchymosis, and tenderness at injection site.

INTERACTIONS
Drug-drug. *Nephrotoxic drugs:* Additive nephrotoxicity. Monitor patient closely.
Probenecid: High doses of 1 or 2 g/day may enhance hepatic clearance of ceftriaxone and shorten its half-life. Avoid using together.
Drug-lifestyle. *Alcohol use:* Disulfiram-like reaction possible. Advise patient to avoid alcohol consumption.

EFFECTS ON LAB TEST RESULTS
• May increase BUN, ALT, AST, alkaline phosphatase, bilirubin, and LDH levels.
• May increase PT, INR, and eosinophil and platelet counts. May decrease WBC count.
• May elevate serum or urine creatinine level in tests using Jaffe reaction. May cause false-positive results in Coombs' test and in urine glucose tests using cupric sulfate (Benedict's reagent or Clinitest).

ACTION
Inhibits mucopeptide synthesis in the bacterial cell wall, promoting osmotic instability. Its broad spectrum of activity includes gram-positive bacteria, including *Staphylococcus aureus, S. epidermidis, Streptococcus pneumoniae,* group A beta-hemolytic streptococci, and groups B and D streptococci.

Susceptible gram-negative bacteria include *Acinetobacter, Citrobacter, C. freundii, Eikenella corrodens, Enter-*

obacter aerogenes, E. cloacae, Escherichia coli, Haemophilus influenzae including ampicillin-resistant strains, *H. parainfluenzae, Klebsiella pneumoniae, Moraxella, Morganella morganii, Neisseria gonorrhoeae, N. meningitidis, Proteus mirabilis, P. vulgaris, Providencia rettgeri, P. stuartii, Pseudomonas, Salmonella, Serratia marcescens, Shigella,* and *Yersinia enterocolitica.*

Susceptible anaerobic bacteria include *Actinomyces, Borrelia burgdorferi, Fusobacterium, Lactobacillus, Peptococcus, Peptostreptococcus, Propionibacterium,* and *Veillonella.*

PHARMACOKINETICS

Drug level peaks immediately after infusion.

Distribution: Widespread, with therapeutic levels found in myometrium, gallbladder, bone, lungs, prostate, bile, sputum, and peritoneal, ascitic, synovial, pleural, and blister fluids. Higher levels appear in CSF when meninges are inflamed. Drug is 85% to 95% protein bound, readily crosses the placental barrier, and appears in breast milk.

Metabolism: Partly in liver and partly in intestine after biliary excretion.

Excretion: By renal and biliary routes; 33% to 67% excreted unchanged in urine by glomerular filtration, the remainder removed in feces unchanged or as metabolites. Elimination half-life, 6 to 9 hours.

CLINICAL CONSIDERATIONS

● Osmolality: Frozen premixed solutions have osmolalities of 276 to 324 mOsm/kg; 50 mg/ml in D_5W is 352 mOsm/kg; 50 mg/ml in normal saline solution is 364 mOsm/kg.

● Check for previous penicillin or cephalosporin allergy before giving first dose. Negative history doesn't rule out future allergic reaction.

● Obtain specimens for culture and sensitivity testing before giving first dose.

Therapy may start before results are available.

● For patients on sodium restriction, note that ceftriaxone contains 3.6 mEq of sodium per gram of drug.

● *Alert:* Names of some cephalosporins are similar. Use caution when giving.

● High doses and rapid infusion rates increase risk of cholelithiasis.

● If patient experiences symptoms of gallbladder disease, stop drug.

● Monitor PT and INR in patient with impaired vitamin K synthesis or low vitamin K stores. For patients with prolonged PT or INR at risk for vitamin K deficiency, give vitamin K.

● If diarrhea persists during therapy, collect stool specimens to rule out pseudomembranous colitis.

● If patient receives more than 2 g/day; receives other antibiotics, especially aminoglycosides; or has renal impairment, monitor renal function and intake and output because of the risk of nephrotoxicity.

● To avoid inaccurate results when checking urine for glucose, use glucose oxidase methods such as Clinistix or glucose enzymatic test strip.

● If patient is undergoing high-dose or long-term therapy, monitor him for superinfection.

● For patients at risk for gallbladder effects, obtain results of serial abdominal ultrasonography.

● For patients with severe renal impairment and those with both renal and hepatic impairment, monitor drug level.

● Treatment should continue for at least 2 days after symptoms of infection disappear. Usual duration of 4 to 14 days may be prolonged in patients with severe infection.

PATIENT TEACHING

● Advise patient to report diarrhea and other adverse reactions promptly.

● Instruct patient to report discomfort at I.V. site immediately.

Reactions may be *common*, uncommon, *life-threatening*, or COMMON AND LIFE-THREATENING.

• If patient is on a sodium-restricted diet, advise him of the sodium content of the drug.

---

cefuroxime sodium
Zinacef

Pharmacologic class: semi-synthetic second-generation cephalosporin
Therapeutic class: antibiotic
Pregnancy risk category: B
pH: 6 to 8.5 for reconstituted product, 5 to 7.5 for frozen premixed solutions

---

INDICATIONS & DOSAGES
➤ **Uncomplicated UTI, skin and skin-structure infections, disseminated gonococcal infections, and uncomplicated pneumonia caused by susceptible organisms—**
Adults: 750 mg I.V. q 8 hours.
Children older than age 3 months: 50 to 100 mg/kg I.V. daily in divided doses q 6 to 8 hours.
➤ **Severe or complicated infections; bone and joint infections caused by susceptible organisms—**
Adults: 1.5 g I.V. q 8 hours.
Children older than age 3 months: For bone and joint infections, give 150 mg/kg/day I.V. in divided doses q 8 hours.
➤ **Bacterial meningitis—**
Adults: Up to 3 g I.V. q 8 hours.
Children older than age 3 months: Initially, 200 to 240 mg/kg/day I.V. in divided doses q 6 to 8 hours; after clinical improvement, dosage may be reduced to 100 mg/kg/day.
➤ **Life-threatening infections or infections caused by less susceptible organisms—**
Adults: 1.5 g I.V. q 6 hours.
Adjust-a-dose: For adults with a creatinine clearance greater than 20 ml/minute, give 750 mg to 1.5 g I.V. q 8

hours; if clearance is 10 to 20 ml/minute, give 750 mg q 12 hours; and if clearance is less than 10 ml/minute, give 750 mg q 24 hours.
If patient is undergoing hemodialysis, give dose at end of session.
➤ **Preoperative prevention for clean-contaminated or potentially contaminated surgery—**
Adults: 1.5 g I.V. 30 to 60 minutes before surgery and, during prolonged procedures, 750 mg q 8 hours. Continue drug for at least 24 hours afterward. Open-heart surgery patients should receive 1.5 g initially and q 12 hours, to total of 6 g.

ADMINISTRATION
Direct injection: Give directly into vein over 3 to 5 minutes or inject into an I.V. line containing a free-flowing, compatible solution.
Intermittent infusion: Infuse solution over 15 to 60 minutes. Stop primary infusion during cefuroxime administration.
Continuous infusion: Using an established I.V. line, infuse the solution at the ordered rate.

PREPARATION & STORAGE
Available as a sterile powder in 750-mg and 1.5-g vials.
Reconstitute drug in 750-mg vial with 9 ml of sterile water for injection, withdrawing 8 ml for 750 mg dose. For the 1.5-g vial, reconstitute with 16 ml of sterile water for injection, withdrawing the entire volume for a 1.5 g dose. If kept at room temperature, reconstituted solutions maintain potency for 24 hours; if refrigerated, 48 hours; and if properly frozen, up to 6 months. ADD-Vantage vials should be reconstituted according to the manufacturer's directions.
For infusion, dilute 750 mg or 1.5 g in 50 to 100 ml of D_5W for injection. If kept at room temperature, solution maintains potency for 24 hours; if re-

---

frigerated, 7 days. Other compatible solutions include dextrose 5% in 0.2% or half-normal or normal saline solution; dextrose 10% in water; invert sugar 10%; Ringer's injection; lactated Ringer's; normal saline solution; and 1/6 M sodium lactate.

Store vials between 59° and 86° F (15° and 30° C), and protect them from light.

Incompatibilities
Aminoglycosides, doxapram, filgrastim, fluconazole, midazolam, ranitidine, sodium bicarbonate injection, vinorelbine tartrate.

CONTRAINDICATIONS & CAUTIONS
• Contraindicated in those hypersensitive to cephalosporins.
• Use cautiously in those hypersensitive to penicillin or with ulcerative colitis, regional enteritis, or antibiotic-associated colitis because of increased risk of pseudomembranous colitis.
• Use cautiously in those with renal dysfunction because of increased risk of toxic reaction.

ADVERSE REACTIONS
CV: thrombophlebitis.
Hematologic: anemia, eosinophilia, *neutropenia, leukopenia.*

INTERACTIONS
Drug-drug. *Aminoglycosides, diuretics, nephrotoxic drugs:* Additive nephrotoxicity. Monitor patient closely.
Probenecid: Reduces renal excretion of cefuroxime. Drug is sometimes used for this effect.

EFFECTS ON LAB TEST RESULTS
• May increase ALT, AST, alkaline phosphatase, bilirubin, and LDH levels. May falsely elevate serum or urine creatinine levels in tests using Jaffe reaction.
• May increase PT and INR and eosinophil count. May decrease hemo-

globin, hematocrit, and neutrophil and platelet counts.
• May cause false-positive Coombs' test results and false-positive results in urine glucose tests using cupric sulfate (Benedict's reagent or Clinitest).

ACTION
Inhibits mucopeptide synthesis in the bacterial cell wall, promoting osmotic instability. Drug's spectrum of activity includes most gram-positive aerobic cocci, such as *Staphylococcus aureus, S. epidermidis, Streptococcus pneumoniae,* group A beta-hemolytic streptococci, and group B streptococci. Drug is also effective against many gram-negative aerobic bacteria, including *Citrobacter diversus, C. freundii, Enterobacter aerogenes, Escherichia coli,* ampicillin-resistant strains of *Haemophilus influenzae, H. parainfluenzae, Klebsiella pneumoniae, Morganella morganii, Neisseria gonorrhoeae, N. meningitidis, Proteus inconstans, P. mirabilis, P. stuartii, Salmonella, Shigella,* and *Providencia rettgeri.*

Susceptible anaerobic bacteria include *Actinomyces, Borrelia burgdorferi, Clostridium, Eubacterium, Fusobacterium, Lactobacillus, Peptococcus, Peptostreptococcus, Propionibacterium acnes,* and *Veillonella.*

PHARMACOKINETICS
Drug level peaks immediately after infusion.
Distribution: Throughout fluids and tissues, with therapeutic levels found in pleural and synovial fluid, CSF in meningeal inflammation, bile, sputum, bone, and aqueous humor. About 33% to 50% is bound to protein. Drug crosses the placental barrier and appears in breast milk.
Metabolism: None.
Excretion: In urine by glomerular filtration and tubular secretion as unchanged drug; most removed within

6 hours, 90% to 100% within 24 hours. Half-life, 1 to 2 hours.

CLINICAL CONSIDERATIONS

• Osmolality: for frozen premixed cefuroxime, about 300 mOsm/kg; 50 mg/ml in D_5W is 329 mOsm/kg; 50 mg/ml in normal saline solution is 335 mOsm/kg.
• Check for penicillin or cephalosporin hypersensitivity. Negative history doesn't rule out future allergic reaction.
• Obtain specimens for culture and sensitivity testing before giving first dose. Therapy may start before results arrive.
• *Alert:* Names of some cephalosporins are similar. Use caution when giving.
• If diarrhea persists during therapy, collect stool specimens to rule out pseudomembranous colitis.
• For patients who must restrict their sodium intake, include 54.2 mg of sodium per gram of drug in daily count.
• To avoid risk of nephrotoxicity, monitor intake and output and creatinine and BUN levels.
• To avoid inaccurate results when checking urine for glucose, use Clinistix or glucose enzymatic test strip.
• Watch for superinfection when high-dose or long-term therapy is used.
• Assess I.V. site for signs and symptoms of phlebitis and change site, as needed.
• Treat overdose or anaphylaxis symptomatically. Hemodialysis and peritoneal dialysis remove drug.

PATIENT TEACHING

• Advise patient to report diarrhea, rash, and other adverse reactions promptly.
• If patient is on a sodium-restricted diet, advise him of the sodium content of the drug.
• Instruct patient to report discomfort at I.V. site immediately.

chloramphenicol sodium succinate
Chloromycetin Sodium Succinate

Pharmacologic class: dichloroacetic acid derivative
Therapeutic class: antibiotic
Pregnancy risk category: C
pH: 6.4 to 7

INDICATIONS & DOSAGES

➤ **Haemophilus influenzae meningitis, acute Salmonella typhi infection, meningitis, bacteremia, or other severe infections caused by sensitive Salmonella species, Rickettsia, lymphogranuloma, psittacosis, or various sensitive gram-negative organisms—**
Adults: 50 mg/kg I.V. daily, divided q 6 hours. Maximum dose is 100 mg/kg daily.
Infants and children with normal metabolic processes: 50 mg/kg I.V. daily, divided q 6 hours for severe infections. For meningitis or other sever infections caused by *Staphylococcus pneumoniae,* 75 to 100 mg/kg I.V. daily, divided q 6 hours.
Neonates, children, and infants with immature metabolic processes: 25 mg/ kg I.V. daily in divided doses.

ADMINISTRATION

Direct injection: Give by direct I.V. infusion slowly over at least 1 minute.
Intermittent infusion: Not recommended.
Continuous infusion: Not recommended.

PREPARATION & STORAGE

Available as powder for injection in 1-g vials. Reconstitute powder in 1-g vial for injection with 10 ml of sterile water for injection. Concentration will be 100 mg/ml. If kept at room temperature, drug is stable for 30 days; however, it's better to store drug between 59° and 77° F (15° and 25° C). Don't use cloudy solutions.

Incompatibilities
Chlorpromazine, fluconazole, glycopyrrolate, hydroxyzine, metoclopramide, polymyxin B sulfate, prochlorperazine, promethazine, vancomycin.

CONTRAINDICATIONS & CAUTIONS
• Contraindicated in those hypersensitive to the drug.
• Use cautiously in those with impaired hepatic or renal function and in neonates and infants with immature metabolic processes.
• Use cautiously in those during pregnancy at term or during labor and in breast-feeding women because of the potential toxic effects on the child.

ADVERSE REACTIONS
CNS: headache, mild depression, confusion, delirium, peripheral neuropathy with prolonged therapy, fever.
EENT: optic neuritis, glossitis, decreased visual acuity.
GI: nausea, vomiting, stomatitis, diarrhea, enterocolitis.
Hematologic: *aplastic anemia, hypoplastic anemia, granulocytopenia, thrombocytopenia.*
Hepatic: jaundice.
Respiratory: *respiratory distress.*
Skin: rash, urticaria.
Other: *hypersensitivity reactions; anaphylaxis; angioedema; gray syndrome in neonates, which includes abdominal distention, gray cyanosis, vasomotor collapse, death within few hours of onset of symptoms.*

INTERACTIONS
Drug-drug. *Aminoglycosides, penicillin:* Antagonizes bactericidal activity of these drugs. Give these drugs 1 hour or more before chloramphenicol.

Chlorpropamide, dicumarol, phenytoin, tolbutamide: May cause prolonged half-life of these drugs and possible toxicity from increased drug levels. Avoid using together.
Folic acid, iron salts, vitamin B_{12}: Reduces the hematologic response to these substances. Avoid using together.
Myelosuppressives: May cause additive bone marrow toxicity. Avoid using together.
Phenobarbital, rifampin: May decrease level of chloramphenicol. Monitor levels of both drugs.

EFFECTS ON LAB TEST RESULTS
• May decrease hemoglobin and granulocyte and platelet counts.
• May falsely elevate urine PABA level if given during a bentiromide test for pancreatic function. May cause false-positive results on tests for urine glucose using cupric sulfate (Clinitest).

ACTION
Inhibits bacterial protein synthesis by binding to the 50S subunit of the ribosome; bacteriostatic.

PHARMACOKINETICS
Onset, unknown; peak, 1 to 3 hours; duration, unknown.
Distribution: Widely distributed to most body tissues and fluids; 50% to 60% is bound to protein.
Metabolism: Primarily in the liver to inactive metabolites.
Excretion: 8% to 12% is excreted unchanged in the urine. Elimination half-life ranges from 1½ to 4½ hours in adults with normal renal and hepatic function.

CLINICAL CONSIDERATIONS
• Obtain specimen for culture and sensitivity tests before giving first dose. Therapy may begin pending results.
• Don't use for the treatment of mild infections or for indications other than those listed, such as in colds, influenza,

---

Reactions may be *common*, uncommon, *life-threatening*, or COMMON AND LIFE-THREATENING.

infections of the throat, or prophylaxis
against bacterial infections.
• Avoid repeated courses if possible.
• Change to oral dose form as soon as
possible.
• *Alert:* Gray syndrome, a toxic reaction in premature and full-term neonates, may be fatal. In most cases,
therapy was started within the first
48 hours of life and symptoms appeared after 3 to 4 days of high-dose
treatment with chloramphenicol.
Stopping therapy with early symptoms
may reverse the process and allow
complete recovery.
• *Alert:* Serious and fatal blood dyscrasias, such as aplastic anemia, hypoplastic anemia, thrombocytopenia and
granulocytopenia may occur. Don't use
drug when less potentially dangerous
drugs are effective.
• Obtain drug levels. Therapeutic drug
level are as follows: peak, 10 to
20 mcg/ml; trough, 5 to 10 mcg/ml.
• Monitor CBC, platelet and reticulocyte counts, and iron levels before and
every 2 days during therapy. If anemia,
reticulocytopenia, leukopenia, or
thrombocytopenia develops, stop drug
immediately and notify prescriber.
• Monitor patient for superinfection.
• Check injection site daily for
phlebitis and irritation.

PATIENT TEACHING
• Instruct patient to notify prescriber
if he experience adverse reactions,
especially nausea, vomiting, diarrhea,
fever, confusion, sore throat, or mouth
sores.
• Instruct patient to report discomfort
at I.V. site immediately.
• Instruct patient to report symptoms of
superinfection.

chlordiazepoxide hydrochloride
Librium*

Pharmacologic class: benzodiazepine
Therapeutic class: anxiolytic, anticonvulsant, sedative-hypnotic
Pregnancy risk category: D
Controlled substance schedule: IV
pH: About 3 after reconstitution of
100 mg with 5 ml of sterile water
for injection or normal saline solution

INDICATIONS & DOSAGES
➤ **Short-term management of acute
or severe anxiety—**
Adults: 50 to 100 mg I.V. initially, then
25 to 50 mg t.i.d. or q.i.d., p.r.n.
*Elderly patients and children older
than age 12:* 25 to 50 mg I.V. t.i.d. or
q.i.d.
   Don't exceed 300 mg I.V. daily.
➤ **Acute alcohol withdrawal and
management of associated agitation—**
Adults: 50 to 100 mg I.V. initially, then
repeated in 2 to 4 hours if needed.
*Elderly patients and children older
than age 12:* 25 to 50 mg I.V. t.i.d. or
q.i.d.
   Don't exceed 300 mg I.V. daily.

ADMINISTRATION
Direct injection: Inject reconstituted
drug into vein over at least 1 minute.
Or, inject drug into I.V. tubing at a site
directly above needle or cannula insertion site. After injection, flush tubing
with normal saline solution.
Intermittent infusion: Not recommended.
Continuous infusion: Not recommended.

PREPARATION & STORAGE

Available as a dry powder in an amber ampule containing 100 mg of drug.

Don't use the I.M. diluent that the manufacturer provides for I.V. reconstitution because air bubbles will form. Instead, dilute powder with 5 ml of sterile normal saline solution or sterile water for injection to yield a concentration of 20 mg/ml. Gently rotate ampule until powder dissolves.

Give immediately and discard any unused solution. Protect from light.

Incompatibilities

Any I.V. drug.

CONTRAINDICATIONS & CAUTIONS

• Contraindicated in those hypersensitive to the drug or to benzodiazepines.
• Contraindicated in those with a history of drug dependence or emotional instability, glaucoma, hypoalbuminemia, severe depression and myasthenia gravis, or severe COPD.
• Contraindicated in those with shock or unstable blood pressure because of drug's hypotensive effects and in those in a coma because of drug's sedative effects.
• Contraindication in those with acute alcohol intoxication with depressed vital signs because of possible deepened CNS depression and in those with psychosis or hyperkinesis because of possible paradoxical reaction.
• Use cautiously in those with hepatic or renal impairment and in geriatric patients and debilitated patients because of slowed drug metabolism and excretion.

ADVERSE REACTIONS

CNS: ataxia, confusion, *drowsiness, lethargy,* extrapyramidal symptoms, EEG changes.
CV: hypotension, edema.
Hematologic: *agranulocytosis.*
Hepatic: jaundice.

Respiratory: *respiratory depression.*
Skin: *swelling and pain at injection site,* skin eruptions.
Other: altered libido.

INTERACTIONS

Drug-drug. *Antihypertensives:* Potentiates hypotension. Monitor blood pressure closely.
Carbamazepine: May reduce level of either drug. Monitor patient closely.
Cimetidine, disulfiram, erythromycin, hormonal contraceptives: Impairs metabolism of chlordiazepoxide. Monitor patient closely.
CNS depressants, MAO inhibitors: Increases CNS depression. Avoid using together.
Levodopa: Reduces control of parkinsonian symptoms. Avoid using together.
Drug-lifestyle. *Alcohol use:* Increases CNS depression. Discourage use together.
Cigarette smoking: Decreases effectiveness of drug. Monitor patient closely.

EFFECTS ON LAB TEST RESULTS

• May increase liver function test values. May decrease granulocyte count.
• May alter results of urinary 17-ketosteroid (Zimmerman reaction), urine alkaloid (Frings thin-layer chromatography method), and urinary glucose levels (with Chemstrip uG and Diastix).

ACTION

May suppress the limbic subcortical levels of the CNS, resulting in CNS depression ranging from mild sedation to coma. Drug also possesses skeletal muscle relaxant and anticonvulsant properties.

PHARMACOKINETICS

Onset, 1 to 5 minutes; duration, 15 to 60 minutes.

Reactions may be *common,* uncommon, *__life-threatening,__* or COMMON AND LIFE-THREATENING.

Distribution: Throughout body tissues. Drug crosses the blood-brain and placental barriers and appears in breast milk.
Metabolism: In liver to active metabolites.
Excretion: In urine as active and inactive metabolites, with a small amount removed in feces. Half-life, 5 to 30 hours.

CLINICAL CONSIDERATIONS

• *Alert:* Don't stop drug abruptly after long-term administration because patient may experience withdrawal symptoms.
• Initiate drug at lowest dose and increase dose as needed.
• Change to oral dosing as soon as possible.
• Take vital signs before therapy, and monitor them carefully during and after injection. Watch especially for hypotension, respiratory depression, and bradycardia, and immediately report to prescriber. Keep resuscitation equipment readily available.
• Maintain bed rest for at least 3 hours after injection.
• Institute safety measures to prevent falls and injuries caused by hypotension, confusion, or oversedation. Reduce dosage in geriatric or debilitated patients.
• Monitor CBC and liver function studies during prolonged therapy.
• Watch for signs and symptoms of drug dependency.
• If overdose is suspected, provide supportive care. Maintain airway patency and give I.V. fluids. Give norepinephrine or metaraminol for hypotension. Flumazenil may be used to reverse sedative effects. Resedation is possible, however, because the duration of action of chlordiazepoxide is longer than that of flumazenil. Hemodialysis doesn't remove an appreciable amount of drug.

PATIENT TEACHING

• Advise patient to use caution when operating machinery or driving.
• Notify patient of potential for hypotension and stress importance of bed rest after receiving dose.
• Inform patient of potential for drug dependency.

chlorothiazide sodium
Diuril Sodium Intravenous

Pharmacologic class: thiazide diuretic
Therapeutic class: diuretic
Pregnancy risk category: B
pH: 9.2 to 10 for 2.5% solution

INDICATIONS & DOSAGES

➤ **To manage edema—**
Adults: Initially, 0.5 to 2 g I.V. daily or in two divided doses; subsequent dosages reflect patient response. Maximum dose, 2 g/day.

ADMINISTRATION

Direct injection: Inject reconstituted drug directly into vein, using a 21G or 23G needle over 1 to 2 minutes.
Intermittent infusion: Give diluted solution using an intermittent infusion device or piggyback into an I.V. line containing a free-flowing, compatible solution over the prescribed duration.
Continuous infusion: Not recommended.

PREPARATION & STORAGE

Available as a dry white powder in 500-mg vials.
    Reconstitute with at least 18 ml of sterile water for injection. For infusion, further dilute with 0.2% or half-normal or normal saline solution; dextrose 5% in 0.2%, half-normal or normal saline solution; lactated Ringer's; dextran 6%

in normal saline solution; dextran 6% in dextrose 5%; 1/6 M sodium lactate; and invert sugar 5% or 10% in water.

Solutions remain stable for 24 hours at room temperature.

Incompatibilities
Amikacin; chlorpromazine; codeine; hydralazine; insulin (regular); Ionosol B, D, or K and invert sugar 10%; Ionosol B or D-CM and dextrose 5%; Ionosol PSL; levorphanol; methadone; morphine; norepinephrine; Normosol-M (900 calories); Normosol-M in dextrose 5%; Normosol-R in dextrose 5%; polymyxin B; procaine; prochlorperazine; promazine; promethazine hydrochloride; streptomycin; triflupromazine; vancomycin; vitamin B complex with C; whole blood and its derivatives.

CONTRAINDICATIONS & CAUTIONS
• Contraindicated in those hypersensitive to thiazides, sulfonamides, or thimerosal and in those with anuria.
• Use cautiously in those with hepatic impairment or progressive hepatic disease because electrolyte imbalance may precipitate hepatic coma and in those with lupus erythematosus because drug may exacerbate the condition.
• Use cautiously in those with electrolyte imbalance because of possible exacerbation and in those with renal impairment because of possible azotemia.
• Use cautiously in those who have had a sympathectomy because of enhanced antihypertensive effects.
• Use cautiously in those with a history of allergies or with bronchial asthma because of increased risk of sensitivity reactions.

ADVERSE REACTIONS
CNS: vertigo, weakness.
CV: hypotension.
GI: diarrhea, vomiting, *pancreatitis.*
Hepatic: jaundice.

Metabolic: glycosuria, hyperglycemia, hyperuricemia, hypokalemia, hypercalcemia, hypomagnesemia, hyponatremia.
Other: *anaphylaxis.*

INTERACTIONS
Drug-drug. *Amphotericin B (parenteral), corticosteroids, corticotropin, potassium-wasting diuretics:* Increases risk of hypokalemia or other electrolyte disturbances. Monitor blood count closely.
Antidiabetics including insulin: Decreases effectiveness of these drugs. Dosage adjustment of antidiabetics may be required.
CNS depressants (barbiturates, narcotics), antihypertensives: Increases hypotension. Monitor patient closely.
Lithium: Reduces lithium excretion and risk of toxic reaction. Monitor lithium level closely.
Muscle relaxants: Increases responsiveness to muscle relaxant properties. Avoid using together
NSAIDs: Decreases diuretic effect. Monitor patient closely.
Drug-lifestyle. *Alcohol use:* Increases hypotension. Monitor patient closely. Discourage use together.

EFFECTS ON LAB TEST RESULTS
• May increase ammonia, calcium, cholesterol, amylase, blood or urine glucose, and uric acid levels. May decrease potassium, chloride, sodium and magnesium levels.
• May cause false-negative results on the histamine, phentolamine, and tyramine tests for pheochromocytoma. May cause unreliable results in glucose tolerance and parathyroid tests.

ACTION
Alters tubular cell metabolism in the cortical diluting segment of the nephron. It increases excretion of sodium, chloride, and water. Natriuresis is

accompanied by some loss of potassium and bicarbonate.

Direct arteriolar dilation may contribute to the drug's antihypertensive effect.

PHARMACOKINETICS
Onset, 15 minutes; drug effect peaks at 30 minutes; duration, 2 hours.
Distribution: Into extracellular space. Drug crosses the placental barrier and appears in breast milk. Variable protein binding.
Metabolism: None.
Excretion: In urine by glomerular filtration and proximal tubular secretion within 5 hours; 95% excreted unchanged.

CLINICAL CONSIDERATIONS
• Osmolality: 28 mg/ml in sterile water is 344 mOsm/kg.
• Because drug raises glucose and uric acid levels, dosage may need to be adjusted in patients taking antidiabetics or antigout drugs.
• Intermittent scheduling may decrease risk of electrolyte imbalance.
• Carefully monitor intake and output and electrolyte levels. Watch for signs and symptoms of hypokalemia.
• If patient develops dilutional hyponatremia, restrict fluids to 500 ml daily and withdraw drug. This complication commonly occurs in hot weather and in patients with heart failure or hepatic disease.
• Monitor renal function. If progressive disease occurs, stop drug.
• Patients with preexisting hepatic disease are most susceptible to hypokalemic hypochloremic alkalosis.
• Geriatric patients may be more sensitive to drug's effects.
• Overdose is signaled by lethargy progressing to coma without evidence of electrolyte imbalance or dehydration.

PATIENT TEACHING
• Advise diabetic patient that oral antidiabetics may have decreased effectiveness.
• Teach patient signs and symptoms of hypokalemia.

chlorpromazine hydrochloride
Largactil ◇ , Thorazine

Pharmacologic class: aliphatic phenothiazine
Therapeutic class: antipsychotic, antiemetic
Pregnancy risk category: C
pH: 3 to 5, 3.5 to 5.5 for a 10% solution in water

INDICATIONS & DOSAGES
➤ **Severe hiccups—**
Adults: 25 to 50 mg I.V. infused at rate of 1 mg/minute.
➤ **Adjunctive treatment for tetanus—**
Adults: 25 to 50 mg I.V. t.i.d. or q.i.d.
Children ages 6 months and older: 0.55 mg/kg I.V. q 6 to 8 hours. Maximum daily dose: 40 mg for children weighing less than 23 kg and 75 mg for children weighing 23 to 45 kg.
➤ **Vomiting during surgery—**
Adults: 2 mg I.V. q 2 minutes. Total dose, 25 mg.
Children: 1 mg I.V. q 2 minutes. Total dose, 0.275 mg/kg. May repeat dose in 30 minutes if hypotension doesn't occur.
Adjust-a-dose: Dosages in lower range are sufficient for most geriatric patients. Monitor response, adjust dosage accordingly, and increase dosage gradually.

ADMINISTRATION
Direct injection: Slowly inject ordered amount of diluted drug (1 mg/ml concentration) into the tubing of a patent

I.V. line at a rate of no less than 1 mg/minute in adults or 0.5 mg/minute in children. Direct injection is generally used for adjunctive treatment of tetanus and vomiting during surgery.

Intermittent infusion: Not recommended.

Continuous infusion: Slowly infuse ordered dose diluted in 500 to 1,000 ml. Used to treat severe hiccups.

PREPARATION & STORAGE

Available in 1-ml and 2-ml ampules and 10-ml multiple-dose vials containing 25-mg/ml concentration. Store below 104° F (40° C), preferably between 59° and 86° F (15° and 30° C). Protect from light and freezing. Discard if darker than light amber or if precipitate forms.

For direct injection, dilute with normal saline solution to a 1-mg/ml concentration. For infusion, add ordered dose to 500 to 1,000 ml of normal saline solution.

Incompatibilities

Aminophylline, amphotericin B, ampicillin, chloramphenicol sodium succinate, chlorothiazide, cimetidine, dimenhydrinate, furosemide, heparin sodium, melphalan, methohexital, paclitaxel, penicillin, pentobarbital, phenobarbital, solutions having a pH of 4 to 5, thiopental.

CONTRAINDICATIONS & CAUTIONS

• Contraindicated in those hypersensitive to phenothiazines and sulfites.
• Contraindicated in those with severe toxic CNS depression, subcortical brain damage, bone marrow depression, or severe CV disorders because drug may worsen these conditions.
• Avoid use in those with such neurologic disorders as Reye's syndrome, meningitis, encephalopathy, or encephalitis because drug may mask symptoms or confuse diagnosis.

• Use cautiously in those with hypocalcemia because drug may cause dystonic reactions, in alcoholic patients because drug may deepen CNS depression, and those with Parkinson's disease because drug may potentiate extrapyramidal effects.
• Use cautiously in debilitated patients because drug increases risk of toxic reaction, in geriatric patients because drug increases risk of severe adverse effects, and in those with symptomatic prostatic hyperplasia because drug increases risk of urine retention.
• Use cautiously in patients with respiratory disease because of CNS depression and suppression of cough reflex.
• Use cautiously in patients with glaucoma or a predisposition to this disorder because drug may precipitate glaucoma, in those with peptic ulcer disease or urine retention because drug may exacerbate these conditions, and in those with seizure disorders because drug may lower seizure threshold.
• Use cautiously in patients with hepatic or renal disease because they metabolize and excrete drug more slowly, making the risk of toxic reaction greater.
• Use cautiously in those who show severe reactions to electroconvulsive therapy.

ADVERSE REACTIONS

CNS: dizziness, fainting, *seizures,* extrapyramidal effects, *neuroleptic malignant syndrome,* drowsiness.
CV: hypotension, tachycardia.
GI: dry mouth, constipation.
GU: urine retention.
Hematologic: *aplastic anemia, thrombocytopenia, agranulocytosis.*

INTERACTIONS

Drug-drug. *Anticholinergics:* Enhances anticholinergic effects. Use with caution.
Anticonvulsants: Chlorpromazine lowers the seizure threshold, requiring

dosage adjustments of these drugs. Monitor patient closely. Start chlorpromazine therapy at lower doses and increase as needed.

CNS depressants: Enhances CNS depression. Avoid using together.

Epinephrine: Increases risk of severe hypotension and tachycardia, known as epinephrine reversal. Avoid using together.

Guanethidine: Counteract antihypertensive activity. Monitor blood pressure.

Norepinephrine: Decreases pressor effects. Avoid using together.

Phenytoin: Decreases phenytoin metabolism and risk of toxic reaction. Monitor patient closely.

Propranolol: Increases levels of both drugs. Use together cautiously.

Thiazide diuretics: Additive orthostatic hypotension. Monitor patient closely.

Valproic acid: Decreases valproic acid clearance. Monitor patient for toxicity.

Drug-lifestyle. *Alcohol use:* Increases CNS depression. Discourage use together.

Sun exposure: May cause photosensitivity reactions. Advise patient to avoid excessive sunlight exposure.

EFFECTS ON LAB TEST RESULTS

● May increase liver function test values and eosinophil count. May decrease hemoglobin and WBC, granulocyte, and platelet counts.

● May cause false-positive test results for urinary porphyrins, urobilinogen, amylase, and 5-hydroxyindoleacetic acid because of darkening of urine by metabolites and false-positive results for urine pregnancy tests that use human chorionic gonadotropin. May cause false-positive phenylketonuria test result.

ACTION

Inhibits dopamine receptors in the chemoreceptor trigger zone of the medulla.

PHARMACOKINETICS

Onset, within 15 minutes; duration, 6 to 8 hours.

Distribution: Widely distributed to most body fluids, with high levels in the brain, lungs, liver, kidneys, and spleen. Drug readily crosses the placental and blood-brain barriers, appears in breast milk, and is 92% to 97% protein bound.

Metabolism: Extensively metabolized in the liver.

Excretion: Primarily in the urine, but also in feces.

CLINICAL CONSIDERATIONS

● Osmolality: 25 mg/ml is 262 mOsm/kg.

● *Alert:* Because of possible hypotension, give I.V. only to patients on bed rest or to acute ambulatory patients who can be closely monitored. Monitor geriatric patients carefully because they are especially vulnerable to hypotension and extrapyramidal symptoms. Usually, geriatric or debilitated patients require a lower dose.

● Establish baseline blood pressure and heart rate, and monitor patient for tachycardia and hypotension. Keep him supine for at least 30 minutes after injection, and advise him to change position slowly.

● After stopping drug, notify prescriber if patient experiences dizziness, nausea, vomiting, GI upset, pain, trembling of hands or fingers, or controlled, repetitive movements of the mouth, tongue, or jaw.

● Drug's antiemetic effect can obscure diagnosis of a condition with nausea as a primary symptom. Remember that this drug prolongs sleep in postoperative patients.

● Give sugarless gum, sour hard candy, or mouthwash as needed to relieve dry mouth.

● Monitor intake and output for urine retention and constipation.

• To prevent dermatitis, avoid skin contact with drug.
• Geriatric and pediatric patients are at greater risk for hypotensive and extrapyramidal reactions.
• For overdose, anticholinergics may help control extrapyramidal symptoms. Treat severe hypotension with vasopressors, such as norepinephrine or phenylephrine; don't use epinephrine. Acute dystonic reactions may be treated with I.V. diphenhydramine.

PATIENT TEACHING
• Advise patient to report sudden sore throat or other signs or symptoms of infection.
• Advise patient to notify prescriber if he experiences dizziness, nausea, vomiting, GI upset, pain, trembling of hands or fingers, or controlled, repetitive movements of the mouth, tongue, or jaw.
• Advise patient to use caution when operating machinery or driving a motor vehicle.
• Instruct patient to remain recumbent for 30 minutes after injection and change positions slowly.
• Caution women against breast-feeding during therapy.

cidofovir
Vistide

Pharmacologic class: nucleotide analogue
Therapeutic class: antiviral
Pregnancy risk category: C
pH: 6.7 to 7.6

INDICATIONS & DOSAGES
➤ **CMV retinitis in patients with AIDS—**
Adults: Initially, 5 mg/kg I.V. once weekly for 2 weeks; maintenance

dosage, 5 mg/kg given once q 2 weeks. Must be given with 2 g of probenecid P.O. 3 hours before cidofovir, followed by 1 g at 2 and 8 hours after completion of cidofovir infusion.
Adjust-a-dose: For patients with renal impairment, if creatinine level increases 0.3 to 0.4 mg/dl above baseline, reduce dose to 3 mg/kg I.V. at same rate and frequency. If creatinine level increases 0.5 mg/dl or more above baseline, stop drug.

ADMINISTRATION
Direct injection: Not recommended.
Intermittent infusion: Infuse entire volume of diluted solution over 1 hour at a constant rate with an infusion device.
Continuous infusion: Not recommended.

PREPARATION & STORAGE
Because of its mutagenic properties, prepare drug in a class II laminar flow biological safety cabinet, wearing surgical gloves and a closed-front surgical gown with knit cuffs.
    Available in vials containing 75 mg/ml. Dilute with 100 ml of normal saline solution.
    Give diluted solutions within 24 hours of preparation. If not used immediately, refrigerate solution at 36° to 46° F (2° to 8° C) for up to 24 hours.
    Allow solution to reach room temperature before using.

Incompatibilities
None reported.

CONTRAINDICATIONS & CAUTIONS
• Contraindicated in those hypersensitive to the drug or those who have a history of severe hypersensitivity to probenecid or other sulfur-containing drugs.
• Avoid use as an intraocular injection and in breast-feeding women.

• Avoid use in those with baseline creatinine level above 1.5 mg/dl or a calculated creatinine clearance of 55 ml/minute or less unless potential benefits outweigh potential risks.
• Use cautiously in geriatric patients and in those with renal impairment because of risk of toxic reaction.
• Don't exceed recommended dose and frequency and rate of administration because of potential for toxic reaction.
• Safety and efficacy in those with CMV infections, other than AIDS patients with CMV retinitis, haven't been established.

ADVERSE REACTIONS
CNS: *asthenia, headache, fever, pain.*
EENT: ocular hypotony, *decreased intraocular pressure, anterior uveitis or iritis.*
GI: abdominal pain, *nausea, vomiting, diarrhea,* anorexia.
GU: NEPHROTOXICITY, *proteinuria.*
Hematologic: NEUTROPENIA, anemia, *thrombocytopenia.*
Metabolic: metabolic acidosis.
Respiratory: dyspnea, pneumonia, *increased cough.*
Skin: *alopecia, rash.*
Other: *infection, chills.*

INTERACTIONS
Drug-drug. *Nephrotoxic drugs such as amphotericin B, aminoglycosides, foscarnet, and pentamidine:* Increases risk of nephrotoxicity. Avoid using together.
Probenecid: Interacts with the metabolism or renal tubular excretion of many drugs. Monitor patient closely.
Zidovudine: Probenecid decreases zidovudine clearance. Stop or reduce zidovudine therapy by 50% on days when cidofovir is given.

EFFECTS ON LAB TEST RESULTS
• May increase BUN, creatinine, alkaline phosphatase, ALT, AST, and LDH levels. May decrease bicarbonate level.
• May decrease hemoglobin, creatinine clearance, and neutrophil and platelet counts.

ACTION
Suppresses CMV replication by selective inhibition of viral DNA synthesis.

PHARMACOKINETICS
Onset, peak, and duration of drug effect unknown.
Distribution: Unknown.
Metabolism: Converted via cellular enzymes to the pharmacologically active diphosphate metabolite.
Excretion: Unknown.

CLINICAL CONSIDERATIONS
• Osmolality: 382 to 392 mOsm/kg for recommended dilutions in dextrose 5% in half-normal saline solution; 241 to 315 mOsm/kg for recommended dilutions in D_5W or normal saline solution.
• Give 1 L of normal saline solution over 1 to 2 hours immediately before each cidofovir infusion.
• Give probenecid before and after cidofovir infusion.
• Stop zidovudine therapy or reduce dosage by 50% on the days cidofovir is given.
• Monitor WBC counts and differential before each dose.
• Monitor creatinine and urine protein levels before each dose. Adjust dose as needed.
• Monitor neutrophil counts, intraocular pressure, visual acuity, and ocular symptoms periodically.
• If overdose occurs, hemodialysis and hydration may reduce drug level. Probenecid may reduce the potential for nephrotoxicity.

PATIENT TEACHING
• Inform patient that drug isn't a cure for CMV retinitis and that regular oph-thalmologic examinations are needed.
• Alert patient taking zidovudine that drug may need to be stopped or dosage adjusted on days that cidofovir is given.
• Tell patient that he must take pro-benecid with each cidofovir dose to de-crease risk of nephrotoxicity and that he can take it after meals to decrease nausea.
• Advise women of childbearing age not to become pregnant during and within 1 month of cidofovir treatment.

cimetidine hydrochloride
Tagamet

Pharmacologic class: H_2-receptor antagonist
Therapeutic class: antiulcerative
Pregnancy risk category: B
pH: 3.8 to 6 for injection, 5 to 7 for premixed infusion

INDICATIONS & DOSAGES
➤ **To prevent upper GI bleeding in critically ill patients—**
Adults: 50 mg/hour I.V. by continuous infusion for up to 7 days.
Children ◆ : 5 to 10 mg/kg I.V. q 6 to 8 hours.
Adjust-a-dose: For patients with creati-nine clearance less than 30 ml/minute, give half the dose.
➤ **Short-term treatment of duodenal ulcer—**
Adults: 300 mg I.V. q 6 to 8 hours; q 12 hours if creatinine clearance is un-der 30 ml/minute. Maximum daily dose, 2,400 mg. Adjust dosage to main-tain a gastric pH above 5. To increase dosage, give 300-mg doses more fre-quently to maximum daily dose.

Children ◆ : 5 to 10 mg/kg I.V. q 6 to 8 hours.
➤ **Hospitalized patients with in-tractable ulcers or hypersecretory conditions, patients who can't take oral medication, patients with GI bleeding; control of gastric pH in critically ill patients—**
Adults: 300 mg I.V. q 6 to 8 hours. Don't exceed 2,400 mg daily.
Children ◆ : 5 to 10 mg/kg I.V. q 6 to 8 hours.
Adjust-a-dose: For patients with severe renal impairment, give 300 mg I.V. q 8 to 12 hours. Give the dose at the end of hemodialysis. For patients who also have liver impairment, dosage may need to be further reduced.

ADMINISTRATION
Direct injection: Inject diluted drug over at least 5 minutes directly into vein or through an I.V. line containing a free-flowing, compatible solution. Rapid injection may increase the risk of arrhythmias and hypotension.
Intermittent infusion: Give 50 to 100 ml of diluted drug over 15 to 20 minutes, using an intermittent infusion device or infused into an I.V. line containing a free-flowing, compatible solution.
Continuous infusion: Dilute 900 mg of drug in 100 to 1,000 ml of compatible solution. Using an infusion pump, in-fuse at prescribed rate. Patients may re-quire more than 900 mg/day to main-tain pH control. Dosage adjustments should be individualized.

PREPARATION & STORAGE
Available in 2-ml single-dose dispos-able syringes containing 300 mg cime-tidine; in 8-ml multidose vials contain-ing 300 mg/2 ml; and in PVC bags containing 300 mg/50 ml.
   For direct injection, dilute dose (in-cluding the single-dose form) with 20 ml of normal saline injection. For infusion, dilute with 50 to 100 ml of a compatible solution, such as amino

acid solution, D_5W, Ringer's injection, lactated Ringer's, invert sugar 5% in water, normal saline solution, or dextrose 5% in 0.2%, half-normal, or normal saline solution.

Use reconstituted solutions within 48 hours. Check expiration dates.

Protect from light and store at room temperature. Solution becomes cloudy if refrigerated. Discard solutions if discolored or if precipitate appears.

Incompatibilities
Allopurinol, amphotericin B, barbiturates, cephalosporins, chlorpromazine, combination atropine sulfate and pentobarbital sodium, indomethacin sodium trihydrate, pentobarbital sodium, warfarin.

CONTRAINDICATIONS & CAUTIONS
• Contraindicated in those hypersensitive to the drug.
• Use cautiously in geriatric patients and in those with organic brain syndrome or renal or hepatic impairment because of an increased risk of toxic reaction.
• Use cautiously in those with strongyloidosis infection because of the risk of hyperinfection.
• Use cautiously in those younger than age 16. Safe use in these patients hasn't been determined.

ADVERSE REACTIONS
CNS: dizziness, headache, somnolence.
CV: hypotension.
GI: diarrhea.
Skin: rash.
Other: breast soreness, gynecomastia.

INTERACTIONS
Drug-drug. *Benzodiazepines, especially chlordiazepoxide, diazepam, and midazolam; calcium channel blockers; cyclosporine; glipizide; glyburide; lidocaine; methylxanthines such as caffeine and theophylline; metoprolol; metronidazole; oral anticoagulants;*

phenytoin; propranolol; tricyclic antidepressants: Impairs the metabolism of these drugs, increasing the risk of toxic reaction. Monitor patient closely.
Ketoconazole: Decreases absorption of oral ketoconazole. Avoid using together.
Myelosuppressants: Causes additive toxicity. Monitor patient closely.
Procainamide, quinidine: May reduce the clearance of these drugs, increasing the risk of toxic reaction. Monitor patient closely.
Drug-herb. *Guarana:* May increase caffeine level or prolong caffeine half-life. Monitor patient.
Pennyroyal: May change the rate of formation of toxic metabolites of pennyroyal. Monitor patient.
Yerba maté: May decrease clearance of herb's methylxanthines and cause a toxic reaction. Discourage use together.

EFFECTS ON LAB TEST RESULTS
• May increase creatinine, AST, and ALT levels.
• May cause false-negative allergy skin test results. May decrease gastric acid level in gastric acid stimulation test using pentagastrin.

ACTION
Drug reduces gastric acid output and concentration by competitively inhibiting histamine's action on the H_2-receptors of gastric parietal cells, thereby raising gastric pH to 5 or higher. It reduces both basal and stimulated gastric acid production and helps reduce pepsin secretion by decreasing gastric juice volume.

PHARMACOKINETICS
Onset, immediately after I.V. injection; duration, 4 to 5 hours.
Distribution: Throughout body tissues. Drug is 15% to 20% bound to protein, crosses the placental barrier, and appears in breast milk.

Metabolism: In liver to sulfoxide and 5-hydroxymethyl derivatives.

Excretion: In urine, primarily unchanged, with remainder removed as two metabolites; 80% to 90% of drug is excreted in urine in 24 hours. Remainder excreted in feces. Half-life, 2 to 3 hours.

CLINICAL CONSIDERATIONS
● Osmolality: 300 mg/50 ml is 286 mOsm/kg in D_5W and 313 mOsm/kg in normal saline solution; 300 mg/50 ml premixed solution is about 336 mOsm/kg.
● If cimetidine and coumarin anticoagulants must be given together, closely monitor PT and INR and adjust dosage as needed.
● Malignant gastric ulcers have been shown to heal transiently during drug therapy and must be closely monitored.
● Raised gastric pH may permit candidal overgrowth in stomach.
● *Alert:* Geriatric patients may experience drug-induced confusion.
● Because cimetidine alters gastric pH, it may affect the bioavailability of many oral drugs.
● Drug inhibits hepatic microsomal enzymes and may decrease metabolism of many drugs.
● Provide symptomatic treatment for overdose. Treat tachycardia with a beta blocker. Hemodialysis promotes drug clearance.
● Urge patient to avoid smoking and alcohol, which may increase gastric acid secretion and worsen disease.

PATIENT TEACHING
● Advise women of childbearing age to avoid becoming pregnant during drug therapy.
● Caution women against breast-feeding during therapy.

ciprofloxacin
Cipro I.V.

Pharmacologic class: broad-spectrum fluoroquinolone antibiotic
Therapeutic class: antibiotic
Pregnancy risk category: C
pH: 3.3 to 4.6

INDICATIONS & DOSAGES
➤ **UTI**—
Adults: 200 mg I.V. q 12 hours for mild to moderate infection. For severe to complicated UTI, give 400 mg q 12 hours. Continue treatment for 7 to 14 days.
➤ **Infections of the lower respiratory tract, skin, skin structure, bones, and joints**—
Adults: 400 mg I.V. q 12 hours for mild to moderate infections. For severe to complicated infections, 400 mg q 8 hours. Continue treatment for 7 to 14 days. For bone and joint infections, treat for 4 to 6 weeks.
➤ **Nosocomial pneumonia**—
Adults: 400 mg I.V. q 8 hours for 10 to 14 days.
➤ **Intra-abdominal infections, combined with metronidazole**—
Adults: 400 mg I.V. q 12 hours for 7 to 14 days.
➤ **Inhalation anthrax after exposure**—
Adults: 400 mg I.V. q 12 hours. Also use one or two additional antimicrobials. Switch to oral therapy when clinically appropriate. Treat for 60 days (I.V. and P.O. combined).
Children: 10 mg/kg I.V. q 12 hours. Don't exceed 800 to 1,000 mg/day I.V. Also use one or two additional antimicrobials. Switch to oral therapy when clinically appropriate. Treat for 60 days (I.V. and P.O. combined).

Reactions may be *common,* uncommon, *life-threatening,* or COMMON AND LIFE-THREATENING.

Adjust-a-dose: For adults with creatinine clearance below 29 ml/minute, give 200 to 400 mg q 18 to 24 hours.

ADMINISTRATION
Direct infusion: Not recommended.
Intermittent infusion: Infuse diluted solution over 60 minutes into a large vein. Stop flow of any other I.V. solutions temporarily while infusing drug.
Continuous infusion: Not recommended.

PREPARATION & STORAGE
Available as a clear, colorless to slightly yellow solution in 200-mg and 400-mg vials of injection concentrate. Dilute drug before use.

Reconstitute with normal saline injection or dextrose 5% injection to concentrations of 1 to 2 mg/ml. Premixed solution is also available in flexible containers of 200 mg in 100 ml of dextrose 5% or normal saline solution and 400 mg in 200 ml of dextrose 5%.

I.V. dilutions are stable for up to 14 days, whether kept at room temperature or refrigerated.

Incompatibilities
Aminophylline, cefepime, clindamycin phosphate, dexamethasone sodium phosphate, furosemide, heparin sodium, methylprednisolone sodium succinate, phenytoin sodium.

CONTRAINDICATIONS & CAUTIONS
• Contraindicated in those hypersensitive to quinolone antimicrobials, in pregnant or breast-feeding women, and in those younger than age 18.
• Use extremely cautiously in those also receiving theophylline I.V. because the combination may cause a fatal reaction. If both drugs must be given together, closely monitor theophylline level, and adjust dosage accordingly.
• Use cautiously in geriatric patients and in those with renal impairment or CNS disorders.

ADVERSE REACTIONS
CNS: headache, restlessness.
GI: abdominal pain or discomfort, diarrhea, nausea, vomiting.
Hematologic: eosinophilia, anemia, altered platelet count.
Metabolic: hyperglycemia.
Skin: rash, local burning.

INTERACTIONS
Drug-drug. *Cyclosporine:* Increases creatinine level. Monitor cyclosporine level and renal function.
Glyburide: May cause severe hypoglycemia. Monitor glucose levels closely.
Phenytoin: Alters phenytoin level. Monitor level.
Probenecid: Decreases excretion of ciprofloxacin and increases risk of toxic reaction. Monitor patient for toxic reaction.
Theophylline: Decreases metabolism and increases toxic effects of methylxanthines. Monitor theophylline level.
Urine alkalizers: Decreases solubility of ciprofloxacin and risk of crystalluria. Monitor patient closely.
Warfarin: May increase risk of bleeding. Monitor PT and INR.
Drug-herb. *Yerba maté:* May decrease clearance of herb's methylxanthines and cause a toxic reaction. Use together cautiously.
Drug-food. *Caffeine:* Increases effect of caffeine. Monitor patient closely.
Drug-lifestyle. *Sun exposure:* May cause photosensitivity reactions. Advise patient to avoid excessive sunlight exposure.

EFFECTS ON LAB TEST RESULTS
• May increase glucose, BUN, creatinine, ALT, AST, alkaline phosphatase, bilirubin, LDH, and GGT levels.
• May increase eosinophil count. May decrease WBC, neutrophil, and platelet counts.

♦ Off-label use   *May contain benzyl alcohol   ◇ Canada

ACTION

Bactericidal effects may result from inhibition of bacterial DNA replication in
susceptible organisms.

PHARMACOKINETICS

Level peaks immediately after infusion.
Distribution: Throughout body tissues.
Drug crosses the placental barrier and
appears in breast milk.
Metabolism: Chiefly in liver.
Excretion: In normal renal function,
50% to 70% excreted in urine within
24 hours. A small amount is excreted in
bile.

CLINICAL CONSIDERATIONS

• Obtain specimen for culture and sensitivity tests before giving first dose.
• Additional antimicrobials for anthrax
multidrug regimens can include rifampin, vancomycin, penicillin, ampicillin,
chloramphenicol, imipenem, clindamycin, and clarithromycin.
• Follow current Centers for Disease
Control recommendations for anthrax.
• Steroids may be considered as adjunctive therapy for anthrax patients
with severe edema and for meningitis,
based on experience with bacterial
meningitis from other causes.
• Ciprofloxacin or doxycycline is a
first-line therapy for anthrax. Amoxicillin 500 mg P.O. t.i.d. for adults and
80 mg/kg/day divided every 8 hours for
children is an option for completion of
therapy after clinical improvement.
• Make sure patient is adequately hydrated to avoid crystalluria.
• Carefully monitor renal and liver
function tests, eosinophil and platelet
counts, uric acid, glucose, and triglyceride levels.
• If patient is undergoing prolonged
therapy, monitor him for superinfection.

PATIENT TEACHING

• Caution ambulatory patient of risk of
dizziness.
• If patient is breast-feeding, give alternate drug or advise her to stop breast-
feeding during therapy.
• Advise patient that hypersensitivity is
common even after first dose. If rash or
other allergic reaction occurs, notify
prescriber.
• Instruct patient to use caution when
driving or operating heavy machinery
until CNS effects of drug are known.
• Advise patient to drink sufficient fluids to ensure hydration.

cisatracurium besylate
Nimbex

Pharmacologic class: nondepolarizing neuromuscular blocker
Therapeutic class: skeletal muscle
relaxant
Pregnancy risk category: B
pH: 3.3 to 3.7

INDICATIONS & DOSAGES

➤ **As an adjunct to general anesthesia, to facilitate tracheal intubation,
and to provide skeletal muscle relaxation during surgery—**
Adults: 0.15 to 0.2 mg/kg I.V., followed
by maintenance dose of 0.03 mg/kg q
40 to 60 minutes, p.r.n. Or, after initial
dose, 3 mcg/kg/minute maintenance infusion may be given to counteract the
spontaneous recovery of neuromuscular
function, then reduced to 1 to 2 mcg/kg/
minute to maintain neuromuscular
block. Dosage requirements vary
widely.
Children ages 2 to 12: 0.1 mg/kgI.V.,
followed by 3 mcg/kg/minute maintenance infusion, reduced to 1 to 2 mcg/
kg/minute p.r.n. Dosage requirements
vary widely.

➤ **To maintain neuromuscular blockade during mechanical ventilation in ICU—**
Adults— 3 mcg/kg/minute I.V. (range, 0.5 to 10.2 mcg/kg/minute). Dosage requirements vary widely.

ADMINISTRATION
Direct injection: Give reconstituted solution directly into vein or through I.V. line containing a free-flowing compatible solution over 5 to 10 seconds.
Intermittent infusion: Not recommended.
Continuous infusion: Infuse diluted solution through I.V. line containing a compatible solution.

PREPARATION & STORAGE
Available in 2-mg/ml and 10-mg/ml vials. Reconstitute with dextrose 5% injection, normal saline injection, or dextrose 5% and normal saline injection to a concentration of 0.1 to 0.2 mg/ml.

Solutions may be refrigerated or stored at room temperature for 24 hours. Protect from light.

Incompatibilities
Alkaline solutions with pH above 8.5, ketorolac, lactated Ringer's injection, propofol.

CONTRAINDICATIONS & CAUTIONS
• Contraindicated in those hypersensitive to the drug.
• Use cautiously in patients with neuromuscular disease because of risk of prolonged muscular block and in those with burns, hemiparesis, or paraparesis because of possible resistance.

ADVERSE REACTIONS
CV: *bradycardia,* hypotension, flushing.
Respiratory: *bronchospasm.*
Skin: rash.
Other: prolonged recovery.

INTERACTIONS
Drug-drug. *Aminoglycosides, bacitracin, clindamycin, colistin, lincomycin, lithium, local anesthetics, magnesium salts, polymyxins, procainamide, quinidine, tetracyclines, sodium colistimethate:* May enhance neuromuscular blocking action of cisatracurium. Use together cautiously.
Carbamazepine, phenytoin: May cause slightly shorter duration of neuromuscular blockade, requiring a higher infusion rate. Monitor patient closely.
Enflurane or isoflurane given with nitrous oxide or oxygen: May prolong duration of action of cisatracurium. Patient may require less frequent maintenance dosing, lower maintenance doses, or reduced infusion rate of cisatracurium.
Succinylcholine: Time to maximum block of cisatracurium is 2 minutes faster with prior administration of succinylcholine. Monitor patient.

EFFECTS ON LAB TEST RESULTS
None reported.

ACTION
Binds to cholinergic receptors on the motor endplate, antagonizing acetylcholine and blocking neuromuscular transmission.

PHARMACOKINETICS
Onset, 1 to 3.3 minutes; peak, 2 to 5 minutes; duration, 46 to 121 minutes.
Distribution: Volume of distribution limited; binding to protein unknown because of rapid degradation.
Metabolism: Metabolized in liver.
Excretion: 95% of drug recovered in urine, and 4% in feces; less than 10% is unchanged in urine.

CLINICAL CONSIDERATIONS
• *Alert:* Don't give unless personnel and facilities for resuscitation and life support and an antagonist to the drug are immediately available.

• Drug isn't recommended for rapid-sequence endotracheal intubation because of its intermediate onset.

• Drug has no known effect on consciousness, pain threshold, or cerebration. To avoid distress, don't give before patient is unconscious.

• Measure neuromuscular function with a peripheral nerve stimulator during infusion. In patients with hemiparesis or paresis, measure on nonparetic limb.

• Monitor acid-base balance and electrolyte levels.

• Monitor patient for malignant hyperthermia.

• Burn patient may require increased dosages. Give analgesics, if appropriate.

• For overdose, maintain patent airway and control ventilation until normal neuromuscular function is achieved. Once recovery begins, an anticholinesterase and an appropriate anticholinergic may be given.

PATIENT TEACHING

• Reassure patient that he'll be continuously monitored.

• Because patient can still hear, explain all procedures and events to him.

cisplatin (cis-platinum)
Platinol-AQ

Pharmacologic class: alkylating drug (cell cycle–phase nonspecific)
Therapeutic class: antineoplastic
Pregnancy risk category: D
pH: 3.7 to 6 for aqueous injection

INDICATIONS & DOSAGES

➤ **Metastatic testicular cancer—**
Adults: As part of combination therapy, 20 mg/m^2/day I.V. for 5 days q 3 weeks for three or four cycles.

➤ **Metastatic ovarian cancer—**
Adults: As part of combination therapy, 50 to 100 mg/m^2 I.V. q 3 to 4 weeks; as a single drug, 100 mg/m^2 q 4 weeks. Alternative dosages, 30 to 120 mg/m^2 q 3 to 4 weeks.

➤ **Advanced bladder cancer—**
Adults: 50 to 70 mg/m^2 I.V. q 3 to 4 weeks. Patients who have received other antineoplastics or radiation therapy should receive 50 mg/m^2 q 4 weeks.

➤ **Head and neck cancer ♦ —**
Adults: As part of combination therapy, 50 to 120 mg/m^2 I.V. according to hospital protocol; as a single drug, 80 to 120 mg/m^2 q 3 weeks or 50 mg/m^2 on days 1 and 8 of q 4-week cycle.

➤ **Metastatic or recurrent cervical cancer ♦ —**
Adults: 50 to 100 mg/m^2 I.V. q 3 weeks to a maximum of 6 courses.

➤ **Non–small-cell lung cancer ♦ —**
Adults: As part of combination therapy, 75 to 100 mg/m^2 I.V. q 3 to 4 weeks.

➤ **Esophageal cancer ♦ —**
Adults: As part of combination therapy, 75 to 100 mg/m^2 I.V. q 3 to 4 weeks; as a single drug, 50 to 120 mg/m^2 q 3 to 4 weeks.

➤ **Osteogenic sarcoma ♦ , neuroblastoma ♦ —**
Children: 90 mg/m^2 I.V. q 3 weeks or 30 mg/m^2 weekly.

➤ **Recurrent brain tumors ♦ —**
Children: 60 mg/m^2 I.V. once daily for 2 consecutive days q 3 to 4 weeks.
Adjust-a-dose: Patients with mild to moderate renal impairment may receive 50% to 75% of recommended dose.

ADMINISTRATION

Direct injection: Not recommended.
Intermittent infusion: Give diluted solution through a separate I.V. line, using a 21G or 23G needle. Infuse over 6 to 8 hours or follow hospital protocol.
Continuous infusion: Infuse diluted solution over 24 hours or 5 days, according to hospital protocol.

PREPARATION & STORAGE
Available as an aqueous solution of
50 mg/50 ml and 100 mg/100 ml.

To avoid mutagenic, teratogenic, and
carcinogenic risks, use extreme caution
when preparing or giving cisplatin. Use
a biological containment cabinet and
avoid contact with skin. Wear mask and
gloves. If solution comes in contact
with skin or mucosa, immediately wash
thoroughly with soap and water. Dispose of needles, syringes, vials, and
any unused drug carefully.

For intermittent infusion, dilute reconstituted drug in 2 L of 0.33% or
half-normal saline solution along with
37.5 g of mannitol.

Precipitation may cause loss of potency. To avoid this, don't use needles,
syringes, or I.V. kits containing aluminum parts, and don't refrigerate reconstituted solutions.

Reconstituted solutions are stable
for 20 hours at room temperature. Solutions prepared with bacteriostatic
water for injection with benzyl alcohol
or parabens are stable for 72 hours.

Incompatibilities
Aluminum administration sets, amifostine, cefepime, D5W, fluorouracil, mesna, 0.1% sodium chloride solution,
piperacillin sodium with tazobactam
sodium, sodium bicarbonate, sodium
bisulfate, sodium thiosulfate, solutions
with a chloride content less than 2%,
thiotepa.

CONTRAINDICATIONS & CAUTIONS
• Contraindicated in patients hypersensitive to platinum-containing compounds and in those with myelosuppression or hearing impairment.
• Contraindicated in those with renal
disease because of the risk of nephrotoxicity. Renal impairment usually occurs during the second week after infusion but may occur within several days
with high-dose regimens.

• Avoid use in those with existing or recent chickenpox or herpes zoster infections. Immunosuppressive properties
increase the risk of generalized disease.
• Use cautiously in patients who have
received a cytotoxic drug or radiation
therapy, to reduce risk of cumulative
immunosuppression.
• Use cautiously in patients with existing or recent infection to avoid severe
infection and in those with gout or
urate calculi to avoid hyperuricemia.

ADVERSE REACTIONS
CNS: *peripheral neuritis, seizures,*
neuropathy.
EENT: *high frequency hearing loss,*
tinnitus.
GI: *nausea, vomiting,* anorexia.
GU: *severe renal toxicity.*
Hematologic: *leukopenia, thrombocy-
topenia,* anemia.
Metabolic: hyperuricemia, hypocal-
cemia, hypomagnesemia, hypophos-
phatemia, hypokalemia.
Other: *anaphylactoid reaction.*

INTERACTIONS
Drug-drug. *Allopurinol, probenecid,
sulfinpyrazone:* Decreases effectiveness
in lowering uric acid level. Monitor patient closely.
*Myelosuppressants, nephrotoxic drugs,
ototoxic drugs, radiation therapy:* Enhances toxicity. Monitor patient closely.
Phenytoin: Decreases level of phenytoin. Monitor drug level.
Vaccines with killed virus: Decreases
effectiveness. Avoid using together.
Vaccines with live virus: Risk of severe
toxic reaction. Avoid using together.

EFFECTS ON LAB TEST RESULTS
• May increase uric acid level. May decrease magnesium, potassium, calcium,
sodium, phosphate and platelet levels.
• May decrease hemoglobin and WBC
count.

ACTION

Precise mechanism of action unknown. Cross-links strands of DNA material, inhibiting DNA synthesis and leading to cell death.

PHARMACOKINETICS

Level peaks at end of infusion; duration, several days.
Distribution: Throughout body fluids and tissues; highest levels in the liver, kidneys, intestines, and prostate. CSF levels are low. Drug crosses the placental barrier and is extensively bound to protein. It's unknown if drug appears in breast milk.
Metabolism: Rapid nonenzymatic conversion to inactive metabolites.
Excretion: In urine, predominantly by glomerular filtration, with 15% to 50% excreted within 48 hours. Drug's extensive protein binding prolongs excretion. Initial half-life, about 35 minutes; terminal half-life, about 75 hours.

CLINICAL CONSIDERATIONS

• Osmolality: about 285 mOsm/kg for aqueous solution.
• *Alert:* Don't confuse cisplatin with carboplatin.
• *Alert:* Use administration equipment that contains no aluminum.
• Hydrate patient using normal saline solution before giving drug. Maintain urine output of 150 to 400 ml/hour at onset of administration and for 4 to 6 hours thereafter.
• *Alert:* Up to one-third of patients show signs and symptoms of ototoxicity after a single dose. Ototoxicity may be cumulative and more severe in children. To detect high-frequency hearing loss, obtain audiometric test results before each course of therapy.
• Cisplatin raises uric acid level. Monitor level and adjust gout medication appropriately.
• *Alert:* Drug is highly emetogenic. Give antiemetics

• Adequate hydration, allopurinol administration, and alkalization of urine may prevent or minimize uric acid nephropathy from elevated uric acid level.
• Monitor vital signs during infusion.
• Before the first infusion and before each course of therapy, determine magnesium, potassium, calcium, creatinine, and BUN levels and creatinine clearance.
• Maintain urine output of 100 to 200 ml/hour for 18 to 24 hours after therapy.
• Regularly perform neurologic examinations. Stop drug if neurotoxicity occurs.
• Monitor CBC and platelet count weekly; myelosuppression may be cumulative. Leukocyte and platelet nadirs generally occur 18 to 23 days after a single dose. Levels usually return to baseline within 13 to 62 days. Don't repeat dose unless platelet count exceeds $100,000/mm^3$, WBC count is over $4,000/mm^3$, creatinine level is under 1.5 mg/dl, or BUN level is under 25 mg/dl.
• Monitor liver and kidney function. Renal insufficiency, which is generally reversible, usually occurs during the second week of administration.
• Nausea and vomiting may be severe enough to stop treatment.
• Hemodialysis removes only a minimal amount of drug.

PATIENT TEACHING

• Advise women of childbearing age to avoid becoming pregnant during therapy. Suggest consulting with prescriber before making the decision to become pregnant.
• Alert patient that nausea usually begins 1 to 6 hours after administration and may last for 24 hours or more.
• Advise patient to watch for signs and symptoms of infection, such as fever, sore throat, and fatigue, and of bleeding, such as easy bruising, melena,

bleeding gums, and nosebleeds. Tell patient to take temperature daily.

• Advise patient to immediately report tinnitus or numbness in hands or feet.

• Stress importance of adequate fluid intake and urine output to facilitate uric acid excretion.

cladribine (2-chlorodeoxyadenosine)
Leustatin

Pharmacologic class: purine nucleoside analogue
Therapeutic class: antineoplastic
Pregnancy risk category: D
pH: 6 to 6.6

INDICATIONS & DOSAGES

➤ **Active hairy cell leukemia defined by anemia, neutropenia, thrombocytopenia, or disease-related symptoms—**
Adults: 0.09 mg/kg I.V. daily by continuous I.V. infusion for 7 consecutive days, for a total dose of 0.63 mg/kg.

Drug can be given daily over seven consecutive 24-hour periods or as a continuous 7-day infusion. Deviation from this dosage regimen isn't recommended.

ADMINISTRATION

Direct injection: Not recommended.
Intermittent infusion: Infuse daily over seven consecutive 24-hour periods.
Continuous infusion: Infuse continuously over 7 days.

PREPARATION & STORAGE

Available as a preservative-free solution of 1 mg/ml in 10-ml or 10 ml filled in 20-ml single-dose vials.

Drug must be diluted before infusion. For a 24-hour infusion, add the calculated dose to a 500-ml infusion bag of normal saline injection and in-

fuse continuously over 24 hours. Don't use solutions that contain dextrose.

Alternatively, for the 7-day infusion, use bacteriostatic saline injection, which contains benzyl alcohol as a preservative. Because the calculated dose dilutes the benzyl alcohol preservative, in patients weighing more than 187 lb (85 kg), the effectiveness of the preservative may be reduced. To minimize the risk of microbial contamination, calculate the 7-day dose of cladribine and amount of diluent needed to bring the total volume to 100 ml.

First add the calculated dose of cladribine into the infusion reservoir through a sterile 0.22 micron disposable hydrophilic syringe filter; then add the calculated amount of bacteriostatic saline, also through the filter, to bring the total volume to 100 ml. Clamp off the line and disconnect and discard the filter. Using aseptic technique, aspirate any air bubbles from the reservoir using the syringe with a dry sterile filter or sterile vent filter assembly. Reclamp and discard the syringe and filter. Physical and chemical stability have been demonstrated with the Pharmacia Deltec drug cassettes.

Unopened vials should be refrigerated at 36° to 46° F (2° to 8° C) and protected from light. Freezing doesn't adversely affect the solution; however, a precipitate may form at low temperatures. Allowing the solution to warm to room temperature and vigorously shaking the vial cause the precipitate to become soluble again. Don't heat or microwave. Once thawed, the solution is stable until the labeled expiration date if refrigerated. Don't refreeze.

Once diluted, give promptly or store in refrigerator for no more than 8 hours before administration. Discard any unused portion using chemotherapy precautions.

Incompatibilities
Dextrose solutions, other I.V. drugs and additives.

CONTRAINDICATIONS & CAUTIONS
• Contraindicated in those hypersensitive to the drug or to any of its components.
• Use cautiously in those with preexisting bone marrow depression or known or suspected renal or hepatic impairment.

ADVERSE REACTIONS
CNS: acute neurotoxicity with high doses, asthenia, dizziness, fatigue, headache, insomnia, malaise, fever, pain.
CV: tachycardia, edema, phlebitis.
EENT: epistaxis.
GI: abdominal pain, constipation, diarrhea, nausea, vomiting, decreased appetite.
GU: anuria, *acute nephrotoxicity with high doses.*
Hematologic: *myelosuppression, neutropenia, thrombocytopenia,* anemia, thrombosis.
Metabolic: acidosis.
Musculoskeletal: arthralgia, myalgia, trunk pain.
Respiratory: abnormal breath sounds, cough, shortness of breath.
Skin: erythema, petechiae, pruritus, rash, purpura, diaphoresis, injection site pain and swelling.
Other: chills, infection.

INTERACTIONS
Drug-drug. *Myelosuppressants:* Increases myelosuppression. Monitor patient closely.

EFFECTS ON LAB TEST RESULTS
• May increase creatinine, liver function tests, and uric acid levels.
• May decrease hemoglobin, hematocrit, WBC, and platelet counts.

ACTION
Enters tumor cells, is phosphorylated by deoxycytidine kinase, and is subsequently converted to an active triphosphate deoxynucleotide. This metabolite impairs synthesis of new DNA, inhibits repair of existing DNA, and disrupts cellular metabolism.

PHARMACOKINETICS
Mean terminal half-life after 2-hour infusion, about 5½ hours.
Distribution: Crosses membrane of cells with high ratio of deoxycytidine kinase to deoxynucleotidase. It's unknown if drug appears in breast milk. About 20% bound to protein.
Metabolism: Phosphorylated by deoxycytidine kinase and then converted to an active triphosphate deoxynucleotide.
Excretion: Unknown.

CLINICAL CONSIDERATIONS
• Tonicity: isotonic.
• Give drug under supervision of a prescriber experienced in chemotherapy.
• Because drug is a potent antineoplastic, use disposable gloves and protective clothing. If skin or mucous membrane contact occurs, wash with copious amounts of water.
• *Alert:* Don't confuse cladribine with cytarabine.
• If neurotoxicity or renal toxicity occurs, stop or interrupt therapy.
• *Alert:* High doses four to nine times the recommended dose with cyclophosphamide and total body irradiation as preparation for bone marrow transplantation have been linked to irreversible neurologic toxicity or acute renal insufficiency in 45% of patients treated for 7 to 14 days.
• Close monitoring of hematologic function, especially during the first 4 to 8 weeks of therapy, is recommended. Severe bone marrow depression, neutropenia, anemia, and thrombocytopenia commonly occur.

Reactions may be *common*, uncommon, *life-threatening*, or COMMON AND LIFE-THREATENING.

- After peripheral blood counts have returned to normal, bone marrow aspiration and biopsy should be performed to determine response to therapy.
- Monitor renal and hepatic function during therapy. No specific recommendations for dosage adjustments are available.
- During first month of treatment, Monitor patient for fever.

PATIENT TEACHING
- Because of the risk of fetal malformations, advise women of childbearing age to avoid becoming pregnant during therapy.
- Caution women against breast-feed during therapy because of possible infant toxicity.
- Advise patient to watch for signs and symptoms of infection, such as fever, sore throat, and fatigue, and of bleeding, such as easy bruising, nosebleeds, bleeding gums, and melena. Tell patient to take his temperature daily.

clindamycin phosphate
Cleocin Phosphate*, Dalacin C Phosphate ◊ *

Pharmacologic class: lincomycin derivative
Therapeutic class: antibiotic
Pregnancy risk category: B
pH: ranges from 5.5 to 7, but usually 6 to 6.3

INDICATIONS & DOSAGES
➤ **Severe infections caused by susceptible organisms—**
Adults: 600 mg to 2.7 g I.V. daily equally divided q 6, 8, or 12 hours or by continuous infusion to maintain level of 4 to 6 mcg/ml. May increase to 4.8 g daily for life-threatening infections.

Children older than age 1 month: 15 to 40 mg/kg/day I.V. equally divided q 6 to 8 hours. Single dose shouldn't exceed 600 mg.
Children ages 1 month or younger: 15 to 20 mg/kg/day I.V. equally divided q 6 to 8 hours. Maximum dosage, 300 mg daily.

ADMINISTRATION
Direct injection: Not recommended.
Intermittent infusion: Infuse drug diluted to a concentration of 6 mg/ml or less through an intermittent infusion device or into an I.V. line containing a free-flowing, compatible solution. Infuse 300 mg/50 ml over 10 minutes, 600 mg/100 ml over 20 minutes, or 900 mg/150 ml over 30 minutes. Infuse 1,200 mg/100 ml over 40 minutes. Don't infuse more than 1,200 mg over 1 hour.
Continuous infusion: Give as a single, rapid infusion, then follow with a continuous infusion, using a diluted concentration of 6 mg/ml.
   For drug level above 4 mcg/ml, rapidly infuse 10 mg/minute for 30 minutes, and then give maintenance dose of 0.75 mg/minute. For drug level above 5 mcg/ml, rapidly infuse 15 mg/minute for 30 minutes, and then give maintenance dose of 1 mg/minute. For drug level above 6 mcg/ml, rapidly infuse 20 mg/minute for 30 minutes, and then give maintenance dose of 1.25 mg/minute.

PREPARATION & STORAGE
Available in a concentration of 150 mg/ml in 2-ml and 4-ml ampules and 6-ml vials.
   For a concentration of 6 mg/ml or less, add 25 ml of compatible solution to each 150 mg of clindamycin (300 mg/50 ml). Compatible solutions include D_5W or dextrose 10% in water, Isolyte H, Isolyte M and dextrose 5%, Isolyte P and dextrose 5%, Normosol-R, lactated

Ringer's, and normal saline solution. Use solutions within 24 hours.

Store below 104° F (40° C), preferably between 59° and 86° F (15° and 30° C). Protect from freezing.

Incompatibilities
Allopurinol; aminophylline; ampicillin; barbiturates; calcium gluconate; ceftriaxone; ciprofloxacin hydrochloride; filgrastim; fluconazole; idarubicin; magnesium sulfate; phenytoin sodium; rubber closures, such as those on I.V. tubing; tobramycin sulfate.

CONTRAINDICATIONS & CAUTIONS
• Contraindicated in those hypersensitive to the drug or to lincomycin.
• Use cautiously in atopic patients.
• Use cautiously in those with GI disorders because of increased risk of pseudomembranous colitis.
• Use cautiously in those with renal or hepatic impairment because drug may exacerbate these conditions, and in neonates because drug contains benzyl alcohol, which in large doses can cause fatal gasping syndrome.

ADVERSE REACTIONS
GI: abdominal pain, diarrhea, nausea, *pseudomembranous colitis,* vomiting.
GU: *tenesmus.*
Hematologic: eosinophilia, *leukopenia, agranulocytosis, neutropenia, thrombocytopenia.*
Skin: *morbilliform rash, redness,* urticaria.

INTERACTIONS
Drug-drug. *Aminoglycosides:* May antagonize aminoglycoside effects. Monitor patient closely.
Chloramphenicol, erythromycin: Decreases antibiotic effectiveness. Avoid using together.
Inhaled anesthetics, neuromuscular blockers: Enhances neuromuscular blockade. Monitor patient closely.

EFFECTS ON LAB TEST RESULTS
• May increase bilirubin, ALT, AST, and alkaline phosphatase levels.
• May increase eosinophil count. May decrease WBC and platelet counts.

ACTION
Inhibits protein synthesis of susceptible bacteria. Is bactericidal or bacteriostatic, depending on its concentration and the susceptibility of the organism.

Spectrum of activity includes staphylococci, *Streptococcus pneumoniae,* and most other gram-positive cocci. Susceptible gram-negative and gram-positive anaerobic organisms include *Actinomyces, Bacteroides, Clostridium perfringens, C. tetani, Corynebacterium diphtheriae, Eubacterium, Fusobacterium, Mycoplasma, Peptococcus, Peptostreptococcus, Propionibacterium,* and *Veillonella.*

PHARMACOKINETICS
Drug level peaks at end of infusion.
Distribution: Throughout body tissues and fluids, including saliva, bone, bile, and ascitic, pleural, and synovial fluid. About 93% bound to protein. Drug readily crosses the placental barrier and appears in breast milk, but even with inflamed meninges, only small amounts reach CSF.
Metabolism: Partly changed in liver to active and inactive metabolites. Metabolic rate increases in children.
Excretion: In urine, bile, and feces as metabolites. Half-life, 2 to 3 hours.

CLINICAL CONSIDERATIONS
• Osmolality: 795 mOsm/kg or 835 mOsm/kg for undiluted injection; 12 mg/ml in D₅W is 293 mOsm/kg and 309 mOsm/kg in normal saline solution.
• *Alert:* Drug is also incompatible with rubber closures, such as those on I.V. tubing.
• Obtain specimens for culture and sensitivity tests before giving first dose.

Reactions may be *common*, uncommon, *life-threatening*, or COMMON AND LIFE-THREATENING.

Therapy may begin before test results are available.

• If severe, persistent diarrhea occurs, stop drug and obtain a stool specimen for culture.

• Colitis may not develop for several weeks after drug has been stopped.

• To prevent toxin retention, avoid opioids and diphenoxylate when treating drug-induced colitis.

• During long-term therapy, monitor kidney and liver function tests and blood cell counts. Adjust dosage accordingly.

• Monitor clindamycin level during high-dose therapy.

• Observe patient for superinfection with prolonged use.

• Severe anaphylactic reaction requires emergency treatment with epinephrine, oxygen, and corticosteroids.

• Neither hemodialysis nor peritoneal dialysis significantly removes drug.

PATIENT TEACHING

• Notify patient of potential toxic effects. Tell him to report adverse reactions, especially diarrhea, to prescriber and not treat such reactions himself.

• Instruct patient to report discomfort at I.V. site immediately.

codeine phosphate

Pharmacologic class: opioid
Therapeutic class: analgesic, antitussive
Pregnancy risk category: C
Controlled substance schedule: II
pH: 3 to 6

INDICATIONS & DOSAGES

➤ **Mild to moderate pain—**
Adults: 15 to 60 mg I.V. q 4 to 6 hours. Don't exceed 360 mg in 24 hours.
Children: 0.5 mg/kg or 15 mg/m^2 I.V. q 4 to 6 hours.

ADMINISTRATION

Direct injection: Inject diluted drug over 4 to 5 minutes through I.V. tubing containing a free-flowing, compatible solution.
Intermittent infusion: Infuse diluted drug slowly.
Continuous infusion: Not recommended.

PREPARATION & STORAGE

Available in concentrations of 15, 30, and 60 mg/ml in 1-ml vials and 2-ml disposable syringes.

Store below 104° F (40° C), preferably between 59° and 86° F (15° and 30° C). Protect from light and freezing. Don't use solution if it's more than slightly discolored or contains a precipitate.

Incompatibilities

Aminophylline, ammonium chloride, amobarbital, bromides, chlorothiazide, heparin, iodides, pentobarbital, phenobarbital, phenytoin, salts of heavy metals, sodium bicarbonate, sodium iodide, thiopental.

CONTRAINDICATIONS & CAUTIONS

• Contraindicated in those hypersensitive to the drug or to sulfites and in premature neonates.

• Contraindicated in those with acute respiratory depression because drug may exacerbate the condition.

• Contraindicated in those with diarrhea resulting from pseudomembranous colitis or poisoning because elimination of toxins may be slowed.

• Contraindicated in those with pulmonary edema caused by a chemical respiratory irritant. Codeine causes vasodilation, which may produce adverse hemodynamic effects.

• Use cautiously in patients with prostatic hyperplasia, urethral stricture, or recent urinary tract surgery because drug can cause urine retention and in those with arrhythmias because drug can increase response through a vagolytic action.

• Use cautiously in patients with acute abdominal conditions because drug may mask symptoms and in those with head injury or increased intracranial pressure from intracranial lesions because drug may mask changes and elevate CSF pressure.

• Use cautiously in those who have recently had GI surgery because drug may alter GI motility, in those with gallbladder disease because drug may increase biliary contractions, and in those with seizure disorders because drug may induce or exacerbate seizures.

• Use cautiously in patients experiencing drug dependency, emotional instability, or suicidal ideation, because of the potential for abuse.

• Use cautiously in those with inflammatory bowel disease because toxic megacolon may develop.

• Use cautiously in those with hypothyroidism because of the increased risk of respiratory depression and prolonged CNS depression and in geriatric patients, pediatric patients, and those with altered respiratory function because of increased risk of respiratory depression.

• Use cautiously and reduce dosage in patients with hepatic or renal impairment because of increased risk of toxic reaction.

ADVERSE REACTIONS

CNS: light-headedness, dizziness, *sedation.*
CV: *bradycardia,* palpitations, orthostatic hypotension.
GI: nausea, vomiting, constipation.
GU: urine retention, oliguria.
Respiratory: *respiratory depression.*

INTERACTIONS

Drug-drug. *Antidiarrheals, antimuscarinics:* Increases risk of paralytic ileus. Monitor patient closely.

Antihypertensives, diuretics: Increases risk of hypotension. Monitor patient and blood pressure closely.
Aspirin: Causes additive analgesic effects. Monitor patient closely.
CNS depressants, MAO inhibitors: Increases CNS depression. Use together with extreme caution. Monitor patient closely.
Buprenorphine, naloxone, naltrexone: Reduces therapeutic effects of codeine. Avoid using together.
Metoclopramide: Causes antagonistic effect on GI motility. Avoid using together.
Neuromuscular blockers: May increase respiratory depression. Avoid using together.
Drug-lifestyle. *Alcohol use:* Causes additive effects. Discourage use together.

EFFECTS ON LAB TEST RESULTS

• May increase amylase and lipase levels.
• May delay emptying during gastric-emptying studies. May elevate CSF pressure during lumbar puncture and delay visualization during hepatobiliary imaging with technetium-99m disofenin.

ACTION

Codeine binds with stereospecific receptors in the CNS, altering the perception of pain and the emotional response to it.

PHARMACOKINETICS

Drug level peaks immediately; duration, 4 to 5 hours.
Distribution: Rapidly distributed to kidneys, liver, spleen, CNS and lungs. Drug appears in breast milk and is minimally protein bound.
Metabolism: In liver.
Excretion: Excreted mainly in urine; small amounts in feces. Elimination half-life, 2 to 3 hours.

Reactions may be *common*, uncommon, *life-threatening*, or COMMON AND LIFE-THREATENING.

CLINICAL CONSIDERATIONS
• *Alert:* Drug may contain sulfites. Don't use in hypersensitive patients.
• *Alert:* Rapid infusion can cause life-threatening adverse reactions.
• *Alert:* Keep emergency resuscitation equipment available.
• If giving by direct injection, monitor vital signs and respiratory status during injection and q 15 minutes for at least 1 hour after injection. Also monitor vital signs and respiratory status during intermittent infusion.
• To minimize hypotension, give drug with patient in supine position.
• To reverse respiratory depression, give naloxone.
• Drug stimulates vasopressin release and may increase risk of water intoxication.

PATIENT TEACHING
• Instruct patient to change position slowly to lessen dizziness and faintness.
• Advise patient of potential addiction.
• Tell patient to ask for pain medication before pain becomes intense.

colchicine

Pharmacologic class: alkaloid
Therapeutic class: antigout drug
Pregnancy risk category: D

INDICATIONS & DOSAGES
➤ **Acute gout, gouty arthritis—**
Adults: 2 mg I.V., followed by 0.5 mg q 6 hours p.r.n. Maximum daily dose, 4 mg. Don't exceed 4 mg per course of therapy.
➤ **Prophylaxis or maintenance of recurrent or chronic gouty arthritis—**
Adults: 0.5 to 1 mg I.V. once or twice daily.

ADMINISTRATION
Direct injection: Give by slow I.V. push over 2 to 5 minutes directly into vein or through tubing with a free-flowing compatible I.V. solution.
Intermittent infusion: Not recommended.
Continuous infusion: Not recommended.

PREPARATION & STORAGE
Available in 1 mg/2 ml ampules.
   Dilute with normal saline injection or sterile water for injection.
   Store in tight, light-resistant containers away from moisture and high temperatures. Don't use if turbid.

Incompatibilities
Dextrose 5% injection, bacteriostatic normal saline injection.

CONTRAINDICATIONS & CAUTIONS
• Contraindicated in those hypersensitive to drug, blood dyscrasia, or serious CV, renal, or GI disease.
• Avoid use in those with severe renal or hepatic dysfunction because of the increased risk of colchicine toxicity.
• Use cautiously in geriatric patients and debilitated patients and in those with early signs and symptoms of CV, renal, or GI disease because of possible cumulative effects.

ADVERSE REACTIONS
GI: nausea, abdominal pain, vomiting, diarrhea.
Hematologic: *aplastic anemia, thrombocytopenia, agranulocytosis.*
Skin: urticaria, dermatitis, alopecia; severe local reaction if extravasation occurs.

INTERACTIONS
Drug-drug. *CNS depressants, sympathomimetics:* Enhances response to these drugs. Monitor patient closely.

Cyclosporine: Increases GI toxicity when given together. Adjust doses if toxicity occurs. Monitor patient closely.
Loop diuretics: May decrease efficacy of colchicine prophylaxis. Avoid using together.
Vitamin B$_{12}$: Causes reversible malabsorption of vitamin B$_{12}$. Avoid using together.
Drug-lifestyle. *Alcohol use:* Inhibits colchicine. Discourage use together.

EFFECTS ON LAB TEST RESULTS
• May increase alkaline phosphatase, AST, and ALT levels.
• May increase eosinophil count. May decrease hemoglobin and granulocyte and platelet counts. May increase or decrease WBC count.
• May cause false-positive results in urine tests for RBC count or hemoglobin.

ACTION
Drug appears to reduce the inflammatory response to deposition of monosodium urate crystals in joint tissues, possibly by inhibiting polymorphonuclear leukocyte metabolism, mobility, chemotaxis, or leukocyte function. Also, interferes with sodium urate deposition by decreasing lactic acid production.

PHARMACOKINETICS
Distribution: Concentrated in leukocytes but also distributed in kidneys, liver, spleen, and intestinal tract.
Metabolism: Partially in liver.
Excretion: Primarily in feces, with smaller amounts in urine. Plasma half-life, 20 minutes; half-life in leukocytes, about 60 hours.

CLINICAL CONSIDERATIONS
• Don't repeat course of I.V. colchicine for several weeks, to avoid cumulative toxicity.
• Obtain baseline laboratory studies, including CBC, before initiating therapy and periodically thereafter.

• **Alert:** Stop drug if nausea, abdominal pain, vomiting, or diarrhea occur because these are the first signs and symptoms of toxic reaction.
• For overdose, provide symptomatic and supportive treatment, including administration of atropine or morphine for abdominal pain, measures to combat shock, and establishment of adequate respiratory exchange by maintenance of adequate airway, control of respiration, and oxygen administration. Dialysis may be helpful.

PATIENT TEACHING
• Advise patient to report rash, sore throat, fever, unusual bleeding and bruising, tiredness, weakness, numbness, or tingling.
• Tell patient with gout to limit foods high in purine, such as anchovies, liver, sardines, kidneys, sweetbreads, peas, and lentils.

cosyntropin
Cortrosyn

Pharmacologic class: anterior pituitary hormone
Therapeutic class: diagnostic drug
Pregnancy risk category: C

INDICATIONS & DOSAGES
➤ **Rapid screening test of adrenal function—**
Adults and children age 2 and older: 0.25 mg I.V.
Children younger than age 2: 0.125 mg I.V.
Neonates: 0.015 mg/kg/dose I.V.
➤ **Adrenal stimulus—**
Adults: 0.25 mg I.V. at a rate of 0.04 mg/hour for 6 hours.

ADMINISTRATION
Direct injection: Inject reconstituted drug into vein through an intermittent

---

Reactions may be *common,* uncommon, *life-threatening,* or COMMON AND LIFE-THREATENING.

infusion device over 2 minutes. Or, inject drug through an I.V. line containing a free-flowing, compatible solution, but interrupt primary infusion during injection.

Intermittent infusion: Infuse diluted at 0.04 mg/hour over 4 to 8 hours.

Continuous infusion: Not recommended.

PREPARATION & STORAGE

Available in two-vial packets.

To reconstitute, add 1 ml of normal saline injection to vial containing 0.25 mg of cosyntropin to yield a concentration of 250 mcg/ml. For infusion, dilute cosyntropin with D_5W or normal saline solution.

Before reconstitution, store at 59° to 86° F (15° to 30° C), unless manufacturer specifies otherwise. After reconstitution, solution remains stable for 24 hours if kept at room temperature and for 3 weeks if refrigerated at 36° to 46° F (2° to 8° C). Solutions diluted further remain stable for 12 hours at room temperature.

Incompatibilities

Blood products.

CONTRAINDICATIONS & CAUTIONS

• Use cautiously in those hypersensitive to the drug or with allergic disorders.

ADVERSE REACTIONS

CNS: dizziness, *seizures.*
GI: peptic ulcer, nausea, vomiting.
Hepatic: hyperbilirubinemia.
Skin: ecchymoses, pruritus.
Other: *hypersensitivity reactions,* facial edema.

INTERACTIONS

Drug-drug. *Blood, plasma products:* Inactivates cosyntropin. Avoid using together.

Cortisone, hydrocortisone, spironolactone: If taken on test day, causes abnormally high baseline cortisol level, fol-

lowed by a paradoxical decline in level after cosyntropin administration. Avoid using together.

Estrogens: Increases cortisol level before and after administration. Avoid using together.

EFFECTS ON LAB TEST RESULTS

• May increase bilirubin level; may also increase cortisol level if fluorometric methods are used.

ACTION

A synthetic peptide corresponding to amino acids 1 to 24 of human corticotropin, cosyntropin combines with receptors in the adrenal cell plasma membrane to stimulate secretion of cortisol, corticosterone, weak androgenic substances, and a small amount of aldosterone. A cosyntropin dose of 0.25 mg is pharmacologically equal to 25 units of natural corticotropin.

PHARMACOKINETICS

Cortisol level peaks at 1 hour; duration, 2 to 3 hours.

Distribution: Unknown. Drug doesn't cross the placental barrier. It's unknown if it appears in breast milk.

Metabolism: Unknown.

Excretion: Unknown. Half-life, about 15 minutes.

CLINICAL CONSIDERATIONS

• Highest cortisol level occurs 45 to 60 minutes after cosyntropin administration.

• Watch patient closely for signs and symptoms of adverse reactions and allergic reactions, such as rash, dyspnea, wheezing, or anaphylaxis. Keep emergency resuscitation equipment nearby when giving drug because of risk of anaphylaxis.

• More cortisol is secreted if dosage is given slowly I.V.

• Cosyntropin is less antigenic than corticotropin and less likely to produce allergic reactions.

PATIENT TEACHING
• Explain test procedure to patient.
• Tell patient to report to prescriber adverse reactions promptly.
• Inform patient about possible drug interactions.

---

co-trimoxazole (sulfamethoxazole and trimethoprim)
Bactrim I.V.*, Septra I.V.*

Pharmacologic class: sulfonamide and folate antagonist
Therapeutic class: antibiotic
Pregnancy risk category: C
pH: about 10

INDICATIONS & DOSAGES
➤ **Systemic bacterial infections caused by susceptible organisms—**
Adults and children ages 2 months and older: 8 to 10 mg/kg I.V. of trimethoprim in divided doses q 6, 8, or 12 hours. Maximum dosage, 960 mg/day of trimethoprim.
➤ **Pneumocystis carinii** *pneumonitis—*
Adults and children ages 2 months and older: 15 to 20 mg/kg I.V. of trimethoprim in divided doses q 6 to 8 hours.
Adjust-a-dose: For patients with renal impairment, if creatinine clearance is 15 to 30 ml/minute, give half usual adult dose. If clearance is below 15 ml/minute, avoid use.

ADMINISTRATION
Direct injection: Not recommended.
Intermittent infusion: Using a 21G to 23G needle, infuse diluted drug into an I.V. line of free-flowing D_5W over 60 to 90 minutes. If only one site available, flush tubing with 10 ml of sterile water for injection before and after infusion and turn off primary I.V. solution during co-trimoxazole administration.

Continuous infusion: Not recommended.

PREPARATION & STORAGE
Available in 5-ml, 10-ml, 20-ml, and 30-ml vials.
    Before infusion, add 125 ml of D_5W to dilute drug in a 5-ml vial. New concentration contains 0.64 mg/ml of trimethoprim and 3.2 mg/ml of sulfamethoxazole.
    Diluted solution is stable for 6 hours at room temperature. Solutions containing 0.80 mg/ml of trimethoprim and 4 mg/ml of sulfamethoxazole remain stable for 4 hours; those containing 1.1 mg/ml of trimethoprim and 5.3 mg/ml of sulfamethoxazole remain stable for 2 hours.
    Don't refrigerate drug or solutions. Discard cloudy solutions and those that contain precipitates.

Incompatibilities
All I.V. solutions except D_5W, other I.V. drugs.

CONTRAINDICATIONS & CAUTIONS
• Contraindicated in those hypersensitive to sulfonamides or trimethoprim and in pregnant patients or breast-feeding patients.
• Contraindicated in neonates because sulfonamides can cause kernicterus.
• Contraindicated in patients with megaloblastic anemia because of folate deficiency.
• Use cautiously in patients hypersensitive to furosemide, thiazide diuretics, sulfonylureas, or carbonic anhydrase inhibitors because these patients may also be hypersensitive to sulfonamides.
• Use cautiously in those with renal or hepatic impairment, bronchial asthma, G6PD deficiency, folic acid deficiency, or AIDS because of the increased risk of adverse reactions and in those receiving chemotherapy because of increased risk of myelosuppression.

Reactions may be *common*, uncommon, *life-threatening*, or COMMON AND LIFE-THREATENING.

• Use cautiously in mentally disabled children because reduced folate level can worsen psychomotor regression.
• Use cautiously in patients with streptococcal pharyngitis because of risk of organism resistance and in geriatric, malnourished, alcoholic, or debilitated patients because of risk of toxic reaction.

ADVERSE REACTIONS
CNS: headache, *seizures,* depression.
EENT: tinnitus.
GI: nausea, vomiting, anorexia, diarrhea.
GU: *toxic nephrosis with oliguria and anuria.*
Hematologic: *agranulocytosis, aplastic anemia, thrombocytopenia, hemolytic anemia.*
Hepatic: *hepatic necrosis.*
Musculoskeletal: arthralgia, myalgia.
Respiratory: pulmonary infiltrates.
Skin: *erythema multiforme (Stevens-Johnson syndrome),* generalized skin eruptions, *epidermal necrolysis,* exfoliative dermatitis.
Other: *anaphylaxis.*

INTERACTIONS
Drug-drug. *Cyclosporine:* Increases metabolism of cyclosporine and may increase the risk of nephrotoxicity. Avoid using together.
Dapsone: Increases levels of both drugs. Use cautiously together.
Digoxin: Increases digoxin level and risk of toxicity. Monitor digoxin level.
Hydantoins such as phenytoin, methotrexate, oral antidiabetics, warfarin: Increases risk of toxic reaction caused by displacement from protein-binding sites, impaired metabolism, or decreased excretion. Monitor patient and appropriate blood levels closely.
Hormonal contraceptives: Decreases contraceptive effectiveness. Advise patient to use an additional nonhormonal contraceptive during therapy.

Zidovudine: Increases zidovudine level because of decreased renal clearance. Monitor patient closely.
Drug-herb. *Dong quai, St. John's wort:* May increase photosensitivity reactions. Advise patient to avoid excessive sunlight exposure.
Drug-lifestyle. *Sun exposure:* May cause photosensitivity reactions. Advise patient to avoid excessive sunlight exposure.

EFFECTS ON LAB TEST RESULTS
• May increase BUN, creatinine, aminotransferase, and bilirubin levels.
• May prolong PT, PTT, and INR. May decrease hemoglobin and granulocyte, platelet, and WBC counts.

ACTION
Sequentially inhibits enzymes of folic acid pathways and bacterial thymidine synthesis. Drug's spectrum of activity includes many gram-positive aerobic bacteria, including most strains of *Streptococcus pneumoniae,* many strains of *Staphylococcus aureus,* group A and beta-hemolytic streptococci, and *Nocardia.* Susceptible gram-negative aerobic bacteria include *Acinetobacter, Enterobacter, Escherichia coli, Klebsiella pneumoniae, Proteus mirabilis, Salmonella, Shigella, Haemophilus influenzae* including ampicillin-resistant strains, *H. ducreyi, Neisseria gonorrhoeae, Providencia, Serratia,* and many indole-positive strains of *Proteus.* Co-trimoxazole is also active against the protozoa *Pneumocystis carinii.*

PHARMACOKINETICS
Drug level peaks immediately after infusion; duration, 11 to 18 hours.
Distribution: Throughout body tissues and fluids, such as aqueous humor, middle ear fluid, prostatic fluid, bile, and CSF. Trimethoprim is 44% bound to protein; sulfamethoxazole, 70%

bound. Drug crosses the placental barrier and appears in breast milk.
Metabolism: In liver. Trimethoprim is metabolized to oxide and hydroxylated metabolites; sulfamethoxazole is acetylated and conjugated with glucuronic acid.
Excretion: In urine, through glomerular filtration and renal tubular secretion, and in small amounts in feces. About 50% to 60% of trimethoprim is excreted primarily unchanged in 24 hours; 45% to 70% of sulfamethoxazole is excreted within 24 hours.

In adults with normal renal function, trimethoprim has a half-life of 8 to 11 hours; sulfamethoxazole, 10 to 13 hours. Half-life may triple in patients with chronic renal failure. In children younger than age 10, half-life averages almost 7 hours.

CLINICAL CONSIDERATIONS
• Osmolality: sulfamethoxazole-trimethoprim in D_5W at concentrations of 4 + 0.8 mg/ml is 541 mOsm/kg; 5.5 + 1.1 mg/ml is 669 mOsm/kg; 8 + 1.6 mg/ml is 798 mOsm/kg; in normal saline solution at a concentration of 8 + 1.6 mg/ml is 833 mOsm/kg.
• Obtain specimens for culture and sensitivity tests before giving first dose. Therapy may begin before receiving results.
• Monitor BUN, creatinine, and electrolyte levels; CBC; platelet count; PTT; PT; and INR. Also, monitor results of urinalysis.
• Leucovorin can be given for bone marrow depression; folic acid supplements, for hematologic adverse effects.
• Closely monitor patients with AIDS because of increased risk of severe adverse reactions.
• Observe patient for superinfection with prolonged use.
• Dialysis partially removes trimethoprim and active sulfamethoxazole.
• *Alert:* Don't use drug in pregnant patients at full term.

PATIENT TEACHING
• Notify patient to report fever, sore throat, pallor, jaundice, or purpura.
• Advise patient to increase fluid intake to maintain hydration.
• Instruct patient to report any discomfort at the I.V. site.

cyclophosphamide
Cytoxan, Neosar, Procytox ◊

Pharmacologic class: alkylating drug (cell cycle–phase nonspecific)
Therapeutic class: antineoplastic
Pregnancy risk category: D
pH: 3 to 9 for reconstituted solutions

INDICATIONS & DOSAGES
➤ **Lymphomas; leukemia; small cell lung cancer ◆ ; cancer of the brain, breast, or reproductive organs; autoimmune diseases; prevention of graft-versus-host disease in organ transplants ◆** —
Adults: Initially, 40 to 50 mg/kg I.V. in divided doses over 2 to 5 days. Maintenance dosage is 10 to 15 mg/kg q 7 to 10 days or 3 to 5 mg/kg twice weekly.
Children: Initially, 2 to 8 mg/kg or 60 to 250 mg/m² I.V. daily depending on susceptibility of neoplasm. Maintenance dosage depends on patient tolerance and a WBC count of 2,500 to 4,000/mm³.

ADMINISTRATION
Direct injection: Using a 23G to 25G winged-tip needle, inject reconstituted drug directly into vein over 2 to 3 minutes.
Intermittent infusion: Using a 23G to 25G winged-tip needle, infuse diluted drug over 15 to 20 minutes.
Continuous infusion: Not recommended.

PREPARATION & STORAGE

To avoid mutagenic, teratogenic, and carcinogenic risks, use a biological containment cabinet, wear gloves and mask, and use syringes with tight luer-lock fittings to prevent leakage. Dispose of needles, syringes, vials, and unused drug correctly.

Available in 100-mg, 200-mg, 500-mg, 1-g, and 2-g vials.

Reconstitute with sterile water for injection or bacteriostatic water for injection (parabens-preserved only) to a concentration of 20 mg/ml. Powder contains enough saline solution to produce an isotonic solution. Shake vigorously.

Other compatible solutions include dextrose 5% in lactated Ringer's, dextrose 5% in normal saline solution, lactated Ringer's, half-normal or normal saline solution, and 1/6 M sodium lactate.

If prepared with sterile water for injection, use solution within 6 hours. Unreconstituted drug remains stable at room temperature; reconstituted drug remains stable for 24 hours if kept at room temperature and for 6 days if refrigerated. Discard any unused drug after 24 hours.

Incompatibilities
None known.

CONTRAINDICATIONS & CAUTIONS
• Contraindicated in those hypersensitive to the drug.
• Contraindicated in those with existing or recent chickenpox or herpes zoster and in those with severe leukopenia or thrombocytopenia because of increased risk of generalized infection.
• Use cautiously in those with bone marrow depression, tumor infiltration of bone marrow, prior therapy with radiation or other cytotoxic drugs, or impaired hepatic or renal function because of an increased risk of toxic reaction.
• Use cautiously in those with renal or hepatic impairment or a history of gout or urate renal stones because of the risk of hyperuricemia.

ADVERSE REACTIONS
CNS: fainting.
CV: facial flushing, *cardiotoxicity (with very high doses and with doxorubicin).*
GI: *nausea, vomiting,* abdominal discomfort or pain, anorexia, stomatitis.
GU: hematuria, *hemorrhagic cystitis,* amenorrhea.
Hematologic: *leukopenia, thrombocytopenia,* hypoprothrombinemia, hyperuricemia.
Respiratory: *interstitial pulmonary fibrosis.*
Skin: skin pigmentation, *alopecia.*
Other: *hypersensitivity reactions.*

INTERACTIONS
Drug-drug. *Allopurinol:* Increases myelosuppression. Monitor patient for toxicity.
Barbiturates, hepatic enzyme inducers: Increases cyclophosphamide toxicity. Monitor patient closely.
Anticoagulants (oral), aspirin: Increases risk of bleeding. Avoid using together.
Cardiotoxic drugs, myelosuppressives, thiazide diuretics: Increases toxic effects. Monitor patient closely.
Digoxin: May decrease digoxin level. Monitor digoxin level closely.
Immunosuppressants: Increases risk of infection and neoplasms. Monitor patient closely.
Succinylcholine: Prolongs neuromuscular blockade. Avoid using together.

EFFECTS ON LAB TEST RESULTS
• May increase uric acid level. May decrease pseudocholinesterase level.
• May decrease hemoglobin and WBC, RBC, and platelet counts.
• May suppress positive reaction to *Candida,* mumps, *Trichophyton,* and

tuberculin skin test. May cause false-positive result for the Papanicolaou test.

ACTION
Prevents cell division by cross-linking DNA strands or by breaking the DNA molecule itself, thereby interfering with DNA replication and RNA transcription. It also inhibits protein synthesis and acts as a potent immunosuppressant.

PHARMACOKINETICS
Drug level peaks at 2 to 3 hours; duration, 72 hours.
Distribution: Throughout body tissues, with 10% to 50% of alkylating metabolites, but not parent drug, bound to protein. Drug crosses the blood-brain barrier, probably crosses the placental barrier, and appears in CSF and breast milk.
Metabolism: Primarily in liver to active metabolites.
Excretion: In urine, with 5% to 30% excreted unchanged and the rest removed as metabolites; 36% to 99% is excreted in 48 hours.

CLINICAL CONSIDERATIONS
• Osmolality: 352 mOsm/kg for 20 mg/ml for dilutions of saline-containing products; 172 mOsm/kg for 20 mg/ml and 219 mOsm/kg for 25 mg/ml dilutions of lyophilized product.
• *Alert:* Don't confuse cyclophosphamide with ifosfamide.
• Use a new site for each injection or infusion. Heparin or saline locks aren't recommended.
• Infuse slowly to prevent facial flushing.
• High I.V. dose may cause SIADH leading to hyponatremia.
• Drug is sometimes given with mesna, a bladder protectant.
• Monitor CBC, kidney and liver function, and uric acid levels.

• Watch for infection in patients with leukopenia.
• Alkalizing urine, providing good hydration, and giving allopurinol may prevent or minimize hyperuricemia.
• If symptoms of cystitis, such as hematuria and painful urination occur, stop drug immediately.
• If infection occurs, give antibiotics; consider reduced dosage of cyclophosphamide.
• *Alert:* Impaired renal function may preclude high-dose I.V. cyclophosphamide therapy in some chemotherapy protocols; check treatment protocols for details.
• Treat overdose supportively. Dialysis removes drug.

PATIENT TEACHING
• To avoid hemorrhagic cystitis, encourage patient to void q 1 to 2 hours while awake and to drink plenty of fluids before, during, and for 72 hours after treatment.
• Advise patient to watch for signs and symptoms of infection, such as fever, chills, sore throat, and fatigue, and of bleeding, such as easy bruising, bleeding gums, nosebleeds, and melena. Tell patient to take temperature daily.
• Instruct patient to avoid OTC drugs that contain aspirin.
• Advise men and women to practice contraception while taking the drug and for 4 months after because drug is potentially teratogenic.
• Advise women to avoid breast-feeding because of possibility of infant toxicity.
• Drug can cause irreversible toxicity in men and women. Counsel patient of childbearing age before initiating therapy. Also, recommend that patient consult with prescriber before becoming pregnant.
• Inform patient that reversible alopecia is common, usually beginning 3 weeks after initiation of therapy.

Reactions may be *common*, uncommon, *life-threatening*, or COMMON AND LIFE-THREATENING.

• Notify patient that amenorrhea is common and menses will resume a few months after therapy is completed.
• Notify patient of possible interference with wound healing.

cyclosporine
Sandimmune

Pharmacologic class: polypeptide antibiotic
Therapeutic class: immunosuppressant
Pregnancy risk category: C

INDICATIONS & DOSAGES
➤ **To prevent organ tissue rejection—**
Adults and children: 5 to 6 mg/kg I.V. daily, beginning 4 to 12 hours before surgery and continuing after surgery until patient can tolerate oral form. Adjust dose to maintain plasma trough level of 100 to 300 ng/ml.

ADMINISTRATION
Direct injection: Not recommended.
Intermittent infusion: Not recommended.
Continuous infusion: Infuse diluted drug slowly over 2 to 6 hours or up to 24 hours. Significant amounts of drug are lost when given through polyvinyl chloride tubing.

PREPARATION & STORAGE
Available in 5-ml ampules containing a concentration of 50 mg/ml.
For infusion, dilute each milliliter of drug in 20 to 100 ml of normal saline solution or D_5W.
Reconstituted solutions remain stable for up to 24 hours in D_5W injection and for 6 to 12 hours in normal saline injection—6 hours in polyvinyl chloride containers and 12 hours in glass containers. Store below 104° F (40° C), preferably at 59° to 86° F (15° to 30° C). Don't freeze or expose to light.

Incompatibilities
None reported.

CONTRAINDICATIONS & CAUTIONS
• Contraindicated in those hypersensitive to the drug or the diluent, polyoxyl 35 castor oil.
• Contraindicated in those with existing or recent chickenpox or herpes zoster infection because of an increased risk of generalized disease.
• Use cautiously in those with hyperkalemia or infection because drug may worsen these conditions.
• Use cautiously in those with hepatic or renal impairment because of an increased risk of toxic reaction.

ADVERSE REACTIONS
CNS: *tremors, headache,* paresthesia, ***seizures.***
CV: *hypertension,* flushing.
EENT: sinusitis.
GI: diarrhea, nausea, vomiting, *gingival hyperplasia.*
GU: ***nephrotoxicity.***
Hematologic: ***leukopenia, thrombocytopenia,*** hyperuricemia.
Hepatic: ***hepatotoxicity.***
Metabolic: hyperkalemia, hypomagnesemia.
Skin: *hirsutism,* acne.
Other: bacterial and fungal infections, gynecomastia.

INTERACTIONS
Drug-drug. *ACE inhibitors, banked blood, potassium-containing products, potassium-sparing diuretics:* Increases risk of hyperkalemia. Monitor potassium level closely.
Allopurinol, amiodarone, antifungals, calcium channel blockers, clarithromycin, colchicine, erythromycin, methylprednisolone, protease inhibi-

tors: Increases cyclosporine level. Use cautiously together and monitor cyclosporine level.

Amphotericin B, cimetidine, gentamicin, ketoconazole, melphalan, NSAIDs, ranitidine, tacrolimus, tobramycin, vancomycin: Increases risk of nephrotoxicity. Avoid using together.

Carbamazepine, nafcillin, octreotide, phenobarbital, phenytoin, rifabutin, rifampin, ticlopidine: Decreases cyclosporine level. Use cautiously together and monitor cyclosporine level.

Digoxin, lovastatin, prednisolone: Reduces clearance of these drugs. Monitor patient closely.

Live vaccines: Vaccination may be less effective. Avoid vaccination if possible.

Drug-herb. *St. John's wort:* Decreases cyclosporine level, possibly causing organ rejection. Warn patient against using together.

Drug-food. *Grapefruit juice:* Slows drug metabolism. Avoid using together.

EFFECTS ON LAB TEST RESULTS
● May increase BUN, creatinine, low-density lipoprotein, bilirubin, AST, ALT, alkaline phosphatase, uric acid, potassium, and glucose levels. May decrease magnesium level.
● May decrease hemoglobin and WBC and platelet counts.

ACTION
Inhibits interleukin-1 and interleukin-2, which play a major role in cell-mediated and humoral immunity.

PHARMACOKINETICS
Drug level peaks at end of infusion.
Distribution: Throughout fluids and tissues, with about 90% bound to protein. Distribution in blood depends on dose; with high drug concentrations, WBCs and RBCs become saturated. Drug crosses the placental barrier and appears in breast milk.
Metabolism: Extensively, in liver.

Excretion: Eliminated primarily in bile, 6% in urine; only 0.1% excreted unchanged. Drug has a biphasic half-life: initial phase, about 70 minutes; terminal phase, 8 to 27 hours.

CLINICAL CONSIDERATIONS
● Drug should always be used with a corticosteroid.
● *Alert:* I.V. administration may cause anaphylaxis, so give only to patients who can't tolerate oral dose.
● *Alert:* Monitor patient continuously for the first 30 minutes and then at frequent intervals because of risk of anaphylaxis. Keep resuscitation equipment nearby.
● Monitor patient for signs and symptoms of infections or other complications of immunosuppression.
● Monitor blood pressure, CBC, uric acid, potassium, lipid, and magnesium levels.
● If infusing drug during home care, protect solution from light.
● Monitor liver and renal function test results routinely.
● Monitor blood pressure; hypertension can develop within a few weeks after therapy is initiated.

PATIENT TEACHING
● Advise patient that hirsutism usually develops within 2 to 4 weeks and may be improved by decreasing the dosage of cyclosporine.
● Inform patient that careful oral hygiene before and after transplantation reduces risk of gingival hyperplasia.
● Tell patient that if he develops gingival hyperplasia, it should resolve 1 to 2 months after drug therapy is stopped.

---

cytarabine (arabinoside, Ara-C, cytarabine arabinoside)
Cytosar ◇ *, Cytosar-U*

Pharmacologic class: antimetabolite (S-phase specific)
Therapeutic class: antineoplastic
Pregnancy risk category: D
pH: 4 to 6

INDICATIONS & DOSAGES
➤ **To induce remission in acute myelogenous or lymphocytic leukemia—**
Adults and children: As a single agent, 200 mg/m² I.V. daily for 5 days by continuous infusion, then 2 weeks off the drug. As combination therapy, 2 to 6 mg/kg daily or 100 to 200 mg/m² daily by continuous I.V. infusion or in two to three divided doses by rapid I.V. injection or infusion, for 5 to 10 days in a course of therapy or daily until remission is attained.

Maintenance dosage, 70 to 200 mg/m² by rapid I.V. injection or continuous infusion daily for 2 to 5 days at monthly intervals. Dosage varies, depending on regimen.
➤ **Refractory leukemia or refractory non-Hodgkin's lymphoma ♦—**
Adults: 3 g/m² I.V. infusion over 1 to 3 hours q 12 hours for up to 12 doses.

ADMINISTRATION
Direct injection: Give directly into vein or through a winged-tip needle, an intermittent infusion device, or an I.V. line containing a free-flowing, compatible solution.
Intermittent infusion: Infuse diluted solution over 1 hour or as ordered.
Continuous infusion: Infuse diluted solution over ordered duration, usually 5 days.

PREPARATION & STORAGE
To avoid mutagenic, teratogenic, and carcinogenic risks, use a biological containment cabinet, wear gloves and mask, and use syringes with luer-lock tight fittings to prevent drug leakage. Dispose of needles, syringes, vials, and unused drug correctly.

Drug is available in 100-mg, 500-mg, 1-g, and 2-g vials. Reconstitute 100-mg vial with 5 ml of bacteriostatic water for injection with benzyl alcohol for a concentration of 20 mg/ml. Reconstitute 500-mg vial with 10 ml of bacteriostatic water for injection with benzyl alcohol for a concentration of 50 mg/ml. Reconstitute 1-g vial with 10 ml of bacteriostatic water for injection with benzyl alcohol for a concentration of 100 mg/ml. Reconstitute 2-g vial with 20 ml of bacteriostatic water for injection with benzyl alcohol for a concentration of 100 mg/ml. Don't use benzyl alcohol as a diluent when preparing high-dose cytarabine. Reconstituted solution remains stable for 48 hours at room temperature. Discard if cloudy.

For infusion, dilute with D_5W or with normal saline solution; solution stays stable for 8 days at room temperature. Other compatible solutions include dextrose 5% in normal saline solution and dextrose 5% in lactated Ringer's.

Incompatibilities
Allopurinol sodium, fluorouracil, ganciclovir sodium, heparin sodium, insulin (regular), methylprednisolone sodium succinate, nafcillin, oxacillin, penicillin.

CONTRAINDICATIONS & CAUTIONS
• Contraindicated in those hypersensitive to the drug.
• Contraindicated in those with existing or recent chickenpox or herpes zoster infection because of an increased risk of generalized disease.

• Use cautiously in those with preexisting myelosuppression because the drug exacerbates this condition.
• Use cautiously in those with hepatic impairment because the liver detoxifies much of the dose and in those with renal impairment because drug excretion is reduced.
• Use cautiously in those with history of gout or urate renal calculi because of increased risk of hyperuricemia.

ADVERSE REACTIONS

CNS: dizziness, *fever,* abnormal gait, confusion, somnolence, *headache, asthenia, pain.*
CV: chest pain, thrombophlebitis, *peripheral edema.*
GI: diarrhea, *nausea, vomiting,* anorexia, oral and anal ulcers, *constipation.*
GU: urine retention, *urinary incontinence.*
Hematologic: THROMBOCYTOPENIA, *anemia,* bleeding, NEUTROPENIA.
Hepatic: *hepatic dysfunction.*
Skin: alopecia, freckling, rash; cellulitis at infusion site.

INTERACTIONS

Drug-drug. *Aminoglycosides:* May alter antibacterial effects. Monitor aminoglycoside level.
Digoxin: Decreases absorption of oral digoxin. Monitor patient and digoxin level closely.
Myelosuppressants: Increases toxic effects. Monitor patient closely.

EFFECTS ON LAB TEST RESULTS

• May increase potassium, phosphorus, bilirubin, AST, ALT, alkaline phosphatase, and uric acid levels.
• May increase megaloblast count. May decrease hemoglobin and WBC, RBC, platelet, and reticulocyte counts.

ACTION

Interferes with DNA synthesis by blocking conversion of cytidine to de-oxycytidine. Affects rapidly dividing cells in S phase. Also suppresses humoral or cell-mediated immune responses. May have antiviral properties.

PHARMACOKINETICS

Drug level peaks immediately after infusion.
Distribution: Rapidly and widely dispersed throughout body tissues, with high levels in GI mucosa and liver. Drug crosses the blood-brain and placental barriers. It's unknown if drug appears in breast milk. Protein binding is low.
Metabolism: Rapidly and extensively changed in liver; also metabolized in kidneys, GI mucosa, granulocytes, and other tissues.
Excretion: 70% to 80% of dose excreted in urine within 24 hours, with about 90% removed as inactive metabolites and 10% as unchanged drug. Drug's biphasic half-life has an initial phase of 10 minutes; terminal phase, 1 to 3 hours.

CLINICAL CONSIDERATIONS

• Osmolality: 150 mOsm/kg for 20 mg/ml in sterile water.
• *Alert:* When giving high-dose cytarabine, perform a thorough neurologic assessment before every dose. Check for nystagmus, ataxia, dysarthria, memory loss, weakness, and vertigo. Note whether patient has an abnormal gait or a weak grasp. Afterward, observe for signs and symptoms of toxic reaction, and ask family members to help.
• Many prescribers order prophylactic ophthalmic corticosteroid solutions and pyridoxine, 100 mg daily, for patients receiving high-dose therapy.
• *Alert:* If patient experiences a toxic reaction, don't give next dose of cytarabine. Notify prescriber. The drug may be withheld for 24 hours if just one sign is present; with multiple signs, the

drug may be stopped because high doses can cause permanent brain damage.
• Monitor kidney and liver function and WBC and platelet counts.
• Watch for signs and symptoms of infection.
• Initial WBC nadir occurs at 7 to 9 days, with level briefly rising at about 12 days; second nadir occurs at 15 to 24 days, with level rapidly rising above baseline in next 10 days. Platelet count declines at 5 days, with a nadir at 12 to 15 days; levels rise above baseline in the next 10 days.
• Treat skin reactions resulting from high-dose cytarabine with drugs used in burn therapy. Reactions most commonly affect the palms, soles, and extensor surfaces.
• If patient develops diarrhea, give meticulous skin care to avoid or treat perirectal abscess. Watch for electrolyte imbalance, malabsorption, and pressure ulcers.
• Treat nausea and vomiting with antiemetics.
• Prevent or minimize uric acid nephropathy by providing good hydration, alkalizing urine, or giving allopurinol.

PATIENT TEACHING

• Tell patient to report to prescriber fever, sore throat, or unusual bleeding or bruising.
• Encourage adequate fluid intake to facilitate urinary excretion of uric acid.
• Advise women of childbearing age to avoid becoming pregnant during treatment.
• Advise women to avoid breast-feeding because of possible infant toxicity.

cytomegalovirus immune globulin intravenous, human (CMV-IGIV)
CytoGam

Pharmacologic class: immune globulin
Therapeutic class: immune serum
Pregnancy risk category: C

INDICATIONS & DOSAGES

➤ **To attenuate primary CMV disease in seronegative kidney transplant recipients who have a CMV-seropositive donor—**
Adults: Within 72 hours of transplant, give 150 mg/kg I.V. Additional 100-mg/kg dosages should be given once every 2 weeks, at 2, 4, 6, and 8 weeks after transplant. Then, give 50 mg/kg at 12 and 16 weeks after transplant. Maximum dose per infusion is 150 mg/kg.
➤ **To prevent CMV disease linked to lung, liver, pancreas, and heart transplants—**
Adults: Within 72 hours of transplant, give 150 mg/kg I.V. Additional 150-mg/kg doses should be given once every 2 weeks at 2, 4, 6 and 8 weeks after transplant. Then, give 100 mg/kg at 12 and 16 weeks after transplant. Maximum dose per infusion is 150 mg/kg.

ADMINISTRATION

Direct injection: Not recommended.
Intermittent infusion: Give initial dose at 15 mg/kg/hour. Increase to 30 mg/kg/hour after 30 minutes if no adverse reactions occur, then increase to 60 mg/kg/hour after another 30 minutes if no adverse reactions occur. Rate shouldn't exceed 75 ml/hour. Subsequent doses may be given at 15 mg/kg/hour for 15 minutes, increasing at 15-minute intervals in a stepwise fashion to 60 mg/kg/hour.

Give through a separate I.V. line with an in-line filter using a continuous infusion pump. When this is impossible, piggyback into preexisting line of normal saline injection, dextrose 2.5% in water, D₅W, dextrose 10% in water, or dextrose 20% in water. Dextrose solutions may or may not have saline added. Don't dilute more than 1:2 with any of the above solutions.

Continuous infusion: Not recommended.

PREPARATION & STORAGE

Available in a single-dose vial containing about 2,500 mg of lyophilized immunoglobulin.

To prepare, remove tab and swab rubber stopper with 70% alcohol or equivalent. Reconstitute with 50 ml sterile water for injection. Final concentration is about 50 mg/ml. Don't shake; avoid foaming. Use a double-ended transfer needle or large syringe to add diluent. If using a double-ended transfer needle, first insert one end into the vial of water because the lyophilized powder is in an evacuated vial and the water will transfer by suction. After the water is transferred, release any residual vacuum to hasten dissolving process.

Gently rotate the container to wet any undissolved powder. Allow 30 minutes for dissolution to occur. Reconstituted solution should appear colorless and translucent. Further dilution isn't recommended. Infusions should begin within 6 hours of reconstitution and end within 12 hours.

Store in refrigerator at 36° to 46° F (2° to 8° C). Don't store reconstituted drug.

Incompatibilities

Other I.V. drugs.

CONTRAINDICATIONS & CAUTIONS

● Contraindicated in those with a history of severe reaction resulting from this or other human immunoglobulin preparations.

● Anaphylactic reactions may result if given to those with selective immunoglobulin A deficiency who may have developed antibodies to immunoglobulin A. Epinephrine should be available for the treatment of acute anaphylaxis.

ADVERSE REACTIONS

CNS: fever.
CV: hypotension, flushing.
GI: nausea, vomiting.
Musculoskeletal: back pain, muscle cramps.
Respiratory: wheezing.
Other: *anaphylaxis,* chills.

INTERACTIONS

Drug-drug. *Vaccines with live virus:* May interfere with the immune response to live-virus vaccines. Postpone vaccination for at least 3 months.

EFFECTS ON LAB TEST RESULTS

None reported.

ACTION

Provides passive immunity by supplying a relatively high level of immunoglobulin G antibodies against CMV. Increasing these antibody levels in CMV-exposed patients may attenuate or reduce the risk of CMV disease.

PHARMACOKINETICS

Rapidly available after infusion.
Distribution: Unknown; other immune globulins distribute between intravascular and extravascular spaces.
Metabolism: Unknown.
Excretion: Unknown.

CLINICAL CONSIDERATIONS

● Monitor vital signs before infusion, midway through infusion, after infusion, and before any increase in infusion rate.

● Adverse reactions are usually related to rate of administration. Slow or stop

infusion if minor adverse reactions occur.

• Monitor patient for hypersensitivity
reactions, drop in blood pressure, and
aseptic meningitis (characterized by severe headache, nuchal rigidity, drowsiness, lethargy, fever, photophobia,
painful eye movements, nausea and
vomiting). Rule out other causes of
meningitis by neurologic examination
and CSF analysis.

PATIENT TEACHING

• Instruct patient to defer live-virus
vaccinations for at least 3 months after
administration.

• Review drug therapy regimen with
patient and stress importance of follow-
up visits.

• Tell patient to immediately report adverse reactions to prescriber.

D

dacarbazine
DTIC ◇, DTIC-Dome

Pharmacologic class: alkylating
drug (cell cycle–phase nonspecific)
Therapeutic class: antineoplastic
Pregnancy risk category: C
pH: 3 to 4

INDICATIONS & DOSAGES
➤ **Metastatic malignant melanoma—**
Adults: 2 to 4.5 mg/kg/day I.V. for 10
days, repeated q 4 weeks; or 250 mg/
m^2/day for 5 days, repeated q 3 weeks.
➤ **Hodgkin's disease as second-line
therapy—**
Adults: 150 mg/m^2/day I.V. for 5 days
combined with other drugs, repeated q
4 weeks; or 375 mg/m^2 on day 1 combined with other drugs, repeated q
15 days.
Adjust-a-dose: Hematopoietic toxicity
(leukocyte count less than 3,000/mm^3
and platelet count less than 100,000/
mm^3) may require stopping therapy.

ADMINISTRATION
Direct injection: Using a 21G or 23G
needle, inject drug directly into vein or
through an intermittent infusion device
over 1 minute. Apply hot packs to injection site to alleviate pain or burning.
Intermittent infusion: Using a 21G or
23G needle, infuse diluted drug over
15 to 30 minutes.
Continuous infusion: Not recommended.

PREPARATION & STORAGE
Use caution when preparing drug to
avoid mutagenic, teratogenic, and carcinogenic risks. Use a biological containment cabinet and wear gloves and
mask. Use syringes with tight luer-
locks to prevent drug leakage, and dispose of needles, syringes, vials, and
unused drug correctly. Avoid contaminating work surfaces.
   Drug comes as a powder in 100-mg
and 200-mg vials.
   Reconstitute by adding 9.9 ml of sterile water to 100-mg vial or 19.7 ml of
sterile water to 200-mg vial. Dilute further for infusion by mixing reconstituted
solution with 250 ml of either D$_5$W or
normal saline solution for infusion.
   Refrigerate vials at 36° to 46° F (2°
to 8° C) and protect from light. Reconstituted drug remains stable for 8 hours
if kept at room temperature and for up
to 72 hours if refrigerated. Diluted solutions remain stable for 8 hours at
room temperature and for up to 24
hours if refrigerated. Protect drug from
light during infusion. If solution turns
pink, it has decomposed.

Incompatibilities
Allopurinol sodium, cefepime, hydrocortisone sodium succinate, piperacillin with tazobactam.

CONTRAINDICATIONS & CAUTIONS
• Contraindicated in those hypersensitive to the drug.
• Contraindicated in those with recent
or existing chickenpox or herpes zoster
infection because of increased risk of
generalized disease.
• Use cautiously in those with myelosuppression or hepatic or renal impairment.

ADVERSE REACTIONS
CNS: confusion, headache, paresthesia, fever, *seizures.*
CV: facial flushing.
EENT: blurred vision.
GI: *anorexia, nausea, vomiting.*
Hematologic: *leukopenia, thrombocytopenia* usually 2 to 4 weeks after dose.
Hepatic: *hepatotoxicity.*
Metabolic: anorexia.
Musculoskeletal: myalgia.
Skin: photosensitivity, alopecia, tissue damage with extravasation, pain and burning at injection site.
Other: *anaphylaxis.*

INTERACTIONS
Drug-drug. *Bone marrow depressants:* Worsens myelosuppression. Monitor patient closely.
Drug-lifestyle. *Sun exposure:* May cause photosensitivity reactions, especially during first 2 days of therapy. Advise patient to avoid excessive sunlight exposure.

EFFECTS ON LAB TEST RESULTS
• May increase BUN and liver enzyme levels.
• May decrease WBC, RBC, and platelet counts.

ACTION
Acts as an alkylating drug; may inhibit DNA and RNA synthesis.

PHARMACOKINETICS
Level peaks immediately after I.V. administration.
Distribution: Localized in some body tissues, probably liver, and slightly bound to protein. Drug enters CSF, reaching about 14% of serum level. Unknown if drug crosses the placental barrier or appears in breast milk.
Metabolism: Extensively metabolized in the liver.
Excretion: In urine by renal tubular secretion, with 40% of drug and metabolites excreted in 6 hours. Biphasic half-life, 19 minutes for initial phase; 5 hours for terminal phase. In renal and hepatic dysfunction, initial phase increased to 55 minutes and terminal phase increased to 7.2 hours.

CLINICAL CONSIDERATIONS
• Osmolality: 10 mg/ml in sterile water is 109 mOsm/kg.
• *Alert:* Don't confuse dacarbazine with procarbazine. Drug is commonly used with other antineoplastics.
• Giving antiemetics before giving dacarbazine may help decrease nausea. Nausea and vomiting may subside after several doses.
• Some prescribers recommend that patient be well hydrated 1 hour before receiving drug.
• When possible, give by infusion; injection can be painful.
• Restrict patient's food and fluids 4 to 6 hours before giving drug to help reduce nausea and vomiting.
• Avoid extravasation. If it occurs, stop drug and give at another site. Apply ice to area for 24 to 48 hours.
• Monitor hematologic status carefully. WBC nadir is 21 to 25 days; platelet nadir, 16 days. Recovery usually occurs in 3 to 5 days.
• Monitor kidney and liver function carefully; dysfunction can delay drug excretion. Avoid I.M. injections when platelet counts are below 100,000/mm^3.
• Monitor daily temperature. Observe patient for signs and symptoms of infection.

PATIENT TEACHING
• Advise ambulatory patient to avoid sunlight and sunlamps for first 2 days of therapy.
• Advise patient to avoid contact with persons with infections.
• Instruct patient to watch for signs and symptoms of infection, such as fever, sore throat, and fatigue, and of bleeding, such as easy bruising, nosebleeds,

bleeding gums, and melena. Tell him to take his temperature daily.
• Reassure patient that hair growth should resume 4 to 8 weeks after treatment has ended, but hair is usually of a different texture and color.
• Inform patient that flu syndrome may be treated with acetaminophen.

daclizumab
Zenapax

Pharmacologic class: humanized immunoglobulin G1 monoclonal antibody
Therapeutic class: transplant immunosuppressant
Pregnancy risk category: C
pH: 6.9

INDICATIONS & DOSAGES
➤ **To prevent acute organ rejection in patients receiving renal transplants (combined with an immunosuppressive regimen that includes cyclosporine and corticosteroids)—**
Adults: 1 mg/kg I.V. for five doses. Give first dose no more than 24 hours before transplantation; remaining four doses are given at 14-day intervals.

ADMINISTRATION
Direct injection: Don't use drug as direct I.V. injection. Dilute before administration.
Intermittent infusion: Give over 15 minutes via a central or peripheral line.
Continuous infusion: Not recommended.

PREPARATION & STORAGE
Supplied as 25 mg/5 ml concentrate in single-use vials.
Dilute in 50 ml of sterile normal saline solution before administration. To avoid foaming, don't shake. Inspect for particulate matter or discoloration

before use. If particulate matter or discoloration is apparent, don't use.
Drug may be refrigerated at 36° to 46° F (2° to 8° C) for 24 hours and is stable at room temperature for 4 hours. Discard solution if not used within 24 hours. Protect undiluted solution from direct light.

Incompatibilities
Other drugs infused simultaneously through same I.V. line.

CONTRAINDICATIONS & CAUTIONS
• Contraindicated in patients hypersensitive to drug or its components.

ADVERSE REACTIONS
CNS: tremor, headache, dizziness, insomnia, generalized weakness, prickly sensation, fatigue, depression, anxiety, fever, pain.
CV: tachycardia, hypertension, hypotension, edema, fluid overload, chest pain, peripheral edema.
EENT: blurred vision, pharyngitis, rhinitis.
GI: constipation, nausea, diarrhea, vomiting, abdominal pain, dyspepsia, pyrosis, abdominal distention, epigastric pain, flatulence, gastritis, hemorrhoids.
GU: *oliguria,* dysuria, *renal tubular necrosis, renal damage,* urine retention, hydronephrosis, urinary tract bleeding, urinary tract disorder, renal insufficiency.
Hematologic: lymphocele; platelet, bleeding, and clotting disorders.
Metabolic: diabetes mellitus, dehydration, hyperglycemia.
Musculoskeletal: musculoskeletal or back pain, arthralgia, myalgia, leg cramps.
Respiratory: dyspnea, coughing, atelectasis, congestion, *hypoxia,* crackles, abnormal breath sounds, pleural effusion, *pulmonary edema.*
Skin: acne, impaired wound healing without infection, pruritus, hirsutism, rash, night sweats, increased sweating.
Other: shivering.

Reactions may be *common*, uncommon, *life-threatening*, or COMMON AND LIFE-THREATENING.

INTERACTIONS
None reported.

EFFECTS ON LAB TEST RESULTS
• May increase glucose levels.

ACTION
An interleukin (IL)-2 receptor antagonist that inhibits IL-2 binding to prevent IL-2-mediated activation of lymphocytes, a critical pathway in the cellular immune response against allografts. Once in circulation, daclizumab impairs the immune system's response to antigenic challenges.

PHARMACOKINETICS
Onset, peak, and duration of drug effects unknown.
Distribution: Not reported.
Metabolism: Not reported.
Excretion: Estimated elimination half-life is 20 days.

CLINICAL CONSIDERATIONS
• Use cautiously and only under supervision of a prescriber experienced in immunosuppressive therapy and management of organ transplantation.
• Drug is used as part of an immunosuppressive regimen that includes corticosteroids and cyclosporine.
• *Alert:* Anaphylactoid reactions have been reported after the administration of proteins. Drugs used in the treatment of anaphylactic reactions should be immediately available.
• Monitor for lipoproliferative disorders and opportunistic infections.

PATIENT TEACHING
• Tell patient to consult prescriber before taking other drugs during therapy.
• Advise patient to take steps to prevent infection.
• Inform patient that neither he nor any household member should receive vaccinations unless medically approved.

• Tell patient to report immediately wounds that fail to heal, unusual bruising or bleeding, or fever.
• Advise patient to drink plenty of fluids during drug therapy, and report painful urination, blood in the urine, or decrease in urine amount.
• Instruct women of childbearing age to use effective contraception before beginning therapy and to continue it until 4 months after completing therapy.

dactinomycin
(actinomycin D, ACT)
Cosmegen

Pharmacologic class: antibiotic antineoplastic (cell cycle–phase nonspecific)
Therapeutic class: antineoplastic
Pregnancy risk category: D
pH: 5.5 to 7 for reconstituted solution

INDICATIONS & DOSAGES
➤ **Choriocarcinoma, Ewing's sarcoma, rhabdomyosarcoma, testicular cancer, Wilms' tumor—**
Adults: 500 mcg/day I.V. for maximum of 5 days.
Children older than age 6 months: 15 mcg/kg/day I.V. for 5 days or total dose of 2.5 mg/m^2 over 1 week. Both adults and children may have a second course after 3 weeks if toxic effects have subsided.

ADMINISTRATION
Direct injection: Inject 500 mcg over a few minutes, preferably through a side port in an I.V. line containing free-flowing D$_5$W or normal saline solution. Assess vein patency frequently. After injection, run the I.V. solution for 2 to 5 minutes or inject 5 to 10 ml of I.V. solution through tubing to remove residual drug. Use of some in-line cellulose es-

ter filters may partially remove active drug from the I.V. solution.
Intermittent infusion: Infuse diluted dose over 10 to 15 minutes into tubing of a free-flowing I.V. solution.
Continuous infusion: Not recommended.

PREPARATION & STORAGE
Because of mutagenic, teratogenic, and carcinogenic risks, use a biological containment cabinet during drug preparation. Wear gloves and mask, use syringes with tight luer-lock fittings to prevent drug leakage, and avoid contamination of work surface. Properly dispose of needles, syringes, vials, and unused drug.

Supplied as powder for injection.

To prepare drug, reconstitute each 500-mcg vial with 1.1 ml of sterile water without preservative to yield 0.5 mg/ml; use 2.2 ml to yield 0.25 mg/ml. For infusion, dilute the clear, gold-colored reconstituted drug with D_5W or normal saline solution. Product doesn't contain any preservative; discard unused portion of reconstituted solution. Store intact vials below 85° F (29° C).

Incompatibilities
Diluents containing preservatives, filgrastim.

CONTRAINDICATIONS & CAUTIONS
• Contraindicated in those with recent or active chickenpox or herpes zoster infection because of risk of generalized disease and in children ages 6 months and younger because of increased risk of toxic reaction.
• Use cautiously in those with gout or history of urate renal calculi because of risk of hyperuricemia and in those with myelosuppression because of increased risk of toxic reaction.

ADVERSE REACTIONS
CNS: fatigue, fever, malaise, lethargy.
GI: abdominal pain, anorexia, diarrhea, ulcers, *nausea, vomiting,* ulcerative stomatitis, dysphagia, esophagitis, glossitis.
GU: *proctitis.*
Hematologic: *pancytopenia,* anemia.
Hepatic: *hepatitis,* veno-occlusive disease, hepatomegaly.
Metabolic: hypocalcemia, hyperuricemia.
Musculoskeletal: myalgia.
Skin: cheilosis, hyperpigmentation of previously irradiated skin, *maculopapular rash,* alopecia, pruritus, injection site pain, erythema.
Other: *anaphylaxis.*

INTERACTIONS
Drug-drug. *Bone marrow depressants:* Worsens myelosuppression. Monitor patient closely.

EFFECTS ON LAB TEST RESULTS
• May increase uric acid level. May decrease calcium level.
• May decrease WBCs, RBCs, granulocytes, platelets, and hemoglobin.
• May alter liver function test results. May interfere with determination of antibiotic drug levels (peak and trough).

ACTION
Has cytotoxic action; forms a complex with DNA to inhibit RNA synthesis. Greatest activity apparently occurs in phase G_1. Drug may also have immunosuppressive and hypocalcemic properties.

PHARMACOKINETICS
Drug level peaks immediately after infusion.
Distribution: Rapidly distributed into tissues, with high levels in bone marrow and nucleated cells. Drug penetrates CSF poorly but apparently crosses placental barrier. Tissue binding is extensive. Unknown if drug appears in breast milk.
Metabolism: Minimal.

Reactions may be *common,* uncommon, *life-threatening,* or **COMMON AND LIFE-THREATENING.**

Excretion: In bile and urine as unchanged drug. Half-life, 36 hours.

CLINICAL CONSIDERATIONS
● Osmolality: 0.5 mg/ml in sterile water is 189 mOsm/kg.
● Give antiemetics before giving drug.
● Dosage varies, depending on patient tolerance, size and location of tumor, and use of other treatments; in obese or geriatric patients, base dosage on body surface area.
● Monitor CBC and platelet count. Severe hematologic toxicity may require supportive measures, antibiotics for secondary infections, and blood transfusions.
● Monitor renal and hepatic function.
● Drug may potentiate radiation therapy effects. Identify and monitor previously irradiated skin for radiation recall, a flare-up of skin irritation, or necrosis.
● Monitor patient for extravasation, which can produce necrosis, cellulitis, phlebitis, and possible muscle contracture. Drug is a vesicant; the longer the duration of the infusion, the higher the risk of extravasation.
● If extravasation occurs, stop infusion and aspirate as much drug as possible. Infiltrate area with 4 ml of isotonic sodium thiosulfate (1 g/10 ml) diluted with 6 ml of sterile water for injection, 50 to 100 mg of hydrocortisone sodium succinate, or ascorbic acid injection. Cover with sterile gauze and apply cold compresses.
● Alkalinizing urine or giving allopurinol may prevent or minimize uric acid nephropathy.
● Drug may be stopped if stomatitis or diarrhea occurs in patients also receiving other antineoplastics.

PATIENT TEACHING
● Encourage patient to maintain adequate hydration.
● Teach and encourage good oral hygiene to reduce risk of stomatitis.

● Warn patient that alopecia may occur but that it's usually reversible.
● Tell patient to watch for signs and symptoms of infection, such as fever, sore throat, and fatigue, and of bleeding, such as easy bruising, nosebleeds, bleeding gums, and melena. Tell him to take his temperature daily and to avoid exposure to others with infection.
● Tell patient who received a course of radiation therapy that he may experience a "radiation recall effect" in the prior treatment field.

dantrolene sodium
Dantrium Intravenous

Pharmacologic class: hydantoin derivative
Therapeutic class: skeletal muscle relaxant
Pregnancy risk category: C
pH: about 9.5 when reconstituted in 60 mg of sterile water

INDICATIONS & DOSAGES
➤ **To prevent malignant hyperthermia crisis in susceptible patients undergoing surgery—**
Adults: 2.5 mg/kg I.V. given over 1 hour, about 1¼ hours before anesthesia.
➤ **Adjunctive treatment of malignant hyperthermia crisis—**
Adults and children: Minimum dose 1 mg/kg I.V. initially; repeat until symptoms subside, or to a maximum total dose of 10 mg/kg. To prevent recurrence, infuse 1 mg/kg or more as clinically indicated for up to 3 days after malignant hyperthermic crisis.

ADMINISTRATION
Direct injection: Rapidly inject drug directly into vein or through an I.V. line containing a free-flowing, compatible solution.

Intermittent infusion: Not recommended.
Continuous infusion: Not recommended.

PREPARATION & STORAGE
Supplied in 20-mg vials. Reconstitute drug with 60 ml of sterile water without a bacteriostatic agent for a concentration of 0.333 mg/ml. Solution remains stable for 6 hours when stored at 59° to 86° F (15° to 30° C). Protect from light.

Incompatibilities
D_5W, normal saline solution, other I. V. drugs mixed in a syringe.

CONTRAINDICATIONS & CAUTIONS
• No contraindications exist for I.V. use.
• Use cautiously in those with COPD or cardiac impairment because of increased risk of pleural effusion or pericarditis.

ADVERSE REACTIONS
CNS: dizziness, drowsiness, lightheadedness, fatigue, malaise.
CV: thrombophlebitis.
GI: diarrhea, nausea.
Musculoskeletal: muscle weakness.
Respiratory: *pulmonary edema.*
Skin: urticaria, erythema.

INTERACTIONS
Drug-drug. *Calcium channel blockers:* Ventricular fibrillation and CV collapse caused by severe hypokalemia. Stop drug before giving dantrolene.
CNS depressants: Excessive depression. Avoid using together.
Vecuronium: Potentiates neuromuscular blocking effects. Use cautiously together.
Drug-lifestyle. *Alcohol use:* Increases CNS depression. Discourage alcohol use.

EFFECTS ON LAB TEST RESULTS
None reported.

ACTION
Interferes with calcium ion release from sarcoplasmic reticulum of skeletal muscle, reducing myoplasmic level of calcium ions, thus helping to inactivate the catabolic processes linked to malignant hyperthermia crisis. Drug produces skeletal muscle relaxation by affecting the muscle beyond the myoneural junction.

PHARMACOKINETICS
Level peaks immediately after administration.
Distribution: Throughout tissues, with substantial amounts reversibly bound to protein, especially albumin. Drug probably appears in breast milk.
Metabolism: In liver to 5-hydroxy derivative, which is less active than parent compound, and to its amino derivative by the liver.
Excretion: In urine, mainly as metabolites. Half-life, 4 to 8 hours.

CLINICAL CONSIDERATIONS
• Signs and symptoms of malignant hyperthermia include muscle rigidity (often the first sign), sudden tachycardia, cardiac arrhythmias, cyanosis, tachypnea, severe hypercarbia, unstable blood pressure, rapidly rising temperature, acidosis, and shock.
• The serious adverse effects caused by long-term P.O. dantrolene (such as hepatitis, seizures, pleural effusion, or periocarditis) haven't been linked to short term I.V. use.
• While giving dantrolene, also provide oxygen, treatments for metabolic acidosis, and cooling measures, as ordered.
• Because of solution's high pH, avoid extravasation.
• Obtain baseline neuromuscular functions for later comparisons.
• Maintain urine output and monitor electrolytes.

PATIENT TEACHING
• Inform patient that he may notice decreased grip strength and increased weakness of leg muscles, especially when walking downstairs.
• Warn patient to avoid driving and other hazardous activities because CNS effects may persist for up to 2 days after I.V. administration.
• Advise patient to report adverse reactions promptly.

darbepoetin alfa
Aranesp

Pharmacologic class: hematopoietic
Therapeutic class: antianemic
Pregnancy risk category: C
pH: 5.7 to 6.4

INDICATIONS & DOSAGES
➤ **Anemia from chronic renal failure—**
Adults: 0.45 mcg/kg I.V. once weekly. Adjust dose so that hemoglobin doesn't exceed 12 g/dl. Dose shouldn't be increased more than once a month. For patients being converted from epoetin alfa, starting dose is based on epoetin alfa dose, as shown below.

Weekly epoetin alfa dose (units/wk)	Weekly darbepoetin alfa dose (mcg/wk)
< 2,500	6.25
2,500-4,999	12.5
5,000-10,999	25
11,000-17,999	40
18,000-33,999	60
34,000-89,999	100
> 90,000	200

Darbepoetin alfa should be given less frequently than epoetin alfa. If patient was receiving epoetin alfa two to three times weekly, give darbepoetin alfa once weekly. If patient was receiving epoetin alfa once weekly, give darbepoetin alfa once every two weeks.
Adjust-a-dose: If hemoglobin approaches 12 g/dl, the dose should be reduced by 25%. If hemoglobin continues to increase, the dose should be withheld until hemoglobin begins to decrease; then, restart at a dose 25% below the previous dose. If hemoglobin increases by more than 1 g/dl over 2 weeks, decrease the dose by 25%. If increase in hemoglobin is less than 1 g/dl over 4 weeks and iron stores are adequate, increase the dose by 25% of previous dose. Further increases can be made at 4-week intervals until target hemoglobin is reached.
Patients who don't need dialysis may need lower maintenance doses. Patients who are marginally dialyzed may need adjustments in dialysis prescriptions.

ADMINISTRATION
Direct injection: Give drug I.V. over ordered rate.
Intermittent infusion: May infuse I.V. via mini-infuser.
Continuous infusion: Not recommended.

PREPARATION & STORAGE
Available as a clear polysorbate or albumin solution in 25-mcg/ml, 40-mcg/ml, 60-mcg/ml, 100-mcg/ml, and 200-mcg/ml single-dose vials.
Give drug undiluted for I.V. injection. Don't shake the single-dose vials because shaking can denature the drug and render it biologically inactive. Also, don't pool unused portions because these single-dose vials don't contain preservatives. Discard solution if discolored or if precipitate appears.

Store drug in the refrigerator and protect drug from light.

Incompatibilities
Other I.V. drugs and solutions.

CONTRAINDICATIONS & CAUTIONS
• Contraindicated in patients hypersensitive to the drug or its components and in patients with uncontrolled hypertension.
• Safety and efficacy haven't been established in patients with underlying hematologic disease, such as hemolytic anemia, sickle cell anemia, thalassemia, or porphyria.
• Use cautiously in elderly patients who may have greater sensitivity to the drug.
• It isn't known whether the drug appears in breast milk. Use cautiously in breast-feeding women.

ADVERSE REACTIONS
CNS: *headache, dizziness, fatigue, fever,* asthenia, *seizures.*
CV: *hypertension, hypotension,* CAR-DIAC ARRHYTHMIA, CARDIAC ARREST, angina, *heart failure, thrombosis, edema,* chest pain, fluid overload, *acute MI.*
GI: *diarrhea, vomiting, nausea, abdominal pain, constipation.*
Metabolic: dehydration.
Musculoskeletal: *myalgia, arthralgia, limb pain,* back pain.
Respiratory: *upper respiratory tract infection, dyspnea, cough,* bronchitis, pneumonia, *pulmonary embolism.*
Skin: hemorrhage at access site, pruritus, rash.
Other: *infection,* flulike symptoms.

INTERACTIONS
None reported.

EFFECTS ON LAB TEST RESULTS
None reported.

ACTION
Simulates erythropoietin, a naturally occurring hormone produced by the kidneys, by the same mechanism as endogenous erythropoietin. Endogenous erythropoietin is released into the bloodstream in response to hypoxia and increases RBC production. Acts on erythroid tissues in bone marrow, stimulating mitotic activity of erythroid progenitor cells and early precursor cells. When RBC production increases, hemoglobin rises. The production of endogenous erythropoietin is impaired in patients with chronic renal failure, and erythropoietin deficiency is the primary cause of their anemia.

PHARMACOKINETICS
Duration, 21 hours.
Distribution: Mostly confined to the vascular space. Distribution half-life is 1½ hours. Bioavailability ranges from 30% to 50%. Steady-state levels achieved within 4 weeks.
Metabolism: Unknown.
Excretion: Drug has a half-life three times longer than that of epoetin alfa.

CLINICAL CONSIDERATIONS
• *Alert:* Patient may experience serious allergic reactions, including skin rash and urticaria. If an anaphylactic reaction occurs, the drug should be stopped and appropriate therapy given.
• *Alert:* Drug may increase blood pressure. Blood pressure should be carefully monitored and controlled before starting therapy and during therapy. Uncontrolled blood pressure has been linked to seizures and hypertensive encephalopathy in patients with chronic renal failure who are undergoing darbepoetin alfa therapy.
• Monitor renal function and electrolytes in predialysis patients.
• Monitor iron status before and during treatment. Provide supplemental iron in patients whose ferritin level is less than

---

100 mcg/L and transferrin saturation is less than 20%.

• *Alert:* Patient may have seizures. Monitor patient closely, especially during the first several months of therapy.

• Drug may increase the risk of CV events. Monitor patient for CV signs and symptoms.

• *Alert:* Monitor hemoglobin weekly until stabilized. Don't exceed the target hemoglobin of 12 g/dl. Decrease dosage if the hemoglobin increases 1 g/dl in any 2-week period. Any rise in hemoglobin greater than the target hemoglobin of 12 g/dl or any rise in hemoglobin greater than 1 g/dl within a 2-week period will increase the risk of CV and neurological events, such as seizures, stroke, hypertension, heart failure, acute MI, fluid overload or edema, or vascular thrombosis, infarction, or ischemia. If any of these symptoms occurs, decrease dose of the drug by 25%.

• Hemoglobin may not increase until 2 to 6 weeks after starting therapy.

• If patient fails to respond to drug therapy, re-evaluate him for other possible causes of inhibited erythropoiesis, such as folic acid or vitamin B_{12} deficiencies, infections, inflammatory or malignant processes, osteofibrosis cystica, occult blood loss, hemolysis, severe aluminum toxicity, and bone marrow fibrosis.

PATIENT TEACHING
• Advise patient of possible adverse effects and allergic reactions.

• Inform patient of the need for frequent monitoring of blood pressure and hemoglobin; emphasize compliance with prescribed antihypertensive drug therapy and dietary restrictions to control blood pressure.

daunorubicin citrate liposomal
DaunoXome

Pharmacologic class: antibiotic antineoplastic (cell cycle–phase nonspecific)
Therapeutic class: antineoplastic
Pregnancy risk category: D
pH: 4.9 to 6

INDICATIONS & DOSAGES
➤ **First-line cytotoxic therapy for advanced Kaposi's sarcoma caused by HIV infection—**
Adults: 40 mg/m² I.V. over 60 minutes once q 2 weeks. Continue treatment until evidence of disease progression or other complications of HIV occur.
Adjust-a-dose: If bilirubin is 1.2 to 3 mg/dl, give three-fourths the normal dose; if bilirubin or creatinine is greater than 3 mg/dl, give one-half the normal dose.

ADMINISTRATION
Direct injection: Not recommended.
Intermittent infusion: After dilution, immediately give I.V. over 60 minutes. Don't use in-line filters for the I.V. infusion.
Continuous infusion: Not recommended.

PREPARATION & STORAGE
Follow procedures for proper handling and disposal of antineoplastics.

Available as 2 mg/ml solution for injection.

Drug should be diluted with D_5W before administration. Withdraw the calculated volume of drug from the vial and transfer it into an equivalent amount of D_5W. The recommended concentration after dilution should be 1 mg/ml.

If unable to use immediately, refrigerate at 36° to 46° F (2° to 8° C) for a maximum of 6 hours.

Incompatibilities
Bacteriostatic agents, other I.V. drugs, saline and other solutions.

CONTRAINDICATIONS & CAUTIONS
• Contraindicated in those who have experienced a severe hypersensitivity reaction to daunorubicin citrate liposomal or any of its components.
• Use cautiously in those with myelosuppression, preexisting cardiac disease, previous radiotherapy encompassing the heart, or hepatic or renal dysfunction and in those who have used more than 300 mg/m^2 of anthracycline or its equivalent of doxorubicin.

ADVERSE REACTIONS
CNS: *neuropathy, fatigue, headache, fever,* depression, dizziness, insomnia, malaise, amnesia, anxiety, ataxia, confusion, ***seizures,*** hallucination, tremor, hypertonia, emotional lability, abnormal gait, hyperkinesia, somnolence, abnormal thinking.
CV: dose-related cardiomyopathy, chest pain, hypertension, palpitation, flushing, edema, tachycardia, ***MI.***
EENT: *rhinitis,* sinusitis, abnormal vision, conjunctivitis, tinnitus, eye pain, deafness, earache.
GI: *abdominal pain, anorexia, diarrhea, nausea, vomiting,* constipation, stomatitis, dry mouth, gingival bleeding, ***GI hemorrhage,*** gastritis, stomatitis, taste disturbances, melena, hemorrhoids, tenesmus, thirst, dental caries.
GU: dysuria, nocturia, polyuria.
Hematologic: ***neutropenia.***
Metabolic: dehydration, hyperuricemia.
Musculoskeletal: *back pain,* arthralgia, myalgia.
Respiratory: *cough, dyspnea,* hemoptysis, hiccups, pulmonary infiltration, increased sputum.
Skin: alopecia, pruritus, *increased sweating,* dry skin, seborrhea, folliculitis, injection site inflammation.

Other: splenomegaly, lymphadenopathy, opportunistic infections, *allergic reactions,* influenza-like symptoms, *rigors.*

INTERACTIONS
None reported.

EFFECTS ON LAB TEST RESULTS
• May increase uric acid level.
• May decrease neutrophil and platelet counts.

ACTION
Maximizes the selectivity of daunorubicin for solid tumors in situ. Penetrates the tumor, and then is released over time to exert its antineoplastic activity by inhibiting DNA synthesis and DNA-dependent RNA synthesis through intercalation.

PHARMACOKINETICS
Onset, peak, and duration of drug effects unknown.
Distribution: Unknown.
Metabolism: Unknown.
Excretion: Elimination half-life is about 4 hours.

CLINICAL CONSIDERATIONS
• Give only under the supervision of a prescriber specializing in cancer chemotherapy.
• *Alert:* Back pain, flushing, and chest tightness may occur within the first 5 minutes of the infusion. These signs and symptoms subside after stopping the infusion and generally don't recur when the infusion is given at a slower rate.
• Because local tissue necrosis is possible, monitor I.V. site closely to avoid extravasation.
• Monitor patient closely for signs of opportunistic infections, especially because patients with HIV infection are immunocompromised.
• Monitor and assess cardiac function before giving each dose because of

potential risk for cardiac toxicity and heart failure. Determine left ventricular ejection fraction at total cumulative doses of 320 mg/m^2 and every 160 mg/m^2 thereafter.
• Careful hematologic monitoring is needed because severe myelosuppression may occur. Repeat and evaluate blood counts before each dose. If absolute granulocyte count is less than 750 cells/mm^3, stop treatment.
• Monitor renal and hepatic function and uric acid level.
• *Alert:* Don't confuse daunorubicin with doxorubicin.

PATIENT TEACHING
• Inform patient that alopecia may occur but that it's usually reversible.
• Instruct patient to report sore throat, fever, or any other signs or symptoms of infection. Tell patient to avoid exposure to people with infections.
• Tell patient to report back pain, flushing, and chest tightness during the infusion.
• Advise patient to tell prescriber if she is or might be pregnant during therapy.
• Tell any woman of childbearing age that she shouldn't become pregnant during treatment.

daunorubicin hydrochloride
Cerubidine

Pharmacologic class: antibiotic antineoplastic (cell cycle–phase nonspecific)
Therapeutic class: antineoplastic
Pregnancy risk category: D
pH: 4.5 to 6.5 for reconstituted solution

INDICATIONS & DOSAGES
➤ **To induce remission of acute non-lymphocytic leukemia (combined with other chemotherapeutic drugs)—**
Adults: 45 mg/m^2/day I.V. on days 1, 2, and 3 of first course. For subsequent courses, drug is given for 2 days. Total dosage shouldn't exceed 500 to 600 mg/m^2.
Elderly patients age 60 and older: 30 mg/m^2/day I.V. for 3 days of first course. Subsequent courses are given daily for 2 days.
➤ **To induce remission in acute lymphocytic leukemia (combined with other chemotherapeutic drugs)—**
Adults: 45 mg/m^2/day I.V. daily on days 1 to 3.
Children ages 2 and older: 25 to 45 mg/m^2/day I.V. on day 1, weekly for up to 6 weeks.
Children younger than age 2 or with a body surface area less than 0.5 m^2: Calculate dose based on weight.
➤ **To induce remission of acute myelogenous leukemia ♦ —**
Adults: 60 mg/m^2/day I.V. for 3 days, repeated q 3 to 4 weeks as single-agent therapy. Maximum total lifetime dose, 550 mg/m^2. Previous chest radiation therapy requires a limit of 450 mg/m^2.
Adjust-a-dose: For patients with bilirubin level of 1.2 to 3 mg/dl, give 75% of usual daily dose; for those with bilirubin or creatinine level higher than 3 mg/dl, 50% of usual dose.

ADMINISTRATION
Direct injection: Give drug through the side port of a newly started I.V. line, preferably using a 23G or 25G winged-tip needle. Inject a 10- to 15-ml solution over 2 to 3 minutes. After administration, flush vein with primary I.V. solution.
  Closely monitor patient for signs and symptoms of infiltration, and instruct the patient to promptly report changes in sensation, such as burning at the I.V. site. Extravasation can cause slow, progressive necrosis of skin and painful ulcers. If it occurs, stop injec-

tion and aspirate as much of drug as possible. Then immediately infiltrate the area with 50 to 100 ml of hydrocortisone sodium succinate or sodium bicarbonate and apply cold compresses.
Intermittent infusion: Infuse a 100-ml solution over 30 to 45 minutes. Flush and monitor site as above.
Continuous infusion: Not recommended.

PREPARATION & STORAGE
Because of mutagenic, teratogenic, and carcinogenic risks, use a biological containment cabinet and wear gloves and mask. Use syringes with tight luer-locks to prevent drug leakage, and dispose of needles, syringes, vials, and unused drug correctly. Avoid contaminating work surfaces.

Available in 20-mg glass vials.

Reconstitute with 4 ml of sterile water for injection; then withdraw desired dose into syringe containing 10 to 15 ml of normal saline solution.

Reconstituted solution remains stable for 48 hours if refrigerated and for 24 hours if kept at room temperature protected from direct sunlight.

Incompatibilities
Other I.V. drugs.

CONTRAINDICATIONS & CAUTIONS
• Contraindicated in those with existing or recent chickenpox or herpes zoster infection because of increased risk of generalized disease.
• Use cautiously in those with preexisting myelosuppression or cardiac disease and in those who have had prior therapy with doxorubicin, cyclophosphamide, dacarbazine, dactinomycin, or mitomycin because of increased risk of cardiomyopathy.
• Use cautiously in those with a history of gout or urate renal calculi because of increased risk of hyperuricemia and in those with hepatic or renal impairment

because of increased risk of toxic reaction. Dosage may need to be adjusted.

ADVERSE REACTIONS
CNS: fever.
CV: *reversible cardiomyopathy,* cardiotoxicity.
GI: esophagitis, stomatitis, abdominal pain, mouth ulcers, diarrhea, *acute nausea and vomiting.*
GU: red urine.
Hematologic: *myelosuppression.*
Hepatic: *hepatotoxicity.*
Metabolic: hyperuricemia.
Skin: *alopecia,* contact dermatitis, pigmentation of fingernails and toenails, rash, urticaria, severe cellulitis and tissue sloughing if drug extravasates.
Other: *anaphylactoid reaction,* chills.

INTERACTIONS
Drug-drug. *Bone marrow depressants:* Worsens myelosuppression. May need to adjust daunorubicin dosage.
Cyclophosphamide, doxorubicin: Increases risk of cardiotoxicity. Monitor patient closely.
Dexamethasone, heparin: May form a precipitate. Don't mix together.
Hepatotoxic drugs (methotrexate): Increases risk of hepatotoxicity. Monitor patient closely.

EFFECTS ON LAB TEST RESULTS
• May increase uric acid, AST, bilirubin, and alkaline phosphatase levels.
• May decrease hemoglobin, hematocrit, and WBC and platelet counts.

ACTION
Binds with the DNA molecule, interfering with DNA and DNA-dependent RNA synthesis. Although most cytotoxic in the S phase, drug isn't cell cycle–phase specific. Drug has immunosuppressant and antibacterial properties.

PHARMACOKINETICS

Onset, immediate; half-life, 45 minutes to 18 hours.

Distribution: Rapid and throughout body tissues. Highest levels in spleen, kidneys, liver, lungs, and heart. Crosses placental barrier but probably not the blood-brain barrier. Unknown if drug appears in breast milk.

Metabolism: Slow and extensive in liver.

Excretion: Primarily in bile, with 14% to 23% removed in urine. Its biphasic half-life consists of an initial phase of 40 minutes and a terminal phase of 18 hours.

CLINICAL CONSIDERATIONS

• Osmolality: 5 mg/ml in sterile water is 141 mOsm/kg.

• *Alert:* Monitor pulse rate closely. Light resting pulse rate is a sign of cardiac adverse reactions. Notify prescriber immediately.

• Monitor ECG before treatment and monthly during therapy, CBC, and hepatic function.

• *Alert:* If patient develops signs or symptoms of heart failure or cardiomyopathy, stop drug immediately and notify prescriber.

• Give antiemetic before treatment to prevent nausea and vomiting.

• Using a scalp tourniquet to prevent or minimize alopecia increases risk of micrometastatic scalp lesions.

• Monitor patient for infections that develop during myelosuppression.

• Drug can reactivate radiation-induced skin lesions. If this occurs, reduce dosage.

• Keep patient well hydrated. Alkalizing urine and giving allopurinol may prevent or minimize uric acid nephropathy.

• Limit cumulative dose in adults to 500 mg/m^2 or less (400 to 450 mg/m^2 if patient has received other cardiotoxic drugs or radiation therapy that encompasses the heart).

• *Alert:* Don't confuse daunorubicin with doxorubicin.

• *Alert:* Avoid extravasation, which can cause tissue necrolysis, severe cellulitis, thrombophlebitis, and induration at injection site.

PATIENT TEACHING

• Instruct patient to avoid exposure to people with infections.

• Encourage patient to drink plenty of fluids.

• Warn patient that alopecia may occur but that it's usually reversible.

• Tell patient to watch for signs and symptoms of infection, such as fever, sore throat, and fatigue, and of bleeding, such as easy bruising, nosebleeds, bleeding gums, and melena. Tell him to take his temperature daily.

• Advise any woman of childbearing age to avoid becoming pregnant during therapy and to consult a prescriber before becoming pregnant.

• Warn patient that urine may appear red for 1 to 2 days but that it doesn't indicate presence of blood in the urine.

deferoxamine mesylate
Desferal, Desferrioxamine mesilate ◇, PMS-Deferoxamine ◇

Pharmacologic class: chelate
Therapeutic class: heavy metal antagonist
Pregnancy risk category: C

INDICATIONS & DOSAGES

➤ **Acute iron intoxication—**
I.M. administration is preferred and should be used for all patients not in shock. Slow I.V. infusion should be used only for patients in CV collapse.
Adults and children: Initially, 1 g I.V., at a rate not exceeding 15 mg/kg/hour. This may be followed by 500 mg over 4 hours for two doses, at a rate not ex-

ceeding 125 mg/hour. Depending on response, may give 500 mg I.V. over 4 to 12 hours. Maximum dose, 6 g in 24 hours.

➤ **Chronic iron overload—**
Adults and children: 0.5 to 1 g I.M. daily. Give an additional 2 g I.V. with, but separate from, each unit of blood. I.V. rate must not exceed 15 mg/kg/hour.

ADMINISTRATION
Direct injection: Not recommended.
Intermittent infusion: Infuse diluted solution directly into vein or through an I.V. line containing a free-flowing, compatible solution at an hourly rate not exceeding 15 mg/kg for initial dose.
Continuous infusion: Same rate as intermittent infusion.

PREPARATION & STORAGE
Available in 500-mg and 2-g vials.
   Reconstitute by adding 2 ml of sterile water for injection to each vial. Further dilute for I.V. infusion by adding normal saline solution, D_5W, or lactated Ringer's solution.
   Reconstituted solutions remain stable for 1 week when protected from light. Store below 25º C.

Incompatibilities
All other I.V. drugs.

CONTRAINDICATIONS & CAUTIONS
• Contraindicated in those with severe renal disease or anuria because ferrioxamine and deferoxamine are excreted by the kidneys and in those with primary hemochromatosis because phlebotomy is more effective.
• Use cautiously in those with pyelonephritis to avoid exacerbating this disorder.

ADVERSE REACTIONS
CNS: *seizures,* fever.
CV: hypotension, flushing.
EENT: ocular and auditory disturbances, cataracts.

GI: abdominal discomfort, diarrhea.
GU: red urine.
Skin: erythema, urticaria, pruritus, injection site pain and induration.
Other: *anaphylaxis, shock,* infection.

INTERACTIONS
Drug-drug. *Ascorbic acid:* Small doses may enhance chelating action of deferoxamine. High doses may impair CV function. Use together with extreme caution; monitor patient closely.

EFFECTS ON LAB TEST RESULTS
• May falsely lower result of colorimetric iron test. May cause distorted imaging result in gallium scintigraphy.

ACTION
Chelates iron, forming ferrioxamine, a stable water-soluble compound easily excreted by the kidneys, and chelates aluminum. Drug can remove iron from ferritin and hemosiderin in the body.

PHARMACOKINETICS
Onset, immediate; drug level peaks immediately after infusion.
Distribution: Throughout body tissues. Unknown if drug appears in breast milk.
Metabolism: Rapid, by plasma enzymes via unknown pathways.
Excretion: In urine, as the iron chelate ferrioxamine, giving urine a red tint; some removed through bile in feces.

CLINICAL CONSIDERATIONS
• Drug is most effective when given early in treatment of iron intoxication. It's used only in potentially fatal intoxication, with iron level above 400 mcg/dl, and in patients with severe symptoms such as coma, seizures, or CV collapse; it isn't intended as a substitute for standard measures used in iron intoxication.
• If giving I.V., change to I.M. route as soon as possible.
• Have epinephrine 1:1,000 readily available in case of allergic reaction.

Reactions may be *common,* uncommon, *life-threatening,* or COMMON AND LIFE-THREATENING.

• Dialysis removes ferrioxamine.

PATIENT TEACHING
• Warn patient that urine may appear red.
• Instruct patient to report adverse reactions promptly, such as changes in hearing or vision.
• Advise patient to have regular eye examinations during prolonged therapy because drug may cause cataracts.

desmopressin acetate
DDAVP Injection, Octostim ◇

Pharmacologic class: posterior pituitary hormone
Therapeutic class: antidiuretic, hemostatic
Pregnancy risk category: B
pH: about 4

INDICATIONS & DOSAGES
➤ **Nonnephrogenic diabetes insipidus—**
Adults and children age 12 and older: Usual maintenance dosage is 2 to 4 mcg I.V. daily, given in two divided doses. Dosage adjustment depends on changes in urine volume and osmolality.
➤ **Hemophilia A and von Willebrand disease—**
Adults and children ages 3 months and older: 0.3 mcg/kg by slow I.V. infusion.

ADMINISTRATION
Direct injection: Not recommended.
Intermittent infusion: Infuse diluted drug over 15 to 30 minutes. Rapid administration may produce hypotension.
Continuous infusion: Not recommended.

PREPARATION & STORAGE
Available in 10-ml multidose vials and 1-ml ampules with a concentration of 4 mcg/ml.

For infusion, dilute the appropriate dose in 50 ml of normal saline solution for adults and children weighing over 10 kg (22 lb) or in 10 ml of normal saline solution for children weighing 10 kg or less.

Store at 39° F (4° C) unless manufacturer specifies otherwise; protect from freezing.

Incompatibilities
None reported.

CONTRAINDICATIONS & CAUTIONS
• Contraindicated in those hypersensitive to the drug.
• Avoid use in those with type IIB form of von Willebrand disease or pseudo–von Willebrand disease because of risk of thrombocytopenia and platelet aggregation.
• Use cautiously in those with coronary artery insufficiency or hypertensive CV disease.

ADVERSE REACTIONS
CNS: transient headache.
CV: hypotension, facial flushing, slight rise in blood pressure, tachycardia, edema.
GI: mild abdominal cramps, nausea.
GU: vulval pain, increased urine osmolality.
Metabolic: hyponatremia, water intoxication.
Skin: local erythema, swelling and burning at injection site.
Other: *anaphylaxis.*

INTERACTIONS
Drug-drug. *Carbamazepine, chlorpropamide, fludrocortisone:* May potentiate antidiuretic effect. Avoid using together.
Clofibrate: May potentiate and prolong antidiuretic effect. Monitor patient carefully.
Demeclocycline, large doses of epinephrine, heparin, lithium: May reduce

---

antidiuretic effect. Monitor patient closely.

Pressor agents: Large doses of desmopressin may potentiate pressor effects. Use cautiously.

Drug-lifestyle. *Alcohol use:* Increased risk of adverse effects. Discourage using together.

EFFECTS ON LAB TEST RESULTS

None reported.

ACTION

As an antidiuretic, promotes reabsorption of water by renal collecting ducts, resulting in increased urine osmolality and diminished urine flow. As an antihemorrhagic, temporarily raises levels of factor VIII:C, factor VIII:R (von Willebrand factor), and other components of factor VIII complex.

PHARMACOKINETICS

Level peaks at 90 minutes to 3 hours.
Distribution: Unknown if drug crosses the placental or blood-brain barrier. Drug appears in breast milk.
Metabolism: Possibly in kidneys.
Excretion: Exact mechanism unknown. Plasma levels decline biphasically, with half-lives of 8 and 76 minutes after I.V. administration.

CLINICAL CONSIDERATIONS

• I.V. desmopressin has 10 times the antidiuretic effect of the same dose given intranasally.
• Decrease fluid intake to avoid water intoxication and hyponatremia.
• Drug has been successfully used to reduce blood loss during cardiac surgery.
• During infusion, monitor patient's blood pressure and pulse. After infusion, monitor intake and output and sodium level.
• If patient has a hemorrhagic disorder, monitor factor VIII, factor VIII:R cofactor, factor VIII antigen levels, and APTT.

• If patient has diabetes insipidus, monitor urine volume and osmolality. Also, periodically monitor osmolality.
• Measure response to antidiuretic therapy by volume and frequency of urination and by duration of sleep.
• If overdose occurs, reduce desmopressin dosage. If fluid overload is severe, give furosemide.

PATIENT TEACHING

• Tell patient to drink only enough to satisfy his thirst to reduce risk of water intoxication and hyponatremia if he doesn't need drug for its antidiuretic effect.
• Inform patient of possible oxytocic reaction.
• Tell patient to report nasal congestion, allergic rhinitis, or upper respiratory tract infections to prescriber promptly.

dexamethasone sodium phosphate*
Dalalone*, Decadron Phosphate, Decaject, Dexasone, Dexone*, Hexadrol Phosphate*, Solurex

Pharmacologic class: corticosteroid, synthetic glucocorticoid
Therapeutic class: anti-inflammatory
Pregnancy risk category: C
pH: 7 to 8.5

INDICATIONS & DOSAGES

➤ **Adjunctive treatment of shock—**
Adults: 1 to 6 mg/kg I.V. in a single dose, 40 mg q 2 to 6 hours, or 20 mg in a single dose followed by 3 mg/kg over 24 hours in a continuous infusion.
➤ **Adjunctive treatment of cerebral edema—**
Adults: 10 mg I.V. initially, then 4 mg I.M. q 6 hours. For inoperable or recurrent brain tumors, 2 mg I.V. maintenance dose may be given b.i.d. or t.i.d.

ADMINISTRATION

Direct injection: Give undiluted drug over at least 1 minute.
Intermittent infusion: Give diluted drug, as ordered.
Continuous infusion: Infuse diluted drug over 24 hours.

PREPARATION & STORAGE

Available in concentrations of 4 mg/ml, 10 mg/ml, 20 mg/ml, and 24 mg/ml in vials and syringes in a range of sizes. The solution is clear but may appear yellow at higher concentrations.

Dilute drug in D_5W or normal saline solution for intermittent or continuous infusion.

Protect from light and freezing.

Incompatibilities

Ciprofloxacin, daunorubicin, diphenhydramine, doxapram, doxorubicin, glycopyrrolate, idarubicin, midazolam, vancomycin.

CONTRAINDICATIONS & CAUTIONS

• Contraindicated in those with sensitivity to any component of the drug, including sulfites. Sodium bisulfites can cause severe allergic reactions.
• Contraindicated in those with peptic ulcers, except if life threatening, because of increased risk of GI bleeding.
• Use cautiously in those with diverticulitis or nonspecific ulcerative colitis if risk of perforation, abscess, or other pyogenic infection exists.
• Use cautiously in patients with hypothyroidism or cirrhosis because of risk of an exaggerated drug response and in those with cardiac disease, heart failure, renal insufficiency, or hypertension because of risk of fluid retention.
• Use cautiously in patients with hepatic impairment or hypoalbuminemia because of risk of toxic reaction and in those with ocular herpes simplex because of risk of corneal perforation.
• Use cautiously in those with thromboembolic disease because drug increases blood coagulability and risk of intravascular thrombosis.
• Use cautiously in those with a history of tuberculosis or with positive skin test results because drug may reactivate disease, in those with glaucoma because the drug may raise intraocular pressure, and in those with hyperlipidemia because drug may raise cholesterol or fatty acid level
• Use cautiously in patients with recent intestinal anastomoses, seizure disorders, diabetes mellitus, osteoporosis, or bacterial, viral, or fungal infections because drug may exacerbate these disorders or mask their signs.
• Use cautiously in those with hyperthyroidism because accelerated metabolism may reduce drug effect and in those with hypothyroidism because slowed metabolism may enhance drug effect.

ADVERSE REACTIONS

CNS: *euphoria,* psychotic behavior; increased intracranial pressure may cause abducens or oculomotor paralysis, headache, *insomnia,* weakness.
CV: *heart failure,* hypertension, edema, *thromboembolism.*
EENT: cataracts, glaucoma, papilledema, vision loss in children.
GI: irritation, increased appetite, *pancreatitis and pancreatic destruction, peptic ulcer.*
Hematologic: altered platelet count.
Metabolic: hyperglycemia, hypokalemia, hypercholesterolemia, hyperuricemia, hypernatremia, hypocalcemia.
Musculoskeletal: growth suppression in children.
Skin: acne, delayed wound healing, increased sweating, hirsutism.
Other: *anaphylaxis,* increased susceptibility to infection, *acute adrenal insufficiency after increased stress,* cushingoid state.

INTERACTIONS
Drug-drug. *Anticholinesterases:* Causes severe weakness in patients with myasthenia gravis. Use together cautiously.

Antidiabetics: Increases glucose levels. Dosage of antidiabetic therapy may need to be adjusted.

Cardiac glycosides: Increases risk of arrhythmias. Monitor patient closely.

Estrogen: Enhances dexamethasone effects. Monitor patient closely.

Hepatic enzyme inhibitors: Increases glucocorticoid metabolism. Avoid using together.

^{131}I: Reduces uptake. Avoid using together.

Indomethacin, other ulcerogenic drugs: Increases risk of GI ulcers. Use together cautiously.

Potassium-wasting diuretics, other potassium-wasting drugs: May increase potassium loss. Monitor potassium level.

Salicylates: Enhances salicylate clearance. May require dosage increase.

Vaccines with killed virus: Diminishes response. Avoid using together.

Vaccines with live virus: Increases risk of neurologic toxicity. Avoid using together.

EFFECTS ON LAB TEST RESULTS
• May increase glucose and cholesterol levels. May decrease potassium, calcium, T_3, T_4, urine 14-ketosteroid, and urine 17-hydroxycorticosteroid levels.
• May suppress reactions to skin tests, causes false-negative results in the nitro-blue tetrazolium test for systemic bacterial infections, and decreases ^{131}I uptake and protein-bound iodine level in thyroid function tests.

ACTION
Decreases inflammation by stabilizing leukocyte lysosomal membranes. It also suppresses pituitary release of corticotropin, thereby halting adrenocortical secretion of corticosteroids and sti-fling the immune response. Drug also influences protein, fat, and carbohydrate metabolism.

PHARMACOKINETICS
Rapid onset and varied duration, depending on dose, frequency of administration, and length of therapy.

Distribution: Throughout muscles, liver, skin, intestines, and kidneys. Drug crosses the placental barrier and appears in breast milk.

Metabolism: Primarily in the liver, less so in the kidneys and other tissues to inactive compounds.

Excretion: In urine as inactive metabolites, primarily glucuronides and sulfates but also as unconjugated products. Small amounts of unchanged drug are excreted in urine, negligible amounts in bile.

CLINICAL CONSIDERATIONS
• Osmolality: 356 mOsm/kg for 4 mg/ml Elkins-Sinn product.
• Adjust drug to lowest effective dose.
• I.V. administration is usually followed by use of I.M. or P.O. route.
• Short-term administration is unlikely to cause adverse reactions, even with massive doses. Long-term therapy may retard bone growth in infants and children and should be closely monitored.
• Monitor patient's weight, blood pressure, and electrolyte levels.
• Watch for depression or psychotic episodes, especially in high-dose therapy.
• *Alert:* Because of risk of hypersensitivity reactions, make sure emergency resuscitation equipment is nearby before starting therapy.
• *Alert:* Some products may contain sulfites.

PATIENT TEACHING
• Tell patient to report signs and symptoms of infection, such as sore throat, chills, and fever.

Reactions may be *common*, uncommon, *life-threatening*, or COMMON AND LIFE-THREATENING.

• Advise patient to avoid exposure to infections.

dexmedetomidine hydrochloride
Precedex

Pharmacologic class: selective alpha$_2$-adrenoceptor agonist
Therapeutic class: sedative
Pregnancy risk category: C
pH: 4.5 to 7

INDICATIONS & DOSAGES

➤ **Initial sedation in intubated and mechanically ventilated patients in ICU—**
Adults: Loading infusion of 1 mcg/kg I.V. over 10 minutes; then a maintenance infusion of 0.2 to 0.7 mcg/kg/hour for up to 24 hours, adjusted to achieve the desired level of sedation.
Adjust-a-dose: Consider dosage adjustments in patients with renal or hepatic impairment and in elderly patients.

ADMINISTRATION
Direct injection: Not recommended.
Intermittent infusion: Give loading dose over 10 minutes.
Continuous infusion: Give maintenance infusion of 0.2 to 0.7 mcg/kg/hour for no longer than 24 hours.

PREPARATION & STORAGE
Available as 100 mcg/ml in 2-ml vials and 2-ml ampules.
   To prepare the infusion, withdraw 2 ml of dexmedetomidine and add to 48 ml of sodium chloride injection to a total of 50 ml. Shake gently to mix well.
   Dexmedetomidine infusion is compatible with lactated Ringer's solution, D$_5$W, sodium chloride in water, and 20% mannitol.

   Store at controlled room temperature.

Incompatibilities
Blood, plasma.

CONTRAINDICATIONS & CAUTIONS
• Use cautiously in patients with advanced heart block or renal or hepatic impairment and in elderly patients.

ADVERSE REACTIONS
CNS: pain, fever, agitation.
CV: *hypotension,* **bradycardia, arrhythmias,** *hypertension,* tachycardia.
GI: *nausea,* thirst, vomiting, dry mouth.
GU: oliguria.
Hematologic: anemia, leukocytosis, **hemorrhage.**
Metabolic: hyperglycemia, acidosis.
Respiratory: *hypoxia,* pleural effusion, **pulmonary edema.**
Other: infection, rigors.

INTERACTIONS
Drug-drug. *Anesthetics, hypnotics, opioids, sedatives:* May enhance effects. May need to reduce dexmedetomidine dose.

EFFECTS ON LAB TEST RESULTS
• May increase glucose, AST, and ALT levels.
• May increase WBC count. May decrease hemoglobin.

ACTION
Thought to produce sedation by selective stimulation of alpha$_2$-adrenoceptors in the CNS.

PHARMACOKINETICS
Onset, peak, and duration of drug effects unknown.
Distribution: After I.V. administration, drug is rapidly and widely distributed. Drug is 94% protein bound.

Metabolism: Almost completely hepatically metabolized to inactive metabolites.
Excretion: Inactive metabolites are 95% renally eliminated and 4% fecally eliminated. The elimination half-life is about 2 hours.

CLINICAL CONSIDERATIONS
• Give only by persons skilled in the management of patients in the intensive care setting where the patient's cardiac status can be continuously monitored.
• Bradycardia and hypotension have occurred after administration of drug in patients older than age 65. Dosage reduction may be considered in this group.
• *Alert:* Give using a controlled infusion device at the rate calculated for body weight.
• *Alert:* Don't give infusion for longer than 24 hours.
• Dexmedetomidine has been continuously infused in mechanically ventilated patients before extubation, during extubation, and after extubation. It isn't necessary to stop dexmedetomidine before extubation.
• Continuously monitor cardiac status.
• Determine renal and hepatic function before administration, particularly in elderly patients.
• Some patients receiving dexmedetomidine are arousable and become alert when stimulated. This shouldn't be considered as a lack of the drug's effectiveness, unless other signs and symptoms of alertness also occur.

PATIENT TEACHING
• Tell patient he will be sedated while the drug is given, but that he may arouse when stimulated.
• Tell patient he will be closely monitored and attended while sedated.

dexrazoxane
Zinecard

Pharmacologic class: intracellular chelate
Therapeutic class: cardioprotective drug
Pregnancy risk category: C
pH: 3.5 to 5.5 for reconstituted solutions

INDICATIONS & DOSAGES
➤ **To reduce the incidence and severity of doxorubicin-induced cardiomyopathy in women with metastatic breast cancer who have received a cumulative dose of 300 mg/m^2 but would benefit from continued doxorubicin therapy—**
Adults: Dosage ratio of dexrazoxane to doxorubicin is 10:1; for example, 500 mg/m^2 of dexrazoxane to 50 mg/m^2 of doxorubicin. After reconstitution, give dexrazoxane by slow I.V. push or rapid I.V. infusion. After completion of dexrazoxane administration and before 30 minutes have elapsed from its start, give the I.V. injection of doxorubicin.

ADMINISTRATION
Direct injection: Give by slow I.V. push.
Intermittent infusion: Give by rapid I.V. infusion over 5 to 15 minutes.
Continuous infusion: Not recommended.

PREPARATION & STORAGE
Available as powder for injection in 250 mg and 500 mg vials.
When handling and preparing reconstituted solution, wear gloves and use same precautions as those for handling antineoplastics. If drug powder or solution contacts skin or mucosa, immediately wash affected area thoroughly with soap and water.

Reactions may be *common,* uncommon, *life-threatening,* or COMMON AND LIFE-THREATENING.

Dilute drug with 0.167 M sodium lactate injection, the diluent supplied with drug, to give concentration of 10 mg of dexrazoxane per 1 ml of sodium lactate. Reconstituted drug may be further diluted with either normal saline solution or D_5W to a concentration range of 1.3 to 5 mg/ml in I.V. infusion bags.

Resultant solutions are stable for 6 hours at 59° to 86° F (15° to 30° C). Discard unused solutions.

Incompatibilities
Other I.V. drugs.

CONTRAINDICATIONS & CAUTIONS
• Contraindicated in those not receiving anthracycline as part of their chemotherapy regimen.
• Avoid use in pregnant and breast-feeding women.
• Drug isn't recommended for use until after patient has an accumulated doxorubicin dose of 300 mg/m² and continuation of doxorubicin therapy is desired. For those receiving combination therapy, give dexrazoxane before doxorubicin.
• Use cautiously in all patients because administration with cytotoxic drugs may cause additive effects of immuno-suppression.

ADVERSE REACTIONS
CNS: *neurotoxicity, fatigue, malaise, fever.*
CV: phlebitis.
GI: *nausea, vomiting, anorexia, stomatitis, diarrhea,* esophagitis, dysphagia.
Hematologic: *immunosuppression, hemorrhage.*
Skin: *alopecia,* local I.V. site reaction, erythema, extravasation, *injection pain.*
Other: *infection, **sepsis.***

INTERACTIONS
Drug-drug. *Cytotoxic drugs:* Increases risk of myelosuppression. Monitor patient and blood counts closely.

EFFECTS ON LAB TEST RESULTS
None reported.

ACTION
A cyclic derivative of EDTA that readily penetrates cell membranes. May be converted to ring-opened chelate that interferes with iron-mediated free radical generation thought to be partly responsible for anthracycline-induced cardiomyopathy.

PHARMACOKINETICS
Drug level peaks in 15 minutes.
Distribution: Not bound to protein.
Metabolism: Unknown.
Excretion: Urine excretion plays an important role in elimination.

CLINICAL CONSIDERATIONS
• Monitor CBC closely. Institute infection control and bleeding precautions as indicated by CBC results.
• ***Alert:*** Doxorubicin shouldn't be given before dexrazoxane. Also, dexrazoxane isn't recommended for use with the initiation of doxorubicin therapy, but only after a cumulative dosage of doxorubicin of 300 mg/m² has been reached and continuation of doxorubicin is desired.
• Therapy doesn't eliminate the possibility of cardiac toxicity. Carefully monitor cardiace function.

PATIENT TEACHING
• Explain purpose of drug to patient.
• Instruct patient to report signs and symptoms of infection, such as fever, sore throat, and fatigue, and of bleeding, such as easy bruising, nosebleeds, bleeding gums, hematuria, and melena. Tell him to take his temperature daily.
• Inform patient that alopecia is usually reversible.

---

dextran

Low–molecular-weight dextran 40:
10% Dextran 40 in 5% Dextrose Injection, 10% Dextran 40 in Normal Saline Injection, 10% Gentran 40 in 5% Dextrose Injection, 10% Gentran 40 in Normal Saline Injection, 10% LMD in 5% Dextrose Injection, 10% LMD in Normal Saline Injection, 10% Rheomacrodex in 5% Dextrose Injection, 10% Rheomacrodex in Normal Saline Injection

High–molecular-weight dextran 70 and 75: 6% Dextran 70 in 5% Dextrose Injection, 6% Dextran 70 in Normal Saline Injection, 6% Dextran 75 in 5% Dextrose Injection, 6% Dextran 75 in Normal Saline Injection, 6% Gentran 70 in Normal Saline Injection, Macrodex in Normal Saline Injection

Pharmacologic class: glucose polymer
Therapeutic class: plasma volume expander
Pregnancy risk category: C
pH: 3 to 7 for dextran 40 10% solution in D_5W, 3.5 to 7 for dextran 40 10% solution in normal saline solution

INDICATIONS & DOSAGES

➤ **Adjunctive treatment of shock from hemorrhage, burns, surgery, or other trauma—**
Adults and children: Dosage reflects fluid loss and resultant hemoconcentration. Total dose of 10% low–molecular-weight solution shouldn't exceed 2 g/kg (20 ml/kg) I.V. for first 24 hours, then 1 g/kg (10 ml/kg) daily for 4 days. Total dose of 6% high–molecular-weight solution shouldn't exceed 1.2 g/kg (20 ml/kg) I.V. for first 24 hours, then 0.6 g/kg (10 ml/kg) daily, p.r.n.

Adjust-a-dose: For children, the best guide for determining dosage is body weight or surface area; the total dose shouldn't exceed 20 ml/kg.
➤ **To prevent venous thrombosis and pulmonary embolism—**
Adults: 50 to 100 g (500 to 1,000 ml) of 10% low–molecular-weight solution I.V. during surgery, then 50 g daily for 2 to 3 days, followed by 50 g q 2 or 3 days for up to 2 weeks.

ADMINISTRATION

Direct injection: Not recommended.
Intermittent infusion: Rapidly infuse first 500 ml of low–molecular-weight dextran over 15 to 30 minutes. Slowly infuse remainder based on patient response. In an emergency, infuse high–molecular-weight dextran at 1.2 to 2.4 g (20 to 40 ml)/minute. In normovolemic patient, don't exceed 0.24 g (4 ml)/minute.
Continuous infusion: Infuse over 24 hours based on patient condition and response.

PREPARATION & STORAGE

Low–molecular-weight dextran is available in 500-ml bottles as a 10% solution diluted in normal saline solution or D_5W. High–molecular-weight dextran comes in 500-ml bottles as a 6% solution diluted in normal saline solution or D_5W. Store solutions at a constant temperature, preferably 77° F (25° C). Crystals may form at low temperatures. If this occurs, submerge bottle in warm water to dissolve crystals before infusing. Don't give cloudy solutions. Preparation has no preservatives; discard partially used containers.

Incompatibilities

Any other I.V. drug added to a bottle of dextran, ascorbic acid, phytonadione, promethazine, protein hydrolysate.

Reactions may be *common*, uncommon, ***life-threatening***, or COMMON AND LIFE-THREATENING.

CONTRAINDICATIONS & CAUTIONS

• Contraindicated in those hypersensitive to the drug.

• Contraindicated in those with pulmonary edema because drug may worsen the condition.

• Contraindicated in those with marked thrombocytopenia, a coagulation defect, or a bleeding disorder because of increased risk of prolonged bleeding time and in those with renal disease and severe oliguria or anuria because of increased risk of circulatory overload.

• Avoid use of low–molecular-weight dextran in those who are extremely dehydrated because renal failure can occur.

• Use cautiously, especially saline solutions, in those with heart failure or cardiac decompensation because of increased risk of pulmonary edema.

• Use cautiously in patients who are hemorrhaging because increased perfusion pressure and improved microvascular flow can cause additional blood loss.

ADVERSE REACTIONS

CNS: fever.
CV: chest tightness, thrombophlebitis, hypotension, bradycardia.
GI: nausea, vomiting.
Hematologic: anemia.
Metabolic: hypovolemia.
Musculoskeletal: arthralgia.
Respiratory: wheezing.
Skin: urticaria, extravasation of I.V. solution.
Other: *anaphylaxis.*

INTERACTIONS

None reported.

EFFECTS ON LAB TEST RESULTS

• May increase sodium, glucose, ALT and AST levels. May increase or decrease bilirubin and protein levels.

• May increase bleeding time. May decrease hemoglobin and hematocrit.

• May interfere with analyses of blood grouping and cross-matching.

ACTION

A short-acting plasma volume expander, low–molecular-weight dextran increases plasma volume by twice its own volume. It helps to restore normal circulatory dynamics, increasing arterial and pulse pressure, central venous pressure (CVP), and cardiac output. It also improves microcirculatory flow to prevent venous stasis and mobilizes water from body tissues to increase urine output.

High–molecular-weight dextran has colloidal properties similar to those of human albumin. It expands plasma volume by slightly more than its own volume; then the volume decreases over 24 hours. It improves hemodynamic status for at least 24 hours. A glucose polymer, it's degraded to glucose and excreted in urine.

PHARMACOKINETICS

Onset and peak effects of dextran are immediate.

Distribution: Throughout the vascular system.

Metabolism: Dextran molecules with molecular weights above 50,000 are enzymatically degraded by dextrinase to glucose at a rate of about 70 to 90 mg/kg/day. Process is variable.

Excretion: Dextran molecules with molecular weights below 50,000 are eliminated by renal excretion, with 40% of dextran 70 appearing in urine within 24 hours. About 50% of dextran 40 is excreted in urine within 3 hours, 60% within 6 hours, and 75% within 24 hours. Remaining 25% is partially excreted in urine and feces and partially oxidized.

CLINICAL CONSIDERATIONS

• Osmolarity: dextran 40 10% in D_5W is 255 mOsm/L and 310 mOsm/L in normal saline solution.

• *Alert:* Stop infusion at first sign of an allergic reaction, but maintain I.V. access. Give antihistamines, ephedrine, or epinephrine, as needed. Keep resuscitation equipment available.

• Maintain hydration with additional I.V. fluids. Dextran is a colloid hypertonic solution that attracts water from the extravascular space and causes tissue dehydration.

• Monitor pulse, blood pressure, CVP, and urine output every 5 to 15 minutes for first hour and then hourly. Watch for signs of fluid overload or hypersensitivity.

• Slow or stop the infusion if CVP rises rapidly or if patient is anuric or oliguric after receiving 500 ml of dextran. Normal CVP is 7 to 14 cm H_2O. Give mannitol to help increase urine flow.

• Dextran can impair coagulation, possibly leading to additional blood loss. Notify prescriber if bleeding increases or if hematocrit drops below 30%.

• Change I.V. tubing or flush well with normal saline solution before transfusing blood. Dextran may cause blood to coagulate in the tubing.

• Use high–molecular-weight dextran only when whole blood or blood products aren't available. It isn't a substitute for whole blood or protein because it has no oxygen-carrying ability.

• *Alert:* Don't confuse dextran with dextrose.

PATIENT TEACHING
• Tell patient to report adverse reactions promptly.
• Explain use and administration of drug to patient and family.

dextrose in sodium chloride solutions

Pharmacologic class: carbohydrate
Therapeutic class: caloric drug, fluid volume replacement
Pregnancy risk category: C
pH: 3.2 to 6.5 for commercially prepared solutions

INDICATIONS & DOSAGES
➤ **Temporary treatment of circulatory insufficiency and shock when plasma volume expander isn't available; fluid replacement in burned, dehydrated, and other patients—**
Adults and children: Concentration and infusion rate reflect patient's age, weight, condition, and fluid, electrolyte, and acid-base balance.

ADMINISTRATION
Direct injection: Not recommended.
Intermittent infusion: Not recommended.
Continuous infusion: Infuse through a peripheral or central vein at ordered rate.

PREPARATION & STORAGE
Available in 250-ml, 500-ml, and 1,000-ml bottles and polyvinyl chloride bags. Dextrose 5% in 0.2% sodium chloride solution also comes in 150-ml containers. Concentrations include dextrose 2.5% in half-normal saline solution; dextrose 5% in 0.11%, 0.2%, 0.225%, 0.3%, half-normal or normal saline solution; and dextrose 10% in 0.2% or normal saline solution.

Store solutions in a cool, dry place, and protect from freezing or extreme heat. Don't give cloudy solutions.

Incompatibilities
Amphotericin B, ampicillin sodium, diazepam, erythromycin lactobionate, mannitol, phenytoin.

Reactions may be *common,* uncommon, *life-threatening,* or COMMON AND LIFE-THREATENING.

CONTRAINDICATIONS & CAUTIONS
• Contraindicated in those in a diabetic coma or with an allergy to corn or corn products.
• Use extremely cautiously in those receiving corticosteroid therapy and in those with heart failure, severe renal insufficiency, urinary obstruction, or edema with sodium retention because of increased risk of circulatory overload.
• Use cautiously in those with renal impairment because of increased risk of sodium retention.
• Use cautiously in those with diabetes mellitus or carbohydrate intolerance because drug may exacerbate hyperglycemia.

ADVERSE REACTIONS
CNS: fever.
CV: phlebitis, thrombosis, *exacerbated hypertension.*
Metabolic: fluid overload, hypernatremia, hypervolemia, hypokalemia, hypovitaminosis, metabolic acidosis or alkalosis.
Skin: extravasation.

INTERACTIONS
None reported.

EFFECTS ON LAB TEST RESULTS
• May increase ammonia, sodium, and liver enzyme levels. May decrease phosphate, magnesium, and potassium levels. May increase or decrease glucose levels.

COMPOSITION
These solutions contain combinations of hypotonic or isotonic concentrations of dextrose and sodium chloride solution. Solutions of dextrose 2.5% or 5% and half-normal saline solution are hypotonic. Others are isotonic.

ACTION
A rapidly metabolized source of calories and fluids in patients with inadequate oral intake. Dextrose increases glucose levels and may decrease body protein and nitrogen losses, promote glycogen deposition, decrease or prevent ketosis, and induce diuresis. Parenterally injected doses of dextrose undergo oxidation to carbon dioxide and water. A 5% solution is isotonic and is administered peripherally. Concentrated dextrose infusions provide increased caloric intake with less fluid volume; they may be irritating if given by peripheral infusions. Give solutions over 10% only by central venous catheters.

PHARMACOKINETICS
Distribution: As a source of calories and water for hydration, dextrose solutions expand plasma volume.
Metabolism: Metabolized to carbon dioxide and water.
Excretion: In some patients, dextrose solutions may produce diuresis.

CLINICAL CONSIDERATIONS
• Give electrolyte supplements as needed.
• Monitor changes in fluid balance, electrolyte levels, and acid-base balance during prolonged parenteral therapy.
• *Alert:* Watch closely for fluid overload, indicated by exacerbated hypertension, signs of heart failure, or pulmonary edema, especially in geriatric patients or those with renal or cardiac disease.

PATIENT TEACHING
• Tell patient to report adverse reactions promptly.
• Explain use and administration of I.V. fluids to patient and family.

dextrose in water solutions (glucose solutions)

Pharmacologic class: carbohydrate
Therapeutic class: TPN component, caloric drug, fluid volume replacement
Pregnancy risk category: C
pH: 4 with a range of 3.3 to 6.5 for D_5W or dextrose 10% in water

INDICATIONS & DOSAGES
➤ **To provide calories and water to meet metabolic and hydration needs—**
Adults and children: 2.5%, 5%, or 10% solution I.V.
➤ **Hyperkalemia and conditions that require adequate calories but little water—**
Adults and children: 20% solution I.V.
➤ **To promote diuresis—**
Adults and children: 20% to 50% solution I.V.
➤ **Base solution for I.V. hyperalimentation—**
Adults and children: 10% to 70% solution I.V.
➤ **Adjunctive treatment of shock—**
Adults and children: 40% to 70% solution I.V.
➤ **Cerebral edema, pregnancy-induced hypertension, renal disease, acute hypoglycemia, and as a sclerosing drug—**
Adults and children: 50% solution I.V.
➤ **Acute symptomatic hypoglycemia—**
Infants and neonates: 10% to 25% solution I.V.

ADMINISTRATION
Direct injection: Give 50 ml of 50% solution at 3 ml/minute.
Intermittent infusion: Not recommended.
Continuous infusion: Give isotonic solutions through a peripheral vein, hypertonic solutions through a central venous line. Rate depends on solution's concentration and patient's age and condition. An hourly rate above 0.5 g/kg may cause glycosuria in healthy people. Maximum rate shouldn't exceed 0.8 g/kg/hour.

PREPARATION & STORAGE
Available in 50-ml, 100-ml, 150-ml, 250-ml, 500-ml, and 1,000-ml bottles or polyvinyl chloride bags in the following concentrations: 2.5%, 5%, 7.7%, 10%, 11.5%, 20%, 25%, 30%, 38%, 38.5%, 40%, 50%, 60%, and 70%. Because dextrose is an excellent medium for bacterial growth, store solutions in a cool, dry place. Protect from freezing and extreme heat. Don't give cloudy solutions.

Incompatibilities
Ampicillin sodium, cisplatin, diazepam, erythromycin lactobionate, 10% and 25% fat emulsion solutions, phenytoin, procainamide, solutions of 10% thiopental and above, whole blood.

CONTRAINDICATIONS & CAUTIONS
• Hypertonic solutions are contraindicated in those undergoing neurosurgical procedures.
• Hypertonic solutions are contraindicated in those with delirium tremens with dehydration or intracranial or intraspinal hemorrhage because the solutions may cause hyperosmolar syndrome and in those with anuria because of risk of circulatory overload.
• All dextrose solutions are contraindicated in those in a diabetic coma because of risk of exacerbation and in those with allergies to corn or corn products because solution is made from corn sugar.
• Use dextrose solutions cautiously in patients with renal disease, cardiac disease, or hypertension because of risk of

circulatory overload and in those with urinary obstruction because of excretion difficulty.

• Use dextrose solutions cautiously in those with diabetes mellitus because solution may worsen hyperglycemia, and in those with carbohydrate intolerance because solution may cause hyperosmolar syndrome.

ADVERSE REACTIONS

CNS: hyperosmolar syndrome, confusion, unconsciousness caused by rapid administration of hypertonic solution, fever from contaminated solution.
CV: thrombosis.
Metabolic: glycosuria or hyperglycemia from prolonged infusion, hypertonic solution, or metabolic insufficiency; hypervolemia; hypokalemia; hypovitaminosis; metabolic acidosis or alkalosis; water intoxication from prolonged infusion of hypotonic or isotonic solution.
Skin: extravasation, infusion site reactions including local pain, phlebitis, or sclerosed veins with prolonged infusion of hypertonic solution.

INTERACTIONS

None reported.

EFFECTS ON LAB TEST RESULTS

• May increase ammonia and liver enzyme levels. May decrease phosphate, magnesium, and potassium levels. May increase or decrease glucose levels.

COMPOSITION

These solutions contain glucose and water and vary in tonicity and concentration. Solutions of 2.5% are hypotonic, solutions of 5% are isotonic, and solutions over 10% are hypertonic.

ACTION

A rapidly metabolized source of calories and fluids in patients with inadequate oral intake. Dextrose increases glucose levels and may decrease body protein and nitrogen losses, promote glycogen deposition, decrease or prevent ketosis, and induce diuresis. Parenterally injected doses of dextrose undergo oxidation to carbon dioxide and water. A 5% solution is isotonic and is administered peripherally. Concentrated dextrose infusions provide increased caloric intake with less fluid volume; they may be irritating if given by peripheral infusions. Give solutions over 10% only by central venous catheters.

PHARMACOKINETICS

Distribution: Dextrose solutions expand plasma volume.
Metabolism: Metabolized to carbon dioxide and water.
Excretion: In some patients, dextrose solutions may produce diuresis.

CLINICAL CONSIDERATIONS

• Osmolarity: 126 mOsm/L for dextrose 2.5 in water, 250 mOsm/L for D_5W; 505 mOsm/L for dextrose 10% in water; 1,010 mOsm/L for dextrose 20% in water; 1,330 mOsm/L for dextrose 25% in water; 1,515 mOsm/L for dextrose 30% in water; 1,920 mOsm/L for dextrose 38% in water; 2,020 mOsm/L for dextrose 40% in water; 2,525 mOsm/L for dextrose 50% in water; 3,030 mOsm/L for dextrose 60% in water; 3530 mOsm/L for dextrose 70% in water.
• *Alert:* Avoid extravasation because tissue sloughing and necrosis can occur. Never infuse hypertonic solutions rapidly because this can cause hyperglycemia and fluid shift.
• The maximum rate at which dextrose can be infused without producing glycosuria is 0.5 g/kg/hour. About 95% is retained when infused at 0.8 g/kg/hour.
• Expect osmotic diuresis when giving hypertonic solutions.
• To avoid rebound hypoglycemia, substitute dextrose 5% or 10% after stopping hypertonic solutions.

• Monitor intake and output and weight, and watch for signs of fluid overload, such as exacerbated hypertension, signs of heart failure, or pulmonary edema, especially in geriatric patients or those with renal or cardiac disease.

• Monitor glucose levels; hypertonic solutions especially can alter insulin requirements, and prolonged infusion of nutrients can diminish insulin production and secretion. Watch for signs of hyperglycemia. If they occur, reduce infusion rate and give insulin.

• Monitor electrolyte level and acid-base balance during prolonged administration.

• Give electrolyte supplements, as needed.

PATIENT TEACHING

• Tell patient to report adverse reactions promptly.

• Explain use and administration of I.V. fluids to patient and family.

diazepam
Diazemuls ◇ , Valium*

Pharmacologic class: benzodiazepine
Therapeutic class: anxiolytic, skeletal muscle relaxant, amnestic, anticonvulsant, sedative-hypnotic
Pregnancy risk category: D
Controlled substance schedule: IV
pH: 6.2 to 6.9

INDICATIONS & DOSAGES

➤ **Short-term, symptomatic relief from acute anxiety; skeletal muscle relaxant in patients who can't take oral form of the drug—**
Adults and children older than age 12: 2 to 10 mg (0.4 to 2 ml) I.V. q 3 to 4 hours. May repeat in 1 hour, with maximum of 30 mg in 8 hours. Give 2 to 5 mg to geriatric patients or when another sedative has been given.

➤ **Cardioversion—**
Adults: 5 to 15 mg (1 to 3 ml) I.V. just before procedure as amnestic drug.

➤ **Endoscopy—**
Adults: Up to 20 mg I.V. before procedure, then titrated to achieve desired effect. May produce anterograde amnesia.

➤ **Tetanus—**
Adults and children ages 5 and older: 5 to 10 mg I.V. May repeat dose in 3 to 4 hours.
Infants older than age 1 month: 1 to 2 mg I.V. q 3 to 4 hours.

➤ **Status epilepticus and recurrent seizures—**
Adults: 5 to 10 mg by slow I.V. push at 2 to 5 mg/minute. May repeat dose q 5 to 10 minutes up to maximum of 30 mg. Give 2 to 5 mg to geriatric or debilitated patients; in recurrent seizures, dose may be repeated in 20 to 30 minutes.
Children ages 5 and older: 0.5 to 1 mg I.V. q 2 to 5 minutes up to total dose of 10 mg. May be repeated in 2 to 4 hours.
Infants older than age 1 month: 0.1 to 0.5 mg I.V. q 2 to 5 minutes up to a total dose of 5 to 10 mg. May be repeated in 2 to 4 hours.

ADMINISTRATION

Direct injection: Slowly inject undiluted drug into large vein or catheter at a rate of less than 5 mg/minute for adults and 0.25 mg/kg of body weight over 3 minutes for children. Avoid extravasation. If drug is injected into tubing, choose a site directly above the needle or catheter insertion site. Afterward, flush with normal saline solution.
Intermittent infusion: Not used. Drug precipitates in any solution.
Continuous infusion: Not used.

PREPARATION & STORAGE
Available in 10-ml vials (5 mg/ml), prefilled syringes, and 2-ml ampules. Protect vials from light.

Because of incompatibility, the manufacturer warns against diluting drug before administration. However, diazepam infusions may be prepared using normal saline injection. The concentration shouldn't exceed 10 mg/ 100 ml, and only glass bottles should be used. Avoid polyvinyl chloride infusion sets, and use an in-line filter. Don't store in plastic syringes. Check with a pharmacist for more information.

Incompatibilities
All other I.V. drugs, most I.V. solutions.

CONTRAINDICATIONS & CAUTIONS
• Contraindicated in those hypersensitive to the drug.
• Contraindicated in those with acute angle-closure glaucoma or untreated chronic open-angle glaucoma because of drug's possible anticholinergic effect and in those who are in shock or in a coma because drug's hypotensive or hypnotic effects may be prolonged or worsened.
• Contraindicated in those with acute alcohol intoxication because drug deepens CNS depression.
• Contraindicated in pregnant women because of possible fetal malformations and in infants younger than age 30 days because of slow drug metabolism.
• Use extremely cautiously in those with limited pulmonary reserve because of risk of apnea and cardiac arrest.
• Use extremely cautiously for endoscopy, keeping emergency resuscitation equipment readily available in case of laryngospasm.
• Use cautiously in psychotic patients because of possible paradoxical reaction, in depressed patients because of possible worsened depression, and in

those with myasthenia gravis or porphyria because of possible exacerbation.
• Use cautiously in those with renal or hepatic impairment because of delayed drug elimination, in those with hypoalbuminemia because of increased risk of adverse effects, in geriatric or debilitated patients because of increased CNS effects, and in patients prone to addiction.

ADVERSE REACTIONS
CNS: ataxia, confusion, dizziness, *drowsiness,* dysarthria, headache, nightmares, slurred speech, syncope, tremors, vertigo, depression, fatigue, lethargy.
CV: *bradycardia, CV collapse,* hypotension, phlebitis.
EENT: nystagmus, blurred or double vision.
GI: nausea, vomiting.
GU: urine incontinence or retention.
Respiratory: *respiratory depression.*
Skin: desquamation, rash, urticaria, injection site pain and phlebitis.
Other: hangover, *acute withdrawal syndrome* after sudden discontinuation in physically dependent persons.

INTERACTIONS
Drug-drug. *Anesthetics (general), barbiturates, narcotics, phenothiazines:* Intensifies CNS depression. Avoid using together.
Antihypertensives: Potentiates effects. Monitor patient closely.
Cimetidine: Elevates diazepam level resulting from diminished hepatic metabolism. Monitor patient carefully.
Digoxin: Reduces digoxin excretion and increases digoxin level. Monitor patient for signs and symptoms of toxicity.
Isoniazid: May increase diazepam level. Monitor patient closely.
Ketamine: Heightens risk of hypotension or respiratory depression. Avoid using together.

Levodopa: Diminishes therapeutic effects. Avoid using together.
Magnesium sulfate: Potentiates CNS effects. Avoid using together.
MAO inhibitors, other antidepressants: Deepens CNS depression. Avoid using together.
Neuromuscular blockers: Deepens respiratory depression. Monitor respirations closely.
Rifampin: Decreases diazepam effectiveness. Monitor patient closely.
Drug-lifestyle. *Alcohol use:* Increases CNS depression. Discourage use together.
Smoking: Decreases effectiveness of benzodiazepine. Monitor patient closely; discourage use together.

EFFECTS ON LAB TEST RESULTS
● May increase liver function test values. May decrease neutrophil count.

ACTION
May enhance or facilitate the action of the neurotransmitter gamma-aminobutyric acid, which depresses the CNS at the limbic, thalamic, and hypothalamic levels of the CNS, producing an anxiolytic effect.

As an anticonvulsant, drug suppresses the spread of impulses from irritable foci in the cortex, thalamus, and limbic structures. As a skeletal muscle relaxant, it purportedly inhibits polysynaptic afferent pathways. As an amnestic drug, its mechanism of action is unknown.

PHARMACOKINETICS
Onset, 1 to 5 minutes; duration, 15 to 60 minutes.
Distribution: Throughout body tissues, with 80% to 99% bound to protein. Drug crosses the blood-brain and placental barriers and appears in breast milk.
Metabolism: In the liver.
Excretion: In urine as metabolites; small amounts in feces. Half-life, 20 to 50 hours.

CLINICAL CONSIDERATIONS
● Osmolality: 7,775 mOsm/kg for Roche product and 349 mOsm/kg for Kabi product.
● *Alert:* Always keep emergency resuscitation equipment nearby when giving I.V. diazepam.
● Obtain baseline respiratory rate before administration, and notify prescriber if rate falls below 12 breaths/ minute. Also obtain baseline blood pressure, and monitor carefully during and after administration.
● Monitor respiratory rate for 1 hour after administration. If rate falls below 8 breaths/minute, arouse patient and encourage him to breathe at rate of 10 to 12 breaths/minute. If you can't arouse patient, maintain airway patency and use a handheld ventilator to maintain rate of 10 to 12 breaths/minute. Notify prescriber; intubation may be needed.
● Observe infusion site for signs of phlebitis.
● If patient is receiving a narcotic, reduce its dosage by at least one-third.
● Discontinue drug if a paradoxical reaction occurs, including anxiety, acute excitation, hallucinations, increased muscle spasticity, insomnia, and rage.
● *Alert:* Abrupt withdrawal after high doses or extended use can cause seizures and delirium.
● If overdose occurs, provide supportive care. Maintain airway patency and give I.V. fluids. Give dopamine, norepinephrine, and metaraminol for hypotension. Flumazenil is a benzodiazepine antagonist that's used to reverse sedative and respiratory depressant effects. Hemodialysis doesn't remove an appreciable amount of the drug.

PATIENT TEACHING
● Instruct patient to maintain bed rest for 3 hours after parenteral administration.
● Warn patient to avoid activities that require alertness and good psychomo-

tor skills until CNS effects of drug are known.
• Tell patient to report adverse reactions promptly.
• Explain use and administration of drug to patient and family.

diazoxide
Hyperstat IV

Pharmacologic class: peripheral vasodilator
Therapeutic class: antihypertensive
Pregnancy risk category: C
pH: 11.6

INDICATIONS & DOSAGES
➤ **Emergency treatment of severe malignant and nonmalignant hypertension—**
Adults and children: 1 to 3 mg/kg up to 150 mg I.V., as a single injection, repeated q 5 to 15 minutes, p.r.n. Maintenance doses given q 4 to 24 hours up to 1.2 g daily.

ADMINISTRATION
Direct injection: Inject undiluted drug directly into peripheral vein or peripheral I.V. line over 10 to 30 seconds. Avoid extravasation because drug is extremely alkaline. If extravasation occurs, infiltrate the area with sodium chloride solution, then apply warm compresses. Relieve pain by infiltrating a local anesthetic.
Intermittent infusion: Not recommended.
Continuous infusion: Not recommended.

PREPARATION & STORAGE
Available in 20-ml ampules of 300 mg.
   Store between 36° and 86° F (2° and 30° C), and protect from freezing, heat, and light.

Incompatibilities
Hydralazine, propranolol.

CONTRAINDICATIONS & CAUTIONS
• Contraindicated in those hypersensitive to thiazide diuretics or sulfonamide-type drugs because of the risk of cross-sensitivity to diazoxide.
• Contraindicated in those with hypertension caused by aortic coarctation or arteriovenous shunt because therapy should treat underlying condition.
• Use cautiously during labor because drug can stop uterine contractions.
• Use cautiously in those with impaired cerebral or cardiac function because drug can cause transient myocardial or cerebral ischemia and in those with diabetes because drug can aggravate hyperglycemia, requiring a dosage adjustment in insulin or oral drugs.
• Use cautiously in those with uremia because of potentiated hypotensive effect and in those who could be harmed by fluid and sodium retention, rapid blood pressure reduction, tachycardia, decreased perfusion, or renal impairment.

ADVERSE REACTIONS
CNS: anxiety, confusion, dizziness, drowsiness, headache, light-headedness, paralysis, paresthesia, *seizures,* unconsciousness, weakness.
CV: *heart failure,* excessive hypotension from overdose, facial flushing or redness, angina, *arrhythmias,* chest pain, orthostatic hypotension, tachycardia, edema.
EENT: altered taste, dry mouth, salivation, tinnitus.
GI: abdominal discomfort, anorexia, constipation, diarrhea, ileus, nausea, vomiting.
GU: retention of nitrogenous wastes, urine retention.
Hematologic: anemia.
Metabolic: diabetic ketoacidosis in renal impairment, generalized or local-

ized warmth, hyperglycemia, weight gain, hypernatremia, hyperuricemia. **Musculoskeletal:** back pain, severe muscle cramps. **Skin:** pruritus, sweating, injection site pain. **Other:** *anaphylaxis.*

INTERACTIONS

Drug-drug. *Allopurinol, colchicine, probenecid, sulfinpyrazone:* May decrease effectiveness, resulting from elevated uric acid levels. Monitor patient closely.
Anticoagulants: May enhance effect of anticoagulant. Monitor PT and INR closely.
Antidiabetics (oral), insulin: Reverses hyperglycemic effects of diazoxide. Monitor glucose levels closely.
Antihypertensives: May intensify hypotensive effect if given within 6 hours of diazoxide. Use together cautiously.
Anti-inflammatory analgesics, especially indomethacin: Antagonizes hypotensive effects of diazoxide. Avoid using together.
Phenytoin: May decrease phenytoin level or increase phenytoin toxicity and risk of hyperglycemia because of altered metabolism or protein binding. Use together cautiously.
Thiazide and loop diuretics: May increase antihypertensive, hyperglycemic, and hyperuricemic effects of diazoxide. Use together cautiously.

EFFECTS ON LAB TEST RESULTS

• May increase glucose, sodium, IgG, renin, and uric acid levels. May decrease cortisol and glucose-stimulated insulin levels.
• May cause false-negative insulin response to glucagon.

ACTION

Acts directly on arterial smooth muscle, causing vasodilation. It also reduces peripheral resistance by inhibiting alpha receptors.

PHARMACOKINETICS

Onset, 1 minute; duration, 30 minutes to 72 hours.
Distribution: Highest levels found in kidneys, liver, and adrenal glands with about 90% bound to protein. Drug crosses the placental and blood-brain barriers. Unknown if drug appears in breast milk.
Metabolism: In the liver by oxidation and conjugation.
Excretion: In urine by glomerular filtration, with about 50% excreted unchanged. Half-life, 21 to 45 hours; longer in patients with renal impairment and possibly shorter in children.

CLINICAL CONSIDERATIONS

• Osmolality: 130 mOsm/kg.
• Keep patient supine during infusion and for 15 to 30 minutes afterward. If he becomes hypotensive, keep him supine for at least 1 hour. If he receives furosemide along with diazoxide, keep him supine for 8 to 10 hours.
• Give drug rapidly; slow injection causes a reduced response because of drug's extensive protein binding.
• I.V. diazoxide therapy usually lasts no longer than 5 days and is followed by oral antihypertensive therapy. Don't give drug for more than 10 days.
• Record blood pressure during and after rapid infusion to monitor rapid fall. Monitor patient every 5 minutes until blood pressure is stable, then hourly.
• Monitor intake and output for fluid retention. Weigh patient daily.
• Watch diabetic patient for signs of severe hyperglycemia or hyperosmolar hyperglycemic nonketotic syndrome. Give insulin, as needed.
• If overdose occurs, treat symptomatically. For excessive hypotension, give vasopressors such as norepinephrine or metaraminol. For acute hyperglycemia or ketoacidosis, give insulin and restore fluid and electrolyte balance. Hemodialysis removes only a small amount of the drug and its metabolites.

Reactions may be *common,* uncommon, *life-threatening,* or COMMON AND LIFE-THREATENING.

PATIENT TEACHING
• Advise patient to change positions slowly to avoid dizziness.
• Tell patient to alert nurse if discomfort occurs at I.V. site.
• Tell patient to report adverse reactions promptly.

---

digoxin
Lanoxin

Pharmacologic class: cardiac glycoside
Therapeutic class: antiarrhythmic, inotropic
Pregnancy risk category: C
pH: 6.8 to 7.2

INDICATIONS & DOSAGES
➤ **Heart failure, atrial flutter and fibrillation, atrial tachycardias including paroxysmal atrial tachycardia—**
Adults and children older than age 10: Loading dose, 0.5 to 1 mg I.V.; alternatively, 0.008 to 0.012 mg/kg; maintenance dose, 0.125 to 0.5 mg daily; usual dose, 0.25 mg daily.
Children ages 5 to 10: Loading dose, 0.015 to 0.03 mg/kg I.V.; maintenance dose, 25% to 35% of loading dose.
Children ages 2 to 5: Loading dose, 0.025 to 0.035 mg/kg I.V.; maintenance dose, 25% to 35% of loading dose.
Children ages 1 month to 2 years: Loading dose, 0.03 to 0.05 mg/kg I.V.; maintenance dose, 25% to 35% of loading dose.
Full-term neonates younger than age 1 month: Loading dose, 0.02 to 0.03 mg/kg I.V.; maintenance dose, 25% to 35% of loading dose.
Premature infants: Loading dose, 0.015 to 0.025 mg/kg I.V.; maintenance dose, 20% to 30% of loading dose.
Adjust-a-dose: Digoxin clearance may be decreased in geriatric patients with decreased renal function. A lower maintenance dose of digoxin may be needed.

ADMINISTRATION
Direct injection: Inject drug over at least 5 minutes as close to I.V. insertion site as possible.
Intermittent infusion: Not recommended.
Continuous infusion: Not recommended.

PREPARATION & STORAGE
Available in 1-ml and 2-ml ampules (0.25 mg/ml) for adults and in 1-ml ampules (0.1 mg/ml) for children. Store drug at room temperature.
Dilute with 10 ml of D_5W, normal saline solution, or sterile water, or give undiluted. Drug can precipitate if less than a fourfold dilution is used. Give diluted drug immediately.

Incompatibilities
Dobutamine, doxapram, drugs or solutions given through the same I.V. line, fluconazole, foscarnet, other I.V. drugs.

CONTRAINDICATIONS & CAUTIONS
• Contraindicated in those with digitalis toxicity because of risk of additive toxicity and in those with ventricular fibrillation.
• Use extremely cautiously in those with renal impairment or heart failure because of increased risk of toxic reaction.
• Use cautiously in geriatric patients and in those with an acute MI, incomplete AV block, severe heart failure, hypothyroidism, or chronic constrictive pericarditis because of increased risk of cardiac glycoside–induced arrhythmias.
• Use cautiously in those who have received a cardiac glycoside within the past 3 weeks and in those with acute myocarditis, renal insufficiency, severe pulmonary disease, hypoxia, sick sinus syndrome, myxedema, or

---

♦ Off-label use.   *May contain benzyl alcohol   ◇ Canada.

Wolff-Parkinson-White syndrome with atrial fibrillation because of increased risk of arrhythmias.
• Use cautiously in those with hypokalemia, hypomagnesemia, or hypercalcemia because of risk of digitalis toxicity and in those with hypertrophic cardiomyopathy because of risk of increased left ventricular outflow obstruction.
• Use cautiously in patients with increased carotid sinus sensitivity because digoxin increases vagal tone.

ADVERSE REACTIONS

CNS: agitation, dizziness, hallucinations, headache, light flashes, paresthesia, stupor, vertigo, fatigue, generalized weakness, malaise.
CV: *AV block, profound sinus bradycardia, ventricular tachycardia,* atrial and junctional tachycardia, hypotension, PVCs.
EENT: blurred vision, diplopia, photophobia, yellow-green halos around visual images.
GI: anorexia, diarrhea, nausea, vomiting.
Skin: rash, urticaria.
Other: *anaphylaxis,* gynecomastia.

INTERACTIONS

Drug-drug. *Amiodarone, captopril, diltiazem, nifedipine, quinidine, spironolactone, verapamil:* Increases digoxin level. Monitor patient closely.
Amphotericin B, corticosteroids, diuretics, ticarcillin: May cause digoxin toxicity caused by hypokalemia. Monitor potassium level.
Bretylium: Aggravates arrhythmias caused by digitalis toxicity. Avoid using together.
Calcium salts: Causes severe arrhythmias from effects on cardiac contractility and excitability. Avoid using together.
Edrophonium: May cause excessive slowing of heart rate. Avoid using together.

Heparin: Partially counteracts anticoagulant effect. Monitor PTT closely.
Pancuronium, rauwolfia alkaloids, succinylcholine, sympathomimetics: May increase risk of arrhythmias. Monitor patient closely.
Drug-herb. *Betel palm, fumitory, goldenseal, lily-of-the-valley, motherwort, rue, shepherd's purse:* May enhance cardiac effects. Discourage use together.
Licorice, oleander, Siberian ginseng, squill: May enhance toxic effect. Monitor patient closely; discourage use together.
St. John's wort: May decrease level and therapeutic effect of digoxin. Warn patient not to use together.

EFFECTS ON LAB TEST RESULTS
None reported.

ACTION
Depresses the SA node and increases the refractory period of the AV node. Also indirectly increases intracellular calcium by inhibiting sodium-potassium activated adenosine triphosphatase.

PHARMACOKINETICS
Onset, 5 to 30 minutes; peak, 1 to 5 hours.
Distribution: Throughout body tissues, with high levels in skeletal muscle, liver, heart, brain, and kidneys. About 20% to 30% bound to protein. Drug doesn't accumulate in adipose tissue, but it crosses the placental barrier and appears in breast milk.
Metabolism: In the liver and biliary tract, although variable among patients.
Excretion: In urine by glomerular filtration and active renal tubular secretion, with 50% to 70% excreted unchanged and remainder excreted as metabolites. Small amounts of drug and metabolites also excreted in bile. Half-life, 34 to 44 hours in normal renal function; longer in renal impairment.

Reactions may be *common*, uncommon, *life-threatening*, or COMMON AND LIFE-THREATENING.

CLINICAL CONSIDERATIONS

• Osmolality: digoxin pediatric injection is 9,105 mOsm/kg by freezing point depression and 5,885 mOsm/kg by vapor pressure.

• Digoxin has a low therapeutic index, requiring an individualized dosage based on patient's ideal body weight and response to drug.

• Divide the loading dose over 24 hours. First dose is 50% of total loading dose; the next two doses, given 4 to 8 hours apart, are 25% of loading dose. Loading dose may be omitted in patients with heart failure and reduced in those with renal failure.

• *Alert:* Geriatric patients may suffer hallucinations, delusions, and anxiety from digoxin toxicity. Immediately report these symptoms. Protect patient by raising the bed rails, helping him walk, using restraints if needed, and reorienting, reassuring, and observing him frequently.

• Check patient's apical pulse for 1 minute before each dose. Report significant changes, such as irregular beats or pulse rate below 60 beats/minute or above 100 beats/minute. A pulse rate below 60 beats/minute may indicate toxic reaction. Also report blood pressure changes and anticipate an order for a 12-lead ECG.

• Use a continuous ECG to monitor patients on I.V. digoxin for development or improvement of arrhythmias. If arrhythmias, which are a symptom of toxic reaction, develop, notify prescriber immediately and then treat the toxic reaction.

• Therapeutic levels are 0.5 to 2 ng/ml. Measure peak level at least 4 hours after a dose and trough level just before the next dose.

• Stop drug at first sign or symptom of toxic reaction, such as anorexia, diarrhea, nausea, and vomiting in adults or cardiac arrhythmias in children. Monitor ECG continuously and maintain patient's potassium level between 3.5 and 5 mEq/L. Treat bradycardia with 0.5 to 1 mg of I.V. atropine; treat ventricular arrhythmias with lidocaine or procainamide. If symptomatic bradycardia or AV block occurs, patient may need temporary transvenous pacing. Digoxin-immune FAB can be used to bind with digoxin and reduce the toxic effects of the drug in life-threatening overdose.

PATIENT TEACHING

• Tell patient to report promptly adverse reactions, especially nausea, vomiting, anorexia, and visual disturbances.

• Explain use and administration of drug to patient and family.

digoxin immune FAB
Digibind, DigiFab

Pharmacologic class: antibody fragment
Therapeutic class: cardiac glycoside antidote
Pregnancy risk category: C
pH: 6 to 8

INDICATIONS & DOSAGES

➤ **Potentially life-threatening digoxin toxicity—**
Adults and children: Dosage based on ingested amount or level of digoxin. When calculating amount of antidote, round up to the nearest whole number.

For digoxin tablets, find the number of antidote vials by multiplying the ingested amount in milligrams by 0.8; divide answer by 0.5. For example, if patient takes 25 of 0.25-mg tablets, the ingested amount is 6.25 mg. Multiply 6.25 mg by 0.8 and divide answer by 0.5 to obtain 10 vials of antidote.

For digoxin capsules, find the number of antidote vials by dividing the ingested dose in milligrams by 0.5. For example, if patient takes 50 of 0.2-mg capsules, the ingested amount is 10 mg. Divide 10 mg by 0.5 to obtain 20 vials of antidote.

If the digoxin level is known, determine the number of antidote vials as follows: multiply the digoxin level in nanograms per milliliter by patient's weight in kilograms; divide by 100. For example, if digoxin is 4 ng/ml, and patient weighs 60 kg, multiply together to obtain 240. Divide by 100 to obtain 2.4 vials; then round up to 3 vials.

➤ **Acute toxicity, or if ingested amount or digoxin level is unknown—**
Adults and children: 10 vials of digoxin immune FAB I.V., then observe patient's response. Follow with another 10 vials if needed. Dosage should be effective in most life-threatening ingestions in adults and children but may cause volume overload in young children.

ADMINISTRATION
Direct injection: If cardiac arrest is imminent, rapidly inject directly into vein or I.V. line containing a free-flowing, compatible solution, using a 0.22-micron filter needle.
Intermittent infusion: Not recommended.
Continuous infusion: Infuse diluted solution over 15 to 30 minutes through a 0.22-micron filter needle.

PREPARATION & STORAGE
Available in 38-mg vials (Digibind) and 40-mg vials (DigiFab). Reconstitute with 4 ml of sterile water for injection. For infusion, further dilute solution with normal saline solution. For children or other patients who need small doses, reconstitute Digibind in 38-mg vial with 38 ml of normal saline solution for 1 mg/ml concentration; reconstitute DigiFab in 40-mg vial with 40 ml of normal saline solution for

1 mg/ml concentration. Use reconstituted solution promptly. If not used immediately, refrigerate for up to 4 hours.

Incompatibilities
None reported.

CONTRAINDICATIONS & CAUTIONS
• Experience with this drug is limited. Use only in life-threatening situations.
• Use cautiously in those with heart failure; cardiac glycoside level may fall below effective inotropic level.
• Use cautiously in those with renal impairment. Excretion of the FAB fragment–digoxin complex from the body is probably delayed. Monitor these patients closely for a prolonged period.

ADVERSE REACTIONS
CV: worsening of low cardiac output states or heart failure, rapid ventricular response in patients with atrial fibrillation, *heart failure.*
Metabolic: hypokalemia.

INTERACTIONS
Drug-drug. *Cardiac glycosides:* Reverses effects of cardiac glycosides. Redigitalization should be postponed until the FAB fragments have been eliminated from the body, which may take at least several days.

EFFECTS ON LAB TEST RESULTS
• May decrease potassium level.
• May interfere with digoxin immunoassay measurement.

ACTION
Prevents or reverses toxic effects of cardiac glycosides. Specific antigen-binding fragments bind with free digoxin intravascularly or in extracellular spaces, making them unavailable for binding at site of action.

PHARMACOKINETICS
Peaks at end of infusion.
Distribution: Appears to be rapidly distributed throughout extracellular space.
Metabolism: None.
Excretion: In urine by glomerular filtration, principally as cardiac glycoside–FAB fragment complex. Elimination half-life, 14 to 20 hours.

CLINICAL CONSIDERATIONS
• Osmolality: 349 to 359 mOsm/kg for reconstituted product.
• If patient is allergic to sheep proteins or has previously reacted to digoxin immune FAB and his condition isn't life-threatening, consider skin testing. Dilute 0.1 ml of reconstituted drug in 10 ml of sterile sodium chloride solution. Inject 0.1 ml of this solution I.D., and examine site after 20 minutes. Urticarial wheal surrounded by erythema indicates positive result.
• Obtain digoxin level before giving digoxin immune FAB because drug level studies are difficult to interpret afterward.
• Closely monitor vital signs, ECG, and potassium level during and after administration.
• Don't attempt redigitalization until antidote has been eliminated, which can take up to 1 week.
• If hypokalemia occurs, give potassium supplements cautiously to avoid hyperkalemia. Allergic reactions, though rare, can occur.
• Overly high doses can cause allergic reaction, febrile reaction, or delayed serum sickness.
• Digoxin doses above 10 mg in healthy adults or 4 mg in healthy children can cause cardiac arrest.

PATIENT TEACHING
• Tell patient to report adverse reactions promptly.
• Explain use and administration of drug to patient and family.

dihydroergotamine mesylate
D.H.E. 45

Pharmacologic class: ergot alkaloid
Therapeutic class: vasoconstrictor
Pregnancy risk category: X
pH: 3.2 to 4

INDICATIONS & DOSAGES
➤ **Rapid control of vascular headaches, including migraine and cluster headaches—**
Adults: 1 mg I.M. at start of attack, then 1 mg I.M. in 1 hour, p.r.n. until relief of headache; not to exceed 3 mg/day. When more rapid response is needed, drug may be given I.V. to maximum of 2 mg. Don't exceed I.M. or I.V. dose of 6 mg weekly.

ADMINISTRATION
Direct injection: I.M. or I.V. at the first warning sign of a headache.
Intermittent infusion: Not recommended.
Continuous infusion: Not recommended.

PREPARATION & STORAGE
Available as a colorless solution in 1-mg/ml vials. Drug doesn't need dilution for I.V. use. Protect from light, freezing, and heat. Store at 59° to 86° F (15° to 30° C). Don't give discolored solutions.

Incompatibilities
None reported.

CONTRAINDICATIONS & CAUTIONS
• Contraindicated in those hypersensitive to ergot alkaloids.
• Contraindicated in children, pregnant women, and breast-feeding women because safety and efficacy haven't been determined.

◆ Off-label use.   *May contain benzyl alcohol   ◇ Canada.

• Contraindicated in patients with peripheral vascular disease, coronary artery disease, or severe hypertension because drug can increase vasoconstriction and induce vasospasm.
• Contraindicated in those with hepatic or renal impairment because impaired drug metabolism can lead to ergot poisoning and in those with infection or sepsis because these conditions may enhance the drug's vasoconstrictive effects.
• Contraindicated in patients taking concurrent CYP3A4 inhibitors (azole antifungals, macrolides, protease inhibitors).
• Use cautiously in geriatric patients who may be predisposed to peripheral vascular disease and have slowed drug clearance.

ADVERSE REACTIONS

CNS: *seizures (with overdose),* dizziness, headache, paresthesia.
CV: *coronary vasospasm,* peripheral ischemia, precordial distress and pain, tachycardia, *bradycardia.*
GI: nausea, vomiting.
Musculoskeletal: muscle pain in extremities, weakness in legs.
Other: *anaphylaxis;* localized edema in legs and feet; pale, cold hands and feet.

INTERACTIONS

Drug-drug. *CYP 3A4 inhibitors (azole antifungals, macrolides, protease inhibitors):* Causes serious and life-threatening peripheral and cerebral ischemia. Avoid using together.
Propranolol, other beta blockers: May block vasodilation activity of epinephrine, resulting in excessive vasoconstriction and cold extremities. Monitor patient closely.
SSRIs: May cause weakness, hyperreflexia, and incoordination. Monitor patient closely.

Sumatriptan: Causes additive effect. May also cause coronary artery vasospasm. Avoid using together.
Peripheral vasoconstrictors: Causes synergistic elevation of blood pressure. Avoid using together.
Drug-lifestyle. *Nicotine:* May provoke vasoconstriction in some patients, predisposing to a greater ischemic response to ergot therapy. Discourage use together.

EFFECTS ON LAB TEST RESULTS
None reported.

ACTION
Causes peripheral vasoconstriction by stimulating alpha receptors. Directly affects cranial vessels, causing vasoconstriction and reduction in amplitude of pulsations caused by vascular headaches. Also causes vasodilation in hypertonic vessels and may reduce catecholamine and serotonin levels.

PHARMACOKINETICS
Onset, less than 5 minutes; duration, 1 to 4 hours.
Distribution: Throughout body tissues, with 90% bound to protein. Drug crosses the blood-brain and placental barriers.
Metabolism: In the liver.
Excretion: In urine and feces, primarily as metabolites.

CLINICAL CONSIDERATIONS
• Give drug when prodromal signs occur or as soon as possible after headache begins. Dosage and speed of relief may be directly related to prompt administration.
• *Alert:* Don't confuse dihydroergotamine with dihydroergotoxine.
• Monitor patient for signs and symptoms of peripheral or central vasoconstriction or vasospasm.
• Watch for ergotamine rebound or increase in headache, which may occur when drug is stopped.

Reactions may be *common*, uncommon, *life-threatening*, or COMMON AND LIFE-THREATENING.

• If overdose occurs, treat symptomatically. Treat seizures with I.V. diazepam or barbiturates, as ordered. Support respirations as needed. For severe vasospasm, apply warmth to ischemic extremities to prevent tissue damage. Carefully give vasodilators, such as nitroprusside, prazosin, or tolazoline, because they can cause hypotension.

PATIENT TEACHING
• After initial dose, advise patient to lie down and relax in a quiet, darkened room.
• Instruct patient to immediately report symptoms such as numbness or tingling in extremities, weakness, chest pain, changes in heart rate, edema, or itching.
• Advise patient to avoid exposure to cold, which also increases vasoconstriction.
• Teach patient to protect extremities from injury if paresthesia occurs.

diltiazem hydrochloride
Apo-Diltiaz ◇ , Cardizem Injectable

Pharmacologic class: calcium channel blocker
Therapeutic class: antianginal
Pregnancy risk category: C
pH: 3.7 to 4.1 for vials, 4 to 7 for lyophilized product

INDICATIONS & DOSAGES
➤ **Temporary control of rapid ventricular rate in atrial fibrillation or atrial flutter; rapid conversion of paroxysmal supraventricular tachycardia—**
Adults: Initially, 0.25 mg/kg I.V. as a bolus given over 2 minutes; if inadequate, a second bolus dose of 0.35 mg/kg may be given after 15 minutes. Subsequent I.V. bolus doses should be individualized. For low–body-weight patient, base dosage on body weight. Some may respond to 0.15 mg/kg; however, duration of action is shorter. For continued reduction of heart rate, a continuous infusion of 10 mg/hour may be started immediately after the bolus dose. The initial infusion rate may be increased by 5 mg/hour up to a maximum rate of 15 mg/hour, p.r.n. Infusions continued beyond 24 hours or at a rate exceeding 15 mg/hour aren't recommended.

ADMINISTRATION
Direct injection: Give ordered dose via patent I.V. line. Don't inject with incompatible drugs or solutions.
Intermittent infusion: Not recommended.
Continuous infusion: Give via an infusion control device. Infuse over 24 hours at rate not exceeding 15 mg/hour.

PREPARATION & STORAGE
Available as a 5 mg/ml solution in 5-ml and 10-ml single-dose vials and 100-mg vial for I.V. infusion. Refrigerate at 36° to 46° F (2° to 8° C). Drug may be stored at room temperature for up to 1 month; after 1 month it must be destroyed.

To prepare bolus injection, withdraw calculated dose from vial. To prepare continuous infusion, aseptically transfer calculated dose to desired volume of normal saline solution, D_5W, or dextrose 5% in half-normal saline solution. Mix thoroughly and use within 24 hours.

Refrigerate until ready to use.

Incompatibilities
Acetazolamide, acyclovir, aminophylline, ampicillin, cefoperazone, diazepam, furosemide, heparin, hydrocortisone, insulin (regular), methylprednisolone, nafcillin, phenytoin, rifampin, sodium bicarbonate, thiopental.

CONTRAINDICATIONS & CAUTIONS
• Contraindicated in those hypersensitive to drug.

• Contraindicated in those with sick sinus syndrome; second- or third-degree AV block, except if the patient has a functioning ventricular pacemaker; severe hypotension; cardiogenic shock; atrial fibrillation; or atrial flutter caused by Wolff-Parkinson-White syndrome.

• Use cautiously in those with impaired hepatic, renal, or ventricular function and in those taking other drugs that decrease peripheral resistance, intravascular volume, myocardial contractility, or conduction. Dosage may need to be decreased.

ADVERSE REACTIONS

CNS: headache, dizziness, paresthesia, somnolence, insomnia, asthenia.
CV: *heart failure, arrhythmias, bradycardia, first-degree AV block,* hypotension, vasodilation, *ventricular fibrillation.*
GI: constipation, nausea, vomiting.
GU: polyuria.
Hepatic: acute hepatic injury.
Skin: *erythema multiforme,* exfoliative dermatitis, sweating, rash, pruritus, injection site reactions.
Other: *anaphylaxis.*

INTERACTIONS

Drug-drug. *Anesthetics:* Decreases cardiac contractility, conductivity, automaticity; possible potentiated vascular dilation. Monitor patient.
Beta blockers, cardiac glycosides: May cause bradycardia, AV block. Use together cautiously.
Carbamazepine: Elevates carbamazepine level. Monitor patient closely.
Cimetidine, ranitidine: Increases diltiazem level. Monitor patient for signs and symptoms of toxic reaction and additive AV node conduction slowing.
Cyclosporine: Increases cyclosporine level; reduce cyclosporine dose in renal and cardiac transplant patients. Monitor cyclosporine level closely.
Digoxin: May increase digoxin level. Monitor patient for toxicity.

EFFECTS ON LAB TEST RESULTS

• May increase AST and alkaline phosphatase levels.

ACTION

Inhibits calcium ion influx across cardiac and smooth-muscle cells, decreasing myocardial contractility and oxygen demand, and dilates coronary arteries and peripheral arterioles. Electrophysiologic effects include decreased AV nodal conduction time and prolonged AV refractory period. These effects slow the ventricular response to atrial fibrillation or flutter or act to break reentry circuit and restore normal sinus rhythm in paroxysmal supraventricular tachycardia.

PHARMACOKINETICS

Elimination half-life, about 3.5 hours. After rapid I.V. injection, onset is within 3 minutes; effect peaks in 2 to 7 minutes; duration, 1 to 3 hours. Duration after continuous infusion, 7 to 10 hours.
Distribution: 70% to 80% bound to protein; 35% to 40% bound to albumin. Drug appears in breast milk.
Metabolism: Extensively in the liver.
Excretion: Biliary and renal; 2% to 4% excreted unchanged in urine.

CLINICAL CONSIDERATIONS

• Make sure duration of infusion doesn't exceed 24 hours. Patient should then be given other antiarrhythmics.
• Don't give I.V. diltiazem and I.V. beta blockers together or within a few hours of each other.
• Stop drug if dermatologic events progressing to erythema multiforme or exfoliative dermatitis occur or persist.
• When using continuous infusion, continuously monitor ECG. Frequently monitor blood pressure. Have a defibrillator and emergency equipment readily available.
• If systolic blood pressure is below 90 mm Hg or heart rate is below

---

60 beats/minute, withhold dose and notify prescriber.
• If overdose or exaggerated response occurs, use supportive measures. For bradycardia and first-degree AV block, consider atropine, isoproterenol, or cardiac pacing. For cardiac failure, use inotropics and diuretics. For hypotension, give vasopressors. Dialysis doesn't appear to remove diltiazem.

PATIENT TEACHING
• Tell patient to report adverse reactions promptly.
• Explain use and administration of drug to patient and family.

dimenhydrinate
Dinate*, Dramanate*, Dymenate*, Gravol ◊ *, Hydrate*

Pharmacologic class: ethanol amine-derivative antihistamine
Therapeutic class: antihistamine (H$_1$-receptor antagonist), antiemetic, antivertigo drug
Pregnancy risk category: B
pH: 6.4 to 7.2

INDICATIONS & DOSAGES
➤ **To prevent and treat nausea and vomiting—**
Adults: 50 mg diluted in 10 ml of solution, given I.V. slowly over 2 minutes; repeat q 4 hours, p.r.n.

ADMINISTRATION
Direct injection: Inject diluted drug into vein or into a previously established I.V. line over 2 minutes.
Intermittent infusion: Not recommended.
Continuous infusion: Not recommended.

PREPARATION & STORAGE
Available in 1-ml, 5-ml and 10-ml vials and 1-ml ampules of 50 mg/ml.
Dilute each 50 mg (1 ml) with 10 ml of normal saline solution before injection.
Store diluted solution at 59° to 86° F (15° to 30° C); avoid freezing.

Incompatibilities
Aminophylline, ammonium chloride, amobarbital, butorphanol, chlorpromazine, glycopyrrolate, heparin, hydrocortisone sodium succinate, hydroxyzine hydrochloride, midazolam, pentobarbital sodium, phenobarbital sodium, phenytoin, prochlorperazine edisylate, promazine, promethazine hydrochloride, and thiopental.

CONTRAINDICATIONS & CAUTIONS
• Contraindicated in those hypersensitive to the drug or its components.
• Contraindicated in children younger than age 2 because safety and efficacy haven't been determined.
• Use cautiously in those with prostatic hyperplasia, stenosing peptic ulcer, pyloroduodenal obstruction, bladder neck obstruction, angle-closure glaucoma, bronchial asthma, seizures, or arrhythmias because drug may exacerbate these conditions.

ADVERSE REACTIONS
CNS: confusion, *drowsiness,* hallucinations, headache, restlessness, insomnia, malaise.
CV: chest tightness, hypotension, palpitations, tachycardia.
EENT: blurred vision; diplopia; nasal stuffiness; dry mouth, nose, and throat.
GI: anorexia, constipation, diarrhea, epigastric distress, nausea.
GU: difficult or painful urination.
Hematologic: hemolytic anemia.
Respiratory: *respiratory depression* with massive overdose, thickened bronchial secretions, wheezing.

Skin: photosensitivity, urticaria.
Other: *anaphylaxis.*

INTERACTIONS
Drug-drug. *Tricyclic antidepressants:* Increases anticholinergic effect. Monitor patient closely.
Barbiturates, CNS depressants: May cause additive effects, precipitating overdose. Avoid using together.
Ototoxic drugs such as cisplatin and vancomycin: Masks ototoxic symptoms. Monitor patient closely; use together with caution.
Drug-lifestyle. *Alcohol use:* Causes additive CNS depression. Discourage use together.

EFFECTS ON LAB TEST RESULTS
• May cause false-negative results in tests using allergen extracts.

ACTION
Competes with histamine at H_1-receptors to prevent, but not reverse, the actions of histamine. Also, inhibits acetylcholine, which in turn inhibits the vestibular and reticular systems, and depresses the CNS.

PHARMACOKINETICS
Onset, immediate; duration, 3 to 6 hours.
Distribution: Probably throughout body tissues. Drug crosses the placental and blood-brain barriers and appears in breast milk in small amounts.
Metabolism: In the liver.
Excretion: In urine, primarily as metabolites.

CLINICAL CONSIDERATIONS
• **Alert:** Most I.V. products contain benzyl alcohol, which has been linked to a fatal "gasping syndrome" in premature and low-birth-weight infants.
• Keep patient supine during drug administration.
• CNS depression and hypotension are more common in geriatric patients.

• Drug can interfere with diagnosis of appendicitis.
• Like other antiemetics, drug may mask symptoms of ototoxicity, brain tumor, or intestinal obstruction. Closely monitor patients at risk.
• In adults, 500 mg or more of dimenhydrinate may cause initial sedation followed by difficulty swallowing and speaking, psychosis, CNS excitation, seizures, and postictal depression. Signs and symptoms in children include dilated pupils, flushed face, excitation, hallucinations, confusion, ataxia, intermittent clonic convulsions, coma, and cardiorespiratory collapse, which can lead to death. Treat symptomatically. For respiratory depression, provide mechanical ventilation and oxygen. Treat seizures with diazepam.

PATIENT TEACHING
• Warn patient to avoid activities that require alertness and psychomotor skills until CNS effects of drug are known.
• Tell patient to report adverse reactions promptly.
• Explain use and administration of drug to patient and family.

diphenhydramine hydrochloride
Benadryl, Hyrexin-50, PMS-Diphenhydramine ◇

Pharmacologic class: ethanol amine-derivative antihistamine
Therapeutic class: antihistamine (H_1-receptor antagonist), antiemetic, antivertigo drug, sedative-hypnotic, antidyskinetic
Pregnancy risk category: B
pH: 5 to 6

INDICATIONS & DOSAGES
➤ **Parkinsonism and drug-induced extrapyramidal reaction in geriatric**

patients unable to tolerate more potent drugs; mild cases of parkinsonism, including drug-induced parkinsonism, with centrally acting anticholinergics; allergic reactions, nausea, and vertigo—
Adults: 10 to 50 mg I.V., up to 100 mg if needed. Maximum daily dose, 400 mg.
Children: 5 mg/kg/day or 150 mg/m²/ day I.V. divided into four doses. Maximum daily dose, 300 mg.

ADMINISTRATION
Direct injection: Inject drug over 3 to 5 minutes, not to exceed 25 mg/minute, directly into vein or into an I.V. line containing a free-flowing, compatible solution.
Intermittent infusion: After diluting appropriate dosage, infuse slowly.
Continuous infusion: Not recommended.

PREPARATION & STORAGE
Available in 10- mg/ml and 50-mg/ml vials.
  Further dilution isn't needed for direct injection.
  Store in light-resistant containers at 59° to 86° F (15° to 30° C), and avoid freezing.
  Compatibility depends on several factors, including concentration of drugs, specific diluents, pH, and temperature. Consult specialized references for compatibility information.

Incompatibilities
Allopurinol, amobarbital, amphotericin B, cefepime, cefmetazole, dexamethasone, foscarnet, haloperidol lactate, pentobarbital, phenytoin, phenobarbital, thiopental.

CONTRAINDICATIONS & CAUTIONS
• Contraindicated in those hypersensitive to antihistamines.
• Contraindicated in neonates and premature infants because of increased

risk of seizures and antimuscarinic effects, such as CNS excitation.
• Use cautiously in those with lower respiratory tract symptoms, including asthma, because drug thickens and dries secretions, making expectoration difficult.
• Use cautiously in those with angle-closure glaucoma, stenosing peptic ulcer, pyloroduodenal obstruction, symptomatic prostatic hyperplasia, bladder neck obstruction, CV disease, or hypertension because drug can worsen symptoms.
• Use cautiously in geriatric patients because drug is more likely to have CNS effects and cause hypotension. It may also cause paradoxical stimulation. Dosage may need to be reduced.

ADVERSE REACTIONS
CNS: confusion, euphoria, excitation, headache, hysteria, neuritis, insomnia, nightmares, paresthesia, *seizures,* tremor, fatigue, *drowsiness, sedation, dizziness, incoordination.*
CV: chest tightness, extrasystoles, hypotension, palpitations, tachycardia.
EENT: acute labyrinthitis; blurred vision; diplopia; dry nose and throat; nasal congestion; tinnitus.
GI: anorexia, constipation, diarrhea, nausea, vomiting, *dry mouth.*
GU: urine retention.
Hematologic: *agranulocytosis, hemolytic anemia, thrombocytopenia.*
Respiratory: thickened bronchial secretions, wheezing.
Skin: diaphoresis, photosensitivity, rash, urticaria.
Other: *anaphylaxis,* chills.

INTERACTIONS
Drug-drug. *Antimuscarinics:* May potentiate effects. Monitor patient closely.
CNS depressants, hypnotics, sedatives, tranquilizers: Deepens CNS depression. Use together cautiously.

MAO inhibitors: Prolongs and intensifies anticholinergic effects. Avoid using together.

Other products containing diphenhydramine (including topical forms): Increases risk of adverse reactions. Avoid using together.

Ototoxic drugs such as cisplatin and vancomycin: Masks signs of ototoxicity. Monitor patient closely.

Stimulants: May cause seizures. Avoid using together.

Drug-lifestyle. *Alcohol use:* Increases CNS depression. Discourage use together.

Sun exposure: May cause photosensitivity reaction. Advise patient to avoid excessive sunlight exposure.

EFFECTS ON LAB TEST RESULTS

- May decrease hemoglobin and platelet and granulocyte counts.
- May cause false-positive results in tests using allergen extracts.

ACTION

Competes with histamine for H_1-receptor sites on effector cells to prevent, but not reverse, the actions of histamine. Drug's anticholinergic properties are probably responsible for antiemetic and sedative effects.

PHARMACOKINETICS

Onset, 15 to 20 minutes; duration, 4 to 6 hours.

Distribution: Highest levels appear in lungs, spleen, and brain; lower levels in heart, muscles, and liver; 82% is bound to proteins. Drug crosses the placental barrier and appears in breast milk in small amounts.

Metabolism: In the liver, where drug apparently undergoes first-pass metabolism.

Excretion: Mainly in urine, primarily as metabolites, in 24 hours. Half-life averages 5 hours.

CLINICAL CONSIDERATIONS

- Osmolality: 50 mg/ml is 240 mOsm/kg; 10 mg/ml is 65 mOsm/kg.
- *Alert:* Don't confuse diphenhydramine with diphenoxylate or dimenhydrinate.
- Keep patient supine during drug administration.
- Stop drug 4 days before skin tests.
- Signs and symptoms of overdose vary from CNS depression in geriatric patients to CNS stimulation in children. Others include dry mouth, flushing, GI symptoms, and fixed, dilated pupils.
- If overdose occurs, treat symptomatically with oxygen and I.V. fluids. Give vasopressors for hypotension.

PATIENT TEACHING

- Tell patient that coffee and tea may reduce drowsiness and that sugarless gum, sour hard candy, or ice chips may relieve dry mouth.
- Warn patient to avoid activities that need alertness and psychomotor skills until CNS effects of drug are known.
- Tell patient to report adverse reactions promptly.

dobutamine hydrochloride
Dobutrex

Pharmacologic class: adrenergic, beta$_1$ agonist
Therapeutic class: inotropic drug
Pregnancy risk category: B
pH: 2.5 to 5.5 for 12.5-mg/ml vials and premixed infusion solutions

INDICATIONS & DOSAGES

➤ **Short-term treatment of cardiac decompensation resulting from depressed contractility in heart disease or cardiac surgery—**
Adults: 2.5 to 15 mcg/kg/minute I.V.

ADMINISTRATION
Direct infusion: Not used.
Intermittent infusion: Not used.
Continuous infusion: Give through a central I.V. line, using an infusion pump for most accurate titration.

PREPARATION & STORAGE
Supplied in 20-ml vials containing 250 mg of drug.

Reconstitute with 10 ml of sterile water or D₅W (25 mg/ml).

Before administration, further dilute with at least 50 ml of solution, using one of the following as diluent: D_5W, dextrose 5% in half-normal saline solution, dextrose 5% in lactated Ringer's solution, dextrose 5% in normal saline solution, normal saline solution, 10% dextrose injection, Isolyte M with 5% dextrose injection, Ringer's injection, Normosol-M in D_5W, 20% Osmitrol in water for injection, or sodium lactate injection. For a concentration of 250 mcg/ml, mix 250 mg of drug in 1,000 ml of solution; for 500 mcg/ml, mix 250 mg in 500 ml of solution; for 1 mg/ml, mix 250 mg in 250 ml of solution. Maximum concentration for infusion is 5 mg/ml.

Before reconstitution, store at room temperature. Reconstituted solution remains potent for 6 hours at room temperature and for 48 hours if refrigerated. Use diluted solution within 24 hours. Solution may turn pink from slight drug oxidation, but this doesn't significantly affect its potency. Avoid freezing; solution may crystallize.

Incompatibilities
Acyclovir, alkaline solutions, alteplase, aminophylline, bretylium, bumetanide, calcium chloride, calcium gluconate, cefepime, cefmetazole, diazepam, digoxin, doxapram, furosemide, heparin, indomethacin, insulin (regular), magnesium sulfate, midazolam, piperacillin with tazobactam, phenytoin, phytonadione, potassium chloride, sodium bicarbonate, thiopental, verapamil, warfarin.

CONTRAINDICATIONS & CAUTIONS
● Contraindicated in those hypersensitive to the drug or to sulfites.
● Contraindicated in those with hypertrophic cardiomyopathy because drug may exacerbate symptoms.
● Use cautiously in those with atrial fibrillation because drug facilitates AV conduction and rapid ventricular response.
● Use cautiously in patients after an MI because high doses may intensify oxygen demand, increasing ischemia, and in those with PVCs because drug may worsen arrhythmia.
● Use cautiously in patients with hypertension because of risk of an exaggerated pressor response.
● Use cautiously in patients with hypovolemia because therapy should aim to correct the condition.

ADVERSE REACTIONS
CNS: headache, paresthesia.
CV: angina, hypertension, *tachycardia,* palpitations, ventricular ectopy, phlebitis.
GI: nausea, vomiting.
Musculoskeletal: mild leg cramps.
Respiratory: dyspnea, asthmatic episodes.

INTERACTIONS
Drug-drug. *Anesthetics, such as cyclopropane and halothane:* Increases risk of ventricular arrhythmias. Monitor ECG closely.
Beta blockers: Antagonizes beta₁ receptor effects of dobutamine. Avoid using together.
Guanadrel, guanethidine: Elevates blood pressure and arrhythmias, resulting from diminished hypotensive effects of these drugs and potentiated pressor effects of dobutamine. Monitor patient closely.

Insulin: Increases requirements in diabetics. Monitor glucose levels closely.

MAO inhibitors, tricyclic antidepressants: Enhances pressor effects of dobutamine. Use together with caution.

Nitroprusside: Additive effects, including higher cardiac output and lower pulmonary artery wedge pressure. Monitor patient closely.

Rauwolfia alkaloids: Prolongs effect of dobutamine because these drugs prevent its uptake into storage granules. Avoid using together.

Drug-herb. *Rue:* Increases inotropic potential. Use together cautiously.

EFFECTS ON LAB TEST RESULTS
• May decrease potassium level.

ACTION
Stimulates beta$_1$ receptors in the heart to increase myocardial contractility and stroke volume, thereby increasing cardiac output. Preload decreases because of reduced ventricular filling pressure; afterload declines because of reduced systemic vascular resistance. Drug also produces mild chronotropic, hypertensive, arrhythmogenic, vasodilative effects.

PHARMACOKINETICS
Onset, 1 to 2 minutes, or up to 10 minutes with slow infusion; duration, a few minutes.

Distribution: In plasma. Unknown if drug crosses the placental barrier or appears in breast milk.

Metabolism: In the liver and other tissues. Drug also undergoes conjugation with glucuronic acid.

Excretion: Primarily in urine as metabolites, with small amounts in feces. Half-life, about 2 minutes.

CLINICAL CONSIDERATIONS
• Osmolality: 273 mOsm/kg for vials; 260 to 284 mOsm/kg for the four available premixed infusion solutions.

• Before treatment, correct hypovolemia with a volume expander and, as ordered, digitalize patient who has a rapid ventricular response to atrial fibrillation.

• Monitor blood pressure and heart rate and rhythm continuously. Also monitor cardiac output and pulmonary artery wedge pressure.

• Monitor electrolyte levels, especially potassium.

• *Alert:* Drug may contain sulfites, which can cause allergic reactions in some patients.

• Signs of overdose include tachycardia or excessive alteration in blood pressure. If overdose occurs, reduce infusion rate or stop therapy until patient's condition is stable. Because drug has a short half-life, other measures usually aren't needed.

PATIENT TEACHING
• Tell patient to promptly report adverse reactions, especially dyspnea and drug-induced headache.

• Explain use and administration of drug to patient and family.

• Tell the patient to alert nurse if discomfort occurs at I.V. site.

docetaxel
Taxotere

Pharmacologic class: taxoid
Therapeutic class: antineoplastic
Pregnancy risk category: D

INDICATIONS & DOSAGES
➤ **Patients with locally advanced or metastatic breast cancer that has progressed during anthracycline-based therapy or patients who have relapsed during anthracycline-based adjuvant therapy—**
Adults: 60 to 100 mg/m^2 I.V. over 1 hour q 3 weeks.

Adjust-a-dose: In patients initially given 100 mg/m^2 who have febrile neutropenia, neutrophil count under 500 cells/mm^3 for more than 1 week, or severe or cumulative cutaneous reactions, dose should be decreased to 75 mg/m^2. If reactions continue, decrease dose to 55 mg/m^2 or stop therapy. In patients initially given 60 mg/m^2 who don't have any of the reactions stated above, including severe peripheral neuropathy, dose may be increased. Therapy is stopped in those who develop grade 3 peripheral neuropathy.

➤ **Locally advanced or metastatic non–small-cell lung cancer after failure of platinum-based chemotherapy—**
Adults: 75 mg/m^2 I.V. over 1 hour q 3 weeks. Premedicate with dexamethasone 16 mg daily for 3 days, starting 1 day before docetaxel therapy.
Adjust-a-dose: For patients with febrile neutropenia, neutrophil count under 500 cells/mm^3 for more than 1 week, severe or cumulative cutaneous reactions, or other grade 3 or 4 nonhematologic toxicities during therapy, stop docetaxel until toxicity is resolved, then restart at 55 mg/m^2. For patients who develop grade 3 or higher peripheral neuropathy, stop docetaxel entirely.

➤ **Patients with unresectable, locally advanced or metastatic non–small-cell lung cancer who haven't previously received chemotherapy for this condition (combined with cisplatin)—**
Adults: 75 mg/m^2 docetaxel I.V. over 1 hour, immediately followed by cisplatin 75 mg/m^2 I.V. over 30 to 60 minutes q 3 weeks.
Adjust-a-dose: In patients whose platelet count nadir during the previous course of therapy is under 25,000 cells/mm^3, those with febrile neutropenia, and those with serious nonhematologic toxicities, decrease docetaxel dosage to 65 mg/m^2. In patients who require a further dose reduction, a dose of 50 mg/m^2 is recommended. For cisplatin dosage adjustments, see manufacturers' prescribing information.

ADMINISTRATION
Direct injection: Not recommended.
Intermittent infusion: Give as 1-hour infusion at room temperature and under ambient light.
Continuous infusion: Not recommended.

PREPARATION & STORAGE
Available as a 20-mg vial with diluent vial of 1.83 ml and 80-mg vial with diluent vial of 7.33 ml.

Wear gloves during preparation and administration. If solution gets on skin, wash immediately and thoroughly with soap and water. If drug comes in contact with mucous membranes, flush thoroughly with water.

Reconstitute drug in vials with entire contents of their respective diluent vials, yielding a concentration of 10 mg/ml. Allow drug and diluent to stand at room temperature 5 minutes before mixing. After mixing, allow foam to dissipate before proceeding to next step.

Solution is further diluted for infusion in 250 ml of either normal saline solution solution or 5% dextrose to produce a final concentration of 0.3 to 0.9 mg/ml.

If a dose greater than 240 mg is desired, use a larger volume of infusion solution. Don't exceed a concentration exceeding 0.9 mg/ml of solution. Mix infusion thoroughly by manually rotating the vial.

Store unopened vials at 36° to 46° F (2° to 8° C). Protect from light.

Incompatibilities
None reported.

CONTRAINDICATIONS & CAUTIONS
• Contraindicated in patients severely hypersensitive to the drug or other formulations containing polysorbate 80.
• Contraindicated in those with neutrophil counts below 1,500 cells/mm^3.
• Avoid use in patient with bilirubin level above upper limit of normal. Patients with ALT or AST level above 1.5 times upper limit of normal and alkaline phosphatase level above 2.5 times upper limit of normal generally shouldn't receive drug.

ADVERSE REACTIONS
CNS: asthenia, dysesthesia, pain.
CV: fluid retention, hypotension, flushing.
GI: *stomatitis, nausea, vomiting, diarrhea.*
Hematologic: *anemia,* NEUTROPENIA, MYELOSUPPRESSION, LEUKOPENIA, *thrombocytopenia.*
Musculoskeletal: back pain, myalgia, arthralgia.
Respiratory: dyspnea, chest tightness.
Skin: *alopecia,* skin eruptions, desquamation, *nail pigmentation alterations,* nail pain, rash.
Other: *hypersensitivity reactions, sepsis, infection,* drug fever.

INTERACTIONS
Drug-drug. *Compounds that induce, inhibit, or are metabolized by the cytochrome P-450 3A4 system, such as cyclosporine, erythromycin, ketoconazole, and troleandomycin:* May modify metabolism of docetaxel. Use together cautiously.

EFFECTS ON LAB TEST RESULTS
• May increase ALT, AST, bilirubin, and alkaline phosphatase levels.
• May decrease hemoglobin and WBC and platelet counts.

ACTION
Disrupts the microtubular network essential for cellular functions.

PHARMACOKINETICS
Drug effects are immediate.
Distribution: Rapidly distributed to peripheral tissue compartments; 94% is protein bound.
Metabolism: In the liver.
Excretion: Primarily in the urine and feces. Triphasic half-life (alpha, beta, gamma) of 4 minutes, 36 minutes, and 11 hours, respectively.

CLINICAL CONSIDERATIONS
• *Alert:* Patients with elevated bilirubin level or abnormal transaminase and alkaline phosphatase levels are at increased risk for developing grade 4 neutropenia, febrile neutropenia, infections, severe thrombocytopenia, severe stomatitis, severe skin toxicity, and toxic death. Patients with isolated elevated transaminase level greater than 1.5 times upper limit of normal also had a higher rate of grade 4 febrile neutropenia.
• Premedicate all patients with oral corticosteroids, such as 8 mg of dexamethasone twice daily for 3 days, starting 1 day before docetaxel administration, to reduce incidence and severity of fluid retention and hypersensitivity reactions.
• *Alert:* Don't confuse Taxotere with Taxol.
• Bone marrow toxicity is the most common, dose-limiting toxicity. Frequent blood count monitoring is needed during therapy.
• Monitor patient closely for hypersensitivity reactions, especially during the first and second infusions.
• Monitor bilirubin, AST, ALT, and alkaline phosphatase levels regularly and before start of each new cycle of docetaxel.
• If overdose occurs, monitor vital signs closely. Expect bone marrow suppression, peripheral neurotoxicity, and mucositis. No specific antidote is available.

PATIENT TEACHING
• Advise patient of childbearing age to avoid pregnancy.
• Advise women not to breast-feed during therapy.
• Warn patient that alopecia occurs in almost 80% of patients.
• Instruct patient to promptly report such signs and symptoms as sore throat, fever, unusual bruising or bleeding, swelling, or dyspnea.

dolasetron mesylate
Anzemet

Pharmacologic class: selective serotonin 5-HT$_3$ receptor antagonist
Therapeutic class: antinauseant, antiemetic
Pregnancy risk category: B
pH: 3.2 to 3.8

INDICATIONS & DOSAGES
➤ **To prevent nausea and vomiting caused by cancer chemotherapy—**
Adults: 1.8 mg/kg, or a fixed dose of 100 mg, as a single I.V. dose given 30 minutes before chemotherapy.
Children ages 2 to 16: 1.8 mg/kg, as a single I.V. dose given 30 minutes before chemotherapy. Maximum dose of 100 mg.
➤ **To prevent and treat postoperative nausea and vomiting—**
Adults: 12.5 mg, as a single I.V. dose given about 15 minutes before stopping anesthesia or as soon as nausea or vomiting occurs.
Children ages 2 to 16: 0.35 mg/kg, up to 12.5 mg, as a single I.V. dose given about 15 minutes before stopping anesthesia or as soon as nausea or vomiting occurs.

ADMINISTRATION
Direct injection: Direct injection can be infused as rapidly as 100 mg/30 seconds.
Intermittent infusion: Diluted in 50 ml compatible solution and infused over 15 minutes.
Continuous infusion: Not recommended.

PREPARATION & STORAGE
Available as 20 mg/ml injection in single-use 0.625-ml ampules and 5-ml vials.
May be given undiluted or further diluted in 50 ml of normal saline solution, D$_5$W, dextrose 5% in half-normal saline solution, or dextrose 5% in lactated Ringer's injection.
After dilution, drug should be discarded after 24 hours if stored at room temperature and 48 hours if refrigerated.
Store unopened drug at controlled room temperature and protect from light.

Incompatibilities
Injection shouldn't be mixed with other drugs.

CONTRAINDICATIONS & CAUTIONS
• Contraindicated in those hypersensitive to the drug.
• Avoid use in children younger than age 2.
• Use cautiously in patients who have or who may develop prolonged cardiac conduction intervals, such as those with electrolyte abnormalities or a history of arrhythmia and those receiving cumulative high-dose anthracycline therapy.
• Use cautiously in breast-feeding women.

ADVERSE REACTIONS
CNS: *headache,* dizziness, drowsiness, fatigue, fever.

◆ Off-label use.   *May contain benzyl alcohol   ◇ Canada.

CV: *arrhythmias,* ECG changes, hypotension, hypertension, tachycardia.
GI: *diarrhea,* dyspepsia, abdominal pain, constipation, anorexia.
GU: oliguria, urine retention.
Skin: pruritus, rash, injection site pain.
Other: chills, *anaphylaxis.*

INTERACTIONS

Drug-drug. *Drugs that prolong ECG intervals, such as antiarrhythmics:* Increases risk of arrhythmia. Monitor patient closely.
Drugs that induce the P-450 enzymes, such as rifampin: Decreases dolasetron's metabolite levels. Monitor patient for decreased efficacy of antiemetic.
Drugs that inhibit the P-450 enzymes, such as cimetidine: Increases dolasetron's metabolite levels. Monitor patient for adverse reactions.

EFFECTS ON LAB TEST RESULTS

● May increase bilirubin, ALT, and AST levels.
● May increase PTT.

ACTION

Blocks the action of serotonin, preventing serotonin from stimulating the vomiting reflex.

PHARMACOKINETICS

Onset, rapid; peak, 36 minutes; duration, 7 hours.
Distribution: Widely distributed, with 69% to 77% bound to protein.
Metabolism: A ubiquitous enzyme, carbonyl reductase, mediates the reduction of dolasetron to hydrodolasetron. Cytochrome P-450 (CYP) 2D6 and CYP 3A4 coenzyme systems are responsible for its metabolism.
Excretion: Elimination half-life of hydrodolasetron is 7.3 hours; 67% of the drugs is excreted in urine and 33% in feces.

CLINICAL CONSIDERATIONS

● *Alert:* Don't confuse Avandamet (rosiglitazone maleate and metformin HCl) with Anzemet (dolasetron mesylate).
● ECG changes are related to elevated drug levels and are self-limiting as levels decline.
● Monitor patient for nausea and vomiting.

PATIENT TEACHING

● Tell patient about potential adverse effects.
● Tell patient to report nausea or vomiting.

dopamine hydrochloride
Intropin, Revimine ◇

Pharmacologic class: adrenergic
Therapeutic class: inotropic, vasopressor
Pregnancy risk category: C
pH: 3.3 for vials, 3.6 for premixed infusion

INDICATIONS & DOSAGES

➤ **Adjunctive treatment of shock that persists after adequate fluid volume replacement or in which oliguria is refractory to other vasopressors; to increase cardiac output, blood pressure, and urine flow—**
Adults: Initially, 1 to 5 mcg/kg/minute I.V., increased by 1 to 4 mcg/kg/minute or less at 10- to 30-minute intervals until desired response is achieved. Maintenance dosage, usually under 20 mcg/kg/minute.
    In severely ill patients, give 5 mcg/kg/minute I.V. initially, increased by 5 to 10 mcg/kg/minute at 10- to 30-minute intervals up to 50 mcg/kg/minute until desired response is achieved.

Carefully adjust infusion to patient response.

➤ **Chronic refractory heart failure—**
Adults: 0.5 to 2 mcg/kg/minute I.V. until desired response is achieved.

Carefully adjust infusion to patient response.

ADMINISTRATION
Direct injection: Not used.
Intermittent infusion: Not used.
Continuous infusion: Use an infusion-control device to avoid inadvertent bolus administration of dopamine. Using an appropriately diluted concentration, give dopamine through a long I.V. catheter in a large vein, such as the antecubital fossa, rather than in a hand or ankle vein because of risk of extravasation. Continuously observe the infusion site for extravasation, which can lead to gangrene. If extravasation occurs, use a small-gauge needle to promptly infiltrate the area with 10 to 15 ml of normal saline solution containing 5 to 10 mg of phentolamine.

PREPARATION & STORAGE
Available in 5-ml vials, single-dose vials, and prefilled syringes of 200 mg (40 mg/ml), 400 mg (80 mg/ml), and 800 mg (160 mg/ml). Because injectable solution is light-sensitive, it's available in protective vials. Dopamine also comes premixed with D_5W for infusion in concentrations of 0.8, 1.6, and 3.2 mg/ml in 250-ml and 500-ml glass or polyvinyl chloride containers. Don't use discolored solutions or those darker than light yellow.

Dilute dopamine concentrate to 200 mg/250 ml or 200 mg/500 ml using normal saline solution, D_5W, dextrose 5% in normal saline solution, lactated Ringer's solution, dextrose 5% in lactated Ringer's solution, or 1/6 M sodium lactate. Dilution with 250 ml yields an 800-mcg/ml solution. Protect the diluted concentration from light. It's stable for 24 hours.

Incompatibilities
Acyclovir sodium, additives with a dopamine and dextrose solution, alteplase, amphotericin B, cefepime, furosemide, gentamicin, indomethacin sodium trihydrate, iron salts, insulin (regular), oxidizing agents, penicillin G potassium, sodium bicarbonate or other alkaline solutions, thiopental.

CONTRAINDICATIONS & CAUTIONS
• Contraindicated in those hypersensitive to the drug or to sulfites.
• Contraindicated in those with pheochromocytoma because of risk of severe hypertension.
• Use cautiously in those with tachyarrhythmias or ventricular arrhythmias because drug may worsen these conditions and in those with occlusive disease, Raynaud's disease, or arterial embolism because drug may impair circulation.

ADVERSE REACTIONS
CNS: anxiety, headache.
CV: conduction abnormalities, *hypotension, **ventricular arrhythmias with high doses,*** angina, ectopic heartbeats, hypertension, tachycardia, widened QRS complex.
GI: nausea, vomiting.
Metabolic: azotemia, mild hypokalemia.
Respiratory: dyspnea, asthmatic episodes.
Skin: piloerection, necrosis and tissue sloughing with extravasation.
Other: allergic reactions, gangrene in extremities with high doses in occlusive vascular disease.

INTERACTIONS
Drug-drug. *Alpha blockers, such as phenoxybenzamine:* Decreases peripheral vasoconstriction with high dopamine doses. Avoid using together.
Anesthetics, such as chloroform, cyclopropane, halothane, or trichloroethylene: Intensifies risk of severe arrhyth-

mias or hypertension. Use with extreme caution; monitor patient carefully.

Antihypertensives: Reduces antihypertensive effect if dopamine is given in sufficient amounts to produce alpha-adrenergic effects. Monitor patient closely.

Beta blockers, sympathomimetics: Decreases cardiac effects. Monitor patient closely.

Cardiac glycosides, levodopa: May increase risk of arrhythmias. Monitor patient closely.

Diuretics: Enhances diuresis. Monitor patient closely.

Doxapram, oxytocin: Increases vasopressor effects. Use cautiously.

Ergonovine, ergotamine, methylergonovine, methysergide: May increase vasopressor effects and enhance vasoconstriction. Avoid using together.

Guanadrel, guanethidine, mecamylamine, methyldopa, methylphenidate, trimethaphan: May increase vasopressor effects. Monitor patient closely.

MAO inhibitors: Prolongs and intensifies dopamine effects. Avoid using together if possible.

Maprotiline, tricyclic antidepressants: May potentiate dopamine's CV effects. Higher doses of dopamine may be needed.

Nitrates: May reduce antianginal effects. Monitor patient closely.

Phenytoin: May cause hypotension and bradycardia. Monitor patient carefully.

Radio contrast dyes (diatrizoate, iothalamate, ioxaglate): If given after dopamine, increases neurologic effects during aortography. Monitor patient closely.

Thyroid hormones: May heighten effects of these hormones or of dopamine. Monitor patient carefully.

EFFECTS ON LAB TEST RESULTS
• May increase glucose and urine urea levels.

ACTION
Stimulates dopamine receptors in the renal, mesenteric, coronary, and intracerebral vascular beds. As dosage increases, dopamine activates other adrenergic receptors. At 2 to 10 mcg/kg/minute, $beta_1$ receptors are stimulated; at dosages above 10 mcg/kg/minute, alpha receptors are stimulated.

PHARMACOKINETICS
Onset, 5 minutes; duration, 3 to 10 minutes.

Distribution: Throughout body but not across blood-brain barrier. Unknown if drug crosses the placental barrier.

Metabolism: In the liver, kidneys, and plasma by MAO and catechol *O*-methyltransferase to inactive compounds. About 25% is metabolized to norepinephrine in adrenergic nerve terminals.

Excretion: Primarily in urine, with about 80% removed in 24 hours as metabolites; small amount is excreted unchanged. Half-life, about 2 minutes.

CLINICAL CONSIDERATIONS
• Osmolality: 581 to 619 mOsm/kg for 40 mg/ml vials.
• Osmolarity: For premixed infusion in D_5W, it's 269 mOsm/L, 277 mOsm/L, and 294 mOsm/L for 0.8-mg/ml, 1.6-mg/ml, and 3.2-mg/ml concentrations, respectively.
• Before and during therapy, monitor heart rate, blood pressure, urine output, peripheral perfusion, central venous pressure or pulmonary artery wedge pressure, and cardiac output.
• Correct hypovolemia before dopamine therapy.
• When stopping drug, reduce infusion rate gradually to prevent severe hypotension.
• Infusion rates of 50 mcg/kg/minute have been used safely in patients with advanced circulatory decompensation. High doses of dopamine can increase

renal vasoconstriction and peripheral resistance.
• During infusion, monitor ECG, blood pressure, cardiac output, central venous pressure, pulmonary artery wedge pressure, pulse rate, urine output, and color and temperature of extremities.
• If extravasation occurs, stop infusion and infiltrate site promptly with a 10- to 15-ml normal saline injection containing 5 to 10 mg of phentolamine. Use syringe with a fine needle, and infiltrate area liberally with phentolamine solution. In children, 0.1 to 0.2 mg/kg, up to 10 mg per dose, is recommended.
• *Alert:* Drug may contain sulfites, which may cause allergic reactions in some patients.
• If overdose occurs, reduce infusion rate or temporarily stop infusion. If this won't lower blood pressure, give a short-acting alpha blocker, such as phentolamine.

PATIENT TEACHING
• Tell patient to promptly report adverse reactions.
• Explain use and administration of drug to patient and family.
• Tell patient to report discomfort at I.V. site.

doxacurium chloride
Nuromax*

Pharmacologic class: nondepolarizing neuromuscular blocker
Therapeutic class: skeletal muscle relaxant
Pregnancy risk category: C
pH: 3.9 to 5

INDICATIONS & DOSAGES
➤ **To relax skeletal muscle during surgery as an adjunct to general anesthesia—**
Adults: Dosage is highly individualized. Considerable variation is normal.

Rapid I.V. infusion of 0.05 mg/kg allows endotracheal intubation in 5 minutes in about 90% of patients when used as part of a thiopental and opioid induction technique. Lower doses may require longer times before intubation is possible. Neuromuscular blockade at this dose will last for an average of 100 minutes. Higher doses (0.8 mg/kg) will produce intubating conditions more rapidly, within 4 minutes, but neuromuscular blockade will last for 160 minutes or more. If given during anesthesia with enflurane, halothane, or isoflurane, consider reducing the dose by 33%.
Children older than age 2: Initially, 0.03 mg/kg I.V. given during halothane anesthesia produces a block with an onset of 7 minutes and duration of 30 minutes; 0.05 mg/kg produces a block in 4 minutes lasting 45 minutes.
➤ **To maintain skeletal muscle paralysis during general anesthesia—**
Adults and children older than age 2: After 60 to 100 minutes, follow initial dose with 0.005 to 0.01 mg/kg I.V. q 30 to 45 minutes. In general, children require more frequent maintenance doses.

ADMINISTRATION
Direct injection: Inject ordered dose directly into a vein or tubing of a free-flowing I.V. solution.
Intermittent infusion: Not recommended.
Continuous infusion: Not recommended.

PREPARATION & STORAGE
Available in 5-ml vials containing 1 mg/ml.
  Reconstitute with D_5W, normal saline injection, dextrose 5% in normal saline injection, lactated Ringer's injec-

tion, or dextrose 5% in lactated Ringer's injection.

Diluted solutions are stable for 24 hours at room temperature, but because the preservative is diluted, a risk of contamination exists. Give immediately after reconstituting. Discard unused solution after 8 hours.

Incompatibilities
Alkaline solutions, such as barbiturate solutions, given through the same I.V. line.

CONTRAINDICATIONS & CAUTIONS
• Contraindicated in patients hypersensitive to the drug, in those requiring prolonged mechanical ventilation in the intensive care unit, and in those who have received other nondepolarizing neuromuscular blockers.
• Contraindicated during cesarean section because safety to the neonate hasn't been established and drug's long duration exceeds that of the procedure.
• Contraindicated in neonates because drug contains benzyl alcohol. Safety and efficacy in children younger than age 2 haven't been determined.
• Use cautiously and reduce dosage in debilitated patients, obese patients, those in whom difficulty with reversal is anticipated, and those with metastatic cancer, severe electrolyte disturbances, or neuromuscular diseases.
• Use cautiously in those with end-stage kidney disease because drug has a longer half-life in these patients, and they may be more sensitive to the neuromuscular-blocking effects of the drug.
• Use cautiously in breast-feeding women because it's unknown if drug appears in breast milk.
• Use cautiously in those with myasthenia gravis or myasthenic syndrome (Eaton-Lambert syndrome) because these patients are particularly sensitive

to the effects of nondepolarizing relaxants. Shorter-acting drugs are recommended for such patients.

ADVERSE REACTIONS
CNS: fever.
CV: *MI,* hypotension, flushing.
EENT: diplopia.
Musculoskeletal: prolonged muscle weakness.
Respiratory: apnea, *respiratory depression, respiratory insufficiency, bronchospasm,* dyspnea, wheezing.
Skin: urticaria.

INTERACTIONS
Drug-drug. *Aminoglycosides, such as gentamicin, kanamycin, neomycin, and streptomycin; bacitracin; colistin; polymyxin B; sodium colistimethate; tetracyclines:* Increases muscle weakness. Use together cautiously.
Carbamazepine, phenytoin: May prolong time to maximal block or shorten the duration of block. Monitor patient closely.
Inhalation anesthetics, magnesium salts, quinidine, procainamide: May enhance activity, or increase duration of action, of nondepolarizing neuromuscular blockers. Monitor patient closely.

EFFECTS ON LAB TEST RESULTS
• May increase glucose and urine urea levels.

ACTION
Competes with acetylcholine for receptor sites at the motor end plate.

PHARMACOKINETICS
Onset, 3.5 to 9 minutes; duration, 55 to 160 minutes; half-life, 100 minutes.
Distribution: Rapid; extent of protein binding unknown.
Metabolism: Not metabolized.
Excretion: In urine and bile as unchanged drug.

CLINICAL CONSIDERATIONS

• Drug has no effect on consciousness or pain threshold. Don't give drug until the general anesthetic dulls the patient's consciousness.
• Higher initial doses may be needed in patients with burns and in those with severe liver disease.
• Give only under direct medical supervision and only if familiar with the use of neuromuscular blockers and techniques involved in maintaining a patent airway. Don't give drug unless the equipment for artificial respiration, mechanical ventilation, oxygen therapy, intubation, and antagonist are available.
• Adjust dosage to ideal body weight in obese patients because prolonged neuromuscular block may occur.
• When diluted as directed, drug is compatible with alfentanil, fentanyl citrate, and sufentanil.
• Monitor patient for signs and symptoms of bradycardia during anesthesia; drug has minimal vagolytic action.
• Adjust dosage as needed for patients with renal or hepatic insufficiency who exhibit prolonged neuromuscular blockade.
• A nerve stimulator and train-of-four monitoring is recommended to assess recovery of muscle strength. Don't attempt pharmacologic reversal with neostigmine without evidence of spontaneous recovery.
• Acid-base or electrolyte imbalance may influence action of drug. Alkalosis may counteract the paralysis, and acidosis may enhance it.
• If overdose occurs, maintain patent airway and control ventilation. As ordered, give an anticholinesterase and an anticholinergic.

PATIENT TEACHING

• Tell patient to report adverse reactions promptly.

• Explain use and administration of drug to patient and family.
• Reassure patient and family that he'll be monitored at all times and his needs anticipated.

doxapram hydrochloride
Dopram*

Pharmacologic class: analeptic
Therapeutic class: CNS and respiratory stimulant
Pregnancy risk category: B
pH: 3.5 to 5

INDICATIONS & DOSAGES

➤ **Postanesthesia respiratory depression or apnea unrelated to muscle relaxants—**
Adults and children older than age 12: 0.5 to 1 mg/kg I.V., repeated, if needed, q 5 minutes up to a total dose of 2 mg/kg.
When desired response is obtained or if adverse effects appear, reduce infusion rate to 1 to 3 mg/minute. Recommended total dose by infusion, 4 mg/kg or 300 mg.
➤ **Drug-induced CNS depression—**
Adults and children older than age 12: Initially, 1 to 2 mg/kg I.V., repeated in 5 minutes, then 1 to 2 mg/kg q 1 to 2 hours until patient awakens or up to maximum daily dose of 3 g.
➤ **COPD caused by acute hypercapnia—**
Adults: 1 to 2 mg/minute I.V. for up to 2 hours. Maximum infusion rate, 3 mg/minute. Infusion beyond the single maximum of 2 hours, or additional infusions, aren't recommended.

ADMINISTRATION

Direct injection: Inject drug into a vein or into an I.V. line containing a free-flowing, compatible solution.

Intermittent infusion: Give diluted solution at ordered rate, usually 1 to 2 mg/minute, but not exceeding 3 mg/minute, for up to 2 hours. If needed, repeat in 30 minutes to 2 hours. Rapid infusion may cause hemolysis. Avoid extravasation or extended use of a single injection site; either may lead to thrombophlebitis or local skin irritation.
Continuous infusion: Not used.

PREPARATION & STORAGE
Available in 20-ml multidose vials with a concentration of 20 mg/ml.

Compatible with most I.V. fluids. For use in postanesthesia or drug-induced CNS depression, add 250 mg of drug to 250 ml of D_5W, dextrose 10% in water, or normal saline solution. In COPD, add 400 mg of drug to 180 ml of D_5W, dextrose 10% in water, or normal saline solution.

Store between 59° and 86° F (15° and 30° C); avoid freezing.

Incompatibilities
Aminophylline, ascorbic acid, cefoperazone, cefotaxime, cefotetan, cefuroxime sodium, dexamethasone sodium phosphate, diazepam, digoxin, dobutamine, folic acid, furosemide, hydrocortisone sodium phosphate, hydrocortisone sodium succinate, ketamine, methylprednisolone sodium succinate, minocycline, thiopental, ticarcillin disodium.

CONTRAINDICATIONS & CAUTIONS
● Contraindicated in patients hypersensitive to the drug.
● Contraindicated in neonates and in those with ventilatory incompetence caused by mechanical disorders of ventilation such as airway obstruction, pneumothorax, muscle paresis, or flail chest.
● Contraindicated in patients with pulmonary embolism, acute asthma, restrictive respiratory disorders, or respiratory failure brought on by neuromuscular disorders.
● Contraindicated in those with seizure disorders because drug may trigger seizures.
● Avoid use in patients with severe hypertension, CVA, or head injury because drug may raise blood pressure and exacerbate these conditions and in those with coronary artery disease or frank uncompensated heart failure because drug may increase cardiac workload and oxygen consumption.
● Use extremely cautiously in those with cerebral edema, asthma, hyperthyroidism, severe tachycardia, cardiac disease, or pheochromocytoma because drug's cardiac and pressor effects may worsen these conditions.
● Use cautiously in those receiving a sympathomimetic or MAO inhibitor.

ADVERSE REACTIONS
CNS: apprehension, bilateral Babinski's signs, disorientation, dizziness, *headache,* hyperactivity, increased deep tendon reflexes, involuntary movements, paresthesia especially in genitalia and perineum, fever, *seizures.*
CV: *arrhythmias, chest pain and tightness, heart rate variations,* lowered T waves, *hypertension,* flushing, thrombophlebitis at injection site.
EENT: *laryngospasm,* pupillary dilation.
GI: diarrhea, nausea, vomiting.
GU: incontinence, albuminuria, urine retention.
Hematologic: hemolysis, anemia.
Musculoskeletal: muscle spasticity.
Respiratory: cough, dyspnea, rebound hypoventilation, tachypnea, wheezing, *bronchospasm,* hiccups.
Skin: pruritus, sweating.
Other: *anaphylaxis.*

INTERACTIONS
Drug-drug. *CNS stimulants:* May cause additive effects. Monitor patient closely.

Reactions may be *common,* uncommon, *life-threatening,* or COMMON AND LIFE-THREATENING.

General anesthetics: May cause arrhythmias. Monitor patient closely.
MAO inhibitors, sympathomimetics: May increase pressor effects. Use together cautiously.
Neuromuscular blockers: May temporarily mask residual effects. Use together cautiously.

EFFECTS ON LAB TEST RESULTS
• May increase BUN level.
• May decrease hemoglobin, hematocrit, and erythrocyte, WBC, and RBC counts.

ACTION
Stimulates the entire CNS. Is thought to stimulate respiration through its effects on peripheral carotid chemoreceptors and the medullary respiratory center.

PHARMACOKINETICS
Onset, 20 to 40 seconds; duration, 5 to 12 minutes.
Distribution: Probably dispersed throughout body tissues. Unknown if drug crosses the placental barrier or appears in breast milk.
Metabolism: Probably metabolized rapidly.
Excretion: In urine and feces in 24 to 48 hours.

CLINICAL CONSIDERATIONS
• Osmolality: 20 mg/ml is 159 mOsm/kg.
• Establish an adequate airway before giving drug; prevent aspiration of vomitus by placing patient on his side.
• Delay giving drug for at least 10 minutes after stopping general anesthetics, which are known to sensitize the myocardium.
• Drug has a narrow margin of safety. Don't use as an analeptic or with mechanical ventilation.
• Monitor blood pressure, pulse rate, and deep tendon reflexes.

• If sudden hypotension or dyspnea develops, stop drug.
• In COPD patients, draw samples for blood gas analysis before doxapram and oxygen administration, then at least every 30 minutes.
• Early signs of overdose include excessive pressor effects and skeletal muscle activity, tachycardia, and hyperactive deep tendon reflexes. Such signs may indicate that dosage or infusion rate needs to be adjusted. Seizures, a more serious sign, don't usually occur at the recommended dosage; nevertheless, keep anticonvulsants, oxygen, and resuscitation equipment available.

PATIENT TEACHING
• Instruct patient to report promptly all musculoskeletal adverse reactions and shortness of breath.
• Explain use and administration of drug to patient and family.
• Encourage patient and family to ask questions and express concerns.

doxorubicin hydrochloride (hydroxydaunomycin hydrochloride)
Adriamycin PFS, Adriamycin RDF, Rubex

Pharmacologic class: antineoplastic antibiotic (cell cycle–phase nonspecific)
Therapeutic class: antineoplastic
Pregnancy risk category: D
pH: 2.5 to 4.5 for solution products, 3.8 to 6.5 for lyophilized product reconstituted with normal saline solution

INDICATIONS & DOSAGES
➤ **Solid tumors, including carcinomas, soft-tissue and osteogenic sarcomas, breast carcinoma, ovarian, transitional cell bladder carcinoma,**

small-cell lung carcinoma, gastric carcinoma, neuroblastoma, Wilms' tumor, lymphomas, acute lymphocytic leukemia, acute myelocytic leukemia—

Adults: 60 to 75 mg/m² I.V. as a single dose at 21-day intervals; 20 mg/m² weekly; or 25 to 30 mg/m²/day for 2 or 3 consecutive days q 3 to 4 weeks. Total lifetime dose shouldn't exceed 550 mg/m² because of risk of cumulative cardiotoxicity.

Children: 30 mg/m² I.V. for 3 consecutive days q 4 weeks.

Adjust-a-dose: Reduce dosage in hepatic impairment. If bilirubin level is 1.2 to 3 mg/dl, reduce dosage by 50%; if above 3 mg/dl, reduce dosage by 75%.

ADMINISTRATION

Direct injection: Using a 21G or 23G winged-tip needle, inject drug into a large vein over 3 to 5 minutes. Or, inject drug into tubing of free-flowing I.V. line containing normal saline solution or D₅W. Avoid injecting into veins over joints or extremities with compromised venous return or impaired lymphatic drainage. Flush administration set with normal saline solution after use.

Intermittent infusion: Not recommended.

Continuous infusion: Not recommended.

PREPARATION & STORAGE

To avoid mutagenic, teratogenic, and carcinogenic risks when preparing doxorubicin, use a biological containment cabinet during preparation, wear a mask to avoid inhaling drug particles or solution, and put on gloves to avoid skin contact. If drug comes in contact with skin or mucosa, immediately wash the area with soap and water.

Dispose of needles, vials, and unused drug correctly. Use syringes with luer-lock fittings to prevent drug leakage. Avoid contamination of work surfaces. Clean spills with 5% sodium hypochlorite (household bleach) to inactivate drug.

Doxorubicin is supplied as a powder in 10-mg, 20-mg, 50-mg, 100-mg, and 150-mg vials. Drug is also supplied as aqueous solution in 10 mg, 20 mg, 50 mg, 75 mg, 150 mg and 200 mg in preservative-free vials. Reconstitute with normal saline solution, D₅W, or sterile water for injection. Avoid using diluents containing preservatives or having a pH less than 3 or greater than 7.

To reconstitute drug, add 5 ml of diluent to 10-mg vial, 10 ml to 20-mg vial, 25 ml to 50-mg vial, 50 ml to the 100-mg vial, or 75 ml to the 150-mg vial. When using sterile water injection, add 2 to 3 volumes of normal saline solution to drug to make solution isotonic. Shake vial to help dissolve drug.

Store in a dry place, away from sunlight. Reconstituted drug remains stable for 24 hours at room temperature and for 48 hours at 39° to 50° F (4° to 10° C). For best results, use within 8 hours of reconstitution. Discard unused drug.

Incompatibilities

Allopurinol, aluminum, aminophylline, bacteriostatic diluents, cefepime, dexamethasone sodium phosphate, diazepam, fluorouracil, furosemide, ganciclovir, heparin sodium, hydrocortisone sodium succinate, piperacillin with tazobactam.

CONTRAINDICATIONS & CAUTIONS

● Contraindicated in patients with myelosuppression and in those who have received a total lifetime dose of 550 mg/m². Avoid giving a lifetime dose exceeding 400 mg/m² to those who have received chest radiation therapy, a related tetracyclic chemotherapeutic drug such as daunorubicin, or cyclophosphamide. Data suggest that cardiotoxicity may occur at doses lower than recommended cumulative limit.

• Contraindicated in those with chickenpox or herpes zoster infection because of risk of severe generalized disease.

• Use cautiously in patients with gout or a history of urate stones because of increased risk of hyperuricemia, in those with heart disease because of increased risk of cardiotoxicity, and in those with bone marrow depression because of increased risk of myelosuppression.

ADVERSE REACTIONS
CNS: fever, peripheral neuropathy, dizziness, depression, anxiety, confusion, *asthenia.*
CV: *acute cardiotoxicity, heart failure (dose-related),* phlebosclerosis, tachycardia, facial flushing.
EENT: conjunctivitis, sore throat.
GI: *anorexia, diarrhea,* esophagitis, *GI bleeding,* nausea, vomiting, ulceration and necrosis of colon in patient with acute myelocytic leukemia who is receiving cytarabine, *stomatitis, constipation.*
Hematologic: anemia, secondary acute myeloid leukemia, *leukopenia with nadir 10 to 14 days after administration, thrombocytopenia, myelosuppression.*
Metabolic: hyperuricemia.
Musculoskeletal: joint pain.
Respiratory: dyspnea.
Skin: *alopecia,* hyperpigmented nail beds, radiation recall—darkened or reddened skin and severe dermatitis or mucositis in previously irradiated areas, urticaria, severe soft-tissue damage from extravasation.
Other: swollen feet and legs, chills, *anaphylaxis.*

INTERACTIONS
Drug-drug. *Cyclophosphamide, dactinomycin, daunorubicin, mito-*

mycin: Increases risk of cardiotoxicity. Monitor patient closely.
Cyclosporine: May induce coma or seizures. Avoid using together.
Digoxin: May decrease digoxin level. Monitor level closely.
Hepatotoxic drugs: Increases risk of toxic reaction. Monitor patient closely.
Myelosuppressants, radiation therapy: Increases risk of bone marrow depression or, if chest has been irradiated, of cardiomyopathy. Monitor patient closely.
Phenytoin: May decrease phenytoin level. Monitor level closely.
Streptozocin: May prolong half-life of doxorubicin. May need to adjust dosage.
Vaccines with live virus: Increases risk of neurotoxicity. Avoid using together.
Drug-herb. *Green tea:* May enhance the antitumorigenic activity of doxorubicin. Monitor patient.

EFFECTS ON LAB TEST RESULTS
• May increase uric acid level.
• May decrease WBC and platelet counts.

ACTION
Decreases DNA, RNA, and protein synthesis by binding to DNA through intercalation between base pairs. Acts in the S phase of the cell cycle.

PHARMACOKINETICS
Peaks at 90% at 24 hours.
Distribution: Throughout plasma and tissues, especially in the heart, liver, kidneys, and lungs. Drug doesn't cross blood-brain barrier or concentrate in CSF. It may cross the placental barrier and does appear in breast milk.
Metabolism: Rapidly in liver and other tissues, a first-pass effect. The major metabolite, doxorubicinol, has antineoplastic effects.
Excretion: Primarily in bile. 10% to 20% in feces in 24 hours and 40% to 50% in 7 days; 6% in urine after 5 days.

Half-life is multiphasic after I.V. injection; initial phase, about 5 minutes, with a terminal half-life of 20 to 48 hours.

CLINICAL CONSIDERATIONS
● Osmolality: 2 mg/ml in sterile water is 280 mOsm/kg.
● *Alert:* Don't confuse doxorubicin with daunorubicin.
● Prevent or minimize uric acid nephropathy through hydrating patient, alkalizing urine, or giving allopurinol.
● Give antibiotics to patients with leukopenia or neutropenia who develop infection.
● Avoid extravasation, which may be asymptomatic. If extravasation occurs, stop infusion, apply ice to area, notify prescriber, and consider use of local corticosteroids. Restart infusion at another site.
● If patient develops facial flushing or local erythema, reduce administration rate.
● Some degree of toxic reaction occurs with a therapeutic response.
● Regularly monitor ECG in patients who have received 300 mg/m² or more of drug. Also monitor CBC and liver function test results for signs of toxic reaction.
● Watch for early signs of heart failure; many drug-induced conditions don't respond to therapy. If heart failure occurs, give cardiac glycosides, diuretics, and peripheral vasodilators, as ordered.
● Cardiotoxicity may be more common in children younger than age 2, in geriatric patients, in patients who have received chest radiation therapy, and in those whose cumulative dose exceeds 550 mg/m².
● Signs and symptoms of overdose include mucositis, leukopenia, and thrombocytopenia.
● If overdose occurs, give antibiotics, platelets, and granulocyte transfusions, as ordered. Treat mucositis symptomatically.

PATIENT TEACHING
● Advise patient to avoid exposure to people with infections.
● Tell patient that urine and stools may be red for 1 to 2 days and that reversible alopecia may occur.
● Tell patient to report adverse reactions promptly.
● Explain use and administration of drug to patient and family.
● Encourage patient and family to ask questions and express concerns.
● Tell patient to report discomfort at I.V. site.
● Tell patient to watch for signs and symptoms of infection, such as fever, sore throat, and fatigue, and of bleeding, such as easy bruising, nosebleeds, bleeding gums, and melena. Tell him to take his temperature daily.

doxorubicin hydrochloride liposomal
Caelyx ◇ , Doxil

Pharmacologic class: anthracycline
Therapeutic class: antineoplastic
Pregnancy risk category: D
pH: 6.5

INDICATIONS & DOSAGES
➤ **Metastatic carcinoma of the ovary in patients with disease that's refractory to both paclitaxel- and platinum-based chemotherapy regimens—**
Adults: 50 mg/m² (doxorubicin equivalent) I.V. at an initial infusion rate of 1 mg/minute once every 4 weeks for a minimum of four courses. Continue treatment as long as the patient doesn't progress, shows no evidence of cardiotoxicity, and continues to tolerate treatment. If no infusion-related ad-

verse events are observed, increase infusion rate to complete administration over 1 hour.

➤ **AIDS-related Kaposi's sarcoma in patients with disease that has progressed on prior combination chemotherapy or in patients who are intolerant of such therapy—**
Adults: 20 mg/m² (doxorubicin equivalent) I.V. over 30 minutes, once q 3 weeks, for as long as patient responds satisfactorily and tolerates treatment.
Adjust-a-dose: For patients with impaired hepatic function, reduce dosage as follows: If bilirubin is 1.2 to 3 mg/dl, give one-half normal dose; if bilirubin is greater than 3 mg/dl give one-fourth normal dose.

The recommended dosage changes for managing palmar-plantar erythrodysesthesia, hematologic toxicity, and stomatitis follow.

Palmar-plantar erythrodysesthesia

Grade 1

Symptoms: Mild erythema, swelling, or desquamation not interfering with daily activities

Dosage adjustment: Give previous dose unless patient has experienced a previous grade 3 or 4 skin toxicity. If so, delay up to 2 weeks and decrease dose by 25%. Return to original dose interval.

Grade 2

Symptoms: Erythema, desquamation, or swelling interfering with, but not precluding, normal physical activities; small blisters or ulcerations less than 2 cm in diameter

Dosage adjustment: Delay therapy up to 2 weeks or until resolved to grade 0 to 1. If no resolution after 2 weeks, stop drug.

Grade 3

Symptoms: Blistering, ulceration, or swelling interfering with walking or normal daily activities; patient unable to wear regular clothing

Dosage adjustment: Delay therapy up to 2 weeks or until resolved to grade 0 to 1. Decrease dose by 25% and return to original dose interval. If no resolution after 2 weeks, stop drug.

Grade 4

Symptoms: Diffuse or local disease causing infectious complications, a bedridden state, or hospitalization

Dosage adjustment: Delay therapy up to 2 weeks or until resolved to grade 0 to 1. Decrease dose by 25% and return to original dose interval. If no resolution after 2 weeks, stop drug.

Hematologic toxicity

Grade 1

Absolute neutrophil count (ANC) (cells/mm³): 1,500-1,900
Platelets (cells/mm³): 75,000-150,000

Dosage adjustment: Resume treatment with no dosage reduction.

Grade 2

ANC (cells/mm³): 1,000-1,500
Platelets (cells/mm³): 50,000-75,000

Dosage adjustment: Wait until ANC ≥ 1,500 and platelets ≥ 75,000; resume treatment with no dosage reduction.

Grade 3

ANC (cells/mm³): 500-999
Platelets (cells/mm³): 25,000-50,000

Dosage adjustment: Wait until ANC ≥ 1,500 and platelets ≥ 75,000; resume treatment with no dosage reduction.

Grade 4

ANC (cells/mm³): < 500
Platelets (cells/mm³): < 25,000

Dosage adjustment: Wait until ANC ≥ 1,500 and platelets ≥ 75,000; reduce dose by 25% or continue full dose with cytokine support.

Stomatitis

Grade 1

Symptoms: Painless ulcers, erythema, or mild soreness

Dosage adjustment: Give previous dose unless patient has experienced previous grade 3 or 4 toxicity. If so, delay therapy up to 2 weeks and decrease dose by 25%. Return to original dose interval.

Grade 2

Symptoms: Painful erythema, edema, or ulcers; patient can eat

Dosage adjustment: Delay therapy up to 2 weeks or until resolved to grade 0 to 1. If no resolution after 2 weeks, stop drug.

Grade 3

Symptoms: Painful erythema, edema, or ulcers; patient can't eat

Dosage adjustment: Delay therapy up to 2 weeks or until resolved to grade 0 to 1. Reduce dose by 25% and return to original dose interval. If no resolution after 2 weeks, stop drug.

Grade 4

Symptoms: Requires parenteral or enteral support

Dosage adjustment: Delay therapy up to 2 weeks or until resolved to grade 0 to 1. Decrease dose by 25% and return to original dose interval. If no resolution after 2 weeks, stop drug.

ADMINISTRATION

Don't use with in-line filters.
Direct injection: Don't give I.M., S.C., or I.V. push.
Intermittent infusion: Infuse I.V. over 30 to 60 minutes, depending on the dose.
Continuous infusion: Not recommended.

PREPARATION & STORAGE

Follow procedures for proper handling and disposal of antineoplastics.

Available as 20-mg injection in 10-ml vials.

Dilute appropriate dose, up to a maximum of 90 mg, in 250 ml of D_5W using aseptic technique. Carefully check the label on the I.V. bag before giving. Accidental substitution of Doxil for conventional doxorubicin hydrochloride has resulted in severe adverse effects.

If signs or symptoms of extravasation occur, stop infusion immediately and restart in another vein. Application of ice over the site of extravasation for about 30 minutes may help alleviate local reaction.

Diluted solution should be refrigerated at 36° to 46°F (2° to 8°C) and given within 24 hours.

Incompatibilities
Other I.V. drugs.

CONTRAINDICATIONS & CAUTIONS

● Contraindicated in patients with a history of hypersensitivity reactions to the conventional formulation of the drug or any component in the liposomal formulation.
● Contraindicated in patients who have marked myelosuppression, in those who have received a lifetime cumulative dosage of 550 mg/m^2 or 400 mg/m^2, and in those who have received radiotherapy to the mediastinal area or therapy with other cardiotoxic drugs such as cyclophosphamide.
● Use cautiously in those who have received other anthracyclines. When determining total dosage, figure in any therapy with related compounds such as daunorubicin. Heart failure and cardiomyopathy may occur after therapy is stopped.
● Use in those with history of CV disease only when the benefit outweighs the risk to the patient.

ADVERSE REACTIONS

CNS: *asthenia,* paresthesia, headache, somnolence, dizziness, depression, insomnia, anxiety, malaise, emotional lability, fatigue, fever.

CV: chest pain, hypotension, tachycardia, peripheral edema, cardiomyopathy, *heart failure, arrhythmias,* pericardial effusion.

EENT: *mucous membrane disorder,* mouth ulceration, pharyngitis, rhinitis, conjunctivitis, retinitis, optic neuritis.

GI: *nausea, vomiting, constipation, anorexia, diarrhea,* abdominal pain, dyspepsia, oral candidiasis, enlarged abdomen, esophagitis, dysphagia, *stomatitis,* taste perversion, glossitis.

GU: albuminuria.

Hematologic: *leukopenia, neutropenia, thrombocytopenia, anemia.*

Metabolic: dehydration, weight loss, hypocalcemia, hyperglycemia, hyperbilirubinemia.

Musculoskeletal: myalgia, back pain.

Respiratory: dyspnea, increased cough, pneumonia.

Skin: *rash, alopecia,* dry skin, pruritus, skin discoloration, skin disorder, exfoliative dermatitis, sweating, *palmar-plantar erythrodysesthesia.*

Other: allergic reaction, chills, infection, infusion-related reactions, herpes zoster.

INTERACTIONS

None reported.

EFFECTS ON LAB TEST RESULTS

- May increase PT, INR, bilirubin, and glucose levels. May decrease calcium level.
- May decrease hemoglobin and WBC, neutrophil, platelet counts.

ACTION

Thought to be related to its ability to bind DNA and inhibit nucleic acid synthesis.

PHARMACOKINETICS

Onset, peak, and duration of drug effects unknown.

Distribution: Distributed mostly to vascular fluid. The percentage of drug that's bound to protein is unknown.

Metabolism: Doxorubicinol, the major metabolite of doxorubicin, is detected at very low level in the plasma.

Excretion: Plasma elimination is slow and described as biphasic; half-life about 5 hours in first phase, 55 hours in second phase at doses of 10 to 20 mg/m^2.

CLINICAL CONSIDERATIONS

- *Alert:* Drug exhibits unique pharmacokinetic properties compared to conventional doxorubicin hydrochloride and shouldn't be substituted on a milligram-per-milligram basis.
- Drug may potentiate the toxic effects of other antineoplastics. Evaluate patient's hepatic function before therapy, and adjust dosage accordingly.
- Monitor cardiac function closely by endomyocardial biopsy, echocardiography, or gated radionuclide scans. If results indicate possible cardiac injury, the benefit of continued therapy must be weighed against the risk of myocardial injury.
- Monitor CBC, including platelets, before each dose and frequently throughout therapy. Leukopenia is usually transient. Hematologic toxicity may require that dosage be reduced or suspended or therapy be delayed. Persistent severe myelosuppression may result in superinfection or hemorrhage. Patient may require granulocyte colony-stimulating factor or granulocyte-macrophage colony-stimulating factor to support blood counts.
- Monitor patient carefully during drug infusion. Acute infusion-associated reactions, such as flushing, shortness of breath, facial swelling, headache, chills, back pain, tightness in the chest

or throat, or hypotension, may occur. These reactions resolve over several hours to a day once the infusion is stopped. The reaction may resolve by slowing the infusion rate.

PATIENT TEACHING
● Tell patient to notify prescriber if he experiences symptoms of hand-foot syndrome, such as tingling or burning, redness, flaking, bothersome swelling, small blisters, or small sores on the palms of his hands or soles of his feet.
● Advise patient to report signs and symptoms of stomatitis, such as painful redness, swelling, or sores in his mouth.
● Advise patient to avoid exposure to people with infections. Tell him to report fever of 100.5° F (38° C) or higher.
● Tell patient to report nausea, vomiting, tiredness, weakness, rash, or mild hair loss.
● Advise any woman of childbearing age to avoid pregnancy during therapy.

---

doxycycline hyclate
Doxy 100, Doxy 200

Pharmacologic class: tetracycline
Therapeutic class: antibiotic
Pregnancy risk category: D
pH: 1.8 to 3.3 for reconstituted solutions

INDICATIONS & DOSAGES
➤ **Infections caused by susceptible organisms when oral route can't be used**—
Adults and children older than age 8 weighing more than 45 kg (99 lb): 100 mg I.V. q 12 hours on day 1, then 100 to 200 mg/day, depending on severity of infection.
Children older than age 8 weighing 45 kg or less: 2.2 mg/kg I.V. q 12 hours on day 1, then 2.2 to 4.4 mg/kg/day, depending on severity of infection.
➤ **Acute pelvic inflammatory disease when *Neisseria gonorrhoeae* or *Chlamydia trachomatis* infection is suspected**—
Adults: 100 mg I.V. q 12 hours, plus cefoxitin 2 g q 6 hours, daily for at least 4 days and then substitute P.O. doxycycline.
➤ **Adjunct to other antibiotics for inhalation, GI, and oropharyngeal anthrax**—
Adults: 100 mg I.V. q 12 hours, initially, until susceptibility test results are known. Switch to 100 mg P.O. b.i.d. when appropriate. Treat for 60 days total.
Children older than age 8 weighing more than 45 kg: 100 mg I.V. q 12 hours, then switch to 100 mg P.O. b.i.d. when appropriate. Treat for 60 days total.
Children older than age 8 weighing 45 kg or less: 2.2 mg/kg I.V. q 12 hours, then switch to 2.2 mg/kg P.O. b.i.d. when appropriate. Treat for 60 days total.
Children age 8 and younger: 2.2 mg/kg I.V. q 12 hours, then switch to 2.2 mg/kg P.O. b.i.d. when appropriate. Treat for 60 days total.

ADMINISTRATION
Direct injection: Not used.
Intermittent infusion: Infuse 100 mg (0.5 mg/ml) over 1 to 4 hours, depending on dose. Watch for evidence of extravasation.
Continuous infusion: Not used.

PREPARATION & STORAGE
Available as sterile powder in 100-mg and 200-mg vials.
    Reconstitute with sterile water for injection or other compatible solution. Use 10 ml/100 mg of drug. Further dilute to a concentration of 0.1 to 1 mg/ml using suitable diluent, such as normal saline solution, D_5W, Ringer's in-

jection, invert sugar 10% in water, lactated Ringer's injection, dextrose 5% in lactated Ringer's injection, Normosol-M in dextrose 5%, Normosol-R in dextrose 5%, Plasma-Lyte 56 in dextrose 5%, or Plasma-Lyte 148 in dextrose 5%.

Before reconstitution, store at room temperature. After reconstitution, dilutions using normal saline solution or D_5W remain stable for 48 hours at room temperature when protected from direct sunlight. Other appropriately diluted solutions retain potency for 12 hours if kept at room temperature and for up to 72 hours if refrigerated and protected from light. To ensure stability, complete infusions within 6 hours.

When frozen immediately after reconstitution, solutions at concentrations of 10 mg/ml are stable for 8 weeks. Once solution is thawed, don't refreeze.

Incompatibilities
Allopurinol; cefmetazole; drugs unstable in acidic solutions, such as barbiturates; erythromycin lactobionate; heparin; meropenem; nafcillin; penicillin G potassium; piperacillin with tazobactam; riboflavin; and sulfonamides.

CONTRAINDICATIONS & CAUTIONS
• Contraindicated in those hypersensitive to tetracyclines.
• Contraindicated during bone and tooth development, that is, in the last half of pregnancy and in children younger than age 8, because drug may cause permanent tooth discoloration and enamel defects and may retard bone growth.
• Use cautiously in those exposed to direct sunlight because of risk of photosensitivity.

ADVERSE REACTIONS
CNS: *benign intracranial hypertension in adults, which resolves when drug is stopped;* bulging fontanels in infants; dizziness.
CV: thrombophlebitis.
EENT: darkened or discolored tongue, dysphagia, glossitis, unusual thirst.
GI: abdominal discomfort, anorexia, bulky and loose stools, diarrhea, flatulence, nausea, pseudomembranous colitis.
GU: itching and inflammatory anogenital lesions, urinary frequency.
Hematologic: eosinophilia, hemolytic anemia, *neutropenia, thrombocytopenia.*
Skin: exfoliative dermatitis, discolored nails, *maculopapular rash, erythematous rash,* photosensitivity.
Other: superinfection, *anaphylaxis,* Jarisch-Herxheimer reaction in brucellosis or spirochetal infections.

INTERACTIONS
Drug-drug. *Anticoagulants:* Depresses plasma prothrombin activity. Monitor PT and INR; anticoagulant dosage may need to be adjusted.
Barbiturates, carbamazepine, phenytoin: Decreases doxycycline level. Monitor patient closely.
Hormonal contraceptives: Decreases effectiveness with breakthrough bleeding. Recommend use of a nonhormonal form of birth control.
Penicillins: Impairs bactericidal action. Give penicillin 2 to 3 hours before doxycycline.
Drug-lifestyle. *Alcohol use:* Decreases antibiotic effect. Discourage use.
Sun exposure: May cause photosensitivity reactions. Advise patient to avoid excessive sunlight exposure.

EFFECTS ON LAB TEST RESULTS
• May increase BUN and liver enzyme levels.

● May increase eosinophil count. May decrease hemoglobin and platelet, neutrophil, and WBC counts.

● May falsely elevate results of fluorometric test for urine catecholamines. May cause false-negative results in urine glucose tests using glucose oxidase reagent (Diastix or Chemstrip uG). Parenteral form may cause false-positive Clinitest result.

ACTION

Primarily bacteriostatic, doxycycline inhibits protein synthesis by preventing transfer RNA from binding to its messenger RNA complex. Its broad spectrum of activity includes many gram-positive bacteria, such as *Actinomyces israelii, Arachnia propionica, Bacillus anthracis, Clostridium perfringens, C. tetani, Listeria monocytogenes, Nocardia, Propionibacterium acnes,* and some strains of staphylococci and streptococci.

Drug is effective against the gram-negative bacteria *Bartonella bacilliformis, Bordetella pertussis, Brucella, Calymmatobacterium granulomatis, Campylobacter fetus, Francisella tularensis, Haemophilus ducreyi, H. influenzae, Legionella pneumophila, Leptotrichia buccalis, Neisseria gonorrhoeae, N. meningitidis, Pasteurella multocida, Pseudomonas mallei, P. pseudomallei, Shigella, Spirillum minus, Streptobacillus moniliformis, Vibrio cholerae, V. parahaemolyticus, Yersinia enterocolitica, Y. pestis,* and some strains of *Acinetobacter, Bacteroides, Enterobacter aerogenes, Escherichia coli,* and *Klebsiella.*

Drug is also effective against *Borrelia recurrentis, Chlamydia psittaci, C. trachomatis, Coxiella burnetii, Fusobacterium nucleatum, Leptospira, Mycobacterium fortuitum, Mycoplasma hominis, M. pneumoniae, Rickettsia akari, R. prowazekii, R. rickettsii, R. tsutsugamushi, R. typhi, Treponema pallidum, T. pertenue,* and *Ureaplasma urealyticum.*

PHARMACOKINETICS

Drug level peaks immediately after infusion.

Distribution: Widespread to most body fluids and bound to protein in varying degrees. Drug tends to localize in reticuloendothelial cells of the liver, spleen, and bone marrow. It crosses the blood-brain barrier; the CSF level reaches about 25% of the serum level, the prostatic level about 60%. Therapeutic levels appear in the eye. Drug crosses the placental barrier and appears in breast milk.

Metabolism: Not metabolized, but partly deactivated in the intestine by chelate formation.

Excretion: Within 48 hours, 20% to 26% of drug is eliminated in urine via glomerular filtration and 20% to 40% is removed in feces. In normal renal function, half-life is 14 to 17 hours after a single dose and 22 to 24 hours after multiple doses.

CLINICAL CONSIDERATIONS

● Osmolality: 10 mg/ml in sterile water is 507 mOsm/kg; 1 mg/ml is 292 mOsm/kg in D_5W and 310 mOsm/kg in normal saline solution.

● Obtain specimens for culture and sensitivity before giving first dose. Therapy may begin before results are available.

● If syphilitic infection is suspected when treating other venereal diseases, perform a dark-field examination before therapy. Repeat blood serology monthly for at least 4 months.

● Cutaneous anthrax with signs of systemic involvement, extensive edema, or lesions on the head or neck require I.V. therapy and a multidrug approach.

● Additional antimicrobials for anthrax multidrug regimens can include rifampin, vancomycin, penicillin, ampicillin,

chloramphenicol, imipenem, clindamycin, and clarithromycin.
• Steroids may be considered as adjunctive therapy for anthrax patients with severe edema and for meningitis, based on experience with bacterial meningitis of other etiologies.
• If meningitis is suspected, doxycycline would be less optimal than ciprofloxacin because of poor CSF penetration.
• Ciprofloxacin or doxycycline is first-line therapy for anthrax. Amoxicillin 500 mg P.O. t.i.d. for adults and 80 mg/kg/day divided every 8 hours for children is an option for completion of therapy after clinical improvement. Follow current Centers for Disease Control and Prevention recommendations for anthrax.
• If diarrhea persists during therapy, collect stool specimens to detect possible pseudomembranous colitis.
• Watch for signs of overgrowth. Check patient's tongue for signs of *Candida* infection, and stress good oral hygiene.
• Pregnant women and immunocompromised patients should receive the usual doses and regimens for anthrax.
• In pregnant women adverse effect on fetus' developing teeth and bones are dose-limited; therefore, doxycycline might be used for a short time (7 to 14 days) before 6 months' gestation.
• Hemodialysis doesn't remove drug.

PATIENT TEACHING
• Advise patient to report discomfort at I.V. site.
• Tell patient to report signs and symptoms of superinfection.
• If patient is being treated for a sexually transmitted disease, counsel him regarding the indication for HIV antibody testing.

droperidol
Inapsine

Pharmacologic class: butyrophenone derivative
Therapeutic class: tranquilizer
Pregnancy risk category: C
pH: 3.3 to 3.8

INDICATIONS & DOSAGES
➤ **Adjunct in regional anesthesia—**
Adults: 2.5 to 5 mg.
➤ **Nausea and vomiting during surgical or diagnostic procedure—**
Adults: 2.5 mg I.V. Additional doses of 1.25 mg may be given if needed.
Children ages 2 to 12 years: 0.1 mg/kg I.V.
Adjust-a-dose: Reduce initial dose in geriatric, debilitated, or high-risk patients. Adjust dose based on patient's response.

ADMINISTRATION
Direct injection: Inject directly into vein in small incremental boluses or into an established I.V. line containing a free-flowing solution.
Intermittent infusion: Not recommended.
Continuous infusion: Not recommended.

PREPARATION & STORAGE
Available in concentrations of 2.5 mg/ml in 1-ml, 2-ml, and 5-ml ampules and in 10-ml multidose vials.
Drug is compatible with all I.V. solutions.
Protect from light and store at room temperature.

Incompatibilities
Allopurinol, barbiturates, cefepime, cefmetazole, fluorouracil, foscarnet, furosemide, heparin, leucovorin,

methotrexate sodium, nafcillin, piperacillin with tazobactam.

CONTRAINDICATIONS & CAUTIONS
• Contraindicated in those hypersensitive to the drug.
• Contraindicated in patients with prolonged QT interval, including those with congenital long QT interval syndrome.
• Use cautiously in those at risk of developing QT interval prolongation syndrome (heart failure, bradycardia, cardiac hypertrophy, hypokalemia, hypomagnesemia, or use of diuretic or other drug that prolongs QT interval).
• Use cautiously in geriatric, debilitated, and other high-risk patients. As ordered, reduce the dosage, titrating slowly according to patient response.
• Use cautiously in those with hepatic or renal impairment because of increased risk of toxic reaction.
• Use cautiously in hypotensive or hypovolemic patients because drug may exacerbate hypotension.

ADVERSE REACTIONS
CNS: *neuroleptic malignant syndrome,* akathisia, anxiety, depression, dizziness, dystonia, emergence delirium, nightmares, hallucinations, hyperactivity, oculogyric crisis with extended neck, flexed arms, fine tremors, postoperative drowsiness, restlessness.
CV: severe hypotension with high doses, tachycardia, mild to moderate transient hypotension, *prolonged QT interval, torsades de pointes, cardiac arrest, ventricular tachycardia.*
EENT: upward rotation of eyes.
Respiratory: *respiratory depression with high doses, bronchospasm, laryngospasm.*
Skin: facial sweating.
Other: chills.

INTERACTIONS
Drug-drug. *CNS depressants:* Deepens CNS depression. Dosage may need to be reduced.
Drugs that prolong QT interval (class I or III antiarrhythmics, certain antihistamines, antimalarials, calcium channel blockers, certain neuroleptics, antidepressants): Increases risk of prolonged QT interval. Avoid using together.
Epinephrine: Paradoxically lowers blood pressure because of droperidol's alpha-blocking action. Monitor patient closely.
Opioid analgesics: Prolongs narcotic effect and respiratory depression. Use together cautiously.

EFFECTS ON LAB TEST RESULTS
• May cause abnormal EEG patterns for up to 12 hours. May reduce pulmonary artery pressure.

ACTION
Blocks central dopaminergic receptors, producing sedation and antiemetic effects, and alpha receptors.

PHARMACOKINETICS
Onset, 3 to 10 minutes; duration, 2 to 4 hours for sedation.
Distribution: Crosses the blood-brain and placental barriers.
Metabolism: In the liver.
Excretion: In urine and feces.

CLINICAL CONSIDERATIONS
• *Alert:* Use drug only in patients who have failed to respond to other drugs.
• Keep resuscitation equipment available during administration.
• *Alert:* Obtain 12-lead ECG on all patients before administration. Don't give drug if QTc exceeds 440 msec (males) or 450 msec (females). Monitor ECG for 2 to 3 hours after completing therapy to detect signs and symptoms of arrhythmias.

Reactions may be *common,* uncommon, ***life-threatening,*** or COMMON AND LIFE-THREATENING.

• When used as an anesthetic, drug should be given only by staff specially trained in giving I.V. anesthetics and managing their adverse reactions.
• Move and position patient slowly during anesthesia to avoid orthostatic hypotension.
• Watch for signs of an extrapyramidal reaction, such as akathisia or dystonia. Call prescriber immediately if such signs occur.
• When giving an opioid analgesic with droperidol, reduce opioid dosage by one-fourth to one-third for up to 12 hours or until patient becomes fully alert.
• Drug has been used experimentally to prevent or reduce nausea and vomiting caused by chemotherapeutic drugs, especially cisplatin.
• If overdose occurs, provide supportive care. Maintain airway patency and give vasopressors to correct hypotension. Observe patient for 24 hours, maintain warmth, and give fluids.

PATIENT TEACHING
• Tell patient to report adverse reactions promptly.
• Explain use and administration of drug to patient and family.

drotrecogin alfa (activated)
Xigris

Pharmacologic class: recombinant serine protease of human activated protein C
Therapeutic class: antithrombotic
Pregnancy risk category: C

INDICATIONS & DOSAGES
➤ **To reduce risk of death in patients with severe sepsis (from acute organ dysfunction)—**
Adults: 24 mcg/kg/hour I.V. infusion for 96 hours.

ADMINISTRATION
Direct injection: Not recommended.
Intermittent infusion: Not recommended.
Continuous infusion: Give via a dedicated I.V. line or a central venous catheter. Infuse at 24 mcg/kg/hour for 96 hours.

PREPARATION & STORAGE
Available as a sterile, white to off-white powder contained in 5- and 20-mg single-use vials.
    Reconstitute 5-mg vials with 2.5 ml sterile water for injection and 20-mg vials with 10 ml of sterile water for injection. The resulting concentration is about 2 mg/ml. Gently swirl each vial until powder is completely dissolved; don't shake or invert the vial. Further dilute the reconstituted solution with sterile normal saline injection. If the reconstituted vial isn't used immediately, it may be held at room temperature 59° to 86° F (15° to 30° C), but must be used within 3 hours.
    When adding the drug to the I.V bag, direct the stream to the side of the bag to minimize agitation of the solution. Gently invert the infusion bag to obtain a homogenous solution. Don't transport the infusion bag between locations using mechanical delivery systems. I.V. administration must be completed within 12 hours after the I.V. solution is prepared. Inspect for particulate matter and discoloration before giving.
    When using an I.V. pump to give the drug, the solution of reconstituted drotrecogin alfa is typically diluted into an infusion bag containing sterile normal saline injection to a final concentration between 100 mcg/ml and 200 mcg/ml. When using a syringe pump to give the drug, the reconstituted solution is typically diluted with sterile normal saline injection to a final concentration between 100 mcg/ml and 1,000 mcg/ml. When giving at low con-

centrations (less than about 200 mcg/ml) at low flow rates (less than about 5 ml/hour), the infusion set must be primed for about 15 minutes at a flow rate of about 5 ml/hour.

Store in a refrigerator at 35° to 46° F (2° to 8° C). Don't freeze. Avoid exposing drug to heat or direct sunlight.

Incompatibilities
Other I.V. drugs.

CONTRAINDICATIONS & CAUTIONS
• Contraindicated in patients with active internal bleeding, recent (within 3 months) hemorrhagic stroke, recent (within 2 months) intracranial or intraspinal surgery, severe head trauma, trauma with an increased risk of life-threatening bleeding, presence of an epidural catheter, intracranial neoplasm or mass lesion, or evidence of cerebral herniation.
• *Alert:* The only other solutions that can be given through the same line are normal saline injection, lactated Ringer's injection, dextrose, or dextrose and saline mixtures.
• Drug is also contraindicated in patients hypersensitive to drotrecogin alfa (activated) or any of its components.
• Use cautiously with other drugs that affect hemostasis.
• Consider the increased risk of bleeding in patients taking heparin (15 units/kg/hour or more) and in those with a platelet count less than 30,000 × 10^6/L (even if the platelet count is increased after transfusions), an INR greater than 3, recent (within 6 weeks) GI bleeding, recent administration (within 3 days) of thrombolytic therapy, recent administration (within 7 days) of oral anticoagulants or glycoprotein IIb/IIIa inhibitors, recent administration (within 7 days) of aspirin (more than 650 mg/day) or other platelet inhibitors, recent (within 3 months) ischemic stroke, intracranial arteriovenous malformation or aneurysm, bleeding diathesis, chron-

ic severe hepatic disease, any other condition in which bleeding constitutes a significant hazard (such as severe coagulopathy or severe thrombocytopenia) or would be particularly difficult to manage because of its location.
• Use drug in pregnant women only if clearly needed.
• It isn't known whether the drug appears in breast milk or is absorbed systemically after ingestion. Advise women not to breast-feed during therapy.

ADVERSE REACTIONS
Hematologic: *hemorrhage.*

INTERACTIONS
Drug-drug. *Drugs that affect hemostasis:* Increases risk of bleeding. Use together cautiously.

EFFECTS ON LAB TEST RESULTS
• May prolong PTT.
• May cause falsely reduced factor VIII, IX, and XI levels.

ACTION
The antisepsis action of drotrecogin alfa is unknown. The drug is thought to produce dose-dependent reductions in D-dimer and IL-6. Also thought to exert an anti-inflammatory effect by inhibiting human tumor necrosis factor production and by limiting the thrombin-induced inflammatory responses.

PHARMACOKINETICS
Onset, rapid.
Distribution: Steady-state levels achieved within 2 hours after starting infusion.
Metabolism: No information available.
Excretion: No information available.

CLINICAL CONSIDERATIONS
• If the infusion is interrupted, restart at the 24 mcg/kg/hour infusion rate. Dose escalation, bolus doses, and dose ad-

justment based on clinical or laboratory findings aren't recommended.

• Stop drug 2 hours before invasive surgery. After hemostasis is achieved, consider restarting drug 12 hours after major invasive procedures or surgery or immediately after uncomplicated less invasive procedures.

• Because drug may prolong PTT, it can't be reliably used to assess coagulopathy status during infusion. Drug has minimal effect on the PT, however, so PT can be used to monitor coagulopathy status in these patients.

• Monitor patient for allergic reactions.

• Monitor patient closely for bleeding. If significant bleeding occurs, immediately stop the infusion.

PATIENT TEACHING

• Inform patient of the potential adverse reactions.

• Instruct patient to promptly report signs of bleeding.

• Advise patient that bleeding may occur for up to 28 days after treatment.

E

edetate calcium disodium (calcium EDTA)
Calcium Disodium Versenate

Pharmacologic class: chelate
Therapeutic class: heavy metal antagonist
Pregnancy risk category: B
pH: 6.5 to 8

INDICATIONS & DOSAGES
➤ **To diagnose lead poisoning (calcium EDTA mobilization test)—**
Adults and children: 500 mg/m² I.V. Maximum dosage, 1 g by I.V. infusion over 1 hour.
➤ **Acute and chronic lead poisoning and lead encephalopathy—**
Adults and children with lead level exceeding 70 mcg/dl: 50 mg/kg/day I.V. over several hours or by continuous infusion, with dimercaprol, for 3 to 5 days. Second course may be necessary.
Asymptomatic children with lead level of 45 to 69 mcg/dl: 1 g/m² daily I.V. by continuous infusion or intermittent infusion. Second course may be necessary.
➤ **Lead nephropathy—**
Adults: If creatinine level is 2 mg/dl or less, give 1 g I.V. daily for 5 days; if creatinine level is 2 to 3 mg/dl, give 500 mg I.V. q 24 hours for 5 days; if creatinine level is 3 to 4 mg/dl, give 500 mg I.V. q 48 hours for three doses; and if creatinine level exceeds 4 mg/dl, give 500 mg I.V. once weekly. May need to repeat at 1-month intervals.

➤ **Manganese intoxication ◆—**
Adults: 1 g in 500 ml of D₅W or normal saline solution I.V. over 5 hours once daily for 3 days.

ADMINISTRATION
Direct injection: Not used.
Intermittent infusion: Infuse diluted drug into an established I.V. line at a rate guided by patient's condition. In asymptomatic patients, infuse half the daily dose over at least 1 hour q 12 hours. In symptomatic patients, infuse half the daily dose over at least 2 hours and give the second dose after 6 or more hours.
Continuous infusion: Infuse the single daily dose over 8 to 24 hours.

PREPARATION & STORAGE
Available in 5-ml ampules containing 200 mg/ml.
For infusion, dilute with D₅W or normal saline solution to yield 2 to 4 mg/ml.
Store at room temperature.

Incompatibilities
Amphotericin B, dextrose 10% in water, hydralazine hydrochloride, invert sugar 10% in normal saline solution, invert sugar 10% in water, lactated Ringer's solution, Ringer's injection, 1/6 M sodium lactate.

CONTRAINDICATIONS & CAUTIONS
• Contraindicated in those with severe oliguria or anuria because of drug's nephrotoxic effects.
• Don't use drug to diagnose lead poisoning if patient's lead level exceeds 55 mcg/dl.
• Use extremely cautiously in those with renal impairment because of risk

of nephrotoxicity. Reduce dosage, if needed.
• Use cautiously in those with hypercalcemia because drug may worsen it, and in those with lead encephalopathy because rapid administration may produce a sudden, lethal rise in intracranial pressure (ICP).

ADVERSE REACTIONS
CNS: *suddenly increased ICP in cerebral edema,* headache, fatigue, paresthesia.
CV: *arrhythmias,* hypertension, hypotension, thrombophlebitis.
EENT: nasal congestion, cheilosis.
GI: anorexia, nausea, excessive thirst, vomiting.
GU: hematuria, proteinuria, *renal tubular necrosis leading to fatal nephrosis,* urinary frequency and urgency.
Hematologic: *transient bone marrow depression with prolonged use.*
Metabolic: hypercalcemia, zinc deficiency.
Musculoskeletal: myalgia.
Other: sneezing, sudden fever and chills within 8 hours after infusion, skin and mucous membrane lesions that subside when infusion stops.

INTERACTIONS
Drug-drug. *Adrenocorticosteroids:* Increases risk of nephrotoxicity. Monitor patient closely.
Zinc-insulin preparations: Shortens action because of zinc chelation. Avoid using together.

EFFECTS ON LAB TEST RESULTS
• May increase AST, ALT, and calcium levels.
• May decrease hemoglobin.
• May cause T-wave inversion on ECG.

ACTION
Divalent and trivalent metals, especially lead, displace calcium from edetate calcium disodium to form stable soluble complexes.

PHARMACOKINETICS
Onset, 1 hour; duration, unknown.
Distribution: Mainly in extracellular fluid. Drug doesn't penetrate erythrocytes or enter CSF in appreciable amounts. Unknown if drug crosses the placental barrier or if it appears in breast milk.
Metabolism: None.
Excretion: Rapidly removed from urine by glomerular filtration. About 50% is eliminated in 1 hour, 95% in 24 hours. Drug is excreted unchanged or as metal chelates. Half-life, 20 to 60 minutes.

CLINICAL CONSIDERATIONS
• Strict adherence to dosage schedule is essential because of potentially fatal drug effects. Each course of therapy should last no more than 7 days, with a 2-week interval between courses.
• To avoid toxic reaction, use with dimercaprol.
• Before first dose, establish urine flow by giving I.V. dextrose 10% with mannitol if needed. If urine flow isn't established after 3 hours of fluid infusion, use edetate calcium disodium with hemodialysis. Once urine flow is established, maintain infusion rate to supply basal fluid and electrolyte requirements only. Stop drug when urine flow ceases.
• If drug is given by continuous infusion, stop for 1 hour before checking lead level.
• Monitor liver function test results and electrolyte levels.
• Monitor BUN level before and during therapy to detect renal impairment.
• Monitor ECG during therapy to detect arrhythmias.
• Perform urinalysis daily. Check for increased protein levels, erythrocytes, or large renal epithelial cells to help determine if drug should be stopped.

• *Alert:* Don't confuse calcium EDTA with EDTA.

PATIENT TEACHING
• Explain use and administration of drug to patient and family.
• To facilitate lead excretion, encourage patient to drink fluids unless he has lead encephalopathy.

edetate disodium (EDTA)
Endrate

Pharmacologic class: chelate
Therapeutic class: heavy metal antagonist
Pregnancy risk category: C
pH: 6.5 to 7.5

INDICATIONS & DOSAGES
➤ **Emergency treatment of hypercalcemia—**
Adults: 50 mg/kg/day I.V. to maximum of 3 g/day.
Children ◆ *:* 40 to 70 mg/kg/day or 50 mg/kg I.V. in single dose.
➤ **Cardiac glycoside–induced arrhythmias—**
Adults: 15 mg/kg I.V. hourly, not to exceed 60 mg/kg/day.
Children ◆ *:* 15 mg/kg I.V. hourly, not to exceed 60 mg/kg/day.

ADMINISTRATION
Direct injection: Not recommended.
Intermittent infusion: Not recommended.
Continuous infusion: Infuse diluted solution over 4 to 6 hours or, if necessary, over 3 to 4 hours. Take care not to exceed patient's cardiac reserve. Watch for irritation and infiltration; extravasation can cause tissue damage and necrosis.

PREPARATION & STORAGE
Available in 20-ml ampules containing 150 mg/ml.
Dilute in 500 ml of D_5W or normal saline solution. Don't exceed 3% concentration (30 mg/ml).
Store at room temperature, and protect from freezing.

Incompatibilities
None reported.

CONTRAINDICATIONS & CAUTIONS
• Contraindicated in those with renal disease or reduced glomerular filtration because of risk of nephrotoxicity.
• Contraindicated in those with seizures or intracranial lesions because drug-induced hypocalcemia may reduce seizure threshold.
• Avoid use in those with active tuberculosis or healed calcified tubular lesions because drug may worsen these conditions.
• Use cautiously in those with cardiac disease because drug affects myocardial contractility.
• Use cautiously in those with diabetes mellitus because drug may reduce glucose levels and in those with hypokalemia or hypocalcemia because drug may worsen these conditions.

ADVERSE REACTIONS
CNS: headache, fatigue, weakness, malaise, transient circumoral paresthesia, fever, *seizures.*
CV: hypotension, thrombophlebitis.
GI: abdominal cramps, unusual thirst, anorexia, diarrhea, nausea, vomiting.
GU: glycosuria, hyperuricemia, *nephrotoxicity.*
Hematologic: anemia.
Metabolic: *severe hypocalcemia.*
Musculoskeletal: back pain, muscle cramps.
Skin: erythematous skin eruptions, *exfoliative dermatitis,* pain or burning at infusion site.

Reactions may be *common,* uncommon, *life-threatening,* or COMMON AND LIFE-THREATENING.

Other: calcium embolization, chills, numbness.

INTERACTIONS
Drug-drug. *Zinc-insulin preparations:* Shortens duration because of zinc chelation. Avoid using together.

EFFECTS ON LAB TEST RESULTS
• May decrease calcium, glucose, magnesium, and alkaline phosphatase levels.
• May decrease hemoglobin and hematocrit.

ACTION
By forming chelates with calcium and divalent and trivalent metals, drug increases urinary excretion of calcium, magnesium, zinc, and other trace elements. Also exerts a negative inotropic effect on the heart.

PHARMACOKINETICS
Drug level peaks immediately after drug is given.
Distribution: Unknown. Drug doesn't enter CSF in appreciable amounts. It's unknown if drug appears in breast milk.
Metabolism: None.
Excretion: Rapidly excreted in urine. About 95% is excreted in 24 hours as calcium chelate. Half-life, 20 to 60 minutes.

CLINICAL CONSIDERATIONS
• Before infusion, evaluate renal function. Monitor BUN levels periodically and urinalysis daily.
• After infusion, keep patient in supine position to avoid orthostatic hypotension.
• Monitor ECG, especially when treating ventricular arrhythmias caused by digitalis toxicity.
• Monitor calcium levels after each dose. Watch for a sudden drop.
• Monitor electrolyte levels in patients with hypokalemia or hypocalcemia.

• **Alert:** Don't confuse EDTA with calcium EDTA.
• Overdose may cause tetany, seizures, severe arrhythmias, and respiratory arrest. If overdose occurs, give I.V. calcium.

PATIENT TEACHING
• Teach patient to report symptoms of electrolyte imbalances, such as muscle cramps, irregular heart rate, and muscle weakness.
• Tell patient to report adverse reactions promptly.
• Explain use and administration of drug to patient and family.

edrophonium chloride
Enlon, Reversol, Tensilon

Pharmacologic class: anticholinesterase
Therapeutic class: cholinergic agonist, diagnostic
Pregnancy risk category: C
pH: 5.4

INDICATIONS & DOSAGES
➤ **Diagnosis of myasthenia gravis—**
Adults and children weighing more than 34 kg (75 lb): Initially, 2 mg I.V.; then up to an additional 8 mg I.V., depending on response.
Children weighing up to 34 kg: Initially, 1 mg I.V.; then up to an additional 5 mg I.V., depending on response.
➤ **Evaluation of anticholinesterase therapy in myasthenia gravis—**
Adults: 1 to 2 mg I.V. given 1 hour after last oral dose of anticholinesterase.
➤ **Differentiation of myasthenic from cholinergic crisis—**
Adults: Initially, 1 mg I.V.; may repeat dose once if bradycardia or hypotension fails to occur. Don't exceed total dose of 2 mg I.V. Patients with myas-

thenic crisis show improved muscle strength.

➤ **Antagonism of neuromuscular blockers, such as curare, after surgery—**
Adults: Initially, 10 mg I.V.; may repeat dose p.r.n. q 5 to 10 minutes. Maximum total dose, 40 mg I.V.

ADMINISTRATION

Direct injection: To diagnose myasthenia gravis, draw 10 mg (1 ml) of drug into a tuberculin syringe with a 21G or 23G needle. Inject 2 mg (0.2 ml) directly into vein or into the tubing of a free-flowing I.V. line over 30 to 45 seconds. If patient shows no cholinergic effects after 45 seconds, give remaining 8 mg slowly in 2-mg increments. If cholinergic response occurs, stop drug and give atropine.

To evaluate anticholinesterase therapy in patients with myasthenia gravis or to differentiate myasthenic from cholinergic crisis, draw 2 mg (0.2 ml) into a tuberculin syringe and give slowly over 30 to 45 seconds in 1-mg increments.

To antagonize neuromuscular blockers, inject drug over 30 to 45 seconds.
Intermittent infusion: Not recommended.
Continuous infusion: Not recommended.

PREPARATION & STORAGE

Available in 1-ml ampules and 10-ml and 15-ml vials with a concentration of 10 mg/ml.

Compatible with D_5W, dextrose 5% in lactated Ringer's solution, lactated Ringer's solution, and normal saline solution.

Incompatibilities
None reported.

CONTRAINDICATIONS & CAUTIONS

• Contraindicated in those hypersensitive to anticholinesterases and in those with mechanical obstruction of urinary or GI tract.
• Don't give drug to patients receiving the ganglionic blocking agent, mecamylamine.
• Use cautiously in those with arrhythmias or bronchial asthma because drug may worsen these conditions.

ADVERSE REACTIONS

CNS: incoordination, weakness, *seizures.*
CV: *cardiac arrest, bradycardia,* hypotension, *AV block.*
EENT: blurred or double vision, excessive salivation, lacrimation, pupillary constriction.
GI: abdominal cramps, diarrhea, nausea, vomiting.
GU: urinary frequency.
Musculoskeletal: fasciculations, arthralgia.
Respiratory: *bronchospasm, respiratory paralysis,* increased bronchial secretions.
Skin: diaphoresis.

INTERACTIONS

Drug-drug. *Aminoglycosides, nondepolarizing neuromuscular blockers:* Antagonizes effects. Avoid using together.
Cardiac glycosides: Worsens bradycardia and AV block. Use together with caution.
Cholinergic drugs: May lead to additive toxicity. Avoid use together.
Corticosteroids: May decrease the cholinergic effects of edrophonium; when corticosteroids are stopped, however, cholinergic effects may increase, possibly affecting muscle strength. Watch for lack of drug effect.
Depolarizing neuromuscular blockers, such as succinylcholine: Increases neuromuscular blocking effects. Provide respiratory support as needed if drugs must be used together.
Ganglionic blockers, such as mecamylamine: May lead to a critical blood

pressure decrease. Avoid using together.

Magnesium: May have a direct depressant effect on skeletal muscle. Avoid using together.

Other anticholinesterases, such as ambenonium, neostigmine, and pyridostigmine: Enhances risk of cholinergic crisis, including paralysis, resulting from increased effects. Avoid using together.

Quinidine: May block cholinergic effects of edrophonium. Avoid using together.

Drug-herb. *Jaborandi tree, pill-bearing spurge:* May cause an additive effect and increase risk of toxicity. Advise patient to use together cautiously.

EFFECTS ON LAB TEST RESULTS
None reported.

ACTION
Inhibits or inactivates acetylcholinesterase at sites of cholinergic transmission, allowing acetylcholine to accumulate at cholinergic synapses. Acetylcholine, in turn, causes bronchial constriction, bradycardia, miosis, and increased skeletal and intestinal muscle tone and salivary and sweat gland secretion.

PHARMACOKINETICS
Onset, 30 to 60 seconds; duration, 5 to 10 minutes.
Distribution: Throughout body. Drug crosses the blood-brain barrier only at high doses. Probably crosses the placental barrier in limited amounts.
Metabolism: Unknown.
Excretion: In urine, but not well understood.

CLINICAL CONSIDERATIONS
• Osmolality: 329 mOsm/kg.
• Drug should be given under close medical supervision.
• Before giving drug, have 1 mg atropine available for immediate injection. Keep suction, endotracheal intu-

bation, and mechanical ventilation equipment readily available.
• Establish baseline blood pressure, heart rate, and respiratory rate and quality. Keep patient on cardiac monitor during administration. Watch for hypotension, bradycardia, and respiratory distress.
• Evaluate vital capacity and muscle strength before and during administration.
• If drug is being used to differentiate myasthenic from cholinergic crisis or to antagonize neuromuscular blockers, start mechanical ventilation before administration.
• For patients older than age 50, give 0.4 to 0.6 mg of atropine with edrophonium because of increased risk of bradycardia and hypotension.
• In patients sensitive to edrophonium, give small doses with atropine.
• Before giving drug to diagnose myasthenia gravis, stop all other anticholinesterases for at least 8 hours.
• Drug has also been used to treat paroxysmal atrial tachycardia.
• *Alert:* Drug may contain sulfites, which may cause an allergic reaction in some patients.
• Some patients with myasthenia gravis show a myasthenic response—a marked but transient improvement in muscle strength—which indicates an insufficient anticholinesterase dosage. Other patients show a cholinergic response—increased weakness, fasciculations, and other adverse muscarinic effects—which indicates an excessive anticholinesterase dosage.
• When you differentiate myasthenic from cholinergic crisis, use the same guidelines as when you evaluate anticholinesterase therapy. It may be difficult to distinguish myasthenic from cholinergic crisis in myasthenia gravis patients because muscarinic reactions and fasciculations may be diminished or absent.

• Some patients with myasthenia gravis experience effects lasting up to 30 minutes when receiving drug for first time.
• With an overdose, weakness usually appears first in masticatory, swallowing, and neck muscles and then in shoulder, arm, pelvic, eye, and leg muscles. If overdose occurs, protect patient's airway; intubate if needed. Give 0.4 to 0.5 mg of atropine by direct I.V. injection to antagonize muscarinic effects of edrophonium.

PATIENT TEACHING

• Tell patient to promptly report adverse reactions.
• Explain use and administration of drug to patient and family.
• Tell patient to alert nurse if discomfort occurs at I.V. site.

enalaprilat*

Pharmacologic class: ACE inhibitor
Therapeutic class: antihypertensive
Pregnancy risk category: C; D in second and third trimesters
pH: 6.5 to 7.5

INDICATIONS & DOSAGES

➤ **Mild to severe hypertension in patients not receiving a diuretic—**
Adults: 1.25 mg I.V. over a 5-minute period q 6 hours.
➤ **Hypertension in patients receiving diuretic therapy—**
Adults: 0.625 mg I.V. over a 5-minute period q 6 hours. If after 1 hour clinical response is inadequate, dose may be repeated.
Adjust-a-dose: For adults with a creatinine clearance below 30 ml/minute, initial dose is 0.625 mg I.V. Gradually adjust dose based on response. Patients undergoing hemodialysis should receive a supplemental dose on dialysis days.

ADMINISTRATION

Direct injection: Give as provided or dilute with up to 50 ml of a compatible diluent. Infuse slowly over at least 5 minutes.
Intermittent infusion: Not recommended.
Continuous infusion: Not recommended.

PREPARATION & STORAGE

Available as a clear, colorless solution in 1-ml and 2-ml vials containing 1.25 mg/ml.
   May be diluted with up to 50 ml. Compatible solutions include D_5W, normal saline injection, dextrose 5% in normal saline injection, dextrose 5% in lactated Ringer's injection, and Isolyte E.
   Diluted solutions maintain full activity for 24 hours at room temperature. Store below 86° F (30° C).

Incompatibilities

Amphotericin B, phenytoin sodium.

CONTRAINDICATIONS & CAUTIONS

• Contraindicated in patients hypersensitive to drug or those with a history of angioedema caused by ACE inhibitor treatment.
• Use cautiously in those with collagen vascular disease, immune system disorders, or renal impairment and in those taking drugs that may depress immune function or decrease WBC count.
• Use cautiously in those taking potassium-sparing diuretics, potassium supplements, and salt substitutes because of risk of hyperkalemia.
• Use cautiously in those with vascular insufficiency, a recent MI, or cerebrovascular disease because of risk of adverse effects linked to hypotension.
• Use cautiously in breast-feeding women because trace amounts of drug appear in breast milk.

Reactions may be *common*, uncommon, *life-threatening*, or COMMON AND LIFE-THREATENING.

ADVERSE REACTIONS
CNS: dizziness, headache, fever, fatigue.
CV: *cardiac arrest, MI,* hypotension.
GI: nausea, constipation.
Hematologic: *agranulocytosis.*
Respiratory: cough.
Skin: rash.
Other: *angioedema.*

INTERACTIONS
Drug-drug. *Antihypertensives, diuretics:* Increases hypotensive effect. Monitor blood pressure closely.
Lithium: Decreases renal clearance of lithium. Monitor patient; may need to adjust lithium dose.
NSAIDS: Decreases enalaprilat effect and may decrease renal function. Monitor blood pressure and renal function.
Potassium-sparing diuretics, potassium supplements: Increases risk of hyperkalemia. Monitor potassium level.
Rifampin: Decreases enalaprilat effect. Monitor therapeutic effect.
Drug-herb. *Capsaicin:* Increases risk of cough. Discourage use together.
Drug-food. *Potassium-containing salt substitutes:* Increases risk of hyperkalemia. Discourage use together.

EFFECTS ON LAB TEST RESULTS
• May increase BUN, creatinine, bilirubin, liver enzyme, and potassium levels. May decrease sodium level.
• May decrease hemoglobin, hematocrit, and WBC and granulocyte counts.

ACTION
Inhibits ACE, the enzyme that catalyzes the conversion of angiotensin I to the vasoconstrictor substance angiotensin II. Reduced angiotensin II levels decrease peripheral arterial resistance, thus lowering blood pressure, and decrease aldosterone secretion, thus reducing sodium and water retention.

PHARMACOKINETICS
Onset occurs in 5 to 15 minutes; effect peaks in 1 to 4 hours.
Distribution: 50% to 60% protein bound. Drug crosses the placental barrier, and trace amounts appear in breast milk. Drug doesn't appear to cross the blood-brain barrier.
Metabolism: None.
Excretion: In urine and feces. Half-life, 11 hours. Removed by hemodialysis and peritoneal dialysis.

CLINICAL CONSIDERATIONS
• Drug is usually used only when oral therapy with enalapril maleate isn't feasible.
• *Alert:* I.V. and oral doses aren't interchangeable.
• If hypotension occurs, place patient in a supine position and infuse normal saline solution, as ordered.
• Geriatric patients may need lower dose because of impaired drug clearance.
• *Alert:* Observe patient for facial swelling and difficulty breathing, which may indicate angioedema. Stop treatment immediately if angioedema of the face, extremities, lips, tongue, glottis, or larynx occurs. Give epinephrine solution 1:1,000 (0.3 to 0.5 ml) S.C. and ensure a patent airway. Monitor patient carefully until signs and symptoms disappear.
• Monitor WBC count and liver and kidney function.
• Because drug may reduce WBC count, observe patient for signs and symptoms of infection, such as sore throat, fever, and malaise.
• The most common sign of overdose is hypotension. Usual treatment is I.V. infusion of normal saline solution.

PATIENT TEACHING
• Because safe use of drug during pregnancy hasn't been established, advise patient in the second or third trimester

---

of potential hazards to the fetus; recommend ultrasound examinations.
● Advise patient that light-headedness may occur and that sudden position changes may cause dizziness.
● Tell patient to report adverse reactions promptly, especially signs and symptoms of angioedema.

ephedrine sulfate

Pharmacologic class: adrenergic
Therapeutic class: bronchodilator, vasopressor (parenteral form), nasal decongestant
Pregnancy risk category: C
pH: 4.5 to 7

INDICATIONS & DOSAGES
➤ **Bronchospasm—**
Adults: 12.5 to 25 mg I.V. Subsequent doses based on patient response. Maximum dosage, 150 mg I.V. q 24 hours.
➤ **Hypotension and temporary support of ventricular rate in bradycardia, AV block, carotid sinus syndrome, or Stokes-Adams syndrome—**
Adults: 10 to 25 mg I.V., repeated in 5 to 10 minutes p.r.n. Maximum dosage, 150 mg I.V. q 24 hours.
Children: 2 to 3 mg/kg or 67 to 100 mg/m^2 I.V. daily in four to six divided doses.

ADMINISTRATION
Direct injection: Slowly inject drug directly into vein or into an I.V. line containing a free-flowing, compatible solution.
Intermittent infusion: Not recommended.
Continuous infusion: Not recommended.

PREPARATION & STORAGE
Available in 1-ml vials containing 50 mg/ml. Discard unused, cloudy, or precipitated solutions.
Drug is compatible with most common I.V. fluids.
Store at 59° to 86° F (15° to 30° C) in light-resistant containers; drug gradually decomposes and darkens on exposure to light.

Incompatibilities
Fructose 10% in normal saline solution; hydrocortisone sodium succinate; Ionosol B, D-CM, and D solutions; pentobarbital sodium; phenobarbital sodium; thiopental.

CONTRAINDICATIONS & CAUTIONS
● Contraindicated in those hypersensitive to drug.
● Contraindicated in those with angle-closure glaucoma because of risk of increased ocular pressure and in those with psychoneurosis because of aggravating CNS effects.
● Contraindicated in those with cardiac disease because drug increases oxygen consumption, thus stimulating the heart, and in those receiving cyclopropane or halothane anesthesia.
● Use extremely cautiously in those with hypertension or hyperthyroidism because of increased risk of adverse reactions.
● Use cautiously in geriatric patients with prostatic hyperplasia because of risk of urine retention, and in patients with CV disease or pheochromocytoma because of pressor effects.
● Use cautiously in diabetic patients because drug raises glucose levels.

ADVERSE REACTIONS
CNS: agitation, anxiety, confusion, delirium, dizziness, distress, euphoria, fear, hallucinations, headache, hyperactive reflexes, insomnia, irritability, restlessness, *seizures,* talkativeness, tremor.

Reactions may be *common,* uncommon, *life-threatening,* or COMMON AND LIFE-THREATENING.

CV: *extrasystoles, potentially fatal arrhythmias, including ventricular fibrillation,* palpitations, tachycardia, precordial pain.
EENT: dry nose and throat.
GI: anorexia, nausea, vomiting.
GU: acute urine retention, painful urination.
Respiratory: breathing difficulty.
Skin: pallor.
Other: *anaphylaxis.*

INTERACTIONS

Drug-drug. *Alpha blockers, antihypertensives, nitrates:* May reduce antihypertensive effects. Monitor therapeutic effects closely.
Atropine, doxapram, ergot alkaloids, guanadrel, guanethidine, MAO inhibitors, sympathomimetics: Enhances pressor response to ephedrine. Monitor patient closely.
Beta blockers: May reduce ephedrine effects, increase risk of hypertension, and cause excessive bradycardia with heart block. Monitor patient closely.
Cardiac glycosides, general anesthetics such as cyclopropane, halogenated hydrocarbons: Sensitizes myocardium to sympathomimetic effects. Monitor cardiac status.
CNS stimulants: May cause excessive CNS stimulation. Monitor patient closely.
Corticosteroids: May increase metabolic clearance. Monitor patient closely.
Ionic radio contrast dyes (such as diatrizoate, iothalamate, and ioxaglate): May enhance CNS toxicity. Monitor patient closely.
Levodopa: May increase risk of arrhythmias. Use together cautiously.
Mazindol, methylphenidate: May enhance CNS stimulation and potentiate pressor effects. Monitor patient closely.
Mecamylamine, methyldopa, trimethaphan: May diminish hypotensive effects of these drugs and enhance pressor effects of ephedrine. Monitor patient closely.
Thyroid hormones: May heighten thyroid hormone or ephedrine effects and enhance risk of coronary insufficiency in coronary artery disease. Monitor patient closely. Evaluate for possible dosage adjustment.
Tricyclic antidepressants: Decreases pressor response. Monitor patient closely.
Urinary alkalizers such as sodium bicarbonate, carbonic anhydrase inhibitors: Prolongs ephedrine effects. Monitor patient closely.
Xanthines: May increase adverse reactions. Use together cautiously.
Drug-herb. *Dietary supplements containing ephedrine alkaloids:* May have serious adverse effects. Discourage use together.

EFFECTS ON LAB TEST RESULTS
None reported.

ACTION
Stimulates alpha and beta receptors, relaxing bronchial smooth muscle and producing a positive inotropic effect; dilates coronary vessels and constricts renal arteries.

PHARMACOKINETICS
Drug level peaks immediately after administration; duration, 1 hour.
Distribution: Unknown. Drug may cross placental barrier and appears in breast milk.
Metabolism: Slowly, in liver.
Excretion: In urine within 48 hours, mostly as unchanged drug and its metabolites. Half-life, 3 to 6 hours.

CLINICAL CONSIDERATIONS
● Correct hypovolemia before giving drug.
● Monitor blood pressure and cardiac status before, during, and after therapy. Hypoxia, hypercapnia, and acidosis may reduce drug's effectiveness.

• A sedative or tranquilizer may combat CNS stimulation.
• Overdose may cause CV collapse. As ordered, give beta blockers for arrhythmias, phentolamine for hypertension, diazepam or paraldehyde for seizures, and cold applications and I.V. dexamethasone for fever. Don't give vasopressors.

PATIENT TEACHING
• Inform patient and family about underlying disease.
• Tell patient to report adverse reactions promptly.
• Explain use and administration of drug to patient and family.

epinephrine hydrochloride
Adrenalin Chloride

Pharmacologic class: adrenergic
Therapeutic class: bronchodilator, vasopressor, cardiac stimulant, sympathomimetic
Pregnancy risk category: C
pH: 2.5 to 5

INDICATIONS & DOSAGES
➤ **Bronchospasm and hypersensitivity reaction—**
Adults: 0.1 to 0.25 mg I.V. (1 to 2.5 ml of 1:10,000 dilution) slowly over 5 to 10 minutes. May be followed by an infusion of 1 to 4 mcg/minute.
Children: 0.1 mg I.V. (10 ml of 1:100,000 dilution) slowly over 5 to 10 minutes. Don't exceed 0.5 mg/dose. May be followed by an infusion of 0.1 mcg/kg/minute, increased p.r.n. to a maximum of 1.5 mcg/kg/minute.
➤ **Cardiac arrest—**
Adults: 0.1 to 1 mg I.V. (1 to 10 ml of 1:10,000 dilution), repeated q 3 to 5 minutes p.r.n. May be followed by an infusion of 1 mcg/minute, increased p.r.n. to 4 mcg/minute.

Children: 0.01 mg/kg I.V. (0.1 ml/kg of a 1:10,000 dilution), repeated q 3 to 5 minutes p.r.n. May be followed by an I.V. infusion of 0.1 mcg/kg/minute, increased p.r.n. by 0.1 mcg/kg/minute to a maximum of 1 mcg/kg/minute.
Neonates: 0.01 to 0.03 mg/kg I.V. (0.1 to 0.3 ml/kg of 1:10,000 dilution), repeated q 3 to 5 minutes p.r.n.

ADMINISTRATION
Direct injection: Slowly inject drug directly into a vein or into an I.V. line containing a free-flowing, compatible solution.
Intermittent infusion: Using an appropriately diluted solution, piggyback drug into a compatible solution and infuse over 5 to 10 minutes.
Continuous infusion: Using an appropriately diluted solution, infuse drug at ordered rate using an infusion pump.

PREPARATION & STORAGE
Available in 1-ml and 30-ml vials containing 0.1 mg/ml (1:10,000), 0.5 mg/ml (1:2,000), or 1 mg/ml (1:1,000). Also available in prefilled syringes containing 1 or 2 ml of 1 mg/ml concentration, 10 ml of 0.1 mg/ml, or 5 ml of 0.01 mg/ml.
To obtain a solution of 4 mcg/ml, add 1 mg of drug to 250 ml of D_5W or normal saline solution, dextrose 10% in water, dextrose 5% in lactated Ringer's injection, or dextrose 5% in Ringer's injection.
Compatible with most other I.V. solutions. Rapidly destroyed by alkalies or oxidizing drugs, including halogens, nitrates, nitrites, permanganates, sodium bicarbonate, and salts of easily reducible metals, such as iron, copper, and zinc.
Protect epinephrine from light. Keep ampules in carton until ready to use. Discard brown solutions or solutions that contain a precipitate.

Reactions may be *common*, uncommon, *life-threatening*, or COMMON AND LIFE-THREATENING.

Incompatibilities

Aminophylline; ampicillin sodium; cephapirin; furosemide; Ionosol D-CM, PSL, and T solutions with D_5W; mephentermine.

CONTRAINDICATIONS & CAUTIONS

• Contraindicated in those with shock (except anaphylactic shock) because of increased myocardial oxygen demand, and in those with angle-closure glaucoma because of risk of increased intra-ocular pressure.

• Contraindicated in those with organic brain damage, cerebral arteriosclerosis, organic heart disease, cardiac dilation, coronary insufficiency, and most arrhythmias because drug may worsen these conditions.

• Use cautiously in those with hyperthyroidism (especially geriatric patients) because of increased risk of adverse reactions, and in those with sensitivity to sulfites or sympathomimetic amines because of increased risk of hypersensitivity.

• Use cautiously in those with psychoneurosis or CV disorders—such as angina pectoris, tachycardia, heart failure, coronary artery disease, and hypertension—because drug may worsen these conditions.

• Use cautiously in those with diabetes mellitus because drug causes hyperglycemia, requiring an increased dosage of insulin or an antidiabetic, and in those with Parkinson's disease because drug temporarily increases rigidity or tremors.

ADVERSE REACTIONS

CNS: agitation, fever, anxiety, weakness, disorientation, dizziness, excitability, hallucinations, headache, impaired memory, insomnia, lightheadedness, mood changes, restlessness, tremors, *cerebral hemorrhage.*
CV: *ventricular arrhythmias, bradycardia,* chest pain, hypertension, palpitations, tachycardia.

EENT: blurred vision.
GI: nausea, vomiting.
Musculoskeletal: muscle cramps.
Respiratory: breathing difficulty.
Skin: pallor, sweating.
Other: *anaphylaxis,* chills.

INTERACTIONS

Drug-drug. *Alpha blockers:* Antagonizes vasoconstrictive and hypertensive effects. Monitor patient closely.
Antihistamines, MAO inhibitors, sympathomimetics, tricyclic antidepressants, thyroid hormones: Potentiates epinephrine effects. Monitor patient closely.
Beta blockers: Causes hypotension. Monitor blood pressure.
Cardiac glycosides: Sensitizes heart to arrhythmias. Avoid using together.
CNS stimulants, mazindol, methylphenidate, methylxanthines: May increase CNS stimulation and pressor effects of epinephrine. Use together cautiously.
Diuretics: May decrease vascular response to epinephrine. Monitor patient closely.
Doxapram, guanadrel, guanethidine: May increase pressor effects. Adjust doses of these drugs.
Ergot alkaloids: May enhance vasoconstriction, peripheral ischemia, and pressor effects, resulting in severe hypertension. Monitor patient closely.
General anesthetics (such as cyclopropane and halogenated hydrocarbons), levodopa: Increases risk of ventricular arrhythmias. Avoid using together.
Ionic radio contrast dyes (such as diatrizoate, iothalamate, and ioxaglate): May increase CNS toxicity. Monitor patient closely.
Methyldopa: May decrease antihypertensive effects and heighten pressor effects of epinephrine. Avoid using together.

EFFECTS ON LAB TEST RESULTS
• May increase BUN, glucose, and lactic acid levels.

ACTION
Stimulates alpha and beta receptors and the heart, relaxes bronchial smooth muscle, and dilates skeletal muscle vasculature.

PHARMACOKINETICS
Onset, immediate; duration, brief.
Distribution: Rapid and widespread. Crosses placental barrier but not the blood-brain barrier. Drug appears in breast milk.
Metabolism: In sympathetic nerve endings, liver, and other tissues.
Excretion: In urine.

CLINICAL CONSIDERATIONS
• Osmolality: 273 to 348 mOsm/kg.
• *Alert:* Drug may contain sulfites, which can cause allergic reactions in some patients.
• Monitor vital signs. Drug can widen pulse pressure.
• *Alert:* Overdose may cause renal shutdown and circulatory collapse. Overdose or prolonged use can produce severe metabolic acidosis because of elevated lactic acid levels. If overdose occurs, alpha or beta blockers may be given to treat symptoms. Rapid-acting vasodilators such as nitrites or sodium nitroprusside may counteract marked pressor effects.

PATIENT TEACHING
• Provide information regarding underlying disease process to patient and family.
• Tell patient to report adverse reactions promptly.
• Explain use and administration of drug to patient and family.

epirubicin hydrochloride
Ellence

Pharmacologic class: anthracycline
Therapeutic class: antineoplastic
Pregnancy risk category: C
pH: 3

INDICATIONS & DOSAGES
➤ **Adjuvant therapy in patients with evidence of axillary node tumor involvement after resection of primary breast cancer—**
Adults: 100 to 120 mg/m² I.V. infusion over 3 to 5 minutes through a free-flowing I.V. solution on day 1 of each cycle or divided equally in two doses on days 1 and 8 of each cycle; repeat cycle q 3 to 4 weeks for six cycles; used with regimens containing cyclophosphamide and fluorouracil.

After the first cycle, dose should be modified based on toxic reaction. For patients with platelet count less than 50,000/mm³, absolute neutrophil count (ANC) less than 250/mm³, neutropenic fever, or grade 3 or 4 nonhematologic toxicity, reduce the day 1 dose in subsequent cycles to 75% of the day 1 dose given in the current cycle. Day 1 therapy in subsequent cycles should be delayed until platelet count is 100,000/mm³ or more, ANC is 1,500/mm³ or more, and nonhematologic toxicities recover to grade 1.

For patients receiving divided doses (days 1 and 8), the day 8 dose should be 75% of the day 1 dose if platelet count is 75,000 to 100,000/mm³ and ANC is 1,000 to 1,499/mm³. If day 8 platelet count is less than 75,000/mm³, ANC is less than 1,000/mm³, or grade 3 or 4 nonhematologic toxicity has occurred, omit the day 8 dose.
Adjust-a-dose: For patients with bone marrow dysfunction, as in heavily pretreated patients, those with bone mar-

row depression, or those with neoplastic bone marrow infiltration, start at lower doses of 75 to 90 mg/m^2.

For patients with a bilirubin level of 1.2 to 3 mg/dl or an AST level of two to four times upper limit of normal, give half of the recommended starting dose. If the bilirubin level is above 3 mg/dl or the AST level is greater than four times the upper limit of normal, give a quarter of the recommended starting dose.

For patients with a creatinine level greater than 5 mg/dl, consider a lower dose.

ADMINISTRATION

Direct injection: Not recommended.
Intermittent infusion: Give through free-flowing I.V. solution of normal saline solution or D$_5$W over 3 to 5 minutes.
Continuous infusion: Not recommended.

PREPARATION & STORAGE

Available in ready-to-use single-dose vials. Discard any portion not used within 24 hours after vial is penetrated.

Store refrigerated at 36° to 46° F (2° to 8° C) and protected from light before use.

Incompatibilities

Fluorouracil, heparin, other I.V. drugs.

CONTRAINDICATIONS & CAUTIONS

• Contraindicated in those hypersensitive to this drug, other anthracyclines, or anthracenediones.
• Contraindicated in those with baseline neutrophil counts of fewer than 1,500 cells/mm^3, in those with severe myocardial insufficiency or a recent MI, in those who were previously treated with anthracyclines to total cumulative doses, and in those with severe hepatic dysfunction.
• Use cautiously in those with active or dormant cardiac disease and in those

with prior or concurrent radiotherapy to the mediastinal and pericardial area, previous therapy with other anthracyclines or anthracenediones, or other cardiotoxic drugs.
• Advise women to avoid pregnancy during treatment.

ADVERSE REACTIONS

CNS: *lethargy,* fever.
CV: *cardiomyopathy, hot flashes, **heart failure.***
EENT: *conjunctivitis, keratitis.*
GI: *nausea, vomiting, diarrhea,* anorexia, *mucositis.*
GU: *amenorrhea.*
Hematologic: LEUKOPENIA, NEUTROPENIA, *febrile neutropenia,* anemia, THROMBOCYTOPENIA.
Skin: *alopecia,* rash, itch, skin changes.
Other: *infection, local toxic reaction.*

INTERACTIONS

Drug-drug. *Calcium channel blockers, cardioactive compounds:* May increase risk of heart failure. Monitor cardiac function closely.
Cimetidine: May increase levels of epirubicin by 50%. Avoid using together.
Cytotoxic drugs: Causes additive toxicities, especially hematologic and GI. Monitor patient closely.
Radiation therapy: May enhance effects. Monitor patient carefully.
Drug-lifestyle. *Sun exposure:* May increase risk of photosensitivity reactions. Advise patient to avoid excessive sunlight exposure.

EFFECTS ON LAB TEST RESULTS

• May decrease hemoglobin and WBC, neutrophil, and platelet counts.

ACTION

Thought to form a complex with DNA, thereby inhibiting DNA, RNA, and protein synthesis; cytocidal effects result from DNA cleavage. Drug may also interfere with replication and transcription of DNA, and it generates cytotoxic free radicals.

PHARMACOKINETICS

Onset, peak, and duration of drug effects unknown.

Distribution: Rapidly and widely distributed into tissues with 77% protein bound. Drug is twice as concentrated in RBCs as in plasma.

Metabolism: Extensively and rapidly by the liver.

Excretion: Primarily through biliary excretion. About 35% is in feces and 27% in urine.

CLINICAL CONSIDERATIONS

• Epirubicin administration should be supervised by a health care provider experienced in cancer chemotherapy. Pregnant nurses shouldn't handle this drug.

• Wear protective clothing, goggles, gown, and disposable gloves when handling this drug.

• Facial flushing and local erythematous streaking along the vein may indicate excessively rapid administration.

• An antiemetic may be given before epirubicin to reduce nausea and vomiting.

• Obtain baseline total bilirubin and AST levels, creatinine level, and CBC including ANC; evaluate cardiac function by measuring left ventricular ejection fraction (LVEF) before therapy.

• Monitor LVEF regularly during therapy, and stop drug at the first sign of impaired cardiac function.

• Early signs of cardiac toxicity include sinus tachycardia, ECG abnormalities, tachyarrhythmias, bradycardia, AV block, and bundle-branch block.

• Obtain total and differential WBC, RBC, and platelet counts before and during each cycle of therapy.

• Avoid veins over joints or in arms or legs with compromised venous or lymphatic drainage.

• Immediately stop infusion if burning or stinging occurs and restart in another vein.

• Patients receiving 120 mg/m^2 of epirubicin should also receive prophylactic antibiotic therapy with trimethoprim-sulfamethoxazole or a fluoroquinolone.

• The WBC count usually reaches its nadir 10 to 14 days after drug is given and returns to normal by day 21.

• Anthracycline-induced leukemia may occur.

• Administration of drug after previous radiation therapy may induce an inflammatory cell reaction at the radiation site.

• Monitor uric acid, potassium, calcium phosphate, and creatinine levels immediately after initial chemotherapy administration in patients susceptible to tumor lysis syndrome.

• Hydration, urine alkalization, and prophylaxis with allopurinol may prevent hyperuricemia and minimize potential complications of tumor lysis syndrome.

• Cardiac toxicity, as indicated by reduced LVEF and signs and symptoms of heart failure (such as tachycardia, dyspnea, pulmonary edema, dependent edema, hepatomegaly, ascites, pleural effusion, and gallop rhythm), may be delayed until 2 or 3 months after treatment is completed. Delayed cardiac toxicity depends on the cumulative dose of epirubicin, which shouldn't exceed 900 mg/m^2.

PATIENT TEACHING

• Advise patient to report nausea, vomiting, inflammatory conditions of the mouth, dehydration, fever, evidence of infection, or signs and symptoms of heart failure, such as rapid heart beat, shortness of breath, and swelling.

- Tell patient to immediately report pain, stinging, or burning at infusion site.
- Inform patient of the risk of cardiac damage and treatment-related leukemia with use of drug.
- Advise the use of effective contraception during treatment.
- Advise women that irreversible absence of menstrual periods or premature menopause may occur.
- Tell patient that hair usually grows back within 2 or 3 months after therapy ends.

epoetin alfa (erythropoietin)
Epogen*, Eprex ◊ *, Procrit*

Pharmacologic class: glycoprotein
Therapeutic class: antianemic
Pregnancy risk category: C
pH: 5.8 to 7.2

INDICATIONS & DOSAGES
➤ **Anemia linked to chronic renal failure—**
Adults: Initially, 50 to 100 units/kg three times weekly. Patients receiving dialysis should be given drug I.V.; those with chronic renal failure not on dialysis may receive drug S.C.
Reduce dosage when target hematocrit is reached or if hematocrit rises more than 4 points within 2-week period. Increase dosage if hematocrit doesn't rise by five to six points after 8 weeks of therapy and target range of 30% to 33% hasn't been reached. Individualize dosage for maintenance range.
➤ **Anemia linked to zidovudine therapy in patients infected with HIV who have low endogenous erythropoietin levels—**
Adults: Initially, 100 units/kg I.V. three times weekly for 8 weeks. If response is inadequate, increase to 150 or 200 units/kg I.V. three times weekly.

Reevaluate response q 1 or 2 months and increase by 50 to 100 units/kg I.V. three times weekly, p.r.n.
Response to drug is unlikely with dosages above 300 units/kg I.V. three times weekly. Adjust doses cautiously based on infections or changes in zidovudine therapy.

ADMINISTRATION
Direct injection: May give through the I.V. access site after dialysis session.
Intermittent infusion: Not recommended.
Continuous infusion: Not recommended.

PREPARATION & STORAGE
Available in vials of 2,000 units/ml; 3,000 units/ml; 4,000 units/ml; 10,000 units/ml; and 40,000 units/ml. Vials also contain 2.5 mg/ml of human albumin. Single-dose vials don't contain preservative. Use only one dose per vial. Also available as 2-ml multidose vials containing 10,000 units/ml or 20,000 units/ml, which contain preservative.
Don't shake; doing so may denature glycoprotein. Don't dilute solution.
Refrigerate at 36° to 46° F (2° to 8° C).

Incompatibilities
Other I.V. drugs.

CONTRAINDICATIONS & CAUTIONS
- Contraindicated in those hypersensitive to products derived from mammal cells or to human albumin.
- Contraindicated in those with uncontrolled hypertension.

ADVERSE REACTIONS
CNS: *headache,* fatigue, asthenia, dizziness, **seizures if hematocrit rises too rapidly,** *pyrexia.*
CV: *hypertension,* chest pain, edema.
GI: diarrhea, *nausea,* vomiting.
Musculoskeletal: *arthralgias.*

Respiratory: *cough in those taking zidovudine.*
Skin: *rash in those taking zidovudine.*

INTERACTIONS
None reported.

EFFECTS ON LAB TEST RESULTS
• May increase BUN, creatinine, uric acid, potassium, and phosphate levels.
• May increase hemoglobin and hematocrit.

ACTION
An amino acid glycoprotein synthesized using recombinant DNA technology, drug mimics naturally occurring erythropoietin (which is produced by the kidneys). Drug stimulates the division and differentiation of cells within the bone marrow to produce RBCs.

PHARMACOKINETICS
Onset, immediate; half-life, 4 to 13 hours; duration, 24 hours.
Distribution: Throughout plasma; also to bone marrow, kidneys, spleen, and liver.
Metabolism: Unknown.
Excretion: Half-life ranges from 4 to 13 hours, depending on dose. Higher doses have a longer half-life. Less than 5% of drug is eliminated by renal excretion, and end-stage renal disease doesn't affect half-life.

CLINICAL CONSIDERATIONS
• Tonicity: isotonic.
• Determine endogenous erythropoietin levels in patient receiving drug for zidovudine-induced anemia before therapy. Patient is unlikely to respond to drug therapy if endogenous levels exceed 500 milliunits/ml.
• Monitor hematocrit at least twice weekly when therapy starts and during dosage adjustment. A rapid rise in hematocrit can lead to uncontrolled blood pressure. During initial therapy when hematocrit is increasing, about

25% of patients require antihypertensive therapy or dosage adjustment in current therapy. Reduce dosage so hematocrit doesn't increase by more than four points in 2 weeks. Drug may have to be withheld until blood pressure is controlled. New dosage may take 2 to 6 weeks to change hematocrit.
• Routine monitoring of CBC with differential and platelet counts is recommended.
• If hematocrit isn't carefully monitored and dosage appropriately adjusted, drug therapy can cause polycythemia. Stop drug if hematocrit rises beyond target range of 30% to 33%. If polycythemia is of concern, phlebotomy may be considered to decrease hematocrit.
• Although maximum safe dosage hasn't been established, doses up to 1,500 units/kg have been given three times weekly for 3 weeks without causing direct toxic effects.
• If patient fails to respond to therapy, consider the following causes: vitamin deficiency, especially of folate or vitamin B_{12}; iron deficiency; underlying inflammatory disease or infection; occult blood loss; underlying hematologic disease, including thalassemia, refractory anemia, or myelodysplastic disorders; hemolysis; aluminum intoxication; osteitis fibrosa cystica; or cancer.
• Drug may increase hematocrit and decrease plasma volume, which may reduce effectiveness of dialysis treatments.
• Hemodialysis patients being treated with epoetin alfa may require increased heparin dosage to reduce risk of clotting dialysis machine.
• Most patients require supplemental iron therapy. Before and during therapy, monitor patient's iron stores, including ferritin level and transferrin saturation.

PATIENT TEACHING

• Explain to patient and family the importance of regularly monitoring blood pressure.

• Explain that patient may feel an improved sense of well-being.

• Advise patient to follow dietary restrictions and to report as directed for dialysis sessions during therapy.

• Remind dialysis patient that taking this drug won't affect the course of renal failure.

• When treatment begins, instruct patient to avoid driving or operating heavy machinery because of possible increased risk of seizures.

epoprostenol sodium
Flolan

Pharmacologic class: naturally occurring prostaglandin
Therapeutic class: vasodilator, platelet aggregation inhibitor
Pregnancy risk category: B

INDICATIONS & DOSAGES

➤ **Long-term I.V. treatment of primary pulmonary hypertension and pulmonary hypertension linked to the scleroderma spectrum of disease in New York Heart Association Class III and IV patients who don't respond adequately to conventional therapy—**
Adults: Initially, 2 ng/kg/minute by continuous I.V. infusion. Increase dosage by 2 ng/kg/minute I.V. q 15 minutes or more until dose-limiting effects occur or a tolerance limit is established and further increases are no longer warranted.
Adjust-a-dose: If symptoms of pulmonary hypertension persist or recur after improving, increase I.V. infusion by 1- to 2-ng/kg/minute increments at intervals of at least 15 minutes. If dose-limiting effects occur, decrease dosage gradually in 2-ng/kg/minute decrements q 15 minutes or longer until dose-limiting effects resolve. Avoid abrupt withdrawal or sudden large reductions in infusion rate.

ADMINISTRATION

Direct injection: Not recommended.
Intermittent infusion: Not recommended.
Continuous infusion: Give by ambulatory infusion pump via a central catheter. Peripheral infusion may be done on a temporary basis until central access is established.

PREPARATION & STORAGE

Available as sterile freeze-dried powder in 17-ml vials.

Reconstitute drug only as directed, using sterile diluent provided. The prescribed concentration should be compatible with the infusion pump's minimum and maximum flow rates and reservoir capacity, and with other criteria the manufacturer has recommended. When used for maintenance infusion, drug should be prepared in a drug delivery reservoir appropriate for the infusion pump, with a total reservoir volume of at least 100 ml. Prepare drug using two vials of sterile diluent for use during 24 hours. Don't reconstitute or mix with other parenteral drugs or solutions before or during administration.

Protect reconstituted solutions from light and refrigerate at 36° to 46° F (2° to 8° C); don't freeze. Discard frozen solution or solution that has been refrigerated longer than 48 hours.

Incompatibilities

Other I.V. drugs or solutions.

CONTRAINDICATIONS & CAUTIONS

• Contraindicated in those hypersensitive to the drug or to structurally related compounds.

• Long-term use is contraindicated in those with heart failure caused by severe left ventricular systolic dysfunction, and in those who develop pulmonary edema during initial dosing.
• Use cautiously in geriatric, pregnant, or breast-feeding patients.

ADVERSE REACTIONS

CNS: *headache, anxiety, nervousness, agitation, dizziness, hypesthesia, paresthesia, tremor, fever.*
CV: *hypotension, chest pain,* **bradycardia, tachycardia,** *flushing.*
GI: *nausea, vomiting,* abdominal pain, dyspepsia, *diarrhea.*
Hematologic: *thrombocytopenia.*
Musculoskeletal: *myalgia, nonspecific muscle pain.*
Respiratory: *dyspnea.*
Skin: *flushing,* sweating.
Other: *jaw pain, flulike syndrome,* **sepsis,** *chills.*

INTERACTIONS

Drug-drug. *Anticoagulants, antiplatelet drugs:* May increase risk of bleeding. Monitor patient closely.
Antihypertensives, diuretics, vasodilators: Causes additional reduction in blood pressure. Monitor blood pressure closely.

EFFECTS ON LAB TEST RESULTS

• May decrease potassium level.
• May decrease platelet count.

ACTION

Directly vasodilates pulmonary and systemic arterial vascular beds and inhibits platelet aggregation.

PHARMACOKINETICS

In vitro half-life in human blood, about 6 minutes.
Distribution: Unknown.
Metabolism: Extensive.
Excretion: Mainly in urine.

CLINICAL CONSIDERATIONS

• *Alert:* Drug should be used only by health care providers experienced in the diagnosis and treatment of primary pulmonary hypertension. The dosage must be determined in a setting with adequate personnel and equipment for monitoring and emergency care.
• Avoid abrupt withdrawal of drug or sudden large reductions in infusion rate.
• Have backup infusion pump and infusion set available to prevent interruptions in therapy.
• To facilitate extended use at temperatures above 77° F (25° C), use a cold pouch with frozen gel packs. The pouch must be able to maintain a temperature of 36° to 46° F (2° to 8° C) for 12 hours. When you use such a pouch, use the reconstituted solution for no longer than 24 hours.
• If other I.V. therapies are routinely given, consider using a multilumen catheter.
• Give anticoagulant therapy during maintenance infusion unless contraindicated. Monitor PT and INR closely.
• Check patient's blood pressure when he's standing and supine, and monitor heart rate for several hours to ensure tolerance.

PATIENT TEACHING

• Discuss patient's long-term need for therapy, and determine if he or a family member can provide catheter and infusion pump care.
• Instruct patient or caregiver how to reconstitute, give, and store drug; operate the infusion pump; and replace a failing pump.
• Advise patient to promptly report adverse effects.
• Provide patient and family with telephone numbers of needed resources, such as a home care company, 24-hour contact person, or support group for patients and families with chronic illness.

Reactions may be *common,* uncommon, *life-threatening,* or COMMON AND LIFE-THREATENING.

eptifibatide
Integrilin

Pharmacologic class: glycoprotein IIb/IIIa receptor blocker
Therapeutic class: antiplatelet drug
Pregnancy risk category: B
pH: 5.3

INDICATIONS & DOSAGES
➤ **Acute coronary syndrome (unstable angina or non–Q-wave MI) in patients being managed medically and in those undergoing percutaneous coronary intervention (PCI)—**
Adults with creatinine level less than 2 mg/dl: 180-mcg/kg I.V. bolus as soon as possible after diagnosis, followed by a continuous I.V. infusion of 2 mcg/kg/minute until hospital discharge or initiation of coronary artery bypass graft surgery, up to 72 hours. If patient undergoes PCI, continue infusion until hospital discharge or for up to 18 to 24 hours after the procedure, whichever comes first, up to 96 hours. For patients weighing more than 121 kg (266 lb), the maximum bolus is 22.6 mg and the maximum infusion rate is 15 mg/hour.
Adults with creatinine level of 2 to 4 mg/dl: 180-mcg/kg I.V. bolus as soon as possible after diagnosis, followed by an infusion rate of 1 mcg/kg/minute. For patients weighing more than 121 kg, the maximum bolus dose is 22.6 mg and the maximum infusion rate is 7.5 mg/hour.
➤ **Patients undergoing PCI—**
Adults with creatinine level less than 2 mg/dl started at the time of PCI: 180-mcg/kg I.V. bolus given immediately before the procedure, followed by an infusion of 2 mcg/kg/minute and a second I.V. bolus of 180 mcg/kg given 10 minutes after the first bolus. Continue infusion until hospital discharge or

for up to 18 to 24 hours (whichever comes first); at least 12 hours of eptifibatide infusion is recommended. For patients weighing more than 121 kg, the maximum bolus dose is 22.6 mg and the maximum infusion rate is 15 mg/hour.
Adults with creatinine level of 2 to 4 mg/dl started at the time of PCI: 180-mcg/kg I.V. bolus given immediately before the procedure, followed by an infusion of 1 mcg/kg/minute and a second I.V. bolus of 180 mcg/kg given 10 minutes after the first bolus. For patients weighing more than 121 kg, the maximum bolus dose is 22.6 mg and the maximum infusion rate is 7.5 mg/hour.

ADMINISTRATION
Direct injection: Bolus given as I.V. push over 1 to 2 minutes.
Intermittent infusion: Not recommended.
Continuous infusion: Give undiluted directly from 100-ml vial by continuous I.V. infusion, using an infusion pump, for 24 to 72 hours, depending on indication.

PREPARATION & STORAGE
Available as 2-mg/ml injection for I.V. bolus and 0.75-mg/ml injection for infusion.
Withdraw bolus dose from 10-ml vial into a syringe or use a ready-to-use syringe. Inspect solution for particulate matter before administration. If particles are visible, discard solution.
Drug may be given in same I.V. line as alteplase, atropine, dobutamine, heparin, lidocaine, meperidine, metoprolol, midazolam, morphine, nitroglycerin, or verapamil and in the same I.V. line as normal saline solution or dextrose 5% in normal saline solution. Drug also may contain up to 60 mEq/L of potassium chloride.
Refrigerate vials at 36° to 46° F (2° to 8° C). Protect from light until drug is given.

Incompatibilities
Furosemide.

CONTRAINDICATIONS & CAUTIONS
• Contraindicated in those hypersensitive to the drug or its ingredients and in those with a platelet count below 100,000/mm³.
• Contraindicated in those with a history of CVA or bleeding diathesis or evidence of active abnormal bleeding within the previous 30 days.
• Contraindicated in those with blood pressure above 200/110 mm Hg who are inadequately controlled with antihypertensives and in those with current or planned use of another parenteral glycoprotein (GP) IIb/IIIa inhibitor.
• Contraindicated in those who have had major surgery within the previous 6 weeks and in those on renal dialysis.
• Use cautiously in those at increased risk for bleeding and in those weighing more than 143 kg (315 lb).

ADVERSE REACTIONS
CV: hypotension.
GU: hematuria.
Hematologic: *bleeding, thrombocytopenia.*
Other: bleeding at femoral artery access site.

INTERACTIONS
Drug-drug. *Clopidogrel, dipyridamole, NSAIDs, oral anticoagulants, thrombolytics, ticlopidine:* Increases risk of bleeding. Monitor patient closely.
Inhibitors of platelet receptor GP IIb/IIIa: May cause serious bleeding. Avoid using together.

EFFECTS ON LAB TEST RESULTS
• May decrease platelet count.

ACTION
Inhibits platelet aggregation by reversibly binding to the GP IIb/IIIa receptor on platelets.

PHARMACOKINETICS
Onset, immediate; peak, immediate; duration, 4 to 6 hours after end of infusion.
Distribution: 25% bound to protein, primarily albumin.
Metabolism: Rapidly degraded in bladder after elimination from plasma.
Excretion: Half-life is about 2½ hours, with 50% excreted in urine.

CLINICAL CONSIDERATIONS
• Drug is intended for use with heparin and aspirin.
• Perform baseline laboratory tests before starting drug therapy, including hematocrit, platelet count, hemoglobin, creatinine levels, PT, INR, and aPTT.
• If patient is to undergo coronary artery bypass graft surgery, stop infusion before surgery.
• Minimize use of arterial and venous punctures, I.M. injections, urinary catheters, nasotracheal tubes, and NG tubes.
• When obtaining I.V. access, avoid using noncompressible sites (such as subclavian or jugular veins).
• Monitor patient for bleeding.
• If patient's platelet count is below 100,000/mm³, stop eptifibatide and heparin.
• Stop eptifibatide and heparin and achieve sheath hemostasis by standard compression techniques at least 4 hours before hospital discharge.

PATIENT TEACHING
• Explain that drug prevents blood clotting and is used to prevent chest pain and heart attack.
• Explain that the benefits of the drug far outweigh the risk of serious bleeding.
• Instruct patient to immediately report chest discomfort or other adverse reactions.
• Caution patient to avoid activities that might cause bleeding or bruising.

ertapenem sodium
Invanz

Pharmacologic class: carbapenem
Therapeutic class: anti-infective
Pregnancy risk category: B
pH: 7.5

INDICATIONS & DOSAGES
➤ **Complicated intra-abdominal infections caused by** *Escherichia coli, Clostridium clostridiiforme, Eubacterium lentum, Peptostreptococcus* species, *Bacteroides fragilis, B. distasonis, B. ovatus, B. thetaiotaomicron, B. uniformis*—
Adults: 1 g I.V. once daily for 5 to 14 days.
➤ **Complicated skin and skin-structure infections caused by** *Staphylococcus aureus* (methicillin-susceptible strains), *Streptococcus pyogenes, E. coli, Peptostreptococcus* species—
Adults: 1 g I.V. once daily for 7 to 14 days.
➤ **Community-acquired pneumonia caused by** *S. pneumoniae* (penicillin-susceptible strains), *Haemophilus influenzae* (beta-lactamase–negative strains), *Moraxella catarrhalis;* **complicated UTIs, including pyelonephritis caused by** *E. coli, Klebsiella pneumoniae*—
Adults: 1 g I.V. once daily for 10 to 14 days. If patient improves after at least 3 days of treatment, appropriate oral therapy may be used to complete the full course.
➤ **Acute pelvic infections including postpartum endomyometritis, septic abortion, and postsurgical gynecologic infections caused by** *Streptococcus agalactiae, E. coli, B. fragilis, Porphyromonas asaccharolyticus,*

Peptostreptococcus **species,** *Prevotella bivia*—
Adults: 1 g I.V. once daily for 3 to 10 days.
Adjust-a-dose: For patients with creatinine clearance of 30 ml/minute or less, give 500 mg I.V. daily. When patients receiving hemodialysis are given the recommended daily dose of 500 mg I.V. less than 6 hours before the hemodialysis session, a supplementary dose of 150 mg I.V. is recommended after the session. If ertapenem is given at least 6 hours before hemodialysis, no supplementary dose is needed.

ADMINISTRATION
Direct injection: Not recommended
Intermittent infusion: Not recommended.
Continuous infusion: Infuse at a constant rate over 30 minutes. Complete the infusion within 6 hours of reconstitution.

PREPARATION & STORAGE
Available as a lyophilized, white to off-white crystalline powder in a 1-g single-dose vial.
 Reconstitute the contents of 1-g vial with 10 ml of water for injection, normal saline solution, or bacteriostatic water for injection. Shake well to dissolve and immediately transfer contents of the reconstituted vial to 50 ml of normal saline injection. Reconstituted solutions may range from colorless to pale yellow. Variations in color don't affect the potency of the drug.
 Don't store lyophilized powder above 77° F (25° C). The reconstituted solution, immediately diluted in normal saline injection, may be stored at 77° F and used within 6 hours or refrigerated for 24 hours at 41° F (5° C) and used within 4 hours after removal from refrigerator. Don't freeze solutions.

Incompatibilities
Diluents containing dextrose (alpha-D-glucose), other I.V. drugs.

CONTRAINDICATIONS & CAUTIONS
• Contraindicated in patients hypersensitive to any component of the drug or to other drugs in the same class and in patients who have had anaphylactic reactions to penicillins, cephalosporins, and other beta-lactams.
• Drug can also be given I.M.; however, I.M. use is contraindicated in patients hypersensitive to local anesthetics of the amide type because of the use of lidocaine hydrochloride as a diluent.
• Use cautiously in patients with CNS disorders, compromised renal function, or both, because drug may cause seizures.
• Use in pregnant women only if clearly needed.
• Drug appears in breast milk. Give drug to breast-feeding women only when the expected benefit outweighs the risk.
• Use caution when selecting dose in geriatric patients with renal impairment.

ADVERSE REACTIONS
CNS: asthenia, fatigue, anxiety, altered mental status, dizziness, headache, insomnia, fever.
CV: edema, swelling, chest pain, hypertension, hypotension, tachycardia, infused vein complication, phlebitis, thrombophlebitis.
EENT: pharyngitis.
GI: abdominal pain, acid regurgitation, oral candidiasis, constipation, *diarrhea,* dyspepsia, nausea, vomiting.
GU: vaginitis, renal dysfunction.
Hematologic: coagulation abnormalities, eosinophilia, anemia, ***neutropenia, leukopenia, thrombocytopenia,*** *thrombocytosis.*
Hepatic: jaundice.
Metabolic: hyperglycemia, hyperkalemia.

Musculoskeletal: leg pain.
Respiratory: cough, dyspnea, rales, rhonchi, respiratory distress.
Skin: erythema, pruritus, rash, extravasation.

INTERACTIONS
Drug-drug. *Probenecid:* Reduces renal clearance and increases half-life. Don't give together with probenecid to extend half-life.

EFFECTS ON LAB TEST RESULTS
• May increase albumin, ALT, AST, alkaline phosphatase, bilirubin, creatinine, glucose, and potassium levels.
• May increase PT and eosinophil and urinary RBC counts. May decrease hemoglobin, hematocrit, and segmented neutrophil count. May increase or decrease platelet and WBC counts.

ACTION
Inhibits cell-wall synthesis and binds to penicillin-binding proteins. Drug is active against susceptible gram-positive, gram-negative, and anaerobic bacteria.

PHARMACOKINETICS
Onset, immediate; peak, ½ hour; duration, 24 hours.
Distribution: Highly bound to protein, primarily albumin.
Metabolism: Doesn't inhibit metabolism mediated by cytochrome P-450 isoforms.
Excretion: Mostly in the kidneys. Mean half-life, about 4 hours; 80% excreted in urine, 10% in feces.

CLINICAL CONSIDERATIONS
• *Alert:* Check for previous penicillin, cephalosporin, or other beta-lactam hypersensitivity before giving first dose.
• Obtain specimens for culture and sensitivity testing before giving first dose. Therapy may start before results are available.

Reactions may be *common,* uncommon, *life-threatening,* or COMMON AND LIFE-THREATENING.

• If diarrhea persists during therapy, stop drug and collect stool specimen for culture to rule out pseudomembranous colitis.

• If allergic reaction occurs, stop drug immediately. Serious anaphylactic reactions require immediate emergency treatment with epinephrine, oxygen, I.V. corticosteroids, and airway management.

• Continue anticonvulsants in patients with seizure disorders. If focal tremors, myoclonus, or seizures occur, evaluate patient neurologically and give anticonvulsants if not done earlier. Reexamine the dosage to determine whether it should be decreased or the drug stopped.

• Methicillin-resistant staphylococci and *Enterococcus* species are resistant to ertapenem.

• Monitor renal, hepatic, and hematopoietic function during prolonged therapy.

• Be alert for any signs and symptoms of superinfection during prolonged therapy.

• *Alert:* Don't confuse Avinza (morphine sulfate) with Invanz (ertapenem).

• Signs and symptoms of overdose may include nausea, diarrhea, and dizziness. If an overdose occurs, stop ertapenem and treat supportively until drug has been eliminated renally. Ertapenem can be removed by hemodialysis.

PATIENT TEACHING

• Inform patient of potential adverse reactions and tell him to report them immediately.

• Tell patient to contact prescriber immediately if he develops diarrhea.

• Tell patient to report discomfort at injection site.

erythromycin lactobionate
Erythrocin Lactobinate I.V.*

Pharmacologic class: erythromycin
Therapeutic class: antibiotic
Pregnancy risk category: B
pH: 6.5 to 7.5

INDICATIONS & DOSAGES

➤ **Acute pelvic inflammatory disease caused by** *Neisseria gonorrhoeae*—
Adults: 500 mg I.V. q 6 hours for 3 days, followed by 250 mg base, estolate, or stearate or 400 mg ethylsuccinate P.O. q 6 hours for 7 days.

➤ **Mild to moderately severe respiratory tract, skin, and soft-tissue infections caused by sensitive group A beta-hemolytic streptococci,** *Streptococcus pneumoniae, Mycoplasma pneumoniae, Corynebacterium diphtheriae,* **or** *Bordetella pertussis*—
Adults: 15 to 20 mg/kg I.V. daily as continuous infusion or in divided doses q 6 hours for 10 days, or for 3 weeks for *Mycoplasma* infection.
Children: 15 to 20 mg/kg I.V. daily, in divided doses q 4 to 6 hours for 10 days or 3 weeks for *Mycoplasma* infection.

➤ **Pneumonia in infants caused by** *Chlamydia trachomatis*—
Infants: 15 to 20 mg/kg/day I.V. as a continuous infusion or in four divided doses.

ADMINISTRATION

Direct injection: Not recommended.
Intermittent infusion: Infuse over 20 to 60 minutes at intervals not greater than every 6 hours. Drug should be diluted enough to minimize pain and vein irritation.
Continuous infusion: Preferred method because of slower infusion rate and lower concentration of erythromycin.

Drug should be diluted enough to minimize pain and vein irritation.

PREPARATION & STORAGE
Available as vials of 500 mg or 1,000 mg as powder for injection.

Add 10 ml of sterile water for injection to a 500-mg vial or 20 ml to a 1,000-mg vial. Use only sterile water for injection for initial reconstitution. Dilute drug further with normal saline solution to yield a concentration of 1 to 5 mg/ml. Use at least 100 ml of diluent. D_5W may be used as a diluent only if it's buffered by adding 1 ml of 4% sodium bicarbonate to each 100 ml of diluent. Inspect product for particulate matter and discoloration before giving. After reconstituting drug, give it completely within 8 hours.

Store unopened vials at 59° to 86° F (15° to 30° C).

Incompatibilities
Ampicillin sodium, ascorbic acid injection, colistimethate, dextrose 2.5% in half-strength Ringer's lactate, dextrose 5% in lactated Ringer's solution, dextrose 5% in normal saline solution, D_5W, dextrose 10% in water, heparin sodium, metoclopramide, dextrose 5% in Normosol-M , Normosol R, Ringer's injection, vitamin B complex with C.

CONTRAINDICATIONS & CAUTIONS
• Contraindicated in patients hypersensitive to drug or other macrolides.
• Contraindicated in patients with hepatic disease.

ADVERSE REACTIONS
CNS: fever.
CV: *ventricular arrhythmias, vein irritation, thrombophlebitis.*
EENT: hearing loss with high I.V. doses.
GI: abdominal pain and cramping, nausea, vomiting, diarrhea, *pseudomembranous colitis.*
Skin: urticaria, rash, eczema.

Other: overgrowth of nonsusceptible bacteria or fungi, *anaphylaxis.*

INTERACTIONS
Drug-drug. *Carbamazepine:* Increases carbamazepine levels and risk of toxic reaction. Monitor patient closely.
Clindamycin: May cause antagonistic effects. Avoid using together.
Cyclosporine: Increases cyclosporine level. Monitor patient closely.
Digoxin: Increases digoxin level. Monitor patient for digoxin toxicity.
Disopyramide: Increases disopyramide levels, in some cases causing arrhythmias and increasing QT intervals. Monitor ECG.
Midazolam, triazolam: Increases effects of these drugs. Monitor patient closely.
Oral anticoagulants: Increases anticoagulant effect. Monitor PT and INR closely.
Theophylline: Decreases erythromycin level and increases theophylline toxicity. Use together cautiously.
Drug-herb. *Pill-bearing spurge:* May inhibit CYP3A enzymes, affecting drug metabolism. Advise patient to use together cautiously.

EFFECTS ON LAB TEST RESULTS
• May falsely elevate AST and ALT levels. May interfere with fluorometric determination of urine catecholamines and with colorimetric assays.

ACTION
Inhibits bacterial protein synthesis by binding to the 50S subunit of the ribosome. May be bacteriostatic or bactericidal, depending on concentration.

PHARMACOKINETICS
Onset, unknown; peak, immediate; duration, unknown.
Distribution: In most body tissues and fluids, especially liver and bile. Drug is 73% to 81% protein bound. It crosses the placental barrier, and fetal levels

are 5% to 20% as high as those of the mother. It appears in breast milk in levels about half those of the mother.
Metabolism: Partly changed in the liver to inactive metabolites.
Excretion: In bile, mainly as unchanged drug, and in urine with 12% to 15% excreted unchanged. In normal renal function, plasma half-life is 1 to 3 hours; in anuria, it may extend to 6 hours.

CLINICAL CONSIDERATIONS
● Osmolality: 223 to 313 mOsm/kg.
● Obtain specimens for culture and sensitivity tests before giving first dose.
● Dialysis removes only a small amount of drug.
● Oral therapy should replace I.V. therapy as soon as possible.
● Minimize the pain of venous irritation by diluting drug, infusing drug slowly, or applying ice to infusion site.
● Monitor renal and hepatic function test results.
● Monitor patient for superinfection.
● Drug may cause overgrowth of nonsusceptible bacteria or fungi.

PATIENT TEACHING
● Instruct patient to report adverse effects, especially injection site pain, nausea, abdominal pain, and fever.

esmolol hydrochloride
Brevibloc

Pharmacologic class: beta$_1$ blocker
Therapeutic class: antiarrhythmic
Pregnancy risk category: C
pH: 3.5 to 5.5

INDICATIONS & DOSAGES
➤ **Supraventricular tachycardia; to lower heart rate and blood pressure in patients with acute myocardial ischemia ◆ —**
Adults: Loading dose is 500 mcg/kg/minute by I.V. infusion over 1 minute, followed by a 4-minute maintenance infusion of 50 mcg/kg/minute. If patient doesn't respond adequately within 5 minutes, repeat the loading dose and follow it with a maintenance infusion of 100 mcg/kg/minute for 4 minutes. Repeat loading dose and increase maintenance infusion in a stepwise fashion p.r.n. Maximum maintenance infusion for tachycardia is 200 mcg/kg/minute.
➤ **To manage perioperative hypertension and tachycardia—**
Adults: For immediate intraoperative control, inject 80 mg over 30 seconds. If needed, follow with an infusion of 150 mcg/kg/minute. For gradual control of hypertension, follow dosing schedule for supraventricular tachycardia.

ADMINISTRATION
Direct injection: Inject intraoperative dose over 30 seconds; don't use 250-mg/ml ampule.
Intermittent infusion: Not recommended.
Continuous infusion: Using an I.V. catheter and an infusion pump, give loading dose over 1 minute and maintenance dose over 4 minutes. If reaction occurs at infusion site, stop infusion and resume at another site. Don't use a winged infusion needle or inject into very small veins.

PREPARATION & STORAGE
Available in 10-ml ampules containing 250 mg/ml. Concentrations of 20 mg/ml or higher are linked to venous irritation and thrombophlebitis. A ready-to-use formulation containing 10 mg/ml in a 10-ml single-dose vial is also available.
　Remove 20 ml from a 500-ml container of compatible solution and add

contents of two ampules to yield a concentration of 10 mg/ml.

Compatible solutions include D_5W, dextrose 5% in lactated Ringer's solution, lactated Ringer's solution, dextrose 5% in half-normal saline solution; potassium chloride 40 mEq in D_5W injection, and half-normal or normal saline solution.

Diluted solution is stable for 24 hours at room temperature. Although freezing doesn't alter the drug's effect, avoid exposing the drug to high temperatures.

Incompatibilities
Furosemide, procainamide, warfarin sodium.

CONTRAINDICATIONS & CAUTIONS
• Contraindicated in those with sinus bradycardia or second- or third-degree heart block because of chronotropic effects of beta blockade, and in those with cardiogenic shock or overt heart failure because beta blockade further depresses myocardial contractility.
• Use cautiously in those with bronchospastic disease because drug may worsen the condition; use cautiously in those with diabetes mellitus or hypoglycemia because drug may mask tachycardia during hypoglycemia.
• Use cautiously in geriatric patients and in those with renal impairment because of increased risk of toxic reaction; base dosage on clinical response.

ADVERSE REACTIONS
CNS: agitation, confusion, fatigue, dizziness, somnolence, *seizures,* headache.
CV: hypotension, *peripheral ischemia, bradycardia, heart block.*
GI: nausea, vomiting.
Respiratory: *bronchospasm,* dyspnea, *pulmonary edema.*
Skin: *sweating,* inflammation and induration at injection site.

INTERACTIONS
Drug-drug. *Antihypertensives:* May potentiate effects. Monitor patient closely.
Cardiac glycosides: Increases digoxin levels. Monitor cardiac status and assess for dosage adjustment.
Catecholamine-depleting drugs, such as reserpine: May enhance effects of both drugs. Dosage may need to be adjusted.
Insulin: May mask symptoms of hypoglycemia, except sweating and dizziness. Monitor patient closely.
Morphine I.V.: Increases esmolol levels by 50%. Dosage may need to be adjusted.
Nondepolarizing neuromuscular blockers: May cause prolonged action. Monitor patient closely.

EFFECTS ON LAB TEST RESULTS
• May increase LDH level.
• May decrease hemoglobin.

ACTION
Ultra short-acting cardioselective beta blocker with no sympathomimetic activity. Blocks the agonist effect of sympathetic neurotransmitters.

PHARMACOKINETICS
Onset, 2 minutes; duration, 10 to 20 minutes.
Distribution: Rapidly into plasma; 55% protein bound. Drug probably crosses the placental barrier.
Metabolism: Rapid hydrolysis by RBC esterases.
Excretion: 75% to 90% excreted in urine in 24 to 48 hours. Half-life, about 9 minutes. Renal dysfunction prolongs elimination.

CLINICAL CONSIDERATIONS
• Osmolarity: 1,063 mOsm/L.
• Monitor ECG and blood pressure continuously during infusion. Up to 25% of patients develop hypotension. Monitor patient closely, especially if

his blood pressure before treatment was low.
- Hypotension can usually be reversed within 30 minutes by decreasing the dose or, if needed, by stopping the infusion.
- Once patient's heart rate has stabilized, you may substitute a longer-acting antiarrhythmic, as ordered. After starting new drug, gradually reduce esmolol infusion over 1 hour.
- If overdose occurs, stop drug. As needed, give atropine or another anticholinergic for severe bradycardia, a theophylline derivative or B_2 adrenergic agonist for bronchospasm, and a diuretic or a cardiac glycoside for cardiac failure. Closely monitor blood pressure and heart rate and rhythm, and frequently check for signs of neurologic deficit.

PATIENT TEACHING
- Instruct patient to promptly report breathing or heart symptoms and other adverse effects.
- Explain use and administration of drug to patient and family.
- Tell patient to report discomfort at I.V. site.

estrogens, conjugated
Premarin Intravenous*

Pharmacologic class: hormone
Therapeutic class: estrogen replacement
Pregnancy risk category: X

INDICATIONS & DOSAGES
➤ **Abnormal uterine bleeding from hormonal imbalance in the absence of disease—**
Adults: 25 mg I.V., repeated in 6 to 12 hours, if needed.

ADMINISTRATION
Direct injection: Inject reconstituted drug directly into a vein over 1 to 5 minutes or into an established I.V. line containing a free-flowing, compatible solution; inject just distal to the infusion needle.
Intermittent infusion: Not recommended.
Continuous infusion: Not recommended.

PREPARATION & STORAGE
Available in package containing 25-mg vial of drug and 5-ml ampule of sterile water for injection and 2% benzyl alcohol.
   To reconstitute, withdraw air from vial and slowly inject provided diluent against inside wall of vial. Swirl gently; don't shake vigorously. Compatible with dextrose, saline, and invert sugar solutions.
   Intact vial remains stable for 5 years if refrigerated. Reconstituted drug remains stable for 60 days if refrigerated and protected from light, but manufacturer recommends immediate use.
   Don't use if drug darkens or precipitate forms.

Incompatibilities
Ascorbic acid, solutions with an acidic pH.

CONTRAINDICATIONS & CAUTIONS
- Contraindicated in those with known or suspected estrogen-dependent neoplasia or breast cancer, except for those being treated for metastatic disease, and in those with undiagnosed vaginal bleeding or active or past thrombophlebitis or thromboembolic disorders because estrogen may worsen these conditions.
- Avoid use in pregnant patients because of increased risk of fetal cancers and abnormalities.
- Use cautiously in those with metastatic bone disease linked to hypercalcemia

because drug affects calcium and phosphorus metabolism and in those with hepatic impairment because drug may be poorly metabolized.

ADVERSE REACTIONS

CNS: headache, dizziness, chorea, depression, *seizures.*
CV: thrombophlebitis; *thromboembolism;* hypertension; edema; *increased risk of CVA, pulmonary embolism, MI.*
EENT: worsening of myopia or astigmatism, intolerance of contact lenses.
GI: *nausea,* vomiting, abdominal cramps, bloating, anorexia, increased appetite, *pancreatitis,* gallbladder disease.
GU: breakthrough bleeding, altered menstrual flow, dysmenorrhea, amenorrhea, *increased risk of endometrial cancer, increased risk of breast cancer,* cervical erosion, altered cervical secretions, enlargement of uterine fibromas, vaginal candidiasis.
Hepatic: cholestatic jaundice, *hepatic adenoma.*
Metabolic: weight changes.
Skin: melasma, urticaria, flushing (with rapid administration), hirsutism or hair loss, erythema nodosum, dermatitis.
Other: breast tenderness, enlargement, or secretion.

INTERACTIONS

Drug-drug. *Anticoagulants:* Reduces anticoagulant effects. Monitor patient closely.
Corticosteroids: Reduces clearance and increases elimination half-life. Monitor patient closely; dosage may need to be adjusted.
Drugs that induce hepatic metabolism, such as carbamazepine and primidone: Reduces estrogen's effectiveness because of altered metabolism. Monitor patient closely.

Hepatotoxic drugs such as dantrolene: Increases risk of hepatotoxicity. Monitor hepatic status.
Insulin, oral antidiabetics: May increase or decrease glucose levels. Dosage may be adjusted, as needed.
Tricyclic antidepressants: Increases toxic effects. Monitor patient for toxic reaction.
Drug-herb. *Red clover:* May interfere with hormone therapy. Discourage use together.
Drug-food. *Caffeine:* May increase caffeine level. Discourage use together.
Drug-lifestyle. *Smoking:* Increases risk of adverse CV effects. Advise patient to avoid smoking.

EFFECTS ON LAB TEST RESULTS

• May increase total T_4, thyroid-binding globulin, phospholipid, fibrinogen, plasminogen, glucose, triglyceride, and factor VII, VIII, IX, and X levels. May decrease folate, antifactor Xa, and antithrombin III levels.
• May increase PT and norepinephrine-induced platelet aggregation.

ACTION

Conjugated estrogenic substances bind to cytoplasmic proteins, forming a complex that promotes synthesis of DNA, RNA, and other proteins in responsive tissues. They also reduce pituitary gonadotropin production, curtailing release of follicle-stimulating hormone and luteinizing hormone.

PHARMACOKINETICS

Drug level peaks at end of injection.
Distribution: In cells of female genitalia, breasts, hypothalamus, and pituitary. Drug is moderately to highly protein bound; it crosses the placental barrier and appears in breast milk.
Metabolism: Primarily in the liver.
Excretion: Primarily in the urine.

Reactions may be *common,* uncommon, *life-threatening,* or COMMON AND LIFE-THREATENING.

CLINICAL CONSIDERATIONS
• Osmolality: exceeds 2,000 mOsm/kg.
• If pathology specimens are taken, indicate that patient is undergoing estrogen therapy.
• Give direct I.V. injection slowly to avoid flushing reaction.
• Monitor glucose level when giving drug to a diabetic patient.
• *Alert:* Estrogens and progestins shouldn't be used to prevent CV disease. The Women's Health Initiative study reported an increased risk of MI, stroke, invasive breast cancer, pulmonary emboli, and deep vein thrombosis in postmenopausal women during 5 years of combination therapy. Because of these risks, estrogens and progestins should be prescribed at the lowest effective doses and for the shortest duration consistent with treatment goals and risks for each patient.

PATIENT TEACHING
• Instruct patient to immediately report adverse reactions.
• Teach women how to perform breast self-examination.
• Explain use and administration of drug to patient and family.

ethacrynate sodium
Sodium Edecrin

Pharmacologic class: loop diuretic
Therapeutic class: diuretic
Pregnancy risk category: B
pH: 6.3 to 7.7

INDICATIONS & DOSAGES
➤ **Edema linked to heart failure, cirrhosis, renal disease, ascites in cancer, lymphedema, or nephrotic syndrome; when rapid diuresis is needed, such as in acute pulmonary edema—**
Adults: 50 mg or 0.5 to 1 mg/kg I.V.; may be repeated in 2 to 4 hours if needed, then in 4 to 6 hours. In emergency use, may repeat hourly. Maximum, 100 mg/dose.

ADMINISTRATION
Direct injection: Inject drug directly into vein over several minutes, or infuse slowly over 20 to 30 minutes through I.V. tubing of free-flowing, compatible solution. In repeated doses, change I.V. sites to reduce risk of thrombophlebitis.
Intermittent infusion: Not recommended.
Continuous infusion: Not recommended.

PREPARATION & STORAGE
Supplied in 50-mg vials.
    Reconstitute with 50 ml of normal saline solution or D_5W to a concentration of 1 mg/ml. Don't use cloudy solution, a sign of pH below 5. Compatible solutions include dextrose 5% in normal saline solution, D_5W, Normosol-R, Ringer's injection, lactated Ringer's solution, and normal saline solution.
    Store at room temperature and discard unused solution after 24 hours.

Incompatibilities
Hydralazine, Normosol-M, procainamide, ranitidine, reserpine, solutions or drugs with pH below 5, tolazoline, triflupromazine, whole blood and its derivatives.

CONTRAINDICATIONS & CAUTIONS
• Contraindicated in infants and children or those hypersensitive to ethacrynate or thimerosal (a preservative).
• Contraindicated in those with electrolyte imbalance, hypotension, dehydration with low sodium levels, and metabolic alkalosis with hypokalemia because drug worsens these conditions.

• Avoid use in those with anuria, azotemia, or oliguria because of increased risk of toxic reaction.
• Use cautiously in those with diabetes mellitus because drug may impair glucose tolerance, and in those with hyperuricemia or gout because drug may raise uric acid level.
• Use cautiously in those with hepatic impairment because possible dehydration and electrolyte imbalance may precipitate hepatic coma, and in those with an acute MI because diuresis may precipitate shock.
• Use cautiously in those with a history of pancreatitis or lupus erythematosus because drug may worsen these conditions.

ADVERSE REACTIONS
CNS: fever, apprehension, confusion, fatigue, vertigo, headache, malaise.
EENT: feeling of fullness in the ears, ototoxicity.
GI: *acute necrotizing pancreatitis,* anorexia, nausea, vomiting, diarrhea, dysphagia, GI bleeding, discomfort, pain.
GU: hematuria, *profound diuresis.*
Hematologic: *severe neutropenia, thrombocytopenia, agranulocytosis.*
Hepatic: *hepatic coma.*
Metabolic: fluid and electrolyte depletion, acute gout, hyperglycemia.
Skin: rash.
Other: chills, local irritation.

INTERACTIONS
Drug-drug. *Aminoglycosides, amphotericin B, ototoxic and nephrotoxic drugs:* Increases risk of ototoxicity and nephrotoxicity and intensifies electrolyte imbalance. Use together with caution.
Amiodarone, cardiac glycosides: Increases risk of arrhythmias linked to hypokalemia. Monitor potassium level.
Anticoagulants, thrombolytics: Enhances anticoagulant effects and risk of GI bleeding. Monitor patient closely.

Antidiabetics, insulin: Interferes with hypoglycemic effects. Monitor patient for possible dose adjustment.
Antigout drugs: May increase uric acid levels. Monitor patient closely.
Antihistamines, antivertigo drugs, phenothiazines, thioxanthenes, trimethobenzamide: Masks symptoms of ototoxicity. Avoid using together.
Antihypertensives: Enhances hypotensive and diuretic effects. Monitor blood pressure closely.
Corticosteroids: May decrease natriuretic and diuretic effects and intensify electrolyte imbalance. Monitor electrolyte levels.
Lithium: Increases risk of toxic reaction because of reduced clearance. Monitor patient for toxic reaction.
Neuromuscular blockers: Prolongs blockade resulting from hypokalemia. Monitor potassium level.
NSAIDs, probenecid: May antagonize natriuresis and diuresis and increase risk of renal failure. Monitor renal status.
Sodium bicarbonate: Increases risk of hypochloremic alkalosis. Monitor patient closely.
Sympathomimetics: Reduces antihypertensive effects of ethacrynate. Monitor blood pressure closely.
Drug-lifestyle. *Alcohol use:* Enhances hypotensive and diuretic effects. Discourage use together.

EFFECTS ON LAB TEST RESULTS
• May increase glucose and uric acid levels. May decrease potassium, sodium, calcium, and magnesium levels.
• May decrease granulocyte, neutrophil, and platelet counts.

ACTION
Inhibits reabsorption of electrolytes, including sodium and chloride, in the proximal tubule and ascending loop of Henle and increases potassium excretion in the distal tubule. Also, may di-

---

rectly affect electrolyte transport at the proximal tubule.

PHARMACOKINETICS
Onset, 5 minutes; duration, 2 hours.
Distribution: Readily dispersed, but probably accumulates only in the liver. Highly protein bound; doesn't cross the blood-brain barrier. It's unknown if drug crosses placental barrier or appears in breast milk.
Metabolism: Primarily in the liver.
Excretion: 30% to 65% secreted by proximal renal tubules and excreted in urine. Drug is 35% to 40% excreted in bile.

CLINICAL CONSIDERATIONS
● Osmolality: 268 mOsm/kg.
● In those with renal edema and hypoproteinemia, give salt-poor albumin, as ordered, to enhance response to ethacrynate sodium.
● In those at high risk for metabolic alkalosis, give ammonium chloride or arginine chloride, as ordered.
● Drug may be used in hypertensive crisis, in nephrogenic diabetes insipidus unresponsive to vasopressin or chlorpropamide, in hypercalcemia to promote calcium excretion, in bromide intoxication to promote bromide excretion, and with mannitol in ethylene glycol poisoning.
● Drug may increase risk of GI bleeding when used with corticosteroids.
● If patient experiences severe, watery diarrhea, drug may need to be stopped.
● Signs of overdose include excessive diuresis with dehydration and electrolyte depletion.
● If overdose occurs, correct fluid and electrolyte imbalance and treat symptomatically.
● Monitor blood pressure, BUN and electrolyte levels, intake and output, and weight.

PATIENT TEACHING
● Advise patient to rise slowly and avoid sudden posture changes to limit dizziness.
● Tell patient to report adverse reactions promptly.

etidronate disodium
Didronel IV

Pharmacologic class: bisphosphonate
Therapeutic class: antihypercalcemic
Pregnancy risk category: C
pH: 4 to 5.5

INDICATIONS & DOSAGES
➤ **Hypercalcemia linked to malignant neoplasms—**
Adults: 7.5 mg/kg by I.V. infusion over at least 2 hours for three consecutive days. If hypercalcemia recurs, retreatment may be needed. Allow at least 7 days between courses of therapy. Safety and efficacy of more than two courses of therapy haven't been established.

ADMINISTRATION
Direct injection: Not recommended.
Intermittent infusion: Infuse each dose over at least 2 hours.
Continuous infusion: Not recommended.

PREPARATION & STORAGE
Available in 6-ml ampules containing 300 mg (50 mg/ml).
   Dilute in at least 250 ml of normal saline solution. Store at 59° to 86° F (15° to 30° C).
   Diluted solutions may be stored at controlled room temperature for 48 hours.

Incompatibilities
Other I.V. drugs.

CONTRAINDICATIONS & CAUTIONS
• Contraindicated in those hypersensitive to drug and in those with creatinine
level of 5 mg/dl or more.
• In patients with creatinine level of 2.5
to 4.9 mg/dl, use cautiously and only if
potential benefits outweigh risks of
worsening renal function. May need to
reduce dosage.

ADVERSE REACTIONS
GI: nausea; metallic, altered, or loss of
taste.
GU: *abnormal renal function.*
Metabolic: hypocalcemia.
Skin: rash.

INTERACTIONS
Drug-drug. *Warfarin:* Increases PT.
Monitor patient carefully.

EFFECTS ON LAB TEST RESULTS
• May decrease calcium level.

ACTION
Inhibits normal and abnormal bone resorption, reducing the flow of calcium
into the blood from reabsorbing bone
and decreasing total and ionized calcium levels in patients with hypercalcemia caused by cancer.

PHARMACOKINETICS
After 24 hours, reduces urine calcium
excretion and bone reabsorption.
Distribution: About 50% of dose distributed to bone in areas of elevated osteogenesis.
Metabolism: None.
Excretion: 40% to 60% of dose excreted unchanged in urine. Half-life,
6 hours.

CLINICAL CONSIDERATIONS
• Drug doesn't interfere with the effects
of parathyroid hormone at the renal

tubule, alter renal tubular reabsorption
of calcium, or affect hypercalcemia in
hyperparathyroidism.
• Although some patients may be
treated for up to 7 consecutive days,
risk of hypocalcemia is increased after
3 days.
• On first day after the last dose of I.V.
therapy, start 20 mg/kg of oral etidronate daily for 30 to 90 days.
• I.V. administration at doses and rates
higher than those recommended have
been linked to renal insufficiency.
• Hydration with sodium chloride solution and use of a loop diuretic increases
renal excretion of calcium and reduces
calcium levels in patient treated for
hypercalcemia from malignant neoplasms.
• Avoid overhydration in patients with
heart failure.
• Rapid I.V. administration may produce ECG changes and bleeding problems caused by rapid decreases in ionized calcium levels. If these occur, they
can be reversed with calcium gluconate.
• Monitor albumin and calcium levels
periodically during therapy.
• Geriatric patients may be more prone
to overhydration when treated with
etidronate and hydration. Monitor electrolyte levels carefully.

PATIENT TEACHING
• Inform patient that improvement may
continue for months after drug is
stopped.
• Emphasize the importance of good
nutrition, especially adequate intake of
foods high in calcium and vitamin D.

Reactions may be *common*, uncommon, *life-threatening*, or COMMON AND LIFE-THREATENING.

etoposide (VP-16, VP-16-213)
Toposar*, VePesid*

etoposide phosphate
Etopophos

___

Pharmacologic class: podophyllo-toxin (specific to the G_2 and late S phases)
Therapeutic class: antineoplastic
Pregnancy risk category: D
pH: 3 to 4

___

INDICATIONS & DOSAGES
Dosages are for etoposide; use equivalent dosages for etoposide phosphate.
➤ **To induce remission in refractory testicular cancer—**
Adults: 50 to 100 mg/m²/day I.V. on days 1 to 5, or 100 mg/m²/day I.V. on days 1, 3, and 5. Repeat q 3 to 4 weeks.
➤ **Small-cell lung cancer—**
Adults: 35 mg/m²/day I.V. for 4 days or 50 mg/m²/day I.V. for 5 days, repeated q 3 to 4 weeks.

ADMINISTRATION
Direct injection: Not used because of delayed and possibly fatal toxic reaction.
Intermittent infusion: Give diluted etoposide over at least 30 to 60 minutes through a 21G or 23G needle. Watch for irritation and infiltration; extravasation can cause tissue damage and necrosis. Etoposide phosphate may be given over 5 to 210 minutes.
Continuous infusion: Not recommended.

PREPARATION & STORAGE
Supplied in vials of 100 mg, 150 mg, 200 mg, 250 mg, and 500 mg, each containing 20 mg/ml. Etoposide phosphate is supplied as 113.6-mg vials equivalent to 100 mg etoposide.

Dilute etoposide with D_5W or normal saline solution to 0.2 mg/ml or 0.4 mg/ml. Discard discolored or precipitated solution. Reconstitute etoposide phosphate in each vial with 5 ml or 10 ml of sterile water for injection, D_5W injection, normal saline injection, bacteriostatic water for injection with benzyl alcohol, or bacteriostatic saline for injection with benzyl alcohol. Reconstitution with 5 ml diluent yields a concentration equivalent to 20 mg/ml; using 10 ml diluent yields a concentration of 10 mg/ml.

After reconstitution, etoposide phosphate may be given without further dilution or can be further diluted to as low as 0.1 mg/ml using D_5W injection or normal saline injection. Discard discolored or precipitated solution.

Unopened ampules of etoposide remain stable at room temperature for 2 years; diluted solutions remain stable up to 48 hours. After reconstitution, etoposide phosphate can be stored at room temperature—68° to 77° F (20° to 25° C)—or refrigerated at 36° to 46° F (2° to 8° C) for 24 hours. If refrigerated, use immediately upon return to room temperature.

Incompatibilities
Cefepime hydrochloride, filgrastim, gallium nitrate, idarubicin.

CONTRAINDICATIONS & CAUTIONS
• Contraindicated in those hypersensitive to drug and in those with known or recent chickenpox or herpes zoster infection because of risk of generalized infection.
• Contraindicated in those with platelet counts below 50,000/mm³ or with neutrophil counts below 500/mm³ because drug increases myelosuppression.
• Use cautiously in those with hepatic or renal impairment because of increased risk of toxic reaction.

___

ADVERSE REACTIONS

CNS: *fever,* peripheral neuropathy, *asthenia,* malaise.
CV: hypotension from too-rapid infusion.
GI: abdominal pain, *anorexia, diarrhea, nausea, vomiting, mucositis, stomatitis,* constipation, taste alteration.
Hematologic: LEUKOPENIA, THROMBOCYTOPENIA, NEUTROPENIA, *anemia.*
Hepatic: *hepatotoxicity.*
Skin: *alopecia.*
Other: *anaphylaxis, chills.*

INTERACTIONS

Drug-drug. *Cyclosporine in high doses:* Increases etoposide levels. Monitor patient closely.
Drugs causing myelosuppression or blood dyscrasia: Worsens bone marrow depression. Avoid using together.
Vaccines with live virus: Potentiates virus replication. Avoid using together.
Warfarin: May prolong PT and INR. Monitor patient closely.

EFFECTS ON LAB TEST RESULTS

• May decrease hemoglobin and WBC, RBC, platelet, and neutrophil counts.

ACTION

Inhibits or alters DNA synthesis. It arrests the cell cycle at G_2 phase, killing cells in that phase or in late S phase.

PHARMACOKINETICS

Drug level peaks at end of infusion.
Distribution: Minimally, into pleural fluid; drug is 94% protein bound. Drug crosses the placental barrier, but it's unknown if it appears in breast milk.
Metabolism: Unknown, but probably in the liver.
Excretion: Primarily in urine as unchanged drug and metabolites.

CLINICAL CONSIDERATIONS

• Osmolality of etoposide: exceeds 2,000 mOsm/kg. Osmolality of etoposide phosphate: 62 mOsm/kg.
• *Alert:* Be extremely cautious when preparing or giving drug to avoid mutagenic, teratogenic, and carcinogenic risks. Use a biological containment cabinet and avoid contact with skin. Wear mask and gloves. If solution contacts skin or mucosa, immediately wash thoroughly with soap and water. Use syringes with luer-lock fittings to handle concentrate for injection. Dispose of needles, syringes, ampules, and unused drug correctly. Avoid contaminating work surfaces.
• Etoposide is usually given with other chemotherapeutic drugs.
• Obtain baseline blood pressure before starting therapy. Monitor blood pressure every 15 minutes during infusion. If systolic blood pressure falls below 90 mm Hg, stop infusion and notify prescriber. Give fluids and other supportive treatment, as ordered.
• *Alert:* Have diphenhydramine, hydrocortisone, epinephrine, and emergency equipment available to establish an airway if anaphylaxis occurs.
• Don't give through a membrane-type in-line filter because diluent may dissolve it.
• To control nausea and vomiting, give an antiemetic. As ordered, treat anaphylaxis with pressors, adrenocorticosteroids, antihistamines, or volume expanders.
• Anticipate need for blood transfusions to treat anemia.
• Drug has been used investigationally to treat refractory acute myelogenous and lymphocytic leukemia.
• Therapeutic response to drug is usually linked to toxic effects.
• Patients with low albumin levels may be at increased risk for toxic reaction.
• Monitor CBC at least weekly.
• Observe oral cavity for ulcerations.

Reactions may be *common*, uncommon, *life-threatening*, or COMMON AND LIFE-THREATENING.

PATIENT TEACHING

• Instruct patient to promptly report signs and symptoms of infection (such as fever, chills, and sore throat) or evidence of bleeding (such as easy bruising, nosebleeds, bleeding gums, and bloody stools). Also, tell patient to take his temperature daily.

• Teach patient good oral care to reduce mouth inflammation.

• Provide anticipatory guidance to patient regarding hair loss.

• Advise any woman of childbearing age to avoid pregnancy and breastfeeding during therapy.

F

factor IX
AlphaNine SD, Bebulin VH,
BeneFix, Mononine, Profilnine SD,
Proplex T

Pharmacologic class: blood
derivative
Therapeutic class: systemic
hemostatic
Pregnancy risk category: C

INDICATIONS & DOSAGES
➤ **Hemostasis in factor IX deficiency
(hemophilia B)—**
Adults and children: Specific dosage
depends on patient and type of bleeding episode. To find number of IUs
needed to raise recombinant factor IX
level percentages, multiply 1.2 IU/kg
by body weight (kg) by desired increase (percent of normal). To find
number of IUs needed to raise human-
derived factor IX level percentages,
multiply 1 IU/kg by body weight (kg)
by desired increase (percent of normal). About 15 minutes after giving
2 IU/kg of factor IX, plasma levels rise
by about 3% and factor VII levels by
about 4%. Minor bleeding episodes
need a circulating factor IX level of
20% to 40% of normal; major bleeding
episodes, 20% to 60% of normal. Give
doses q 24 hours.
➤ **Hemostasis in patients with factor
VIII inhibitors—**
Adults and children: 75 IU/kg; repeat q
12 hours, p.r.n.
➤ **Hemostasis in factor VII
deficiency—**
Adults and children: To find the appropriate number of IUs of Proplex T, multiply 0.5 × body weight (kg) by the desired percentage of increase. Repeat
dose in 4 to 6 hours, p.r.n.

ADMINISTRATION
Direct injection: Using a 21G or 23G
winged infusion set, inject slowly;
don't exceed 3 ml/minute. Slow injection minimizes the risk of thrombosis.
If facial flushing or tingling occurs during infusion, stop momentarily and resume at a slower rate.
Intermittent infusion: Not recommended.
Continuous infusion: Not recommended.

PREPARATION & STORAGE
Available in kit that includes concentrate, diluent (from 10 to 30 ml, depending on manufacturer), and filter
needle. Number of IUs of factor IX per
vial appears on label.

After warming concentrate and diluent to room temperature, reconstitute
using aseptic technique. Add diluent,
and swirl bottle to dissolve contents.
Using the filter needle, draw concentrate into syringe. Give within 3 hours.

Refrigerate, but avoid freezing; diluent bottle will break. Don't refrigerate
after reconstitution.

Incompatibilities
All I.V. drugs and solutions, except
normal saline solution.

CONTRAINDICATIONS & CAUTIONS
• Contraindicated in those hypersensitive to mouse protein (Mononine).
• Contraindicated in those with hepatic
disease who show signs of intravascular coagulation or fibrinolysis.

• Contraindicated in those undergoing elective surgery, especially if predisposed to thrombosis, because of the risk of postoperative thrombosis. If drug must be used, prophylactic anticoagulant should be given.

• Use cautiously in patients receiving multiple infusions of blood or plasma products for first time because of the risk of transmitting a virus, especially hepatitis C. Also, note that factor IX contains trace amounts of blood groups A and B hemagglutinins. Intravascular hemolysis may occur with large or frequent doses.

ADVERSE REACTIONS
CNS: headache, fever.
CV: *thrombosis, especially in those with hepatic disease;* pulse changes; blood pressure changes.
GI: nausea, vomiting.
Hepatic: *viral hepatitis.*
Skin: facial flushing, urticaria.
Other: chills, *anaphylaxis,* tingling.

INTERACTIONS
Drug-drug. *Aminocaproic acid:* Increases risk of thrombotic complications if given within 12 hours of factor IX infusion. Avoid giving within 12 hours of drug infusion.

EFFECTS ON LAB TEST RESULTS
None reported.

COMPOSITION
Derived from pooled plasma, this sterile, dried concentrate contains vitamin K–dependent coagulation factors II, IX, and X and low levels of factor VII (higher levels in Proplex T). One IU of factor IX concentrate equals the amount of factor IX in 1 ml of normal plasma.

CLINICAL CONSIDERATIONS
• Obtain coagulation assays before and during treatment.
• Prepared from pooled plasma and treated to minimize viral transmission, factor IX concentrate still carries the risk of transmitting severe infection, especially hepatitis C. Before giving drug, weigh its benefits and risks against those of single-donor fresh frozen plasma.

• To reduce risk of thrombosis, the International Committee on Thrombosis and Hemostasis recommends adding 5 units of heparin/ml of diluent when treating factor IX–deficient patients. This practice isn't recommended for patients with factor VIII inhibitors.

PATIENT TEACHING
• Educate patient about AIDS, and encourage immunization against hepatitis B in those who test negative for hepatitis B surface antigen. Explain that the risk of infection with HIV is low in patients receiving heat-treated factor IX concentrate from screened donors.
• Tell patient to report adverse reactions promptly.
• Explain use and administration of drug to patient and family.
• Encourage patient and family to ask questions and express concerns.

famotidine
Pepcid I.V.

Pharmacologic class: H$_2$-receptor antagonist
Therapeutic class: antiulcerative
Pregnancy risk category: B
pH: 5 to 5.6

INDICATIONS & DOSAGES
➤ **Active duodenal and gastric ulcers; hypersecretory conditions; patients unable to take oral drugs—**
Adults: 20 mg q 12 hours.
Children ages 1 to 16: 0.25 mg/kg q 12 hours, up to 40 mg/day.

ADMINISTRATION

Direct injection: Inject 5 ml or 10 ml of reconstituted drug over at least 2 minutes, no faster than 10 mg/minute.
Intermittent infusion: Infuse drug diluted in 100 ml over 15 to 30 minutes.
Continuous infusion: Not recommended.

PREPARATION & STORAGE

Available in 2-ml single-dose vials and 4-ml and 20-ml multidose vials with a concentration of 10 mg/ml. Also available premixed as 20 mg/50 ml in normal saline solution.

For injection, reconstitute with 5 or 10 ml of diluent; for infusion, use 100 ml of diluent.

Compatible with sterile water for injection, normal saline solution, D_5W, dextrose 10% in water, lactated Ringer's solution, or 5% sodium bicarbonate.

Diluted solution remains stable for 48 hours at room temperature. Refrigerate vials, but avoid freezing.

Incompatibilities

Cefepime, piperacillin with tazobactam.

CONTRAINDICATIONS & CAUTIONS

● Contraindicated in those hypersensitive to drug.
● Contraindicated in patients who are breast-feeding.
● Use cautiously in severe renal or hepatic impairment because of decreased plasma clearance.

ADVERSE REACTIONS

CNS: *seizures,* asthenia, hallucinations, headache, confusion, agitation, depression, anxiety, decreased libido, paresthesia, fatigue, pain, insomnia, fever, dizziness.
CV: *arrhythmias,* AV block, palpitations, chest tightness.
EENT: conjunctival infection, tinnitus, taste disorder.

GI: dry mouth, vomiting, nausea, abdominal discomfort, anorexia, constipation, diarrhea.
Hematologic: *agranulocytosis, pancytopenia, leukopenia, thrombocytopenia.*
Hepatic: cholestatic jaundice.
Musculoskeletal: muscle cramps, arthralgia.
Respiratory: *bronchospasm.*
Skin: *toxic epidermal necrolysis,* alopecia, acne, pruritus, dry skin, flushing.

INTERACTIONS

None reported.

EFFECTS ON LAB TEST RESULTS

● May increase BUN, creatinine, and liver enzyme levels.
● May decrease WBC, RBC, platelet, and granulocyte counts.
● May cause false-positive skin test results.

ACTION

Inhibits H_2 receptors, suppressing acid concentration and gastric secretion.

PHARMACOKINETICS

Drug effect peaks at 30 minutes.
Distribution: About 15% to 20% protein bound. Drug probably crosses the placental barrier and may appear in breast milk.
Metabolism: In the liver.
Excretion: In urine, with 65% to 70% excreted as unchanged drug and 30% to 35% as metabolites. Half-life is about 3 hours; in those with moderate renal impairment, half-life is 11 hours; in those with severe renal impairment, more than 20 hours.

CLINICAL CONSIDERATIONS

● Osmolarity: 217 to 290 mOsm/L.
● Check I.V. site for irritation.
● Stop drug for 24 hours before diagnostic skin tests.

Reactions may be *common,* uncommon, *life-threatening,* or COMMON AND LIFE-THREATENING.

• Drug may treat or prevent stress ulcers, hemorrhagic gastritis, and other upper-GI hemorrhage.
• Have gastric cancer ruled out before starting famotidine therapy.
• Closely monitor patient with gastric ulcers.

PATIENT TEACHING

• Warn patient that smoking may increase gastric acid secretion.
• Explain use and administration of drug to patient and family.

fat emulsions
Intralipid 10%, Intralipid 20%, Intralipid 30% ◇, Liposyn II 10%, Liposyn II 20%, Liposyn III 10%, Liposyn III 20%

Pharmacologic class: lipid
Therapeutic class: total parenteral nutrition
Pregnancy risk category: C

INDICATIONS & DOSAGES
➤ **Source of calories and fatty acids in I.V. hyperalimentation—**
Adults: Up to 500 ml I.V. 10% solution on day 1, gradually increasing on following days to 60% of daily caloric intake. Or, up to 500 ml I.V. of Intralipid 20% or up to 250 ml I.V. of Liposyn 20% on day 1, gradually increasing on following days. Maximum daily dose for Intralipid is 2.5 g/kg I.V.; for Liposyn, 3 g/kg I.V.
Children: 1 g/kg I.V. of Intralipid 10% or 100 ml/hour of Liposyn 10% on day 1, gradually increasing to 5 to 10 ml/kg I.V. daily. Or, 1 g/kg I.V. of Intralipid 20% over 4 hours on day 1, gradually increasing to 3 g/kg I.V. daily, or 100 ml/hour I.V. of Liposyn 20% on day 1, gradually increasing to 2.5 to 5 ml/kg I.V. daily.

Neonates: Maximum dosage, 1 g/kg I.V. given over 4 hours.
➤ **Fatty acid deficiency—**
Adults and children: 8% to 10% of caloric intake.

ADMINISTRATION
Direct injection: Not recommended.
Intermittent infusion: Give once daily as part of I.V. hyperalimentation. See guidelines for continuous infusion.
Continuous infusion: Give the solution through the nonphthalate infusion set that the manufacturer provides. Fat emulsions may extract phthalates from phthalate-plasticized polyvinyl chloride tubing. Don't use an in-line filter when giving drug because fat particles, which are 0.5-micron in diameter, are larger than the 0.22-micron in-line filter.
Use a new I.V. line for each bottle of fat emulsion, infusing solution through a peripheral or central venous line. Control flow rates by infusion pump, using a separate pump for solutions running simultaneously.
Infuse fat emulsions intermittently, alternating with a protein-calorie solution for I.V. hyperalimentation. Or infuse fat emulsions into same vein with carbohydrate–amino acid solution, using a Y-connector near the infusion site. To facilitate flow, hang the fat emulsion container higher than the other one.
In adults, begin infusing 10% fat emulsion at 0.1 ml/minute or 20% emulsion at 0.5 ml/minute. In children, for the 20% emulsion, give 0.05 ml/minute for the first 15 minutes. If tolerated, increase infusion rate to allow no more than 1 g of fat/kg in the first 4 hours. Closely monitor patient; if no adverse reactions occur within 15 minutes, increase infusion rate. For adults, infuse 500 ml of 10% solution or 250 ml of 20% solution over 4 to 6 hours. If patient develops fever, chills, or other reactions, especially in first 15 minutes, or if infusion bottle shows evidence of conta-

mination or instability, stop infusion and notify prescriber.

PREPARATION & STORAGE

Ready-to-use, sterile, nonpyrogenic emulsions are available in single-dose glass bottles. Intralipid 10% comes in 50-, 100-, and 500-ml bottles; Intralipid 20%, in 100-, 250-, and 500-ml bottles; Intralipid 30%, in 333-ml bottles. Liposyn 10% is supplied in 25-, 50-, 100-, 200-, and 500-ml bottles; Liposyn 20%, in 200- and 500-ml bottles.

Store fat emulsions at room temperature and discard if accidentally frozen. Inspect bottle for cracks or separation at the seams; check expiration date and integrity of closure. Discard bottle for any problem.

Only the Intralipid brand can be mixed in the same I.V. container with amino acid solution, dextrose, electrolytes, or vitamins.

Incompatibilities

Additives, aminophylline, amphotericin B, ampicillin sodium, ascorbic acid injection, calcium chloride, calcium gluconate, electrolytes, gentamicin, I.V. drugs, magnesium chloride, penicillin G, phenytoin sodium, potassium chloride, sodium bicarbonate, sodium chloride solution, vitamins.

CONTRAINDICATIONS & CAUTIONS

• Contraindicated in those who are hypersensitive to solution components or have severe egg allergy. Product contains egg yolk phospholipids.
• Contraindicated in those with impaired fat metabolism—for example, those with hyperlipemia, lipoid nephrosis, or acute pancreatitis with hyperlipemia.
• Contraindicated in those with bone marrow dyscrasias because fat emulsions may induce blood dyscrasias, and in infants with hyperbilirubinemia be-

cause fat emulsions may worsen jaundice.
• Use cautiously in those with severe hepatic or pulmonary disease, coagulation disorders, anemia, thrombocytopenia, diabetes mellitus, gastric ulcer, or a risk of fat embolism because the solution may worsen these conditions.
• Use cautiously in premature infants and infants who are small for their age.

ADVERSE REACTIONS

CNS: fever, agitation, drowsiness, *focal seizures,* headache.
CV: chest pain, flushing, cyanosis, *cardiac arrest, shock.*
EENT: dilated, nonreactive pupils; pressure over eyes.
GI: nausea, vomiting.
Hematologic: anemia, bleeding, *leukopenia, thrombocytopenia,* hypercoagulability, leukocytosis.
Hepatic: hepatosplenomegaly.
Metabolic: hyperlipidemia, hyperthermia, metabolic acidosis.
Musculoskeletal: back pain.
Respiratory: *pulmonary edema,* hyperventilation.
Skin: diaphoresis, I.V. fat pigment syndrome, pruritus, urticaria, irritation at injection site.
Other: overhydration, *sepsis.*

INTERACTIONS

None reported.

EFFECTS ON LAB TEST RESULTS

• May increase lipid, bilirubin, and liver enzyme levels.
• May decrease platelet count. May increase or decrease WBC count.

COMPOSITION

Although the percentage of components varies, fat emulsions contain soybean oil (Intralipid) or safflower oil (Liposyn) and provide neutral triglycerides and primarily unsaturated fatty acids—linoleic, oleic, palmitic, stearic, and linolenic. Fatty acids are an energy source, essential to the normal structure and function of cell membranes.

Preparations also contain glycerol to adjust tonicity and 1.2% egg yolk to emulsify fat particles. The 10% solutions contain 1.1 calories/ml; the 20% solutions, 2 calories/ml. All fat emulsions are isotonic.

CLINICAL CONSIDERATIONS

• Osmolarity: 260 to 292 mOsm/L.
• Before administration, perform a complete nutritional assessment.
• Fat emulsions, along with total parenteral nutrition, are commonly given at night to provide more patient freedom during the day.
• Obtain baseline CBC, platelet count, coagulation studies, liver function tests, and lipid levels, especially triglycerides and cholesterol.
• After 4 to 6 hours of infusion, obtain triglyceride and cholesterol determination samples because transient lipemia must clear after each daily dose. In long-term therapy, monitor liver function test results and repeat other baseline studies once or twice weekly.
• Check the infusion site frequently during administration for signs of inflammation or infection.
• Neonates and premature infants receive fat emulsions over 24 hours because they metabolize fats more slowly than adults. Monitor triglyceride and free fatty acid levels daily. Also, obtain daily platelet counts during the first week of therapy because neonates are susceptible to thrombocytopenia. In succeeding weeks, obtain platelet counts on alternate days.

PATIENT TEACHING

• If patient is to take drug at home, teach patient and caregiver about I.V. site care and proper administration techniques to prevent infection and complications.
• Tell patient to promptly report adverse reactions.

• Explain use and administration of drug to patient and family.

fenoldopam mesylate
Corlopam

Pharmacologic class: dopamine D_1–like receptor agonist
Therapeutic class: antihypertensive
Pregnancy risk category: B
pH: 2.8 to 3.8

INDICATIONS & DOSAGES

➤ **In-hospital management of severe hypertension for up to 48 hours when rapid but quickly reversible reduction of blood pressure is indicated, including malignant hypertension with deteriorating end-organ function—**
Adults: Give by continuous I.V. infusion. Start at 0.03 to 0.1 mcg/kg/minute and titrate up or down no more than q 15 minutes to achieve desired blood pressure. Recommended increments for titration are 0.05 to 0.1 mcg/kg/minute. Doses up to 1.6 mcg/kg/minute have been used.

ADMINISTRATION
Direct injection: I.V. bolus not recommended.
Intermittent infusion: Not recommended.
Continuous infusion: Infusion may be increased every 15 minutes if needed to maintain desired blood pressure.

PREPARATION & STORAGE
Available as 10-mg/ml single-dose ampules.

Dilute drug in normal saline solution or D_5W to a final concentration of 4 mcg/ml. Infuse drug with a calibrated mechanical infusion pump. May abruptly stop or gradually taper.

Store ampules at 36° to 86° F (2° to 30° C). Diluted solution is stable at room temperature for at least 24 hours. Discard unused portion.

Incompatibilities
None reported.

CONTRAINDICATIONS & CAUTIONS
• Use cautiously in those with glaucoma or ocular hypertension; drug can cause dose-dependent increases in intraocular pressure.
• Use cautiously in those who have had acute cerebral infarction or hemorrhage; drug may cause symptomatic hypotension.
• Use cautiously in breast-feeding women; drug may appear in breast milk.
• Use during pregnancy only if needed.

ADVERSE REACTIONS
CNS: dizziness, headache, insomnia, fever, anxiety.
CV: hypotension, palpitations, ***bradycardia,*** tachycardia, angina, *MI,* T-wave inversion, nonspecific chest pain, flushing.
EENT: nasal congestion.
GI: nausea, vomiting, abdominal pain, constipation, diarrhea.
GU: oliguria, UTI.
Hematologic: leukocytosis, bleeding.
Metabolic: hypokalemia.
Musculoskeletal: limb cramps, back pain.
Respiratory: dyspnea.
Skin: injection site reaction, sweating.

INTERACTIONS
Drug-drug. *Antihypertensives:* May cause hypotension. Avoid using together.

EFFECTS ON LAB TEST RESULTS
• May increase creatinine, BUN, glucose, LDH, and transaminase levels. May decrease potassium level.
• May increase WBC count.

ACTION
A rapid-acting vasodilator; an agonist for D_1-like dopamine receptors that binds to alpha$_2$ adrenoreceptors.

PHARMACOKINETICS
Onset, 15 minutes; peak, 20 minutes; duration, unknown.
Distribution: Not reported.
Metabolism: Primarily through conjugation, with little involvement of cytochrome P-450 coenzyme system.
Excretion: 90% in urine, 10% in feces. Half-life, 5 minutes.

CLINICAL CONSIDERATIONS
• Drug causes a dose-related tachycardia that diminishes over time but remains substantial at higher doses.
• Monitor blood pressure and heart rate every 15 minutes until patient's condition is stable.
• *Alert:* Drug contains sodium metabisulfite, which may cause allergic-type reactions, including anaphylactic symptoms and severe asthmatic episodes, in susceptible individuals. Sulfite sensitivity is common in asthmatic patients.
• Oral antihypertensives can be added once blood pressure is stable.
• Monitor electrolyte levels and watch for hypokalemia.

PATIENT TEACHING
• Tell patient that drug causes dose-related decreases in blood pressure and increases in heart rate.
• Advise patient to change positions slowly to avoid dizziness.
• Encourage patient to report adverse reactions promptly.

Reactions may be *common*, uncommon, *life-threatening*, or COMMON AND LIFE-THREATENING.

fentanyl citrate
Sublimaze

Pharmacologic class: opioid agonist
Therapeutic class: analgesic adjunct to anesthesia, anesthetic
Pregnancy risk category: C
Controlled substance schedule: II
pH: 4 to 7.5

INDICATIONS & DOSAGES
Dosage depends on other drugs being given, especially anesthetics, type and anticipated length of surgery, and patient's age, weight, body size, physical status, underlying disorder, and response to drug.
➤ **Short-term perioperative analgesia—**
Adults: Up to 2 mcg/kg I.V. in divided doses.
➤ **General anesthesia, as sole drug with 100% oxygen—**
Adults: 50 to 100 mcg/kg I.V.; up to 150 mcg/kg I.V.
➤ **To induce and maintain general anesthesia—**
Children ages 2 to 12: 1.7 to 3.3 mcg/kg I.V.
➤ **Adjunct in general anesthesia—**
Adults: Low dose, 2 mcg/kg I.V. in divided doses; moderate dose before major surgery, 2 to 20 mcg/kg I.V. initially, then 25 to 100 mcg p.r.n.; high dose before complicated surgery, 20 to 50 mcg/kg I.V. initially, then 25 mcg to half initial dose p.r.n.
➤ **Adjunct in regional anesthesia—**
Adults: 50 to 100 mcg.

ADMINISTRATION
Direct injection: Inject drug over at least 1 minute to avoid muscle rigidity. If rapid injection is needed, give a neuromuscular blocker first to prevent rigidity.

Intermittent infusion: Not recommended.
Continuous infusion: Sometimes used for induction of general anesthesia. Use high-dose concentrations to rapidly and smoothly achieve initial induction dose.

PREPARATION & STORAGE
Available in 2-, 5-, 10-, 20-, 30-, and 50-ml containers.
Drug is compatible with most common I.V. solutions.
Store at room temperature, avoid excessive heat or freezing, and protect from light.

Incompatibilities
Fluorouracil, methohexital, pentobarbital sodium.

CONTRAINDICATIONS & CAUTIONS
• Contraindicated in those hypersensitive to fentanyl derivatives.
• Use cautiously in those with bradyarrhythmia because drug may exacerbate the condition; and in those with poor pulmonary reserve because drug may further diminish respiratory drive and increase airway resistance.
• Use cautiously in patients with head injury and increased intracranial pressure because drug may interfere with neurologic assessment. Drug may also raise intracranial pressure by causing hypoventilation and hypercarbia.
• Use cautiously in those with hepatic, renal, or respiratory dysfunction because of increased risk of toxic reaction; in those with hypothyroidism because of risk of prolonged respiratory and CNS depression; and in geriatric, young, or debilitated patients because of increased sensitivity to drug effects.

ADVERSE REACTIONS
CNS: headache, apathy, *dizziness,* euphoria, paresthesia, *sedation.*
CV: *bradycardia,* hypertension, flushing, ventricular extrasystole.

EENT: vision abnormalities.
GI: nausea, vomiting, constipation.
Respiratory: *apnea, hypoventilation.*
Skin: pallor, pruritus, *rash.*

INTERACTIONS
Drug-drug. *Antihypertensives:* May potentiate hypotension. Monitor blood pressure.
Benzodiazepines: Decreases induction time when given for preoperative sedation. Avoid using together.
Beta blockers: Decreases frequency and severity of hypertensive response to surgery. Monitor patient closely.
Buprenorphine, other partial agonists: Decreases therapeutic effects of fentanyl. Avoid using together.
Cimetidine: May increase CNS toxicity. Monitor patient closely.
CNS depressants: Deepens CNS and respiratory depression. Avoid using together.
MAO inhibitors: May cause unpredictable, severe hypertension and tachycardia if given within 14 days of fentanyl citrate. Separate doses by at least 14 days.
Naloxone, naltrexone: Antagonizes analgesic, hypotensive, CNS, and respiratory effects of fentanyl. Avoid using together.
Neuromuscular blockers: Deepens respiratory depression and alleviates muscle rigidity. Avoid using together.
Nitrous oxide: Causes CV depression when combined with high-dose fentanyl. Use together cautiously.

EFFECTS ON LAB TEST RESULTS
None reported.

ACTION
An agonist at stereospecific opioid receptor sites in the CNS, probably the mu receptors. Drug alters perception of and emotional response to pain.

PHARMACOKINETICS
Onset, immediate; duration, 30 to 60 minutes, depending on dose.
Distribution: Rapidly dispersed to inactive tissue sites, such as skeletal muscle, and lungs; more slowly distributed to fat compartments. Drug is highly protein bound. It probably crosses the placental barrier and readily crosses the blood-brain barrier. It's unknown if drug appears in breast milk.
Metabolism: Extensively, in the liver. Rate depends on hepatic blood flow and release from body tissues.
Excretion: By the kidneys, with 10% to 25% excreted in urine as unchanged drug; 70% of dose is excreted within 4 days.

CLINICAL CONSIDERATIONS
● Only staff trained in giving I.V. anesthetics and managing their adverse effects should give drug.
● Monitor patient's respiratory, CV, and neurologic status before, during, and after surgery.
● When high doses of drug are used, respiratory depression may persist for several hours after the patient awakens, necessitating ventilatory support.
● Patient who receives repeated doses or is tolerant of other opioids may become tolerant of fentanyl.
● Drug may cause muscle rigidity in the chest wall, leading to problems with ventilation. These problems may occur when patient emerges from anesthesia. A neuromuscular blocker may be needed.
● After recovery from anesthesia, patient may experience delayed respiratory depression, respiratory arrest, bradycardia, asystole, arrhythmias, and hypotension.
● If overdose occurs, continue supportive therapy until drug is metabolized. For hypoventilation or apnea, give oxygen and positive-pressure ventilation via bag and mask or endotracheal tube to maintain a patent airway and ventila-

tion. To reverse respiratory depression, give naloxone in divided doses.

PATIENT TEACHING
• Tell patient before surgery about the type of monitoring and anticipated postanesthesia effects.
• Explain use and administration of drug to patient and family.

filgrastim
Neupogen

Pharmacologic class: cytokine glycoprotein
Therapeutic class: neutrophil production stimulant
Pregnancy risk category: C
pH: 3.8 to 4.2

INDICATIONS & DOSAGES
➤ **To decrease risk of infection caused by myelosuppressive effects of cancer chemotherapy used for nonmyeloid tumors**—
Adults and children: 5 mcg/kg/day I.V. given as a single daily injection. If needed, increase dose by 5 mcg/kg/day for each cycle. Begin at least 24 hours after the last dose of chemotherapy and continue beyond nadir until neutrophil count reaches 10,000/mm^3. Stop at least 24 hours before next dose of chemotherapy.
➤ **To reduce duration of neutropenia and neutropenia-related effects in patients with nonmyeloid malignancies undergoing myeloablative chemotherapy followed by bone marrow transplant**—
Adults: After bone marrow transplant, 10 mcg/kg/day given as an I.V. infusion over 4 to 24 hours or as a continuous, 24-hour, S.C. infusion. Give first dose at least 24 hours after chemotherapy

and at least 24 hours after bone marrow infusion.
➤ **To reduce the risk and duration of the effects of neutropenia in symptomatic patients with congenital, cyclic, or idiopathic neutropenia**—
Adults: 2 to 60 mcg/kg/day infused I.V. over 30 minutes for congenital neutropenia; for idiopathic or cyclic neutropenia, 0.5 to 11.5 mcg/kg daily infused I.V. over 30 minutes. Long-term administration is needed to maintain clinical benefit.
➤ **AIDS ♦**—
Adults: 0.3 to 3.6 mcg/kg/day I.V.
➤ **Aplastic anemia ♦**—
Adults: 800 to 1,200 mcg/m^2/day I.V.
➤ **Hairy cell leukemia, myelodysplasia ♦**—
Adults: 15 to 500 mcg/m^2/day I.V.

ADMINISTRATION
Direct injection: Not recommended.
Intermittent infusion: Infuse over 15 to 30 minutes using an established I.V. line containing dextrose solution.
Continuous infusion: Infuse over 24 hours or at 10 mcg/kg/day.

PREPARATION & STORAGE
Available in 1- and 1.6-ml single-dose vials (300 mcg/ml).
   For infusion, may dilute drug in D$_5$W to yield 5 to 15 mcg/ml. Add albumin to a final concentration of 2 mg/ml to prevent adsorption to plastic.
   Store in refrigerator; don't freeze. Stable at room temperature for 24 hours. Don't shake.

Incompatibilities
Amphotericin B, cefepime, cefonicid, cefotaxime, cefoxitin, ceftizoxime, ceftriaxone, cefuroxime, clindamycin, dactinomycin, etoposide, fluorouracil, furosemide, heparin sodium, mannitol, methylprednisolone sodium succinate, metronidazole, mitomycin, piperacillin,

prochlorperazine edisylate, sodium solutions, thiotepa.

CONTRAINDICATIONS & CAUTIONS
• Contraindicated in patients hypersensitive to products derived from *Escherichia coli.*

ADVERSE REACTIONS
Most adverse reactions result from underlying malignancy or cytotoxic chemotherapy.
CNS: headache, *fatigue, fever,* pain.
CV: *arrhythmias,* chest pain, *MI.*
EENT: sore throat, stomatitis.
GI: *nausea, vomiting, diarrhea, mucositis,* anorexia, constipation.
Hematologic: *neutropenic fever, thrombocytopenia.*
Musculoskeletal: skeletal pain, generalized weakness, *medullary bone pain.*
Respiratory: *adult respiratory distress syndrome,* dyspnea, cough.
Skin: *alopecia,* rash.

INTERACTIONS
Drug-drug. *Chemotherapy, radiation therapy:* Safety and efficacy haven't been established. Avoid using together.
Lithium, other drugs that may potentiate release of neutrophils: May increase neutrophil count. Use together cautiously.

EFFECTS ON LAB TEST RESULTS
• May increase creatinine, uric acid, alkaline phosphatase, and LDH levels.
• May increase WBC count. May decrease platelet count.

ACTION
Produced by recombinant DNA technology. Stimulates proliferation, differentiation, and functional activity of neutrophils, causing a rapid rise in WBC counts in 2 or 3 days in patients with normal bone marrow function and 7 to 14 days in those with bone marrow depression. Blood counts usually return to pretreatment levels within 1 week after therapy ends.

PHARMACOKINETICS
Neutrophil counts exceed baseline levels within 24 hours.
Distribution: Throughout body into bone marrow.
Metabolism: Unknown.
Excretion: By kidneys; half-life, 3½ hours.

CLINICAL CONSIDERATIONS
• Obtain CBC and platelet count before therapy and twice weekly during therapy. Regularly monitor hematocrit.
• Before injection, allow vial to reach room temperature for a maximum of 24 hours. Discard after 24 hours. Use only one dose per vial; don't reenter vial.
• Mild to moderate bone pain is the most frequent adverse reaction and may be controlled with nonnarcotic analgesics or with opioid analgesics if severe.
• *Alert:* Adult respiratory distress syndrome may occur in septic patients because of the influx of neutrophils at inflammation site. An MI or an arrhythmia may occur; closely monitor patients with cardiac conditions.

PATIENT TEACHING
• Instruct patient to promptly report signs and symptoms of infection, such as fever, chills, and sore throat.
• Explain use and administration of drug to patient and family.
• Explain the importance of having blood tested regularly and keeping all scheduled appointments for follow-up care.

fluconazole
Diflucan

Pharmacologic class: triazole
derivative
Therapeutic class: antifungal
Pregnancy risk category: C
pH: 4 to 8

INDICATIONS & DOSAGES
➤ **Oropharyngeal candidiasis—**
Adults: 200 mg I.V. on day 1, followed
by 100 mg I.V. once daily. Continue
treatment for 2 weeks.
Children: 6 mg/kg I.V. on day 1, followed by 3 mg/kg I.V. once daily.
➤ **Esophageal candidiasis—**
Adults: 200 mg I.V. on day 1, followed
by 100 mg I.V. once daily. Higher doses
of up to 400 mg/day I.V. have been
used, depending on patient's condition
and tolerance of treatment. Continue
treatment for at least 3 weeks, or 2
weeks after symptoms resolve.
Children: 6 mg/kg I.V. on day 1, followed by 3 mg/kg I.V. once daily. May
give up to 12 mg/kg/day I.V.
➤ **Systemic candidiasis—**
Adults: 400 mg I.V. on day 1, followed
by 200 mg I.V. once daily. Continue
treatment for at least 4 weeks, or 2
weeks after symptoms resolve.
Children: 6 to 12 mg/kg/day I.V.
➤ **Cryptococcal meningitis—**
Adults: 400 mg/day I.V. Continue treatment for 10 to 12 weeks after CSF cultures are negative.
Children: 12 mg/kg/day I.V. on day 1,
followed by 6 mg/kg I.V. once daily.
➤ **To suppress cryptococcal meningitis relapse in patients with HIV infection—**
Adults: 200 mg/day I.V.
Children: 6 mg/kg/day I.V.
Adjust-a-dose: For adults and children
with renal impairment, give an initial
loading dose of 50 to 400 mg I.V. If

creatinine clearance is 21 to 50 ml/
minute, reduce dosage by 50%; if creatinine clearance is 11 to 20 ml/minute,
reduce dosage by 75%.
　　Patients receiving regular hemodialysis treatment should receive the usual
dose after each dialysis session. Additional dosage adjustments may be needed, depending on the patient's condition.

ADMINISTRATION
Direct injection: Not recommended.
Intermittent infusion: Give ordered
dose at 200 mg/hour.
Continuous infusion: Not recommended.

PREPARATION & STORAGE
Available in glass bottles or plastic I.V.
bags with 200 mg/100 ml or 400 mg/
200 ml.
　　Store glass bottles at 41° to 86° F
(5° to 30° C) and plastic bags at 41° to
77° F (5° to 25° C). Protect from freezing. Brief exposure of plastic containers
to temperatures up to 104° F (40° C)
won't adversely affect drug. I.V. bags of
fluconazole are shipped with a protective overwrap that shouldn't be removed
until just before use to help ensure
product sterility. The plastic container
may be opaque from moisture absorbed
during sterilization, but this doesn't affect drug and diminishes over time.

Incompatibilities
Amphotericin B, ampicillin sodium, calcium gluconate, cefotaxime sodium,
ceftazidime, ceftriaxone, cefuroxime
sodium, chloramphenicol sodium succinate, clindamycin phosphate, cotrimoxazole, diazepam, digoxin, erythromycin lactobionate, furosemide,
haloperidol lactate, hydroxyzine hydrochloride, imipenem and cilastatin sodium, other I.V. drugs, pentamidine,
piperacillin sodium, ticarcillin disodium.

CONTRAINDICATIONS & CAUTIONS
• Contraindicated in those hypersensitive to drug.
• Use cautiously in those hypersensitive to other antifungal azole compounds because no information exists regarding cross-sensitivity.
• Use cautiously in those with abnormal liver function test results. Evaluate patient for serious liver injury, and stop drug if liver function continues to deteriorate.

ADVERSE REACTIONS
CNS: headache.
GI: abdominal pain, diarrhea, nausea, vomiting.
Hepatic: *hepatotoxicity.*
Skin: *Stevens-Johnson syndrome*, rash.

INTERACTIONS
Drug-drug. *Buspirone, cyclosporine, oral sulfonylureas, phenytoin, tacrolimus, theophylline, tricyclic antidepressants, zidovudine, zolpidem:* May increase levels of these drugs. Monitor patient closely.
Cimetidine: Decreases fluconazole level. Monitor patient closely.
Hormonal contraceptives: May increase or decrease hormone levels. Advise patient to use backup contraceptive method.
Hydrochlorothiazide: May decrease renal clearance of fluconazole. Monitor patient closely.
Rifampin: Enhances fluconazole metabolism. Monitor patient closely.
Vinca alkaloids: Increases risk of alkaloid toxicity, causing constipation, myalgia, and neutropenia. Monitor patient closely.
Warfarin: Increases PT and INR. Monitor patient closely.

EFFECTS ON LAB TEST RESULTS
• May increase alkaline phosphatase, ALT, AST, bilirubin, and GGT levels.
• May decrease WBC and platelet counts.

ACTION
Alters fungal cell membranes, causing increased membrane permeability, leakage of essential elements, and impaired uptake of precursor molecules. Selectively inhibits fungal cytochrome P-450 sterol C-14 alpha-demethylase, thus preventing production of normal sterols.

PHARMACOKINETICS
Onset of drug effect is immediate.
Distribution: Penetrates all compartments well at steady state, including CNS. Apparent volume of distribution is similar to that of total body water; 11% to 12% protein bound.
Metabolism: 11% of drug appears in urine as metabolites.
Excretion: Primarily by kidneys. Elimination half-life, about 30 hours; range, 20 to 50 hours.

CLINICAL CONSIDERATIONS
• Osmolarity: 300 to 315 mOsm/L.
• Drug's oral bioavailability is more than 90% and is unaffected by gastric pH. Dosage is the same for P.O. or I.V. use.
• Don't use I.V. bags in series connections to prevent air embolism resulting from residual air being drawn from primary container before infusion of fluid from secondary container is complete.
• When preparing I.V. bag, check for leaks by squeezing the inner bag firmly. If a leak is present, discard the solution, which may not be sterile.
• Risk of adverse reactions appears to be greater in patients with severe underlying disease, including cancers, and in those with HIV infection, especially if they're taking other drugs that are hepatotoxic or linked to exfoliative skin disorders.
• Closely monitor patient who develops a rash. Stop drug if rash worsens.
• Monitor liver function test results.
• Overdose may cause hallucinations and paranoid behavior. Provide supportive and symptomatic treatment.

Reactions may be *common*, uncommon, *life-threatening*, or COMMON AND LIFE-THREATENING.

PATIENT TEACHING
● Advise women who are receiving drug to use something other than hormonal contraceptives for birth control.
● Tell patient to promptly report adverse reactions.

---

fludarabine phosphate
Fludara

Pharmacologic class: antimetabolite
Therapeutic class: antineoplastic
Pregnancy risk category: D
pH: 7.2 to 8.2

INDICATIONS & DOSAGES
➤ **B-cell chronic lymphocytic leukemia in patients who either haven't responded or have responded inadequately to at least one standard alkylating drug regimen—**
Adults: 25 mg/m² I.V. daily over 30 minutes for 5 consecutive days. Repeat cycle q 28 days.
Adjust-a-dose: For patients with creatinine clearance 30 to 70 ml/minute, decrease dose by 20%.

ADMINISTRATION
Direct injection: Not recommended.
Intermittent infusion: Infuse 25 mg/m² over 30 minutes.
Continuous infusion: Not recommended.

PREPARATION & STORAGE
Available as a 50-mg single-dose vial of lyophilized solid cake.
    To prepare, add 2 ml of sterile water for injection to the solid cake of fludarabine. Dissolution should occur within 15 seconds. Each milliliter will contain 25 mg of drug. Use within 8 hours of reconstitution. Can be diluted in 100 or 125 ml of D₅W or normal saline solution.

Store in refrigerator at 36° to 45° F (2° to 8° C).

Incompatibilities
Acyclovir sodium, amphotericin B, chlorpromazine, daunorubicin, ganciclovir, hydroxyzine hydrochloride, prochlorperazine edisylate.

CONTRAINDICATIONS & CAUTIONS
● Contraindicated in those hypersensitive to drug or its components. Not recommended for patients with creatinine clearance less than 30 ml/minute.
● Use cautiously and with dosage adjustments in geriatric patients and in patients with renal insufficiency or bone marrow impairment because of possible increased or excessive toxic effects.

ADVERSE REACTIONS
CNS: fever, *coma with high doses,* headache, sleep disorders, depression, cerebellar syndrome, impaired mental activity, fatigue, malaise, paresthesia, *TIA, CVA, aneurysm.*
CV: *arrhythmias, heart failure,* edema, *DVT,* thrombophlebitis.
EENT: visual disturbances, hearing loss, sinusitis, pharyngitis, epistaxis, mucositis.
GI: esophagitis, hemoptysis, *nausea, vomiting, diarrhea,* anorexia, stomatitis, GI bleeding, constipation, dysphagia.
GU: dysuria, UTI, hematuria, *renal failure,* proteinuria, urinary hesitancy.
Hematologic: *hemorrhage, myelosuppression.*
Hepatic: *liver failure,* cholelithiasis.
Metabolic: hyperglycemia, dehydration.
Musculoskeletal: *pain,* weakness.
Respiratory: *cough, pneumonia,* dyspnea, upper respiratory tract infection, allergic pulmonitis, bronchitis, *hypoxia.*
Skin: diaphoresis, alopecia, rash, pruritus, seborrhea.
Other: *anaphylaxis, death with high doses,* chills, infection, tumor lysis syndrome.

INTERACTIONS
Drug-drug. *Cytarabine:* May decrease metabolism of fludarabine when cytarabine is given first. Avoid giving cytarabine before fludarabine phosphate.
Other myelosuppressants: Increases toxic effects. Avoid using together.
Pentostatin: May cause severe or fatal pulmonary toxicity. Avoid using together.

EFFECTS ON LAB TEST RESULTS
• May increase uric acid, glucose, potassium, phosphate, creatinine, and BUN levels. May decrease calcium level.
• May increase liver function test values. May decrease hemoglobin and RBC, WBC, and platelet counts.

ACTION
After conversion to its active metabolite, drug may interfere with DNA synthesis by inhibiting DNA polymerase alpha, ribonucleotide reductase, and DNA primase.

PHARMACOKINETICS
Drug level peaks in 2 to 4 minutes after rapid I.V. injection and in 2 hours after infusion.
Distribution: Preferentially, into malignant cells; widely distributed with highest levels in liver, kidney, and spleen; extent of distribution into CNS is undetermined, but drug is probably absorbed and distributed into CSF.
Metabolism: Dephosphorylated in serum; transported intracellularly and converted by deoxycytidine kinase to fludarabine triphosphate.
Excretion: 23% in urine as unchanged drug.

CLINICAL CONSIDERATIONS
• Osmolality: 352 mOsm/kg.
• Drug has been used experimentally to treat malignant lymphoma, macroglobulinemic lymphoma, prolymphocytic leukemia or prolymphocytoid variant of chronic lymphocytic leukemia, mycosis fungoides, hairy cell leukemia, and Hodgkin's disease.
• Treating acute leukemia with high doses causes severe neurologic effects. High doses are linked to irreversible CNS toxicity characterized by delayed blindness, coma, and death.
• Closely monitor hematologic function during and after therapy. Most toxic effects are dose dependent.
• Tumor lysis syndrome (hyperuricemia, hyperphosphatemia, hypocalcemia, metabolic acidosis, hyperkalemia, hematuria, urate crystalluria, and renal failure) has occurred in chronic lymphocytic leukemia patients with large tumors.

PATIENT TEACHING
• Instruct patient to promptly report signs and symptoms of infection (such as chills, fever, cough, and sore throat) or of bleeding (such as hematuria, bleeding gums, easy bruising, and tarry stools).
• Advise women of childbearing age to avoid becoming pregnant during therapy and to consult a prescriber before becoming pregnant.
• Advise women not to breast-feed during therapy because of possible toxic effects on infant.

flumazenil
Anexate ◇, Romazicon

Pharmacologic class: benzodiazepine antagonist
Therapeutic class: antidote
Pregnancy risk category: C
pH: 4

INDICATIONS & DOSAGES
➤ **To completely or partially reverse the sedative effects of benzodiazepines after anesthesia or short diag-**

Reactions may be *common,* uncommon, *life-threatening,* or COMMON AND LIFE-THREATENING.

nostic procedures (conscious sedation)—

Adults: Initially, 0.2 mg I.V. over 15 seconds. If patient doesn't reach the desired level of consciousness after 45 seconds, repeat dose. If needed, repeat at 1-minute intervals until a cumulative dose of 1 mg I.V. has been given—that is, an initial dose plus four additional doses. Most patients respond after 0.6 to 1 mg I.V. of drug. In case of resedation, dosage may be repeated after 20 minutes; however, no more than 1 mg should be given at any one time, and no more than 3 mg/hour.

➤ **To manage suspected benzodiazepine overdose—**

Adults: Initially, 0.2 mg I.V. over 30 seconds. If patient doesn't reach desired level of consciousness after 30 seconds, give 0.3 mg I.V. over 30 seconds. If patient still doesn't respond adequately, give 0.5 mg I.V. over 30 seconds; repeat 0.5-mg I.V. doses at 1-minute intervals until a cumulative dose of 3 mg I.V. has been given. Most patients suffering from benzodiazepine overdose respond to cumulative doses between 1 and 3 mg I.V.; rarely, patients who respond partially after 3 mg may require additional doses. Don't give more than 5 mg over 5 minutes initially. Sedation that persists after this dosage is unlikely to be caused by benzodiazepines. In case of resedation, dosage may be repeated after 20 minutes; however, no more than 1 mg should be given at any one time, and no more than 3 mg/hour.

ADMINISTRATION

Direct injection: Inject over 15 to 30 seconds into an I.V. line in a large vein with free-flowing I.V. solution.
Intermittent infusion: Not recommended.
Continuous infusion: Not recommended.

PREPARATION & STORAGE

Available as a 0.1-mg/ml solution in 5-ml and 10-ml vials.

Flumazenil is compatible with D_5W, lactated Ringer's solution, and normal saline solution. If drawn into a syringe or mixed with any of these solutions, discard after 24 hours.

Incompatibilities

None reported.

CONTRAINDICATIONS & CAUTIONS

• Contraindicated in patients hypersensitive to flumazenil or benzodiazepines.
• Contraindicated in those who have been given a benzodiazepine for a potentially life-threatening condition, such as to control intracranial pressure or status epilepticus, and in those who show signs of serious cyclic antidepressant overdose.
• Don't use drug during labor and delivery.
• Don't use drug to treat benzodiazepine dependence or manage protracted benzodiazepine abstinence syndromes.
• Use cautiously in those with hepatic impairment because clearance is reduced to 40% to 60% in mild to moderate impairment and to 25% in severe impairment and in psychiatric patients because the drug has caused panic attacks in those with panic disorder.
• Use cautiously in those at high risk for seizures, including those withdrawing from sedative hypnotics; in those displaying some signs of seizure activity, such as myoclonus; and in those who may be at risk for unrecognized benzodiazepine dependence, such as those in the ICU.
• Use cautiously in those who have recently received multiple doses of a parenteral benzodiazepine and in those who have received neuromuscular blockers.
• Use cautiously in those with alcohol or other drug dependence because of increased risk of benzodiazepine toler-

ance and in those with head injury because of the risk of causing seizures.

ADVERSE REACTIONS
CNS: headache, *dizziness,* agitation, insomnia, emotional lability, confusion, *seizures,* somnolence, tremor, paresthesia, fatigue.
CV: cutaneous vasodilatation, *arrhythmias, bradycardia,* tachycardia, hypertension, palpitations.
EENT: dry mouth, speech disorder, diplopia, blurred vision, abnormal hearing.
GI: nausea, vomiting.
Respiratory: dyspnea, hyperventilation.
Skin: diaphoresis.

INTERACTIONS
Drug-drug. *Overdose of antidepressants:* Causes seizures or arrhythmias after the effects of benzodiazepine overdose are treated. Don't use to treat mixed overdose, especially when seizures are likely to occur.
Drug-food. *Any food:* May increase drug clearance by 50%. Monitor patient closely if he eats food during infusion.

EFFECTS ON LAB TEST RESULTS
None reported.

ACTION
Competitively inhibits the actions of benzodiazepines on the gamma-aminobutyric acid benzodiazepine receptor complex.

PHARMACOKINETICS
Onset within 1 to 2 minutes after injection; within 3 minutes, 80% response is reached; effect peaks at 6 to 10 minutes.
Distribution: 50% protein bound; no preferential partitioning into RBCs.
Metabolism: In liver.
Excretion: 90% to 95% in urine; 5% to 10% in feces. Half-life, 54 minutes.

CLINICAL CONSIDERATIONS
● To control the reversal of sedation to the desired end point and to minimize the risk of adverse effects, give flumazenil as a series of small injections, not as a single bolus dose.
● Patients should have a secure airway and I.V. access before drug is given and should be awakened gradually.
● To minimize pain at injection site, give through a free-flowing I.V. solution into a large vein.
● Drug may cause dose-dependent signs and symptoms of withdrawal in patients with established physical dependence on benzodiazepines.
● Monitor patient closely for resedation after reversal of benzodiazepine effects, which may occur because the duration of action of flumazenil is shorter than that of all benzodiazepines.
● Duration of monitoring depends on the specific drug being reversed. Monitor patient closely after long-acting benzodiazepines, such as diazepam, or after high doses of short-acting benzodiazepines, such as midazolam.
● Resedation is unlikely in patients who fail to show signs of it 2 hours after a 1-mg dose of flumazenil.
● Excessively high doses of flumazenil may produce anxiety, agitation, and seizures. Treat these reactions with barbiturates, benzodiazepines, and phenytoin.

PATIENT TEACHING
● Provide written instructions to patient or family members.
● Warn patient not to perform hazardous activities for 24 hours after the procedure because of risk of resedation.
● Advise patient to avoid alcohol, CNS depressants, and OTC drugs for 24 hours after administration.

Reactions may be *common,* uncommon, *life-threatening,* or COMMON AND LIFE-THREATENING.

fluorouracil (5-FU)
Adrucil

Pharmacologic class: antimetabolite (S phase–specific)
Therapeutic class: antineoplastic
Pregnancy risk category: D
pH: 9.2

INDICATIONS & DOSAGES
➤ **Palliative treatment of colorectal, stomach, pancreatic, and advanced breast cancer—**
Adults: Initially, 12 mg/kg/day I.V. for 4 days. Maximum dosage, 800 mg/day. If patient doesn't have a toxic reaction, give 6 mg/kg I.V. on days 6, 8, 10, and 12. Give no therapy on days 5, 7, 9, or 11, and stop therapy on day 12. For maintenance, give initial dose, repeat in 30 days; then give 10 to 15 mg/kg I.V. weekly.

Dosage depends on protocol and patient weight.
High-risk adults: Initially, 6 mg/kg/day I.V. for 3 days. Maximum dosage, 400 mg/day. If patient doesn't have a toxic reaction, give 3 mg/kg I.V. on days 5, 7, and 9. Give no therapy on days 4, 6, or 8. Reduce maintenance dosage.

Dosage depends on protocol and patient weight.

ADMINISTRATION
Direct injection: Give by a 23G or 25G winged infusion set at any convenient rate. Consider using distal rather than major veins to allow for repeated venipunctures, if needed. Use a new site for each injection.
Intermittent infusion: Not recommended.
Continuous infusion: Infuse appropriately diluted drug via central line over 2 to 24 hours.

PREPARATION & STORAGE
Available in 10-ml glass ampules containing 500 mg of drug in a clear yellow aqueous solution and in 10-, 20-, and 100-ml vials containing 50-mg/ml solution. Don't use dark-yellow solutions; potency may be affected.

For injection, drug requires no further dilution. For infusion, dilute with D_5W or normal saline solution in an appropriate volume based on the patient's condition. Use a filtered needle to prevent injection of glass particles that may enter the solution when opening the ampule.

Store at room temperature and protect from direct sunlight.

Incompatibilities
Carboplatin, cisplatin, cytarabine, diazepam, doxorubicin, droperidol, epirubicin, fentanyl citrate, filgrastim, gallium nitrate, leucovorin calcium, metoclopramide, morphine sulfate, ondansetron, vinorelbine tartrate.

CONTRAINDICATIONS & CAUTIONS
• Contraindicated in those with serious infection, especially recent or existing chickenpox or herpes zoster, because of increased risk of severe generalized disease.
• Contraindicated in patients who have had surgery within the previous month.
• Use cautiously in those with hepatic or renal impairment because of increased risk of toxic reaction.
• Use cautiously in those with previous metastasis to the bone marrow, high-dose radiation therapy, or use of alkylating drugs because of heightened risk of hematologic toxicity.

ADVERSE REACTIONS
CNS: lethargy, malaise, weakness, acute cerebellar syndrome, headache, disorientation, confusion, euphoria, fever.
CV: *ischemia,* angina.
EENT: photophobia, lacrimation, pharyngitis, decreased vision, nystag-

mus, diplopia, lacrimal duct stenosis, visual changes, epistaxis.
GI: stomatitis, esophagopharyngitis, diarrhea, anorexia, nausea, vomiting, *enteritis,* cramps, duodenal ulcer, watery stool, duodenitis, gastritis, glossitis, *GI bleeding.*
Hematologic: *leukopenia, thrombocytopenia, pancytopenia, agranulocytosis,* anemia.
Skin: alopecia, dermatitis, rash, photosensitivity, nail changes, dry skin, fissuring, vein pigmentation.
Other: generalized allergic reactions, *anaphylaxis.*

INTERACTIONS

Drug-drug. *Myelosuppressants, drugs causing blood dyscrasias:* May worsen bone marrow depression. Avoid using together.
Thiazide diuretics: May increase hematologic toxicity. Avoid using together.
Vaccines with live virus: May cause virus replication. Avoid using together.

EFFECTS ON LAB TEST RESULTS

● May increase alkaline phosphatase, AST, ALT, bilirubin, and LDH levels. May decrease albumin level.
● May decrease hemoglobin and WBC, RBC, platelet, and granulocyte counts.

ACTION

Interferes with DNA synthesis and to a lesser extent, RNA synthesis, which most affects cells that grow rapidly and take up fluorouracil at a faster pace.

PHARMACOKINETICS

Drug level peaks immediately after injection.
Distribution: By diffusion to all areas of body water, such as tumors, intestinal mucosa, bone marrow, liver, CNS, and other tissues. Drug crosses the placental barrier, but it's unknown if it appears in breast milk.
Metabolism: In the liver. Up to 80% is rapidly detoxified to an active metabolite.

Excretion: 60% to 80% eliminated through the lungs as carbon dioxide. 15% is removed unchanged in urine, mostly in the first hour. Half-life is 10 to 20 minutes, up to 20 hours for metabolites.

CLINICAL CONSIDERATIONS

● Osmolality: 650 mOsm/kg.
● Be extremely careful when preparing fluorouracil to avoid mutagenic, teratogenic, and carcinogenic risks. Use a biological containment cabinet and wear gloves and mask. Use syringes with luer-lock tips to avoid drug leakage. Correctly dispose of needles, ampules, and unused drug, and avoid contaminating work surfaces. Manufacturer recommends cleaning spills with sodium hypochlorite 5% (household bleach) to inactivate drug.
● Fluorouracil may be used with other chemotherapeutic drugs.
● Monitor CBC and liver and kidney function test results. If platelet count is less than 100,000/mm^3 or if WBC count is less than 3,500/mm^3 or decreases rapidly, therapy should be stopped.
● WBC count usually reaches its nadir from days 9 to 14 after treatment, possibly up to day 25. Recovery usually occurs by day 30.
● Antibiotics should be given if myelosuppressed patient develops an infection.
● Therapeutic doses of fluorouracil will cause toxic effects.
● Anything that increases stress, interferes with nutrition, or depresses bone marrow function increases the toxic effects of fluorouracil.
● Treat anorexia and nausea with an antiemetic. Stop drug if patient develops intractable vomiting or diarrhea or GI bleeding.
● Examine patient's mouth for ulceration before each dose.

PATIENT TEACHING

● Inform patient of expected adverse effects.

- Advise patient to avoid exposure to people with infections and to report unusual bleeding or bruising.
- Advise women not to become pregnant while undergoing drug therapy.
- Advise women not to breast-feed during therapy.
- Teach both men and women to use reliable contraception during drug therapy.

folic acid
Folvite*

___

Pharmacologic class: folic acid derivative
Therapeutic class: vitamin supplement
Pregnancy risk category: A; C if greater than RDA
pH: 5 to 6

___

INDICATIONS & DOSAGES
➤ **Megaloblastic and macrocytic anemias as seen in tropical sprue, anemia of nutritional origin, pregnancy, infancy, or childhood—**
Adults and children: 250 mcg to 1 mg I.V. daily.

ADMINISTRATION
Direct injection: Slowly inject dose directly into vein or into the tubing of a free-flowing, compatible I.V. solution.
Intermittent infusion: Not recommended.
Continuous infusion: Not recommended.

PREPARATION & STORAGE
Available in 10-ml vials containing 5 mg/ml.
    Dilute 1 ml of 5-mg/ml concentration with 49 ml of sterile water for injection to yield 0.1 mg/ml.
    Store between 59° and 86° F (15° and 30° C). Protect from light and freezing.

Incompatibilities
Calcium gluconate, dextrose 40% in water, dextrose 50% in water, doxapram, oxidizing and reducing drugs, heavy metal ions.

CONTRAINDICATIONS & CAUTIONS
- Contraindicated in neonates and immature infants because benzyl alcohol contained in preparation may lead to fatal toxic reaction.
- Use cautiously in patients who have vitamin B_{12} deficiency. Folic acid can mask the diagnosis of pernicious anemia by improving hematologic values. Neurologic damage, however, will progress. Don't use as sole treatment of pernicious anemia.

ADVERSE REACTIONS
CNS: fever, altered sleep, malaise, difficulty concentrating, irritability, overactivity, excitement, depression, confusion, impaired judgment.
GI: anorexia, nausea, abdominal distention, flatulence, bitter taste.
Other: *anaphylaxis,* allergic sensitization.

INTERACTIONS
Drug-drug. *Aminosalicylic acid:* Decreases folate level. Avoid using together.
Hormonal contraceptives: Decreases folate level. Avoid using together.
Methotrexate, pyrimethamine, triamterene, trimethoprim: Reduces dihydrofolate reductase, resulting in antagonized folic acid effect. Monitor patient closely.
Phenytoin: May increase phenytoin metabolism, resulting in decreased phenytoin level and more seizures. Avoid using together.
Sulfasalazine: Causes folate deficiency. Avoid using together.

EFFECTS ON LAB TEST RESULTS
- May decrease vitamin B_{12} and serum and RBC folate levels.

___

ACTION
Tetrahydrofolic acid is needed for normal erythropoiesis and nucleoprotein synthesis.

PHARMACOKINETICS
Drug is rapidly cleared from plasma.
Distribution: To all body tissues, especially the liver, CNS, and erythrocytes. Drug crosses placental barrier and appears in breast milk.
Metabolism: In the liver to metabolically active tetrahydrofolic acid by dihydrofolate reductase.
Excretion: In urine as metabolites and small amounts of unchanged drug. With higher doses, larger amounts of unchanged drug are removed in the urine.

CLINICAL CONSIDERATIONS
• Osmolality: 186 mOsm/kg.
• Use I.V. administration only when oral administration isn't feasible.
• Monitor CBC to measure effectiveness of drug treatment.

PATIENT TEACHING
• Tell patient to report adverse reactions promptly.
• Explain use and administration of drug to patient and family.

---

foscarnet sodium
Foscavir

Pharmacologic class: pyrophosphate analogue
Therapeutic class: antiviral
Pregnancy risk category: C
pH: 7.4

INDICATIONS & DOSAGES
➤ **CMV retinitis in patients with AIDS—**
Adults: Initially, 60 mg/kg by I.V. infusion over at least 1 hour as induction treatment q 8 hours, or 90 mg/kg over

1½ to 2 hours q 12 hours for 2 or 3 weeks based on clinical response. Then maintenance infusion of 90 mg/kg/day given over 2 hours. May increase dose 120 mg/kg/day if disease shows signs of progression.
➤ **Herpes simplex virus infection—**
Adults: 40 mg/kg I.V. infusion over at least 1 hour, q 8 or 12 hours for 2 or 3 weeks or until infection resolved.
➤ **Varicella-zoster infection in immunocompromised patients ◆—**
Adults: 40 mg/kg I.V. q 8 hours for 10 to 12 days or until complete healing occurs.
Adjust-a-dose: For patients with renal impairment, see package insert for complete dosage information.

ADMINISTRATION
Direct injection: Not recommended.
Intermittent infusion: 60 mg/kg or less infused over at least 1 hour; higher doses, over at least 2 hours. Give undiluted solutions through a central line and diluted solutions through a peripheral line. Foscarnet must be given at a constant rate by an infusion pump.
Continuous infusion: Not recommended.

PREPARATION & STORAGE
Available as a 24-mg/ml solution for infusion in 250- and 500-ml glass bottles.
    To prevent venous irritation, give undiluted drug only through a central line. For peripheral administration, dilute with an equal amount (1:1) of dextrose 5% injection or normal saline injection to yield 12 mg/ml. To avoid accidental overdose, calculate dose, and then remove and discard any excess before starting infusion.
    Store at 59° to 86° F (15° to 30° C). Undiluted drug is stable for 24 months at 77° F (25° C). At a concentration of 12 mg/ml in normal saline solution, foscarnet is stable for 30 days at 41° F

Reactions may be *common*, uncommon, *life-threatening*, or COMMON AND LIFE-THREATENING.

(5° C). Don't freeze; precipitation is likely. Discard any frozen product.

Incompatibilities
Acyclovir; amphotericin B; co-trimoxazole; dextrose 30%; diazepam; digoxin; diphenhydramine; dobutamine; droperidol; ganciclovir; haloperidol; lactated Ringer's solution; leucovorin; lorazepam; midazolam; pentamidine; phenytoin; prochlorperazine; promethazine; solutions containing calcium, such as total parenteral nutrition; trimetrexate; vancomycin.

CONTRAINDICATIONS & CAUTIONS
• Contraindicated in those hypersensitive to drug.
• Use cautiously in those with abnormal renal function because it may result in drug accumulation and enhanced toxic drug effects. Because drug is nephrotoxic, it may worsen renal impairment. Some degree of nephrotoxicity occurs in most patients treated with this drug. To avoid renal toxicity, adjust dose according to renal function and hydrate patient well before and during foscarnet therapy.
• Use cautiously in anemic patients because foscarnet can decrease hemoglobin.

ADVERSE REACTIONS
CNS: *fever, cerebral edema, coma, neurotoxicity, headache,* SEIZURES, cerebrovascular disorder, depression, confusion, anxiety, asthenia, fatigue, malaise, paresthesia, dizziness, involuntary muscle contractions, hypoesthesia, neuropathy.
CV: chest pain, edema, hypertension, palpitations, tachycardia, *first-degree AV block,* ST-segment and T-wave changes, hypotension.
EENT: vision abnormalities.
GI: *pancreatitis,* anorexia, *nausea, diarrhea, vomiting,* abdominal pain.
GU: *nephrotoxicity.*

Hematologic: BONE MARROW DEPRESSION, *anemia, granulocytopenia, leukopenia.*
Metabolic: *electrolyte imbalances.*
Musculoskeletal: rigors, pain.
Respiratory: *bronchospasm,* coughing, dyspnea.
Skin: rash, diaphoresis, injection site pain and inflammation.
Other: infection, *sepsis.*

INTERACTIONS
Drug-drug. *Nephrotoxic drugs, such as amphotericin B and aminoglycosides; ritonavir; saquinavir:* Increases risk of nephrotoxicity. Avoid using together.
Pentamidine: Increases risk of nephrotoxicity and severe hypocalcemia. Monitor calcium level; avoid using together.
Zidovudine: May increase risk or severity of anemia. Monitor CBC values.

EFFECTS ON LAB TEST RESULTS
• May increase creatinine, BUN, ALT, AST, alkaline phosphatase, and bilirubin levels. May decrease calcium, magnesium, potassium, and sodium levels. May increase or decrease phosphate levels.
• May increase platelet count. May decrease hemoglobin and granulocyte, WBC, and platelet counts.

ACTION
Inhibits all herpes viruses, including CMV, Epstein-Barr virus, and varicella zoster virus, in vitro, by blocking the pyrophosphate binding site on DNA polymerases and reverse transcriptases.

PHARMACOKINETICS
Drug level peaks at end of infusion.
Distribution: About 14% to 17% protein bound; may accumulate in bone, but the extent is unknown; variable penetration into CSF.
Metabolism: Minimal.
Excretion: About 80% to 90% unchanged in urine.

CLINICAL CONSIDERATIONS

• Osmolality: 271 mOsm/kg.
• Drug is highly toxic. Because toxic effects are probably dose-related, use the lowest effective maintenance dose.
• Foscarnet may be active against certain CMV strains resistant to ganciclovir.
• Anemia occurs in up to 33% of patients treated. Transfusion may be needed.
• Don't exceed the recommended infusion rate or frequency of administration. All doses must be individualized according to each patient's renal function.
• Check creatinine clearance two to three times weekly during induction and at least once every 1 or 2 weeks during maintenance. A 24-hour creatinine clearance test is recommended periodically to assess proper dosing. If creatinine clearance falls below 0.4 ml/kg/minute, stop drug.
• Monitor electrolyte levels (including calcium, magnesium, phosphorus, and potassium) on a schedule similar to that for creatinine clearance. Monitor patient for tetany and seizures linked to abnormal electrolyte levels.
• Regular ophthalmologic examinations are needed.
• No specific treatment for overdose exists. Hemodialysis and hydration may help reduce drug levels, but their effectiveness hasn't been evaluated. Observe patient for signs of renal impairment and electrolyte imbalance, and treat as needed.

PATIENT TEACHING

• Because laboratory tests don't always show decreased calcium levels, advise patient to report tingling around the mouth, numbness in the extremities, and paresthesia.
• Tell patient to report discomfort at I.V. site.
• Explain to patient the importance of drinking plenty of fluids during therapy.

fosphenytoin
Cerebyx

Pharmacologic class: hydantoin derivative
Therapeutic class: anticonvulsant
Pregnancy risk category: D
pH: 8.6 to 9

INDICATIONS & DOSAGES
Fosphenytoin should always be prescribed and dispensed in phenytoin sodium–equivalent units (PE).
➤ **Status epilepticus—**
Adults: 15 to 20 mg PE/kg I.V. at 100 to 150 mg PE/minute as loading dose; then 4 to 6 mg PE/kg/day I.V. as maintenance dose. Phenytoin may be used instead of fosphenytoin as maintenance, using the appropriate dose.
➤ **To prevent and treat seizures during neurosurgery as nonemergent loading or maintenance dose—**
Adults: Loading dose of 10 to 20 mg PE/kg I.M. or I.V. at infusion rate not exceeding 150 mg PE/minute. Maintenance dose is 4 to 6 mg PE/kg/day I.V. or I.M.
➤ **Short-term substitution for oral phenytoin therapy—**
Adults: Same total daily dose equivalent as oral phenytoin sodium therapy given as a single daily dose I.M. or I.V., at an infusion rate not exceeding 150 mg PE/minute. Some patients may require more frequent dosing.

ADMINISTRATION
Direct injection: Not recommended; can be given I.M. Don't use I.M. administration for patients with status epilepticus because therapeutic levels may not be reached as quickly as with I.V. administration.
Intermittent infusion: Infuse drug diluted to 1.5 to 25 mg PE/ml at no more than 150 mg PE/minute. Typical infu-

---

sion for a 50-kg patient takes 5 to 7 minutes.

Continuous infusion: Not recommended.

PREPARATION & STORAGE

Available as 2-ml vial containing fosphenytoin sodium 150 mg equivalent to 100 mg of phenytoin sodium and 10-ml vial containing fosphenytoin sodium 750 mg equivalent to 500 mg of phenytoin sodium.

Before I.V. infusion, dilute drug in D_5W or normal saline solution for injection to yield 1.5 to 25 mg PE/ml.

Refrigerate unopened vials at 36° to 46° F (2° to 8° C). Don't store at room temperature for longer than 48 hours. Discard vial containing particulate matter.

Incompatibilities

Other I.V. drugs.

CONTRAINDICATIONS & CAUTIONS

• Contraindicated in those hypersensitive to phenytoin, fosphenytoin, or other hydantoins.

• Contraindicated in those with sinus bradycardia, SA block, second- or third-degree AV block, or Stokes-Adams syndrome.

• Use cautiously in those hypersensitive to drugs that have a structure similar to fosphenytoin—such as barbiturates, oxazolidinediones, and succinimides—and in those with porphyria.

ADVERSE REACTIONS

CNS: abnormal thinking, agitation, asthenia, *ataxia,* brain edema, decreased reflexes, *dizziness,* dysarthria, headache, extrapyramidal syndrome, fever, hypoesthesia, increased reflexes, incoordination, **intracranial hypertension,** nervousness, paresthesia, speech disorder, *somnolence,* stupor, vertigo.
CV: hypotension, hypertension, tachycardia, tremor, vasodilation.

EENT: amblyopia, deafness, diplopia, *nystagmus,* tinnitus.
GI: constipation, dry mouth, nausea, taste perversion, tongue disorder, vomiting.
Metabolic: hypokalemia.
Musculoskeletal: back pain, myasthenia, pelvic pain.
Respiratory: pneumonia.
Skin: ecchymosis, injection-site reaction, injection-site pain, *pruritus,* rash.
Other: accidental injury, chills, facial edema, infection.

INTERACTIONS

Drug-drug. *Amiodarone, chloramphenicol, chlordiazepoxide, cimetidine, disulfiram, estrogens, ethosuximide, fluoxetine, H_2 antagonists, halothane, isoniazid, methylphenidate, phenothiazines, salicylates, succinimides, sulfonamides, tolbutamide, trazodone:* May increase fosphenytoin level. Use together cautiously.
Carbamazepine, reserpine: May decrease fosphenytoin level. Dose may need to be adjusted.
Coumarin, doxycycline, estrogens, furosemide, hormonal contraceptives, quinidine, rifampin, theophylline, vitamin D: Decreases efficacy caused by increased hepatic metabolism. Dose may need to be adjusted.
Phenobarbital, valproic acid, valproate sodium: May increase or decrease levels of either drug. Dose may need to be adjusted.
Tricyclic antidepressants: May lower seizure threshold, requiring adjustment in fosphenytoin dose. Avoid using together.
Drug-lifestyle. *Alcohol use:* Acute alcohol use may increase drug levels; chronic alcohol use may decrease drug levels. Discourage use together.

EFFECTS ON LAB TEST RESULTS

• May increase alkaline phosphatase, GGT, and glucose levels. May decrease folate, potassium, and T_4 levels.

ACTION
Fosphenytoin's anticonvulsant action is the same as phenytoin's. Phenytoin is believed to stabilize neuronal membranes and limit seizure activity by modulating sodium channels, inhibiting calcium flux across neuronal membranes, modulating voltage-dependent calcium channels of neurons, and enhancing sodium-potassium ATPase activity in neurons and glial cells.

PHARMACOKINETICS
Drug level peaks at the end of I.V. administration or about 30 minutes after I.M. administration.
Distribution: 95% to 99% protein bound.
Metabolism: Conversion half-life, about 15 minutes. Mechanism is unknown.
Excretion: Unknown.

CLINICAL CONSIDERATIONS
• If rapid phenytoin loading is a primary goal, I.V. administration is preferred because therapeutic phenytoin levels are achieved quicker than with I.M. administration.
• The phosphate load that fosphenytoin supplies (0.0037 mmol phosphate/mg PE fosphenytoin) affects patients who must significantly restrict their phosphate intake, such as those with renal impairment. Monitor phosphate levels.
• Severe CV complications occur most commonly in geriatric or very ill patients. Administration rate may need to be reduced or the drug stopped.
• Patients receiving 20 mg PE/kg at 150 mg PE/minute will likely have sensory discomfort, usually in the groin. This can be lessened by slowing or temporarily stopping the infusion.
• Abrupt withdrawal of drug may precipitate status epilepticus.
• Monitor vital signs and ECG continuously during period when maximum phenytoin levels occur—that is, 10 to 20 minutes after fosphenytoin infusion ends.

• If rash occurs, stop infusion and notify prescriber.
• Monitor liver function test results. Stop drug in patients with acute hepatotoxicity.
• Don't check phenytoin levels until fosphenytoin has completely converted to phenytoin—that is, about 2 hours after I.V. administration.
• For patients with renal or hepatic disease or hypoalbuminemia, consider obtaining free phenytoin levels, as opposed to serum levels. These patients may have more frequent and severe adverse reactions because more of the drug is unbound.
• No known antidote for fosphenytoin or phenytoin overdose exists. Closely monitor respiratory and CV function and provide supportive care. Consider hemodialysis because phenytoin isn't completely protein bound.

PATIENT TEACHING
• Warn patient of sensory disturbances that may occur with I.V. administration.
• Instruct patient to immediately report all adverse effects, especially rash.
• Instruct patient never to abruptly stop or adjust drug dosage.
• Inform women that breast-feeding isn't recommended.

furosemide
Lasix, Lasix Special ◇

Pharmacologic class: loop diuretic
Therapeutic class: diuretic, antihypertensive
Pregnancy risk category: C
pH: 8 to 9.3

INDICATIONS & DOSAGES
➤ **Edema—**
Adults: Initially, 20 to 40 mg I.V., increased in 20-mg increments q 2 hours until desired response is achieved. Ef-

fective dose given once or twice daily p.r.n.

➤ **Pulmonary edema—**
Adults: Initially, 40 mg I.V., increased to 80 mg I.V. in 1 hour, if needed.
Infants and children: Initially, 1 mg/kg, increased by 1 mg/kg q 2 hours, if needed. Maximum daily dose, 6 mg/kg I.V.

➤ **Hypertensive crisis with pulmonary edema—**
Adults: 40 to 80 mg I.V. In patients with reduced renal function, give higher doses.

➤ **Heart failure and chronic renal failure—**
Adults: For bolus injection, don't exceed 1 g/day I.V. given over 30 minutes.
Infants and children ♦ *:* Initially, 1 mg/kg I.V., increased by 1 mg/kg I.V. q 2 hours, if needed. Maximum daily dose, 6 mg/kg I.V.

➤ **Hypercalcemia** ♦ **—**
Adults: 80 to 100 mg I.V. q 1 to 2 hours.

ADMINISTRATION
Direct injection: Inject directly into vein or through tubing of a free-flowing, compatible solution over 1 to 2 minutes.
Intermittent infusion: Infuse diluted drug at appropriate rate, but not exceeding 4 mg/minute.
Continuous infusion: Not recommended.

PREPARATION & STORAGE
Available in 2-, 4-, and 10-ml ampules and single-use vials and in syringes containing 10 mg/ml.

For infusion, dilute in D_5W, lactated Ringer's solution, dextrose 5% in lactated Ringer's solution, dextrose 5% in Ringer's injection, or normal saline solution. Filter solution to remove any glass particles from ampules.

Store at room temperature and protect from light. Discard yellow, discolored solution or solution that contains a precipitate.

Incompatibilities
Acidic solutions, aminoglycosides, amiodarone, bleomycin, buprenorphine, chlorpromazine, diazepam, dobutamine, doxapram, doxorubicin, droperidol, erythromycin, esmolol, fluconazole, fructose 10% in water, gentamicin, hydralazine, idarubicin, invert sugar 10% in electrolyte #2, isoproterenol, meperidine, metoclopramide, milrinone, morphine, netilmicin, ondansetron, prochlorperazine, promethazine, quinidine, vinblastine, vincristine.

CONTRAINDICATIONS & CAUTIONS
● Contraindicated in those hypersensitive to furosemide or sulfonamides and in those with anuria or worsening azotemia or oliguria.
● Use cautiously in those with diabetes mellitus because drug may impair glucose tolerance; in those with hyperuricemia or gout because drug may raise uric acid levels; and in those with pancreatitis or lupus erythematosus because drug may worsen these disorders.
● Use cautiously in those with hepatic impairment because potential dehydration and electrolyte imbalance may precipitate hepatic coma and in those with acute MI because diuresis may precipitate shock.

ADVERSE REACTIONS
CNS: fever, vertigo, headache, dizziness, restlessness, paresthesia.
CV: *cardiac arrest,* orthostatic hypotension, chronic aortitis, thrombophlebitis, *necrotizing angiitis.*
EENT: blurred vision, hearing loss, yellowish appearance of objects.
GI: anorexia, nausea, vomiting, diarrhea, oral or gastric irritation, constipation.

GU: interstitial nephritis, urinary bladder spasm, hyperuricemia.

Hematologic: anemia, *leukopenia, aplastic anemia, thrombocytopenia, agranulocytosis.*

Hepatic: *pancreatitis,* jaundice, *ischemic hepatitis.*

Metabolic: glycosuria, hyperglycemia.

Musculoskeletal: muscle spasm, weakness.

Skin: purpura, photosensitivity, urticaria, pruritus, *exfoliative dermatitis,* erythema multiforme, rash.

INTERACTIONS

Drug-drug. *Aminoglycosides, amphotericin B, nephrotoxic or ototoxic drugs:* May increase risk of nephrotoxicity and ototoxicity and intensifies electrolyte imbalance. Avoid using together.

Amiodarone, cardiac glycosides: May enhance risk of arrhythmias because of hypokalemia. Monitor potassium level.

Anticoagulants, thrombolytics: May increase anticoagulant effects and risk of GI bleeding. Monitor patient closely.

Antidiabetics, insulin: May interfere with hypoglycemic effects. Dosage may need to be adjusted.

Antigout drugs: May elevate uric acid level. Monitor patient closely.

Antihistamines, antivertigo drugs, phenothiazines, thioxanthenes, trimethobenzamide: May mask signs of ototoxicity. Avoid using together.

Antihypertensives: May enhance hypotensive and diuretic effects. Avoid using together.

Chloral hydrate: May cause diaphoresis, hot flashes, and variable blood pressure. Monitor patient for adverse reactions.

Corticosteroids: May increase natriuretic and diuretic effects and intensify electrolyte imbalance. Monitor patient closely.

Dopamine: May enhance diuresis. Monitor patient closely.

Lithium: May increase risk of toxic reaction because of reduced clearance. Monitor patient for toxic reaction. Use together with caution.

Neuromuscular blockers: May antagonize or potentiate these drugs, depending on dose. Monitor patient closely.

NSAIDs, probenecid: Antagonizes natriuresis and diuresis and increases risk of renal impairment. Avoid using together.

Sympathomimetics: May reduce antihypertensive effects of furosemide. Monitor patient closely.

Drug-lifestyle. *Alcohol use:* May enhance hypotensive and diuretic effects. Discourage use together.

EFFECTS ON LAB TEST RESULTS

● May increase glucose, cholesterol, and uric acid levels. May decrease potassium, sodium, calcium, and magnesium levels.

● May decrease hemoglobin and granulocyte, WBC, and platelet counts.

ACTION

Inhibits reabsorption of electrolytes, including sodium and chloride, in the ascending loop of Henle; increases excretion of potassium in the distal tubule; and affects electrolyte transport at the proximal tubule. Drug also may cause renal vasodilation and a transient rise in GFR.

PHARMACOKINETICS

Onset, 5 minutes; duration, 2 hours.

Distribution: 95% protein bound. Drug crosses the placental barrier and appears in breast milk.

Metabolism: Small amount metabolized in the liver.

Excretion: 80% to 88% in urine in 24 hours, mostly in first 4 hours; about 12% in bile, some as unchanged drug. Half-life is 1½ hours.

Reactions may be *common*, uncommon, *life-threatening*, or COMMON AND LIFE-THREATENING.

CLINICAL CONSIDERATIONS

• Osmolality: 287 to 291 mOsm/kg.
• Drug may cause hypochloremic metabolic alkalemia and a compensatory respiratory acidemia—that is, increased partial pressure of carbon dioxide.
• Give slowly; overly rapid injection or infusion can cause ototoxicity.
• Signs and symptoms of overdose include excessive diuresis with dehydration and electrolyte depletion.
• Monitor BUN, uric acid, glucose, and electrolyte levels as well as liver and kidney function test results; also monitor patient's weight, intake and output, and vital signs.
• If overdose occurs, correct fluid and electrolyte imbalance and treat symptomatically.

PATIENT TEACHING

• Encourage patient to eat potassium-rich foods, such as citrus fruits, bananas, tomatoes, dates, and apricots.
• Advise patient to change position slowly to avoid dizziness.
• Instruct patient to immediately report changes in hearing, abdominal pain, sore throat, or fever, which may indicate furosemide toxicity.

G

ganciclovir sodium
Cytovene

Pharmacologic class: synthetic nucleoside
Therapeutic class: antiviral
Pregnancy risk category: C
pH: 11

INDICATIONS & DOSAGES
➤ **CMV retinitis—**
Adults: Initially, 5 mg/kg I.V. q 12 hours for 14 to 21 days, then maintenance dose of 5 mg/kg/day for 7 days/week or 6 mg/kg/day for 5 days/week.
➤ **To prevent CMV disease in transplant recipients—**
Adults: Initially, 5 mg/kg I.V. q 12 hours for 7 to 14 days, then 5 mg/kg/day for 7 days/week or 6 mg/kg/day for 5 days/week. Duration of therapy depends on degree and duration of immunosuppression.
➤ **Other CMV infections (GI infections, pneumonitis) ♦—**
Adults: 5 mg/kg I.V. over 1 hour q 12 hours for 14 to 21 days; or 2.5 mg/kg I.V. q 8 hours for 14 to 21 days. Maintenance doses similar to other indications have been used.
➤ **To prevent CMV disease recurrence in HIV patients ♦—**
Adults and children: 5 to 6 mg/kg I.V. once daily for 5 to 7 days/week.
Adjust-a-dose: For adults receiving hemodialysis, give 1.25 mg/kg I.V. three times a week, initially; then give maintenance dosage of 0.625 mg/kg three times a week. For adults with renal impairment, adjust dosages according to the following table.

I.V. induction dosages

Creatinine clearance (ml/min)	Dose (mg/kg)	Interval
50-69	2.5	12 hr
25-49	2.5	24 hr
10-24	1.25	24 hr
< 10	1.25	3 times/wk

I.V. maintenance dosages

Creatinine clearance (ml/min)	Dose (mg/kg)	Interval
50-69	2.5	24 hr
25-49	1.25	24 hr
10-24	0.625	24 hr
< 10	0.625	3 times/wk

ADMINISTRATION
Direct injection: Not recommended.
Intermittent infusion: Give drug over 1 hour.
Continuous infusion: Not recommended.

PREPARATION & STORAGE
Available in 500-mg vials.
   Add 10 ml of sterile water without preservative to one 500-mg vial to produce 50 mg/ml. Shake vial until solution is clear to ensure that all particles are completely dissolved. Dilute further to a final concentration of 10 mg/ml with 100 ml of normal saline solution, D₅W, Ringer's injection, or lactated Ringer's injection.
   Store vials between 59° and 86° F (15° and 30° C). After reconstitution,

solutions with a concentration of 50 mg/ml retain potency for 12 hours at room temperature; don't refrigerate. Use fully diluted solutions within 24 hours; keep refrigerated until use; don't freeze.

Incompatibilities

Aldesleukin, amifostine, aztreonam, cefepime, cytarabine, doxorubicin hydrochloride, fludarabine, foscarnet, ondansetron, other I.V. drugs, parabens (bacteriostatic agent), piperacillin sodium with tazobactam, sargramostim, vinorelbine.

CONTRAINDICATIONS & CAUTIONS

• Contraindicated in those hypersensitive to ganciclovir or acyclovir.
• Because ganciclovir solutions are alkaline with a pH of about 11, be careful when handling and preparing drug. Latex gloves and safety glasses are recommended. If solution contacts skin or mucous membranes, wash area thoroughly with soap and water; irrigate eyes with plain water.

ADVERSE REACTIONS

CNS: *fever,* neuropathy, paresthesia.
GI: *abdominal pain, diarrhea, nausea, anorexia, vomiting.*
Hematologic: *granulocytopenia,* LEU-KOPENIA, *anemia,* **thrombocytopenia, neutropenia.**
Hepatic: *hepatotoxicity.*
Respiratory: pneumonia.
Skin: rash, *diaphoresis,* pruritus, photosensitivity reactions.
Other: *infection, chills,* SEPSIS.

INTERACTIONS

Drug-drug. *Imipenem and cilastatin sodium:* Causes generalized seizures. Avoid using together.
Immunosuppressants: Causes additional bone marrow depression. Monitor patient closely.
Nephrotoxic drugs: Increases creatinine level. Monitor patient closely.

Probenecid: Reduces renal clearance of ganciclovir. Monitor patient for toxic reaction.
Zidovudine: Increases risk of neutropenia. Monitor patient closely.
Drug-lifestyle. *Sun exposure:* Photosensitivity reactions may occur. Advise patient to avoid excessive sunlight exposure.

EFFECTS ON LAB TEST RESULTS

• May increase creatinine, ALT, AST, GGT, and alkaline phosphatase levels.
• May decrease hemoglobin and granulocyte, platelet, neutrophil, and WBC counts.

ACTION

Competitively inhibits viral DNA polymerase and may be incorporated in viral DNA to cause early termination of DNA replication.

PHARMACOKINETICS

Onset, immediate; peak, within 1 hour; half-life, 4 to 30 hours.
Distribution: Drug concentrates in cells infected with CMV because of the preferential phosphorylation in these cells. Drug crosses the blood-brain barrier, but it's unknown if drug appears in breast milk.
Metabolism: More than 90% of drug is excreted unchanged.
Excretion: By kidneys. Elimination half-life, about 3 hours. Hemodialysis removes drug.

CLINICAL CONSIDERATIONS

• Osmolality: 320 mOsm/kg.
• *Alert:* Because ganciclovir should be considered a carcinogen, handle it according to institutional guidelines developed for cytotoxic drugs.
• Patients receiving hemodialysis should receive their dose of ganciclovir after the dialysis session because treatment substantially reduces drug levels.
• About 40% of patients experience some hematologic toxicity, including

granulocytopenia or thrombocytopenia. Granulocytopenia usually occurs during the first week but may occur anytime during therapy. Patients with drug-induced immunosuppression seem more likely to develop thrombocytopenia than those infected with HIV. Cell counts usually recover 3 to 7 days after the drug is stopped.

• Monitor CBC to detect neutropenia, which may occur in up to 40% of patients, usually after about 10 days of therapy. Neutropenia is reversible but may require stopping therapy. Patient therapy can restart when CBC returns to normal.

• Patients with HIV infection and patients with organ and bone marrow transplants may be at increased risk for CMV infections. Gancyclovir is being tested for other forms of CMV infections, including pneumonitis and GI disease.

• If overdose occurs, dialysis may be useful in reducing drug levels. Make sure patient is adequately hydrated. Consider use of hematopoietic growth factors.

PATIENT TEACHING

• Tell patient that maintenance infusions are needed to prevent disease recurrence.

• Advise patient to immediately report signs and symptoms of infection (such as fever, chills, and sore throat) or of bleeding (such as easy bruising, bleeding gums, blood in urine, or tarry stools).

• Instruct patient to take extra care when brushing teeth and when using dental floss or toothpicks.

• Advise women not to breast-feed during treatment and for at least 72 hours after last ganciclovir treatment.

• Advise patient to use effective birth control during therapy.

gatifloxacin
Tequin

Pharmacologic class: fluoroquinolone
Therapeutic class: antibiotic
Pregnancy risk category: C
pH: 3.5 to 5.5

INDICATIONS & DOSAGES

➤ **Acute bacterial exacerbation of chronic bronchitis caused by** *Streptococcus pneumoniae, Haemophilus influenzae, H. parainfluenzae, Moraxella catarrhalis,* **or** *Staphylococcus aureus*—
Adults: 400 mg I.V. daily for 5 days.
➤ **Complicated UTI caused by** *Escherichia coli, Klebsiella pneumoniae,* **or** *Proteus mirabilis;* **acute pyelonephritis caused by** *E. coli;* **uncomplicated skin and skin structure infection caused by** *S. aureus* **(methicillin-susceptible strains only) or** *Streptococcus pyogenes*—
Adults: 400 mg I.V. daily for 7 to 10 days.
➤ **Acute sinusitis caused by** *S. pneumoniae* **or** *H. influenzae*—
Adults: 400 mg I.V. daily for 10 days.
➤ **Community-acquired pneumonia caused by** *S. pneumoniae, H. influenzae, H. parainfluenzae, M. catarrhalis, S. aureus, Mycoplasma pneumoniae, Chlamydia pneumoniae,* **or** *Legionella pneumophila*—
Adults: 400 mg I.V. daily for 7 to 14 days.
Adjust-a-dose: For patients with creatinine clearance less than 40 ml/minute, those receiving hemodialysis, and those receiving continuous peritoneal dialysis, initial dosage is 400 mg I.V. daily and subsequent dosage is 200 mg I.V. daily. For patients receiving hemodialysis, give dose after hemodialysis session.

➤ **Uncomplicated urethral gonorrhea in men and cervical gonorrhea or acute uncomplicated rectal infections in women caused by** *Neisseria gonorrhoeae*—
Adults: 400 mg I.V. as single dose.
➤ **Uncomplicated UTI caused** *by E. coli, K. pneumoniae, or P. mirabilis*—
Adults: 400 mg I.V. as single dose, or 200 mg I.V. daily for 3 days.

ADMINISTRATION
Direct injection: Should be avoided.
Intermittent infusion: Infuse over 60 minutes.
Continuous infusion: Not recommended.

PREPARATION & STORAGE
Available as 200-mg/20-ml vial, 400-mg/40-ml vial, 200 mg in 100 ml D₅W, and 400 mg in 200 ml D₅W.

Dilute drug in single-use vials with either D₅W or normal saline solution to 2 mg/ml before administration.

Diluted solutions are stable for 14 days at room temperature or refrigerated. Frozen solutions are stable for up to 6 months except for 5% sodium bicarbonate solutions. Thaw at room temperature. After being thawed, solutions are stable for 14 days when stored at room temperature or under refrigeration. Discard any unused portion of the single-dose vials.

Incompatibilities
Other I.V. drugs.

CONTRAINDICATIONS & CAUTIONS
Contraindicated in patients hypersensitive to fluoroquinolones. Don't use in patients with prolonged QTc interval or with uncorrected hypokalemia.

Use cautiously in patients with bradycardia, acute myocardial ischemia, known or suspected CNS disorders, or renal insufficiency.

Safety in children younger than age 18 and in pregnant or breast-feeding women hasn't been established.

ADVERSE REACTIONS
CNS: fever, headache, dizziness, abnormal dreams, insomnia, paresthesia, tremor, vertigo.
CV: palpitations, chest pain, peripheral edema.
EENT: tinnitus, abnormal vision, pharyngitis.
GI: nausea, diarrhea, abdominal pain, constipation, dyspepsia, oral candidiasis, glossitis, stomatitis, mouth ulcer, vomiting, taste perversion.
GU: dysuria, hematuria, vaginitis.
Musculoskeletal: back pain, arthralgia, myalgia.
Respiratory: dyspnea.
Skin: rash, sweating, redness at injection site.
Other: allergic reaction, chills.

INTERACTIONS
Drug-drug. *Antidiabetics (glyburide, insulin):* May cause symptomatic hypoglycemia or hyperglycemia. Monitor glucose level.
Antipsychotics, erythromycin, tricyclic antidepressants: May prolong QTc interval. Use together cautiously.
Class IA antiarrhythmics (quinidine, procainamide), class III antiarrhythmics (amiodarone, sotalol): May prolong QTc interval. Avoid using together.
Digoxin: May increase digoxin levels. Watch for signs of digoxin toxicity.
NSAIDs: May increase risk of CNS stimulation and seizures. Use together cautiously.
Probenecid: Increases gatifloxacin levels and prolongs its half-life. Monitor patient closely.
Warfarin: May enhance effects of warfarin. Monitor PT and INR.
Drug-herb. *Dong quai, St. John's wort:* May cause photosensitivity reac-

tions. Advise patient to avoid excessive sunlight exposure.
Drug-lifestyle. *Sun exposure:* May cause photosensitivity reactions. Advise patient to avoid excessive sunlight exposure.

EFFECTS ON LAB TEST RESULTS
None reported.

ACTION
Inhibits DNA gyrase and topoisomerase, preventing cell replication and division. Gatifloxacin is active against gram-positive and gram-negative organisms.

PHARMACOKINETICS
Onset, peak, and duration of drug effects unknown.
Distribution: 20% protein bound; widely distributed into many tissues and fluids.
Metabolism: Limited biotransformation.
Excretion: More than 70% by the kidneys. Half-life is 7 to 14 hours.

CLINICAL CONSIDERATIONS
● Pseudomembranous colitis may occur in patients taking antibiotics
● Stop drug if patient has seizures, increased intracranial pressure, psychosis, or CNS stimulation leading to tremors, restlessness, lightheadedness, confusion, hallucinations, paranoia, depression, nightmares, and insomnia.
● In patients being treated for gonorrhea, test for syphilis at time of diagnosis.
● Stop drug for skin rash or other sign of hypersensitivity.
● Stop drug if patient experiences pain, inflammation or rupture of a tendon.
● Signs and symptoms of overdose include decreased respiratory rate, vomiting, tremors, and seizures. Provide symptomatic and supportive treatment, monitor ECG, and maintain hydration.

Gatifloxacin isn't removed by hemodialysis or peritoneal dialysis.

PATIENT TEACHING
● Advise patient to use sunblock and protective clothing when exposed to excessive sunlight.
● Warn patient to avoid hazardous tasks until adverse CNS effects of drugs are known.
● Advise diabetic patient to monitor glucose levels and notify prescriber if hypoglycemia occurs.
● Advise patient to immediately report palpitations; fainting spells; rash; hives; difficulty swallowing or breathing; swelling of the lips, tongue, or face; tightness in throat; hoarseness; or other symptoms of allergic reaction.
● Advise patient to stop drug, refrain from exercise, and notify prescriber if pain, inflammation, or rupture of a tendon occur.

gemcitabine hydrochloride
Gemzar

Pharmacologic class: nucleoside analogue
Therapeutic class: antineoplastic
Pregnancy risk category: D

INDICATIONS & DOSAGES
➤ **Locally advanced or metastatic adenocarcinoma of the pancreas and in patients treated previously with fluorouracil—**
Adults: 1,000 mg/m^2 I.V. over 30 minutes once weekly for up to 7 weeks, unless toxicity occurs. Treatment course of 7 weeks is followed by 1 week of rest. Subsequent dosage cycles consist of 1 infusion weekly for 3 of 4 consecutive weeks.
Adjust-a-dose: If absolute granulocyte count (AGC) is 500 to 999/mm^3 or platelet count is 50,000 to 99,999/mm^3,

give 75% of dose. Withhold dose if AGC is below 500/mm^3 or platelet count is below 50,000/mm^3. Dosage adjustments for subsequent cycles are based on AGC and platelet count nadirs and degree of nonhematologic toxicity.

➤ **With cisplatin as first-line treatment of inoperable, locally advanced, or metastatic non–small-cell lung cancer—**

Adults: For 4-week course, 1,000 mg/m^2 I.V. over 30 minutes on days 1, 8, and 15 of each 28-day cycle. Cisplatin 100 mg/m^2 on day 1 after gemcitabine infusion.

For 3-week course, 1,250 mg/m^2 I.V. over 30 minutes on days 1 and 8 of each 21-day cycle. Cisplatin 100 mg/m^2 on day 1 after gemcitabine infusion.

ADMINISTRATION

Direct injection: Not recommended.
Intermittent infusion: Infuse over 30 minutes; don't prolong infusion time beyond 60 minutes because of increased toxicity.
Continuous infusion: Not recommended.

PREPARATION & STORAGE

Available as 200-mg powder in 10-ml single-use vial and as 1-g powder in 50-ml single-use vial.

To reconstitute, add 5 ml normal saline injection to the 200-mg vial or 25 ml to the 1-g vial to yield 40 mg/ml. Higher concentrations may result in incomplete dissolution. Shake vials to assist dissolution. Reconstituted drug may be further diluted with normal saline injection to as low as 0.1 mg/ml. Inspect solution before administration and discard if discolored or contains particulates.

When reconstituted, solutions are stable at room temperature of 68° to 77° F (20° to 25° C) for 24 hours. Don't refrigerate because crystallization may occur. Discard unused solutions.

Incompatibilities

None reported.

CONTRAINDICATIONS & CAUTIONS

• Contraindicated in those hypersensitive to drug.
• Drug isn't recommended for pregnant or breast-feeding patients.
• Use cautiously in those with renal or hepatic impairment.

ADVERSE REACTIONS

CNS: *fever, somnolence, paresthesia, pain.*
CV: *edema, peripheral edema.*
GI: *stomatitis, nausea, vomiting, diarrhea, constipation.*
GU: *proteinuria, hematuria.*
Hematologic: *anemia,* **leukopenia, neutropenia, thrombocytopenia, hemorrhage.**
Respiratory: *dyspnea,* **bronchospasm.**
Skin: *alopecia, rash.*
Other: *flulike syndrome, infection.*

INTERACTIONS

None reported.

EFFECTS ON LAB TEST RESULTS

• May increase BUN, creatinine, ALT, AST, and bilirubin levels.
• May decrease hemoglobin and WBC, neutrophil, and platelet counts.

ACTION

Drug is cytotoxic, primarily killing cells undergoing DNA synthesis and blocking progression of cells.

PHARMACOKINETICS

Duration, 1.7 to 19.4 hours.
Distribution: Protein binding is negligible.
Metabolism: Intracellularly by nucleoside kinases to the active diphosphate and triphosphate nucleosides.
Excretion: Primarily in urine.

CLINICAL CONSIDERATIONS

• Prepare and handle gemcitabine solutions with caution. Wear gloves. If the solution contacts skin or mucosa, immediately wash skin with soap and water, and flush mucosa with copious amounts of water. Dispose of empty vials, infusion bags and sets, and syringes according to facility policy for disposing of chemotherapeutic waste.

• Obtain baseline and periodic renal and hepatic function tests.

• Prolonging infusion time for longer than 60 minutes or giving drug more than once weekly has been linked to increased toxic effects.

• Expect to modify dosage according to degree of toxic reaction and extent of myelosuppression. Age, sex, and renal impairment may predispose a patient to a toxic reaction.

• Obtain patient's CBC, including differential and platelet count, before each infusion and adjust dosage if needed. Hold the infusion if the AGC is below 500/mm³ or the platelet count is below 50,000/mm³.

PATIENT TEACHING

• Instruct patient to promptly report signs and symptoms of infection (such as fever, chills, and sore throat) or of bleeding (such as easy bruising, bleeding gums, blood in urine, and tarry stools).

• Instruct patient to take temperature daily.

• Advise women of childbearing age to avoid pregnancy and breast-feeding during therapy.

gemtuzumab ozogamicin
Mylotarg

Pharmacologic class: antibody-cytotoxic antitumor antibiotic conjugate
Therapeutic class: antineoplastic
Pregnancy risk category: D

INDICATIONS & DOSAGES

➤ **Patients with CD33-positive acute myeloid leukemia in first relapse who aren't candidates for cytotoxic chemotherapy—**
Adults age 60 or older: 9 mg/m² by I.V. infusion over 2 hours q 14 days for two doses total. Premedicate with diphenhydramine 50 mg P.O. and acetaminophen 650 to 1,000 mg P.O. 1 hour before infusion.

ADMINISTRATION

Direct injection: Not recommended.
Intermittent infusion: Give over 2 hours.
Continuous infusion: Not recommended.

PREPARATION & STORAGE

Available as 20-ml vial of 5-mg powder for injection.

The drug product is light sensitive and must be protected from direct and indirect sunlight and unshielded fluorescent light during preparation and administration.

Give in 100 ml of normal saline injection. Place the 100-ml I.V. bag into an ultraviolet-protectant bag. Give drug immediately. A separate I.V. line equipped with a low-protein–binding 1.2-micron terminal filter must be used for administration. May be infused by central or peripheral line.

Admixed solution should be used immediately. Vials should be stored in refrigerator at 36° to 47° F (2° to 8° C).

Incompatibilities
None reported.

CONTRAINDICATIONS & CAUTIONS
• Contraindicated in patients hypersensitive to gemtuzumab ozogamicin or any of its components.
• Use cautiously in patients with hepatic impairment.

ADVERSE REACTIONS
CNS: *fever, asthenia, depression, dizziness, headache, insomnia, pain.*
CV: *hypertension, hypotension, tachycardia, peripheral edema.*
EENT: *epistaxis, pharyngitis, rhinitis.*
GI: *enlarged abdomen, abdominal pain, anorexia, constipation, diarrhea, dyspepsia, nausea, stomatitis, vomiting.*
GU: *hematuria,* **vaginal hemorrhage.**
Hematologic: *anemia,* HEMORRHAGE, LEUKOPENIA, NEUTROPENIA, NEUTROPENIC FEVER, THROMBOCYTOPENIA.
Hepatic: *hepatotoxicity, increased liver enzyme levels.*
Metabolic: hyperglycemia, hypokalemia, hypomagnesemia.
Musculoskeletal: *arthralgia, back pain.*
Respiratory: *increased cough, dyspnea,* **hypoxia,** *pneumonia.*
Skin: *ecchymosis, local reaction, petechiae, rash.*
Other: *herpes simplex, chills,* SEPSIS.

INTERACTIONS
None reported.

EFFECTS ON LAB TEST RESULTS
• May increase ALT, AST, LDH, and glucose levels. May decrease potassium and magnesium levels.
• May decrease hemoglobin and WBC, neutrophil, and platelet counts.

ACTION
Thought to bind to the CD33 antigen expressed on the surface of leukemic blasts in more than 80% of patients with acute myeloid leukemia.

PHARMACOKINETICS
Onset, peak, and duration of drug effects unknown.
Distribution: Unknown.
Metabolism: Unknown. Studies suggest that liver microsomal enzymes are involved.
Excretion: The elimination half-lives of total and unconjugated calicheamicin are about 45 and 100 hours, respectively, after the first dose. After the second dose, the elimination half-life of total calicheamicin is increased to 60 hours.

CLINICAL CONSIDERATIONS
• Drug should be used only under the supervision of a prescriber experienced in the use of cancer chemotherapeutic drugs.
• Gemtuzumab can produce a postinfusion symptom complex of chills, fever, hypotension, hypertension, hyperglycemia, hypoxia, and dyspnea that may occur during the first 24 hours after administration.
• Premedicate with diphenhydramine and acetaminophen. Additional doses of acetaminophen 650 to 1,000 mg P.O. can be given every 4 hours, as needed.
• Tumor lysis syndrome may occur. Provide adequate hydration and treat with allopurinol to prevent hyperuricemia.
• *Alert:* Protect drug from light during preparation and administration.
• Monitor vital signs during infusion and for 4 hours after infusion.
• Severe myelosuppression will occur in all patients given the recommended dose of this drug. Careful hematologic monitoring is required.
• Monitor electrolyte levels, hepatic function, CBC, and platelet count during therapy.

PATIENT TEACHING
• Advise patient to immediately report signs and symptoms of infection (such as fever, sore throat, and fatigue) or of bleeding (such as easy bruising, nosebleeds, bleeding gums, and tarry stools).

• Advise patient about postinfusion symptoms. Tell patient he can take acetaminophen every 4 hours as needed to relieve fever.

gentamicin sulfate
Garamycin

Pharmacologic class: aminoglycoside
Therapeutic class: antibiotic
Pregnancy risk category: D
pH: 3 to 5.5

INDICATIONS & DOSAGES
➤ **Life-threatening infections caused by susceptible organisms—**
Adults: 5 mg/kg/day I.V. in divided doses q 6 to 8 hours. Adjust dosage based on drug levels; decrease dosage to 3 mg/kg/day in divided doses as soon as possible.
➤ **Severe infections caused by susceptible organisms—**
Adults: 3 mg/kg I.V. q 8 hours.
Children age 1 and older: 2 to 2.5 mg/kg I.V. q 8 hours.
Infants and neonates: 2.5 mg/kg I.V. q 8 hours.
Neonates age 1 week and younger: 2.5 mg/kg I.V. q 12 hours.
➤ **Endocarditis prophylaxis in GI or GU procedures, usually given with ampicillin—**
Adults: 1.5 mg/kg I.V. of gentamicin with 2 g of ampicillin, given separately 30 minutes before surgery. Give P.O. ampicillin after procedure.
Children: 2 mg/kg of gentamicin and 50 mg/kg of ampicillin 30 minutes before procedure. Give P.O. ampicillin, as ordered, after procedure.
Adjust-a-dose: For patients with renal failure, calculate dose adjustments by monitoring peak and trough levels. If patient is undergoing hemodialysis, measure drug levels after each session;

dialysis may remove half of the drug. If drug levels aren't measured, give 1 to 1.7 mg/kg for adults and 2 to 2.5 mg/kg for children, depending on severity of infection.

ADMINISTRATION
Direct injection: Not recommended, but used for adults if needed. Inject drug directly into vein or an established I.V. line over 30 minutes. Don't use infusion units.
Intermittent infusion: Infuse solution, with a concentration not exceeding 1 mg/ml, over 30 minutes to 2 hours.
Continuous infusion: Not used.

PREPARATION & STORAGE
Available as a clear, colorless to slightly yellow aqueous solution in 2-ml vials containing 10 or 40 mg/ml, in 20-ml vials containing 40 mg/ml, and in 1.5- and 2-ml disposable syringes containing 40 mg/ml. Also available in 60-, 80-, and 100-ml containers with a concentration of 1 mg/ml diluted with D_5W for intermittent infusion and in 50- and 100-ml bags containing 0.4 to 2.4 mg/ml diluted with normal saline solution for intermittent infusion.
    Containers and bags have no preservatives and must be used promptly once the seal is broken. Discard unused portions. Don't use discolored or precipitated solution.
    Store solution between 36° and 86° F (15° and 30° C). Stable for 24 hours at room temperature.

Incompatibilities
Allopurinol, amphotericin B, ampicillin, cefazolin, cefepime, cefuroxime, cephapirin, certain parenteral nutrition formulations, cytarabine, dopamine, fat emulsions, furosemide, heparin, hetastarch, indomethacin sodium trihydrate, nafcillin, other I.V. drugs, propofol, ticarcillin, warfarin.

Reactions may be *common*, uncommon, *life-threatening*, or COMMON AND LIFE-THREATENING.

CONTRAINDICATIONS & CAUTIONS
• Contraindicated in those hypersensitive to aminoglycosides or previous severe toxic reaction.
• Use cautiously in those with renal impairment because of risk of nephrotoxicity, and in geriatric patients, infants, neonates, and those who have had previous aminoglycoside therapy because of increased risk of nephrotoxicity and ototoxicity.
• Use cautiously in patients with hearing impairment or history of noise exposure or ear infections because of an increased risk of further cranial nerve VIII damage.
• Use cautiously in infants with botulism and those with neuromuscular disorders, especially myasthenia gravis, because of risk of further weakness.
• Use cautiously in those with hypomagnesemia, hypocalcemia, and hypokalemia to avoid exacerbation.

ADVERSE REACTIONS
CNS: headache, *encephalopathy,* confusion, lethargy, *seizures,* dizziness, vertigo, myasthenia gravis–like syndrome, numbness, peripheral neuropathy, tingling.
CV: hypotension.
EENT: tinnitus, roaring in ears, hearing loss, blurred vision.
GI: vomiting, nausea.
GU: oliguria, proteinuria, casts.
Hematologic: anemia, eosinophilia, *leukopenia, thrombocytopenia, granulocytopenia.*
Metabolic: hyponatremia, hypocalcemia, hypokalemia, hypomagnesemia.
Musculoskeletal: twitching.
Respiratory: *apnea.*
Skin: rash, urticaria, itching.
Other: *anaphylaxis.*

INTERACTIONS
Drug-drug. *Antihistamines, phenothiazines, thioxanthenes:* May mask symptoms of ototoxicity. Monitor patient closely.

Beta-lactam antibiotics, vancomycin: May cause synergistic effect against certain organisms. Monitor therapeutic effect.
Chloramphenicol, clindamycin, tetracycline: Antagonizes bactericidal effects of gentamicin. Monitor therapeutic effect.
General anesthetics, neuromuscular blockers, opioid analgesics, parenteral polymyxin B: May potentiate neuromuscular blockade and respiratory paralysis. Use together cautiously, and monitor patient closely.
Indomethacin I.V.: Increases risk of gentamicin toxicity in neonates. Monitor patient closely.
Nephrotoxic, neurotoxic, ototoxic drugs: Increases risk of toxic reaction. Avoid using together.

EFFECTS ON LAB TEST RESULTS
• May increase BUN, creatinine, nonprotein nitrogen, sodium, ALT, AST, bilirubin, and LDH levels. May decrease calcium, potassium, and magnesium levels.
• May increase eosinophil count. May decrease hemoglobin and WBC, platelet, and granulocyte counts.

ACTION
Inhibits protein synthesis by binding to the 30S ribosomal subunit. The ribosomes separate from the messenger RNA and cells die. Drug's spectrum of action includes susceptible gram-negative aerobic bacteria and susceptible gram-positive bacteria.

PHARMACOKINETICS
Drug level peaks within 30 to 60 minutes.
Distribution: Mostly in extracellular fluid; also found in sputum and in abscess, pleural, synovial, peritoneal, and pericardial fluids. Small amounts appear in bile, inner ear, kidneys, and ocular tissue. Drug crosses the placental barrier. It's unknown if drug appears in breast milk.

Metabolism: Not metabolized.
Excretion: In urine, principally unchanged by glomerular filtration; 70% removed within 24 hours in adults. About 10% excreted within 12 hours in neonates younger than age 3 days. In adults, half-life is 2 to 3 hours; in adults with renal impairment, 24 to 60 hours; in children, 6 to 12 hours; in infants between ages 1 week and 6 months, about 3 hours; and in younger neonates, nearly 6 hours.

CLINICAL CONSIDERATIONS
● Osmolality: 116 to 320 mOsm/kg.
● Osmolarity: 284 to 308 mOsm/L.
● Collect specimens for culture and sensitivity tests before giving first dose; therapy may begin before results are available.
● Weigh patient and test renal function before therapy.
● During therapy, monitor renal function and intake and output. Keep patient well hydrated to minimize risk of toxicity and chemical irritation of renal tubules.
● Obtain peak and trough drug levels and adjust dosage, as ordered, especially in patients with renal impairment. Coordinate specimen collection times with laboratory. Peak levels above 10 mcg/ml and trough levels above 2 mcg/ml increase risk of toxic reaction.
● Beta-lactam antibiotics and cephalosporins may inactivate aminoglycosides when admixed. Ticarcillin and carbenicillin have the most significant beta-lactam effect. Separate these infusions by several hours.
● Risk of neuromuscular blockade is greatest after rapid, direct injection or if given soon after anesthesia or muscle relaxants.
● *Alert:* Drug may contain sulfites, which can cause allergic reactions in some patients.
● If overdose occurs, support respiratory and renal function. Hemodialysis or peritoneal dialysis may help remove

drug. Provide adequate hydration and monitor fluid balance, creatinine clearance, and plasma drug levels. In neonates, exchange transfusions may be used.

PATIENT TEACHING
● Ask patient if he has ringing in the ears or hearing loss. An audiogram may be ordered if hearing problems are suspected.
● Tell patient to promptly report adverse reactions.

glucagon

Pharmacologic class: antihypoglycemic
Therapeutic class: antihypoglycemic, diagnostic aid
Pregnancy risk category: B
pH: 2.5 to 3

INDICATIONS & DOSAGES
➤ **Severe hypoglycemia—**
Adults and children weighing 20 kg (44 lb) or more: 1 mg I.V. Larger doses may be needed.
Children weighing less than 20 kg: 0.5 mg I.V. or dose equivalent to 20 to 30 mcg/kg I.V. If patient doesn't respond, may repeat dose twice.
➤ **Diagnostic aid for GI, urologic, and radiologic examinations—**
Adults: 0.25 to 2 mg I.V., depending on desired onset time and duration of effect.

ADMINISTRATION
Direct injection: Give directly into vein or into I.V. tubing of a free-flowing, compatible solution over 2 to 5 minutes. Interrupt primary infusion during glucagon injection if you're using the same I.V. line.
Intermittent infusion: Not recommended.

Reactions may be *common,* uncommon, *life-threatening,* or COMMON AND LIFE-THREATENING.

Continuous infusion: Not recommended.

PREPARATION & STORAGE
Available as a powder in 1-unit vials.

Reconstitute with provided diluent, which is clear, sterile, and contains 0.2% phenol as a preservative and 1.6% glycerin. Preparation contains lactose.

Store vials at room temperature. Use reconstituted solution immediately.

Incompatibilities
Sodium chloride solution, solutions with a pH of 3 to 9.5.

CONTRAINDICATIONS & CAUTIONS
• Contraindicated in those hypersensitive to glucagon.
• Use cautiously in those who are allergic to proteins because they also may be allergic to glucagon.
• Use cautiously in those with a history of insulinoma because severe hypoglycemia may occur and in those with pheochromocytoma because of risk of a marked increase in blood pressure.

ADVERSE REACTIONS
CV: hypotension.
GI: nausea, vomiting.
Respiratory: *respiratory distress.*
Skin: urticaria.

INTERACTIONS
Drug-drug. *Anticoagulants:* May potentiate anticoagulant effects. Monitor PT and INR closely.
Epinephrine: Enhances and prolongs hyperglycemic effect. Dose may need to be adjusted. Monitor therapeutic effect.

EFFECTS ON LAB TEST RESULTS
• May decrease potassium level.

ACTION
Promotes hepatic glycogenolysis and gluconeogenesis, raising glucose levels. It also relaxes GI smooth muscle and produces a positive inotropic and chronotropic myocardial effect.

PHARMACOKINETICS
For diagnostic use, 0.25 to 0.5 mg has an onset of action within 1 minute and a duration of 9 to 17 minutes, depending on dose. When 2 mg are used, onset of action is within 1 minute and duration of effect is 22 to 25 minutes. For hypoglycemic use, onset is 5 to 30 minutes; duration, 1 to 2 hours.
Distribution: To most tissues and plasma. It's unknown if drug crosses the placental barrier or appears in breast milk.
Metabolism: Primarily in the liver and kidneys.
Excretion: By the kidneys, mostly as metabolites. Half-life, 3 to 6 minutes.

CLINICAL CONSIDERATIONS
• Potency of glucagon is expressed in USP units. One USP unit equals 1 IU and about 1 mg.
• If hypoglycemic patient doesn't respond to glucagon, give I.V. dextrose. Glucagon may fail to relieve coma because of markedly depleted hepatic stores of glycogen or irreversible brain damage caused by prolonged hypoglycemia.
• Glucagon causes a smooth, gradual termination of insulin coma. When used to terminate insulin shock therapy in a psychiatric patient, give dose 1 hour after coma induction.
• Monitor patient's blood pressure. Rapid glucagon administration can reduce blood pressure.
• Monitor glucose levels. Once hypoglycemia resolves, give carbohydrate- and protein-containing foods to prevent recurrence.
• If drug is given to patient who is taking warfarin, monitor PT and INR.
• Drug has been used as a cardiac stimulant in managing toxicity resulting from use of beta blockers, quinidine, and tricyclic antidepressants.

PATIENT TEACHING
• Teach hypoglycemic patient's family how to give glucagon in an emergency. Instruct them to use a standard insulin syringe and a 90-degree approach, rather than the usual S.C. one, to deliver a deeper injection and achieve a faster response.
• Explain use and administration of drug to patient and family.

glycopyrrolate
Robinul*

Pharmacologic class: anticholinergic
Therapeutic class: antimuscarinic, GI antispasmodic
Pregnancy risk category: B
pH: 2 to 3

INDICATIONS & DOSAGES
➤ **Adjunctive treatment of peptic ulcers—**
Adults and children age 12 and older: 0.1 to 0.2 mg I.V. q 6 to 8 hours; maximum, four doses daily.
➤ **Antiarrhythmias during surgery—**
Adults: 0.1 mg I.V., repeated q 2 to 3 minutes, p.r.n.
Children: 0.004 mg/kg I.V., maximum 0.1 mg per dose. Repeat q 2 to 3 minutes, p.r.n.
➤ **Blockage of adverse muscarinic effects of neostigmine or pyridostigmine—**
Adults and children: 0.2 mg I.V. for each 1 mg of neostigmine or 5 mg of pyridostigmine. Give in same syringe.

ADMINISTRATION
Direct injection: Inject drug at ordered rate into vein or into an I.V. line containing a free-flowing, compatible solution.

Intermittent infusion: Infuse at ordered rate or according to facility guidelines.
Continuous infusion: Not recommended.

PREPARATION & STORAGE
Available as a clear, colorless sterile solution in 1-, 2-, 5-, and 20-ml vials containing 0.2 mg/ml. Drug can be given diluted or undiluted. Having a pH of 2 to 3, drug is most stable in acidic solutions and unstable in solutions with pH exceeding 6.
For infusion, solutions containing 0.8 mg/L remain stable at room temperature for 48 hours when mixed with D_5W, dextrose 5% in half-normal saline solution, normal saline solution, or Ringer's injection. When using lactated Ringer's injection, prepare admixture immediately before use.
Store vials at room temperature.

Incompatibilities
Chloramphenicol sodium succinate, dexamethasone sodium phosphate, diazepam, dimenhydrinate, drugs with alkaline pH, methohexital, methylprednisolone sodium succinate, pentazocine lactate, pentobarbital sodium, sodium bicarbonate, thiopental.

CONTRAINDICATIONS & CAUTIONS
• Contraindicated in those hypersensitive to drug.
• Contraindicated in those with severe ulcerative colitis, toxic megacolon, obstructive GI disease, cardiospasm, paralytic ileus, or intestinal atony, because drug diminishes intestinal motility and increases risk of obstruction.
• Contraindicated in those with angle-closure glaucoma because intraocular pressure may be increased, and in those with obstructive uropathy or prostatic hyperplasia because urine retention may worsen.
• Avoid use in infants younger than age 1 month because drug contains benzyl alcohol; avoid using in patients with

acute hemorrhage, unstable CV status, or myasthenia gravis.

• Use cautiously in children, especially those younger than age 2, because of increased risk of adverse reactions. In children with brain damage, CNS effects may worsen.

• Use cautiously in geriatric patients because drug may cause paradoxical excitement, agitation, increased drowsiness, or acute glaucoma.

• Use cautiously in those with coronary artery disease, heart failure, cardiac arrhythmias, hypertension, or hyperthyroidism.

• Use cautiously in those with spastic paralysis because of possible increased response to drug; in those with Down syndrome because of risk of tachycardia; and in febrile patients and those exposed to high temperatures because of risk of hyperthermia.

• Use cautiously in those with hyperthyroidism because tachycardia may worsen; in those with hypertension because of possible aggravation; and in hepatic or renal impairment because of increased risk of adverse reactions.

• Use cautiously in those with tachyarrhythmias, heart failure, or coronary artery disease because drug blocks vagal inhibition of the SA node; and in those with esophageal reflux or hiatal hernia because drug promotes gastric retention and aggravates reflux.

• Use cautiously in those with autonomic or partial obstructive uropathy because drug may aggravate or precipitate urine retention, and in those with COPD because drug may promote mucus plug formation.

• Use cautiously in those with known or suspected GI infection because diminished GI motility prolongs retention of causative organisms and toxins.

• Use cautiously in those with gastric ulcer because delayed gastric emptying may cause antral stasis; in those with diarrhea because this sign may be an early indicator of intestinal obstruction;

and in those with xerostomia because salivary flow may be further curtailed.

• Use cautiously in those with mild or moderate ulcerative colitis because decreased GI motility may produce paralytic ileus or toxic megacolon.

ADVERSE REACTIONS
Most reactions are dose-dependent.
CNS: headache, nervousness, drowsiness, dizziness, confusion, insomnia, fever.
CV: palpitations, flushing, *bradycardia,* tachycardia.
EENT: blurred vision, mydriasis, photophobia, cycloplegia, increased intraocular pressure, dilated pupils, nasal congestion.
GI: xerostomia, nausea, vomiting, heartburn, constipation, paralytic ileus, altered taste, dysphagia.
GU: urinary hesitancy, urine retention, impotence.
Musculoskeletal: weakness.
Respiratory: *respiratory paralysis.*
Skin: urticaria, decreased sweating.
Other: *anaphylaxis,* suppression of lactation.

INTERACTIONS
Drug-drug. *Amantadine, antidyskinetics, antihistamines, antimuscarinics, phenothiazines, quinidine, tricyclic antidepressants:* Has additive anticholinergic effects. Monitor patient closely.
Atenolol: May increase effects. Dosage may need to be adjusted.
Antimyasthenics: May reduce intestinal motility. Monitor GI function.
Antipsychotics, benzodiazepines, disopyramide, glutethimide, MAO inhibitors: Increases anticholinergic effects.
Cyclopropane anesthetics: Causes ventricular arrhythmias. Use together cautiously.
Guanadrel, guanethidine, reserpine: Antagonizes inhibitory action of glycopyrrolate on gastric acid. Monitor patient closely.

Metoclopramide: Antagonizes effect on GI motility. Monitor GI function.
Opioid analgesics: Increases risk of severe constipation and additive anticholinergic effects. Monitor patient closely.
Potassium chloride, wax-matrix preparations, Slow-K: Increases severity of GI mucosal lesions. Monitor patient closely.
Urinary alkalizers, such as antacids and carbonic anhydrase inhibitors: Delays excretion. Avoid using together. Monitor patient for prolonged or toxic effects.

EFFECTS ON LAB TEST RESULTS
None reported.

ACTION
Inhibits the muscarinic effects of acetylcholine on autonomic effectors. Drug stops GI motility and gastric, nasal, bronchial, and oropharyngeal secretions; reduces tone and amplitude of ureteral and bladder contractions; decreases motility; and causes vagal stimulation.

PHARMACOKINETICS
Onset, about 1 minute; duration, 2 to 3 hours for vagal effect, up to 7 hours for salivary inhibition, and 8 to 12 hours for anticholinergic effect.
Distribution: Rapid and widespread, with high levels found in stomach and intestines. Drug crosses the placental barrier and appears in CSF in low levels. It's unknown if drug appears in breast milk.
Metabolism: In small amounts to several metabolites.
Excretion: Removed primarily as unchanged drug in feces and urine. Half-life is less than 5 minutes.

CLINICAL CONSIDERATIONS
• Osmolality: 91 mOsm/kg.
• Geriatric or debilitated patients usually require lower dosages.

• Avoid giving drug for 24 hours before gastric acid secretion tests.
• High doses over a prolonged period may cause CNS stimulation, resulting in a curarelike action.
• Monitor intake, output, vital signs, and bowel habits.
• If overdose occurs, provide symptomatic and supportive care. Physostigmine may be given I.V. to combat CNS effects and neostigmine may be given I.V. to combat peripheral anticholinergic effects, but these uses are controversial.

PATIENT TEACHING
• Encourage good oral hygiene. Provide gum or sugarless candy to help relieve dry mouth.
• Instruct patient to report signs of urinary frequency or urgency.
• Warn patient to avoid activities requiring alertness until he knows how the drug affects his CNS.

gonadorelin hydrochloride
Factrel

Pharmacologic class: hormone
Therapeutic class: fertility drug, hypogonadism diagnostic agent
Pregnancy risk category: B

INDICATIONS & DOSAGES
➤ **To induce ovulation in women with primary hypothalamic amenorrhea and to evaluate functional capacity and response of anterior pituitary gonadotropin to aid diagnosis of hypogonadism—**
Adults and children older than age 12: 100 mcg (0.1 mg) I.V. as single dose. In women, try to give early in follicular phase of the menstrual cycle.

ADMINISTRATION
Direct injection: Inject directly into vein over 3 to 5 minutes, or inject into an I.V. line containing a free-flowing, compatible solution.
Intermittent infusion: Not recommended.
Continuous infusion: Not recommended.

PREPARATION & STORAGE
Available in 100- and 500-mcg vials.
Immediately before use, add 1 ml of diluent provided by manufacturer to 100-mcg vial or 2 ml to 500-mcg vial.
Reconstituted mixture remains stable for 24 hours at room temperature. Discard unused portions.

Incompatibilities
None reported.

CONTRAINDICATIONS & CAUTIONS
● Give cautiously to patients hypersensitive to gonadorelin and to those with other drug allergies or chronic renal failure.

ADVERSE REACTIONS
CNS: headache, light-headedness, dizziness.
CV: flushing.
GI: abdominal discomfort, nausea.
Skin: local injection site reactions.
Other: *anaphylaxis.*

INTERACTIONS
Drug-drug. *Androgen, estrogen, glucocorticoids, progestin:* Affects gonadotropin secretions. Don't conduct tests during drug administration.
Digoxin, hormonal contraceptives: May depress gonadotropin level. Avoid using together.
Levodopa, spironolactone: May elevate gonadotropin level. Avoid using together.
Phenothiazines, dopamine agonists: May blunt response to gonadorelin

caused by increased prolactin. Avoid using together.

EFFECTS ON LAB TEST RESULTS
● May alter androgen, estrogen, glucocorticoid, and progestin levels.

ACTION
A synthetic hormone structurally identical to luteinizing hormone (LH)–releasing hormone. Stimulates release of LH.

PHARMACOKINETICS
Drug effect peaks at 13 to 41 minutes in men and 12 to 60 minutes in premenopausal women; duration, 3 to 5 hours.
Distribution: Unknown.
Metabolism: Unknown.
Excretion: By kidneys as metabolites. Half-life is a few minutes.

CLINICAL CONSIDERATIONS
● Obtain serum samples for LH determinations 15 minutes before gonadorelin injection, immediately before injection, and at regular intervals after injection, usually at 15, 30, 45, 60, and 120 minutes.
● Multidose administration may cause hypersensitivity and anaphylactic reactions.
● To test women, give drug early in follicular phase of the menstrual cycle, between days 1 and 7.
● A subnormal response may indicate impaired function of the pituitary, hypothalamus, or both.

PATIENT TEACHING
● Tell patient to promptly report adverse reactions.
● Explain use and administration of drug to patient and family.
● Encourage patient and family to ask questions and express concerns.

granisetron hydrochloride
Kytril

Pharmacologic class: serotonin
(5-HT$_3$) receptor antagonist
Therapeutic class: antiemetic,
antinauseant
Pregnancy risk category: B
pH: 4.7 to 7.3

INDICATIONS & DOSAGES
➤ **To prevent nausea and vomiting
from emetogenic cancer chemotherapy—**
Adults and children age 2 and older:
10 mcg/kg I.V. undiluted and given by
direct injection over 30 seconds, or diluted and infused over 5 minutes. Begin
giving within 30 minutes before starting chemotherapy.
➤ **Postoperative nausea and vomiting—**
Adults: 1 mg I.V. undiluted and given
over 30 seconds. For prevention, give
before anesthesia induction or immediately before reversal.

ADMINISTRATION
Direct injection: May be given undiluted over 30 seconds.
Intermittent injection: May be diluted
and given over 5 minutes.
Continuous injection: Not recommended.

PREPARATION & STORAGE
Available as 1-mg/ml strength in a 1-ml
single-dose vial.
    Immediately before use, dilute with
normal saline solution or D$_5$W injection to a total volume of 20 to 50 ml.
    Diluted product is stable for up to
24 hours when stored at room temperature. Don't freeze; protect from light.

Incompatibilities
Other I.V. drugs.

CONTRAINDICATIONS & CAUTIONS
• Contraindicated in patients with previous hypersensitivity to drug.
• Safety and efficacy haven't been established for children age 2 and
younger for the treatment of nausea
and vomiting caused by chemotherapy.
Also, safety and efficacy haven't been
established for children for the prevention or treatment of postoperative nausea and vomiting.

ADVERSE REACTIONS
CNS: *headache,* asthenia, somnolence,
agitation, anxiety, CNS stimulation, insomnia, fever, dizziness.
CV: hypertension, hypotension, bradycardia.
GI: *nausea, vomiting,* diarrhea, *constipation,* taste disorder, abdominal pain,
flatulence, dyspepsia.
GU: UTI, oliguria.
Hematologic: anemia, *leukocytosis,
leukopenia, thrombocytopenia.*
Respiratory: cough, sputum increase.
Skin: rash, dermatitis.
Other: *hypersensitivity reactions
(anaphylaxis, urticaria, dyspnea, hypotension), pain,* infection.

INTERACTIONS
Drug-drug. *Cytochrome P-450 inducers or inhibitors:* May alter clearance
and half-life of granisetron. Monitor
therapeutic effect and need for dosage
adjustment.
Ketoconazole: May inhibit metabolism
of granisetron. Monitor patient for toxic reaction.
Drug-herb. *Horehound:* Enhances
serotonergic effects. Discourage use together.

EFFECTS ON LAB TEST RESULTS
• May increase ALT and AST levels.
May alter fluid and electrolyte levels.
• May decrease hemoglobin and WBC
and platelet counts.

ACTION
Blocks serotonin type 3 (5-hydroxy-tryptamine type 3 [5-HT$_3$]) receptors at the chemoreceptor trigger zone in the medulla to prevent activation of the vomiting center. Peripherally, drug acts at vagal nerve terminals to prevent the muscular movement of the abdomen and diaphragm linked to vomiting.

PHARMACOKINETICS
Half-life, about 4 hours in healthy patients; 9 to 11 hours in patients with cancer; and 7½ hours in patients age 65 and older.
Distribution: About 65% protein bound; distributes freely between plasma and RBCs.
Metabolism: Hepatic.
Excretion: About 12% unchanged in urine; remainder as metabolites with 49% in urine and 34% in feces.

CLINICAL CONSIDERATIONS
• Osmolality: 290 mOsm/kg.
• Don't give solution if discolored or if particulate matter is visible.
• Although hepatic impairment may increase drug's half-life, no dosage adjustment is recommended.
• Expect geriatric patients to have a slightly higher risk of adverse CV effects, such as hypotension.
• In patients in whom nausea and vomiting must be avoided postoperatively, granisetron is recommended even if the risk of nausea and vomiting is low.

PATIENT TEACHING
• Warn patient against activities requiring alertness until effects of drug on CNS are known.
• Tell patient to report adverse reactions immediately.
• Explain use and administration of drug to patient and family.
• Encourage patient and family to ask questions and express concerns.

H

heparin sodium
Hepalean ◇ *, Hepalean-Lok ◇ *,
Heparin Leo ◇ *, Heparin Sodium*,
Hep-Lock*, Hep-Lock U/P

Pharmacologic class: anti-coagulant
Therapeutic class: anticoagulant
Pregnancy risk category: C
pH: 5 to 8

INDICATIONS & DOSAGES
Dosage depends on patient's weight, disease, hepatorenal function, and PTT. Use dosages below as a guide.
➤ **Venous thrombosis or pulmonary embolism—**
Adults: 5,000 units I.V. initially; then continuous infusion of 20,000 to 40,000 units in 1,000 ml of normal saline solution over 24 hours. Or, 10,000 units initially; then 5,000 to 10,000 units q 4 to 6 hours.
Children: 50 units/kg I.V. initially; then continuous infusion of 100 units/kg q 4 hours or 20,000 units/m^2 over 24 hours. Or, 100 units/kg initially; then 50 to 100 units/kg q 4 hours.
➤ **DIC—**
Adults: 50 to 100 units/kg I.V. q 4 hours. Stop after 4 to 8 hours if condition doesn't improve.
Children: 25 to 50 units/kg I.V. q 4 hours. Stop after 4 to 8 hours if condition doesn't improve.
➤ **I.V. flush to maintain indwelling catheter patency—**
Adults and children: 10 to 100 units I.V. after catheter use or at designated intervals.
➤ **Cardiac and vascular surgery—**
Adults: Initially, at least 150 units/kg I.V. for open-heart surgery. For procedures lasting less than 1 hour, give 300 units/kg I.V. For procedures lasting more than 1 hour, give 400 units/kg I.V.

ADMINISTRATION
Direct injection: Give diluted or undiluted drug through intermittent infusion device or into I.V. tubing containing a free-flowing, compatible solution.
Intermittent infusion: Give drug undiluted or diluted in 50 to 100 ml of normal saline solution. Using an infusion pump, give through a peripheral or central venous line over prescribed duration.
Continuous infusion: Using an infusion pump, give diluted solution over 24 hours.

PREPARATION & STORAGE
Available in 0.5- to 1-ml ampules, vials, or prefilled syringes and in 1-, 2-, 4-, 5-, 10-, and 30-ml multidose vials, ranging from 1,000 to 40,000 units/ml. Heparin flush ranges from 10 to 100 units/ml.
For infusion, dilute to achieve the prescribed concentration and volume. When diluting for continuous infusion, invert the container at least six times to ensure adequate mixing and to prevent pooling of heparin in the solution.
Compatible with normal saline solution, dextrose and Ringer's combination, dextrose 2.5% in water, D$_5$W, fructose 10%, Ringer's injection, or lactated Ringer's solution.
Store commercially available heparin preparations at room temperature. Avoid exposure to excessive heat. Don't freeze heparin solutions.

Incompatibilities

Alteplase; amikacin; amiodarone; ampicillin sodium; atracurium; chlorpromazine; ciprofloxacin; codeine phosphate; cytarabine; dacarbazine; daunorubicin; dextrose 4.3% in sodium chloride solution 0.18%; diazepam; diltiazem; dobutamine; doxorubicin; doxycycline hyclate; droperidol; ergotamine; erythromycin gluceptate or lactobionate; filgrastim; gentamicin; haloperidol lactate; hydrocortisone sodium succinate; hydroxyzine hydrochloride; idarubicin; kanamycin; labetalol; levorphanol; meperidine; methadone; methotrimeprazine; methylprednisone sodium succinate; morphine sulfate; netilmicin; nicardipine; penicillin G potassium; penicillin G sodium; pentazocine lactate; phenytoin sodium; polymyxin B sulfate; prochlorperazine edisylate; promethazine hydrochloride; quinidine gluconate; 1/6 M sodium lactate; solutions containing a phosphate buffer, sodium carbonate, or sodium oxalate; streptomycin; tobramycin sulfate; trifluoperazine; triflupromazine; vancomycin; vinblastine; warfarin.

CONTRAINDICATIONS & CAUTIONS

● Contraindicated in those hypersensitive to heparin, except in life-threatening situations.
● Contraindicated in those with severe thrombocytopenia because of possible exacerbation; in those with uncontrollable bleeding, except when caused by DIC, because of risk of severe hemorrhage; and in those with severe, uncontrolled hypertension because of increased risk of cerebral hemorrhage.
● Avoid using heparin if coagulation tests can't be performed regularly.
● Avoid using commercially available heparin sodium injections and heparin lock flush solutions that contain benzyl alcohol in neonates because these preparations have caused death in premature infants.

● Use extremely cautiously in those who are or who are at risk for hemorrhaging and in those with GI conditions (such as ulcerative colitis).
● Use extremely cautiously in pregnant women (especially in the last trimester), in women right after giving birth because of risk of maternal hemorrhage, and in women older than age 60 because they're more susceptible to hemorrhage.
● Use extremely cautiously in those with a history of allergies because of possible hypersensitivity reaction; and in those with mild hepatic disease because of increased risk of toxic reaction.
● Use cautiously in those with hypoaldosteronism because of possible hyperkalemia.
● Use cautiously in those with renal insufficiency because of decreased renal clearance.
● Use cautiously in diabetic patients undergoing medical or dental procedures because of risk of bleeding.

ADVERSE REACTIONS

CNS: fever.
GU: priapism.
Hematologic: *severe hemorrhage, acute thrombocytopenia,* new thrombus formation, white clot syndrome.
Metabolic: rebound hyperlipidemia.
Skin: delayed or transient alopecia, local irritation, erythema, urticaria.
Other: *anaphylaxis,* chills, suppressed aldosterone synthesis.

INTERACTIONS

Drug-drug. *Antihistamines, cardiac glycosides, nicotine, tetracyclines:* Diminishes anticoagulant effect. Use together cautiously.
Aspirin, dextran, dipyridamole, hydrochloroquine, NSAIDs: Impairs platelet aggregation and may increase risk of bleeding. Monitor coagulation tests.
Nitroglycerin I.V.: May diminish heparin effects. Monitor patient closely.

Oral anticoagulants: May prolong PT. Wait at least 5 hours after giving I.V. heparin before blood is drawn to measure PT.

Parenteral penicillins and cephalosporins: Alters platelet aggregation and coagulation test results. Monitor patient for bleeding.

Streptokinase, urokinase: May cause resistance to heparin anticoagulation. Monitor patient closely.

Drug-herb. *Dong quai, garlic, ginger, ginkgo, motherwort, red clover:* May increase risk of bleeding. Discourage use together.

EFFECTS ON LAB TEST RESULTS
● May increase ALT and AST levels.
● May increase INR, PT, and PTT. May decrease platelet count.
● May cause false-positive sulfobromophthalein test results.

ACTION
Potentiates the effects of antithrombin, which inhibits conversion of fibrinogen to fibrin. Inhibits the action of factors IX, X, XI, and XII. Inactivates fibrin-stabilizing factor and prevents formation of a stable fibrin clot. Drug doesn't dissolve existing clots.

PHARMACOKINETICS
Drug level steady with continuous infusion.

Distribution: In plasma with extensive protein binding. Drug doesn't cross the placental barrier or appear in breast milk.

Metabolism: Apparently partly metabolized in the liver but mainly removed from circulation by reticuloendothelial system.

Excretion: Metabolites are excreted in the urine. Half-life averages 1 or 2 hours.

CLINICAL CONSIDERATIONS
● Osmolality: 283 to 384 mOsm/kg.

● Before giving drug, inspect heparin for particles or discoloration. Discard solution if it contains precipitate or is markedly discolored. Slight discoloration doesn't affect potency.
● Observe bleeding precautions. Test all exudates for blood, regularly inspect I.V. and wound sites and the skin, and promote safety.
● Major bleeding episodes occur more frequently with intermittent infusion than with continuous infusion.
● Monitor patient for bleeding, which may occur at any site and may be difficult to detect. Frequently monitor hematocrit and check stools for occult blood to detect asymptomatic bleeding.
● Frequently monitor platelet count and coagulation test results, such as PT, PTT, INR, and activated coagulation time. Therapeutic range for PTT is 1½ to 2½ times the control value; for activated coagulation time, two or three times the control value.
● Be careful when transfusing blood collected in heparin sodium and later converted to acid-citrate-dextrose blood because coagulation may be altered.
● If signs of acute adrenal hemorrhage and insufficiency appear, stop heparin, give I.V. corticosteroids, and draw samples for cortisol levels.
● If white clot syndrome or severe thrombocytopenia occurs, promptly stop heparin and substitute a coumarin anticoagulant.
● If overdose occurs, give 1% solution of protamine sulfate by slow infusion. Don't infuse more than 50 mg in a 10-minute period. Hemodialysis doesn't remove the drug.

PATIENT TEACHING
● Teach patient signs and symptoms of bleeding.
● Tell patient to report nosebleeds, tarry stools, and blood in urine.
● Discuss the need for routine monitoring of blood studies.

Reactions may be *common*, uncommon, *life-threatening*, or COMMON AND LIFE-THREATENING.

• Advise patient to avoid taking aspirin during therapy.

hetastarch (HES)
Hespan

Pharmacologic class: amylopectin derivative
Therapeutic class: plasma volume expander
Pregnancy risk category: C
pH: 3.5 to 7

INDICATIONS & DOSAGES
Dosage reflects amount of fluid loss and hemoconcentration.
➤ **Plasma volume expansion and fluid replacement—**
Adults: 500 to 1,000 ml I.V., maximum 20 ml/kg or 1,500 ml daily I.V. In hemorrhagic shock, maximum is 20 ml/kg hourly I.V. Lower dosages are used in burns and septic shock.
Adjust-a-dose: After the initial dose, subsequent doses should be reduced by 50% to 75% for patients with creatinine clearance of less than 10 ml/minute.
➤ **Continuous flow centrifugation leukapheresis—**
Adults: 250 to 700 ml infused I.V. at a fixed ratio of 1 part hetastarch to 8 parts whole blood.

ADMINISTRATION
Direct injection: Not recommended.
Intermittent infusion: Not recommended.
Continuous infusion: Infuse at rate determined by patient's condition and therapeutic response.

PREPARATION & STORAGE
Available in 500-ml, ready-to-use, sterile, and nonpyrogenic bottles. Each bottle contains hetastarch 6% in normal saline injection but no preservative.

Store at room temperature; avoid excess heat or freezing.

Incompatibilities
Amikacin, ampicillin sodium, cefazolin, cefonicid, cefoperazone, cefotaxime, cefoxitin, gentamicin, ranitidine hydrochloride, theophylline, tobramycin sulfate.

CONTRAINDICATIONS & CAUTIONS
• Contraindicated in pregnant patients, especially during the first trimester, unless the potential benefits outweigh the risks.
• Contraindicated in those with thrombocytopenia because drug interferes with platelet function.
• Contraindicated in geriatric patients and in those with pulmonary edema, heart failure, or renal impairment because of increased risk of circulatory overload.
• Use cautiously in those with liver disease because hetastarch can raise indirect bilirubin levels and in those allergic to corn.

ADVERSE REACTIONS
CNS: headache, fever.
CV: *cardiac arrest,* circulatory overload, pulmonary edema, severe hypotension, *ventricular fibrillation.*
EENT: parotid and submaxillary gland swelling.
GI: vomiting.
Respiratory: wheezing.
Skin: pruritus.
Other: chills.

INTERACTIONS
None reported.

EFFECTS ON LAB TEST RESULTS
• May increase amylase and indirect bilirubin levels.
• May increase PT, PTT, and erythrocyte sedimentation rate. May decrease platelet count and hemoglobin.

COMPOSITION
A synthetic hydroxyethyl starch similar to human glycogen, hetastarch consists almost entirely of amylopectin. A hypertonic solution, hetastarch has a pH of 5.5, adjusted with sodium hydroxide, and an average molecular weight of 480,000 daltons. Each commercially prepared bottle contains 77 mEq of sodium and 77 mEq of chloride. The colloidal properties resemble human albumin.

CLINICAL CONSIDERATIONS
● Osmolarity: 310 mOsm/L.
● Normally a clear, pale yellow to amber; don't use the solution if it turns a turbid deep brown or contains a crystalline precipitate. Discard unused solution.
● Continuous flow centrifugation procedures, such as leukapheresis, using hetastarch up to twice weekly for 5 weeks are safe and effective.
● If patient's sodium intake is restricted, keep in mind that each bottle of hetastarch contains 77 mEq of sodium.
● Measure intake and output, and report significant changes in their ratio; also report oliguria.
● Monitor blood pressure and vital signs frequently, and check for signs of circulatory overload.
● Report dyspnea, wheezing, coughing, crackles, chest pressure, increased pulse and respirations, and elevated central venous pressure.
● Observe patient for bruising or bleeding.
● Don't give as a substitute for blood or plasma.
● Monitor CBC, total leukocyte and platelet counts, leukocyte differential count, hemoglobin, hematocrit, PT, PTT, and electrolyte, BUN, and creatinine levels.

PATIENT TEACHING
● Instruct patient to check for allergy or hypersensitivity, which can continue even after drug has been stopped.
● Explain use and administration of drug to patient and family.
● Tell patient to report adverse reactions promptly.

hydralazine hydrochloride
Apresoline

Pharmacologic class: peripheral vasodilator
Therapeutic class: antihypertensive
Pregnancy risk category: C
pH: 3.4 to 4

INDICATIONS & DOSAGES
➤ **Emergency treatment of hypertension—**
Adults: Initially, 10 to 20 mg I.V., repeated p.r.n. Usual dose is 20 to 40 mg I.V. May be increased according to response.
Children ◆ : 0.1 to 0.2 mg/kg I.V. q 4 to 6 hours p.r.n.
➤ **Pregnancy-induced hypertension—**
Adults: 5 mg initially; then 5 to 20 mg q 20 to 30 minutes p.r.n. Consider another drug if therapeutic response isn't achieved after 20 mg.

ADMINISTRATION
Direct injection: Inject undiluted drug directly into vein or as close to I.V. insertion site as possible. Give at rate of 10 mg/minute.
Intermittent infusion: Not recommended.
Continuous infusion: Not recommended.

PREPARATION & STORAGE
Available in 1-ml vials containing 20 mg/ml.

Reactions may be *common*, uncommon, *life-threatening,* or COMMON AND LIFE-THREATENING.

Avoid mixing with other drugs in same container. Avoid contact with metal syringe parts because discoloration and change in stability may result. Prepare just before use. Discard unused portion.

Drug is compatible with D_5W in lactated Ringer's, sodium lactate 1/6 M, half-normal saline, normal saline, lactated Ringer's, Ringer's injection, and Ionosol solutions.

Store vials at room temperature; don't freeze or refrigerate.

Incompatibilities
Aminophylline, ampicillin sodium, chlorothiazide, dextrose 10% in lactated Ringer's solution, dextrose 10% in normal saline solution, D_5W, diazoxide, edetate calcium disodium, ethacrynate, fructose 10% in normal saline solution, fructose 10% in water, furosemide, hydrocortisone sodium succinate, mephentermine, methohexital, nitroglycerin, phenobarbital sodium, verapamil.

CONTRAINDICATIONS & CAUTIONS
• Contraindicated in those hypersensitive to drug.
• Contraindicated in those with dissecting aortic aneurysm or rheumatic disease affecting the mitral valve because drug may worsen these conditions.
• Contraindicated in those with coronary artery disease because of possible myocardial ischemia.
• Use cautiously in those with CVA or increased intracranial pressure because cerebral ischemia may develop or worsen.
• Use cautiously and in reduced amounts in those with renal impairment.
• Drug may cause signs and symptoms similar to those of systemic lupus erythematosus (arthralgia, dermatoses, fever, splenomegaly, glomerulonephritis).

ADVERSE REACTIONS
CNS: anxiety, depression, disorientation, dizziness, *headache,* fever paresthesia.
CV: *angina,* edema, flushing, hypotension, *palpitations, tachycardia.*
EENT: nasal congestion.
GI: *anorexia,* constipation, *diarrhea, nausea,* paralytic ileus, *vomiting.*
GU: urinary difficulty.
Hematologic: *agranulocytosis,* anemia, eosinophilia, *leukopenia.*
Hepatic: lymphadenopathy, splenomegaly.
Musculoskeletal: arthralgia, muscle cramps, tremors.
Respiratory: dyspnea.
Skin: pruritus, purpura, rash, urticaria.
Other: chills, lupuslike syndrome.

INTERACTIONS
Drug-drug. *Antihypertensives, diazoxide, diuretics, MAO inhibitors:* Potentiates hypotensive effects. Monitor blood pressure closely.
Beta blockers: May increase levels of beta blockers or hydralazine. Dosage may need to be adjusted.
Epinephrine: Causes orthostatic hypotension resulting from reduced pressor response. Monitor patient closely.
Indomethacin: May antagonize hydralazine effects. Monitor patient closely.

EFFECTS ON LAB TEST RESULTS
• May decrease hemoglobin and neutrophil, WBC, granulocyte, platelet, and RBC counts.
• May yield positive response on antinuclear antibody test or Coombs' test without signs of rheumatic disorder.

ACTION
A phthalazine-derivative antihypertensive, hydralazine directly relaxes arterial smooth muscle but has little effect on the veins, thereby reducing peripheral vascular resistance. Drug also increases heart rate and cardiac output,

possibly as a compensatory response to decreased peripheral resistance.

PHARMACOKINETICS
Onset, 5 to 20 minutes; duration, 6 to 12 hours.
Distribution: Throughout tissues, with high levels in plasma, liver, kidneys, and arterial walls and low levels in heart, lungs, brain, muscle, and fat; 85% of drug binds to proteins. Drug crosses the placental barrier, and small amounts appear in breast milk.
Metabolism: In the liver and GI mucosa, through acetylation, hydroxylation, and conjugation. Metabolites have no therapeutic effects.
Excretion: Rapidly removed in urine, primarily as metabolites.

CLINICAL CONSIDERATIONS
● Check patient's vital signs every 5 to 10 minutes for 1 hour, every hour for the next 2 hours, and then every 4 hours after injection. Continuously monitor ECG.
● Monitor patient's CBC, lupus erythematosus cell preparation, and antinuclear antibody titer before therapy and at regular intervals during prolonged use to detect lupuslike syndrome. Stop drug if this syndrome develops.
● Withdraw drug gradually in patients with marked reduction in blood pressure to avoid rebound hypertension.
● Control sodium retention and weight gain with a thiazide diuretic.
● Slow acetylation increases risk of adverse reactions.
● Use of a beta blocker and diuretic may prevent myocardial ischemia in patients with coronary artery disease who must receive hydralazine.
● Headache and tachycardia are common 2 to 4 hours after first dose; they can be minimized by starting with a small dose of hydralazine and gradually increasing it.
● Stop drug if blood dyscrasias occur.

● Signs and symptoms of overdose include arrhythmias, headache, hypotension, shock, and tachycardia. If overdose occurs, give volume expanders to support blood pressure; if a vasopressor is needed, select one that doesn't aggravate arrhythmias. Digitalize patient and monitor renal function, as needed. Tachycardia responds to beta blockers.

PATIENT TEACHING
● Instruct patient to report headache or chest pain.
● Instruct patient to change position slowly to minimize dizziness.

hydrocortisone sodium phosphate
Hydrocortone Phosphate

hydrocortisone sodium succinate
A-Hydrocort*, Solu-Cortef*

Pharmacologic class: glucocorticoid, mineralocorticoid
Therapeutic class: adrenocorticoid replacement
Pregnancy risk category: C
pH: 7.5 to 8.5

INDICATIONS & DOSAGES
➤ **Severe inflammation, adrenal insufficiency—**
Adults: Depending on disease, 15 to 240 mg I.V. of hydrocortisone sodium phosphate daily; or 100 to 500 mg I.V. of hydrocortisone sodium succinate initially, repeated q 2 to 6 hours p.r.n.
Children: 0.16 to 1 mg/kg I.V. or 6 to 30 mg/m² I.V. of hydrocortisone sodium succinate given one to two times daily. High-dose therapy should be stopped within 48 to 72 hours.
➤ **Shock—**
Adults: Initially, 50 mg/kg I.V. of hydrocortisone sodium succinate; repeat

in 4 hours or q 24 hours. Or, 0.5 to 2 g I.V. initially; repeat q 2 to 6 hours p.r.n.

ADMINISTRATION
Direct injection: Inject directly into vein or into an I.V. line containing a free-flowing, compatible solution to a concentration of 0.1 to 1 mg/ml over 30 seconds to several minutes.
Intermittent infusion: Give diluted solution over prescribed duration.
Continuous infusion: Infuse diluted solution over 24 hours.

PREPARATION & STORAGE
Hydrocortisone sodium phosphate is available in 2- and 10-ml multidose vials containing 50 mg/ml. Hydrocortisone sodium succinate is available in 100-, 250-, and 500-mg and 1-g vials.

Reconstitute hydrocortisone sodium succinate with no more than 2 ml of bacteriostatic water for injection or bacteriostatic normal saline injection. Larger containers should be diluted with D_5W, normal saline solution, or dextrose 5% in normal saline solution to yield 0.1 to 1 mg/ml.

Store solutions at 77° F (25° C) or below for up to 3 days. Discard thereafter or if solutions aren't clear. Protect from light.

Incompatibilities
Hydrocortisone sodium phosphate: doxapram, mitoxantrone, sargramostim.

Hydrocortisone sodium succinate: amobarbital; ampicillin sodium; bleomycin; ciprofloxacin, colistimethate; cytarabine; dacarbazine; diazepam; dimenhydrinate; ephedrine; ergotamine; furosemide; heparin sodium; hydralazine; idarubicin; Ionosol B with invert sugar 10%; kanamycin; methylprednisolone sodium succinate; midazolam; nafcillin; pentobarbital sodium; phenobarbital sodium; phenytoin; prochlorperazine edisylate; promethazine

hydrochloride; sargramostim; vancomycin; vitamin B complex with C.

CONTRAINDICATIONS & CAUTIONS
• Don't use in patients with left ventricular free wall rupture after a recent MI.
• Use cautiously in those with hypothyroidism or cirrhosis because an exaggerated drug response may occur.
• Use cautiously in those with seizure disorders because of increased risk of seizures, in those with renal insufficiency because of increased risk of edema, in those with osteoporosis because of possible exacerbation, and in those with history of tuberculosis because of possible disease reactivation.
• Use cautiously in those with recent intestinal anastomosis and in those with diverticulitis or nonspecific ulcerative colitis if patient is at risk for perforation, abscess, or other pyogenic infection because drug may mask infection.
• Use cautiously in those with uncontrolled viral or bacterial infections because drug may mask infection and increase susceptibility.
• Use cautiously in children because of possible bone growth retardation, pancreatitis and pancreatic destruction, and increased intracranial pressure, resulting in papilledema, oculomotor or abducens nerve paralysis, vision loss, and headache.
• Use cautiously in those with ocular herpes simplex because of possible corneal perforation.
• Drug may exacerbate fungal infections.
• Drug may activate latent amebiasis and may be harmful to those with chronic active hepatitis who test positive for hepatitis B surface antigen.
• Prolonged use may produce posterior subcapsular cataracts or glaucoma.

ADVERSE REACTIONS

CNS: increased intracranial pressure, insomnia, *seizures*, steroid psychosis, malaise, fatigue, syncopal episodes.
CV: *CV collapse after rapid injection of large doses, heart failure,* hypertension, hypotension, thrombophlebitis.
GI: distention, esophagitis, increased appetite, nausea, *pancreatitis*, peptic ulceration, vomiting.
GU: postmenopausal bleeding, menstrual irregularity, increased or decreased motility and number of sperm.
Hematologic: leukocytosis.
Metabolic: hyperglycemia, hypocalcemia, hypokalemia, metabolic alkalosis, growth suppression, sodium and fluid retention, weight gain.
Musculoskeletal: aseptic necrosis of femoral or humeral heads, myopathy, osteoporosis, spontaneous fractures, weakness.
Skin: impaired wound healing, increased petechiae and ecchymoses, skin thinning.
Other: *adrenal insufficiency with increased stress or abrupt withdrawal, anaphylaxis,* cushingoid appearance, hirsutism.

INTERACTIONS

Drug-drug. *Amphotericin B, carbonic anhydrase inhibitors, potassium-wasting drugs:* May increase potassium loss. Monitor potassium level.
Anticholinesterases: Causes severe weakness in myasthenia gravis patients. Avoid using together.
Anticoagulants: May increase or decrease anticoagulant effects. Monitor patient closely.
Antidiabetics: May cause hyperglycemia. Adjust dosage of antidiabetic.
Cardiac glycosides: Increases risk of toxic reaction or arrhythmias. Use together cautiously.
Drugs that contain sodium: May cause hypernatremia. Avoid using together.
Drugs that induce hepatic microsomal enzymes (barbiturates, phenytoin, rifampin, ephedrine): May increase hydrocortisone metabolism. Monitor response.
Estrogens, estrogen-containing hormonal contraceptives: Enhances therapeutic and toxic effects of hydrocortisone. Monitor patient for toxic reaction.
Immunosuppressants: Increases risk of infection, lymphomas, and lymphoproliferative disorders. Monitor patient closely.
Isoniazid: Decreases isoniazid levels. Monitor patient closely.
Nondepolarizing neuromuscular blockers: May affect neuromuscular blockade. Use together cautiously.
NSAIDs, ulcerogenic drugs: Increases risk of GI ulcers. Avoid using together. Monitor patient closely.
Toxoids, vaccines: Diminishes response and may cause neurologic complications. Avoid using together.
Drug-food. *Foods that contain sodium:* May cause hypernatremia. Discourage use together.
Drug-lifestyle. *Alcohol use:* Increases risk of GI ulcers. Discourage use together.

EFFECTS ON LAB TEST RESULTS

● May increase glucose and cholesterol levels. May decrease T_3, T_4, potassium, and calcium levels.
● May increase WBC count.
● May falsely suppress skin test reaction and decrease ^{131}I uptake and protein-bound iodine levels in thyroid function tests. May cause false-negative results in the nitroblue tetrazolium test for systemic bacterial infections. May alter gonadorelin test results.

ACTION

A naturally occurring corticosteroid that affects virtually all body systems. Decreases inflammation by stabilizing leukocyte lysosomal membranes and suppresses pituitary release of corticotropin, which causes the adrenal cortex to stop secreting corticosteroids.

PHARMACOKINETICS
Onset, rapid; duration, varies with dosage and duration of therapy.
Distribution: Rapidly dispersed to muscles, liver, skin, intestines, and kidneys. Reversibly bound to corticosteroid-binding albumin. Drug appears in breast milk.
Metabolism: Metabolized in the liver to inactive compounds; also in the kidneys and in most tissues.
Excretion: Inactive metabolites removed by kidneys as glucuronides and sulfates. Small amounts of unmetabolized drug are excreted in urine and negligible amounts in bile.

CLINICAL CONSIDERATIONS
• Osmolality: 533 mOsm/kg.
• Before long-term therapy, evaluate baseline ECGs, blood pressure, chest and spinal X-rays, glucose tolerance tests, potassium level, and hypothalamic and pituitary function.
• Diabetic patients may need their antidiabetic dosage adjusted because of hydrocortisone's hyperglycemic effects.
• Increased protein intake may be needed to keep pace with drug-induced protein catabolism.
• Give phenothiazine or lithium for depression or psychotic behavior.
• Don't stop high-dose therapy abruptly.
• Monitor patient for signs of adrenal insufficiency. Adrenal recovery may occur within 1 week after short-term therapy.
• *Alert:* Hydrocortone Phosphate contains sulfites.

PATIENT TEACHING
• Instruct patient to report signs of infection for up to 12 months after therapy.
• Tell patient to avoid exposure to chickenpox or measles and to notify prescriber immediately if exposure occurs.
• Tell diabetic patient that drug may increase glucose levels.
• Tell patient to notify prescriber if increased appetite, indigestion, nervousness, or trouble sleeping continues or is bothersome.

hydromorphone hydrochloride
Dilaudid, Dilaudid-HP, Dilaudid-HP-Plus ◇, Dilaudid-XP ◇

Pharmacologic class: opioid
Therapeutic class: analgesic
Pregnancy risk category: C
Controlled substance schedule: II
pH: 4 to 5.5

INDICATIONS & DOSAGES
➤ **Moderate to severe pain—**
Adults: 1 or 2 mg S.C. or I.M. q 4 to 6 hours p.r.n. for moderate pain; 3 to 4 mg q 4 to 6 hours for severe pain. May be given by slow I.V. injection over 2 to 5 minutes.

ADMINISTRATION
Giving drug rapidly has been linked to anaphylaxis, respiratory failure, and cardiac arrest.
Direct injection: Inject directly into a vein or into an I.V. line containing a free-flowing, compatible solution over 2 to 5 minutes, especially if 10-mg/ml preparation is used.
Intermittent infusion: Give diluted drug over prescribed duration.
Continuous infusion: Using an infusion pump, give at the ordered dilution and rate.

PREPARATION & STORAGE
Available in preservative-containing multidose vials and syringes in concentrations of 1, 2, 4, and 10 mg/ml. In Canada, also available in vials as

20 mg/ml and 50 mg/ml. Also available in preservative-free ampules containing 2 mg/ml.

Dilution isn't needed, but most common I.V. solutions may be used as diluents.

Store between 59° and 86° F (15° and 30° C). Protect from freezing and light. Don't refrigerate because of possible precipitation or crystallization. Slight yellowish tint may develop but doesn't indicate loss of potency.

Incompatibilities
Alkalies, ampicillin sodium, bromides, cefazolin, dexamethasone, diazepam, gallium nitrate, iodides, minocycline, phenobarbital sodium, phenytoin sodium, prochlorperazine edisylate, sargramostim, sodium bicarbonate, sodium phosphate, thiopental.

CONTRAINDICATIONS & CAUTIONS
• Contraindicated in those hypersensitive to drug.
• Contraindicated in those with diarrhea caused by poisons or toxins because drug may slow GI motility, decreasing elimination of toxins.
• Contraindicated in those with acute respiratory depression, acute bronchial asthma, status asthmaticus, or upper airway obstruction because of possible exacerbation.
• Avoid use in obstetric analgesia.
• Use only if essential in patients with head injury and increased intracranial pressure (ICP) because drug can mask changes in level of consciousness and further raise ICP.
• Use cautiously in those with respiratory impairment because of reduced respiratory drive and increased airway resistance, in those who have recently undergone GI surgery because of slowed GI motility, and in those with hepatic or renal impairment because of slowed drug clearance.
• Use cautiously in those with gallbladder disease because of drug-induced biliary contraction, in those with severe inflammatory bowel disease because of increased risk of toxic megacolon, in geriatric patients and in those with hypothyroidism or Addison's disease because of risk of respiratory depression and prolonged CNS depression, and in those with a history of drug dependence or emotional instability because of risk of dependence.
• Use cautiously in those with hypovolemia because of possible potentiated hypotension and in those with arrhythmias or history of seizures because of possible exacerbation.
• Use cautiously in those with acute abdominal conditions because assessment findings may be unreliable.
• Use cautiously in those with prostatic hyperplasia or urethral stricture and in those who have recently undergone urinary tract surgery because urine retention can occur.

ADVERSE REACTIONS
CNS: agitation, anxiety, confusion, *clouded sensorium,* **coma,** dependence, dizziness, dysphoria, fear, headache, insomnia, lethargy, mood changes, *sedation,* **seizures,** somnolence, tremors.
CV: **bradycardia, cardiopulmonary arrest,** flushing, chest-wall rigidity, **circulatory depression,** edema, hypertension, *hypotension,* palpitations, **shock,** syncope, tachycardia.
EENT: nystagmus, miosis.
GI: anorexia, biliary spasms, *constipation,* dry mouth, ileus, *nausea, vomiting.*
Respiratory: **bronchospasm, respiratory depression.**
Skin: pruritus, rash.

INTERACTIONS
Drug-drug. *Antidiarrheals, antiperistaltics:* Increases risk of severe constipation and CNS depression. Avoid using together.

Antihypertensives: Increases risk of orthostatic hypotension. Monitor patient closely.

Antimuscarinics: Increases risk of severe constipation, paralytic ileus, and urine retention. Monitor patient closely.

Buprenorphine: May reduce therapeutic effects of hydromorphone if given before it; also, depending on dose, may reverse or potentiate respiratory depression and cause or suppress narcotic withdrawal symptoms. Monitor patient closely.

Cimetidine: May cause CNS toxicity, leading to confusion, disorientation, respiratory depression, apnea, and seizures. Avoid using together.

CNS depressants, hydroxyzine, MAO inhibitors, opioid agonists: May potentiate CNS, respiratory, and hypotensive effects. Avoid using together.

Diuretics: Increases risk of orthostatic hypotension; antagonizes effects in heart failure. Use together with caution.

Metoclopramide: Slows GI motility. Monitor GI status.

Naloxone, naltrexone: Antagonizes analgesic, CNS, and respiratory depressant effects of hydromorphone. Monitor patient closely.

Neuromuscular blockers: May deepen respiratory depression. Avoid using together.

EFFECTS ON LAB TEST RESULTS
● May increase amylase and lipase levels.

ACTION
Binds with opiate receptors throughout the CNS, altering the perception of pain and the emotional response to it.

PHARMACOKINETICS
Onset, 15 to 30 minutes; duration, 4 to 5 hours.
Distribution: Throughout tissues, with highest levels in skeletal muscle, kidneys, liver, intestines, lungs, spleen,

and brain. Drug readily crosses the placental barrier.
Metabolism: Chiefly in the liver but also in the CNS, kidneys, lungs, and placenta to form metabolites.
Excretion: In urine, primarily as unchanged drug. Small amounts of drug and metabolites appear in feces.

CLINICAL CONSIDERATIONS
● Check access site before giving drug by I.V. push. Local tissue irritation can occur with infiltration.
● Give smallest effective dose to reduce tolerance and physical dependence. However, high doses may be needed for severe chronic or cancer pain. Adjust dosage based on patient response and severity of pain.
● Give drug with patient lying down to minimize hypotensive effects.
● Give concentrate (10 mg/ml) only to patients tolerant of opioid agonists who are receiving high doses.
● Monitor respiratory status frequently for at least 1 hour after dose. Keep resuscitation equipment and naloxone readily available. If respiratory rate drops below 8 breaths/minute, arouse patient to stimulate breathing. Notify prescriber provider; naloxone or respiratory support may be ordered.
● Assess bowel function. A stool softener may be indicated.
● Duration of effects lengthens with repeated doses because of drug accumulation.
● Patient may develop habituation and psychological dependence with long-term use.
● If needed, reduce dosage in geriatric patients, in patients with renal or hepatic impairment, and in those receiving other opioid analgesics.
● Atropine may control bradycardia or other cholinergic effects.
● Monitor shock patient because overdose may occur when circulation is restored.

• If overdose occurs, maintain airway patency and provide respiratory support. Give 0.4 mg of naloxone by I.V. push, as needed, to reverse respiratory depression. Give I.V. fluids and vasopressors to maintain blood pressure.

PATIENT TEACHING
• After giving drug, tell patient to get up slowly to reduce dizziness and avoid fainting.
• Instruct patient to lie down if dizziness, nausea, or vomiting occurs.
• Because drug can cause drowsiness, advise patient to avoid activities that require alertness.
• Advise patient to avoid using alcoholic beverages or other CNS depressants while receiving drug.

I

ibritumomab tiuxetan
Zevalin

Pharmacologic class: monoclonal antibody
Therapeutic class: antineoplastic
Pregnancy risk category: D
pH: 7.1

INDICATIONS & DOSAGES
➤ **Relapsed or refractory low-grade, follicular, or transformed B-cell non-Hodgkin's lymphoma, including patients with rituximab-refractory follicular non-Hodgkin's lymphoma—**
Adults: On day 1, give 250 mg/m^2 of rituximab by I.V. infusion; then 5 mCi (1.6 mg total antibody dose) of In-111 ibritumomab I.V. push over 10 minutes within 4 hours of completing rituximab. On days 7 to 9, give 250 mg/m^2 of rituximab by I.V. infusion; then 0.4 mCi/kg of Y-90 ibritumomab I.V. push over 10 minutes within 4 hours of completing rituximab. Maximum dose of Y-90 ibritumomab is 32 mCi (1,184 MBq).
Adjust-a-dose: In patients with mild thrombocytopenia (baseline platelet count between 100,000 and 149,000 cells/mm^3), reduce the Y-90 ibritumomab dose to 0.3 mCi/kg (11.1 MBq/kg).

ADMINISTRATION
Direct injection: Not recommended.
Intermittent infusion: When giving ibritumomab, give I.V. bolus over 10 minutes within 4 hours of rituximab infusion.

Continuous infusion: When giving rituximab, consider giving acetaminophen and diphenhydramine before each infusion, at an initial rate of 50 mg/hour. If hypersensitivity or infusion-related events don't occur, increase the infusion rate in 50-mg/hour increments every 30 minutes to a maximum of 400 mg/hour. If hypersensitivity or an infusion-related event does occur, slow or stop the infusion temporarily. The infusion can continue at half the previous rate when symptoms improve. Give second infusion at an initial rate of 100 mg/hour (50 mg/hour if infusion-related events occurred during first administration) and increase in 100-mg/hour increments every 30 minutes to a maximum of 400 mg/hour as tolerated.

PREPARATION & STORAGE
Available as a 3.2-mg solution in kits containing four vials used to produce either a single dose of In-111 or Y-90 for radiolabeling.
  Dose should be measured by a suitable radioactivity calibration system immediately before administration. Follow institutional guidelines for handling and disposing of radioactive materials. The vial contains a protein solution that may develop translucent particles, which will be removed by filtration before administration. Follow manufacturer's directions for radiolabeling procedure.
  Place the reaction vial in a dispensing shield (prewarmed to room temperature). To avoid buildup of excessive pressure, withdraw 10 ml of air. Determine the amount of each component needed. With a sterile 1-ml syringe,

---

withdraw the calculated volume of 50 mM of sodium acetate and empty into the reaction vial. Coat the inner surface of the reaction vial by gently rolling or inverting the vial. Don't shake, to avoid foaming.

Depending on which radiolabeling the patient receives, transfer 5.5 mCi of In-111 chloride or 40 mCi of Y-90 chloride to the reaction vial with a sterile syringe. Mix the two solutions and coat the entire surface of the vial by gentle inversion or rolling. Allow the reaction of In-111 to occur at room temperature for 30 minutes; Y-90 for 5 minutes.

Then, using a sterile 10-ml syringe, transfer the calculated volume of formulation buffer down the side of the reaction vial and coat the entire vial by gentle inversion or rolling. If necessary, withdraw an equal volume of air to normalize air pressure. Label the reaction vial and shielded reaction vial container.

Using a sterile 10-ml syringe, withdraw the calculated volume from the reaction vial and assay the syringe and its contents in a dose calibrator. In-111 must be given within 12 hours and Y-90 within 8 hours of radiolabeling. The prescribed, measured, and given dose of Y-90 ibritumomab mustn't exceed the absolute maximum allowable dose of 32 mCi (1,184 MBq), regardless of the patient's body weight.

Store drug at 35° to 46° F (2° to 8° C) until used.

Incompatibilities
Other I.V. drugs.

CONTRAINDICATIONS & CAUTIONS
• Contraindicated in patients hypersensitive to murine proteins or to any component of this product, including rituximab, yttrium chloride, and indium chloride.

• Don't use in patients with 25% or more lymphoma marrow involvement, impaired bone-marrow reserve, or a history of failed stem-cell collection.
• Don't treat patients with platelet count less than 100,000 cells/mm^3.
• Don't give Y-90 ibritumomab to patients with altered biodistribution of In-111 ibritumomab.
• Use cautiously in patients with evidence of human antimouse antibodies (HAMA) and patients receiving live-viral vaccines.
• It's unknown if the drug appears in breast milk. Because human IgG appears in breast milk, women should be advised to stop breast-feeding.

ADVERSE REACTIONS
CNS: *asthenia, headache, dizziness,* insomnia, anxiety, *fever, pain, **encephalopathy,** subdural hematoma.*
CV: hypotension, flushing, peripheral edema, tachycardia, ***pulmonary embolism, pulmonary edema.***
EENT: *throat irritation,* epistaxis, rhinitis.
GI: *abdominal pain, nausea, vomiting, diarrhea,* anorexia, abdominal enlargement, constipation, dyspepsia, ***GI hemorrhage,*** melena, *hematemesis.*
GU: ***vaginal hemorrhage.***
Hematologic: ***thrombocytopenia, neutropenia,*** anemia, ***pancytopenia, cytopenia, hemorrhage.***
Musculoskeletal: back pain, arthralgia, myalgia, arthritis.
Respiratory: *dyspnea, increased cough, **bronchospasm, apnea.***
Skin: *pruritus,* rash, ecchymosis, urticaria, petechiae, sweats.
Other: *infection, chills,* allergic reaction, tumor pain, ***angioedema, secondary malignancies.***

INTERACTIONS
Drug-drug. *Drugs that interfere with platelet function or coagulation:* May increase the risk of bleeding. Use to-

gether cautiously, and monitor patient closely for thrombocytopenia.

EFFECTS ON LAB TEST RESULTS
• May decrease hemoglobin, hematocrit, and neutrophil, RBC, WBC, and platelet counts.

ACTION
Ibritumomab binds to the CD20 antigen on B-lymphocytes and induces apoptosis in CD20+ B-cell lines in vitro. The chelate tiuxetan, which tightly bonds In-111 or Y-90, is covalently linked to the amino groups of exposed lysines and arginines contained within the antibody. The beta emission from Y-90 induces cellular damage by the formation of free radicals in the target and neighboring cells.

PHARMACOKINETICS
Onset, peak, and duration of drug effects unknown.
Distribution: Binds to lymphoid cells of the bone marrow, lymph nodes, thymus, spleen, lymphoid follicles of the tonsils, and lymphoid nodules of the large and small intestines.
Metabolism: Unknown.
Excretion: Y-90 mean half-life, 30 hours; Y-90 physical radiochemical half-life, 64 hours.

CLINICAL CONSIDERATIONS
• Only trained health care providers experienced in the safe use of radionuclides should give drug.
• Changing the ratio of any reactants in the radiolabeling process may adversely impact therapeutic results.
• *Alert:* The drug regimen may cause severe and potentially fatal infusion reactions, which typically occur 30 minutes to 1 hour after the start of the first rituximab infusion. Signs and symptoms may include hypotension, angioedema, hypoxia, or bronchospasm and may require interruption of rituximab,

In-111 ibritumomab, and Y-90 ibritumomab. Monitor patient carefully and provide emergency treatment as needed.
• Drugs to treat hypersensitivity reactions should always be available during administration.
• The dose of rituximab is lower when used as part of the ibritumomab regimen than when used alone.
• In-111 and Y-90 shouldn't be used without rituximab.
• The product contains albumin and carries a risk for transmission of viral diseases. A risk for transmission of Creutzfeldt-Jakob disease is considered extremely remote.
• Ibritumomab therapeutic regimen is intended as a single course of treatment.
• The biodistribution of In-111 ibritumomab should be assessed at 2 to 24 hours and 48 to 72 hours after injection.
• Monitor CBC and platelet counts weekly after ibritumomab treatment, and continue until levels recover. Monitor these counts more frequently in patients who develop severe cytopenia.
• Monitor patient for cytopenias and their complications for up to 3 months after drug regimen.

PATIENT TEACHING
• Teach patient side effects of the drug.
• Advise patient to report any episodes of bleeding, fever, or signs and symptoms of infection.
• Explain to patient the importance of monitoring and follow-up for 3 months after treatment.
• Review standard radiation precautions for handling blood or body fluids.

ibutilide fumarate
Corvert

Pharmacologic class: methanesul-
fonanilide derivative
Therapeutic class: Class III antiarrhythmic
Pregnancy risk category: C
pH: 4.6

INDICATIONS & DOSAGES
➤ **Rapid conversion of recent-onset
atrial fibrillation or atrial flutter to
sinus rhythm—**
*Adults weighing 60 kg (132 lb) or
more:* 1 mg I.V. over 10 minutes.
Adults weighing less than 60 kg:
0.1 ml/kg (0.01 mg/kg) I.V. over 10
minutes. Stop infusion if arrhythmia
stops or if patient develops ventricular
tachycardia or marked prolongation of
QT or QTc interval. If arrhythmia
hasn't stopped 10 minutes after infusion ends, prepare to give another 10-
minute infusion of equal strength.

ADMINISTRATION
Direct injection: Undiluted solution
may be injected over 10 minutes.
Intermittent infusion: 50-ml infusion
bag over 10 minutes.
Continuous infusion: Not recommended.

PREPARATION & STORAGE
Available as single-dose 10-ml clear
glass vials (0.1 mg/ml).
    Give undiluted or diluted in 50 ml of
diluent, which forms admixture of
about 0.017 mg/ml. Ibutilide may be
diluted with normal saline injection or
D₅W injection before infusion. May be
used with polyvinyl chloride plastic
bags or polyolefin bags. Inspect for
particulate matter and discoloration before administration.

Store vials at controlled room temperature of 68° to 77° F (20° to 25° C).
Store vials in carton until used. After
dilution, product is stable for 24 hours
at room temperature (59° to 86° F [15°
to 30° C]) and 48 hours refrigerated
(36° to 46° F [2° to 8° C]).

Incompatibilities
None reported.

CONTRAINDICATIONS & CAUTIONS
• Contraindicated in those hypersensitive to the drug or its components.
• Drug isn't recommended for patients
with history of polymorphic ventricular
tachycardia.
• Use cautiously in those with hepatic
or renal dysfunction.

ADVERSE REACTIONS
CNS: headache.
CV: *AV block, bradycardia,* bundle-
branch block, hypotension, nonsustained monomorphic and polymorphic
ventricular tachycardia, palpitations,
prolonged QT interval, *sustained polymorphic ventricular tachycardia,
tachycardia,* ventricular extrasystoles.
GI: nausea.

INTERACTIONS
Drug-drug. *Class Ia and class III antiarrhythmics:* Prolongs refractoriness.
Avoid using within 4 hours after infusion.
Digoxin: Arrhythmias may mask the
cardiotoxicity of excessive digoxin levels. Use cautiously together, especially
when digoxin level is above therapeutic
levels.
*Drugs that prolong the QT interval,
phenothiazine, tricyclic and tetracyclic
antidepressants, certain antihistamines
such as H₁-receptor antagonists:* Increases potential for arrhythmias. Monitor patient closely.

EFFECTS ON LAB TEST RESULTS
None reported.

ACTION
Prolongs action potential and increases atrial and ventricular refractoriness.

PHARMACOKINETICS
May convert arrhythmia 30 to 90 minutes after infusion starts, with most patients in normal sinus rhythm 24 hours later.
Distribution: Minimal protein binding.
Metabolism: By kidneys. Also undergoes substantial hepatic clearance.
Elimination: 82% excreted in urine, remainder in feces. Elimination half-life ranges from 2 to 12 hours.

CLINICAL CONSIDERATIONS
• Only skilled health care providers should give the drug.
• Make sure that a cardiac monitor, intracardiac pacing, a cardioverter or defibrillator, and a drug for sustained ventricular tachycardia are available.
• Patients with atrial fibrillation lasting more than 2 to 3 days must be adequately anticoagulated, usually for at least 2 weeks.
• Patients with abnormal liver function should be monitored more often than the 4-hour interval usually recommended.
• To reduce potential for proarrhythmia, correct hypokalemia and hypomagnesemia before therapy.
• Monitor ECG continuously during administration and for at least 4 hours afterward or until QTc returns to baseline. Drug can worsen ventricular arrhythmias. Longer monitoring is needed if ECG shows arrhythmia.

PATIENT TEACHING
• Tell patient to promptly report adverse reactions.
• Instruct patient to report discomfort at the injection site.
• Encourage women not to breast-feed during therapy.

idarubicin
Idamycin, Idamycin PFS

Pharmacologic class: antineoplastic antibiotic
Therapeutic class: antineoplastic
Pregnancy risk category: D
pH: 5 to 7

INDICATIONS & DOSAGES
➤ **Combined with other antileukemic drugs to treat acute myeloid leukemia, including French-American-British classes M1 through M7—**
Adults: 12 mg/m² daily for 3 days by slow (10 to 15 minutes) I.V. injection with cytarabine, which may be given as continuous infusion of 100 mg/m² daily for 7 days or as 25-mg/m² bolus followed by continuous infusion of 200 mg/m² daily for 5 days. A second course may be given if needed.
Adjust-a-dose: If patient develops severe mucositis, delay administration until recovery is complete and reduce dose by 25%.

Reduce dosage in patients with hepatic and renal impairment. Don't give idarubicin if bilirubin level is more than 5 mg/dl.

ADMINISTRATION
Direct injection: Give over 10 to 15 minutes into the tubing of a free-flowing I.V. solution of dextrose 5% injection or normal saline solution. The tubing should be attached to a winged-tip needle inserted into a large vein.
Intermittent infusion: Not recommended.
Continuous infusion: Not recommended.

PREPARATION & STORAGE
Available as a powder for injection or as a preservative-free injection in 5-, 10-, and 20-mg single-dose vials.

Reconstitute powder for injection with normal saline injection without preservatives. Add 5 ml to 5-mg vial, 10 ml to 10-mg vial, or 20 ml to 20-mg vial to yield 1 mg/ml. Don't use bacteriostatic saline solution. Vial is under negative pressure. Insert needle carefully, and avoid inhaling any aerosol.

Drug is compatible in dextrose 5% in normal saline solution, D_5W, lactated Ringer's solution, and normal saline solution.

Store vials at room temperature (59° to 86° F [15° to 30° C]) and protect from light. Reconstituted solutions are stable for 72 hours at room temperature and for 7 days if refrigerated. Refrigerate Idamycin PFS and protect from light. Discard unused solutions according to guidelines for disposal of chemotherapeutic drugs.

Incompatibilities
Acyclovir sodium, alkaline solutions, allopurinol, ampicillin sodium with sulbactam, cefazolin, cefepime, ceftazidime, clindamycin phosphate, dexamethasone sodium phosphate, etoposide, furosemide, gentamicin, heparin, hydrocortisone sodium succinate, lorazepam, meperidine, methotrexate sodium, piperacillin sodium with tazobactam, sodium bicarbonate, teniposide, vancomycin, vincristine.

CONTRAINDICATIONS & CAUTIONS
• Don't use drug in those with severe infection, severe myelosuppression, cardiac disease, or severe hemorrhagic conditions.
• Don't use drug if bilirubin level exceeds 5 mg/dl.
• Use cautiously and adjust dosage in patients with hepatic or renal impairment.
• Lysis of leukemic cells may cause hyperuricemia. Monitor patient closely and take appropriate measures to prevent hyperuricemia.

ADVERSE REACTIONS
CNS: *fever, headache, mental status changes, seizures.*
CV: *arrhythmias,* atrial fibrillation, *cardiotoxicity,* chest pain, *heart failure.*
GI: *cramps and pain, diarrhea, mucositis, nausea, vomiting.*
Hematologic: hemorrhage, myelosuppression.
Metabolic: hyperuricemia.
Skin: *alopecia,* palmar erythema, rash, urticaria.
Other: INFECTION, *hypersensitivity reactions.*

INTERACTIONS
None reported.

EFFECTS ON LAB TEST RESULTS
• May increase uric acid levels.
• May decrease hemoglobin, hematocrit, and WBC and platelet counts.
• May alter renal and hepatic function test results.

ACTION
Inhibits nucleic acid synthesis by intercalation and interacts with the enzyme topoisomerase II. It is highly lipophilic, which causes an increased rate of cellular uptake.

PHARMACOKINETICS
Available in nucleated and bone marrow cells within a few minutes after injection.
Distribution: High volume of distribution, preferentially into nucleated blood and bone marrow cells rather than plasma; extensive tissue binding.
Metabolism: Rapid and extensive hepatic and extrahepatic metabolism to the active, equally potent metabolite idarubicinol.
Excretion: Biliary, as the metabolite; less than 5% in urine.

CLINICAL CONSIDERATIONS
• Take precautions—including using gloves, goggles, and protective

---

Reactions may be *common,* uncommon, *life-threatening,* or COMMON AND LIFE-THREATENING.

gowns—when preparing and giving cytotoxic drugs.

• Obtain chest X-ray and ECG study results before and periodically during therapy.

• Control systemic infections before starting therapy.

• Give an antiemetic to prevent or treat nausea and vomiting.

• Hyperuricemia may result from rapid lysis of leukemic cells. Monitor uric acid levels before and during therapy. Take appropriate measures, including making sure patient is adequately hydrated before starting therapy. Allopurinol may be given.

• Check CBC frequently. Monitor total and differential leukocyte counts; platelet count; hematocrit; hemoglobin; and ALT, AST, bilirubin, creatinine, and LDH levels before and periodically during therapy.

• Examine patient's mouth for ulceration before giving each dose.

• *Alert:* Watch for irritation and infiltration; extravasation can cause tissue damage and necrosis. If signs of extravasation occur, stop infusion immediately and notify prescriber. Treat with intermittent cold packs. Immediately apply ice pack for 30 minutes, and then for 30 minutes four times a day for 3 days.

• Cardiotoxicity may be more common in patients older than age 60 and in those who have heart disease or have received prior therapy with anthracycline compounds.

PATIENT TEACHING

• Tell patient to avoid immunizations.

• Stress importance of adequate fluid intake to increase urine output and help excrete uric acid.

• Tell patient to use toothbrush, floss, or toothpicks cautiously. Remind patient to notify prescriber before having dental work done.

• Tell patient to report unusual bruising or bleeding, tarry stools, or blood in urine.

• Tell patient to use caution when shaving and cutting nails.

• Advise patient to avoid contact sports where bruising or injury may occur.

ifosfamide
Ifex

Pharmacologic class: alkylating drug (cell cycle phase–nonspecific)
Therapeutic class: antineoplastic
Pregnancy risk category: D
pH: 6

INDICATIONS & DOSAGES

➤ **Germ-cell testicular cancers—**
Adults: 1,200 mg/m^2 I.V. daily for 5 consecutive days. Repeat q 3 weeks or after recovery from hematologic toxicity, with platelet count of 100,000/mm^3 or more and WBC count above 4,000/mm^3. Give with mesna, a protective drug used to prevent hemorrhagic cystitis. Extensive hydration needed with at least 2 L of oral or I.V. fluid daily to prevent bladder toxicity. Usually four courses of therapy are given.

➤ **Cervical cancer ♦, ovarian cancer ♦, sarcomas ♦, small-cell lung cancer ♦, uterine cancer ♦—**
Adults: Consult published protocols. 1,200 to 2,500 mg/m^2 I.V. daily for 3 to 5 days. Repeat cycles as necessary.

ADMINISTRATION

Direct injection: Not recommended.
Intermittent infusion: Using a 23G or 25G winged-tip needle, infuse solution over at least 30 minutes. Use a new I.V. site for each infusion, if possible.
Continuous infusion: Not recommended.

PREPARATION & STORAGE

Drug is available as an off-white powder in 1- and 3-g vials.

Reconstitute drug with sterile water for injection or bacteriostatic water for injection. Add 20 ml diluent per gram of drug. Final concentration, 50 mg/ml.

For intermittent infusion, drug may be added to D_5W, dextrose 2.5% in water, half-normal saline injection, normal saline injection, or lactated Ringer's injection.

Intact vials should be stored at room temperature and protected from temperatures above 104° F (40° C). Drug may liquefy at temperatures above 95° F (35° C). Dilutions not prepared with bacteriostatic water for injection should be refrigerated and used within 6 hours. Admixtures with compatible solutions are stable for 1 week at 86° F (30° C) or for 6 weeks at 41° F (5° C).

Incompatibilities
Cefepime, methotrexate sodium.

CONTRAINDICATIONS & CAUTIONS
• Use cautiously in those hypersensitive to drug and in those with renal impairment, severely depressed bone marrow, or current or previous radiation therapy.

ADVERSE REACTIONS
CNS: fever, *coma, seizures, confusion, depression, hallucinations, somnolence.*
CV: phlebitis.
GI: *nausea, vomiting.*
GU: *hematuria, hemorrhagic cystitis,* renal impairment.
Hematologic: anemia, *leukopenia, thrombocytopenia.*
Hepatic: liver dysfunction.
Metabolic: *metabolic acidosis.*
Musculoskeletal: phlebitis.
Skin: *alopecia.*
Other: infection.

INTERACTIONS
Drug-drug. *Allopurinol:* May worsen myelosuppression. Monitor patient closely.
Chloral hydrate, phenobarbital, phenytoin: Enhances ifosfamide conversion

to active and toxic metabolites. Monitor patient closely.
Cisplatin: May have synergistic effect. Monitor patient closely.
Corticosteroids: May impair metabolism and diminish effectiveness of ifosfamide. Monitor patient closely.
Succinylcholine: May increase effects. Monitor patient closely.

EFFECTS ON LAB TEST RESULTS
• May increase BUN, creatinine, and liver enzyme levels. May decrease electrolyte levels.
• May decrease WBC and platelet counts.

ACTION
Interferes with cell division primarily by cross-linking strands of DNA.

PHARMACOKINETICS
Drug level peaks immediately.
Distribution: Throughout body. Drug crosses placental barrier. It's unknown if drug appears in breast milk.
Metabolism: In the liver by microsomal enzymes. Drug must be metabolized to be active.
Excretion: In urine, with 50% to 60% removed unchanged and the remainder excreted as metabolites. Half-life is about 15 hours for high doses and 6 to 7 hours for low ones.

CLINICAL CONSIDERATIONS
• Use caution when preparing and giving drug because of mutagenic, teratogenic, and carcinogenic risks. Use a biological containment cabinet; wear gloves and mask. If drug contacts skin, immediately wash the area with soap and water. If it contacts mucosa, flush with copious amounts of water. Use syringes with tight luer-lock fittings to prevent the solution from leaking, and correctly dispose of needles, syringes, vials, and unused drug. Avoid contaminating work surfaces.

Reactions may be *common*, uncommon, *life-threatening,* or COMMON AND LIFE-THREATENING.

• Maintain daily fluid intake of at least 2 L during and for at least 3 days after therapy to reduce risk of urologic toxicity. Along with giving more fluids, give 250 mg of oral ascorbic acid three times daily and 500 mg of oral ascorbic acid at bedtime to reduce risk of toxic reaction further.

• Drug may impair wound healing.

• Drug has been used to treat bladder cancer, breast cancer, recurrent or advanced lymphomas, gastric or pancreatic cancers, and acute leukemias (except acute myelocytic leukemia.)

PATIENT TEACHING

• Warn patient to immediately report blood in urine or pain or burning during urination.

• Remind patient to urinate frequently because this minimizes contact of drug and its metabolites with the bladder lining.

• Tell patient to use toothbrush, floss, or toothpicks cautiously and to notify prescriber before having dental work done.

• Instruct patient to contact prescriber if he develops unusual bruising or bleeding, tarry stools, or blood in urine.

• Tell patient to use caution when shaving and cutting nails.

imiglucerase
Cerezyme

Pharmacologic class: glycosidase
Therapeutic class: replacement enzyme
Pregnancy risk category: C
pH: 6.1

INDICATIONS & DOSAGES

➤ **Long-term endogenous enzyme replacement therapy in confirmed type I Gaucher's disease—**
Adults: Dosage is individualized; initially, 2.5 to 60 units/kg I.V. over 1 or

2 hours. Dosing typically is once q 2 weeks but may range from three times weekly to once monthly, depending on severity of disease. Dosage may be reduced for maintenance therapy, at intervals of 3 to 6 months, while response is carefully monitored.

ADMINISTRATION
Direct injection: Not recommended.
Intermittent infusion: Infuse diluted solution over 1 to 2 hours.
Continuous infusion: Not recommended.

PREPARATION & STORAGE
Vials of lyophilized powder contain 212 units of enzyme, which provides a withdrawal dose of 200 units.

Reconstitute drug in each vial with 5.1 ml of sterile water for injection. Vials may be gently swirled to mix; avoid excessive agitation. Inspect solution for particulate matter and discoloration before use; if either is present, don't use. Withdraw 5 ml (amount in vial after reconstitution is 5.3 ml) of the reconstituted solution and dilute solution further with normal saline solution to a final volume of 100 to 200 ml. Because imiglucerase is preservative free, use immediately.

Vials should be refrigerated at 36° to 46° F (2° to 8° C). Allow to warm to room temperature before reconstitution. When diluted to 50 ml, drug is stable for up to 24 hours when stored at 36° to 46° F (2° to 8° C).

Incompatibilities
None reported.

CONTRAINDICATIONS & CAUTIONS

• Reevaluate treatment if patient becomes hypersensitive to the drug.

• Use cautiously in those who were previously treated with the drug and have developed antibodies to it or who have signs or symptoms of hypersensitivity.

• Use cautiously in breast-feeding women because it's unknown if drug appears in breast milk.

ADVERSE REACTIONS
CNS: dizziness, headache.
CV: mild hypotension.
GI: abdominal discomfort, nausea.
GU: decreased urinary frequency.
Skin: pruritus, rash.
Other: *hypersensitivity reaction.*

INTERACTIONS
None significant.

EFFECTS ON LAB TEST RESULTS
None reported.

ACTION
Catalyzes the hydrolysis of glucocerebroside to glucose and ceramide, to prevent the effects of Gaucher's disease, which normally result from glucocerebroside accumulation.

PHARMACOKINETICS
Onset and duration unknown. Drug level peaks in 1 hour.
Distribution: Serum; steady-state enzymatic activity within 30 minutes.
Metabolism: No information available.
Excretion: Half-life ranges from 3.6 to 10.4 minutes.

CLINICAL CONSIDERATIONS
• Obtain blood samples to monitor patient's response to drug.
• Monitor response parameters—including improvement in hemoglobin level, hematocrit, and erythrocyte and platelet counts—so that prescriber can determine the lowest effective dosage.
• Monitor patient for reduction of hepatosplenomegaly, regression of cachexia, and improvement in other Gaucher's disease–related signs and symptoms.
• Monitor patient for signs and symptoms of hypersensitivity.

PATIENT TEACHING
• Explain the use and administration of drug to patient and his family. Stress the importance of compliance with administration schedule.
• Tell patient to promptly report persistent or severe adverse reactions.
• Instruct patient to consult prescriber before taking other drugs.

imipenem and cilastatin sodium
Primaxin I.V.

Pharmacologic class: carbapenem (thienamycin class), beta-lactam antibiotic
Therapeutic class: antibiotic
Pregnancy risk category: C
pH: 6.5 to 7.5

INDICATIONS & DOSAGES
➤ **Lower respiratory tract, urinary tract, intra-abdominal, gynecologic, bone and joint, and skin and skin-structure infections; bacterial septicemia; endocarditis; and polymicrobic infections involving susceptible organisms—**
Adults weighing more than 70 kg (154 lb): 250 to 500 mg I.V. q 6 hours for mild infections; 500 mg or 1 g I.V. q 6 to 8 hours for moderate to severe infections. Maximum daily dose, 4 g or 50 mg/kg, whichever is lower.
Children age 3 months and older: 15 to 25 mg/kg I.V. q 6 hours. Maximum daily dose is 2 to 4 g.
Infants ages 4 weeks to 3 months, weighing 1.5 kg (3.3 lb) or more: 25 mg/kg I.V. q 6 hours.
Neonates ages 1 to 4 weeks, weighing 1.5 kg or more: 25 mg/kg I.V. q 8 hours.
Neonates younger than age 1 week, weighing 1.5 kg or more: 25 mg/kg I.V. q 12 hours.

Adjust-a-dose: For children older than age 12, patients weighing less than 70 kg, and those who are renally impaired, refer to package insert for dosage adjustments based on weight, creatinine clearance, and severity of infection.

ADMINISTRATION
Direct injection: Not recommended.
Intermittent infusion: Give diluted solution into an I.V. line containing a free-flowing, compatible solution. For adults, infuse 250- or 500-mg doses over 20 to 30 minutes and 750-mg or 1-g doses over 40 to 60 minutes. For children, doses of 500 mg or less should be infused over 15 to 30 minutes. Doses greater than 500 mg should be infused over 40 to 60 minutes. Reduce rate if nausea, vomiting, hypotension, dizziness, or sweating occurs.
Continuous infusion: Not recommended.

PREPARATION & STORAGE
Available as dry powder in vials and infusion bottles. These contain 250 mg of imipenem and 250 mg of cilastatin or 500 mg of imipenem and 500 mg of cilastatin.

　　Reconstitute drug in vial with 100 ml of compatible diluent.

　　Compatible solutions are normal saline solution, D_5W, dextrose 10% in water, dextrose 5% in normal saline solution, or dextrose 5% with potassium chloride 0.15%.

　　Most solutions are stable for 4 hours if kept at room temperature or 24 hours if refrigerated. Solutions prepared in normal saline solution with a final concentration no greater than 5 mg/ml remain stable for 10 hours if kept at room temperature or 48 hours if refrigerated. Solution is still stable if it turns deep yellow; discard if solution turns brown.

Incompatibilities
Antibiotics, dextrose 5% in lactated Ringer's injection, other I.V. drugs.

CONTRAINDICATIONS & CAUTIONS
● Contraindicated in those hypersensitive to either imipenem or cilastatin.
● Use cautiously in those hypersensitive to cephalosporins or penicillins and in those with a history of seizure disorders or multiple allergies.
● Use cautiously in geriatric patients and those with renal impairment or CNS disorders because of increased risk of toxic reaction and in those with GI disorders, particularly colitis, because of increased risk of pseudomembranous colitis.

ADVERSE REACTIONS
CNS: confusion, *encephalopathy,* lethargy, *seizures.*
CV: chest discomfort, hypotension, thrombophlebitis.
GI: diarrhea, nausea, vomiting, *pseudomembranous colitis.*
Hematologic: eosinophilia, *leukopenia, neutropenia, agranulocytosis, pancytopenia, bone marrow depression, hemolytic anemia, thrombocytopenia,* thrombocytosis.
Metabolic: hyperkalemia, hyperchloremia, hyponatremia.
Respiratory: dyspnea.
Skin: pruritus, rash, urticaria.
Other: *anaphylaxis,* superinfection.

INTERACTIONS
Drug-drug. *Aminoglycosides:* May have synergistic effect. Monitor patient closely.
Cyclosporine: Increases CNS side effects of both drugs due to additive or synergistic toxicity. Monitor patient closely.
Ganciclovir: Causes generalized seizures. Avoid using together.
Probenecid: Decreases excretion of imipenem and cilastatin sodium. Monitor patient for toxic reaction.

EFFECTS ON LAB TEST RESULTS
● May increase BUN, creatinine, ALT, AST, alkaline phosphatase, bilirubin,

LDH, potassium, and chloride levels. May decrease sodium level.
• May increase eosinophil count. May decrease WBC, RBC, granulocyte, and neutrophil counts. May increase or decrease platelet count, PT, and INR.
• May falsely alter glucose level in tests using Benedict's solution or Clinitest. May produce positive Coombs' test results.

ACTION

Imipenem joins with penicillin-binding proteins to inhibit bacterial cell wall synthesis. The broadest-spectrum antibiotic available, it's effective against most gram-positive cocci and many gram-positive and gram-negative organisms.

Cilastatin inhibits renal hydrolysis of imipenem, thus raising urine levels of active imipenem. Cilastatin has no antibacterial activity and doesn't affect imipenem's action.

PHARMACOKINETICS

Drug level peaks in about 20 minutes.
Distribution: Widely and rapidly distributed throughout the body. Low levels appear in CSF. Both imipenem and cilastatin cross the placental barrier. It's unknown if drugs appear in breast milk.
Metabolism: Cilastatin is partly metabolized by the kidneys but prevents imipenem metabolism.
Excretion: 70% to 76% is excreted by kidneys, 20% to 25% by an unknown nonrenal mechanism, and up to 2% in bile. Elimination half-life, about 1 hour.

CLINICAL CONSIDERATIONS

• Check for previous penicillin or cephalosporin hypersensitivity before first dose.
• Obtain specimens for culture and sensitivity testing before giving first dose. Therapy may start before results are available.

• When giving with aminoglycosides, use separate solution containers. However, drug can be infused through same I.V. line.
• If patient is undergoing hemodialysis, give a supplemental dose after treatment unless the next dose is scheduled within 4 hours.
• If diarrhea persists during therapy, stop drug and obtain stool specimens for culture to rule out pseudomembranous colitis.
• If patient has history of seizures, monitor anticonvulsant drug levels carefully. The risk of seizures rises when imipenem dosages exceed 2 g daily.
• Monitor BUN and creatinine levels to assess renal function.
• When drug is used with other anti-infectives, monitor patient for signs and symptoms of bacterial or fungal superinfection.
• Use Clinistix or glucose enzymatic test strip for urine glucose testing to avoid inaccurate results.
• Each gram of imipenem and cilastatin sodium contains 3.2 mEq (75.2 mg) of sodium, so patients who must restrict their sodium intake should figure this into their daily sodium count.
• If overdose occurs, treat symptomatically. Hemodialysis can reduce drug levels.

PATIENT TEACHING

• Stress importance of adhering to dosing schedule.
• Tell patient to report discomfort at I.V. site.
• Tell patient to promptly report adverse reactions.

immune globulin (IGIV)
Carimune, Gamimune N,
Gammagard S/D, Gammar-P I.V.,
Iveegam EN, Panglobulin, Polygam
S/D, Venoglobulin-S

Pharmacologic class: immune
serum
Therapeutic class: antibody
production stimulant
Pregnancy risk category: C
pH: 4 to 5

INDICATIONS & DOSAGES
➤ **Primary immunodeficiency—**
Adults and children: 200 mg/kg
Carimune or Panglobulin I.V. monthly.
May increase to 300 mg/kg or give
more frequently to produce desired
effect.
Adults and children: 100 to 200 mg/kg
Gamimune N I.V. monthly. Maximum
dosage is 400 mg/kg.
Adults and children: Initially, 200 to
400 mg/kg Gammagard S/D I.V.; then
monthly doses of 100 mg/kg I.V.
Adults and children: 200 mg/kg
Iveegam EN I.V. monthly. May increase
dose to 800 mg/kg or give more fre-
quently to produce desired effect.
Adults and children: Initially, 200 to
400 mg/kg Polygam S/D I.V.; then
monthly doses of 100 mg/kg I.V.
➤ **Primary defective antibody syn-
thesis, such as agammaglobulinemia
or hypogammaglobulinemia, in patients at increased risk of infection—**
Adults: 200 to 400 mg/kg Gammar-P
I.V. infused q 3 to 4 weeks.
Adolescents and children: 200 mg/kg
Gammar-P I.V. infused q 3 to 4 weeks.
Adjust dosage according to clinical ef-
fect and to maintain IgG at desired level.
Adults and children: 200 mg/kg
Venoglobulin-S I.V. monthly. May in-
crease to 300 to 400 mg/kg and give

more often if adequate IgG levels
haven't been reached.
➤ **Idiopathic thrombocytopenic purpura—**
Adults and children: 400 mg/kg
Carimune or Panglobulin I.V. daily for
2 to 5 consecutive days. Maximum
dosage is 1 g/kg/day.
Adults and children: 400 mg/kg
Gamimune N 5% solution I.V. for 5
days; or 1,000 mg/kg 5% or 10% solution I.V. for 1 to 2 days, with maintenance dose of 5% or 10% solution at
400 to 1,000 mg/kg I.V. single infusion to maintain platelet count of
30,000/mm^3.
Adults and children: 1 g/kg Gammagard S/D or Polygam S/D I.V. Additional doses depend on response. Up to
three doses may be given on alternate
days if needed.
Adults and children: 2,000 mg/kg
Venoglobulin-S I.V. divided over 5 days
or less. Maintenance dose is 1,000 mg/
kg I.V. p.r.n. to maintain a platelet
count of 30,000/mm^3 in children and
20,000/mm^3 in adults.
➤ **Bone marrow transplant—**
Adults older than age 20: 500 mg/kg
Gamimune N 5% or 10% solution I.V.
on days 7 and 2 before transplantation;
then weekly until 90 days after transplantation.
➤ **B-cell chronic lymphocytic
leukemia—**
Adults: 400 mg/kg Gammagard S/D or
Polygam S/D I.V. q 3 to 4 weeks.
➤ **Kawasaki syndrome to prevent
coronary artery aneurysms—**
Adults and children: Single 1-g/kg dose
Gammagard S/D or Polygam S/D I.V.
Or, 400 mg/kg/day I.V. for 4 consecu-
tive days, beginning within 7 days of
onset of fever. Give with aspirin 80 to
100 mg/kg/day in four divided doses.
Adults and children: Single 2-g/kg
dose Iveegam EN or Venoglobulin-S
I.V. over 10 hours. Or, 400 mg/kg/day
I.V. for 4 consecutive days, beginning
within 10 days of onset of fever. Give

with aspirin 100 mg/kg/day through 14 days of illness, then 3 to 10 mg/kg/day thereafter for 5 weeks.
➤ **Pediatric HIV infection—**
Children: 400 mg/kg Gamimune N 5% or 10% solution I.V. q 28 days.

ADMINISTRATION

Direct injection: Not recommended.
Intermittent infusion: For Carimune or Panglobulin, use 15-micron in-line filter. Infusion rate is 0.5 to 1 ml/minute for 3% solution. After 15 to 30 minutes, increase rate to 1.5 to 2.5 ml/minute.

For Gamimune N, start infusion at 0.01 to 0.02 ml/kg/minute for 30 minutes. If no problems, rate can be slowly increased to maximum of 0.08 ml/kg/minute.

For Gammagard S/D or Polygam S/D, infuse with administration set provided or with 15-micron in-line filter. Initiate infusion at 0.5 ml/kg/hour and increase to maximum of 4 ml/kg/hour. Patients who tolerate 5% concentration at 4 ml/kg/hour can be switched to 10% concentration at 0.5 ml/kg/hour and can be increased to 8 ml/kg/hour if tolerated.

For Gammar-P I.V., use 15-micron in-line filter. Initiate infusion at 0.01 ml/kg/minute and increase to 0.02 ml/kg/minute after 15 to 30 minutes if no problems. Maximum infusion rate is 0.06 ml/kg/minute.

For Iveegam EN, use 15-micron in-line filter. Infusion rate is 1 to 2 ml/minute for 5% solution.

For Venoglobulin-S, begin infusion at 0.01 to 0.02 ml/kg/minute for 30 minutes; then increase 5% solutions to 0.04 ml/kg/minute and 10% solutions to 0.05 ml/kg/minute, if tolerated.
Continuous infusion: Not recommended.

PREPARATION & STORAGE

Injection: 5% and 10% in 10-, 50-, 100-, and 200- vials and 5% in 250-ml

vials for Gamimune N; 5% and 10% in 5-, 10-, and 20-g vials for Venoglobulin-S.
Powder for injection: 1-, 3-, 6-, and 12-g vials for Carimune, 50 mg protein/ml in 2.5-, 5-, and 10-g vials for Gammagard S/D; 1-, 2.5-, 5-, and 10-g vials for Gammar-P I.V.; 500-mg and 1-, 2.5-, and 5-g vials for Iveegam EN; 6- and 12-g vials for Panglobulin; 2.5-, 5-, and 10-g vials for Polygam S/D.

After reconstitution, Gammagard S/D and Polygam S/D contain about 50 mg of protein/ml for 5% solution or 100 mg of protein/ml for 10% solution, and both contain no less than 90% IgG; Gamimune N contains 50 mg of protein/ml for 5% solution or 100 mg of protein/ml for 10% solution, and both contain no less than 98% IgG; Gammar-P I.V. and Iveegam EN contain 50 mg of IgG/ml; Carimune and Panglobulin contain no less than 96% IgG; Venoglobulin-S contains about 50 mg of protein/ml for 5% solution or 100 mg of protein/ml for 10% solution, and both contain no less than 99% IgG.

Reconstitute Carimune and Panglobulin with normal saline solution, D_5W, or sterile water.

Gamimune N 5% and 10% are incompatible with saline solutions; they may be diluted with D_5W, if needed.

Reconstitute Gammagard S/D and Polygam S/D using sterile water for injection as diluent and the transfer device provided. Warm powder and sterile water for injection to room temperature before reconstitution. Give within 2 hours of reconstitution.

Reconstitute Gammar-P I.V. with sterile water for injection diluent provided. Warm powder and diluent to room temperature before reconstitution. After adding diluent, keep vial in upright position and undisturbed for 5 minutes. Gently swirl vial after 5 minutes. Don't shake. Dissolution may take up to 20 minutes. Start infusion within 3 hours of reconstituting.

Reconstitute Iveegam EN with sterile water for injection diluent provided.

Before use, refrigerate Gamimune N and Iveegam EN at 36° to 46° F (2° to 8° C). Before reconstitution, refrigerate Gammagard S/D at 36° to 46° F. Before reconstitution, store Gammagard S/D, Gammar-P I.V., Polygam S/D, and Venoglobulin-S at room temperature, not to exceed 77° F (25° C). Before reconstitution, store Carimune and Panglobulin at room temperature, below 86° F (30° C).

Incompatibilities
Other I.V. drugs or fluids.

CONTRAINDICATIONS & CAUTIONS
• Contraindicated in those hypersensitive to immune globulin or thimerosal.
• Contraindicated in those with certain IgA deficiencies because of increased risk of anaphylaxis.
• Use Gamimune N cautiously in those with compromised acid-base compensatory mechanisms.
• IGIV administration may be linked to thrombotic events. The exact cause is unknown; caution should be used in prescribing and administering IGIV for patients with a history of cardiovascular disease or thrombotic episodes.
• Use with caution if patient has severe thrombocytopenia or any bleeding disorder.

ADVERSE REACTIONS
CNS: fever, burning sensation in head, dizziness, fatigue, pain, malaise, headache; *severe headache requiring hospitalization (Gammagard S/D).*
CV: hypotension, tachycardia; *chest pain, MI, congestive cardiac failure (Gammagard S/D).*
GI: nausea, vomiting.
Musculoskeletal: back, chest, or hip pain; muscle stiffness at injection site.

Respiratory: dyspnea; *pulmonary embolism, transfusion-related acute lung injury (Gammagard S/D).*
Skin: urticaria.
Other: chills, *anaphylaxis, angioedema,* chest tightness, tenderness.

INTERACTIONS
Drug-drug. *Vaccine for measles, mumps, rubella (MMR) with live virus:* May impair response. Don't give vaccine within 3 months of IGIV

EFFECTS ON LAB TEST RESULTS
• May cause false-positive IgG antibody screening test results.

ACTION
Provides passive immunity by increasing antibody titer and antigen-antibody reaction potential.

PHARMACOKINETICS
Highly variable: onset, 1 to 5 days; duration, 2 to 4 weeks.
Distribution: Appears immediately. Drug probably crosses the placental barrier, and it appears in breast milk.
Metabolism: Not metabolized.
Excretion: Not excreted; cleared by the spleen. Half-life, 21 to 29 days.

CLINICAL CONSIDERATIONS
• Osmolarity: 192 to 1,074 mOsm/L.
• Osmolality: 274 to 309 mOsm/kg.
• If a risk of a thrombotic event exists, the Gammagard S/D infusion concentration shouldn't exceed 5%, and the infusion rate should be started no faster than 0.5 ml/kg/hour; it should be advanced slowly only if well tolerated to a maximum rate of 4 ml/kg/hour.
• No discernible risk of transmitting HIV exists with currently available preparations of immune globulin.
• Monitor vital signs continuously during infusion.
• Most adverse reactions are related to infusion rate. If patient becomes symptomatic, reduce rate. A corticosteroid

given before infusion may prevent adverse reactions.
• Signs of an allergic reaction may occur 30 to 60 minutes after start of infusion.
• Don't give live-virus MMR vaccines for 2 weeks before or 3 months after giving immune globulin.

PATIENT TEACHING
• Inform patient of potential adverse effects, especially labored breathing, dizziness, fatigue, and rapid heartbeat.
• Tell patient to notify prescriber if back pain, headache, or malaise continues and is bothersome.

---

inamrinone lactate

Pharmacologic class: bipyridine derivative
Therapeutic class: inotropic, vasodilator
Pregnancy risk category: C
pH: 3.2 to 4

INDICATIONS & DOSAGES
➤ **Short-term management of heart failure, primarily in patients unresponsive to cardiac glycosides, diuretics, and vasodilators—**
Adults: Initially, 0.75 mg/kg I.V. over 2 to 3 minutes, followed by 200 mg in 100 ml of normal saline solution I.V. at 5 to 10 mcg/kg/minute. If needed, additional bolus of 0.75 mg/kg I.V. can be given 30 minutes after therapy starts. Individualize dosage based on patient response. Maximum daily dose is 10 mg/kg. Maintain steady-state plasma level at 3 mcg/ml.
➤ **Advanced cardiac life support when other drugs can't be used for severe heart failure or cardiogenic shock ♦ —**
Adults: Initially, 0.75 mg/kg I.V. over 2 to 3 minutes, followed by an infusion

of 5 to 15 mcg/kg/minute. An additional bolus may be given in 30 minutes.
Children: Initially, 0.75 to 1 mg/kg I.V. over 5 minutes. If this dose is tolerated, may repeat up to two times to a total loading dose of 3 mg/kg; followed by an infusion of 5 to 10 mcg/kg/minute.

ADMINISTRATION
Direct injection: Over 2 to 3 minutes, inject diluted or undiluted drug into vein or I.V. tubing containing a free-flowing, compatible solution. Watch for irritation and infiltration; extravasation can cause tissue damage and necrosis. After injection, flush tubing and cannula with normal saline solution.
Intermittent infusion: Not recommended.
Continuous infusion: Dilute only with saline solution to 1 to 3 mg/ml. May be piggybacked into line close to insertion site containing D_5W. Infusion rate is usually controlled by pump at 5 to 10 mcg/kg/minute.

PREPARATION & STORAGE
Available in 20-ml ampules of clear yellow solution containing 5 mg/ml. Protect ampules from light and store at room temperature. Don't use if solution is discolored or has precipitates. Give undiluted or dilute in half-normal or normal saline solution. Concentrations of 1 to 3 mg/ml remain stable for 24 hours.

Incompatibilities
Bicarbonate, furosemide, glucose, solutions that contain dextrose.

CONTRAINDICATIONS & CAUTIONS
• Contraindicated in those hypersensitive to amrinone or sulfites.
• Contraindicated in those with an acute MI or ischemic coronary artery disease without heart failure because experience using the drug in these patients is limited; in those with severe

aortic or pulmonary valve disease because surgery is needed to relieve the obstruction; and in those with hypertrophic cardiomyopathy because of aggravated outflow tract obstruction.

ADVERSE REACTIONS
CNS: fever.
CV: hypotension, *arrhythmias,* chest pain.
GI: abdominal pain, anorexia, diarrhea, nausea, vomiting.
Hematologic: *thrombocytopenia.*
Hepatic: *hepatotoxicity.*
Skin: burning at injection site.
Other: *anaphylaxis.*

INTERACTIONS
Drug-drug. *Cardiac glycosides:* Increases inotropic effect. Use cautiously together.
Disopyramide: Causes excessive hypotension. Avoid using together.

EFFECTS ON LAB TEST RESULTS
• May increase liver enzyme levels. May decrease potassium level.
• May decrease platelet count.

ACTION
A noncatecholamine, nonglycoside cardiotonic drug that produces a positive inotropic effect by increasing cellular levels of cAMP through phosphodiesterase inhibition. It also acts as a vasodilator. The resulting decreases in central venous pressure, pulmonary artery wedge pressure, and systemic and peripheral vascular resistance reduce preload and afterload.

PHARMACOKINETICS
Onset, 2 to 5 minutes; peak level, 10 minutes; duration, 30 minutes to 2 hours. Action is dose dependent.
Distribution: Unknown, but probably throughout body tissues, with 10% to 49% protein bound. It's unknown if drug crosses placental or blood-brain barriers; also unknown if drug appears in breast milk.
Metabolism: In liver, which produces several metabolites from acetylation, glucuronidation, and addition of glutathione.
Excretion: Primarily in urine, with 10% to 40% excreted unchanged in 24 hours. In rapid I.V. administration, half-life averages 4 hours. In controlled infusion for heart failure, it averages 6 hours.

CLINICAL CONSIDERATIONS
• Because inamrinone may increase ventricular response rate, patients with atrial fibrillation or flutter may also require cardiac glycosides.
• Carefully monitor fluid and electrolyte levels, hepatic and renal function, and platelet count. Expect to decrease dosage if platelet count drops below 150,000/mm^3.
• During infusion, check vital signs every 5 to 15 minutes. If blood pressure drops, slow or stop infusion and notify prescriber.
• Each vial contains sodium metabisulfite 0.25 mg/ml.
• *Alert:* Because of confusion with amiodarone, the generic name amrinone was changed to inamrinone.

PATIENT TEACHING
• Explain to patient and family the use and administration of drug.
• Tell patient to report adverse reactions promptly.
• Instruct home care patient and family on administration procedure.
• Tell patient to report discomfort at I.V. site promptly.

indomethacin sodium trihydrate
Indocid PDA ◇ , Indocin I.V.

Pharmacologic class: NSAID
Therapeutic class: anti-inflammatory
Pregnancy risk category: B; D in last trimester
pH: 6 to 7.5

INDICATIONS & DOSAGES
➤ **Patent ductus arteriosus—**
Infants older than age 7 days: Initially, 0.2 mg/kg I.V.; then one or two doses of 0.25 mg/kg q 12 to 24 hours if needed.
Infants ages 2 to 7 days: Initially, 0.2 mg/kg I.V.; then one or two doses of 0.2 mg/kg q 12 to 24 hours if needed.
Infants younger than age 2 days: Initially, 0.2 mg/kg I.V.; then one or two doses of 0.1 mg/kg q 12 to 24 hours if needed.
Adjust-a-dose: If anuria or urine output below 0.6 ml/kg/hour is evident at time of second or third dose, don't give additional doses until laboratory tests indicate that renal function has returned to normal.
➤ **To prevent patent ductus arteriosus in premature neonates ♦ —**
Premature neonates younger than age 7 days: Initially, 0.2 mg/kg I.V.; then two doses of 0.1 mg/kg q 12 hours.

ADMINISTRATION
Direct injection: Give drug over 5 to 10 seconds through the tubing of a compatible I.V. solution. Watch for irritation and infiltration; extravasation can cause tissue damage and necrosis.
Intermittent infusion: Not recommended.
Continuous infusion: Not recommended.

PREPARATION & STORAGE
Available as a white or yellow powder in single-dose vials containing indomethacin sodium trihydrate equivalent to 1 mg of indomethacin. Reconstitute with 1 ml of preservative-free sterile normal saline solution or preservative-free sterile water for injection to yield 1 mg/ml. Or, reconstitute with 2 ml to yield 0.5 mg/ml. Don't dilute drug. Discard unused portion.

Protect from sunlight and store below 86° F (30° C). Although 1-mg/ml solution remains stable for 16 days, prepare just before use because diluent is preservative free.

Incompatibilities
Amino acid injection, calcium gluconate, cimetidine, dextrose injection, dobutamine, dopamine, gentamicin, solutions with pH less than 6, tobramycin sulfate.

CONTRAINDICATIONS & CAUTIONS
• Contraindicated in those with intracranial hemorrhage, GI bleeding, thrombocytopenia, or coagulation defects because of possible worsened bleeding and in those with infection or necrotizing enterocolitis because of possible masked signs and symptoms, which could lead to unrecognized, overwhelming sepsis.
• Contraindicated in those with severe renal impairment because of risk of hypercalcemia, and in infants who need a patent ductus arteriosus to maintain pulmonary or systemic blood flow.
• Use cautiously in premature infants because of risk of intraventricular hemorrhage.
• Use cautiously in those with cardiac dysfunction or hypertension because of possible fluid retention and peripheral edema, in those with heart failure because of possible exacerbation, and in those with volume depletion or hepatic dysfunction because of increased risk of acute renal failure.

Reactions may be *common,* uncommon, *life-threatening,* or COMMON AND LIFE-THREATENING.

• Drug may suppress water excretion more than sodium excretion. Monitor electrolyte levels and renal function during therapy.

ADVERSE REACTIONS
CNS: *intracranial bleeding.*
CV: *bradycardia.*
EENT: retrolental fibroplasia.
GI: abdominal distention, *bleeding, necrotizing enterocolitis,* transient ileus, vomiting.
GU: *oliguria.*
Hematologic: *DIC,* prolonged bleeding time.
Metabolic: acidosis or alkalosis, fluid retention, hypoglycemia, hyponatremia, hyperkalemia.
Respiratory: *apnea,* exacerbated pulmonary infection, pulmonary hypertension.

INTERACTIONS
Drug-drug. *ACE inhibitors, potassium-sparing diuretics, potassium supplements:* Increases risk of hyperkalemia. Monitor patient closely.
Aminoglycosides, cardiac glycosides: Reduces renal clearance of these drugs. Dosage may need to be adjusted. Monitor patient closely.
Anticoagulants: Increases risk of bleeding. Monitor PT and INR.
Antihypertensives, especially beta blockers, diuretics: May reduce antihypertensive effects. Monitor blood pressure.
Aspirin, other salicylates: May cause severe GI bleeding. Use together with caution.
Cyclosporine, methotrexate, nephrotoxic drugs: Increases risk of renal failure. Avoid using together.
Diflunisal, probenecid: Decreases indomethacin excretion, leading to increased risk of indomethacin toxicity. Monitor patient for signs and symptoms of toxicity.
Dipyridamole: May increase water retention. Use together cautiously.

Furosemide: Decreases effect on plasma renin activity and increases urine output, sodium and chloride excretion, and GFR. Monitor patient closely.
Lithium: May reduce renal clearance. Monitor lithium level.
Phenytoin: Increases phenytoin level. Monitor patient for signs and symptoms of toxicity.
Drug-herb. *Senna:* May block diarrheal effects. Discourage use together.
Drug-lifestyle. *Alcohol use:* Increases risk of GI bleeding. Discourage use together.

EFFECTS ON LAB TEST RESULTS
• May increase potassium, creatinine, BUN, and liver enzyme levels. May decrease sodium, glucose, urine sodium, chloride, and potassium levels.
• May decrease hemoglobin, hematocrit, urine osmolality, and WBC, platelet, and granulocyte counts.

ACTION
Inhibits the enzyme cyclooxygenase, thereby inhibiting prostaglandin synthesis.

PHARMACOKINETICS
Drug level peak varies according to infant's age and weight. Duration may be especially long for a single dose given shortly after birth.
Distribution: Throughout body tissues, with 99% bound to plasma proteins. Drug readily crosses the blood-brain and placental barriers and appears in breast milk.
Metabolism: In the liver.
Excretion: About 60% in urine by renal tubular secretion within 48 hours, primarily as metabolites. About 33% excreted in feces, primarily as metabolites. In premature infants, plasma half-life ranges from 15 to 21 hours, declining with increasing age and weight.

CLINICAL CONSIDERATIONS

• If renal function declines significantly after dose, hold next dose until urine volume or renal studies indicate a return to normal function.

• Carefully monitor hemodynamic indicators, such as vital signs, central venous pressure, cardiac output, pulmonary artery wedge pressure, and pulmonary artery pressure.

• Closely monitor urine output and BUN and creatinine levels. Restrict fluids and compare output with fluid intake.

• If severe hepatic reactions occur, stop drug.

• Check for changes in coagulation studies, such as PT, PTT, and fibrinogen level.

• If infant doesn't respond to two courses of therapy with three doses per course, surgery may be indicated.

• Ductus may reopen, possibly requiring additional indomethacin or surgery. However, spontaneous reclosure commonly occurs.

• Watch for signs of infection.

• Hemodialysis doesn't remove drug.

PATIENT TEACHING

• Explain to family the advantages and possible adverse reactions related to drug use.

• Tell family to report adverse reactions promptly.

infliximab
Remicade

Pharmacologic class: chimeric IgG$_1$k monoclonal antibody
Therapeutic class: antineoplastic
Pregnancy risk category: B
pH: 7.2

INDICATIONS & DOSAGES

➤ **To reduce signs and symptoms and induce and maintain clinical remis-** sion in patients with moderately to severely active Crohn's disease who have responded inadequately to conventional therapy; to reduce the number of draining enterocutaneous and rectovaginal fistulas and maintain fistula closure in patients with fistulizing Crohn's disease—
Adults: 5 mg/kg by I.V. infusion over at least 2 hours, given as an induction regimen at 0, 2, and 6 weeks, followed by a maintenance regimen of 5 mg/kg I.V. q 8 weeks thereafter. For patients who respond and then lose their response, may increase to 10 mg/kg I.V. Patients who don't respond by week 14 are unlikely to respond with continued dosing; these patients may be considered for discontinuation of infliximab.

➤ **To reduce signs and symptoms, inhibit progression of structural damage, and improve physical function in patients with moderately to severely active rheumatoid arthritis who have had an inadequate response to methotrexate—**
Adults: 3 mg/kg by I.V. infusion over at least 2 hours, with methotrexate. Give additional doses of 3 mg/kg I.V. at 2 and 6 weeks after initial infusion and q 8 weeks thereafter. Dose may be increased to 10 mg/kg I.V., or initial dose may be given q 4 weeks if response is inadequate.

➤ **Crohn's disease in pediatric patients ♦—**
Children age 6 and older: 5 mg/kg I.V. over at least 2 hours. May receive one to three doses over a 12-week period.

➤ **Moderate to severe ulcerative colitis unresponsive to other therapies ♦—**
Adults: 5 mg/kg, 10 mg/kg, or 20 mg/kg I.V. as a single dose; may receive a second 5-mg/kg dose I.V. 5 months after the first dose.

ADMINISTRATION
Direct injection: Not recommended.

Intermittent infusion: Not recommended.

Continuous infusion: Infuse over at least 2 hours using an inline, nonpyrogenic, low–protein-binding filter with a pore size of 1.2 mm or less.

PREPARATION & STORAGE
Available as 100 mg in a 20-ml vial. Vials don't contain antibacterial preservatives.

Reconstitute with 10 ml sterile water for injection, using a syringe with a 21G or smaller needle; don't re-enter the vial. Don't shake; gently swirl to dissolve powder and let stand for at least 5 minutes. Solution should be colorless to light yellow and opalescent and may develop a few translucent particles.

Further dilute drug in 250 ml of normal saline injection, and gently mix. Infusion concentration range is 0.4 to 4 mg/ml. Begin infusion within 3 hours of preparation, giving drug over 2 or more hours. Don't use if other particles or discoloration are present.

Refrigerate drug at 36° to 46° F (2° to 8° C).

Incompatibilities
Other I.V. drugs.

CONTRAINDICATIONS & CAUTIONS
• Contraindicated in those hypersensitive to murine proteins or other components of drug.
• Don't give drug to patients with New York Heart Association class III or IV heart failure.
• Don't give to those with active infection.
• Use cautiously in patients with New York Heart Association class I or II heart failure.
• Use cautiously in geriatric patients and in those with chronic infection or a history of recurrent infections.

ADVERSE REACTIONS
CNS: *fever, headache, fatigue,* dizziness, malaise, pain, insomnia, depression.
CV: *hypertension,* flushing, hypotension, tachycardia, chest pain, peripheral edema, hot flashes.
EENT: *pharyngitis, rhinitis, sinusitis,* conjunctivitis.
GI: *nausea, abdominal pain,* vomiting, constipation, *dyspepsia,* flatulence, intestinal obstruction, oral pain, ulcerative stomatitis, *diarrhea.*
GU: dysuria, increased urinary frequency, *UTI.*
Hematologic: anemia, hematoma, ecchymosis.
Musculoskeletal: myalgia, *arthralgia,* arthritis, *back pain.*
Respiratory: *upper respiratory tract infection,* bronchitis, *coughing,* dyspnea, respiratory tract allergic reaction.
Skin: *rash,* pruritus, candidiasis, acne, alopecia, eczema, erythema, erythematous rash, maculopapular rash, papular rash, dry skin, increased sweating, urticaria.
Other: flulike syndrome, chills, toothache, abscess.

INTERACTIONS
Drug-drug. *Vaccines with live virus:* May transmit infection. Avoid using together.

EFFECTS ON LAB TEST RESULTS
• May increase liver enzyme levels.
• May decrease hemoglobin and hematocrit.

ACTION
Binds to human tumor necrosis factor (TNF)-alpha to neutralize its activity and inhibit its binding with receptors, reducing the infiltration of inflammatory cells and TNF-alpha production in inflamed areas of the intestine.

PHARMACOKINETICS

Onset, peak, and duration of drug effects unknown.
Distribution: Unknown.
Metabolism: Unknown.
Excretion: Elimination half-life is 8 to 9.5 days.

CLINICAL CONSIDERATIONS

● Drug may affect normal immune responses. Stop drug if patient develops antinuclear antibodies or lupuslike syndrome. Expect symptoms to resolve.
● Tuberculosis (frequently disseminated or extrapulmonary), invasive fungal infections, and other opportunistic infections have been observed in patients receiving infliximab. Some of these infections have been fatal.
● Re-evaluate therapy for patients with heart failure, a heart weakened by age, or damage from an MI or some other condition. Treatment should stop if patient develops new or worsening symptoms of heart failure.
● Evaluate patient for latent tuberculosis infection with a tuberculin skin test. Treatment of latent tuberculosis infection should be started before therapy with infliximab.
● *Alert:* Patients receiving this drug may develop histoplasmosis, listeriosis, pneumocystosis, and tuberculosis. For patients in regions where histoplasmosis is endemic, the benefits and risks of infliximab therapy should be carefully considered.
● Monitor patient for infusion-related reactions, such as fever, chills, pruritus, urticaria, dyspnea, hypotension, hypertension, and chest pain. If an infusion reaction occurs, stop drug, notify prescriber, and be prepared to give acetaminophen, an antihistamine, a corticosteroid, or epinephrine, as ordered.
● Stop drug if patient develops serious infection or sepsis.
● Monitor patient for lymphomas and infection. Patients with a history of Crohn's disease or with long-term exposure to immunosuppressant therapies are more prone to develop lymphomas and infections.
● Drug has also been used to treat plaque psoriasis and ankylosing spondylitis.

PATIENT TEACHING

● Tell patient about infusion and postinfusion adverse reactions, and instruct him to report them promptly if they occur.
● Inform women not to breast-feed during therapy.

insulin, regular
Humulin-R, Iletin II Regular, Novolin R, Velosulin BR

Pharmacologic class: pancreatic hormone
Therapeutic class: antidiabetic
Pregnancy risk category: B
pH: 7 to 7.8

INDICATIONS & DOSAGES

➤ **Moderate to severe diabetic ketoacidosis or hyperosmolar hyperglycemia**—
Adults older than age 20: Give loading dose of 0.15 unit/kg I.V. by direct injection, followed by 0.1 unit/kg/hour as a continuous infusion. Decrease to 0.05 to 0.1 unit/kg/hour when glucose level reaches 250 to 300 mg/dl. Start infusion of dextrose 5% in half-normal saline solution separately from the insulin infusion when glucose level is between 150 and 200 mg/dl in diabetic ketoacidosis patients or between 250 and 300 mg/dl in hyperosmolar hyperglycemia patients. Give dose of insulin S.C. 1 to 2 hours before stopping insulin infusion; intermediate-acting insulin is recommended.
Adults and children age 20 or younger: Loading dose isn't recommended. Be-

gin therapy at 0.1 unit/kg/hour by I.V. infusion. Once condition improves, decrease to 0.05 unit/kg/hour. Start infusion of dextrose 5% in half-normal saline solution separately from the insulin infusion when glucose level is 250 mg/dl.
➤ **Mild diabetic ketoacidosis—**
Adults older than age 20: Give loading dose of 0.4 to 0.6 unit/kg divided in two equal parts, with half the dose given by direct I.V. injection and the other half given I.M. or S.C. Subsequent doses can be based on 0.1 unit/kg/hour I.M. or S.C.
➤ **Hyperkalemia ♦—**
Adults: 50 ml of dextrose 50% given over 5 minutes, followed by 5 to 10 units of regular insulin by I.V. push.

ADMINISTRATION
Adding insulin (regular) injection to an I.V. infusion solution may result in absorption of insulin in the container and tubing. The amount of an insulin dose lost by absorption to an I.V. infusion system is highly variable, and depends on the insulin concentration, the duration of contact time, and the infusion flow rate.
Direct injection: Inject directly into vein, through an intermittent infusion device, or into a port close to I.V. access site at ordered rate.
Intermittent infusion: Not recommended.
Continuous infusion: Infuse drug diluted in normal saline solution at a rate sufficient to reverse ketoacidosis.

PREPARATION & STORAGE
Available in 10-ml vials containing 100 units/ml. Iletin II Regular insulin is derived from pork; all others are human derivatives.
   Don't use cloudy, discolored, or unusually viscous preparations. Use only syringes calibrated for the specific insulin concentration being given.

Can be added to most I.V. and hyperalimentation solutions.
   Store insulin at 36° to 46° F (2° to 8° C); avoid freezing.

Incompatibilities
Aminophylline, amobarbital, chlorothiazide, cytarabine, digoxin, diltiazem, dobutamine, dopamine, methylprednisolone sodium succinate, nafcillin, norepinephrine, pentobarbital sodium, phenobarbital sodium, phenytoin sodium, sodium bicarbonate, thiopental.

CONTRAINDICATIONS & CAUTIONS
• Use I.V. insulin cautiously. Prolonged, severe hypoglycemia can result in irreversible brain damage.

ADVERSE REACTIONS
CNS: aphasia, anxiety, blurred vision, concentration difficulty, confusion, drowsiness, headache, unconsciousness, weakness, paresthesia, irritability, personality change.
CV: tachycardia.
GI: excessive hunger, nausea.
Metabolic: *hypoglycemia.*
Skin: cool and pale skin; itching, redness, and swelling at the injection site.
Other: chills, cold sweats.

INTERACTIONS
Drug-drug. *ACE inhibitors, anabolic steroids, antidiabetic agents, beta blockers, calcium, chloroquine, clonidine, disopyramide, fluoxetine, guanethidine, lithium, MAO inhibitors, mebendazole, octreotide, pentamidine, propoxyphene, pyridoxine, salicylates, sulfinpyrazone, sulfonamides, tetracyclines:* May enhance the hypoglycemic effects of insulin. Monitor glucose level.
Acetazolamide, adrenocorticosteroids, AIDS antivirals, albuterol, asparaginase, calcitonin, cyclophosphamide, danazol, diazoxide, diltiazem, diuretics, dobutamine, epinephrine, estrogen-containing hormonal contraceptives,

estrogens, ethacrynic acid, isoniazid, lithium, morphine, niacin, nicotine, phenothiazines, phenytoin, somatropin, terbutaline, thyroid hormones: May decrease the insulin response. Monitor glucose level.

Rosiglitazone: Increases risk of CV effects, including heart failure. Monitor patient closely.

Drug-herb. *Basil, bay, bee pollen, burdock, ginseng, glucomannan, horehound, marsh mallow, myrrh, sage:* May affect glycemic control. Monitor glucose level carefully and discourage using together.

Drug-food. *Unregulated diet:* May cause hyperglycemia or hypoglycemia. Monitor diet.

Drug-lifestyle. *Alcohol use:* May prolong hypoglycemic effect. Advise patient to avoid alcohol.

Marijuana use: May increase insulin requirements. Inform patient of this interaction.

Smoking: Decreases absorption of insulin given S.C. Advise patient to avoid smoking within 30 minutes of insulin injection.

EFFECTS ON LAB TEST RESULTS

• May decrease glucose, magnesium, and potassium levels.

ACTION

Stimulates carbohydrate metabolism in skeletal and cardiac muscle and adipose tissue, aiding glucose transport to these cells. Drug stimulates protein synthesis and lipogenesis and inhibits lipolysis and release of free fatty acids from adipose tissue; also promotes intracellular shifts of potassium and magnesium, temporarily reducing elevated electrolyte levels.

PHARMACOKINETICS

Onset, immediately after injection.
Distribution: Rapid, throughout extracellular fluids.

Metabolism: Rapid, primarily in the liver and, to a lesser extent, in the kidneys and muscles.
Excretion: Only small amounts excreted in the urine unchanged.

CLINICAL CONSIDERATIONS

• For patients with high fever, hyperthyroidism, severe infections, trauma, or recent surgery, dosage may need to be increased.
• For those with diarrhea, hepatic or renal impairment, hypothyroidism, nausea, or vomiting, dosage may need to be decreased.
• Monitor serum and urine glucose and ketone levels before starting insulin therapy.
• During insulin therapy, monitor glucose level by reflectance meter every hour; also monitor acetone or ketone level every 1 or 2 hours.
• Monitor electrolyte levels and acid-base balance during therapy.
• Assess patient for signs of hypoglycemia and dehydration.
• Large single doses of insulin aren't recommended because of their short half-life.
• Insulin has been added to dextrose infusions to promote intracellular potassium shift in hyperkalemia.
• If overdose occurs and patient is conscious, give him orange juice, sugar, or candy. If patient has severe hypoglycemia or if he's in a coma, give 10 to 30 ml of dextrose 50%. Or, give 1 unit of glucagon if hepatic glycogen stores are adequate. Severe, untreated hypoglycemia can cause irreversible brain damage.

PATIENT TEACHING

• Describe the different types of insulin, and make sure the patient recognizes the type ordered for him and understands his dosage regimen.
• Explain the importance of frequent laboratory and urine analyses.

interferon alfa-2b, recombinant (IFN-alpha 2b)
Intron A

Pharmacologic class: biological response modifier
Therapeutic class: antineoplastic
Pregnancy risk category: C
pH: 6.9 to 7.5

INDICATIONS & DOSAGES
➤ **Adjuvant to surgical treatment in patients with malignant melanoma who are free from disease immediately after surgery but at high risk for systemic recurrence for up to 8 weeks after surgery—**
Adults: Initially 20 million IU/m² daily by I.V. infusion 5 consecutive days weekly for 4 weeks, followed by maintenance dose of 10 million IU/m² S.C. three times weekly for 48 weeks.

ADMINISTRATION
Direct injection: Not recommended; solution for injection shouldn't be used for I.V. treatment of melanoma.
Intermittent infusion: Infuse appropriate dose, diluted to not less than 100,000 units/ml, over 20 minutes.
Continuous infusion: Not recommended.

PREPARATION & STORAGE
Available as powder for injection at 3 million, 5 million, 10 million, 18 million, 25 million, and 50 million IU/vial.
Reconstitute with recommended amount of diluent according to manufacturer's instructions. Further dilute appropriate dose with 100 ml of normal saline injection to yield not less than 100,000 IU/ml.
Store powder, both before and after reconstitution, between 36° and 46° F (2° and 8° C); stable for 30 days.

Incompatibilities
Dextrose solutions.

CONTRAINDICATIONS & CAUTIONS
• Avoid use in those with decompensated liver disease or immunosuppression after transplant.
• Rule out autoimmune chronic active hepatitis before giving interferon alfa-2b because this drug may cause life-threatening exacerbation of this condition.
• Use cautiously in those with debilitating diseases such as cardiac disease, pulmonary disease, or diabetes mellitus and in those with severe renal disease, seizure disorders, thyroid disorders, brain metastases, or compromised CNS.
• Patients with underlying massive hemangiomas may be at increased risk for substantial hemodynamic changes during therapy.

ADVERSE REACTIONS
CNS: *amnesia,* anxiety, *confusion, depression, suicidal behavior, difficulty in thinking or concentrating, dizziness, fatigue, hypoesthesia, insomnia, malaise,* nervousness, *paresthesia, somnolence,* weakness.
CV: *arrhythmias,* cardiomyopathy, flushing, *chest pain,* edema, hypotension.
EENT: hearing disorders, *nasal congestion,* pharyngitis, rhinitis, *sinusitis,* stye, visual disturbances.
GI: abdominal pain, *anorexia,* constipation, *diarrhea, dry mouth, dyspepsia,* eructation, *nausea,* stomatitis, *vomiting.*
GU: transient impotence.
Hematologic: anemia, *leukopenia, thrombocytopenia.*
Musculoskeletal: *arthralgia, asthenia, back pain.*
Respiratory: *coughing, dyspnea.*
Skin: *alopecia,* dermatitis, *dryness,* candidiasis, *pruritus, increased diaphoresis, rash.*

Other: *flulike signs and symptoms* (including *chills, fatigue, fever, headache,* hypothyroidism, gynecomastia, hyperthyroidism, and *muscle aches*), *rigors.*

INTERACTIONS

Drug-drug. *Aminophylline, theophylline:* May reduce theophylline clearance. Monitor patient for toxic reaction.
CNS depressants: Enhances CNS effects. Avoid using together.
Myelosuppressants, such as zidovudine: May cause synergistic adverse effects. Monitor complete blood counts closely.
Vaccines with live virus: May enhance adverse reaction to vaccine or decrease antibody response. Avoid using together.

EFFECTS ON LAB TEST RESULTS

• May increase calcium, phosphate, AST, ALT, LDH, alkaline phosphatase, triglycerides, and fasting glucose levels.
• May increase PT, INR, and PTT. May decrease hemoglobin and WBC and platelet counts.

ACTION

Appears to involve direct antiproliferative action against tumor or viral cells, inhibiting replication. Also thought to modulate host immune response by enhancing activity of macrophages and augmenting cytotoxicity of lymphocytes.

PHARMACOKINETICS

Onset and duration unknown; drug level peaks in 3 to 12 hours.
Distribution: Thought to be widely and rapidly distributed into body tissues with the highest levels in the spleen, kidney, liver, and lung; may bind to tumors; unknown if it crosses the placental barrier.
Metabolism: Primarily by the kidneys.

Excretion: Rapidly cleared after I.V. administration; half-life ranges from 3.7 to 8.5 hours.

CLINICAL CONSIDERATIONS

• Drug is isotonic.
• In patient with heart disease, monitor ECG, especially during start of therapy.
• In patient with underlying massive hemangiomas, monitor hemodynamic status closely, including blood pressure, urine output, and heart rate.
• To minimize flulike signs and symptoms, premedicate patient with acetaminophen.
• Patients should be well hydrated during therapy.
• If pulmonary function is impaired, monitor serial chest X-rays.
• Check temperature frequently. Fever is common, so report any sudden changes.
• Monitor liver function studies.
• Periodically observe for adverse CNS reactions, especially in geriatric patients.
• If patient has thrombocytopenia, inspect skin frequently for bruising; watch for signs of bleeding.
• *Alert:* Alfa interferons cause or aggravate life-threatening neuropsychiatric, autoimmune, ischemic, and infectious disorders. Patients should be monitored closely with periodic clinical and laboratory evaluations. Patients with persistently severe or worsening conditions may need to be withdrawn from therapy.

PATIENT TEACHING

• Advise patient to avoid contact with those who have a viral illness.
• Instruct patient how to maintain proper oral hygiene during treatment because the bone marrow suppressant effects may lead to microbial infection, delayed healing, and bleeding gums.
• Tell patient to have his blood tested regularly to monitor drug's effect.

Reactions may be *common,* uncommon, *life-threatening,* or COMMON AND LIFE-THREATENING.

• Advise patient to report fever, chills, unusual bleeding and bruising, chest pain, and changes in mental status.
• Instruct patient to drink 2 to 3 quarts (2 to 3 L) of fluid per day.
• Warn patient against performing tasks that require complete mental alertness, such as operating machinery or driving a motor vehicle.
• Warn patient not to change brands of interferon without consulting his prescriber because not all brands are interchangeable.

irinotecan hydrochloride
Camptosar

Pharmacologic class: topoisomerase inhibitor
Therapeutic class: antineoplastic
Pregnancy risk category: D
pH: 3 to 3.8

INDICATIONS & DOSAGES
➤ **Single agent treatment of metastatic carcinoma of the colon or rectum that has recurred or progressed after fluorouracil therapy—**
Adults: Initially, 125 mg/m² by I.V. infusion over 90 minutes. Recommended treatment is 125 mg/m² I.V. once weekly for 4 weeks, followed by 2-week rest period. Additional courses of treatment may be given q 6 weeks, with 4 weeks on and 2 weeks off therapy. Subsequent doses may be adjusted to a minimum of 50 mg/m² or a maximum of 150 mg/m² in 25- to 50-mg/m² increments, depending on patient tolerance.
➤ **First-line therapy for metastatic colorectal cancer with 5-fluorouracil (5-FU) and leucovorin—**
Regimen 1
Adults: 125 mg/m² I.V. over 90 minutes on days 1, 8, 15, and 22; then leucovorin 20 mg/m² I.V. bolus on days 1, 8,

15, and 22 and 5-FU 500 mg/m² I.V. bolus on days 1, 8, 15, and 22.
Adjust-a-dose: During a course of therapy, for patients with absolute neutrophil count (ANC) of 1,000 to 1,499/mm³ or four to six more stools per day than baseline, decrease irinotecan dose to 100 mg/m² and 5-FU dose to 400 mg/m² and continue leucovorin at 20 mg/m².
For patients with ANC of 500 to 999/mm³ or seven to nine more stools per day than baseline, omit one dose; then decrease irinotecan dose to 100 mg/m² and 5-FU dose to 400 mg/m² and continue leucovorin at 20 mg/m² once ANC increases to 1,000/mm³ or more and stools decrease to less than seven per day.
For patients with ANC less than 500/mm³ or 10 or more stools per day than baseline, omit one dose; then decrease irinotecan dose to 75 mg/m² and 5-FU dose to 300 mg/m² and continue leucovorin at 20 mg/m² once ANC increases to 1,000/mm³ or more and stools decrease to less than seven per day.
For patients with neutropenic fever, omit one dose; then decrease irinotecan dose to 75 mg/m² and 5-FU dose to 300 mg/m² and continue leucovorin at 20 mg/m² once neutropenic fever is resolved.
At the beginnning of subsequent courses of therapy, for patients with ANC of 500 to 999/mm³ or seven to nine more stools per day than baseline, decrease irinotecan dose to 100 mg/m² and 5-FU dose to 400 mg/m² and continue leucovorin at 20 mg/m². For patients with ANC less than 500/mm³, neutropenic fever, or 10 or more stools per day than baseline, decrease irinotecan dose to 75 mg/m² and 5-FU dose to 300 mg/m² and continue leucovorin at 20 mg/m².
Regimen 2
Adults: 180 mg/m² I.V. over 90 minutes on days 1, 15, and 29; then leucovorin

200 mg/m^2 I.V. over 2 hours on days 1, 2, 15, 16, 29, and 30; then 5-FU 400 mg/m^2 I.V. bolus on days 1, 2, 15, 16, 29, and 30 and 5-FU 600 mg/m^2 I.V. infusion over 22 hours on days 1, 2, 15, 16, 29, and 30.

Adjust-a-dose: During a course of therapy, for patients with ANC of 1,000 to 1,499/mm^3 or four to six more stools per day than baseline, decrease irinotecan dose to 150 mg/m^2, 5-FU bolus dose to 320 mg/m^2, and 5-FU infusion dose to 480 mg/m^2, and continue leucovorin at 200 mg/m^2.

For patients with ANC of 500 to 999/mm^3 or seven to nine more stools per day than baseline, omit one dose; then decrease irinotecan dose to 150 mg/m^2, 5-FU bolus dose to 320 mg/m^2, and 5-FU infusion to 480 mg/m^2, and continue leucovorin at 200 mg/m^2 once ANC increases to 1,000/mm^3 or more and stools decrease to less than seven per day.

For patients with ANC less than 500/mm^3 or 10 or more stools per day than baseline, omit one dose; then decrease irinotecan dose to 120 mg/m^2, 5-FU bolus dose to 240 mg/m^2, and 5-FU infusion to 360 mg/m^2, and continue leucovorin at 200 mg/m^2 once ANC increases to 1,000/mm^3 or more and stools decrease to less than seven per day.

For patients with neutropenic fever, omit one dose; then decrease irinotecan dose to 120 mg/m^2, 5-FU bolus to 240 mg/m^2, and 5-FU infusion to 360 mg/m^2; then continue leucovorin at 200 mg/m^2 once neutropenic fever is resolved.

At the beginning of subsequent courses of therapy, for patients with ANC of 500 to 999/mm^3 or seven to nine more stools per day than baseline, decrease irinotecan dose to 150 mg/m^2, 5-FU bolus dose to 320 mg/m^2, and 5-FU infusion to 480 mg/m^2, and continue leucovorin at 200 mg/m^2. For patients with ANC less than 500/mm^3,

neutropenic fever, or 10 or more stools per day than baseline, decrease irinotecan dose to 120 mg/m^2, 5-FU bolus dose to 240 mg/m^2, and 5-FU infusion to 360 mg/m^2, and continue leucovorin at 200 mg/m^2.

ADMINISTRATION
Direct injection: Not recommended.
Intermittent infusion: Infuse appropriate dose, diluted to 0.12 to 2.8 mg/ml, over 90 minutes.
Continuous infusion: Not recommended.

PREPARATION & STORAGE
Available as 2-ml or 5-ml vials. Each milliliter contains 20 mg irinotecan.

Dilute irinotecan for injection (5-ml vial containing 20 mg/ml) with D$_5$W injection or normal saline injection to 0.12 to 2.8 mg/ml. Most commonly, irinotecan has been given in 500 ml of D$_5$W.

Solution is stable for up to 24 hours at room temperature and in ambient fluorescent lighting. If diluted in D$_5$W, protect from light. Refrigerated at 36° to 46° F (2° to 8° C), the solution is stable for 48 hours. Because of possible microbial contamination during dilution, the manufacturer recommends use within 24 hours if refrigerated and 6 hours if at room temperature. Don't freeze. Store the undiluted vial at room temperature (59° to 86° F [15° to 30° C]), protect from light, and leave packaged in plastic blister backing in the carton.

Incompatibilities
Other I.V. drugs.

CONTRAINDICATIONS & CAUTIONS
• Contraindicated in those hypersensitive to the drug.
• Use cautiously in geriatric patients and in those who have acute infection, a GI disorder, or diarrhea.

• Use cautiously in those with renal or hepatic function impairment because safety and efficacy in these patients haven't been established.
• Use cautiously in those who have received pelvic or abdominal irradiation because they're at increased risk for myelosuppression.

ADVERSE REACTIONS

CNS: *fever, akathisia, asthenia, dizziness, headache, pain, insomnia.*
CV: *edema, vasodilation.*
EENT: *rhinitis.*
GI: *abdominal cramping and pain, abdominal enlargement, anorexia, constipation,* DIARRHEA, *dyspepsia, flatulence, nausea, stomatitis, vomiting.*
Hematologic: *anemia, **leukopenia, neutropenia.***
Metabolic: *dehydration, weight loss.*
Musculoskeletal: *back pain.*
Respiratory: *coughing, dyspnea.*
Skin: *alopecia, rash, sweating.*
Other: *chills, minor infection.*

INTERACTIONS

Drug-drug. *Antineoplastics:* May cause additive adverse effects, such as myelosuppression and diarrhea. Monitor patient closely.
Dexamethasone: May increase risk of lymphocytopenia and hyperglycemia. Monitor patient closely.
Diuretics: Increases risk of dehydration secondary to vomiting and diarrhea. Consider holding diuretics during irinotecan dosing and during active vomiting and diarrhea.
Laxatives: Worsens diarrhea. Avoid using together.
Drug-herb. *St. John's wort:* May decrease blood levels of irinotecan by about 40%.

EFFECTS ON LAB TEST RESULTS

• May increase alkaline phosphatase and AST levels.
• May decrease hemoglobin and WBC and neutrophil counts.

ACTION

Interacts with the enzyme topoisomerase I, which relieves torsional strain in DNA by inducing reversible single-strand breaks. Irinotecan and its active metabolite bind to the topoisomerase I-DNA complex and prevent religation of these single-strand breaks.

PHARMACOKINETICS

Maximum metabolite levels generally occur within 1 hour after the end of a 90-minute infusion.
Distribution: 30% to 60% protein bound (albumin), whereas its metabolite, SN-38, is 95% bound.
Metabolism: Conversion to SN-38 is mediated by carboxylesterase enzymes and occurs primarily in the liver.
Excretion: In urine, 11% to 20% of drug is unchanged, less than 1% is SN-38, and 3% is an SN-38 glucuronide; terminal half-life, about 10 hours.

CLINICAL CONSIDERATIONS

• Wear gloves when handling and preparing infusion solutions. If drug contacts skin, wash thoroughly with soap and water. If it contacts mucous membranes, flush thoroughly with water.
• Watch for irritation and infiltration; extravasation can cause tissue damage and necrosis. If extravasation occurs, flush site with sterile water and apply ice.
• Premedicate patient with antiemetics, starting at least 30 minutes before giving irinotecan.
• Monitoring of WBC count with differential, hemoglobin, and platelet count is recommended before each dose is given. If absolute neutrophil count drops below 500/mm^3, adjust dosage as recommended. If WBC count falls below 2,000/mm^3, neutrophil count is below 1,000/mm^3, hemoglobin is below 8 g/dl, or platelet

count is below 100,000/mm³, reduce
dosage.
• Drug can induce severe diarrhea.
Diarrhea occurring within 24 hours of
administration may be preceded by
diaphoresis and abdominal cramping.
If not contraindicated, may treat with
0.25 to 1 mg of atropine I.V.
• Pleural effusion or ascites may increase
the risk of neutropenia or diarrhea.
• Promptly treat late diarrhea (occurring more than 24 hours after irinotecan administration) with loperamide.
Monitor patient for dehydration, electrolyte imbalance, or sepsis and treat
appropriately. Delay subsequent
irinotecan treatments until normal bowel function returns for at least 24 hours
without antidiarrhea medication. If
grade 2, 3, or 4 late diarrhea occurs,
decrease subsequent doses of irinotecan within the current cycle.
• Observe I.V. site carefully.
• Routine administration of a colony-
stimulating factor is unnecessary, but it
may be helpful in patients experiencing
significant neutropenia.
• Diuretic therapy may be withheld to
decrease risk of dehydration.
• Signs and symptoms of overdose are
similar to those with recommended
dosage and regimen.

PATIENT TEACHING
• Advise any woman of childbearing
age to avoid pregnancy and breast-
feeding during treatment.
• Instruct patient to report any of the
following: diarrhea for the first time
during treatment; black or bloody
stools; symptoms of dehydration, such
as light-headedness, dizziness, or faintness; inability to take fluids by mouth
because of nausea or vomiting; inability to control diarrhea within 24 hours;
or fever or evidence of infection.
• Warn patient that alopecia may occur.

iron dextran injection
DexFerrum, InFeD

Pharmacologic class: parenteral
iron supplement
Therapeutic class: hematinic
Pregnancy risk category: C
pH: 5.2 to 6.5

INDICATIONS & DOSAGES
➤ **Iron-deficiency anemias—**
Adults and children: See manufacturer's dosage table.
➤ **Iron replacement resulting from
blood loss—**
Adults and children: Replacement iron
(in milligrams) equals blood loss (in
milliliters) multiplied by hematocrit.

ADMINISTRATION
Direct injection: After initial test dose,
give undiluted dose of 2 ml (or less)
over at least 2 minutes.
Intermittent infusion: Not recommended.
Continuous infusion: Not recommended.

PREPARATION & STORAGE
Available as a dark brown, slightly viscous liquid in 2-ml ampules containing
a 50-mg/ml concentration. Give undiluted.
    Store at room temperature, 59° to
86° F (15° to 30° C).

Incompatibilities
Other I.V. drugs, parenteral nutrition
solutions for I.V. infusion.

CONTRAINDICATIONS & CAUTIONS
• Contraindicated in those hypersensitive to iron and in infants age 4 months
or younger.
• Contraindicated in those with hemochromatosis or hemosiderosis because
existing iron load may increase; in

those with acute renal infection because of impaired metabolism; and in those who have had multiple blood transfusions because erythrocytes contain considerable iron.

● Avoid use with oral iron preparations because of possible overdose.

● Avoid use in those with anemia that isn't caused by iron deficiency because drug won't help.

● Use extremely cautiously in those with hepatic impairment because of delayed metabolism, and in those with rheumatoid arthritis because drug may cause fever and trigger or worsen joint pain and swelling.

● Use cautiously and only after test dose in those with a history of significant allergies or asthma because of possible hypersensitivity.

ADVERSE REACTIONS

CNS: disorientation, dizziness, headache, numbness, paresthesia, *seizures,* syncope, unresponsiveness.

CV: *arrhythmias,* chest pain or tightness, hypertension, hypotension, *shock,* tachycardia.

GI: abdominal pain, diarrhea, *nausea, vomiting.*

GU: hematuria.

Hematologic: leukocytosis, *lymphadenopathy.*

Musculoskeletal: arthralgia, *arthritis.*

Respiratory: *bronchospasm,* dyspnea.

Skin: pruritus, purpura, urticaria.

Other: *anaphylaxis, local phlebitis.*

INTERACTIONS

Drug-drug. *Chloramphenicol:* May delay the reticulocyte response to iron dextran injection. Monitor patient closely.

Oral iron: Has additive effects. Monitor patient closely.

Penicillamine: May diminish drug effects. Give 2 hours apart from iron dextran.

Vitamin E: May impair hematologic response in iron-deficiency anemia. May need to increase vitamin dose.

EFFECTS ON LAB TEST RESULTS

● May increase WBC count.

● May cause false increases in bilirubin level. May cause false decreases in calcium level. May yield unreliable bone marrow iron level because residual iron dextran may remain in reticuloendothelial cells.

ACTION

Essential for hemoglobin formation, effective erythropoiesis and, ultimately, the blood's oxygen transport capacity. May promote synthesis of myoglobin or nonhemoglobin heme units.

PHARMACOKINETICS

Levels peak immediately upon administration.

Distribution: In reticuloendothelial system, with high levels in the liver, spleen, and bone marrow. Small amounts of iron cross the placental barrier. Small amounts of drug appear in breast milk.

Metabolism: By reticuloendothelial cells, which separate iron from dextran, allowing iron to become part of body stores. Ferric iron, slowly released into plasma, combines with transferrin for transport to bone marrow, where it's incorporated into hemoglobin.

Excretion: Not easily eliminated. Small amounts are lost in shed skin, hair, and nails and in perspiration. Trace amounts of unmetabolized drug appear in bile, feces, and urine. Half-life, 5 to 20 hours.

CLINICAL CONSIDERATIONS

● Osmolality: 2,000 mOsm/kg.

● *Alert:* Because of the risk of anaphylaxis, inject test dose of 0.5 ml (25 mg) over 5 minutes. Observe patient for 1 hour; if no adverse reactions, proceed with full dose.

• Keep epinephrine and resuscitation equipment readily available to treat possible anaphylaxis.
• Maximum daily dose shouldn't exceed 2 ml undiluted iron dextran.
• Adverse reactions may worsen CV complications in those with CV disease.
• I.V. route is used only when oral route is unsatisfactory or impossible or when iron stores need to be replenished rapidly.
• Make sure diagnosis of iron-deficiency anemia is definitive before giving drug. Otherwise, excess iron storage, hemosiderosis, or iron toxicity may occur.
• Delayed reactions of 1 or 2 days are more common with parenteral administration. Such delayed reactions include arthralgia, backache, chills, dizziness, headache, malaise, moderate to high fever, myalgia, nausea, and vomiting.
• Because toxic reaction may not cause acute signs, monitor ferritin level, hemoglobin, hematocrit, and reticulocyte count. Late-occurring signs and symptoms of toxic reaction include bluish lips, fingernails, and palms; drowsiness; pale, clammy skin; tachycardia; and unusual tiredness or weakness.
• Hemodialysis removes only negligible amounts of drug.
• Acute overdose requires immediate medical treatment.

PATIENT TEACHING
• Warn patient not to take OTC vitamin preparations containing iron.
• Tell patient to keep iron preparations away from children.
• Stress to the patient the importance of complying with his dosage regimen to enhance therapeutic effectiveness.
• Review with the patient the components of a nutritious diet.

iron sucrose injection
Venofer

Pharmacologic class: parenteral iron supplement
Therapeutic class: hematinic
Pregnancy risk category: B
pH: 10.5 to 11.1

INDICATIONS & DOSAGES
➤ **Iron-deficiency anemia in patients undergoing long-term hemodialysis who are receiving supplemental erythropoietin therapy—**
Adults: 100 mg (5 ml) of elemental iron I.V. in the dialysis line, either by slow injection at a rate of 1 ml/minute or by infusion over 15 minutes during the dialysis session, one to three times a week for a total of 1,000 mg in 10 doses; repeat p.r.n.

ADMINISTRATION
Direct injection: Give undiluted directly in the dialysis line, by slow injection at a rate of 1 ml/minute (20 mg elemental iron), not exceeding 1 vial (100 mg elemental iron) per injection.
Intermittent infusion: Infuse into dialysis line at a rate of 100 mg elemental iron over 15 minutes during the dialysis session.
Continuous infusion: Not recommended.

PREPARATION & STORAGE
Available as a 5-ml single-dose vial. Each vial contains 100 mg of elemental iron (20 mg/ml).
   Inspect drug for precipitate and discoloration before administration. For direct injection into the dialysis line, give drug undiluted. For infusion, dilute drug with a maximum of 100 ml normal saline solution immediately before infusion.

Reactions may be *common,* uncommon, *life-threatening,* or COMMON AND LIFE-THREATENING.

Store vials in their original cartons at room temperature. Don't freeze. Discard any unused portions.

Incompatibilities
Other I.V. drugs, parenteral nutrition solutions of I.V. infusion.

CONTRAINDICATIONS & CAUTIONS
• Contraindicated in patients hypersensitive to drug or its components and in those with signs or symptoms of iron overload or anemia not caused by iron deficiency.
• It's unknown if drug appears in breast milk. Use cautiously in breast-feeding women.
• Dose selection in elderly patients should be in the low range because of decreased hepatic, renal, or cardiac function; other diseases; and simultaneous drug therapies.

ADVERSE REACTIONS
CNS: fever, headache, asthenia, malaise, dizziness, pain.
CV: *hypotension,* chest pain, hypertension, fluid retention, *heart failure.*
GI: nausea, vomiting, diarrhea, abdominal pain, taste perversion.
Musculoskeletal: *leg cramps,* bone and muscle pain.
Respiratory: dyspnea, pneumonia, cough.
Skin: pruritus, site reaction.
Other: accidental injury, *anaphylactoid reactions, fatal hypersensitivity reactions, sepsis.*

INTERACTIONS
Drug-drug. *Oral iron preparations:* May reduce absorption of oral iron preparations. Avoid using together.

EFFECTS ON LAB TEST RESULTS
• May increase liver enzyme levels.

ACTION
An exogenous source of iron that is essential to the synthesis of hemoglobin,

which replenishes depleted body iron stores of ferritin and iron.

PHARMACOKINETICS
Duration varies, depending on level of iron deficiency.
Distribution: Mainly in the blood and extravascular fluid. Also in the spleen, liver, and bone marrow. The bone marrow is an iron-trapping compartment and not a reversible source of distribution.
Metabolism: Iron sucrose is dissociated by the reticuloendothelial system into iron and sucrose.
Excretion: The sucrose component and about 5% of the iron component are excreted in urine.

CLINICAL CONSIDERATIONS
• Osmolarity: 1,250 mOsm/L.
• *Alert:* Rare but fatal hypersensitivity reactions characterized by anaphylactic shock, loss of consciousness, collapse, hypotension, dyspnea, or seizure have occurred. Monitor patient for these signs or symptoms.
• *Alert:* Emergency resuscitative equipment must be readily available during administration.
• Giving drug by infusion may reduce the risk of hypotension.
• Withhold dose in patients with signs and symptoms of iron overload.
• Monitor hematocrit and hemoglobin, ferritin, and transferrin saturation levels.
• Transferrin saturation levels increase rapidly after I.V. administration of iron sucrose. Obtain iron levels 48 hours after delivery.
• Overdose may lead to accumulation of iron in storage sites, leading to hemosiderosis. Periodically monitoring ferritin and transferrin saturation will help recognize iron accumulation.
• Signs and symptoms linked to overdose or too-rapid drug infusion include hypotension, headache, vomiting, nausea, dizziness, joint aches, paresthesia, abdominal and muscle pain, edema,

and CV collapse. Stop or reduce drug dosage and offer appropriate treatment if such signs or symptoms occur.

PATIENT TEACHING
• Instruct patient to notify prescriber if headache, nausea, dizziness, joint aches, tingling, or abdominal and muscle pain occurs.

isoproterenol hydrochloride
Isuprel

Pharmacologic class: adrenergic
Therapeutic class: bronchodilator, cardiac stimulant
Pregnancy risk category: C
pH: 2.5 to 4.5

INDICATIONS & DOSAGES
➤ **Bronchospasm during anesthesia—**
Adults: 0.01 to 0.02 mg I.V. (0.5 to 1 ml of a 1:50,000 dilution).
➤ **Arrhythmias—**
Adults: 0.02 to 0.06 mg by I.V. bolus (1 to 3 ml of a 1:50,000 dilution) initially; then 0.01 to 0.2 mg I.V. (0.5 to 10 ml of a 1:50,000 dilution).
Children: 2.5 mcg/minute by I.V. infusion. Adjust subsequent doses based on patient response.
➤ **Shock—**
Adults: 0.5 to 5 mcg/minute by I.V. infusion. In advanced shock, give 5 to 30 mcg/minute.
➤ **Status asthmaticus ♦ —**
Children: 0.08 to 1.7 mcg/kg/minute by I.V. infusion.
➤ **Bradycardia in postoperative cardiac patients ♦ —**
Children: 0.029 mcg/kg/minute by I.V. infusion.
➤ **As an aid in diagnosing the cause of mitral regurgitation ♦ —**
Adults: 4 mcg/minute by I.V. infusion.

➤ **As an aid in diagnosing coronary artery disease or lesions ♦ —**
Adults: 1 to 3 mcg/minute by I.V. infusion.

ADMINISTRATION
Direct injection: Inject diluted solution (1:50,000) directly into vein or into an I.V. line containing a free-flowing, compatible solution. Usual initial dose, 1 to 3 ml (20 to 60 mcg).
Intermittent infusion: Not recommended.
Continuous infusion: Using an infusion pump, give appropriate dose and dilution (1:250,000) at ordered rate. Usual initial dose, 5 mcg/minute (1.25 ml/minute).

PREPARATION & STORAGE
Available in a dilution of 1:5,000 in 1-ml (0.2-mg) and 5-ml (1-mg) ampules and in 5-ml (1-mg) and 10-ml (2-mg) vials.
    For direct injection, add 1 ml of isoproterenol to 10 ml of normal saline solution or D_5W to yield a 1:50,000 dilution (20 mcg/ml). For infusion, dilute 10 ml of isoproterenol with 500 ml of D_5W to yield a dilution of 1:5,000 (2 mg in 500 ml).
    Drug is also compatible with lactated Ringer's solution and dextrose 5% in lactated Ringer's solution.
    Store in a cool place, protect from light, and keep in an opaque container until used. Don't use if pink or brown or if a precipitate forms.

Incompatibilities
Alkalies, aminophylline, furosemide, metals, sodium bicarbonate.

CONTRAINDICATIONS & CAUTIONS
• Contraindicated in those hypersensitive to sympathomimetics or isoproterenol.
• Contraindicated in those with tachyarrhythmias, especially ventricular

---

Reactions may be *common*, uncommon, *life-threatening*, or COMMON AND LIFE-THREATENING.

tachycardia and arrhythmias that require increased inotropic activity.
• Avoid use in shock patients who haven't received fluid replacement.
• Avoid use in those with uncorrected hypoxia, acidosis, hypokalemia, hyperkalemia, or hypercapnia because drug may have reduced effects or may increase risk of adverse reactions.
• Use cautiously in geriatric patients and in those with CV disease, hyperthyroidism, or cardiac glycoside–induced tachycardia because of increased risk of adverse CV effects.
• Use cautiously in those hypersensitive to sulfites if isoproterenol preparation contains this element, in those with Parkinson's disease because drug may temporarily worsen symptoms, and in those with diabetes mellitus. Dosage of insulin or antidiabetic may need to be adjusted.

ADVERSE REACTIONS
CNS: *Stokes-Adams seizures,* dizziness, headache, tremor, weakness.
CV: angina, *arrhythmias,* hypertension, flushing, hypotension, palpitations, tachycardia.
GI: nausea, vomiting.
Skin: sweating.
Other: *anaphylaxis.*

INTERACTIONS
Drug-drug. *Antihypertensives, nitrates:* Reduces effects. Dosage may need to be adjusted.
Beta blockers: Inhibits effects of isoproterenol and beta blockers. Monitor patient closely.
Cardiac glycosides: May increase risk of cardiac arrhythmias. Monitor patient closely.
CNS stimulants: Causes excessive stimulation. Avoid using together.
Epinephrine, sympathomimetics: Causes severe arrhythmias. Separate doses by at least 4 hours.

Inhalation hydrocarbon anesthetics: Causes severe arrhythmias. Avoid using together.
Levodopa: Causes arrhythmias. Monitor patient closely.
MAO inhibitors, tricyclic antidepressants: Causes arrhythmias, tachycardia, severe hypertension. Avoid using together.
Oxytocic drugs: May cause severe, persistent hypertension and cerebral hemorrhage. Monitor patient closely.
Thyroid hormones: May increase effects of both drugs; may increase risk of coronary insufficiency in those with coronary artery disease. Monitor patient closely.
Xanthines: May enhance CNS effects. Monitor patient closely.

EFFECTS ON LAB TEST RESULTS
• May increase glucose level.

ACTION
Sympathomimetic amine acts predominantly on beta$_2$ receptors in smooth muscle and blood vessels. Its direct action on the heart causes tachycardia, elevated systolic pressure from increased contractility and cardiac output, and diminished diastolic pressure from arteriolar dilation and reduced peripheral vascular resistance.
Drug also relaxes bronchial smooth muscle, thereby relieving bronchospasm, increasing vital capacity, and reducing residual volume.

PHARMACOKINETICS
Onset, immediately upon administration; duration, less than 1 hour.
Distribution: Throughout the body. It's unknown if drug appears in breast milk.
Metabolism: Mostly in liver and lungs, and in other tissues by the enzyme catechol *O*-methyltransferase. Metabolized more rapidly and extensively in children.

Excretion: In urine, with 40% to 50% removed unchanged and the remainder excreted as the metabolite 3-*O*-methylisoproterenol. In children, small amounts of unidentified metabolites appear in feces. About 75% of drug is excreted within 15 hours.

CLINICAL CONSIDERATIONS
• Osmolality: 277 to 293 mOsm/kg.
• Adjust infusion rate according to heart rate and blood pressure.
• In those with cardiac arrest, arrhythmias, shock, or heart block, closely observe ECG to help adjust dosage.
• Monitor bicarbonate level and pH. For shock patients, also monitor central venous pressure, heart rate, blood pressure, and urine output.
• With high doses, systolic pressure falls because of marked reduction in peripheral vascular resistance.
• Drug may aggravate ventilation-perfusion abnormalities.
• Consider giving sedatives to reduce CNS stimulation.
• Drug isn't useful if peripheral vascular bed is already dilated.
• Lower dosages are recommended for geriatric patients.
• Signs and symptoms of overdose include severe, persistent chest pain and irregular heartbeat, elevated blood pressure, headache, and dizziness. If any of these occur, stop drug immediately. Cumulative effects haven't been reported.

PATIENT TEACHING
• Discuss signs and symptoms of adverse reactions and have patient report them promptly.
• Explain use and administration of drug to patient and family.

K

kanamycin sulfate
Kantrex, Kantrex Pediatric

Pharmacologic class: aminoglycoside
Therapeutic class: bactericidal antibiotic
Pregnancy risk category: D
pH: 4.5

INDICATIONS & DOSAGES
➤ **Severe infections caused by susceptible organisms—**
Adults, children, and infants with normal renal function: 15 mg/kg I.V. daily in equally divided doses at 8- or 12-hour intervals.
Infants age 7 days or younger, weighing 2 kg (4.4 lb) or less: 15 mg/kg I.V. daily in equally divided doses q 12 hours.
Infants age 7 days or younger, weighing more than 2 kg: 20 mg/kg I.V. daily in equally divided doses q 12 hours.
Adjust-a-dose: In patients with renal impairment, adjust dosage or frequency in response to drug level and the degree of renal impairment. If unable to obtain drug levels, calculate frequency of doses (in hours) by multiplying creatinine level (mg/dl) by 9.
➤ **As part of a multiple-drug regimen to treat *Mycobacterium avium* complex in AIDS patients** ◆ —
Adults: 11 to 13 mg/kg/day I.V.
Adjust-a-dose. In patients receiving hemodialysis or peritoneal dialysis, give supplemental dose of 50% to 75% initial loading dose at the end of dialysis period.

ADMINISTRATION
Direct injection: Not recommended.
Intermittent infusion: Using an appropriate dilution, infuse drug over 30 to 60 minutes.
Continuous infusion: Not recommended.

PREPARATION & STORAGE
Available in 3-ml vials containing 1 g (333 mg/ml), 2-ml vials and disposable syringes containing 500 mg (250 mg/ml), and 2-ml vials containing (pediatric strength) 75 mg (37.5 mg/ml).
 For infusion, mix 100 to 200 ml of D_5W or normal saline solution with contents of 500-mg vial, or mix 200 to 400 ml with contents of 1-g vial. Children require a proportionately smaller diluent volume.
 Store between 59° and 86° F (15° and 30° C). Solution remains stable for 24 hours at room temperature. Protect from freezing. Darkened vial doesn't indicate loss of potency.

Incompatibilities
Amphotericin B, ampicillin sodium, antibacterials, cefotaxime, cefotetan, cephapirin, chlorpheniramine, colistimethate, heparin sodium, hydrocortisone sodium succinate, methohexital, penicillin G sodium, phenobarbital, phenytoin, piperacillin sodium.

CONTRAINDICATIONS & CAUTIONS
• Contraindicated in those hypersensitive to kanamycin or other aminoglycosides.
• Use cautiously in those with myasthenia gravis, infant botulism, or parkinsonism because drug may cause neuromuscular blockade, worsening weakness.

• Use cautiously in patients with renal impairment.

• Use cautiously in geriatric patients—especially those with tinnitus, vertigo, or subclinical deafness—because of increased risk of hearing loss.

• Use cautiously in patients who previously received ototoxic drugs and in those receiving a total dose of 15 g or more.

• Use cautiously in those with cranial nerve VIII dysfunction because of heightened risk of ototoxicity and in those with renal impairment because of risk of nephrotoxicity. Reduce daily dose and lengthen interval between doses.

• Use cautiously in premature infants and neonates because of immature renal function.

ADVERSE REACTIONS

CNS: confusion, disorientation, headache, lethargy, *vertigo.*
CV: hypertension, hypotension, palpitations.
EENT: *ototoxicity, tinnitus,* visual disturbances.
GI: anorexia, diarrhea, nausea, vomiting.
GU: *nephrotoxicity.*
Hematologic: *hemolytic anemia,* leukemic reaction, *pancytopenia.*
Hepatic: *hepatotoxicity,* hepatomegaly.
Metabolic: weight loss.
Other: *anaphylaxis, superinfections.*

INTERACTIONS

Drug-drug. *Antihistamines, loxapine, phenothiazines, thioxanthenes:* May mask signs of ototoxicity. Monitor patient closely.
Antimyasthenics: Antagonizes antimyasthenic effects on skeletal muscles. Adjust dosage.
Beta-lactam antibiotics, vancomycin: Has additive or synergistic effects against certain organisms. Monitor therapeutic effect closely.

Chloramphenicol, clindamycin, tetracycline: May antagonize bactericidal activity. Monitor therapeutic effect closely.
Citrated blood, general anesthetics, neuromuscular blockers, opioid analgesics: Potentiates neuromuscular blockade, causing respiratory depression and paralysis. Avoid using together.
Diuretics (parenteral), such as ethacrynic acid, furosemide, mannitol: May cause rapid loss of hearing and renal impairment. Avoid using together.
Indomethacin (parenteral): Decreases clearance of kanamycin and increases risk of toxic reaction. Monitor patient closely.
Methoxyflurane, polymyxins: May increase risk of nephrotoxicity and neuromuscular blockade. Avoid using together.
Nephrotoxic, neurotoxic, and ototoxic drugs: May increase risk of toxic reaction. Use together cautiously, and monitor patient closely.
Penicillins (broad-spectrum): Has synergistic effects against some *Enterobacteriaceae.* Monitor therapeutic effect closely.

EFFECTS ON LAB TEST RESULTS

• May increase creatinine and BUN levels.
• May decrease RBC, WBC, and platelet counts.

ACTION

Inhibits protein synthesis by binding directly to the 30S ribosomal subunit in susceptible microorganisms. Drug is effective against many susceptible gram-negative and gram-positive aerobic bacteria.

PHARMACOKINETICS

Drug level peaks at about 1 hour.
Distribution: Primarily to extracellular fluids and abscess fluids and tissues. Doesn't bind to protein or reach ocular

tissue. Drug crosses the placental barrier, and small amounts appear in breast milk.

Metabolism: Not metabolized.
Excretion: In urine. Half-life is normally 2 to 4 hours; in those with severe renal impairment, 27 to 80 hours; in premature infants, about 9 hours. In patients with normal renal function, complete elimination takes 10 to 20 days.

CLINICAL CONSIDERATIONS
• Osmolality: 858 to 952 mOsm/kg.
• Check for previous aminoglycoside hypersensitivity before giving first dose.
• Collect specimens for culture and sensitivity testing before giving first dose. Therapy may begin before results are available.
• Obtain a baseline audiogram before therapy, and make sure that audiometric tests are performed during therapy. Stop drug if patient reports tinnitus or hearing difficulty, or if follow-up audiograms show high-frequency hearing loss.
• Monitor BUN and creatinine levels and urinalysis results during therapy. Stop drug if azotemia occurs or urine output declines.
• Provide adequate hydration because drug causes nephrotoxicity.
• Obtain peak and trough drug levels to adjust dosages. Coordinate specimen collection with the laboratory. For systemic infection, desirable peak levels are 15 to 30 mcg/ml and desirable trough levels are 5 to 10 mcg/ml.
• If beta-lactam antibiotics must also be given, give at a separate site. Don't mix with kanamycin or use same I.V. line.
• *Alert:* Drug may contain sulfites.
• Observe patient for superinfections during prolonged use.
• Hemodialysis or peritoneal dialysis aids drug removal. An exchange transfusion may be used in neonates.

PATIENT TEACHING
• Emphasize need for patient to complete full drug regimen.
• Alert patient to adverse reactions.
• Advise breast-feeding patient that drug may pose a risk to the infant.
• Tell patient to report any changes in hearing.

ketamine hydrochloride
Ketalar

Pharmacologic class: dissociative anesthetic
Therapeutic class: general anesthetic
Pregnancy risk category: C
pH: 3.5 to 5.5

INDICATIONS & DOSAGES
➤ **Induction of anesthesia; as sole anesthetic for diagnostic and surgical procedures (especially short ones) that don't require skeletal muscle relaxation; as a preanesthetic; as an adjunct to low-potency anesthetics, such as nitrous oxide—**
Adults: 1 to 4.5 mg/kg I.V. Or, 1 to 2 mg/kg I.V. at 0.5 mg/kg/minute, with 2 to 5 mg I.V. diazepam. Adjust dosage based on patient's response.
➤ **To maintain anesthesia—**
Adults: Slow I.V. infusion of 0.1 to 0.5 mg/minute, when induced with ketamine and augmented with I.V. diazepam.

ADMINISTRATION
Direct injection: Over 1 minute, inject initial dose directly into vein or into I.V. tubing containing a free-flowing, compatible solution.
Intermittent infusion: Not recommended.
Continuous infusion: Infuse diluted drug at 0.1 to 0.5 mg/minute.

PREPARATION & STORAGE

Available in multidose vials containing 10, 50, and 100 mg/ml.

For direct injection, dilute 100-mg/ml concentration with equal volume of sterile water for injection, normal saline solution, or D_5W. For continuous infusion, prepare a 1-mg/ml solution by adding 10 ml from the 50-mg/ml vial or 5 ml from the 100-mg/ml vial to 500 ml of D_5W or dextrose 5% in normal saline solution. If patient must restrict fluids, prepare a 2-mg/ml solution by adding 10 ml of 50 mg/ml or 5 ml of 100 mg/ml of drug to 250 ml of compatible solution.

Store at 59° to 86° F (15° to 30° C). Protect from light.

Incompatibilities

Barbiturates, diazepam, doxapram.

CONTRAINDICATIONS & CAUTIONS

• Contraindicated in those hypersensitive to drug.
• Contraindicated as the sole anesthetic for laryngeal, pharyngeal, or bronchial surgery or for diagnostic procedures because of active laryngeal and pharyngeal reflexes.
• Avoid use in those undergoing intracranial procedures and in those with an intracerebral mass or hemorrhage, increased CSF pressure, or cerebral trauma because it increases intracranial pressure.
• Avoid use in those with hypertension and in those with conditions in which an appreciable rise in blood pressure would be harmful.
• Avoid use in those undergoing eye surgery because drug commonly causes nystagmus and increases intraocular pressure.
• Use cautiously in alcoholic patients because of possible exacerbated withdrawal symptoms.
• Use cautiously in those with psychiatric disorders because of high risk of postoperative hallucinations, and in those with thyrotoxicosis because of increased risk of tachycardia and hypertension.

ADVERSE REACTIONS

CNS: uncontrolled muscle movements, visual illusions, altered body image or mood, delirium, dissociation, *severe emergence reaction* (vivid dreams or hallucinations usually limited to duration of drug effects, but flashbacks may occur for several weeks postoperatively).
CV: *bradycardia,* hypertension, hypotension, *tachycardia.*
GI: vomiting.
Respiratory: bradypnea, dyspnea, *apnea, respiratory depression.*

INTERACTIONS

Drug-drug. *Antihypertensives, CNS depressants:* May increase risk of hypotension or respiratory depression. Avoid using together.
Barbiturates, narcotics: Prolongs recovery time. Monitor patient closely.
Halogenated inhalation anesthetics: Halothane blocks the CV-stimulating effects of ketamine. May decrease cardiac output, blood pressure, and pulse rate. Use together cautiously, and monitor patient closely.
Nondepolarizing muscle relaxants: Increases neuromuscular effects, which prolongs respiratory depression. Monitor patient closely.
Theophylline: Unpredictable extensor-type seizures. Use together cautiously.
Thiopental: Antagonizes hypnotic effects of thiopental. Use together cautiously.
Thyroid hormones: Increases risk of hypertension and tachycardia. Monitor patient closely.

EFFECTS ON LAB TEST RESULTS

• May falsely increase intraocular pressure in ophthalmic examination.

ACTION
Selectively interrupts cerebral pathways, causing dissociative anesthesia.

PHARMACOKINETICS
Onset, 15 to 30 seconds; duration, 5 to 10 minutes.
Distribution: Rapidly dispersed into tissues, including brain. Drug achieves high levels in adipose tissue, liver, and lungs; crosses the placental barrier.
Metabolism: In the liver.
Excretion: About 90% removed in urine as metabolites and about 5% eliminated in feces. Half-life, 2 to 3 hours.

CLINICAL CONSIDERATIONS
• Osmolality: 300 to 387 mOsm/kg.
• Only staff specially trained in giving anesthetics and managing their adverse effects should give ketamine.
• Before giving drug, make sure patient hasn't eaten because of risk of aspirating vomitus.
• Monitor ECG during administration, especially in patients with hypertension or cardiac decompensation.
• Emergence reactions occur in about 12% of patients, but they are least common in young or geriatric patients. If severe, give a small dose of a short-acting sedative.
• Reduce risk of emergence reactions by lowering ketamine dose and giving with I.V. diazepam, and by reducing postoperative sensory stimulation.
• When using ketamine in an outpatient, don't release patient until effects wear off and then only if he's accompanied by a responsible adult.
• If overdose occurs, maintain a patent airway and provide ventilatory support until drug effects subside.

PATIENT TEACHING
• Warn patient not to drive or perform other tasks that require alertness for 24 hours because of risk of psychomotor impairment.

• Tell patient to avoid alcohol within 24 hours of receiving this drug.
• Review signs of adverse reactions with patient.

ketorolac tromethamine
Toradol

Pharmacologic class: NSAID
Therapeutic class: analgesic
Pregnancy risk category: C
pH: 6.9 to 7.9

INDICATIONS & DOSAGES
➤ **Short-term, single-dose treatment of moderately severe, acute pain—**
Adults younger than age 65: 30 mg I.V.
Adjust-a-dose: In adults age 65 and older, in renally impaired patients, and in those weighing less than 50 kg (110 lb), give 15 mg I.V.
➤ **Short-term, multidose treatment of moderately severe, acute pain—**
Adults younger than age 65: 30 mg I.V. q 6 hours, not to exceed 120 mg/day.
Adjust-a-dose: In adults age 65 and older, in renally impaired patients, and in those weighing less than 50 kg (110 lb), give 15 mg I.V. q 6 hours, not to exceed 60 mg/day.

ADMINISTRATION
Direct injection: Give over at least 15 seconds.
Intermittent infusion: Not recommended.
Continuous infusion: Not recommended.

PREPARATION & STORAGE
Available as solution in sterile water for injection and alcohol, containing 15 mg/ml (in 1-ml vial or syringe) or 30 mg/ml (1-ml or 2-ml vial or 1-ml syringe).
    Store at 59° to 86° F (15° to 30° C), and protect from light.

Incompatibilities
Haloperidal lactate; nalbuphine; solutions that result in a relatively low pH, such as hydroxyzine, meperidine, morphine sulfate, and prochlorperazine; thiethylperazine.

CONTRAINDICATIONS & CAUTIONS
• Contraindicated in those hypersensitive to drug.
• Contraindicated in patients with advanced renal impairment or risk for renal impairment caused by volume depletion.
• Contraindicated as prophylactic analgesic before major surgery, intraoperatively when hemostasis is critical, for neuraxial administration, in labor and delivery, in breast-feeding patients, and in patients receiving aspirin or NSAIDs.
• Contraindicated in those with cerebrovascular bleeding, hemorrhagic diathesis, incomplete hemostasis, high risk of bleeding, history of or active peptic ulcer disease, or history of GI bleeding or perforation.
• Use cautiously in geriatric patients or those with heart failure, hepatic or renal dysfunction, history of renal disease, or extracellular fluid depletion.
• Use cautiously in those who may be adversely affected by prolonged bleeding times, in those with a history of hepatic impairment or liver disease, and in those with cardiac decompensation, hypertension, or similar conditions linked to fluid retention.

ADVERSE REACTIONS
CNS: dizziness, *drowsiness, headache, sedation.*
CV: *arrhythmias,* edema, hypertension, palpitations.
GI: constipation, diarrhea, *dyspepsia,* flatulence, GI fullness, *GI pain, nausea,* stomatitis, vomiting, **GI bleeding.**
GU: *acute renal failure.*
Hematologic: decreased platelet adhesion, purpura, *thrombocytopenia.*
Respiratory: *bronchospasm.*

Skin: diaphoresis, pruritus, rash, injection site pain.
Other: *hypersensitivity reactions.*

INTERACTIONS
Drug-drug. *ACE inhibitors:* May increase risk of renal impairment, especially in volume-depleted patients. Avoid using together in these patients.
Anticoagulants: May increase levels of unbound anticoagulants in the blood. Use together cautiously.
Antihypertensives, diuretics: Decreases effectiveness of these drugs. Monitor therapeutic effect.
Lithium: Increases lithium level. Monitor lithium level.
Methotrexate: Decreases methotrexate clearance and increases toxic effects. Avoid using together.
Probenecid: Decreases clearance and increases ketorolac levels. Avoid using together.

EFFECTS ON LAB TEST RESULTS
• May increase ALT and AST levels.
• May increase bleeding time. May decrease platelet count.

ACTION
Is thought to inhibit prostaglandin synthesis.

PHARMACOKINETICS
Onset and peak of drug effect, immediate; duration, up to 8 hours.
Distribution: Not distributed widely. Drug crosses the blood-brain barrier poorly, is more than 99% protein bound, crosses the placental barrier, and appears in small amounts in breast milk.
Metabolism: Undergoes hydroxylation in the liver.
Excretion: Mainly in the urine, with only small amounts excreted in feces; half-life in healthy adults ranges from 2.4 to 9.2 hours.

Reactions may be *common,* uncommon, *life-threatening,* or COMMON AND LIFE-THREATENING.

CLINICAL CONSIDERATIONS

• Drug is isotonic.
• Drug can mask signs and symptoms of infection because of its antipyretic and anti-inflammatory actions.
• The maximum combined duration of therapy is 5 days.
• Monitor renal function closely, including creatinine and BUN levels.
• Monitor bleeding time, and carefully observe patients with coagulopathies and those taking anticoagulants.
• Acute lethal dose is unknown. Metabolic acidosis after intentional overdose has been reported. Dialysis isn't effective in removing drug.
• *Alert:* Don't confuse Toradol (ketorolac) with Foradil (formoterol fumarate).

PATIENT TEACHING

• Teach patient the signs and symptoms of bleeding, and tell him to notify prescriber immediately if they occur.
• Explain use and administration of drug to patient and family.

L

labetalol hydrochloride
Normodyne, Trandate

Pharmacologic class: selective alpha$_1$ blocker, nonselective beta blocker
Therapeutic class: antihypertensive
Pregnancy risk category: C
pH: 3 to 4

INDICATIONS & DOSAGES
➤ **Severe hypertension and hypertensive crisis—**
Adults: Initially, 20 mg by direct I.V. injection; then 40 to 80 mg I.V. q 10 minutes. Or, may give by continuous infusion at initial rate of 2 mg/minute, with the rate of infusion adjusted according to blood pressure response. Usual dosage range is 50 to 200 mg. Maximum dose is 300 mg.
➤ **Hypotension control during halothane anesthesia—**
Adults: 10 to 25 mg I.V. after induction of anesthesia. Hypotension will then be controlled by inspired halothane.
➤ **Hypotension control with use of other anesthetics—**
Adults: Initially, 30 mg I.V.; then 5 to 10 mg I.V. if needed.

ADMINISTRATION
Direct injection: Over 2 minutes, inject directly into vein or into an I.V. line containing a free-flowing, compatible solution.
Intermittent infusion: Not recommended.
Continuous infusion: Give 2 mg/ minute until satisfactory response is obtained; then stop infusion. May repeat in 6 to 8 hours.

PREPARATION & STORAGE
Available as a clear, colorless to light-yellow solution in 20- and 40-ml multidose vials and 4- and 8-ml syringes containing 5 mg/ml.

For infusion, add 200 mg to 160 ml of compatible diluent to yield 1 mg/ml.

Compatible solutions include D_5W, normal saline solution, dextrose 2.5% in half-normal saline solution, dextrose 5% in lactated Ringer's solution, lactated Ringer's solution, dextrose 5% in normal saline solution, Ringer's solution, and dextrose 5% in Ringer's solution.

Store syringes and vials at room temperature. Diluted solutions remain stable for at least 24 hours at room temperature or when refrigerated and must be protected from light.

Incompatibilities
Alkali solutions, cefoperazone, ceftriaxone, furosemide, heparin, nafcillin, sodium bicarbonate, thiopental, warfarin.

CONTRAINDICATIONS & CAUTIONS
• Contraindicated in those with second- or third-degree heart block, overt heart failure, cardiac ischemia, cardiogenic shock, or severe bradycardia because of risk of further myocardial depression.
• Contraindicated in those with asthma or bronchospastic disease because drug may inhibit bronchodilation.
• Use cautiously in those with diabetes mellitus controlled by antidiabetics because drug may mask signs of hypoglycemia.

Reactions may be *common*, uncommon, *life-threatening*, or COMMON AND LIFE-THREATENING.

• Use cautiously in those with myasthenia gravis, depression, or psoriasis because of possible exacerbation, and in those with pheochromocytoma because of possible paradoxical hypertension.
• Use cautiously in those with hepatic impairment because of increased risk of toxic reaction.

ADVERSE REACTIONS
CNS: dizziness, numbness, tingling of skin and scalp, vertigo, paresthesia.
CV: *arrhythmias, intensified AV block, orthostatic hypotension, severe hypotension.*
GI: dyspepsia, *nausea,* vomiting.
Respiratory: *bronchospasm.*

INTERACTIONS
Drug-drug. *Antihypertensives:* Potentiates effects. Monitor patient closely.
Beta-adrenergic agonist: Blunts bronchodilating effect. May need to increase bronchodilator dose.
Halothane anesthetics: Causes synergistic myocardial depression. Use together cautiously.
Insulin, oral antidiabetics: May mask signs of hypoglycemia. May reduce insulin release in response to hyperglycemia. Dosages may need to be altered. Monitor therapeutic effects.
Nitroglycerin: Reduces reflex tachycardia and potentiated hypotension. Monitor patient closely.
Tricyclic antidepressants: Increases risk of tremor. Use together cautiously.

EFFECTS ON LAB TEST RESULTS
• May increase BUN, creatinine, transaminase, and urea levels.
• May cause false-positive evidence of amphetamine in urine and a false-positive increase in urine free and total catecholamine levels when measured by a nonspecific trihydroxyindole fluorometric method. May cause a positive titer for antinuclear antibody test. May alter intraocular pressure. May cause

bradycardia with radionuclide ventriculography.

ACTION
Competitively blocks stimulation of myocardial beta$_2$ receptors, bronchial beta$_2$ receptors, and alpha and beta$_2$ receptors of the vascular smooth muscle. Reduces blood pressure in 5 to 10 minutes and also depresses renin secretion.

PHARMACOKINETICS
Onset, 2 to 5 minutes; duration, 2 to 4 hours.
Distribution: Rapid and widespread into extravascular space, with highest levels in the lungs, liver, and kidneys. Small amounts cross the placental and blood-brain barriers and appear in breast milk.
Metabolism: Primarily in the liver through conjugation to glucuronide metabolites.
Excretion: 55% to 60% eliminated in urine within 24 hours and 30% excreted in feces within 4 days. Less than 5% excreted as unchanged drug.

CLINICAL CONSIDERATIONS
• Osmolality: 287 mOsm/kg.
• Give epinephrine or atropine to treat excessive bradycardia.
• Dialysis removes less than 1% of drug.
• Frequently monitor blood pressure. Avoid reducing blood pressure rapidly. Adjust dosage according to supine blood pressure.
• Steady-state plasma levels aren't attained during infusion. Follow with oral therapy when supine blood pressure begins to rise.
• Adjust dosage as needed in those with severe renal impairment.
• Labetalol is less likely than other beta blockers to decrease heart rate or cardiac output.
• Drug masks common signs of shock and hypoglycemia.

• For orthostatic hypotension, place patient in supine position and elevate his legs.

PATIENT TEACHING
• Advise patient that transient scalp tingling may occur during initial therapy.
• Advise patient to remain lying down for 3 hours after administration to prevent severe dizziness upon standing up.
• Tell patient the symptoms of heart failure and liver dysfunction so he can alert his prescriber if any occur.

---

leucovorin calcium (citrovorum factor, folinic acid)*

Pharmacologic class: formyl derivative (active reduced form of folic acid)
Therapeutic class: vitamin
Pregnancy risk category: C
pH: 8.1

INDICATIONS & DOSAGES
➤ **Methotrexate overdose—**
Adults: Up to 75 mg I.V. within 12 hours or a dosage sufficient to produce leucovorin calcium levels at least equal to methotrexate levels.
➤ **Hematologic toxicity caused by other folic acid antagonists, such as trimethoprim—**
Adults and children: 5 to 15 mg/day I.V.
➤ **To neutralize methotrexate's toxicity or to perform leucovorin rescue—**
Used in various I.V. regimens. Specific dosage depends on extent of systemic toxicity.
Adults and children: 10 mg/m² I.V. given q 6 hours for 10 doses starting 24 hours after the beginning of the methotrexate infusion.

➤ **Palliative treatment of advanced colorectal cancer—**
Adults: 20 mg/m² I.V. followed by 425 mg/m² of I.V. fluorouracil, or 200 mg/m² followed by 370 mg/m² of I.V. fluorouracil, daily for 5 consecutive days. Repeat at 4-week intervals for two additional courses; then repeat at intervals of 4 to 5 weeks if tolerated.

ADMINISTRATION
Direct injection: Using a 21G or 23G needle, inject into vein or into I.V. tubing containing a free-flowing, compatible solution over 5 minutes.
Intermittent infusion: Using a 21G or 23G needle, infuse solution over 15 minutes. Infusion rate shouldn't exceed 16 ml/minute because of the calcium concentration of the solution.
Continuous infusion: Infuse over 24 hours at about 40 ml/hour. Infusion rate shouldn't exceed 16 ml/minute because of the calcium concentration of the solution.

PREPARATION & STORAGE
Available as a yellow-white solution in 1-ml ampule (3 mg/ml) with 0.9% benzyl alcohol; 10 mg/ml in 5-ml vial; 50-mg, 100-mg, and 350-mg vials for reconstitution (containing no preservatives).

Reconstitute powder for injection by adding 5 ml of sterile or bacteriostatic water for injection to 50-mg vial, or 10 ml diluent to 100-mg vial, to yield 10 mg/ml. Or, add 17 ml diluent to 350-mg vial, to yield 20 mg/ml.

When doses exceed 10 mg/m², don't use diluents containing benzyl alcohol.

Compatible solutions include lactated Ringer's solution, D₅W, dextrose 5% in normal saline solution, dextrose 10% in water, and Ringer's solution.

Store ampules and vials at room temperature. Use solutions containing sterile water immediately. Use those containing bacteriostatic water within

---

1 week if refrigerated. Protect from light.

Incompatibilities
Droperidol, fluorouracil, foscarnet, sodium bicarbonate.

CONTRAINDICATIONS & CAUTIONS
• Contraindicated in patients hypersensitive to leucovorin.
• Contraindicated in those with anemia of unknown cause because drug may mask signs of pernicious anemia, leading to severe CNS damage.
• Use cautiously in those with pernicious anemia. Hemolytic remission may accompany progressive neurologic effects.
• For leucovorin rescue, use cautiously in patients with a urine pH less than 7, ascites, dehydration, pleural or peritoneal effusions, or renal dysfunction because of the increased risk of toxic reaction.

ADVERSE REACTIONS
CV: flushing.
Respiratory: wheezing.
Skin: erythema, pruritus, rash, warm sensation.
Other: *anaphylaxis.*

INTERACTIONS
Drug-drug. *Barbiturate and hydantoin anticonvulsants, primidone:* Reduces effects with large leucovorin doses. Monitor patient closely.
CNS depressants: May deepen CNS depression because of alcohol in leucovorin preparation. Avoid using together.

EFFECTS ON LAB TEST RESULTS
None reported.

ACTION
Thought to limit the action of methotrexate and other folic acid antagonists by competing for transport into cells. Rescues bone marrow and GI cells from methotrexate but has no effect on existing methotrexate nephrotoxicity.

PHARMACOKINETICS
Onset, less than 5 minutes; duration, 3 to 6 hours.
Distribution: Throughout body tissues, with highest levels in the liver. Drug crosses the placental barrier; moderate amounts cross the blood-brain barrier. It's unknown if drug appears in breast milk.
Metabolism: More than half metabolized by the liver, primarily to an active metabolite that's the major transport and storage form of folate.
Excretion: In urine, primarily as two metabolites, with 5% to 8% removed in feces.

CLINICAL CONSIDERATIONS
• Osmolality: 274 mOsm/kg.
• Treat overdoses of folic acid antagonists within 1 hour if possible. Drug is usually ineffective after 4-hour delay.
• Begin leucovorin rescue within 24 hours of high-dose methotrexate regimen. If patient's creatinine level is at least 50% of baseline level after 24 hours of leucovorin therapy, increase dosage to 100 mg/m^2 q 3 hours until methotrexate falls below 5×10^{-8} M.
• Monitor methotrexate and creatinine levels, creatinine clearance, and urine pH q 6 to 24 hours during leucovorin rescue.
• If needed, increase leucovorin dosage or lengthen duration of therapy in patients with aciduria, ascites, dehydration, GI obstruction, renal impairment, or pleural or peritoneal effusion. Duration of therapy depends on methotrexate levels.
• Drug may increase the risk of seizures in susceptible children. Adjust dosage of anticonvulsant if needed.
• Don't give drug simultaneously with methotrexate.
• Don't use as the sole antianemic in treating vitamin B$_{12}$ deficiencies.

♦ Off-label use   *May contain benzyl alcohol   ◇ Canada

• **Alert:** Drug may contain benzyl alcohol.

PATIENT TEACHING
• Encourage patient to drink fluids during rescue treatment.
• Explain need for drug use to patient and family.
• Tell patient to report adverse reactions promptly.

---

levofloxacin
Levaquin

Pharmacologic class: fluoroquinolone
Therapeutic class: broad-spectrum antibiotic
Pregnancy risk category: C
pH: 3.8 to 5.8

INDICATIONS & DOSAGES
➤ **Mild, moderate, and severe infections caused by susceptible microorganisms; acute maxillary sinusitis caused by susceptible strains of** *Haemophilus influenzae, Moraxella catarrhalis,* **or** *Streptococcus pneumoniae*—
Adults: 500 mg I.V. daily for 10 to 14 days.
➤ **Acute bacterial exacerbation of chronic bronchitis caused by** *H. influenzae, H. parainfluenzae, M. catarrhalis, Staphylococcus aureus,* **or** *S. pneumoniae*—
Adults: 500 mg I.V. daily for 7 days.
➤ **Community-acquired pneumonia caused by** *Chlamydia pneumoniae, H. influenzae, H. parainfluenzae, Klebsiella pneumoniae, Legionella pneumophila, M. catarrhalis, Mycoplasma pneumoniae, S. aureus,* **or** *S. pneumoniae* **(including penicillin resistant)**—
Adults: 500 mg I.V. daily for 7 to 14 days.

➤ **Mild to moderate uncomplicated skin and skin structure infections caused by** *S. aureus* **or** *Streptococcus pyogenes*—
Adults: 500 mg I.V. daily for 7 to 10 days.
➤ **Chronic bacterial prostatitis due to** *Escherichia coli, Enterococcus faecalis,* **or** *S. epidermidis*—
Adults: 500 mg I.V. daily for 28 days.
Adjust-a-dose: For patients with creatinine clearance of 20 to 49 ml/minute, give initial dose of 500 mg; then 250 mg once daily; if clearance is 10 to 19 ml/minute, or for patients on hemodialysis or chronic ambulatory peritoneal dialysis, give initial dose of 500 mg; then 250 mg q 48 hours.
➤ **Complicated skin and skin-structure infections from methicillin-sensitive** *Staphylococcus aureus, Enterococcus faecalis, Streptococcus pyogenes,* **or** *Proteus mirabilis*—
Adults: 750 mg I.V. infusion over 90 minutes q 24 hours for 7 to 14 days.
➤ **Nosocomial pneumonia**—
Adults: 750 mg once daily for 7 to 14 days.
Adjust-a-dose: For patients with creatinine clearance of 20 to 49 ml/minute, give 750 mg initially; then 750 mg q 48 hours; for patients with clearance of 10 to 19 ml/minute, and for those receiving hemodialysis or chronic ambulatory peritoneal dialysis, give 750 mg initially; then 500 mg q 48 hours.
➤ **Mild to moderate complicated UTI caused by** *Enterobacter cloacae, Enterococcus faecalis, Escherichia coli, K. pneumoniae, Proteus mirabilis,* **or** *Pseudomonas aeruginosa*—
Adults: 250 mg I.V. daily for 10 days.
➤ **Mild to moderate acute pyelonephritis cause by** *E. coli*—
Adults: 250 mg I.V. daily for 10 days.
Adjust-a-dose: If creatinine clearance is 10 to 19 ml/minute, increase dosage interval to q 48 hours.

➤ **Mild to moderate uncomplicated UTI caused by** *E. coli, K. pneumoniae,* **or** *S. saprophyticus*—
Adults: 250 mg P.O. or I.V. daily for 3 days.

➤ **Disseminated gonococcal infection ◆** —
Adults: 250 mg I.V. once daily, continued for 24 to 48 hours after improvement begins. Therapy may be switched to 500 mg P.O. daily to complete at least 1 week of therapy.

➤ **Acute pelvic inflammatory disease ◆** —
Adults: 500 mg I.V. once daily with or without metronidazole 500 mg q 8 hours. Stop parenteral regimen 24 hours after improvement; then begin 100 mg P.O. b.i.d. of doxycycline to complete 14 days of therapy.

ADMINISTRATION

Direct injection: Avoid rapid or bolus I.V. infusion.
Intermittent infusion: Concentration of resulting solution is 5 mg/ml. Infuse 250 mg or 500 mg slowly over at least 60 minutes. Infuse 750 mg over 90 minutes.
Continuous infusion: Not recommended.

PREPARATION & STORAGE

Supplied in single-use 20-ml (500 mg) or 30-ml (750 mg) vials containing 25 mg/ml. Further dilute to 5 mg/ml before I.V. use. Also available as a premixed injection (5 mg/ml) in 50-, 100-, or 150-ml bags containing D_5W.

Withdraw appropriate dose from vial and dilute with a compatible solution to a total volume of 100 ml.

Compatible I.V. solutions include normal saline solution, D_5W, dextrose 5% in normal saline solution, dextrose 5% in lactated Ringer's solution, dextrose 5% in Plasma-Lyte 56, and 1/6 M sodium lactate solution.

Diluted solution is stable for 72 hours when stored below 77° F (25° C)

and for 14 days when stored at 41° F (5° C) in plastic I.V. containers. Solutions frozen in glass bottles or plastic I.V. containers are stable for 6 months at -4° F (-20° C). If frozen, solutions must be thawed at room temperature. Don't thaw by microwave or water bath, and don't refreeze after thawing. Because vials are for single use, discard unused portion. If preparing a 250-mg dose, withdraw entire amount and prepare a second dose for storage. Use careful aseptic technique.

Incompatibilities

Mannitol 20%, multivalent cations (such as magnesium), sodium bicarbonate 5%.

CONTRAINDICATIONS & CAUTIONS

• Contraindicated in those hypersensitive to the drug or its components or to other fluoroquinolones.
• Use cautiously in those with a history of seizure disorders or other CNS diseases because they may have symptoms of excessive CNS stimulation.
• Use cautiously in those with diabetes mellitus because drug may alter glucose levels.
• Adjust dosage for patients with impaired renal function.
• Safety and efficacy in children younger than age 18 and in pregnant or breast-feeding women haven't been established.

ADVERSE REACTIONS

CNS: dizziness, *encephalopathy,* headache, insomnia, pain, paresthesia, *seizures.*
CV: chest pain, palpitations, vasodilation.
GI: abdominal pain, constipation, diarrhea, dyspepsia, flatulence, nausea, *pseudomembranous colitis,* vomiting.
GU: vaginitis.
Hematologic: eosinophilia, hemolytic anemia.

Musculoskeletal: back pain, tendon rupture.
Respiratory: allergic pneumonitis.
Skin: *erythema multiforme,* injection site reaction, photosensitivity, pruritus, rash, *Stevens-Johnson syndrome.*
Other: *anaphylaxis, multisystem organ failure.*

INTERACTIONS
Drug-drug. *Antidiabetics:* May alter glucose level. Monitor glucose level.
NSAIDs: May increase CNS stimulation. Monitor patient closely.
Theophylline: Decreases clearance of theophylline, increasing risk of toxic reaction. Monitor theophylline level.
Warfarin and derivatives: Increases effect of oral anticoagulant with some fluoroquinolones. Monitor patient closely.
Drug-herb. *Dong quai, St. John's wort:* May cause photosensitivity. Advise patient to avoid excessive sunlight exposure.
Drug-lifestyle. *Sun exposure:* Increases photosensitivity. Advise patient to avoid excessive sunlight exposure.

EFFECTS ON LAB TEST RESULTS
• May decrease glucose level.
• May increase eosinophil count. May decrease hemoglobin and WBC count.
• May cause false-positive opiate assay results. May cause abnormal ECG results.

ACTION
Inhibits bacterial DNA gyrase and prevents DNA replication, transcription, repair, and recombination in susceptible bacteria.

PHARMACOKINETICS
Onset and duration unknown; drug level peaks in 1 or 2 hours.
Distribution: Widespread distribution into body tissues; penetration into blister fluid is rapid and extensive; also penetrates well into lung tissue.

Metabolism: Limited.
Excretion: Excreted largely unchanged in the urine, probably through glomerular filtration and tubular secretion. Half-life, 6 to 8 hours after single and multiple doses.

CLINICAL CONSIDERATIONS
• Drug is isotonic.
• Acute hypersensitivity reactions may require treatment with epinephrine, oxygen, antihistamines, corticosteroids, pressor amines, and airway management. Make sure appropriate equipment is available.
• Monitor renal function closely, including creatinine and BUN levels.
• Monitor PT and INR in patients receiving warfarin.
• Monitor glucose level carefully in any patient receiving an antidiabetic.
• Monitor patient for increased CNS stimulation, and take seizure precautions as needed.
• Levofloxacin can cause pseudomembranous colitis. If diarrhea occurs, notify prescriber.
• Neither hemodialysis nor peritoneal dialysis effectively removes drug.
• The potential for acute toxic reaction is low. If overdose occurs, observe patient closely and maintain adequate hydration.

PATIENT TEACHING
• Teach patient the signs and symptoms of excessive CNS stimulation, such as restlessness, tremor, confusion, and hallucinations. Instruct him to notify his prescriber about these or other adverse reactions.
• Warn patient to avoid excessive sunlight.
• Advise diabetic patient of risk of low blood sugar level.

Reactions may be *common,* uncommon, *life-threatening,* or COMMON AND LIFE-THREATENING.

levothyroxine sodium
(T_4, L-thyroxine sodium)
Synthroid

Pharmacologic class: thyroid
hormone
Therapeutic class: thyroid hormone
replacement
Pregnancy risk category: A

INDICATIONS & DOSAGES
➤ **Hypothyroidism—**
Adults: Initially, 25 to 50 mcg I.V. daily. Increase daily dose by 25 mcg q 2 to
4 weeks. Maintenance is 75 to 200 mcg
daily.
Children age 12 and older: More than
150 mcg or 2 to 3 mcg/kg I.V. daily.
Children ages 6 to 12: 100 to 150 mcg
or 4 to 5 mcg/kg I.V. daily.
Children ages 1 to 5: 75 to 100 mcg or
5 to 6 mcg/kg I.V. daily.
Infants ages 6 to 12 months: 50 to
75 mcg or 6 to 8 mcg/kg I.V. daily.
Infants ages 3 to 6 months: 25 to
50 mcg or 8 to 10 mcg/kg I.V. daily.
Infants up to 3 months: 10 to 15 mcg/
kg I.V. daily.
*Premature infants weighing less than
2 kg (4.4 lb) and infants at risk for
heart failure:* Initially, 25 mcg I.V. daily, increased to 37.5 mcg daily after 4
to 6 weeks.
Adjust-a-dose: In elderly patients, give
12.5 to 50 mcg I.V. daily, initially.
Increase daily dose by 12.5 to 25 mcg q
3 to 8 weeks.
➤ **Myxedema coma—**
Adults: Initially, 200 to 500 mcg. Give
100 to 300 mcg on next day to obtain
needed improvement. Maintenance is
50 to 200 mcg daily.

ADMINISTRATION
Direct injection: Inject into vein over 1
to 2 minutes.

Intermittent infusion: Not recommended.
Continuous infusion: Not recommended.

PREPARATION & STORAGE
Available as a buff-colored, odorless
powder in 10-ml vials containing 200
or 500 mcg.
　To reconstitute, add 5 ml of normal
saline injection to the 200- or 500-mcg
vial. Shake to dissolve. The solution
contains 40 or 100 mcg/ml.
　Reconstitute drug immediately before use and discard unused portions.
　Powder remains stable at room temperature. Store in light-resistant containers; otherwise, powder may turn
light pink.

Incompatibilities
Other I.V. solutions.

CONTRAINDICATIONS & CAUTIONS
• Contraindicated in patients hypersensitive to drug or other components of
the injection.
• Contraindicated in those with suppressed TSH level with normal T_3 and
T_4 levels or thyrotoxicosis.
• Contraindicated in those with acute
MI.
• Contraindicated in those with adrenal
insufficiency because thyroid hormones
may increase glucocorticoid clearance,
which may cause an acute adrenal crisis.
• Use cautiously in patients with nontoxic diffuse goiter or nodular thyroid
disease, to prevent thyrotoxicosis.
• Use cautiously in those with CV disease, in elderly patients, and in infants
with congenital hypothyroidism because of possible exacerbation from increased metabolic demands.
• Use cautiously in those undergoing
surgery or emergency treatment because of increased metabolic demands.

• Use cautiously in those with diabetes mellitus because of possible reduced glucose tolerance.

ADVERSE REACTIONS
CNS: severe headache, *insomnia, nervousness,* clumsiness, lethargy, weakness, tremors, fever.
CV: angina, ***heart failure,*** hypertension, ***ischemia,*** tachyarrhythmias.
GI: constipation, diarrhea, nausea.
Metabolic: cold sensation, heat intolerance, weight loss or gain.
Musculoskeletal: accelerated bone growth in infants given high doses, leg cramps.
Respiratory: dyspnea.
Skin: alopecia in children, rash, skin dryness and puffiness, urticaria.

INTERACTIONS
Drug-drug. *Amiodarone, beta blockers, glucocorticoids, propylthiouracil:* May diminish peripheral conversion of T_4 to T_3. May also reduce the effects of beta blockers. Monitor patient closely.
Anticoagulants: Increases anticoagulant effects. Monitor patient closely.
Antidiabetics: Decreases antidiabetic effects. Monitor glucose levels.
Carbamazepine, phenobarbital, phenytoin, rifamycins, and other hepatic enzyme inducers: Enhances hepatic degradation of levothyroxine. Monitor patient closely.
Cardiac glycosides: Decreases cardiac glycoside effects. Monitor levels.
Estrogens: Reduces levothyroxine effectiveness because of increased thyroxine-binding globulin. Monitor therapeutic effect closely.
Ketamine: May cause hypertension and tachycardia. Monitor cardiac status and blood pressure.
Somatrem, somatropin: May accelerate epiphyseal maturation. Avoid using together.
SSRIs: Decreases thyroid hormone levels. Monitor levels closely.

Sympathomimetics, tricyclic and tetracyclic antidepressants: May enhance effects of levothyroxine and these drugs; worsens coronary insufficiency and arrhythmias. Avoid using together.
Theophylline: Decreases theophylline clearance in hypothyroid patients; clearance returns to normal when euthyroid state is reached. Monitor theophylline level.
Drug-herb. *Horseradish:* May cause abnormal thyroid function. Discourage use by patients undergoing thyroid function tests.
Kelp: May cause hyperthyroidism. Discourage use together.
Lemon balm: Has antithyroid effects and inhibits thyroid-stimulating hormone. Discourage use together.

EFFECTS ON LAB TEST RESULTS
• May alter thyroid function test results. May reduce uptake of ^{123}I, ^{131}I, and sodium pertechnetate Tc 99m with radionuclide thyroid scan.

ACTION
Drug's catabolic and anabolic effects are mediated at the cellular level by T_3. T_4 is crucial to normal metabolism, growth, and development.

PHARMACOKINETICS
Onset, 6 to 8 hours; duration, 1 to 3 weeks.
Distribution: Thought to be distributed to most body tissues and fluids, with highest levels in the liver and kidneys. Drug is more than 99% protein bound; doesn't readily cross the placental barrier. Small amounts of drug appear in breast milk.
Metabolism: About 85% deiodinated in peripheral tissues. Smaller amounts are conjugated with glucuronic and sulfate acids in the liver.
Excretion: In feces and urine. Half-life, 6 to 7 days; shorter in those with hyperthyroidism and longer in those with hypothyroidism.

CLINICAL CONSIDERATIONS

• *Alert:* In infants, don't reconstitute with diluent containing benzyl alcohol because of potentially fatal effects.
• In those with myxedema coma, give levothyroxine with hydrocortisone to prevent adrenal crisis. Hydrocortisone dosage starts at 300 mg/day in divided doses and should be tapered over the next 4 to 5 days.
• If adrenal insufficiency occurs during therapy, correct it promptly to prevent adrenal crisis.
• Monitor the ECG for ventricular arrhythmias. Watch for tachyarrhythmias and signs of ischemia.
• Monitor vital signs to detect adverse effects early.
• Monitor thyroid function tests, including levels of serum-free T_4 or serum-free T_4 index, total T_4, T_3 resin uptake, and thyroid-stimulating hormone.
• Regularly assess bone growth and psychomotor development in those with pediatric congenital hypothyroidism.
• For patients older than age 60, reduce adult levothyroxine dosage by about 25%. Also, for those with CV disease and hyperthyroidism, give smaller doses.
• If overdose occurs, withdraw drug for 2 to 6 days. Resume administration at a lower dose.

PATIENT TEACHING

• Tell patient to use drug as his prescriber has instructed and not to alter the brand or amount.
• Advise patient that drug's effects may take a few weeks to become noticeable.
• Discuss signs and symptoms of adverse effects, and advise patient to promptly notify prescriber if needed.
• Emphasize need to notify surgeons, dentists, and other health care providers of the drug regimen.

lidocaine hydrochloride
Xylocaine, Xylocard ◇

Pharmacologic class: amide derivative
Therapeutic class: ventricular antiarrhythmic
Pregnancy risk category: B
pH: 5 to 7 for injection; 3.5 to 6 when premixed in D_5W

INDICATIONS & DOSAGES

➤ **Acute ventricular arrhythmias (PVCs, ventricular tachycardia) linked to acute MI, digitalis toxicity, cardioversion, cardiac manipulation from trauma or surgery, or drug adverse effects—**
Adults: 50 to 100 mg as initial I.V. bolus, repeated after 5 minutes if arrhythmias continue. For maintenance, infuse 20 to 50 mcg/kg/minute (1 to 4 mg/minute in 70-kg adult). Don't exceed 300 mg in 1 hour. Keep rate below 30 mcg/kg/minute in patients with heart failure or liver disease.
Children: 0.5 to 1 mg/kg as initial I.V. bolus, repeated p.r.n. Maximum dose, 5 mg/kg. For maintenance, infuse 10 to 50 mcg/kg/minute.
➤ **Status epilepticus unresponsive to all other measures—**
Adults and children: 1 mg/kg as initial I.V. bolus. If seizure doesn't stop after 2 minutes, give 0.5 mg/kg bolus. For maintenance, infuse 30 mcg/kg/minute.

ADMINISTRATION

Direct injection: Inject undiluted drug into large vein or cannula at 25 to 50 mg/minute.
Intermittent infusion: Not recommended.
Continuous infusion: Using an infusion pump and microdrop tubing, titrate dose according to suppression of ventricular ectopy.

PREPARATION & STORAGE

Available for injection in 5-ml ampules and prefilled syringes, and 5-, 10-, 20-, 30-, and 50-ml vials containing 10 and 20 mg/ml. Drug also comes in pre-mixed 250-ml bottles of 0.4% or 0.8% solution; 500-ml bottles of 0.2%, 0.4%, or 0.8% solution; and 1,000-ml bottle-sof 0.2% solution.

Available for continuous infusion in 40-mg, 1-g, and 2-g single-use 25- or 50-ml vials and in 5- and 10-ml syringes that require mixing with D$_5$W. Dilute 1 or 2 g of drug in 1,000 ml of D$_5$W to obtain a 0.1% or 0.2% solution, respectively.

Store at room temperature. Make sure to use only solutions marked for treating arrhythmias. After dilution with D$_5$W, solution is stable for 24 hours.

Incompatibilities

Amphotericin B, ampicillin sodium, cefazolin, ceftriaxone, hydromorphone, methohexital, phenytoin, sodium bicarbonate.

CONTRAINDICATIONS & CAUTIONS

• Contraindicated in those hypersensitive to lidocaine or amidelike anesthetics.

• Contraindicated in those with Stokes-Adams syndrome, Wolff-Parkinson-White syndrome, or second- or third-degree heart block.

• Use cautiously in children, in geriatric patients, and in those with severe kidney or liver disease, heart failure, or shock because drug may accumulate.

• Use cautiously in those who have sinus bradycardia or incomplete heart block but haven't received isoproterenol or a pacemaker; lidocaine may increase PVCs and ventricular escape beats, leading to ventricular tachycardia.

ADVERSE REACTIONS

CNS: agitation, anxiety, apprehension, *confusion,* dizziness, drowsiness, euphoria, lethargy, *light-headedness,* paresthesia, psychosis, *restlessness,* *seizures,* slurred speech, twitching, unconsciousness.

CV: *bradycardia, cardiac arrest,* hypotension, thrombophlebitis.

EENT: blurred or double vision, tinnitus.

GI: dysphagia, nausea, vomiting.

Musculoskeletal: twitching.

Respiratory: dyspnea, *respiratory arrest.*

Other: *anaphylaxis.*

INTERACTIONS

Drug-drug. *Beta blockers, cimetidine:* Reduces metabolism and increases risk of lidocaine toxicity. Monitor patient closely.

Phenytoin, procainamide, propranolol, quinidine: Potentiates or antagonizes antiarrhythmic effects. Monitor patient closely.

Succinylcholine: Prolongs neuromuscular blockade. Avoid using together.

Tocainide: Increases adverse reactions because these drugs have similar actions. Avoid using together.

EFFECTS ON LAB TEST RESULTS

None reported.

ACTION

A class Ib antiarrhythmic, or a fast sodium channel blocker. Reduces automaticity in the His-Purkinje system and suppresses ventricular depolarization. Also acts as a CNS anesthetic, producing sedative, analgesic, and anticonvulsant effects.

PHARMACOKINETICS

Onset, 45 to 90 seconds; duration, 10 to 20 minutes.

Distribution: Throughout body tissues, with rapid dispersal to the kidneys, lungs, liver, and heart and slower dispersal to skeletal muscle and fat. Drug is 60% to 80% protein bound and crosses the blood-brain and placental barriers. Drug appears in breast milk.

Metabolism: 90% in the liver.

Reactions may be *common,* uncommon, *life-threatening,* or COMMON AND LIFE-THREATENING.

Excretion: In urine, primarily as metabolites. Initial phase half-life, 7 to 30 minutes; terminal phase half-life, 1½ to 2 hours.

CLINICAL CONSIDERATIONS
• Osmolality: 296 to 352 mOsm/kg.
• Use the smallest lidocaine dose possible to control arrhythmias. Therapeutic levels range from 1.5 to 5 mcg/ml; toxic level is greater than 5 mcg/ml.
• Treat underlying causes of ventricular arrhythmias.
• Monitor ECG continuously during administration to titrate continuous infusion and detect prolonged PR interval of more than 0.2 second, widened QRS complex of more than 0.12 second, or worsened ventricular arrhythmias. Keep resuscitation equipment, including a defibrillator, nearby.
• Assess often for signs of toxic reaction.
• Monitor AST, ALT, BUN, and creatinine and electrolyte levels. Report abnormalities to prescriber.
• If overdose occurs, stop infusion immediately and notify prescriber. Ensure an adequate airway and oxygenation. Give oxygen by nasal cannula, if appropriate. Be prepared to start cardiopulmonary resuscitation. Continue to monitor ECG for underlying ventricular arrhythmias, and prepare to give an alternate antiarrhythmic, such as procainamide. Monitor respirations and blood pressure every 5 minutes for 20 minutes. If patient develops bradycardia, give atropine and watch for tachycardia. If seizures occur, give diazepam and monitor the patient carefully for respiratory depression.

PATIENT TEACHING
• If patient is alert, instruct him to report signs and symptoms of toxic reaction during infusion.
• Warn patient not to drive after receiving this drug.
• Discuss signs of adverse reactions with patient and the need to get immediate care if symptoms of a heart attack occur.
• Explain use and administration of drug to patient and family.

lincomycin hydrochloride
Lincocin*, Lincorex*

Pharmacologic class: protein synthesis inhibitor
Therapeutic class: bactericidal drug, bacteriostatic
Pregnancy risk category: NR
pH: 3 to 5.5

INDICATIONS & DOSAGES
➤ **Severe infections caused by susceptible organisms—**
Adults: 600 mg to 1 g q 8 to 12 hours. Maximum dose, 8 g/day.
Children older than age 1 month: 10 to 20 mg/kg daily in two to three divided doses.
Adjust-a-dose: In renally impaired patients, give 25% to 30% of recommended dose.

ADMINISTRATION
Direct injection: Not recommended.
Intermittent infusion: Infuse 100 ml of solution over at least 1 hour. Infuse over 2 to 4 hours for 200- to 400-ml volumes. Rapid infusion may cause cardiac arrest or severe hypotension.
Continuous infusion: Not recommended.

PREPARATION & STORAGE
Available as a clear, colorless to slightly yellow solution in 2- and 10-ml vials containing 300 mg/ml.
    For infusion, dilute drug with 100 to 500 ml of D_5W or dextrose 10% in water, normal saline solution, or Ringer's injection. Drug is also compatible with dextran 6% in normal saline solution, dextran 5% in normal saline solution,

dextrose 10% in normal saline solution, and 1/6 M sodium lactate solution.

Store vials at room temperature; don't freeze. Solution remains stable for 24 hours at room temperature.

Incompatibilities
Ampicillin, colistimethate sodium, kanamycin, penicillin G potassium or sodium, phenytoin.

CONTRAINDICATIONS & CAUTIONS
• *Alert:* Contraindicated in neonates, in those hypersensitive to lincomycin or clindamycin, and in those with hepatic or severe renal disease.
• Avoid drug in breast-feeding women.
• Use cautiously in pregnant, geriatric, debilitated, and renal- or hepatic-impaired patients; in those with GI disorders, especially colitis; and in those with a history of asthma or allergies.

ADVERSE REACTIONS
CNS: headache, syncope, vertigo.
CV: *cardiac arrest, hypotension.*
EENT: glossitis, tinnitus.
GI: abdominal cramps, *diarrhea,* enterocolitis, stomatitis, nausea, unusual thirst, *pseudomembranous colitis,* anal pruritus, vomiting.
GU: oliguria, proteinuria, vaginitis.
Hematologic: *agranulocytosis, aplastic anemia,* azotemia, *leukopenia, neutropenia, pancytopenia, thrombocytopenic purpura.*
Metabolic: weight loss.
Musculoskeletal: myalgia.
Skin: rash, *Stevens-Johnson syndrome,* urticaria, pain at infusion site.
Other: *anaphylaxis, angioneurotic edema, superinfection.*

INTERACTIONS
Drug-drug. *Antimyasthenics:* May antagonize effects. Avoid using together.
Chloramphenicol, erythromycins: May antagonize lincomycin effects. Monitor therapeutic effect.

Hydrocarbon inhalation anesthetics, neuromuscular blockers: Enhances neuromuscular blockade. Avoid using together.
Neurotoxic drugs: Increases risk of toxic reaction. Avoid using together.
Opioid analgesics: May deepen respiratory depression. Avoid using together.

EFFECTS ON LAB TEST RESULTS
• May decrease granulocyte, WBC, neutrophil, RBC, and platelet counts.

ACTION
Bacteriostatic or bactericidal, depending on the organism's susceptibility and the drug's concentration. Inhibits protein synthesis by binding to bacterial ribosomes. Drug is effective against most aerobic gram-positive cocci and many anaerobic and microaerophilic gram-negative and gram-positive organisms.

PHARMACOKINETICS
Drug level peaks in 2 to 4 hours.
Distribution: Rapid and widespread to most body fluids and tissues, with moderate to high protein binding; poor distribution in normal CSF and only up to 18% of drug levels when meninges are inflamed. Drug readily crosses the placental barrier, producing cord levels that are 25% of maternal drug levels. Drug appears in breast milk.
Metabolism: Partly in the liver. Rate rises in children.
Excretion: 2% to 30% in urine and 4% to 14% in feces. Half-life ranges from about 4 to 6 hours; 9 to 13 hours in those with impaired renal or hepatic function.

CLINICAL CONSIDERATIONS
• Use lincomycin only when penicillin is contraindicated or when infection is unresponsive to other antibiotics.
• Obtain specimens for culture and sensitivity testing before giving first dose.

Therapy may start before results are available.

● Frequently monitor blood pressure.

● If diarrhea persists during therapy, stop drug and collect stool specimens for culture to rule out pseudomembranous colitis.

● Monitor CBC, platelet count, and hepatic function. Stop drug if blood dyscrasia develops.

● Observe patient for signs of bacterial or fungal superinfection during prolonged use.

● Check infusion site for signs of phlebitis. Rotate sites regularly.

● If patient has candidiasis, give an antifungal along with lincomycin.

● Neither hemodialysis nor peritoneal dialysis removes an appreciable amount of drug.

PATIENT TEACHING

● Stress to the patient the importance of completing the full course of therapy and of not missing doses.

● Tell patient to contact prescriber if severe diarrhea occurs.

● Alert the patient to those adverse reactions that require a prescriber's immediate attention.

linezolid
Zyvox, Zyvoxam I.V. ◇

Pharmacologic class: oxazolidinone
Therapeutic class: antibiotic
Pregnancy risk category: C
pH: 4.8

INDICATIONS & DOSAGES

➤ **Vancomycin-resistant** *Enterococcus faecium* **infections, including those with concurrent bacteremia**—
Adults and children age 12 and older: 600 mg I.V. q 12 hours for 14 to 28 days.

Neonates age 7 days and older, infants, and children through age 11: 10 mg/kg I.V. q 8 hours for 14 to 28 days.
Neonates younger than age 7 days: 10 mg/kg I.V. q 12 hours for 14 to 28 days. Increase to 10 mg/kg q 8 hours when patient is 7 days old. Consider this dosage increase if neonate has inadequate response.

➤ **Nosocomial pneumonia caused by** *Staphylococcus aureus* **(methicillin-susceptible [MSSA] and methicillin-resistant [MRSA] strains) or** *Streptococcus pneumonia* **(penicillin-susceptible strains only); complicated skin and skin-structure infections caused by** *S. aureus* **(MSSA and MRSA),** *Streptococcus pyogenes,* **or** *Streptococcus agalactiae;* **community-acquired pneumonia caused by** *S. pneumoniae* **(penicillin-susceptible strains only), including those with concurrent bacteremia, or** *S. aureus* **(MSSA only)**—
Adults and children age 12 and older: 600 mg I.V. q 12 hours for 10 to 14 days.
Neonates age 7 days and older, infants, and children through age 11: 10 mg/kg I.V. q 8 hours for 10 to 14 days.
Neonates younger than age 7 days: 10 mg/kg I.V. or q 12 hours for 14 to 28 days. Increase to 10 mg/kg q 8 hours when patient is 7 days old. Consider this dosage increase if neonate has inadequate response.

ADMINISTRATION

Direct injection: Not recommended.
Intermittent infusion: Give over 30 to 120 minutes.
Continuous infusion: Not recommended.

PREPARATION & STORAGE

Available as 2 mg/ml in 100-ml, 200-ml, and 300-ml ready-to-use bags.
    Inspect for particulate matter and leaks.

Linezolid is compatible with D_5W injection, normal saline injection, and lactated Ringer's injection.

Store at room temperature in its protective overwrap. The solution may turn yellow over time but this doesn't affect the drug's potency.

Incompatibilities

Amphotericin B, ceftriaxone sodium, chlorpromazine hydrochloride, diazepam, erythromycin lactobionate, pentamidine isethionate, phenytoin sodium, trimethoprim-sulfamethoxazole.

CONTRAINDICATIONS & CAUTIONS

• Contraindicated in patients hypersensitive to linezolid or any inactive components of the formulation.
• Use cautiously in patients with uncontrolled hypertension, pheochromocytoma, carcinoid syndrome, or untreated hyperthyroidism because linezolid hasn't been studied in these patients.
• Myelosuppression may develop in patients receiving linezolid. Use cautiously and monitor CBC weekly.

ADVERSE REACTIONS

CNS: *headache,* insomnia, dizziness, fever.
GI: *diarrhea, nausea,* constipation, vomiting, elevated amylase and lipase levels, altered taste, tongue discoloration, oral candidiasis, ***pseudomembranous colitis.***
GU: vaginal candidiasis.
Hematologic: anemia, ***leukopenia, neutropenia, thrombocytopenia.***
Skin: rash.
Other: fungal infection.

INTERACTIONS

Drug-drug. *Adrenergic agents, such as dopamine, epinephrine, and pseudoephedrine:* May cause hypertension. Monitor blood pressure and heart rate. Start continuous infusions of dopamine and epinephrine at lower doses and titrate to response.

SSRIs: May cause serotonin syndrome. If patient develops signs and symptoms of serotonin syndrome (confusion, delirium, restlessness, tremors, blushing, diaphoresis, hyperpyrexia), consider stopping the serotoninergic agent.
Drug-food. *Foods and beverages high in tyramine, such as aged cheeses, tap beers, red wines, air-dried meats, soy sauce, sauerkraut:* May increase blood pressure. Tyramine content of meals shouldn't exceed 100 mg.

EFFECTS ON LAB TEST RESULTS

• May increase ALT, AST, bilirubin, alkaline phosphatase, creatinine, BUN, amylase, and lipase levels.
• May decrease hemoglobin and WBC, neutrophil, and platelet counts.

ACTION

Linezolid is bacteriostatic against enterococci and staphylococci, and bactericidal against most strains of streptococci. Exerts antimicrobial effects by interfering with bacterial protein synthesis.

PHARMACOKINETICS

Onset, unknown; peak, 30 minutes; duration, unknown.
Distribution: Readily into well-perfused tissues. Protein binding is about 31%.
Metabolism: Linezolid undergoes oxidative metabolism to two inactive metabolites. Linezolid does not appear to be metabolized by the cytochrome P-450 oxidative system.
Excretion: At steady-state, about 30% of an administered dose appears in the urine as linezolid and about 50% as metabolites. Linezolid undergoes significant renal tubular reabsorption, such that renal clearance is low. Nonrenal clearance accounts for about 65% of the total clearance.

CLINICAL CONSIDERATIONS

• Obtain samples for culture and sensitivity testing before starting linezolid therapy. Sensitivity results should be used to guide subsequent therapy.

• The safety and efficacy of linezolid for longer than 28 days haven't been studied.

• Pseudomembranous colitis may occur. Consider this diagnosis and take appropriate measures in patients with persistent diarrhea.

• Superinfection may occur. Take appropriate measures in patients who develop secondary infections.

• Because the inappropriate use of antibiotics may lead to the development of resistant organisms, carefully consider alternative drugs before starting linezolid therapy, especially in the outpatient setting.

• Linezolid may cause thrombocytopenia. Monitor platelet count in patients at increased risk of bleeding, those with existing thrombocytopenia, those receiving concurrent medications that may cause thrombocytopenia, and those receiving linezolid for more than 14 days.

• Don't adjust dosage when switching from I.V. to P.O. dosage forms.

• **Alert:** Don't confuse Zyvox (linezolid) with Zovirax (acyclovir).

• Symptoms of overdose may include vomiting, tremors, decreased activity, and ataxia. Treatment is supportive, with maintenance of glomerular filtration. Hemodialysis may help increase the elimination of linezolid. Peritoneal dialysis and hemoperfusion haven't been studied.

PATIENT TEACHING

• Stress the importance of completing the entire course of therapy, even if the patient feels better.

• Tell patient to alert prescriber if he has high blood pressure, is taking cough or cold preparations, or is being treated with SSRIs or other antidepressants.

• Tell patient to avoid foods or beverages containing large amounts of tyramine and to keep the amount of tyramine ingested to less than 100 mg per meal. Foods high in tyramine include those that may have undergone protein changes by aging, fermentation, pickling, or smoking to improve flavor, such as aged cheeses, sauerkraut, soy sauce, beer, or red wine.

lorazepam
Ativan*

Pharmacologic class: benzodiazepine
Therapeutic class: sedative-hypnotic
Controlled substance schedule: IV
Pregnancy risk category: D

INDICATIONS & DOSAGES

➤ **Preoperative sedation—**
Adults: 2 mg total dose or 0.044 mg/kg, whichever is smaller, I.V., 15 to 20 minutes before surgery. In patients age 50 and younger, doses up to 0.05 mg/kg—up to 4 mg total—may be given.

➤ **To prevent nausea and vomiting caused by chemotherapy ♦ —**
Adults: 1.5 mg/m^2 (up to 3 mg) I.V. over 5 minutes given 45 minutes before chemotherapy.

➤ **Status epilepticus ♦ —**
Adults and children: 0.05 to 0.1 mg/kg. Repeat at 10- to 15- minute intervals p.r.n. Or, in adults, 4 to 8 mg.

➤ **Delirium ♦ —**
Adults: Initially, give I.V. haloperidol dose of 3 mg, followed by I.V. lorazepam dose of 0.5 to 1 mg. Adjust lorazepam dose p.r.n.

ADMINISTRATION

Direct injection: Inject into vein or I.V. line containing a free-flowing, compati-

ble solution at a maximum rate of 2 mg/minute.
Intermittent infusion: Not recommended.
Continuous infusion: Not recommended.

PREPARATION & STORAGE
Available in 1- and 10-ml vials and 1-ml single-dose prefilled syringes containing 2 and 4 mg/ml. Immediately before administration, dilute drug with an equal volume of sterile water for injection, normal saline solution, or D_5W. Rotate syringe gently to ensure complete mixing. Refrigerate drug, but don't freeze it; protect drug from light. Discard if drug becomes discolored or contains precipitate.

Incompatibilities
Aldesleukin, aztreonam, buprenorphine, foscarnet, idarubicin, imipenem-cilastatin sodium, ondansetron hydrochloride, sargramostim, sufentanil citrate, thiopental.

CONTRAINDICATIONS & CAUTIONS
• Contraindicated in those hypersensitive to benzodiazepines, polyethylene glycol, propylene glycol, or benzyl alcohol, and in those with hepatic or renal failure.
• Contraindicated in those with acute angle-closure glaucoma because of possible anticholinergic effect.
• Contraindicated in those with shock or coma because drug's hypotensive or hypnotic effects may be prolonged or worsened, and in those with acute alcohol intoxication because drug deepens CNS depression.
• Avoid use in those with respiratory depression because of increased risk of airway obstruction.
• Use cautiously in psychotic patients because of possible paradoxical reaction; in depressed patients because of possible worsened depression; and in

those with myasthenia gravis or porphyria because of possible worsening.
• Use cautiously in those with renal or hepatic impairment because of delayed drug elimination; in those with hypoalbuminemia because of increased risk of adverse effects; in geriatric or debilitated patients because of increased CNS effects; and in patients who are prone to addiction.
• Use cautiously in seizure patients because withdrawal may cause seizures.

ADVERSE REACTIONS
CNS: confusion, delirium, dizziness, *drowsiness,* extension of CNS depressant effect.
CV: *cardiac arrest,* hypertension, *hypotension.*
EENT: blurred vision, diplopia.
GI: constipation, dry mouth, gastritis, nausea, sore gums, vomiting.
Respiratory: *apnea,* dyspnea, *partial airway obstruction.*
Skin: rash.

INTERACTIONS
Drug-drug. *Antihypertensives:* Increases risk of severe hypotension. Monitor blood pressure closely.
CNS depressants: Increases effects. Avoid using together.
Digoxin: May enhance effects. Monitor cardiac status closely.
Levodopa: Decreases therapeutic effects of levodopa. Monitor therapeutic effect. Dosage may need to be adjusted.
Drug-herb. *Calendula, catnip, hops, kava, lady's slipper, passionflower, valerian:* May increase sedative effect of the drug. Discourage use together.
Drug-lifestyle. *Alcohol use:* Enhances CNS depression. Discourage use together.
Heavy smoking: Accelerates lorazepam metabolism, thus lowering effectiveness. Discourage smoking.

Reactions may be *common,* uncommon, *life-threatening,* or COMMON AND LIFE-THREATENING.

EFFECTS ON LAB TEST RESULTS

• May increase liver function test values.

ACTION

Thought to enhance or facilitate action of neurotransmitter gamma-aminobutyric acid, which depresses the CNS at the limbic and subcortical levels, producing an anxiolytic effect. Drug also possesses skeletal muscle relaxant, anticonvulsant, and amnesic properties.

PHARMACOKINETICS

Onset, 1 to 5 minutes; duration, usually 6 to 8 hours but sedation may last for up to 24 hours.
Distribution: Widespread, 85% protein bound. Drug crosses the blood-brain and placental barriers and appears in breast milk.
Metabolism: In the liver.
Excretion: In urine as conjugated drug. Half-life, 10 to 20 hours.

CLINICAL CONSIDERATIONS

• Overly rapid infusion can cause apnea, hypotension, bradycardia, or cardiac arrest.
• Always keep emergency resuscitation equipment nearby when giving I.V. lorazepam. Obtain baseline respiratory rate before administration, and notify prescriber if rate falls below 12 breaths/minute. Also, obtain baseline blood pressure, and carefully monitor blood pressure during and after administration.
• Monitor respiratory rate for 1 hour after administration. If rate falls below 8 breaths/minute, arouse the patient and encourage him to breathe at 10 to 12 breaths/minute. If you're unable to arouse the patient, maintain airway patency and manually ventilate to maintain rate of 10 to 12 breaths/minute. Check with prescriber about whether to intubate patient.
• Stop drug if paradoxical reaction occurs. Signs and symptoms include anxiety, acute excitation, hallucinations, increased muscle spasticity, insomnia, and rage.
• Observe infusion site for signs of phlebitis.
• If overdose occurs, maintain a patent airway and adequate ventilation, and give I.V. fluids to enhance drug excretion. Flumazenil may be used to reverse the sedative and respiratory depressant effects of lorazepam. If hypotension occurs, give norepinephrine.

PATIENT TEACHING

• Stress the importance of maintaining bed rest.
• Adjust the bed to lowest position and raise the side rails to prevent falls.
• Warn patient that drug diminishes alertness and coordination.
• Tell patient to avoid use of alcohol and other CNS depressants during therapy.
• Advise patient to use caution if dizziness, drowsiness, light-headedness, or unsteadiness occurs, especially in geriatric patients.

magnesium sulfate

Pharmacologic class: mineral, electrolyte
Therapeutic class: anticonvulsant
Pregnancy risk category: A
pH: 3.5 to 7

INDICATIONS & DOSAGES
➤ **Preeclampsia or eclampsia—**
Adults: 4 g I.V., followed by 1 to 3 g/
hour by continuous I.V. infusion. Dose
over next 24 hours depends on magnesium level and urine output. Maximum
dosage, 30 to 40 g q 24 hours.
Adjust-a-dose: In patients with renal
disease, maximum dosage is 20 g I.V. q
48 hours.
➤ **To control seizures in epilepsy,
glomerulonephritis, or hypothyroidism—**
Adults: 1 g I.V.
➤ **Severe hypertension, encephalopathy, and seizures caused by nephritis—**
Children: 100 to 200 mg/kg I.V. of 1%
to 3% solution. Give total dose within
1 hour, half within the first 15 to 20
minutes.
➤ **Severe magnesium deficiency—**
Adults: 5 g I.V. infused over 3 hours.
➤ **Barium poisoning—**
Adults: 1 to 2 g I.V.
➤ **Sustained ventricular tachycardia
or torsades de pointes—**
Adults: 1 to 6 g I.V. over several minutes, followed by 3 to 20 mg/minute by
I.V. infusion for 5 to 48 hours depending on patient response and magnesium
level.

➤ **Paroxysmal atrial tachycardia—**
Adults: 3 to 4 g I.V. over 30 seconds
with caution.
➤ **To reduce CV morbidity and mortality after MI ♦—**
Adults: 2 g I.V. over 5 to 15 minutes,
then 18 g by I.V. infusion over 24 hours
(about 12.5 mg/minute). Give within
6 hours of symptom onset.
➤ **Acute asthma in children who fail
to respond to traditional
therapy ♦—**
Children: 25 to 50 mg/kg (up to 2 g)
over 10 to 20 minutes by I.V. infusion.
➤ **To prevent hypomagnesemia in
patients who need total parenteral
nutrition—**
Adults: 5 to 8 mEq I.V. daily.
Infants: 0.25 to 0.6 mEq/kg I.V. daily.
➤ **As acute tocolytic drug to manage
preterm labor ♦—**
Adults: 4 to 6 g I.V. infusion over 20
minutes, followed by maintenance infusion of 2 to 4 g/hour for 12 to 24 hours,
as tolerated after contractions have
ceased.

ADMINISTRATION
Direct injection: Inject directly into
vein, not exceeding 150 mg/minute.
Intermittent infusion: Give diluted drug
over 1 to 3 hours.
Continuous infusion: Give by infusion
pump, not exceeding 150 mg/minute
(1.2 mEq/minute).

PREPARATION & STORAGE
Available as a 10% concentration in
20-ml ampules (100 mg/ml) and in 20-
and 50-ml vials; 12.5% concentration
in 8-ml vials (125 mg/ml); and 50%
concentration in 2- and 10-ml ampules
(500 mg/ml), 2-, 5-, 10-, 20-, and
50-ml vials, and 5- and 10-ml syringes.

Also available as 4% (40 mg/ml) and 8% (80 mg/ml) solutions in water for injection, and as 1% (10 mg/ml) and 2% (20 mg/ml) in D_5W.

For seizures, dilute dose in 250 ml of D_5W or normal saline solution. For those with magnesium deficiency, dilute dose in 1 L of D_5W. The most common diluents are 5% dextrose injection or 0.9% sodium chloride injection. For all indications, don't use concentrations over 20% (200 mg/ml).

Store at room temperature and avoid freezing.

Incompatibilities

Alkali carbonates and bicarbonates, amphotericin B, calcium gluconate, cefepime, ciprofloxacin, clindamycin, cyclosporine, dobutamine, heavy metals, I.V. fat emulsion 10%, polymyxin B, procaine, salicylates, sodium bicarbonate, soluble phosphates.

CONTRAINDICATIONS & CAUTIONS

• Contraindicated in those with myocardial damage or heart block because drug depresses cardiac muscle.
• Contraindicated within 2 hours of expected delivery because neonate may show signs of magnesium toxicity.
• Use cautiously in those with renal impairment.

ADVERSE REACTIONS

CNS: *depressed reflexes,* drowsiness, flaccid paralysis.
CV: *cardiac arrest,* prolonged PR interval, *severe bradycardia, severe hypotension,* widened QRS complex, *flushing.*
Metabolic: hypothermia, hypotonia, hypermagnesemia, hypocalcemia.
Respiratory: *respiratory paralysis.*
Skin: diaphoresis.

INTERACTIONS

Drug-drug. *Anesthetics, CNS depressants:* Causes additive CNS depression. Use together cautiously.

Calcium salts: Causes mutual antagonism of effects. Monitor patient closely.
Cardiac glycosides: May exacerbate arrhythmias. Use together cautiously.
Neuromuscular blockers: May cause excessive neuromuscular blockade. Use together cautiously.
Drug-lifestyle. *Alcohol use:* Increases CNS depressant effects. Discourage use together.

EFFECTS ON LAB TEST RESULTS

• May increase magnesium level. May decrease calcium level. May increase or decrease fluid and electrolyte levels.

ACTION

Produces anticonvulsant effects by depressing the CNS; also blocks peripheral neuromuscular transmission.

PHARMACOKINETICS

Onset, immediately after administration; duration, 30 minutes.
Distribution: Widely distributed. Drug crosses the placental barrier and appears in breast milk.
Metabolism: Not metabolized.
Excretion: In urine by glomerular filtration.

CLINICAL CONSIDERATIONS

• Osmolarity: 10% injection, 800 mOsm/L; 12.5% solution, 1,010 mOsm/L; 50% solution, 4,060 mOsm/L.
• Osmolality: 50% solution, 2,620 to 2,875 mOsm/kg.
• Rapid administration causes uncomfortable sensation of heat.
• Monitor vital signs every 15 minutes. Watch for respiratory depression and signs of heart block. Also, monitor intake and output. Before each dose, respirations should be about 16 breaths/minute and urine output should be 100 ml or more for 4 hours.
• Monitor magnesium level. Effective anticonvulsant level is 2.5 to 7.5 mEq/L.

• Observe neonate for signs of magnesium toxicity (such as neuromuscular or respiratory depression), especially when drug has been given to toxemic mothers within 24 hours before delivery.
• Toxicity may cause loss of patellar reflexes signals. Treat with 5 to 10 mEq of calcium (10 to 20 ml of calcium gluconate 10%). In severe overdose, peritoneal dialysis or hemodialysis may be needed.

PATIENT TEACHING
• Teach patient signs and symptoms of an adverse reaction.
• Tell patient to report difficulty breathing or paralysis.

mannitol
Osmitrol

Pharmacologic class: osmotic diuretic
Therapeutic class: diuretic, reduction of intracranial pressure
Pregnancy risk category: C
pH: 4.5 to 7

INDICATIONS & DOSAGES
➤ **Test dose for marked oliguria or inadequate renal function—**
Adults and children older than age 12: 200 mg/kg I.V., or 12.5 g I.V. as a 15% or 20% solution infused over 3 to 5 minutes.
Children age 12 and younger: 0.2 g/kg or 60 g/m² I.V. over 3 to 5 minutes, then 2 g/kg I.V.
➤ **To prevent oliguric phase in acute renal failure—**
Adults: 50 to 100 g I.V., followed by infusion of a 5% or 10% solution.
➤ **Oliguria—**
Adults: 100 g I.V. of a 15% or 20% solution over 90 minutes to several hours.

➤ **To reduce intracranial and intraocular pressure—**
Adults: 1.5 to 2 g/kg I.V. of a 15%, 20%, or 25% solution given over 30 to 60 minutes.
Children age 12 and younger: 2 g/kg I.V. or 60 g/m² I.V. of a 15% or 20% solution given over 30 to 60 minutes.
➤ **To reduce nephrotoxic effects of amphotericin B—**
Adults: 12.5 g I.V. immediately before and after each dose of amphotericin B.
➤ **Adjunctive therapy to promote diuresis in drug intoxication—**
Adults: 50 to 200 g I.V. of a 5% to 25% solution, followed by infusion to maintain urine output at 100 to 500 ml/hour.
➤ **Adjunctive therapy for edema and ascites—**
Adults: 100 g I.V. of a 10% to 20% solution over 2 to 6 hours.
Children age 12 and younger: 2 g/kg I.V. or 60 g/m² I.V. of a 15% or 20% solution over 2 to 6 hours.

ADMINISTRATION
• *Alert:* When giving mannitol solutions with concentrations of 15% or higher, make sure the administration set includes a filter. Rapid administration of large doses may lead to drug accumulation and circulatory overload.
Direct injection: Not recommended.
Intermittent infusion: Infuse appropriate dose and concentration at ordered rate.
Continuous infusion: Infuse appropriate dose and concentration at ordered rate.

PREPARATION & STORAGE
Available in strengths of 5%, 10%, 15%, 20%, and 25% in 250-, 500-, and 1,000-ml glass and plastic I.V. containers. Store at room temperature; avoid freezing. Drug may crystallize in concentrations of 15% or higher, especially if chilled. If crystals form, dissolve according to manufacturer's directions.

Reactions may be *common*, uncommon, *life-threatening*, or COMMON AND LIFE-THREATENING.

Avoid using solution that contains undissolved crystals.

Incompatibilities
Blood products, cefepime, doxorubicin liposomal, filgrastim, imipenem-cilastatin, meropenem, potassium chloride, sodium chloride, strongly acidic or alkaline solutions.

CONTRAINDICATIONS & CAUTIONS
• Contraindicated in patients hypersensitive to the drug, in those with anuria because of possible circulatory overload, and in those with intracranial bleeding, except during craniotomy, because of possible exacerbation.
• Contraindicated in patients with severe dehydration because mannitol worsens the condition, and in those with severe pulmonary congestion and heart failure because increased circulating volume aggravates these conditions.
• Use cautiously in patients with cardiopulmonary impairment because of risk of heart failure, and in those with severe renal impairment because of possible circulatory overload.
• Use cautiously in patients with hyperkalemia or hyponatremia because drug may worsen electrolyte imbalance, and in those with hypovolemia because drug may mask the condition and enhance hemoconcentration.
• Use cautiously in pregnant and breast-feeding women.

ADVERSE REACTIONS
CNS: dizziness, headache, *seizures,* fever.
CV: *arrhythmias,* chest pain, edema, hypertension, hypotension, tachycardia, thrombophlebitis.
EENT: rhinitis, blurred vision.
GI: anorexia, dry mouth, nausea, thirst, *diarrhea.*
GU: *acute renal failure,* diuresis, vacuolar nephrosis, urine retention.

Metabolic: acidosis, fluid and electrolyte imbalance.
Skin: skin necrosis, urticaria, local pain.
Other: chills.

INTERACTIONS
Drug-drug. *Cardiac glycosides:* Enhances risk of hypokalemia-induced toxic reaction. Monitor drug level.
Diuretics, including carbonic anhydrase inhibitors: May potentiate diuretic and intraocular effects. Monitor patient closely.
Lithium: Enhances excretion of lithium. Monitor lithium level.

EFFECTS ON LAB TEST RESULTS
• May alter electrolyte balances and blood ethylene glycol level.

ACTION
Increases osmotic pressure of glomerular filtrate, which inhibits renal tubular reabsorption of water and solutes, thus promoting diuresis. This aids excretion of sodium, potassium, chloride, calcium, phosphates, lithium, magnesium, and some toxins. Also, elevates plasma osmolality, which aids water flow from the brain, CSF, and eyes into interstitial fluid and plasma, thereby reducing CSF, intracranial, and intraocular pressure.

PHARMACOKINETICS
Onset, 15 minutes for reduction of CSF, 30 to 60 minutes for intraocular pressure, and 1 to 3 hours for diuresis; duration, 3 to 8 hours for reduction of CSF or intraocular pressure, 4 to 8 hours for diuresis.
Distribution: Confined to extracellular space. Drug doesn't reach the eye or cross the blood-brain barrier, except in high concentrations or in acidosis. It's unknown if drug crosses the placental barrier.
Metabolism: Metabolized slightly, if at all, to glycogen in the liver.

Excretion: In urine, with about 80% eliminated unchanged in 3 hours. Half-life, about 100 minutes. Clearance decreases in renal disease.

CLINICAL CONSIDERATIONS
• Osmolarity: 5% solution: 275 mOsm/L; 10% solution: 550 mOsm/L; 15% solution: 825 mOsm/L; 20% solution: 1,100 mOsm/L; 25% solution: 1,375 mOsm/L.
• Before giving drug, obtain baseline blood pressure, heart and breath sounds, and ECG.
• Monitor vital signs frequently during first hour of infusion and hourly thereafter or as needed. Also, monitor intake and output and BUN and electrolyte levels, especially sodium and potassium.
• Give test dose of mannitol to determine whether adequate response is possible. Urine flow should increase to at least 30 ml/hour for 2 to 3 hours after giving drug.
• *Alert:* Large doses may cross the blood-brain barrier and cause CNS damage or death.
• Small or debilitated patients may require lower doses.
• Watch for irritation and infiltration; extravasation can cause tissue damage and necrosis.
• Maintain hemostasis with adequate hydration and electrolytes.
• Lower drug concentrations and solutions containing sodium chloride reduce risk of dehydration and electrolyte depletion.
• A rebound increase in intracranial and intraocular pressure may occur about 12 hours after mannitol is given.
• Urine may need to be alkalized with sodium bicarbonate to help treat salicylate or barbiturate poisoning.

PATIENT TEACHING
• Advise patient to change positions slowly to avoid dizziness when standing up quickly.

• Alert patient to report adverse reactions such as dyspnea, apnea, or pain in the chest, back, or legs.

mechlorethamine hydrochloride (nitrogen mustard)
Mustargen

Pharmacologic class: alkylating drug (cell cycle phase–nonspecific)
Therapeutic class: antineoplastic
Pregnancy risk category: D
pH: 3 to 5

INDICATIONS & DOSAGES
➤ **Hodgkin's disease—**
Adults and children: 6 mg/m² I.V. daily on days 1 and 8 of 28-day cycle in combination with other antineoplastics, such as mechlorethamine-vincristine-procarbazine-prednisone (MOPP) regimen. Dosage repeated for six cycles.
    Dosage is based on patient response and degree of toxicity.
Adjust-a-dose: When WBC count is between 3,000 and 3,999/mm³, reduce subsequent doses in MOPP regimen by 50%, and when WBC count is between 1,000 and 2,999/mm³ or platelet count is between 50,000 and 100,000/mm³, reduce subsequent doses by 75%.
➤ **Polycythemia vera, chronic lymphocytic leukemia, chronic myelocytic leukemia, bronchogenic cancer—**
Adults and children: 0.4 mg/kg I.V. as single dose or 0.1 to 0.2 mg/kg I.V. divided in two or four successive daily doses during each course of therapy.
    Dosage is based on patient response and degree of toxicity.

ADMINISTRATION
Direct injection: Use one sterile needle to aspirate reconstituted drug from the vial and another to inject it. Inject reconstituted solution directly into vein

or, preferably, into a free-flowing I.V. solution over a few minutes or according to protocol. After administration, flush tubing and vein with I.V. solution for 2 to 5 minutes.

Intermittent infusion: Not recommended.

Continuous infusion: Not recommended.

PREPARATION & STORAGE

Be cautious when preparing or giving mechlorethamine to avoid mutagenic, teratogenic, and carcinogenic risks. Use a biological containment cabinet, wear gloves and mask, and use syringes with luer-lock fittings to prevent leakage of drug solution. Correctly dispose of needles, vials, and unused drug, and avoid contaminating work surfaces.

Avoid inhaling mechlorethamine dust and vapors, and avoid contact with skin and mucous membranes. If eye contact occurs, irrigate with liberal amounts of water or saline solution and consult an ophthalmologist immediately. If skin contact occurs, irrigate for at least 15 minutes with water and then with sodium thiosulfate solution 2%.

Mechlorethamine is available in 10-mg vials. Store at room temperature. Reconstitute with 10 ml sterile water for injection or normal saline solution for a concentration of 1 mg/ml. Shake vial several times to dissolve drug, and give within 15 minutes. Highly unstable, the solution decomposes while standing. Don't use if it's discolored or if water droplets appear in vial. Discard unused drug.

Incompatibilities

Allopurinol, cefepime, methohexital.

CONTRAINDICATIONS & CAUTIONS

• Contraindicated in those hypersensitive to the drug and in those with chickenpox, herpes, or other infections because of risk of generalized disease.

• Contraindicated in those with acute or chronic suppurative inflammation because drug may contribute to development of amyloidosis.

• Use cautiously in those who are undergoing anticoagulant therapy, radiation therapy, or other chemotherapy, and in those with preexisting myelosuppression or tumor cell infiltration of bone marrow because further myelosuppression may occur.

• Use cautiously in those with gout or history of urate renal stones because of increased risk of hyperuricemia.

ADVERSE REACTIONS

CNS: vertigo, weakness, depression.
CV: thrombophlebitis.
GI: anorexia, diarrhea, jaundice, *nausea, vomiting.*
GU: impaired fertility, menstrual irregularities.
Hematologic: *thrombocytopenia, hemorrhagic diathesis, immunosuppression, myelosuppression,* hemolytic anemia.
Metabolic: hyperuricemia.
Skin: maculopapular skin rash, tissue necrosis with extravasation.
Other: *anaphylaxis, secondary malignant disease,* vesicant thrombosis, precipitation of herpes zoster.

INTERACTIONS

Drug-drug. *Anticoagulants, aspirin, NSAIDs:* Increases risk of bleeding. Avoid using together.
Antigout drugs: Diminishes antigout drug effectiveness. Increased doses may be needed.
Myelosuppressives: Causes additional myelosuppression. Monitor CBC closely.

EFFECTS ON LAB TEST RESULTS

• May increase uric acid levels.
• May decrease hemoglobin, hematocrit, and granulocyte, lymphocyte, RBC, and platelet counts.

ACTION

An alkylating drug that inhibits rapid cell division by interfering with DNA replication and RNA transcription.

PHARMACOKINETICS

Drug level peaks within a few minutes. *Distribution:* Widely distributed to body fluids and tissues. Unknown if drug crosses the placental barrier. *Metabolism:* Rapidly metabolized in body fluids and tissues. *Excretion:* By the kidneys. More than 50% of inactive metabolites are excreted in urine.

CLINICAL CONSIDERATIONS

- Osmolality: 300 mOsm/kg.
- Drug is used almost exclusively in combination chemotherapy. Lower dosages are needed when it is used with other myelosuppressants.
- If infiltration occurs, aspirate as much drug as possible from tissues. Then, inject area with sterile isotonic sodium thiosulfate 1/6 M and apply ice compresses for 6 to 12 hours. Use 4.14 g of sodium thiosulfate per 100 ml of sterile water for injection, or dilute 4 ml of sodium thiosulfate 10% with 6 ml of sterile water for injection.
- Give with hydrocortisone, to reduce risk of phlebitis or painful administration.
- Expect some evidence of toxic reaction with a therapeutic response. Drug is highly toxic and has a low therapeutic index.
- Give an antiemetic to reduce severity of nausea and vomiting, which usually begin 1 to 3 hours after administration.
- Adequate hydration, alkalization of urine, and administration of allopurinol may prevent uric acid nephropathy.
- Monitor WBC and platelet counts and BUN, hematocrit, ALT, AST, bilirubin, creatinine, LDH, and uric acid levels.
- In lymphocytopenia, nadir occurs 1 to 3 weeks after drug administration.

- Interval between courses of therapy is usually 3 to 6 weeks.
- Closely monitor patient for potentially fatal infections or hemorrhagic complications indicated by fever, sore throat, or unusual bruising or bleeding.

PATIENT TEACHING

- Advise patient to avoid exposure to people with infections.
- Tell patient to contact prescriber immediately if unusual bleeding or bruising occurs.
- Tell patient that adequate hydration is important to facilitate excretion of uric acid.
- Advise patient to avoid contact sports.
- Caution patient to use care in dental hygiene with toothbrush, dental floss, and toothpicks.
- Advise patient to take temperature daily and watch for signs and symptoms of infection, such as fever, sore throat, and fatigue.
- Advise any woman of childbearing age to avoid becoming pregnant during therapy and to consult prescriber before becoming pregnant.

melphalan hydrochloride
Alkeran

Pharmacologic class: alkylating drug (cell cycle–phase nonspecific)
Therapeutic class: antineoplastic
Pregnancy risk category: D
pH: 3 to 7

INDICATIONS & DOSAGES

➤ **Palliative treatment of multiple myeloma—**
Adults: 16 mg/m² I.V. as a single infusion over 15 to 20 minutes at 2-week intervals for four doses; then, after adequate recovery from toxic reaction, at 4-week intervals. Adjust dosage based

on blood cell counts at nadir and on day of treatment.

Adjust-a-dose: For patients with a BUN level 30 mg/dl or more, reduce dosage up to 50%.

ADMINISTRATION

Give drug under supervision of a health care provider experienced in the use of chemotherapeutic drugs.

Direct injection: Not recommended.

Intermittent infusion: Give diluted drug over 15 to 20 minutes, within 60 minutes of reconstitution and dilution.

Continuous infusion: Not recommended.

PREPARATION & STORAGE

To avoid mutagenic, teratogenic, and carcinogenic risks, follow facility guidelines for the safe handling, preparation, administration, and disposal of chemotherapeutic drugs.

Available as a 50-mg powder for injection in a single-use vial with a 10-ml vial of sterile water for injection. Protect from light and dispense in glass.

To prepare, reconstitute with 10 ml of the diluent supplied and shake vigorously until solution is clear. The resultant solution contains 5 mg/ml of the drug. Immediately dilute the calculated dose in normal saline injection. Final concentration shouldn't exceed 0.45 mg/ml.

Complete administration within 60 minutes of reconstitution because both reconstituted and diluted solutions are unstable. Don't refrigerate solutions because precipitate will form.

Incompatibilities

Amphotericin B, chlorpromazine, D$_5$W, lactated Ringer's injection. Compatibility with normal saline injection depends on the concentration; don't prepare solutions with a concentration exceeding 0.45 mg/ml.

CONTRAINDICATIONS & CAUTIONS

● Contraindicated in those hypersensitive to drug and in those whose disease is resistant to drug. Patients hypersensitive to chlorambucil may exhibit cross-sensitivity to melphalan.

● Use cautiously in those who have received cytotoxic drugs or radiation therapy within 3 to 4 weeks and in those with renal insufficiency.

ADVERSE REACTIONS

CNS: transient paralysis, peripheral neuritis.

CV: hypotension, tachycardia, edema, *thrombosis,* phlebitis, *pulmonary embolism.*

GI: nausea, vomiting, diarrhea, oral ulceration.

Hematologic: *thrombocytopenia, leukopenia, bone marrow suppression,* hemolytic anemia.

Hepatic: *hepatotoxicity.*

Respiratory: *pneumonitis, pulmonary fibrosis,* dyspnea, *bronchospasm.*

Skin: pruritus, alopecia, urticaria.

Other: *anaphylaxis, hypersensitivity, secondary malignancy,* vesiculation and tissue necrosis.

INTERACTIONS

Drug-drug. *Bone marrow depressants, radiation therapy:* Causes additive bone marrow depression. Monitor hematologic studies closely.

Carmustine: May lower the threshold for carmustine-induced pulmonary toxicity. Monitor patient closely.

Cyclosporine, cisplatin: May increase nephrotoxicity. Monitor renal function closely.

Nalidixic acid: Increases incidence of severe hemorrhagic necrotic enterocolitis in children. Avoid using together.

Vaccines with live virus: May potentiate replication of the vaccine virus or decreased antibody response. Postpone routine immunization for at least 3 months after last dose of melphalan.

EFFECTS ON LAB TEST RESULTS
• May increase urine urea level.
• May decrease hemoglobin, hematocrit, and RBC, WBC, and platelet counts.

ACTION
Cross-links strands of cellular DNA and interferes with RNA transcription, causing an imbalance of growth that leads to cell death.

PHARMACOKINETICS
Onset, peak, and duration of drug effect unknown.
Distribution: Rapidly distributed throughout total body water; 60% to 90% protein-bound; low penetration into CSF. Unknown if drug appears in breast milk.
Metabolism: Chemical hydrolysis to monohydroxy and dihydroxy derivatives.
Excretion: 50% renal (10% to 15% unchanged), 20% to 50% fecal. Initial half-life, 10 minutes; terminal half-life, 75 minutes.

CLINICAL CONSIDERATIONS
• Monitor renal function and adjust dosage as needed.
• Therapeutic effects are commonly accompanied by toxic reaction.
• Perform CBCs before starting therapy and before each subsequent dose. If WBC count falls below 3,000/mm^3, temporarily stop drug or decrease dosage.
• To prevent bleeding, avoid all I.M. injections when patient's platelet count falls below 100,000/mm^3.
• Use anticoagulants and aspirin products cautiously. Watch for signs of bleeding. Advise patient to avoid OTC products containing aspirin.
• Weigh the risks of using the drug against the benefits for patients with bone marrow depression, renal function impairment, tumor cell infiltration

of bone marrow, infection, herpes zoster, or existing or recent exposure to chickenpox.
• Drug may be used in combination with other chemotherapeutic drugs, but dosage may need to be reduced. Altered incidence or increase in severity of adverse effects may occur. For specific protocols, consult specialized sources.
• Appropriate transfusions, antibiotics, and supportive care have been effective in treating drug overdose.

PATIENT TEACHING
• Warn patient to take temperature daily and watch for signs and symptoms of infection such as fever, sore throat, and fatigue, and signs and symptoms of bleeding.
• Advise any woman of childbearing age to avoid becoming pregnant during therapy and to consult a prescriber before becoming pregnant.

meperidine hydrochloride (pethidine hydrochloride)
Demerol

Pharmacologic class: opioid
Therapeutic class: analgesic, adjunct to anesthesia
Pregnancy risk category: C
Controlled substance schedule: II
pH: 3.5 to 6

INDICATIONS & DOSAGES
➤ **Moderate to severe pain**—
Adults: 15 to 35 mg/hour I.V. by infusion. Dosage reflects patient response and severity of pain.
➤ **Adjunct in anesthesia**—
Adults: Fractional doses of a 10 mg/ml solution I.V., repeated p.r.n., or 1 mg/ml by infusion.

ADMINISTRATION
Direct injection: Inject diluted dose over 3 to 5 minutes. Rapid injection increases risk of severe adverse reactions.
Intermittent infusion: Not recommended.
Continuous infusion: Give at rate of 15 to 35 mg/hour, using an infusion control device. Avoid rapid infusion.

PREPARATION & STORAGE
Available in preservative-free ampules and vials and in preservative-containing syringes with strengths of 10, 25, 50, 75, and 100 mg/ml. Store vials and ampules at room temperature. Single doses in syringes remain stable at room temperature for 24 hours.

For direct injection, dilute dose with a compatible solution to a concentration of 10 mg/ml. For infusion, dilute with a compatible solution to a concentration of 1 mg/ml. Compatible I.V. solutions include 5% dextrose in lactated Ringer's solution; dextrose-saline combinations; 2.5%, 5%, or 10% dextrose in water; Ringer's solution; lactated Ringer's solution; 0.45% or 0.9% sodium chloride solution; and 1/6 M sodium lactate solution.

Incompatibilities
Acyclovir, allopurinol, aminophylline, amobarbital, amphotericin B, cefepime, cefoperazone, doxorubicin liposomal, ephedrine, furosemide, heparin, hydrocortisone sodium succinate, idarubicin, imipenem-cilastatin sodium, methylprednisolone sodium succinate, morphine, pentobarbital, phenobarbital sodium, phenytoin, sodium bicarbonate, sodium iodide, thiopental.

CONTRAINDICATIONS & CAUTIONS
• Contraindicated in those hypersensitive to drug.
• Contraindicated in those with diarrhea resulting from poisons, toxins, cephalosporins, or topical clindamycin

until toxic substances clear because meperidine may slow GI motility.
• Contraindicated within 14 days of MAO inhibitor therapy.
• Avoid use in breast-feeding women.
• Avoid use in those with acute respiratory depression because drug may worsen condition.
• Use cautiously in those with seizure disorders because of possibility of exacerbating their condition.
• Use cautiously in pregnant women, taking into consideration the drug's risks versus its benefits.
• Use cautiously in those with head injury and increased intracranial pressure from intracranial lesions because drug can mask changes in level of consciousness and elevate CSF pressure; in those with atrial flutter or other supraventricular tachyarrhythmias because drug can increase ventricular response through a vagolytic action; and in those who have recently undergone GI surgery because drug can alter GI motility.
• Use cautiously in those with prostatic hyperplasia, urethral stricture, or recent urinary tract surgery because drug can cause urine retention; in those with gallbladder disease because drug may increase biliary contractions; and in those with abdominal disorders because drug may obscure diagnosis.
• Use cautiously in those with a history of drug abuse or emotional instability and in those who show evidence of suicide potential because of possible drug abuse.
• Use cautiously in those with hypothyroidism because of risk of prolonged CNS and respiratory depression; in those with altered respiratory function because of risk of respiratory depression; and in those with inflammatory bowel disease because of risk of toxic megacolon.
• Adjust dosage in those with renal or hepatic impairment or renal failure because of slowed drug clearance.

ADVERSE REACTIONS

CNS: agitation, anxiety, delirium, *dizziness,* euphoria, hallucinations, headache, *light-headedness, sedation, seizures,* tremors, syncope.
CV: *bradycardia, cardiac arrest, circulatory depression,* hypertension, hypotension, palpitations, *shock,* tachycardia.
EENT: visual disturbances.
GI: anorexia, biliary tract spasm, constipation, *nausea, vomiting.*
GU: antidiuretic effect, oliguria, urine retention.
Respiratory: *apnea, bronchospasm,* laryngospasm, *respiratory arrest.*
Skin: pruritus, urticaria, *sweating,* pain at injection site.
Other: addiction, *anaphylaxis.*

INTERACTIONS

Drug-drug. *Antidiarrheals:* Increases risk of severe constipation. Monitor closely; encourage fluid intake, as tolerated.
Antihypertensives, diuretics: Potentiates hypotension. Monitor blood pressure closely.
Antimuscarinics: Increases risk of constipation or urine retention. Monitor patient closely.
Chlorpromazine, thioridazine: Increases analgesic effects, possibly causing toxicity. Avoid using together.
Cimetidine: Increases respiratory and CNS depression. Reduce meperidine dose.
CNS depressants: Has additive CNS effects, respiratory depression, and hypotension. Use together cautiously.
HIV protease inhibitors: Increases meperidine level, causing respiratory depression. Avoid using together.
Isoniazid: May potentiate adverse effects of isoniazid. Avoid using together.
MAO inhibitors: Causes severe respiratory depression, cyanosis, hypotension, coma, hyperexcitability, hypertension, hyperpyrexia, seizures, and tachycardia. Don't give meperidine within 2 weeks of MAO inhibitor use.
Naloxone, naltrexone: May block analgesic effect. Avoid using together.
Neuromuscular blockers: Causes additive respiratory depression and severe constipation. Use together cautiously.
Oral anticoagulants: Increases risk of bleeding. Monitor PT and INR closely.
Phenytoin: Decreases meperidine effects. Watch for decreased analgesia.
Drug-herb. *Parsley:* May promote or produce serotonin syndrome. Discourage use together.
Drug-lifestyle. *Alcohol use:* Has additive CNS effects. Discourage use together.

EFFECTS ON LAB TEST RESULTS

● May increase amylase and lipase levels.
● May alter results of gastric emptying study, hepatobiliary imaging, and lumbar puncture.

ACTION

A morphine-like agonist that binds with opiate receptors in the CNS to alter the perception of pain and the emotional response to it. Also exerts mild antitussive action.

PHARMACOKINETICS

Onset, 1 minute; duration, 2 to 4 hours.
Distribution: Widespread. Highly plasma protein-bound, with highest levels in limbic system, thalamus, striatum, hypothalamus, midbrain, and spinal cord. Readily crosses the placental barrier. Drug appears in breast milk.
Metabolism: Occurs primarily in microsomes of the hepatic endoplasmic reticulum. Also occurs in CNS, kidneys, lungs, and placenta. Normeperidine, the primary metabolite, is both active and toxic.
Excretion: Primarily eliminated in urine as metabolites. Small amounts are removed in feces.

Reactions may be *common,* uncommon, *life-threatening,* or **COMMON AND LIFE-THREATENING.**

CLINICAL CONSIDERATIONS

• Osmolality: 50 mg/ml injection, 302 mOsm/kg.
• Check access site before administration. Inadvertent injection around a nerve trunk may cause transient sensorimotor paralysis.
• Give drug with patient in supine position to minimize orthostatic hypotension.
• For improved analgesia, give before patient has intense pain. Initially, a smaller daily dose given on a fixed schedule may help reduce patient anxiety. Once pain control is adequate, scheduling may be individualized.
• Monitor respirations frequently during infusion and every 15 minutes for 1 hour after infusion. Keep resuscitation equipment and naloxone nearby. If respirations drop below 8 breaths/minute, rouse patient to stimulate breathing. Notify prescriber; naloxone or respiratory support may be ordered. To reverse respiratory depression, give 0.4 mg of naloxone by I.V. push; repeat as needed. Maintain blood pressure with I.V. fluids and vasopressors.
• Assess patient's bowel function, and give a stool softener if needed.
• Acidifying urine may enhance excretion of unchanged drug.
• *Alert:* Drug may contain sulfites, which can cause allergic reactions in susceptible individuals.
• Drug may be given to patients allergic to morphine.
• Long-term use can lead to dependence. Withdrawal symptoms may begin 3 to 4 hours after last dose and usually peak within 8 to 12 hours.
• Drug isn't recommended for chronic pain because of potential for toxic reaction.
• Regular use of meperidine during pregnancy can lead to opioid dependence in neonate. Monitor neonate closely.

PATIENT TEACHING

• Tell patient to rise slowly to reduce dizziness.
• Advise patient to avoid alcoholic beverages and other CNS depressants.
• Tell patient to lie down if nausea, vomiting, dizziness, or light-headedness occurs.
• Tell patient to avoid breast-feeding while taking drug.
• Explain risks for a pregnant woman and her fetus.
• Caution patient about drug's CNS effects. Warn patient to avoid activities that require mental alertness until CNS effects of drug are known.
• Advise patient to notify his prescriber or dentist about use of drug if surgery or dental work needs to be done.

meropenem
Merrem I.V.

Pharmacologic class: carbapenem derivative
Therapeutic class: antibiotic
Pregnancy risk category: B
pH: 7.3 to 8.3

INDICATIONS & DOSAGES

➤ **Complicated appendicitis and peritonitis caused by viridans group streptococci,** *Escherichia coli, Klebsiella pneumoniae, Pseudomonas aeruginosa, Bacteroides fragilis, B. thetaiotaomicron,* **and** *Peptostreptococcus* **species; bacterial meningitis, in pediatric patients only, caused by** *Streptococcus pneumoniae, Haemophilus influenzae,* **and** *Neisseria meningitidis—*
Adults: 1 g I.V. q 8 hours. Don't exceed 2 g q 8 hours.
Children ages 3 months and older weighing 50 kg (110 lb) or less: 20 mg/kg I.V. for intra-abdominal infection or 40 mg/kg I.V. for bacterial meningitis q

8 hours; maximum dose is 2 g I.V. q 8 hours.
Children weighing more than 50 kg: 1 g I.V. q 8 hours for intra-abdominal infections and 2 g I.V. q 8 hours for meningitis.
Adjust-a-dose: For adults with creatinine clearance of 26 to 50 ml/minute, give the usual dose q 12 hours. For adults with creatinine clearance of 10 to 25 ml/minute, give half the usual dose q 12 hours. For adults with a creatinine clearance less than 10 ml/minute, give half the usual dose q 24 hours.

ADMINISTRATION

Direct injection: Prescribed dose may be given by direct I.V. injection over about 3 to 5 minutes.
Intermittent infusion: Infuse diluted drug over about 15 to 30 minutes.
Continuous infusion: Not recommended.

PREPARATION & STORAGE

Available in 20- and 30-ml injection vials containing 500 mg and 1 g, respectively. Also supplied in 100-ml infusion vials. ADD-Vantage vials contain 500 mg or 1 g. For I.V. bolus administration, add 10 ml of sterile water for injection to 500 mg/20-ml vial or 20-ml to 1 g/30-ml vial. Shake to dissolve and let stand until clear.

For I.V. infusion, infusion vials of 500 mg or 1 g/100 ml may be directly reconstituted with a compatible infusion fluid. Or, an injection vial may be reconstituted and resulting solution added to an I.V. container for further dilution with the appropriate infusion fluid. Don't use ADD-Vantage vial for this purpose. For ADD-Vantage vials, constitute with only half-normal saline injection, normal saline injection, or D₅W injection in 50-, 100-, or 250-ml Abbott ADD-Vantage flexible diluent containers. Follow manufacturer's guidelines closely. Use freshly prepared solutions immediately, if possible.

Stability of drug varies with type of drug used, that is, injection vial, infusion vial, or ADD-Vantage vial, and type of solution. Consult manufacturer's literature for details.

Dry powder should be stored at controlled room temperature of 68° to 77° F (20° to 25° C).

Incompatibilities

Other I.V. drugs.

CONTRAINDICATIONS & CAUTIONS

● Contraindicated in patients hypersensitive to drug or who have had anaphylactic reactions to beta-lactams.
● Use cautiously in those with previous hypersensitivity to imipenem, penicillins, or cephalosporins.
● Use cautiously in those with asthma or allergies and in those with underlying neurologic disorders.
● Use cautiously in those with renal impairment or liver dysfunction because of possible hepatotoxic effects.
● Use cautiously in breast-feeding patients. It isn't known if drug appears in breast milk.

ADVERSE REACTIONS

CNS: headache, *seizures.*
CV: phlebitis, thrombophlebitis at injection site.
GI: constipation, diarrhea, glossitis, nausea, oral candidiasis, vomiting, *pseudomembranous colitis.*
Respiratory: *apnea.*
Skin: rash; pruritus; injection site inflammation, pain, or edema.
Other: *anaphylactic reaction,* sepsis, shock, superinfection.

INTERACTIONS

Drug-drug. *Probenecid:* Inhibits renal secretion of meropenem. Drug competes with meropenem for active tubular secretion, increasing elimination half-life and extent of systemic exposure. Avoid giving together.

Reactions may be *common,* uncommon, *life-threatening,* or COMMON AND LIFE-THREATENING.

EFFECTS ON LAB TEST RESULTS

• May increase ALT, AST, bilirubin, alkaline phosphatase, LDH, creatinine, and BUN levels.
• May increase eosinophil and urinary RBC counts. May decrease hemoglobin, hematocrit, and WBC count. May increase or decrease PT, PTT, and INR, and platelet count.
• May cause false-positive direct or indirect Coombs' test result.

ACTION

Inhibits cell-wall synthesis in bacteria; readily penetrates cell wall of most gram-positive and gram-negative bacteria to reach penicillin-binding-protein targets.

PHARMACOKINETICS

Onset, unknown; peak levels, 1 hour after start of infusion of a single dose.
Distribution: Penetrates well into most body fluids and tissues, including CSF; plasma protein-binding is about 2%.
Metabolism: Undergoes extrarenal metabolism—20% to 25% of a dose—by dipeptidase or nonspecific degradation.
Excretion: About 70% of drug is excreted unchanged in the urine over 12 hours. Half-life in adults with normal renal function and children ages 2 and older, about 1 hour; in children ages 3 months to 2 years, 1½ hours.

CLINICAL CONSIDERATIONS

• Obtain specimen for culture and sensitivity tests before giving first dose.
• To minimize risk of seizures, closely adhere to dosage regimen, especially in patients predisposed to seizure activity, such as patients with CNS disorders, bacterial meningitis, or compromised renal function.
• *Alert:* Because serious and occasionally fatal hypersensitivity reactions may occur in those receiving therapy with beta-lactams, obtain thorough history and be prepared to treat reactions.

• Monitor patient for signs and symptoms of superinfection. Drug may cause overgrowth of nonsusceptible bacteria or fungi.
• Periodically monitor renal, hepatic, and hematopoietic function.

PATIENT TEACHING

• Instruct patient to report adverse reactions.
• Advise breast-feeding patients that drug may be transmitted to infant through breast milk.

---

mesna
Mesnex*, Uromitexan ◇

Pharmacologic class: thiol derivative
Therapeutic class: uroprotectant
Pregnancy risk category: B
pH: 6.5 to 8.5

INDICATIONS & DOSAGES

➤ **To prevent ifosfamide-induced hemorrhagic cystitis—**
Adults: 60% of ifosfamide dose. Give in three bolus doses, each 20% of ifosfamide dose, the first given at the time of the ifosfamide dose and subsequent doses given 4 and 8 hours later. Or, calculate daily dose as 100% of the ifosfamide dose. Give as a single bolus injection (20%), followed by two P.O. administrations (40% each). Protocols that use 1.2 g/m^2 I.V. ifosfamide would use 240 mg/m^2 I.V. mesna at 0 hours, then 480 mg/m^2 P.O. at 2 and 6 hours.
➤ **To prevent cyclophosphamide-induced hemorrhagic cystitis in bone marrow transplant recipients ♦ —**
Adults: 60% to 160% of cyclophosphamide dose by I.V. injection in three to five divided doses daily or by continuous infusion. For example, give patients receiving cyclophosphamide 50 mg/kg daily 12 mg/kg I.V. mesna

30 minutes before each cyclophos-phamide dose and 3, 6, 9, and 12 hours after each dose. Or, give patients receiving cyclophosphamide 60 mg/kg daily 10 mg/kg I.V. loading dose with cyclophosphamide dose, followed by 60 mg/kg I.V. infusion over 24 hours. Give mesna each day cyclophosphamide is given and continue for at least 24 hours after.

ADMINISTRATION
Direct injection: Using a 21G or 23G needle, inject into vein or into I.V. tubing containing a free-flowing, compatible solution.
Intermittent infusion: Infuse over 15 to 30 minutes.
Continuous infusion: Not recommended.

PREPARATION & STORAGE
Available in 10-ml vials at a concentration of 100 mg/ml.
Dilute the appropriate dose in D_5W, lactated Ringer's solution, or normal saline injection to a concentration of 20 mg/ml.
Diluted solutions are stable for 24 hours at 77° F (25° C), but use within 6 hours is recommended.
Store vials at room temperature.

Incompatibilities
Amphotericin B, carboplatin, cisplatin.

CONTRAINDICATIONS & CAUTIONS
● Contraindicated in those hypersensitive to mesna or other thiol compounds.

ADVERSE REACTIONS
CNS: *fatigue, fever, asthenia,* dizziness, headache, somnolence, anxiety, confusion, insomnia, pain.
CV: chest pain, edema, hypotension, tachycardia, flushing.
GI: *nausea, vomiting,* diarrhea, *constipation, anorexia, abdominal pain,* dyspepsia.
GU: hematuria.

Hematologic: *leukopenia, thrombocytopenia, anemia, granulocytopenia.*
Metabolic: hypokalemia, dehydration.
Musculoskeletal: back pain.
Respiratory: dyspnea, coughing, pneumonia.
Skin: alopecia, increased sweating, injection site reaction, pallor.
Other: *allergy.*

INTERACTIONS
None reported.

EFFECTS ON LAB TEST RESULTS
● May decrease potassium level.
● May decrease hemoglobin, hematocrit, and WBC, platelet, and granulocyte counts.
● May cause false-positive result in test for urinary ketones. May cause falsely elevated glucose and uric acid levels when sequential multiple analyzer is used.

ACTION
Free thiol compound, mesna, reacts with and detoxifies the urotoxic metabolites of ifosfamide.

PHARMACOKINETICS
Onset, peak, and duration of drug effect unknown.
Distribution: Remains intravascular. Unknown if drug appears in breast milk.
Metabolism: Rapidly oxidized to mesna disulfide in blood and reduced to free thiol compound, mesna, in the kidneys.
Excretion: In the kidneys, with 33% of the dose eliminated in the urine in 24 hours. Half-life of mesna, 0.36 hour; for mesna disulfide, 1.17 hours.

CLINICAL CONSIDERATIONS
● Osmolality: 1,563 mOsm/kg.
● Mesna won't prevent or alleviate other adverse reactions to chemotherapy.
● Since mesna is used with chemotherapy drugs, it's difficult to tell which adverse reactions are attributable solely to mesna.

Reactions may be *common*, uncommon, *life-threatening*, or COMMON AND LIFE-THREATENING.

- Hydrate patient with 2 L of oral or I.V. fluid before and during chemotherapy.
- Monitor urine samples for hematuria daily. Monitor BUN, creatinine, and intake and output.

PATIENT TEACHING
- Tell patient to promptly report adverse reactions.
- Explain use and administration of drug to patient and family and encourage them to ask questions and express concerns.
- Advise patient to avoid dehydration on days of chemotherapy administration.

methocarbamol
Robaxin

Pharmacologic class: carbamate derivative of guaifenesin
Therapeutic class: skeletal muscle relaxant
Pregnancy risk category: C
pH: 4 to 5

INDICATIONS & DOSAGES
➤ **Adjunct in severe musculoskeletal pain—**
Adults: 1 g I.V. q 8 hours. Maximum dosage, 3 g I.V. daily for 3 days.
➤ **Tetanus—**
Adults: 1 to 2 g I.V. by direct injection, followed by 1 to 2 g by infusion q 6 hours. Total initial dosage is 3 g I.V. Repeat doses q 6 hours until NG tube can be inserted.
Children age 12 and older: 15 mg/kg or 500 mg/m^2 I.V. q 6 hours. Don't exceed 1.8 g/m^2 I.V. daily for 3 consecutive days.

ADMINISTRATION
Direct injection: Inject drug into vein or through the tubing of free-flowing I.V.

solution at a maximum rate of 300 mg/minute. Slow injection helps to minimize adverse effects. Maximum rate in children is 180 mg/m^2 per minute.
Intermittent infusion: Infuse diluted solution through tubing of free-flowing I.V. line at ordered rate.
Continuous infusion: Not recommended.

PREPARATION & STORAGE
Available in 10-ml vials containing 100 mg/ml.
    Dilute single-dose vial in up to 250 ml of normal saline solution or D$_5$W for infusion.
    Store drug and diluted solution at room temperature; don't refrigerate diluted infusions.

Incompatibilities
None reported.

CONTRAINDICATIONS & CAUTIONS
- Contraindicated in those hypersensitive to drug and in those with renal impairment because polyethylene glycol, the nephrotoxic component used in preparation, may cause increased urea retention and acidosis.
- Use cautiously in those with CNS depression because of risk of exacerbating the condition and in those with epilepsy because of increased risk of seizures.
- Use cautiously in those with hepatic impairment because of decreased drug metabolism.

ADVERSE REACTIONS
CNS: *dizziness, drowsiness,* headache, *light-headedness, seizures,* syncope, vertigo, fever.
CV: *bradycardia,* hypotension, thrombophlebitis, flushing.
EENT: blurred vision, diplopia, conjunctivitis with nasal congestion, nystagmus.
GI: GI upset, metallic taste, nausea.
GU: discolored urine, hematuria.

Hematologic: *leukopenia.*
Musculoskeletal: mild muscular inco-ordination.
Skin: pruritus, rash, extravasation and sloughing at injection site, urticaria.
Other: *anaphylaxis.*

INTERACTIONS
Drug-drug. *CNS depressants:* Deepens CNS depression. Avoid using together.
Pyridostigmine: Causes severe weakness in patients with myasthenia gravis. Use together cautiously.
Drug-lifestyle. *Alcohol use:* Causes additive CNS depression. Discourage use together.

EFFECTS ON LAB TEST RESULTS
• May cause false-positive results in test for urine 5-hydroxyindoleacetic acid using nitrosonaphthol reagent (quantitative method of Udenfriend) and in Gitlow screening test for urine vanillylmandelic acid.

ACTION
Probably related to CNS-depressant effects. Drug has sedative and skeletal muscle-relaxant effects but has no direct action on the contractile mechanism of striated muscle, the nerve fibers, or the motor end-plate.

PHARMACOKINETICS
Onset, immediately after administration; duration, variable.
Distribution: Highest levels probably occur in the liver and kidneys; lowest levels in the lungs, heart, and skeletal muscle. Drug probably crosses the placental barrier, and small amounts appear in breast milk.
Metabolism: Extensively metabolized, presumably in the liver.
Excretion: Rapidly eliminated in urine as unchanged drug and metabolites. Half-life, 1 to 2 hours.

CLINICAL CONSIDERATIONS
• Watch for irritation and infiltration; extravasation can cause tissue damage and necrosis. Solution is hypertonic and may cause thrombophlebitis. Don't give drug for longer than three consecutive days.
• Monitor blood pressure and observe for orthostatic hypotension.
• Keep patient supine during administration and for 10 to 15 minutes afterward.
• Switch to P.O. methocarbamol as soon as possible.
• Although drug may cause seizures, it has been used to stop epileptic seizures.

PATIENT TEACHING
• Inform patient that urine may turn brown, black, or green.
• Warn patient of potential adverse reactions, including blurred vision, dizziness, and drowsiness.
• Advise patient to change positions slowly, particularly from recumbent to upright, and to dangle legs before standing.

methohexital sodium
Brevital Sodium

Pharmacologic class: barbiturate
Therapeutic class: I.V. anesthetic
Pregnancy risk category: B
Controlled substance schedule: IV
pH: 9.5 to 11

INDICATIONS & DOSAGES
➤ To induce anesthesia—
Adults: 1 to 1.5 mg/kg I.V. Dosage must be individualized. Younger adults may require larger doses than middle-aged or geriatric patients.
➤ To maintain general anesthesia—
Adults: About 20 to 40 mg of 1% solution (2 to 4 ml) I.V. as intermittent in-

jection, p.r.n., usually q 4 to 7 minutes;
or infuse 3 ml of 0.2% solution per
minute (1 drop per second).

ADMINISTRATION
Only staff who are trained in giving
anesthetics and managing their adverse
effects should give methohexital. Always keep resuscitation equipment
readily available. Overdose may occur
from overly rapid or repeated injection.
Direct injection: Inject diluted drug directly into vein or into a free-flowing
I.V. solution over 30 seconds. Repeat as
needed to maintain anesthesia.
Intermittent infusion: Not recommended.
Continuous infusion: Give 0.2% solution at prescribed rate, such as 1 gtt/
second.

PREPARATION & STORAGE
Available in 500-mg, 2.5-, and 5-g
vials.
    For a 1% solution for direct injec-
tion, add 50 ml of diluent to the 500-mg
vial, 250 ml to the 2.5-g vial, or 500 ml
to the 5-g vial. For a 0.2% solution for
continuous infusion, add 500 mg of
drug to 250 ml of D_5W or normal saline
solution. Drug is incompatible with sili-
cone present in rubber stoppers or syringe parts.
    Reconstitute with sterile water for
injection, D_5W, or normal saline injection. Don't use lactated Ringer's solution or diluents containing bacteriostatic agents.
    Store vials at room temperature. So-
lutions containing sterile water for injection remain stable at room temperature for 6 weeks; those containing D_5W
or normal saline solution remain stable
for 24 hours. Solutions should remain
clear and colorless; otherwise, discard.

Incompatibilities
Atropine, bacteriostatic diluents, chlorpromazine, cimetidine, clindamycin,
droperidol, fentanyl, glycopyrrolate,
hydralazine, isoproterenol, kanamycin,
lidocaine, mechlorethamine, methyldopate, norepinephrine, penicillin G,
pentazocine lactate, prochlorperazine
mesylate, promazine, promethazine,
scopolamine, streptomycin, succinylcholine, thiamine, tubocurarine.

CONTRAINDICATIONS & CAUTIONS
• Contraindicated in those hypersensitive to drug or barbiturates and in those
for whom general anesthesia is considered hazardous.
• Contraindicated in those with acute
intermittent porphyria, porphyria varie-
gata, or status asthmaticus because
drug may aggravate symptoms.
• Use cautiously in debilitated patients,
in geriatric patients, and in those with
myasthenia gravis or CNS depression
because respiratory depression or hypotension may occur.
• Use cautiously in those with respiratory, circulatory and renal, hepatic, or
endocrine disorders because drug can
cause prolonged depressant and hypnotic effects.

ADVERSE REACTIONS
CNS: emergence delirium, pain, hallucinations, headache, restlessness, anxiety, *seizures.*
CV: *bradycardia, circulatory depression,* hypotension, thrombophlebitis,
tachycardia.
GI: abdominal pain, salivation, nausea,
vomiting.
Musculoskeletal: shivering, muscle
twitching.
Respiratory: *bronchospasm, respiratory depression,* dyspnea, cough, hiccups.
Skin: injection site reaction, including
nerve injury near site; necrosis;
swelling; ulceration; rash.
Other: *anaphylaxis.*

INTERACTIONS
Drug-drug. *Antihypertensives, diuretics:* May cause additive hypotensive effects. Monitor vital signs closely.

Barbiturates, phenytoin: Decreases efficacy of methohexital. Use together cautiously.

CNS depressants, parenteral magnesium sulfate: May deepen CNS depression. Avoid using together.

Ketamine: May increase risk of hypotension or respiratory depression. Monitor vital signs closely.

Opioids: May increase methohexital concentrations. May cause apnea. Use together cautiously.

Phenothiazines: May potentiate hypotensive and CNS excitatory effects. Monitor patient closely.

Probenecid: May extend or achieve anesthetic effects at lower doses. Monitor patient.

Sulfasoxazole: Enhances anesthetic effects. Use together cautiously.

Drug-lifestyle. *Alcohol use:* Potentiates CNS depressant effects. Avoid using together.

EFFECTS ON LAB TEST RESULTS
● May cause falsely elevated sulfobromophthalein levels.
● May decrease ^{123}I and ^{131}I uptake in radioactive iodine test result. May alter liver function test result.

ACTION
Inhibits polysynaptic responses of the reticular-activating system, suppressing its arousal mechanism.

PHARMACOKINETICS
Onset, 10 to 20 seconds; duration, 5 to 7 minutes.

Distribution: Rapidly distributed to the CNS, then redistributed first to lean tissue and eventually to fatty tissue because drug is highly lipid. Also crosses the placental barrier. With large doses, small amounts appear in breast milk.

Metabolism: Probably in the liver; exact metabolism unknown.

Excretion: In urine, although elimination is minimal because of extensive renal tubular reabsorption of drug. About 1% is excreted unchanged in urine, the rest as a by-product of oxidative or conjugative metabolism. Half-life, about 4 hours.

CLINICAL CONSIDERATIONS
● Patient should fast before drug administration to reduce postoperative nausea and to avoid aspiration.
● Effects may be cumulative in continuous I.V. infusion.
● Drug has the potential for abuse.
● Watch for signs and symptoms of extravasation, which may cause local irritation leading to ulceration and necrosis.
● Avoid intra-arterial injection, which can cause platelet aggregation and thrombosis distal to injection site. Intra-arterial injection may lead to necrosis and gangrene, requiring amputation.

PATIENT TEACHING
● Warn patient to avoid tasks that require alertness because psychomotor skills may be impaired for 24 hours.
● Discharge patient to the care of another adult until effects of drug wear off.

methotrexate sodium (amethopterin, MTX)
Methotrexate LPF, Methotrexate Sodium*

Pharmacologic class: antimetabolite (S-phase specific)
Therapeutic class: antineoplastic
Pregnancy risk category: D
pH: 8.5

INDICATIONS & DOSAGES
➤ **Induce remission in lymphoblastic leukemia—**
Adults: 2.5 mg/kg I.V. q 14 days. Dosage varies widely.

➤ **Psoriasis—**
Adults: 10 to 25 mg I.V. once weekly. Up to 100 mg I.V. may be needed; however, manufacturer recommends maximum weekly dose of only 50 mg I.V.

➤ **Adjuvant therapy for osteo-sarcoma—**
Adults: 12 g/m^2 I.V. May be increased to 15 g/m^2 I.V. if lower dose proves insufficient to meet a 1,000 micromolar (10^{-3} mol/L) blood level at end of infusion.

Adjust-a-dose: When treating osteosarcoma, measure creatinine level before each course of therapy. If creatinine level increases by 50% or more over previous levels, measure creatinine clearance to make sure it exceeds 60 ml/minute. If creatinine clearance is below 60 ml/minute, reduce dosage or withhold therapy until renal function improves.

Reduce dosage by 25% if bilirubin level falls between 3 and 5 mg/dl or if AST level is above 180 units/L; and stop therapy if bilirubin level rises above 5 mg/dl.

ADMINISTRATION

Direct injection: Inject directly into vein or into side port of free-flowing I.V. line over prescribed duration.
Intermittent infusion: May be given as a 4-hour infusion.
Continuous infusion: Not recommended.

PREPARATION & STORAGE

Be cautious when preparing and giving methotrexate to avoid mutagenic, teratogenic, and carcinogenic risks. Use a biological containment cabinet, wear gloves and mask, and use syringes with luer-lock fittings. Correctly dispose of needles, vials, and unused drug, and avoid contaminating work surfaces.

Available in 20-, 50-, 100-, 250-, and 1-g vials of lyophilized sterile powder and in 2-, 4-, 8-, and 10-ml vials containing 25 mg/ml solution. Generic preparations may contain benzyl alcohol. Methotrexate LPF is preservative-free.

Reconstitute with sterile water for injection, normal saline solution, or D$_5$W. Reconstituted concentrations range from 2 to 50 mg/ml. Further dilute for injection with normal saline solution or D$_5$W.

Store drug preparations at room temperature and protect from light.

Incompatibilities

Bleomycin, chlorpromazine, dexamethasone sodium phosphate, droperidol, fluorouracil, gemcitabine, idarubicin, ifosfamide, metoclopramide, midazolam, nalbuphine, prednisolone, promethazine, propofol, sodium phosphate, vancomycin.

CONTRAINDICATIONS & CAUTIONS

• Contraindicated in those with preexisting or recent exposure to chickenpox or herpesvirus because of increased risk of generalized disease.
• Use cautiously in psoriasis patients with poor nutrition, renal or hepatic impairment, or blood dyscrasias because of increased risk of toxic reaction, and in those with nausea and vomiting because secondary dehydration increases the risk of toxic reaction.
• Use cautiously in those with GI obstruction, ascites, or peritoneal or pleural effusions because impaired elimination increases risk of toxic reaction.
• Use cautiously in those with gout or a history of urate stones because of increased risk of hyperuricemia, and in those with GI infection, peptic ulcer, ulcerative colitis, myelosuppression, or oral mucositis because drug may exacerbate these conditions.

ADVERSE REACTIONS

CNS: aphasia, dizziness, drowsiness, fatigue, malaise, paresis, fever, *seizures, encephalopathy.*
EENT: blurred vision, pharyngitis.
GI: *abdominal distress, GI hemorrhage,* gingivitis, glossitis, *nausea, ulcerative stomatitis,* vomiting, diarrhea.
GU: cystitis, infertility, *renal failure, spontaneous abortion,* menstrual irregularities.
Hematologic: anemia, *leukopenia, thrombocytopenia, myelosuppression (nadir in 6 to 10 days with rapid recovery).*
Hepatic: *hepatotoxicity.*
Metabolic: diabetes mellitus, hyperuricemia.
Musculoskeletal: osteoporosis, arthralgia, myalgia.
Respiratory: chronic, interstitial obstructive pulmonary disease, *interstitial pneumonitis, pulmonary fibrosis.*
Skin: alopecia, *urticaria, pruritus, hyperpigmentation, erythematous rash, ecchymoses, psoriatic lesions (aggravated by exposure to sun), rash, photosensitivity.*
Other: chills, infection, soft tissue necrosis, osteonecrosis, *septicemia.*

INTERACTIONS

Drug-drug. *Anticoagulants:* Increases risk of bleeding. Monitor PT and INR closely.
Antigout drugs: May increase uric acid level. Dosage may need to be adjusted.
Asparaginase: May block methotrexate effect. Avoid using together.
Aspirin, chloramphenicol, NSAIDs, para-aminobenzoic acid, penicillins, probenecid, protein-bound drugs, pyrimethamine, sulfonamides, sulfonylureas, tetracycline: May increase risk of methotrexate toxicity. Avoid using together.
Folic acid-containing vitamins: May decrease response to methotrexate. Avoid using together.
Hepatotoxic drugs: Increases risk of hepatotoxicity. Monitor liver function tests.
Myelosuppressants, radiation therapy: May increase myelosuppression. Monitor hematologic studies.
Phenytoin: Decreases phenytoin level. Monitor level closely.
Procarbazine: Increases nephrotoxicity. Monitor renal function.
Theophylline: Decreases theophylline clearance. Monitor theophylline level.
Vaccines with live virus: Increases risk of generalized disease. Postpone immunization, if possible.
Drug-lifestyle. *Alcohol use:* May increase hepatotoxicity. Discourage use together.
Sun exposure: May cause photosensitivity reactions. Advise patient to avoid excessive sunlight exposure.

EFFECTS ON LAB TEST RESULTS

• May increase uric acid level.
• May decrease hemoglobin, hematocrit, and WBC, RBC, and platelet counts.

ACTION

Blocks folinic acid's role in DNA synthesis and cell replication. Rapidly proliferating cells, such as bone marrow and malignant cells, are more sensitive to this effect.

PHARMACOKINETICS

Drug level peaks 30 minutes to 2 hours after administration.
Distribution: Widely distributed, with highest levels in the kidneys, gallbladder, spleen, liver, and skin. Drug crosses the placental and blood-brain barriers in minimal amounts. Drug appears in breast milk.
Metabolism: Insignificant.
Excretion: In urine by glomerular filtration and active transport, with 55% to 88% excreted within 24 hours. Small amounts are excreted in feces.

CLINICAL CONSIDERATIONS
• Tonicity is isotonic.
• Expect toxic reactions with therapeutic doses. Drug is highly toxic and has a low therapeutic index.
• Leucovorin calcium is used in high-dose methotrexate therapy to minimize adverse hematologic and GI effects.
• Drug is commonly used with other antineoplastics.
• Administration of large volumes of fluids, alkalization of urine, or use of allopurinol may prevent uric acid neuropathy.
• Monitor patient's intake and output.
• Monitor creatinine and BUN levels daily during high-dose methotrexate therapy.
• Monitor methotrexate level daily during therapy. Continue monitoring until level falls below 5×10^{-8} mol/L (0.05 micromolar).
• *Alert:* Don't repeat drug therapy unless WBC rises above 1,500/mm^3; neutrophil count rises above 200/mm^3; platelet count rises above 75,000/mm^3; bilirubin level is less than 1.2 mg/dl; ALT level is less than 450 units/L; creatinine level is normal; creatinine clearance is at least 60 ml/minute; and patient shows evidence of healing, if he has mucositis. Also, don't repeat therapy if patient experiences pleural effusion.
• Antibiotic therapy may be needed if infection occurs during period of myelosuppression.
• If overdose occurs, give leucovorin calcium as soon as possible, preferably within the first hour. For a massive overdose, urine alkalization and hydration may help prevent precipitation of methotrexate or its metabolites in the renal tubules.

PATIENT TEACHING
• Advise any man receiving the drug to use contraception during therapy and for at least 3 months afterward.

• Warn any woman of childbearing age to avoid becoming pregnant during therapy and for at least one ovulatory cycle after drug therapy ends.
• Advise women not to breast-feed during therapy because of potential for serious adverse effects in the infant.
• Tell patient to notify prescriber if he notices changes in breathing patterns or signs of liver dysfunction, including yellowed eyes or skin, malaise, and nausea.
• Encourage patient to drink more fluids.
• Advise patient to report mouth ulcers, which may be the first sign of toxic reaction.
• Instruct patient to avoid vaccinations.
• Instruct patient on how to check urine pH and to report it if less than 6.5.

methyldopate hydrochloride
Aldomet ◊

Pharmacologic class: centrally acting adrenergic
Therapeutic class: antihypertensive
Pregnancy risk category: C
pH: 3 to 4.2

INDICATIONS & DOSAGES
➤ **Sustained mild to severe hypertension and, in combination therapy, acute hypertensive emergencies**—
Adults: 250 to 500 mg I.V. q 6 hours, p.r.n. Maximum dose, 1 g q 6 hours.
Children: 20 to 40 mg/kg I.V. q 24 hours or 0.15 to 0.3 g/m^2 I.V. q 6 hours. Maximum daily dose, 65 mg/kg, 2 g/m^2, or 3 g I.V., whichever is least.
Adjust-a-dose: Patients with renal impairment may respond to smaller doses.

ADMINISTRATION
Direct injection: Not recommended.

Intermittent infusion: Infuse diluted dose through a patent I.V. line over 30 to 60 minutes.
Continuous infusion: Not recommended.

PREPARATION & STORAGE
Available in concentrations of 50 mg/ml. For infusion, add the needed dose to 100 ml of D_5W or add the required dose to D_5W for a concentration of 100 mg/10 ml. Drug remains stable for 24 hours in most I.V. solutions, but exposure to air may accelerate decomposition. Protect from light and store at room temperature; avoid freezing.

Incompatibilities
Amphotericin B; drugs with poor solubility in acidic media, such as barbiturates and sulfonamides; methohexital; some total parenteral nutrition solutions.

CONTRAINDICATIONS & CAUTIONS
• Contraindicated in those hypersensitive to drug and in those with active hepatitis or cirrhosis.
• Contraindicated in those who have had previous methyldopa therapy linked to liver abnormalities or hemolytic anemia by positive direct Coombs' test because of increased risk of adverse reactions.
• Contraindicated with coadministration of an MAO inhibitor.
• Contraindicated in sulfite-sensitive patients because preparation contains sulfites.
• Use cautiously in dialysis patients because dialysis may remove drug, leading to hypertension.
• Use cautiously in those with pheochromocytoma because drug interferes with urine catecholamine testing and may cause pressor response; and in those with coronary insufficiency or Parkinson's disease because drug may aggravate symptoms.

• Use cautiously in geriatric or debilitated patients who may be more sensitive to drug's hypotensive and sedative effects and in those with renal impairment because of the risk of drug accumulation.

ADVERSE REACTIONS
CNS: asthenia, depression, *headache, sedation,* weakness, *dizziness, decreased mental acuity.*
CV: *bradycardia, myocarditis,* orthostatic hypotension, edema, prolonged carotid sinus hypersensitivity.
GI: constipation, distention, nausea, vomiting, *dry mouth,* **pancreatitis.**
GU: amenorrhea, impotence.
Hematologic: hemolytic anemia, **immune thrombocytopenia, reversible leukopenia.**
Hepatic: **hepatic necrosis, hepatitis.**
Metabolic: *hyperkalemia,* hypernatremia, hyperuricemia.
Other: *anaphylaxis.*

INTERACTIONS
Drug-drug. *Anti-inflammatories, appetite suppressants, beta-blockers (nonselective, such as propranolol), estrogens, phenothiazines, tricyclic antidepressants:* May reduce hypotensive effect. Avoid using together.
CNS depressants: Deepens CNS depression. Monitor patient's mental status.
Diuretics, general anesthetics, hypotensives: Enhances hypotensive effect. Use together cautiously; dosage may need to be adjusted.
Haloperidol: May alter antipsychotic effects. Use together cautiously.
Levodopa: Enhances hypotensive and toxic CNS effects. Monitor blood pressure and neurological status.
Lithium carbonate: Increases risk of lithium toxicity. Monitor lithium level closely.
MAO inhibitors: Causes hyperexcitability, severe hypertension, other CNS disturbances. Avoid using together.

Reactions may be *common,* uncommon, *life-threatening,* or COMMON AND LIFE-THREATENING.

Sympathomimetics: Potentiates pressor effect of these drugs and decreases hypotensive effect of methyldopa. Avoid using together.

Drug-herb. *Capsicum:* May reduce antihypertensive effectiveness. Discourage use together.

EFFECTS ON LAB TEST RESULTS
• May increase BUN, creatinine, potassium, sodium, uric acid, bilirubin, alkaline phosphatase, ALT, and AST levels.
• May decrease hemoglobin, hematocrit, and platelet and WBC counts.
• May cause falsely elevated levels of urine catecholamines, interfering with the diagnosis of pheochromocytoma. May cause false-positive Coombs' test result.

ACTION
Alpha agonist that reduces sympathetic outflow from the CNS, diminishing renin levels and peripheral resistance.

PHARMACOKINETICS
Onset, 4 to 6 hours; duration, 10 to 16 hours.
Distribution: Mostly to the heart, kidneys, and peripheral vessels. Drug and its metabolites are weakly protein bound. Drug crosses blood-brain and the placental barriers.
Metabolism: Hydrolyzed to methyldopa, which is extensively metabolized in the liver.
Excretion: In urine, largely by glomerular filtration, with 20% to 55% removed unchanged. Drug appears in breast milk in levels of 20% to 35% of maternal serum levels. Biphasic elimination has an initial half-life of about 2 hours and a much slower second phase. In impaired renal function, initial half-life is about 3½ hours.

CLINICAL CONSIDERATIONS
• Osmolality: 481 mOsm/kg.
• *Alert:* Drug may contain sulfites.

• Monitor heart rate, cardiac output, blood volume, electrolyte balance, GI motility, renal function, and cerebral activity. To reverse hypotension, give I.V. fluids.
• Monitor hemoglobin, hematocrit, and CBC before and during therapy. If hemolytic anemia develops, stop drug.
• Monitor liver function test results. Stop drug if patient develops fever, abnormal liver function, or jaundice.
• Monitor blood pressure. Once blood pressure is stable, change to oral form of drug, as ordered.
• Monitor patient for signs of drug-induced depression.
• Perform Coombs' test before therapy.
• If overdose occurs, keep patient supine and provide symptomatic care. Dialysis may be helpful in eliminating drug.

PATIENT TEACHING
• Inform patient that drug may cause drowsiness at first. Tell him to rise from bed slowly to prevent dizziness upon standing, and to avoid activities that require alertness.
• Tell patient to report evidence of yellowed skin and eyes immediately.
• Tell patient to report adverse reactions promptly.
• Explain use and administration of drug to patient and family.

methylene blue

Pharmacologic class: thiazine dye
Therapeutic class: antidote
Pregnancy risk category: C
pH: 3 to 4.5

INDICATIONS & DOSAGES
➤ **Methemoglobin and cyanide poisoning—**
Adults and children: 1 to 2 mg/kg I.V. of 1% solution; may repeat in 1 hour.

ADMINISTRATION

Direct injection: Give over several minutes directly into vein or through an I.V. line containing a free-flowing, compatible solution. Overly rapid injection causes additional methemoglobin production. Don't exceed recommended dosage.

Intermittent infusion: Not recommended.

Continuous infusion: Not recommended.

PREPARATION & STORAGE

Available in 1- and 10-ml ampules containing 10 mg/ml. No need to dilute before injection. Store from 59° to 86° F (15° to 30° C).

Incompatibilities

Dichromates, iodides, oxidizing and reducing substances.

CONTRAINDICATIONS & CAUTIONS

• Contraindicated in patients hypersensitive to drug and in those with severe renal impairment.

• Use cautiously in those with G6PD deficiency because drug may cause hemolysis.

• Safe use in pregnant patients hasn't been established.

ADVERSE REACTIONS

CNS: confusion, dizziness, headache.
CV: hypertension, precordial pain.
GI: abdominal pain, nausea, vomiting.
Skin: cyanosis, diaphoresis.
Other: methemoglobin formation.

INTERACTIONS

Drug-lifestyle. *Sun exposure:* May cause photosensitivity reaction. Advise patient to avoid excessive sunlight exposure.

EFFECTS ON LAB TEST RESULTS

• May decrease hemoglobin and hematocrit.

ACTION

High concentrations oxidize the ferrous iron of reduced hemoglobin to ferric iron, forming methemoglobin. Low concentrations increase the conversion rate of methemoglobin to hemoglobin.

PHARMACOKINETICS

Drug level peaks at end of infusion.
Distribution: Unknown if drug crosses the placental barrier or appears in breast milk.
Metabolism: In tissues by reduction to leukomethylene blue.
Excretion: In urine, some unchanged, and bile.

CLINICAL CONSIDERATIONS

• S.C. injection may cause necrotic abscesses.
• In prolonged therapy, monitor for signs of anemia.
• Monitor I.V. site carefully to avoid extravasation.

PATIENT TEACHING

• Tell patient that drug stains skin; stains can be removed with bleach solution.

methylergonovine maleate
Methergine

Pharmacologic class: ergot alkaloid
Therapeutic class: oxytocic
Pregnancy risk category: C
pH: 2.7 to 3.5

INDICATIONS & DOSAGES

➤ **Emergency treatment of severe postpartum and postabortion hemorrhage caused by uterine atony or subinvolution—**
Adults: 0.2 mg I.V. in single dose, repeated q 2 to 4 hours; may give up to five doses, if needed.

ADMINISTRATION

Direct injection: Give directly into vein or into free-flowing, compatible I.V. solution over at least 60 seconds. If desired, use diluted dosage to facilitate slow injection. Overly rapid administration can cause severe CV effects.
Intermittent infusion: Not recommended.
Continuous infusion: Not recommended.

PREPARATION & STORAGE

Available in 1-ml ampules containing 0.2 mg/ml. Store drug below 46° F (8° C) in a light-resistant container. Avoid freezing. Ready-to-use injections are normally clear and colorless. Discard if solution is discolored or contains a precipitate.

Dilute with 5 ml of normal saline solution, if appropriate.

Incompatibilities

None reported.

CONTRAINDICATIONS & CAUTIONS

• Contraindicated in pregnant patients and in patients hypersensitive to drug.
• Contraindicated in patients with hypertension or toxemia.
• Use cautiously in those with occlusive peripheral vascular disease because drug can aggravate symptoms, and in those with sepsis or hepatic or renal impairment because drug can cause ergotism.
• Use cautiously during the second stage of labor and in breast-feeding women.

ADVERSE REACTIONS

CNS: headache, *seizures.*
CV: *hypertension,* hypotension.
GI: nausea, vomiting.
Other: *anaphylaxis.*

INTERACTIONS

Drug-drug. Dopamine, ergot alkaloids, I.V. oxytocin, regional anesthetics, vasoconstrictors: May enhance vasoconstriction. Use together cautiously.

EFFECTS ON LAB TEST RESULTS

• May decrease prolactin level.

ACTION

Produces vasoconstriction, directly stimulates uterine and vascular smooth muscle, and increases cervical contraction.

PHARMACOKINETICS

Onset, immediate; duration, up to 45 minutes.
Distribution: Rapid, into plasma, extracellular fluid, and tissues. Negligible amounts appear in breast milk.
Metabolism: Presumably in the liver.
Excretion: Mostly in feces, some in urine. Elimination may be prolonged in neonates. Half-life is biphasic: initial phase, 1 to 5 minutes; terminal phase, 30 minutes to 2 hours.

CLINICAL CONSIDERATIONS

• Closely monitor blood pressure and pulse. Give I.V. hydralazine or chlorpromazine for hypertension.
• After giving drug, closely monitor uterine activity. Contractions are sustained and uterine tone is high. If appropriate, give analgesics for discomfort.
• Reduce dosage if severe uterine cramping occurs.
• Treatment of overdose is symptomatic and may include maintenance of pulmonary ventilation, correction of hypotension, control of seizures, and control of peripheral vasospasm.

PATIENT TEACHING

• Instruct patient to report shortness of breath, headache, numb or cold fingers or toes, or severe abdominal cramping.

- Discuss importance of taking drug as prescribed, including amount and duration.
- Tell patient to report adverse reactions promptly.
- Explain use and administration of drug to patient and family.

methylprednisolone sodium succinate
A-Methapred*, Solu-Medrol*

Pharmacologic class: glucocorticoid
Therapeutic class: anti-inflammatory, immunosuppressant
Pregnancy risk category: C
pH: 7 to 8

INDICATIONS & DOSAGES
➤ **Severe inflammation or immuno-suppression—**
Adults: 10 mg to 1.5 g I.V. daily. Usual dosage, 10 to 250 mg I.V. q 4 hours.
Children: Individualize dose based on severity of condition. Give at least 0.5 mg/kg I.V. q 24 hours.
➤ **Severe shock—**
Adults: 30 mg/kg I.V. initially, repeated q 4 to 6 hours, p.r.n.; or 100 to 250 mg I.V. initially, repeated q 2 to 6 hours, p.r.n. Initial dose may be followed by 30 mg/kg infusion q 12 hours for 24 to 48 hours.
➤ **Acute exacerbations of multiple sclerosis—**
Adults: 160 mg I.V. daily for 1 week, followed by 64 mg I.V. every other day for 1 month.
➤ **Severe lupus nephritis ◆ —**
Adults: 1 g I.V. by intermittent infusion over 1 hour for 3 days, followed by oral prednisolone or prednisone.
Children: 30 mg/kg I.V. on alternate days for six doses, followed by oral prednisolone or prednisone.

➤ **To decrease residual damage after spinal cord trauma ◆ —**
Adults: 30 mg/kg I.V. as a bolus injection over 15 minutes (within 8 hours of injury), followed in 45 minutes by I.V. infusion of 5.4 mg/kg/hour for next 23 hours.
➤ **Adjunctive treatment of *Pneumocystis carinii* pneumonia ◆ —**
Adults: 30 mg I.V. b.i.d. for 5 days, then 30 mg I.V. daily for 5 days. Finally, give 15 mg I.V. daily for 11 days or until anti-infective therapy is stopped.

ADMINISTRATION
Direct injection: Inject diluted drug into vein or free-flowing, compatible I.V. solution over at least 1 minute. In life-threatening situations, give initial massive dose over 3 to 15 minutes.
Intermittent infusion: Using appropriately diluted dose, adjust flow rate, depending on disorder and patient's response.
Continuous infusion: Using appropriately diluted dose, adjust flow rate, depending on disorder and patient's response.

PREPARATION & STORAGE
Available in container of drug and diluent in the following strengths: 40, 125, 500 mg, and 1 and 2 g. In some preparations, diluent contains benzyl alcohol.

Reconstitute with diluent provided and store at room temperature. Avoid freezing. Don't use solution if cloudy, and discard any unused portion after 48 hours. Dilute for infusion with D_5W or normal saline solution.

Incompatibilities
Allopurinol, aminophylline, calcium gluconate, ciprofloxacin, cytarabine, diltiazem, docetaxel, doxapram, etoposide, gemcitabine, filgrastim, glycopyrrolate, nafcillin, ondansetron, paclitaxel, penicillin G sodium, potassium

chloride, propofol, sargramostim, vinorelbine, vitamin B complex with C.

CONTRAINDICATIONS & CAUTIONS
• Contraindicated in those with systemic fungal infection, sepsis syndrome, or septic shock because drug may mask symptoms and exacerbate these conditions.
• Contraindicated in those hypersensitive to drug or its components and in neonates.
• Use cautiously in those with hyperthyroidism, hypothyroidism, or cirrhosis because of possible exaggerated drug response, and in those with diverticulitis, nonspecific ulcerative colitis, or recent intestinal anastomosis because of possible perforation, abscess, or other pyogenic infection.
• Use cautiously in psychotic patients because drug may precipitate mental disturbances, and in those with a history of tuberculosis because drug may reactivate disease.
• Use cautiously in those with seizure disorders, renal insufficiency, diabetes mellitus, osteoporosis, or ocular herpes simplex infections to prevent exacerbation of symptoms, and in those with hypoalbuminemia to prevent drug toxicity.
• Use cautiously in children because drug may retard bone growth. It may also increase intracranial pressure, resulting in papilledema, oculomotor or abducens nerve paralysis, vision loss, and headache.
• Use cautiously in those with renal dysfunction because of possible severe fluid retention, in those with hepatic dysfunction because of increased risk of toxic reaction, and in those with open-angle glaucoma because of risk of elevated intraocular pressure.

ADVERSE REACTIONS
CNS: depression, *euphoria, insomnia, pseudotumor cerebri, seizures,* fever.

CV: *heart failure, thromboembolism, fatal arrest, circulatory collapse,* bleeding, hypertension, palpitations, facial flushing, tachycardia.
EENT: blurred vision.
GI: GI irritation, nausea, *peptic ulceration,* vomiting, *pancreatitis.*
GU: menstrual irregularities.
Metabolic: fluid and electrolyte imbalance.
Respiratory: dyspnea.
Skin: rash, pain at injection site.
Other: *anaphylaxis,* increased susceptibility to infection, corticosteroid withdrawal syndrome (including anorexia, headache, hypotension, joint pain, lethargy, and weight loss).

INTERACTIONS
Drug-drug. *Anticholinesterases:* Causes severe weakness in patients with myasthenia gravis. Use cautiously and monitor patient.
Asparaginase: May increase risk of neuropathy and disturbances in erythropoiesis. Monitor patient closely.
Barbiturates, phenytoin, rifampin: May increase methylprednisolone metabolism. May need to increase dose of methylprednisolone.
Cardiac glycosides: Increases risk of arrhythmias or digitalis toxicity. Monitor ECG and digoxin level.
Erythromycin, troleandomycin: Potentiates effects of methylprednisolone sodium succinate caused by decreased metabolism. Monitor patient for increased adverse effects.
Estrogen: May potentiate methylprednisolone effects. Monitor patient for increased effects
Indomethacin, NSAIDs, ulcerogenic drugs: Increases risk of GI ulcers. Monitor patient for bleeding.
Isoniazid, mexiletine, salicylates: Glucocorticoids increase the clearance of these drugs, decreasing their effectiveness. Monitor patient for lack of effect.
Potassium-wasting diuretics, other potassium-wasting drugs: Enhances

potassium loss. Monitor potassium level.

Sodium-containing drugs: May cause hypernatremia. Monitor electrolyte level closely.

Streptozocin: Enhances risk of hyperglycemia. Monitor glucose.

Toxoids, vaccines with inactivated virus: Diminishes response. Avoid using together.

Vaccines with live virus: Increases risk of developing systemic diseases. Postpone immunization, if possible.

Drug-food. *Foods containing sodium:* May cause hypernatremia. Monitor electrolyte level closely.

EFFECTS ON LAB TEST RESULTS

• May increase glucose and cholesterol levels. May decrease T_3, T_4, potassium, and calcium levels.

• May decrease ^{131}I uptake and protein-bound iodine levels in thyroid function tests and uptake of contrast medium in radionuclide brain imaging. May cause false-negative result in the nitroblue tetrazolium test for systemic bacterial infections. May alter reactions to skin tests.

ACTION

Suppresses pituitary release of corticotropin, preventing adrenocortical secretion of corticosteroids. As a result, drug suppresses immune responses, stimulates bone marrow, and alters protein, fat, and carbohydrate metabolism. Also decreases inflammation by stabilizing leukocyte lysosomal membranes.

PHARMACOKINETICS

Onset, rapid.

Distribution: Rapidly distributed to muscle, liver, skin, intestines, and kidneys. Drug binds especially with the protein transcortin and crosses the placental barrier. Drug probably appears in breast milk.

Metabolism: In most tissues, but primarily in the liver, to inactive compounds.

Excretion: Primarily in kidneys, with small amounts in urine and negligible amounts in bile. Half-life, 2 to 3½ hours; tissue half-life, up to 36 hours.

CLINICAL CONSIDERATIONS

• Osmolarity: 400 to 500 mOsm/L.

• *Alert:* Because of risk of anaphylaxis, keep resuscitation equipment nearby.

• Before therapy, obtain baseline ECG, blood pressure, chest and spinal X-rays, glucose tolerance test, evaluation of hypothalamic-pituitary-adrenal axis function and, in patients with predisposition to GI disorders, results of upper-GI series.

• Monitor patient for cushingoid effects, including moon-face, buffalo hump, central obesity, thinning hair, hypertension, and increased susceptibility to infection.

• Adjust dosage as needed for patients taking insulin, antithyroid drugs, or thyroid hormones.

• Most adverse reactions to corticosteroids are dose- or duration-dependent.

• Determine whether patient is hypersensitive to other corticosteroids.

• *Alert:* Don't confuse Solu-Medrol with Solu-Cortef (hydrocortisone sodium succinate).

• *Alert:* Don't confuse methylprednisolone sodium succinate with other methylprednisolone salt formulations.

• Adrenal function may recover within 1 week after high-dose therapy lasting for 1 to 5 days.

• During long-term therapy, monitor height, weight, blood pressure, chest and spinal X-rays, and hematopoietic, electrolyte, glucose tolerance, and intraocular pressure test results.

PATIENT TEACHING

• Instruct patient to notify prescriber about signs of infection or injuries received during therapy and for 12 months afterward.

• Patient may need to increase protein intake because drug promotes protein catabolism.

• Explain to patient and family the use and administration of drug.

---

metoclopramide hydrochloride
Octamide PFS, Reglan

Pharmacologic class: para-aminobenzoic acid (PABA) derivative
Therapeutic class: antiemetic, GI stimulant
Pregnancy risk category: B
pH: 3 to 6.5

INDICATIONS & DOSAGES
➤ **Nausea and vomiting during chemotherapy—**
Adults: 2 mg/kg I.V., beginning 30 minutes before chemotherapy; repeat q 2 hours for two doses, then give 1 mg/kg I.V. q 3 hours for three doses. For less emetogenic regimens, 1 mg/kg/dose may be adequate.
➤ **Severe delayed gastric emptying in diabetic gastroparesis in patients unable to take oral dose—**
Adults: 10 mg I.V. q.i.d. 30 minutes before meals and h.s.
➤ **Passage of intestinal tubes for diagnostic tests; radiologic examination of GI tract in delayed gastric emptying that interferes with examination of stomach or intestine—**
Adults: 10 mg I.V.
Children ages 6 to 14: 2.5 to 5 mg I.V.
Children younger than age 6: 0.1 mg/kg I.V.
➤ **Nausea and vomiting during pregnancy and labor ♦—**
Adults: 5 to 20 mg I.V. t.i.d.

Adjust-a-dose: In adults with creatinine clearance less than 40 ml/minute, decrease dosage by 50%.

ADMINISTRATION
Direct injection: Inject over 1 or 2 minutes directly into vein or into I.V. tubing containing a free-flowing, compatible solution. Each 10 mg of drug should be given slowly over 1 to 2 minutes.
Intermittent infusion: Cover solution with a brown paper bag to prevent exposure to light. Infuse over at least 15 minutes. Slow infusion prevents anxiety and restlessness.
Continuous infusion: Not recommended.

PREPARATION & STORAGE
Available with a concentration of 5 mg/ml in 2-, 10-, 30-, 50-, and 100-ml vials and in 2- and 10-ml ampules. For doses greater than 10 mg, dilute with 50 ml of D_5W, normal saline solution, dextrose 5% in half-normal saline solution, Ringer's injection, or lactated Ringer's solution.

Solutions remain stable for 48 hours when stored at 39° to 86° F (4° to 30° C) and protected from light. If diluted with normal saline solution, it may be frozen in polyvinyl chloride bags for up to 4 weeks. Don't use dextrose 5% diluent with polyvinyl chloride bags if solution will be frozen.

Incompatibilities
Allopurinol, ampicillin, amphotericin B, calcium gluconate, cefepime, chloramphenicol sodium succinate, cisplatin, doxorubicin liposomal, erythromycin lactobionate, fluorouracil, furosemide, methotrexate sodium, penicillin G potassium, propofol, sodium bicarbonate.

CONTRAINDICATIONS & CAUTIONS
• Contraindicated in those hypersensitive to or intolerant of metoclopramide.

• Contraindicated when acceleration of GI motility may be hazardous, as in obstruction, hemorrhage, or perforation.

• Contraindicated in patients with epilepsy and those taking drugs that may cause extrapyramidal reactions (such as phenothiazines), which may increase the severity of symptoms.

• Contraindicated in those with pheochromocytoma because drug may cause hypertensive crisis.

• Use cautiously in those with renal impairment because delayed excretion may prolong and intensify drug effects, and in those with Parkinson's disease because drug may exacerbate symptoms.

ADVERSE REACTIONS

CNS: *restlessness, anxiety, drowsiness, fatigue, lassitude,* fever, depression, akathisia, insomnia, confusion, **suicide ideation, seizures, neuroleptic malignant syndrome,** hallucinations, headache, dizziness, extrapyramidal symptoms, tardive dyskinesia, *dystonic reactions.*
CV: transient hypertension, hypotension, **supraventricular tachycardia, bradycardia.**
GI: nausea, bowel disorders, diarrhea.
GU: urinary frequency, incontinence.
Hematologic: *neutropenia, agranulocytosis.*
Skin: rash, urticaria.
Other: loss of libido, porphyria.

INTERACTIONS

Drug-drug. *Anticholinergics, opioid analgesics:* Antagonizes metoclopramide effects on GI motility. Avoid using together.
Cimetidine: Decreases bioavailability of cimetidine. Monitor patient for effect.
CNS depressants: May potentiate sedative effects. Avoid using together.

Cyclosporine: Increases absorption causing toxic effects of cyclosporine. Monitor cyclosporine levels.
Digoxin: Decreases digoxin levels. Monitor digoxin level.
Drugs that cause extrapyramidal reactions: May increase frequency and severity of extrapyramidal effects. Monitor patient closely.
Levodopa: May increase the bioavailability of levodopa. May decrease metoclopramide effects. Don't use metoclopramide in Parkinson's disease patients.
MAO inhibitors: Increases release of catecholamines may lead to toxic reaction. Avoid using together.
Opioid analgesics: Decreases effect. Monitor patient for pain relief.
Oral drugs: Increases GI motility, which may decrease gastric absorption and increase small intestine absorption of drug. Monitor patient for lack of effect.
Succinylcholine: Inhibits cholinesterase, increasing neuromuscular blocking effects. Avoid using together.

EFFECTS ON LAB TEST RESULTS

• May increase aldosterone and prolactin levels.

• May decrease neutrophil, WBC, and granulocyte counts.

ACTION

At the chemoreceptor trigger zone in the CNS to inhibit vomiting. Also enhances gastric emptying and increases GI muscle tone and phasic contractile activity.

PHARMACOKINETICS

Onset, 1 to 3 minutes; duration, 1 to 2 hours.
Distribution: Throughout tissues, with 13% to 22% protein bound. Drug crosses the blood-brain and placental barriers and appears in breast milk.
Metabolism: Minimal, in the liver.

Reactions may be *common,* uncommon, *life-threatening,* or COMMON AND LIFE-THREATENING.

Excretion: In urine and feces. Half-life averages 3 to 6 hours in normal renal function.

CLINICAL CONSIDERATIONS
● Osmolality: 280 mOsm/kg.
● Monitor blood pressure during administration.
● Monitor patient for extrapyramidal effects.
● Adjust insulin dosage, as ordered, in patients with diabetic gastroparesis. Drug affects intestinal food absorption.
● To control extrapyramidal symptoms, give antimuscarinic antiparkinsonians or antihistamines with antimuscarinic properties.

PATIENT TEACHING
● Instruct patient to avoid alcohol, OTC sleep remedies, and sedatives during drug therapy.
● Tell patient to contact prescriber if he experiences involuntary movements in his face, eyes, or limbs.
● Tell patient to promptly report adverse reactions.

metoprolol tartrate
Betaloc ◇, Lopresor ◇, Lopressor

Pharmacologic class: beta$_1$ blocker
Therapeutic class: antihypertensive, adjunctive treatment of acute MI
Pregnancy risk category: C
pH: 7.5

INDICATIONS & DOSAGES
➤ **Early treatment in suspected or definitive acute MI—**
Adults: 5 mg I.V. q 2 minutes for 3 doses, followed by oral maintenance doses if I.V. doses are tolerated.
➤ **Atrial fibrillation after MI ◆—**
Adults: 2.5 to 5 mg I.V. q 2 to 5 minutes to control rate up to 15 mg over a 10- to 15-minute period. May continue therapy with P.O. regimen. Stop when therapeutic effect is achieved or if systolic blood pressure is less than 100 mm Hg or heart rate is less than 50 beats/minute.
➤ **Unstable angina or MI characterized by non–ST-segment elevation MI in patients at high risk for ischemic events ◆—**
Adults: 5 mg I.V. q 5 minutes for 3 doses. May continue therapy with P.O. regimen.
Adjust-a-dose: Dosage may need to be reduced in patients with hepatic dysfunction.

ADMINISTRATION
Direct injection: Rapidly inject bolus into free-flowing I.V. line over 2 to 5 minutes.
Intermittent infusion: Not recommended.
Continuous infusion: Not recommended.

PREPARATION & STORAGE
Available in 5-ml ampules or 1-mg/ml prefilled syringes. Store at room temperature, and protect from light. Discard solution if discolored or if precipitate forms.

Incompatibilities
Amphotericin B.

CONTRAINDICATIONS & CAUTIONS
● Contraindicated in those with first-degree heart block with PR interval greater than 0.2 second; in those with second- or third-degree heart block; in those with bradycardia of less than 45 beats/minute; in those with systolic pressure of less than 100 mm Hg; in those with moderate to severe heart failure; and in those with cardiogenic shock because of increased risk of myocardial depression.
● Use cautiously in those with heart failure controlled with cardiac glyco-

sides and diuretics because drug may exacerbate the condition; in those with bronchospastic disease because drug may aggravate symptoms; and in those with myasthenia gravis because drug may cause muscle weakness.

• Use cautiously in those with diabetes mellitus or hyperthyroidism because drug may mask symptoms, and in those with depression or psoriasis because drug may worsen these conditions.

• Use cautiously in geriatric patients and in those with hepatic or renal disease because of increased risk of toxic reaction and adverse effects.

ADVERSE REACTIONS

CNS: confusion, depression, *dizziness,* hallucinations, headache, insomnia, lethargy, sleep disturbances, *fatigue,* fever.
CV: *severe bradycardia, heart block, heart failure, hypotension, intensified arrhythmias,* palpitations, Raynaud's syndrome.
EENT: sore throat.
GI: abdominal pain, nausea, diarrhea.
Metabolic: hyperglycemia, hypoglycemia, unstable diabetes mellitus.
Respiratory: dyspnea, *respiratory distress with laryngospasm, bronchospasm.*
Skin: rash, alopecia.
Other: cold extremities.

INTERACTIONS

Drug-drug. *Ampicillin, barbiturates, rifampin.* Increases metabolism of metoprolol, decreasing its effectiveness. Monitor patient for decreased effect.
Antihypertensives, calcium channel blockers, cardiac glycosides, catecholamine-depleting drugs such as reserpine, diuretics: May potentiate hypotension or bradycardia. Use together cautiously and monitor vital signs and ECG.

Benzodiazepines: Increases benzodiazepine effects. Monitor patient closely.
Cimetidine: Increases beta blockade resulting from inhibited metoprolol metabolism. Monitor patient closely.
Epinephrine: Causes initial hypertension and then bradycardia. Monitor vital signs and ECG.
Hydrocarbon inhalation anesthetics, phenytoin: Increases risk of myocardial depression and hypotension. Use together cautiously.
Insulin, oral antidiabetics: Amplifies risk of hypoglycemia or hyperglycemia. Monitor glucose level closely.
Lidocaine: Increases effect and risk of toxic reaction, resulting from reduced lidocaine clearance. Monitor patient for toxicity.
MAO inhibitors: Causes severe hypertension if metoprolol is given within 14 days of last dose. Avoid use together within 14 days of MAO inhibitor.
Nondepolarizing neuromuscular blockers: May potentiate and prolong action. Monitor patient closely.
NSAIDs: May decrease antihypertensive effect. Monitor blood pressure.
SSRIs: May cause bradycardia. Monitor heart rate.
Thyroid hormones: May impair metoprolol effect when patient converts to the euthyroid state. Monitor laboratory study results.

EFFECTS ON LAB TEST RESULTS

• May increase transaminase, alkaline phosphatase, LDH, and uric acid levels. May increase or decrease glucose level.

ACTION

Binds to postganglionic receptors in the myocardium and blocks the sympathetic neurotransmitter, norepinephrine. Drug binds to beta$_2$ receptors in bronchial and vascular smooth muscle only when given in high doses.

PHARMACOKINETICS
Drug level peaks 20 minutes after 10-minute infusion.
Distribution: Widely distributed, with highest levels in the heart. Drug is 12% protein bound. It crosses the placental and blood-brain barriers and appears in breast milk.
Metabolism: Primarily in the liver.
Excretion: In urine. About 10% of drug is excreted unchanged, 85% as metabolites. Half-life, 3 to 7½ hours.

CLINICAL CONSIDERATIONS
● Give metoprolol as soon as the MI patient's condition is stable.
● Check apical pulse before giving drug. For heart rate below 60 beats/minute, withhold drug and notify prescriber.
● Continuously monitor hemodynamic status, blood pressure, heart rate, and ECG during infusion.
● If patient develops bradycardia or hypotension before dosage is complete, notify prescriber; injections may be stopped or changed to oral form.
● *Alert:* Don't withdraw drug abruptly. Doing so may exacerbate angina, MI, or ventricular arrhythmia or cause death.
● Observe patient for signs of drug-induced depression.
● If overdose occurs, give atropine, then prepare for temporary pacemaker insertion for bradycardia if atropine is unsuccessful. Further treatment is symptomatic and supportive.

PATIENT TEACHING
● Tell patient that drug shouldn't be stopped without consulting prescriber.
● Instruct patient to avoid operating a motor vehicle or other machinery until the effect of the drug is known.
● Tell patient to contact prescriber if he has difficulty breathing.

metronidazole
Flagyl I.V. RTU

metronidazole hydrochloride
Flagyl I.V.

Pharmacologic class: nitroimidazole
Therapeutic class: antibacterial, antiprotozoal, amebicide
Pregnancy risk category: B
pH: 5 to 7

INDICATIONS & DOSAGES
➤ **Severe infections caused by susceptible bacteria—**
Adults: 15 mg/kg I.V. initially, then 7.5 mg/kg I.V. q 6 hours, beginning 6 hours after loading dose. Maximum dose, 4 g I.V. daily.
➤ **Surgical prophylaxis—**
Adults: 15 mg/kg I.V., completed 1 hour before surgery, then 7.5 mg/kg I.V. q 6 hours for two doses at 6 and 12 hours after initial dose.
➤ **Acute intestinal amebiasis or extraintestinal disease caused by *Entamoeba histolytica*—**
Adults: 500 mg I.V. q 6 hours for 10 days.
➤ **Pelvic inflammatory disease ◆—**
Adults: 500 mg I.V. q 8 hours in combination with levofloxacin I.V.
➤ **Diarrhea and colitis caused by *Clostridium difficile* ◆—**
Adults: 500 to 750 mg I.V. q 6 to 8 hours.
Adjust-a-dose: Dosage may need to be reduced in patients with severe hepatic dysfunction and geriatric patients.

ADMINISTRATION
Direct injection: Not recommended.
Intermittent infusion: Give by slow infusion only, over 1 hour, or when used for surgical prophylaxis, over 30 to 60

minutes. Stop the primary solution during drug administration.
Continuous infusion: Rarely used. Infuse diluted drug over ordered amount of time.

PREPARATION & STORAGE

Flagyl I.V. is supplied as sterile, off-white, lyophilized powder in single-dose vials containing 500 mg of metronidazole and 415 mg of mannitol. Drug requires reconstitution, dilution, and neutralization.

Order of mixing is important. Reconstitute drug with 4.4 ml of sterile water for injection, bacteriostatic water for injection, normal saline injection, or bacteriostatic normal saline injection. Mix thoroughly. Resulting solution provides 5 ml (100 mg/ml) of drug. Solution should be clear; don't use if cloudy or precipitated.

Using a glass or plastic container, dilute further with normal saline injection, dextrose 5% injection, or lactated Ringer's injection. Concentration shouldn't exceed 8 mg/ml.

Neutralize final dilution with 5 mEq of sodium bicarbonate injection for each 500 mg of drug. Because this produces carbon dioxide, the container may require venting.

Reconstituted drug is stable for 96 hours in room light if stored below 86° F (30° C). Don't refrigerate when neutralized because a precipitate may form. Use diluted and neutralized solutions within 24 hours.

Flagyl I.V. RTU is supplied in 100-ml single-dose plastic containers, containing 500 mg of drug. Don't dilute, change pH, or mix any additive with these solutions.

Also avoid using aluminum equipment, such as needles or cannulae, that would come in contact with drug. Although drug may cause opacity of plastic containers, needle hubs, or cannulae, this reaction subsides and doesn't affect solution.

Store at controlled room temperature, 59° to 86° F (15° to 30° C), and protect from light. Don't refrigerate or freeze.

Incompatibilities

Aluminum, amino acid 10%, amphotericin B, aztreonam, ceftriaxone, dopamine, filgrastim, meropenem, other I.V. drugs, warfarin.

CONTRAINDICATIONS & CAUTIONS

• Contraindicated in those hypersensitive to metronidazole or other nitroimidazole derivatives.

• Avoid use in pregnant patients in their first trimester who have trichomoniasis.

• Use cautiously in those with CNS disorders because of risk of CNS toxicity; in those with blood dyscrasias because of possible leukopenia; in those with impaired cardiac function or predisposition to edema because of drug's sodium content; and in those with severe hepatic impairment because of increased risk of toxic reaction.

ADVERSE REACTIONS

CNS: fever, vertigo, *headache,* ataxia, dizziness, syncope, incoordination, confusion, irritability, depression, weakness, insomnia, *seizures,* peripheral neuropathy.
CV: flattened T wave, edema, flushing, thrombophlebitis after I.V. infusion.
EENT: rhinitis, sinusitis, pharyngitis.
GI: abdominal cramping or pain, stomatitis, epigastric distress, *nausea,* vomiting, anorexia, diarrhea, constipation, proctitis, dry mouth, metallic taste.
GU: darkened urine, polyuria, dysuria, cystitis, dyspareunia, dryness of vagina and vulva, vaginal candidiasis, *vaginitis,* genital pruritus.
Hematologic: *transient leukopenia, neutropenia.*
Musculoskeletal: fleeting joint pains.
Respiratory: upper respiratory tract infection.
Skin: rash.

Reactions may be *common*, uncommon, *life-threatening*, or COMMON AND LIFE-THREATENING.

Other: decreased libido, overgrowth of nonsusceptible organisms, especially *Candida.*

INTERACTIONS

Drug-drug. *Barbiturates, phenytoin:* Enhances metronidazole metabolism. Monitor patient closely.

Disulfiram: Causes acute psychosis and confusion. Don't use within 2 weeks of last disulfiram dose.

Drugs that contain alcohol: Causes disulfiram-like reaction. Don't use together or for 3 days after completion of metronidazole therapy.

Drugs that decrease hepatic microsomal enzyme activity: May increase adverse effects of metronidazole. Monitor patient closely.

Drugs that induce hepatic microsomal enzyme activity: Decreases metronidazole levels resulting from accelerated drug excretion. Monitor patient closely.

Neurotoxic drugs: Increases risk of neurotoxicity. Monitor patient closely; use with caution.

Oral anticoagulants: Potentiates action, resulting in prolonged PT. Monitor PT closely.

Phenytoin, lithium: May increase levels of these drugs. Monitor drug levels as indicated.

Drug-lifestyle. *Alcohol use:* Causes disulfiram-like reaction. Avoid using together or for 3 days after completion of metronidazole therapy.

EFFECTS ON LAB TEST RESULTS

• May alter AST, ALT, LDH, triglyceride, and glucose levels.
• May decrease neutrophil and WBC counts.

ACTION

Bactericidal against most gramnegative anaerobic bacteria, *Fusobacterium, Veillonella,* many gram-positive anaerobic bacteria, *E. histolytica, Trichomonas vaginalis, Giardia lamblia,* and *Balantidium coli.*

PHARMACOKINETICS

Drug level peaks immediately after administration.

Distribution: All body tissues. Less than 20% protein bound. Drug crosses the blood-brain and placental barriers and appears in breast milk.

Metabolism: 30% to 60% in the liver.

Excretion: 60% to 80% in urine, 6% to 15% in feces. Half-life, 6 to 12 hours, averaging 8 hours.

CLINICAL CONSIDERATIONS

• Osmolarity: 310 mOsm/L.
• Obtain specimens for culture and sensitivity tests before giving first dose. Therapy may begin before results are available.
• Obtain CBC before and after therapy.
• Because drug action may be altered in geriatric patients, drug levels may need to be monitored so that dosage can be adjusted.
• To minimize risk of thrombophlebitis, avoid prolonged use of I.V. catheters.
• Therapy usually lasts for 7 to 10 days; however, infections of bones and joints, lower respiratory tract, and endocardium may require longer treatment.
• Parenteral therapy may change to oral therapy, depending on severity of disease and patient response.
• RTU form of metronidazole contains 14 mEq (322 mg) of sodium. Neutralized I.V. solution contains 5 mEq (115 mg) of sodium.
• If diarrhea persists during therapy, collect stool specimens for culture to rule out pseudomembranous colitis.
• Observe patient for fungal and bacterial superinfection with prolonged use.

PATIENT TEACHING

• Inform patient that urine may darken.
• Instruct patient being treated for amebiasis about proper hygiene, to avoid infecting others.
• Tell patient to report adverse reactions.

◆ Off-label use   *May contain benzyl alcohol   ◇ Canada

midazolam hydrochloride
Versed*

Pharmacologic class: benzodiazepine
Therapeutic class: preoperative
sedative, drug for conscious
sedation, adjunct for induction of
general anesthesia, amnestic
Pregnancy risk category: D
Controlled substance schedule: IV
pH: 3

INDICATIONS & DOSAGES
➤ **Conscious sedation—**
Adults: Initially, a maximum of 2.5 mg
I.V. given over 2 to 3 minutes (some
patients may respond to 1 mg) then increased in small increments at intervals
of at least 2 minutes until reaching desired effect.
Geriatric or debilitated patients: 1 to
1.5 mg I.V. initially, given over a longer
duration.
    Dosages are highly individualized.
➤ **To sedate intubated and mechanically ventilated patients in critical
care settings—**
Adults: 10 to 50 mcg/kg I.V. over several minutes, repeated at 10 to 15 minute
intervals until adequate sedation is
achieved, then maintenance infusion of
20 to 100 mcg/kg/hour I.V.
Children: Loading dose of 50 to
200 mcg/kg I.V. over 2 to 3 minutes,
followed by continuous infusion of 60
to 120 mcg/kg/hour I.V.
*Term neonates (32 weeks' or more ges-
tation):* 60 mcg/kg/hour as I.V. infusion.
*Preterm neonates (fewer than 32 weeks'
gestation):* 30 mcg/kg/hour as I.V. infusion.
    Dosages are highly individualized.
➤ **To induce general anesthesia without premedication—**
Adults age 55 and older: 300 mcg/kg
I.V.

Adults younger than age 55: 300 to
350 mcg/kg I.V. given over 20 to 30
seconds. Increments of 25% of initial
dose may be needed to complete induction.
*Adults with debilitation or severe sys-
temic disease:* 150 to 250 mcg/kg I.V.
Total dose shouldn't exceed 600 mcg/
kg I.V.
    Dosages are highly individualized.
➤ **To induce anesthesia after premedication with an opioid drug—**
Adults age 55 and older: 200 mcg/kg
I.V. over 20 to 30 seconds.
Adults younger than age 55: 250 mcg/
kg I.V.
*Adults with debilitation or severe sys-
temic disease:* 150 mcg/kg I.V.
    Dosages are highly individualized.
➤ **Status epilepticus ♦—**
Adults: 10 to 15 mg I.V.
    Dosages are highly individualized.

ADMINISTRATION
Only staff trained in giving anesthetics
and managing their adverse reactions
should give midazolam. Also, equipment for respiratory and CV support
should be readily available.
Direct injection: Inject directly into
vein or established I.V. line containing
a compatible solution over 2 to 3 minutes for conscious sedation or over 20
to 30 seconds for anesthesia induction.
Intermittent infusion: Not recommended.
Continuous infusion: Dilute the 5 mg/ml
injection with normal saline solution or
dextrose 5% injection to a concentration
of 0.5 mg/ml.

PREPARATION & STORAGE
Available as 1 mg/ml in 2-, 5-, and
10-ml vials and 2- and 5-ml Carpuject
vials and as 5 mg/ml in 1-, 2-, 5-, and
10-ml vials, 1-, 2-, and 5-ml Carpuject
vials, and 2 ml syringes. Drug may be
given undiluted or diluted with D_5W,
normal saline solution , or lactated
Ringer's solution. Mixtures with D_5W

or normal saline solution at concentrations of 0.5 mg/ml are stable for 24 hours; those with lactated Ringer's solution, for 4 hours.

Store undiluted solution at room temperature and protect from light. Once diluted, solution no longer requires protection from light.

Incompatibilities
Albumin, amphotericin B, ampicillin sodium, bumetanide, butorphanol, ceftazidime, cefuroxime, clonidine, dexamethasone sodium phosphate, dimenhydrinate, dobutamine, foscarnet, fosphenytoin, furosemide, hydrocortisone, imipenem-cilastatin sodium, methotrexate sodium, nafcillin, pentobarbital sodium, perphenazine, prochlorperazine edisylate, ranitidine hydrochloride, sodium bicarbonate, thiopental, some total parenteral nutrition formulations, trimethoprim-sulfamethoxazole.

CONTRAINDICATIONS & CAUTIONS
• Contraindicated in those hypersensitive to drug or to other benzodiazepines.
• Contraindicated in those with severe shock, coma, or acute alcohol intoxication because drug potentiates existing hypotension, and in those with acute angle-closure glaucoma because drug may have an anticholinergic effect.
• Use cautiously in geriatric patients, debilitated patients, and those with COPD because drug depresses the respiratory system; and in those with myasthenia gravis because drug can exacerbate this condition.
• Use cautiously in those with renal impairment because of more rapid induction and prolonged recovery.
• Use cautiously in those with heart failure and hepatic impairment because of increased risk of toxic reaction.

ADVERSE REACTIONS
CNS: agitation, anxiety, ataxia, confusion, dizziness, drowsiness, euphoria, headache, nightmares, oversedation, paresthesia, retrograde amnesia, slurred speech, pain at injection site.
CV: *cardiac arrest,* nodal rhythms, premature ventricular contractions, tachycardia, vasovagal episodes.
EENT: visual disturbances.
GI: dry mouth, nausea, vomiting.
Musculoskeletal: involuntary muscle movement.
Respiratory: *airway obstruction,* APNEA, bradypnea, *bronchospasm,* cough, dyspnea, hiccups, hyperventilation, *hypoxia, laryngospasm, severe respiratory depression,* shallow respirations, tachypnea, wheezing.
Skin: pain, tenderness, and induration at injection site
Other: *anaphylaxis,* prolonged emergence from anesthesia.

INTERACTIONS
Drug-drug. *Antihypertensives:* Worsens hypotension. Monitor blood pressure closely.
Cimetidine, diltiazem, erythromycin, itraconazole, ketoconazole, verapamil: Decreases midazolam metabolism and increases risk of toxic reaction. Avoid using together.
CNS depressants: Causes profound respiratory depression, hypoventilation, or apnea. Prepare to adjust midazolam dosage.
Fentanyl in high doses and other opioids: Causes severe hypotension. Monitor blood pressure closely; give with caution.
Fluvoxamine: Decreases clearance of midazolam. Use cautiously together.
Hormonal contraceptives: Prolongs half-life of midazolam. Use cautiously together.
Indinavir, ritonavir: Increases sedation and respiratory depression. Use cautiously together.

Inhalation anesthetics: Increases effects. Dose of anesthetic may need to be reduced.

Propofol: Increases effects. Monitor patient for adverse effects.

Theophylline: Antagonizes sedative effects of midazolam. Use cautiously together.

Drug-herb. *Catnip, kava, lady's slipper, lemon balm, passion flower, sassafras, skullcap, valerian:* May enhance sedative effects. Discourage use together.

Drug-lifestyle. *Alcohol use:* May increase risk of apnea. Avoid using together.

EFFECTS ON LAB TEST RESULTS
None reported.

ACTION
Short-acting; depresses the CNS at the limbic and subcortical levels by potentiating gamma-aminobutyric acid.

PHARMACOKINETICS
Onset, 1 to 5 minutes; duration, 2 to 6 hours.

Distribution: Rapid and widespread, with highest levels in the liver, kidneys, lungs, heart, and fat. About 97% protein bound. It crosses the blood-brain and placental barriers.

Metabolism: In the liver. Drug undergoes rapid hydroxylation. Its metabolites are conjugated with glucuronic acid.

Excretion: In urine. About 90% excreted in 24 hours.

CLINICAL CONSIDERATIONS
• Osmolality: 385 mOsm/kg.
• *Alert:* Drug may contain benzyl alcohol.
• *Alert:* Before giving drug, have oxygen and resuscitation equipment available in case of severe respiratory depression. Excessive dosage or rapid infusion has been linked to respiratory arrest.
• Drug is three to four times as potent per milligram as diazepam.

• Give drug slowly and in divided doses to titrate to effect. Rapid administration can lead to severe apnea, respiratory arrest, and hypotension, especially in geriatric or debilitated patients.
• Monitor blood pressure, heart rate and rhythm, respirations, airway integrity, and arterial oxygen saturation during administration and throughout procedure.
• Geriatric patients may experience prolonged recovery time.
• Don't give loading doses to neonates. Infusion may be given more rapidly for the first several hours to establish therapeutic drug levels.
• If overdose occurs, give 0.2 mg of flumazenil I.V. to reverse sedative effects. Provide general supportive measures.

PATIENT TEACHING
• Warn patients not to drive or perform other tasks that require alertness until effects subside or until day after drug administration, whichever is longer.
• Because the drug's amnestic effect diminishes patient's recall of perioperative events, provide written information or instructions to patient, and include family in teaching to ensure compliance.

milrinone lactate
Primacor

Pharmacologic class: bipyridine phosphodiesterase inhibitor
Therapeutic class: inotropic vasodilator
Pregnancy risk category: C
pH: 3.2 to 4

INDICATIONS & DOSAGES
➤ **Heart failure—**
Adults: Initial loading dose of 50 mcg/kg I.V. over 10 minutes, fol-

lowed by continuous infusion dose of 0.375 to 0.75 mcg/kg/minute I.V. Adjust dosage to hemodynamic and clinical response.

Adjust-a-dose: For patients with renal impairment, use table below. Don't exceed 1.13 mg/kg/day I.V.

Creatinine clearance (ml/min)	Infusion rate (mcg/kg/min)
50	0.43
40	0.38
30	0.33
20	0.28
10	0.23
5	0.2

ADMINISTRATION

Direct I.V. injection: A loading dose may be given undiluted, but diluting to a total volume of 10 to 20 ml aids with visualization of the injection rate. Give over 10 minutes.

Intermittent infusion: Not recommended.

Continuous infusion: Adjust maintenance dosage if patient responds with increased cardiac output or reduced pulmonary artery wedge pressure.

PREPARATION & STORAGE

Available in 10- and 20-ml vials, 1 mg/ml, and premixed 200 mcg/ml in 5% dextrose (100 ml). Dilute with half-normal or normal saline solution or D_5W only. Store at room temperature (59° to 86° F [15° to 30° C]). Don't use if particulate matter or discoloration is evident.

Incompatibilities

Bumetanide, furosemide, procainamide.

CONTRAINDICATIONS & CAUTIONS

• Contraindicated in those hypersensitive to drug, in those who are in the acute phase of an MI, and in those post-MI.

• Contraindicated in those with severe aortic or pulmonic valvular disease; drug shouldn't be used as a substitute for surgical correction.

• Use cautiously in those with atrial fibrillation or flutter.

ADVERSE REACTIONS

CNS: headache, tremors.
CV: angina, hypotension, nonsustained ventricular tachycardia, *sustained ventricular tachycardia,* VENTRICULAR ARRHYTHMIAS, *ventricular fibrillation,* chest pain.
Hematologic: *thrombocytopenia.*
Metabolic: hypokalemia.
Respiratory: *bronchospasm.*

INTERACTIONS

None reported.

EFFECTS ON LAB TEST RESULTS

• May decrease potassium level.

ACTION

Selective inhibitor of peak III cAMP phosphodiesterase isozyme in cardiac and vascular muscle, it increases myocardial contractility and improves diastolic function.

PHARMACOKINETICS

Distribution: About 70% bound to plasma protein.
Metabolism: About 12% to a glucuronide metabolite.
Excretion: About 90% in urine. Half-life, 2.4 hours.

CLINICAL CONSIDERATIONS

• Correct hypokalemia with potassium supplements before or during use of drug.

• Monitor renal function and fluid and electrolyte changes.

• Monitor blood pressure and heart rate. Continuously monitor ECG, and watch for arrhythmias.
• No specific antidote is available to treat overdose. Lower or temporarily suspend administration until condition stabilizes.

PATIENT TEACHING
• Tell patient to promptly report adverse reactions.
• Tell patient to report discomfort at the I.V. site.

minocycline hydrochloride
Minocin

Pharmacologic class: tetracycline
Therapeutic class: antibiotic
Pregnancy risk category: D
pH: 2 to 2.8

INDICATIONS & DOSAGES
➤ **Severe infections caused by susceptible organisms—**
Adults: Initially, 200 mg I.V., then 100 mg I.V. q 12 hours. Don't exceed 400 mg/day I.V.
Children older than age 8: Initially, 4 mg/kg I.V., then 2 mg/kg I.V. q 12 hours.
Adjust-a-dose: In patients with renal impairment, decrease dose and frequency of administration. Don't exceed 200 mg/day I.V.

ADMINISTRATION
Direct injection: Not recommended.
Intermittent infusion: Infuse over 6 hours.
Continuous infusion: Not recommended.

PREPARATION & STORAGE
Available in 100-mg vials.
Reconstitute with 5 ml of sterile water for injection. Then dilute each 100 mg in 500 to 1,000 ml of compatible I.V. solution for infusion.
Such solutions include dextrose 5% in normal saline solution, D_5W, Ringer's injection, lactated Ringer's solution, and normal saline solution.
Store vials below 104° F (40° C) in light-resistant containers. Reconstituted solution is stable for 24 hours at room temperature.

Incompatibilities
Allopurinol, amifostine, calcium-containing solutions, doxapram, hydromorphone, meperidine, morphine, piperacillin sodium-tazobactam sodium, propofol, rifampin, thiotepa.

CONTRAINDICATIONS & CAUTIONS
• Contraindicated in those hypersensitive to tetracyclines.
• Contraindicated in those who are in the last half of pregnancy because drug interferes with fetal bone and tooth development, and in breast-feeding women.
• Use cautiously in those with hepatic impairment because of increased risk of adverse reactions.

ADVERSE REACTIONS
CNS: *intracranial hypertension,* dizziness, headache, light-headedness, vertigo, fever.
CV: pericarditis, *thrombophlebitis.*
GI: abdominal discomfort, *anorexia, diarrhea, nausea, pseudomembranous colitis,* vomiting, dysphagia, glossitis, oral candidiasis.
Hematologic: *neutropenia, thrombocytopenia,* eosinophilia, hemolytic anemia.
Hepatic: *hepatotoxicity.*
Musculoskeletal: arthralgia.
Skin: exfoliative dermatitis, *hyperpigmentation of skin and mucous membranes, photosensitivity, rash, urticaria.*

Reactions may be *common,* uncommon, *life-threatening,* or COMMON AND LIFE-THREATENING.

Other: *anaphylaxis,* bacterial and fungal superinfection, permanent tooth discoloration, enamel defects.

INTERACTIONS
Drug-drug. *Aminoglycosides, penicillins:* May antagonize bactericidal activity. Avoid using together.
Hormonal contraceptives: Decreases contraceptive effectiveness and causes breakthrough bleeding. Recommend use of nonhormonal form of birth control.
Insulin: May decrease insulin requirements. Monitor glucose level.
Methoxyflurane: Increases risk of nephrotoxicity. Monitor patient carefully.
Oral anticoagulants: Increases risk of bleeding. Monitor PT and INR. May need to adjust dosage.
Drug-lifestyle. *Sun exposure:* Increases risk of photosensitivity reactions. Advise patient to take precautions.

EFFECTS ON LAB TEST RESULTS
• May increase BUN, creatinine, alkaline phosphatase, ALT, AST, and bilirubin levels.
• May increase eosinophil count. May decrease hemoglobin and platelet and neutrophil counts.
• May falsely elevate fluorometric test results for urine catecholamines. May cause false-positive results of copper sulfate test (Clinitest) and false-negative results in urine glucose tests using glucose oxidase reagent (Diastix or Chemstrip uG).

ACTION
Bacteriostatic. May be bactericidal in high concentrations or with susceptible organisms.
Acts against many gram-negative bacteria, many gram-positive bacteria, some strains of staphylococci and streptococci, *Rickettsia* species, *Chlamydia trachomatis, C. psittaci,* and *Mycoplasma pneumoniae.*

PHARMACOKINETICS
Drug level peaks immediately after infusion.
Distribution: Widely distributed, with good penetration in saliva. Drug is more lipid-soluble than other tetracyclines. About 70% to 80% is bound to plasma proteins; drug readily crosses the placental barrier and appears in breast milk.
Metabolism: Partially metabolized in the liver.
Excretion: Mainly removed in feces, with 16% to 22% excreted unchanged in the urine. Half-life, 11 to 18 hours.

CLINICAL CONSIDERATIONS
• Osmolality: 107 mOsm/kg.
• Obtain specimens for culture and sensitivity tests before giving first dose. Therapy may begin before test results are available.
• *Alert:* Check expiration date.
• Monitor renal and liver function.
• Observe patient for fungal and bacterial superinfection with prolonged use.
• If diarrhea persists, collect stool specimen for culture to rule out pseudomembranous colitis.
• Observe I.V. site for signs of thrombophlebitis. Rotate I.V. site every 48 to 72 hours.
• Switch to oral therapy as soon as possible.

PATIENT TEACHING
• If applicable, inform patient that tetracyclines may cause permanent tooth discoloration, enamel hypoplasia, and decreased bone growth in children age 8 or younger and when used during pregnancy.
• Tell patient to use sunscreen and to wear protective clothing to avoid photosensitivity reactions.
• Advise any woman using a hormonal contraceptive to use an alternative form of birth control while taking drug.
• Inform patient that adverse CNS effects—such as dizziness, headache, and

vertigo—are more common with this drug than other available tetracyclines.
• Caution patient against driving vehicles and operating hazardous machinery during therapy until he knows how the drug affects him.

mitomycin
Mitozytrex, Mutamycin

Pharmacologic class: antineoplastic antibiotic (cell cycle–phase nonspecific)
Therapeutic class: antineoplastic
Pregnancy risk category: NR
pH: 6 to 8

INDICATIONS & DOSAGES
➤ **Disseminated adenocarcinoma of stomach or pancreas—**
Adults: 15 mg/m^2 Mitozytrex or 20 mg/m^2 Mutamycin as a single I.V. dose. Repeat cycle after 6 to 8 weeks when WBC and platelet counts have returned to normal.
Adjust-a-dose: Adjust dosage in those with myelosuppression. Give 70% of dose when WBC count is between 2,000/mm^3 and 3,000/mm^3 and platelet count is between 25,000/mm^3 and 75,000/mm^3. Give 50% when WBC count is below 2,000/mm^3 and platelet count is below 25,000/mm^3.

ADMINISTRATION
Direct injection: Give through a new I.V. site, preferably using a 23G or 25G winged-tip needle or an I.V. catheter. Use distal rather than major veins to allow for repeated venipunctures.
Intermittent infusion: Infuse diluted drug through a newly started I.V. line.
Continuous infusion: Not recommended.

PREPARATION & STORAGE
Be cautious when preparing and giving mitomycin to avoid carcinogenic, teratogenic, and mutagenic risks. Use a biological containment cabinet, wear gloves and mask, and use syringes with luer-lock fittings. Dispose of vials, needles, syringes, and unused drug carefully.

Available in 5-, 20-, and 40-mg vials.
To reconstitute 5-mg vial of Mitozytrex, use 8.5 ml of sterile water for injection. For 5-mg vial of Mutamycin, use 10 ml; for 20-mg vial, use 40 ml; and for 40-mg vial, use 80 ml of sterile water for injection, to yield a concentration of 0.5 mg/ml. Shake to dissolve; don't use until completely dissolved.

Mitozytrex reconstituted with sterile water for injection is stable for 24 hours. When diluted, drug is stable in D$_5$W for 4 hours, in normal saline solution for 48 hours, and in sodium lactate solution for 24 hours.

Mutamycin reconstituted with sterile water for injection is stable for 14 days refrigerated or 7 days at room temperature. When diluted, it's stable in D$_5$W for 3 hours, in normal saline solution for 12 hours, and in sodium lactate solution for 24 hours. Before reconstitution, store at room temperature. Protect diluted solutions from light. Store at less than 104° F (40° C).

Incompatibilities
Aztreonam, bleomycin, cefepime, etoposide, filgrastim, gemcitabine, piperacillin sodium-tazobactam sodium, sargramostim, vinorelbine.
The combination of 5 to 15 mg mitomycin and 1,000 to 10,000 units heparin in 30 ml of 0.9% sodium chloride solution for injection is stable at room temperature for 48 hours for Mutamycin and 72 hours for Mitozytrex.

CONTRAINDICATIONS & CAUTIONS
• Contraindicated in patients with existing or recent chickenpox or herpes

zoster infection because of risk of generalized disease.
• Contraindicated in those with a platelet count below 75,000/mm³, a WBC count below 3,000/mm³, or a creatinine level above 1.7 mg/dl because of enhanced risk of toxic reaction.
• Use cautiously in those hypersensitive to drug.
• Use cautiously in those with coagulation disorders; prolonged PT, INR, or bleeding time; or increased bleeding from other causes because of increased risk of bleeding.
• Use cautiously in those with renal impairment because of increased risk of toxic reaction, in those with bone marrow depression because of increased myelosuppression, and in those with infection because of risk of generalized disease.

ADVERSE REACTIONS
CNS: confusion, drowsiness, headache, syncope, fatigue, malaise, pain, *fever.*
CV: edema, thrombophlebitis.
EENT: blurred vision.
GI: *anorexia,* diarrhea, hematemesis, *nausea,* stomatitis, *vomiting.*
GU: hemolytic uremic syndrome, *renal toxicity.*
Hematologic: *myelosuppression, thrombocytopenia, leukopenia, microangiopathic hemolytic anemia characterized by thrombocytopenia, renal failure, and hypertension.*
Respiratory: *acute bronchospasm,* dyspnea, nonproductive cough, *pulmonary toxicity, adult respiratory distress syndrome.*
Skin: alopecia, cellulitis *or pain at infusion site.*
Other: *septicemia.*

INTERACTIONS
Drug-drug. *Bone marrow depressants:* Increases myelosuppression. Monitor hematologic studies closely.

Doxorubicin: Enhances cardiotoxicity. Monitor patient closely.
Vaccines with killed virus: Decreases effectiveness of vaccination. Postpone vaccination, if possible.
Vaccines with live virus: Increases risk of generalized infection. Postpone vaccination, if possible.
Vinca alkaloids: Causes acute shortness of breath and severe bronchospasm. Monitor respiratory status closely.

EFFECTS ON LAB TEST RESULTS
• May increase BUN and creatinine levels.
• May decrease hemoglobin, hematocrit, and WBC and platelet counts.

ACTION
Although drug is cell cycle nonspecific, it's most active in G and S phases of cell division. Drug causes cross-linking of DNA and inhibits DNA synthesis. In high concentrations, it may also inhibit RNA and protein synthesis.

PHARMACOKINETICS
Drug level peaks at end of infusion.
Distribution: Throughout tissues, mostly in kidneys, muscles, eyes, lungs, intestines, stomach, and cancer cells. Drug crosses the placental barrier.
Metabolism: Primarily in liver but also in kidneys, spleen, and heart.
Excretion: In urine; smaller amounts in feces. Plasma half-life, 17 minutes; elimination half-life, 50 minutes.

CLINICAL CONSIDERATIONS
• Osmolality: 9 mOsm/kg.
• Avoid extravasation because of the potential for severe ulceration and necrosis. If extravasation occurs, immediately stop infusion and restart at another site.
• *Alert:* Give drug only under constant supervision of health care provider experienced in use of chemotherapy.

• Expect toxic effects with therapeutic doses. Evaluate patient before each course of therapy.
• In leukopenia, nadir occurs in 8 weeks; in thrombocytopenia, in 4 weeks. Onset is 2 to 4 weeks.
• Assess patient for renal dysfunction.
• Monitor pulmonary function during therapy.
• Give antibiotics for infection during myelosuppression.
• If patient shows no response after two courses of therapy, stop drug.

PATIENT TEACHING
• Tell patient to report blood in urine, painful urination, , or urinary frequency.
• Inform patient that drug-related hair loss is usually reversible.
• Advise patient to avoid exposure to people with infections.
• Tell patient to watch for signs and symptoms of infection (including fever, sore throat, and fatigue) and signs and symptoms of bleeding (such as easy bruising, nosebleeds, bleeding gums, and tarry stools) and to take his temperature daily.

mitoxantrone hydrochloride
Novantrone

Pharmacologic class: antibiotic, antineoplastic
Therapeutic class: antineoplastic
Pregnancy risk category: D
pH: 3 to 4.5

INDICATIONS & DOSAGES
➤ **Combination therapy with cytarabine for acute nonlymphocytic leukemia—**
Adults: Initial therapy, 12 mg/m^2 I.V. on days 1 and 3, followed by 1 to 7 days of I.V. therapy with cytarabine; consolidation therapy, 12 mg/m^2 I.V. on days 1 and 2 and cytarabine given as continuous infusion on days 1 to 5.
➤ **To reduce neurologic disability and frequency of relapse in chronic progressive, progressive relapsing, or worsening relapsing-remitting multiple sclerosis—**
Adults: 12 mg/m^2 I.V. over 5 to 15 minutes q 3 months.
➤ **Advanced hormone-refractory prostate cancer—**
Adults: 12 to 14 mg/m^2 as a short I.V. infusion q 21 days, in combination with corticosteroids.

ADMINISTRATION
Direct injection: Not recommended.
Intermittent infusion: Infuse diluted solution slowly into a free-flowing I.V. line of normal saline solution or D$_5$W over at least 3 minutes, usually 15 to 30 minutes.
Continuous infusion: Not recommended.

PREPARATION & STORAGE
Use caution when preparing or administering drug to avoid mutagenic, teratogenic, and carcinogenic risks. Use a biological containment cabinet, wear gloves and mask, and use syringes with luer-lock fittings to prevent leakage of drug solution. Correctly dispose of needles, vials, and unused drug, and avoid contaminating work surfaces. Avoid inhalation of dust or vapors or contact with skin or mucous membranes.

Available as an aqueous solution of 2 mg/ml in volumes of 10, 12.5, and 15 ml.

Dilute dose in at least 50 ml of normal saline injection or dextrose 5% injection. May be further diluted in D$_5$W, normal saline solution, or dextrose 5% in normal saline solution. Use immediately and discard unused solution.

Store undiluted solution at room temperature. Avoid freezing diluted and undiluted solutions.

Incompatibilities

Amphotericin B, aztreonam, cefepime, doxorubicin liposomal, heparin sodium, hydrocortisone, other I.V. drugs, paclitaxel, piperacillin sodium and tazobactam sodium, propofol, sargramostim.

CONTRAINDICATIONS & CAUTIONS

• Contraindicated in patients hypersensitive to drug.
• Contraindicated in those with significant myelosuppression, unless the benefits outweigh the risks, and in hepatically impaired patients with multiple sclerosis.
• Use cautiously in those with previous exposure to anthracyclines or other cardiotoxic drugs.
• Use cautiously in those with severe hepatic dysfunction because drug clearance may be reduced.

ADVERSE REACTIONS

CNS: *seizures, headache, fever.*
CV: *arrhythmias,* asymptomatic changes in left ventricular ejection fraction, ECG changes, *heart failure,* hypotension, phlebitis, tachycardia.
EENT: conjunctivitis, blue discoloration of the sclera.
GI: *abdominal pain, diarrhea, nausea, stomatitis, vomiting, bleeding, mucositis.*
GU: *renal failure.*
Hematologic: *myelosuppression,* anemia.
Hepatic: *hepatotoxicity,* jaundice.
Metabolic: hyperuricemia.
Respiratory: *cough, dyspnea.*
Skin: *alopecia,* urticaria, local irritation or phlebitis, petechiae, ecchymoses.
Other: allergic reaction, secondary infection, *fungal infections,* **sepsis.**

INTERACTIONS

Drug-drug. *Allopurinol, colchicine, probenecid, sulfinpyrazone:* Decreases effectiveness in controlling hyperuricemia. Monitor patient closely.
Daunorubicin, doxorubicin, radiation therapy: Increases risk of toxic reaction. Monitor patient for toxicity.
Myelosuppressives: Increases risk of hematologic abnormalities. Monitor blood counts closely.
Vaccines with killed virus: Decreases effectiveness. Postpone vaccination, if possible.
Vaccines with live virus: Increases risk of generalized infection. Postpone vaccination, if possible.

EFFECTS ON LAB TEST RESULTS

• May increase ALT, AST, bilirubin, GGT, and uric acid levels.
• May decrease hemoglobin, hematocrit, and leukocyte and granulocyte counts.

ACTION

Reacts with DNA to produce cytotoxic effect and is probably cell cycle nonspecific.

PHARMACOKINETICS

Duration, 2 to 13 days.
Distribution: Rapidly and extensively to tissues; probably not well distributed into the CSF. About 78% protein bound. Unknown if drug appears in breast milk.
Metabolism: In the liver.
Excretion: 11% in kidneys, 25% in feces. Mean half-life, 6 days.

CLINICAL CONSIDERATIONS

• Osmolality: 270 mOsm/kg.
• Treat secondary infections with antibiotics.
• Monitor hematology and chemistry laboratory values and liver function test results closely.
• Monitor left ventricular ejection fraction during administration.

• Monitor uric acid levels during therapy. Keeping patient well hydrated, alkalizing urine, and giving allopurinol may prevent uric acid nephropathy.
• If severe nonhematologic toxicity occurs during first course of therapy, delay second course until patient recovers.
• Only prescribers experienced in chemotherapy should prescribe mitoxantrone.

PATIENT TEACHING
• Inform patient that urine may appear blue-green within 24 hours after administration. Some bluish discoloration of the sclera may also occur.
• If drug comes in contact with the eyes, tell patient to irrigate with water or saline solution and call an ophthalmologist.
• If drug comes in contact with the skin, tell patient to rinse the area well with water. Drug isn't a vesicant.

mivacurium chloride
Mivacron*

Pharmacologic class: nondepolarizing neuromuscular blocker
Therapeutic class: skeletal muscle relaxant
Pregnancy risk category: C
pH: 3.5 to 5

INDICATIONS & DOSAGES
➤ **As an adjunct to anesthesia, to facilitate endotracheal intubation, and to relax skeletal muscles during surgery or mechanical ventilation—**
Adults: Dosage is individualized; 0.15 mg/kg I.V. push over 5 to 15 seconds, 2.5 minutes before intubation. Supplemental doses of 0.1 mg/kg I.V. q 15 minutes. Continuous infusion of 4 mcg/kg/minute begun simultaneously with initial dose, maintains neuromus-

cular blockade. Alternately, 9 to 10 mcg/kg/minute started after spontaneous recovery from initial dose is noted. Dosage is reduced up to 40% when used with isoflurane or enflurane anesthesia.
Children ages 2 to 12: 0.2 mg/kg I.V. push given over 5 to 15 seconds. Maintenance doses are usually needed more frequently in children. Neuromuscular blockade can be maintained with a continuous infusion titrated to effect. Most children respond to 5 to 31 mcg/kg/minute; average, 14 mcg/kg/minute.
Adjust-a-dose: To prevent prolonged neuromuscular blockade, adjust dosage to ideal body weight in those who are 30% or more above their ideal weight. Decrease dosage in those with renal or hepatic insufficiency by as much as 50%.

ADMINISTRATION
Direct injection: Rapid I.V. bolus, 5 to 15 seconds.
Intermittent infusion: Not recommended.
Continuous infusion: Titrate drip to peripheral nerve stimulation and clinical criteria.

PREPARATION & STORAGE
Available as 2 mg/ml in 5- and 10-ml vials, in 20- and 50-ml multidose vials containing benzyl alcohol, and as an infusion of 0.5 mg/ml in 50- and 100-ml D_5W. Protect from ultraviolet light and from freezing. Drug is stable for 24 hours if diluted to a concentration of 0.5 mg/ml in D_5W, dextrose 5% in normal saline solution, lactated Ringer's solution, dextrose 5% in lactated Ringer's solution, or normal saline solution and stored at 41° to 77° F (5° to 25° C).

Incompatibilities
Other I.V. drugs.

CONTRAINDICATIONS & CAUTIONS

• Contraindicated in those hypersensitive to drug. Because multidose vials contain benzyl alcohol as a preservative, this formulation is contraindicated in those hypersensitive to benzyl alcohol.
• Use cautiously in those with significant CV disease and in those who may be adversely affected by release of histamine, such as asthmatics. To avoid hypotension, lower the initial dose or give the drug over a longer period.
• Use cautiously, possibly at a reduced dosage, in debilitated patients and in those with metastatic cancer, severe electrolyte disturbances, or neuromuscular diseases.
• Use cautiously in patients in whom neuromuscular blockade may be potentiated or difficult to reverse, such as those with myasthenia gravis or myasthenic syndrome. Test dose of 0.015 to 0.02 mg/kg may be used to assess patient's sensitivity to drug.
• Use cautiously in breast-feeding women.
• Use cautiously, if at all, in patients who are homozygous for the atypical plasma pseudocholinesterase gene. Drug is metabolized to inactive compound by plasma pseudocholinesterase.

ADVERSE REACTIONS

CNS: dizziness.
CV: *arrhythmias, bradycardia, flushing,* hypotension, tachycardia, phlebitis.
Musculoskeletal: prolonged muscle weakness, spasms.
Respiratory: *apnea, bronchospasm, respiratory insufficiency,* wheezing.
Skin: erythema, rash, urticaria.

INTERACTIONS

Drug-drug. *Alkaline solutions, such as barbiturate solutions:* May form precipitate because drugs are physically incompatible. Don't give drugs through same I.V. line.

Aminoglycosides, bacitracin, colistimethate, colistin, polymyxin B sulfate, tetracyclines: Potentiates neuromuscular blockade, leading to prolonged effect. Use together cautiously.
Carbamazepine, phenytoin: Shortens the duration of neuromuscular blockade, and infusion rate may be high. Monitor patient closely.
Inhalation anesthetics, especially isoflurane or enflurane: May enhance or prolong action of drug. Monitor patient for excessive weakness.
Lithium, local anesthetics, magnesium salts, procainamide, quinidine: May enhance neuromuscular blockade. Monitor patient for excessive weakness.

EFFECTS ON LAB TEST RESULTS

None reported.

ACTION

Nondepolarizing neuromuscular blocker, reducing response to acetylcholine; has no significant effect on consciousness or pain threshold.

PHARMACOKINETICS

Onset, within 1 to 2 minutes; effects peak within 2 to 5 minutes.
Distribution: Short-acting skeletal muscle relaxant. Unknown if drug appears in breast milk.
Metabolism: Enzymatic hydrolysis by cholinesterase.
Excretion: Primarily in urine and bile; also in kidney.

CLINICAL CONSIDERATIONS

• Osmolarity: 260 mOsm/L.
• *Alert:* Use only under direct supervision by staff skilled in use of neuromuscular blockers and techniques to maintain a patent airway. Don't use unless an antagonist and equipment for artificial respiration, mechanical ventilation, oxygen therapy, and intubation are within reach.

• *Alert:* Multidose vials contain benzyl alcohol.
• To avoid patient distress, don't give drug until patient has received a general anesthetic and his consciousness is dulled because drug has no effect on consciousness or pain threshold.
• Dosage requirements for children are higher on a milligram-per-kilogram basis than for adults. Onset and recovery occur more rapidly in children.
• Duration of drug effect is increased about 150% in patients with end-stage renal disease and 300% in patients with hepatic dysfunction.
• Maintain airway and control ventilation until recovery of normal neuromuscular function is ensured.
• Monitor respirations closely until patient is fully recovered, as evidenced by tests of muscle strength, including hand grip, head lift, and ability to cough.
• When mivacurium is given I.V. push to adults receiving anesthetic combinations of nitrous oxide and opiates, neuromuscular blockade usually lasts 15 to 20 minutes; most patients recover 95% of muscle strength in 25 to 30 minutes.
• Provide nerve stimulator and train-of-four monitoring to document antagonism of neuromuscular blockade and recovery of muscle strength. Some evidence of spontaneous recovery should be evident before reversal with neostigmine methylsulfate or edrophonium chloride is attempted.
• Acid-base and electrolyte balance may affect action of and response to nondepolarizing neuromuscular blockers. Alkalosis may counteract paralysis; acidosis may enhance it.

PATIENT TEACHING
• Explain the use of drug to patient.
• Reassure the patient and family that the patient will be monitored continuously.

morphine sulfate
Astramorph PF, Duramorph

Pharmacologic class: opioid
Therapeutic class: opioid analgesic
Pregnancy risk category: C
Controlled substance schedule: II
pH: 2.5 to 7

INDICATIONS & DOSAGES
➤ **Severe pain—**
Adults: 2.5 to 15 mg I.V. q 4 hours, p.r.n.
Children: 50 to 100 mcg/kg I.V. Maximum single dose, 10 mg I.V.
➤ **Pain from MI—**
Adults: 2 to 15 mg I.V., followed by smaller doses q 3 to 4 hours, p.r.n.
➤ **Severe chronic pain—**
Adults: 1 to 10 mg/hour I.V. by continuous infusion. Maintenance dosage, 20 to 150 mg/hour I.V.
Children: 0.025 to 2.6 mg/kg/hour I.V.

ADMINISTRATION
Direct injection: Inject diluted drug over 4 to 5 minutes through I.V. tubing containing a free-flowing, compatible solution. Monitor vital signs and respiratory status for at least 1 hour after injection.
Intermittent infusion: Not recommended.
Continuous infusion: Infuse diluted drug at 1 to 10 mg/hour initially, increasing rate until reaching effective dosage. Monitor vital signs and respiratory status.

PREPARATION & STORAGE
Available with preservatives in concentrations of 1, 2, 4, 5, 8, 10, 15, 25, and 50 mg/ml; 1-mg/ml solutions. Available without preservatives in concentrations of 0.5, 1, 15, and 25 mg/ml; 50-mg/ml solutions.

For direct injection, dilute with 4 to 5 ml of D_5W. Dilute in larger volumes of D_5W to a concentration of 0.1 to 1 mg/ml for slow infusion. Morphine is compatible with most common I.V. solutions. Store below 104° F (40° C), and protect from light and freezing.

Incompatibilities
Aminophylline, amobarbital, cefepime, chlorothiazide, fluorouracil, haloperidol, heparin sodium, meperidine, pentobarbital, phenobarbital sodium, phenytoin sodium, prochlorperazine, promethazine hydrochloride, sodium bicarbonate, thiopental.

CONTRAINDICATIONS & CAUTIONS
• Contraindicated in those hypersensitive to morphine.
• Contraindicated in those with diarrhea resulting from pseudomembranous colitis or poisoning because drug may slow the elimination of toxins; and in those with acute respiratory depression because drug may exacerbate condition.
• Avoid use in those with pulmonary edema caused by a chemical respiratory irritant because drug causes vasodilation and may produce adverse hemodynamic effects.
• Use cautiously in those with altered respiratory function because of increased risk of respiratory depression; in those with hypothyroidism because of increased risk of respiratory depression and prolonged CNS depression; and in those with hepatic or renal impairment because of increased risk of toxic reaction.
• Use cautiously in those with history of drug dependence or emotional instability and in those who show evidence of suicidal ideation because of the potential for abuse.
• Use cautiously in those with inflammatory bowel disease because toxic megacolon may develop.

• Use cautiously in those with arrhythmias because drug can increase response through a vagolytic action; in those with seizure disorders because drug may induce or exacerbate seizures; and in those with head injury or increased intracranial pressure from intracranial lesions because drug may mask clinical changes and elevate CSF pressure.
• Use cautiously in those with acute abdominal conditions because drug may mask symptoms; in those with gallbladder disease because drug may increase biliary contractions; and in those who have recently undergone GI surgery because drug may alter GI motility.
• Use cautiously in patients with prostatic hyperplasia, urethral stricture, or recent urinary tract surgery because drug can cause urine retention.

ADVERSE REACTIONS
CNS: agitation, *coma,* decreased mental acuity or depression, delirium, dizziness, dysphoria, euphoria, insomnia, nervousness, sedation, *seizures,* weakness.
CV: *bradycardia, cardiac arrest, circulatory collapse,* flushing, chest wall rigidity, hypotension, tachycardia, edema.
EENT: visual disturbances.
GI: *constipation, nausea, vomiting.*
GU: oliguria, urine retention.
Hematologic: *thrombocytopenia.*
Respiratory: *respiratory depression, apnea, respiratory arrest.*
Skin: pruritus, sweating, urticaria, pain at infusion site.
Other: *anaphylaxis,* decreased libido, physical dependence.

INTERACTIONS
Drug-drug. *Anticoagulants:* Potentiates anticoagulant effects. Monitor coagulation test results.

Antidiarrheals, antiperistaltics: Increases risk of constipation and CNS depression. Monitor patient closely.

Antihypertensives, diuretics: May increase risk of hypotension. Use together with caution, and reduce morphine dose.

Antimuscarinics: Increases risk of constipation, paralytic ileus, and urine retention. Monitor patient for abdominal pain and distention.

Buprenorphine: May cause respiratory depression and reduced therapeutic morphine effect. May precipitate withdrawal symptoms in drug-dependent patients. Use together with caution, and monitor patient for withdrawal.

Cimetidine: Increases respiratory and CNS depression. Reduce dosage of morphine.

CNS depressants: Deepens CNS depression, respiratory depression, and risk of habituation. Use together with caution, and reduce morphine dose.

MAO inhibitors: Causes severe, unpredictable adverse reactions when given within 14 days of morphine. Reduce morphine dose.

Metoclopramide: May antagonize effect on GI motility. Monitor patient closely.

Neuromuscular blockers: Deepens respiratory depression. Use together with caution, and reduce morphine dose.

Opioid-agonist analgesics: May worsen CNS and respiratory depression and hypotension. Use together with caution, and reduce morphine dose.

Opioid antagonists: Blocks therapeutic morphine effect and may cause withdrawal symptoms in drug-dependent patients. Use together with caution, and reduce morphine dose.

Drug-lifestyle. *Alcohol use:* May have additive effects. Discourage use together.

EFFECTS ON LAB TEST RESULTS

• May increase amylase and lipase levels.

• May decrease platelet count and hemoglobin. May alter liver function test values.

ACTION

Binds with stereospecific receptors in the CNS, altering the perception of pain and the emotional response to it.

PHARMACOKINETICS

Drug level peaks at 20 minutes; duration, 4 to 5 hours.

Distribution: Rapidly to parenchyma. Minimally protein bound. Drug crosses placental barrier and appears in breast milk.

Metabolism: Primarily in liver.

Excretion: Primarily in urine, with 7% to 10% in feces. Half-life, 2 to 3 hours, or longer in patients with hepatic or renal dysfunction.

CLINICAL CONSIDERATIONS

• Osmolality: 54 mOsm/kg.

• Keep emergency resuscitation equipment available.

• Respiratory depression is more common in geriatric and pediatric patients.

• Morphine is the drug of choice in relieving pain of MI; it may cause transient decrease in blood pressure.

• Controlled, around-the-clock scheduling is beneficial in severe, chronic pain.

• To minimize hypotension, give drug with patient in supine position.

• *Alert:* Rapid infusion can cause life-threatening adverse reactions. Ambulatory patients and patients who aren't experiencing severe pain have a higher risk of adverse reactions.

• Monitor respirations frequently during infusion and every 15 minutes for 1 hour after infusion. If respirations fall below 8 breaths/minute, rouse patient to stimulate breathing. Notify prescriber.

• Because opioid agonists stimulate vasopressin release, their use may increase risk of water intoxication in postoperative patients.

• Dose may need to be increased in patients with severe chronic pain who have become tolerant to analgesic effects of opioids.

• Morphine may be used in PCA.

• Assess bowel function frequently; patient may need a stool softener.

• Lumbar puncture may show increased CSF pressure caused by respiratory depression-induced carbon dioxide retention. Gastric emptying may be delayed.

• *Alert:* Generic preparations may contain sulfites. Use cautiously in hypersensitive patients.

• If overdose occurs, treat symptomatically and give naloxone to reverse respiratory depression.

PATIENT TEACHING

• Tell patient to get up slowly to lessen dizziness and faintness.

• With long-term use, patient may develop habituation and physical dependence. Withdrawal symptoms may begin in 24 hours and peak 36 to 72 hours after drug is stopped. Most observable symptoms disappear in 5 to 14 days.

moxifloxacin hydrochloride
Avelox I.V.

Pharmacologic class: fluoro-quinolone
Therapeutic class: antibiotic
Pregnancy risk category: C
pH: 4.1 to 4.6

INDICATIONS & DOSAGES

➤ Acute bacterial sinusitis caused by *Streptococcus pneumoniae, Haemophilus influenzae,* or *Moraxella catarrhalis*—
Adults: 400 mg I.V. once daily for 10 days.

➤ Acute bacterial exacerbation of chronic bronchitis caused by *S. pneumoniae, H. influenzae, H. parainfluenzae, Klebsiella pneumoniae, Staphylococcus aureus,* or *M. catarrhalis*—
Adults: 400 mg I.V. once daily for 5 days.

➤ Community-acquired pneumonia caused by *S. pneumoniae* (including penicillin-resistant strains), *H. influenzae, Mycoplasma pneumoniae, Chlamydia pneumoniae, M. catarrhalis, Staphylococcus aureus,* or *Klebsiella pneumoniae*—
Adults: 400 mg I.V. once daily for 7 to 14 days.

➤ Uncomplicated skin and skin structure infections caused by *Staphylococcus aureus* or *S. pyogenes*—
Adults: 400 mg I.V. once daily for 7 days.

ADMINISTRATION

Direct injection: Not recommended.
Intermittent infusion: Infuse the drug over 60 minutes by direct infusion or through a Y-type I.V. infusion set. Avoid rapid or bolus infusion.
Continuous infusion: Not recommended.

PREPARATION & STORAGE

Supplied as a premixed solution of 400 mg in 250 ml sodium chloride injection. No further dilution is necessary. Drug is compatible at ratios of 1:10 and 10:1 in 0.9% sodium chloride injection, 1M sodium chloride injection, 5% dextrose injection, sterile water for injection, 10% dextrose for injection, or lactated Ringer's solution for injection. Store between 59° and 86° F (15° and 30° C). Don't refrigerate.

Incompatibilities
Other I.V. drugs or additives.

CONTRAINDICATIONS & CAUTIONS

• Contraindicated in patients hypersensitive to drug or its components or fluoroquinolone antimicrobials.

• Safety and efficacy haven't been documented in children, adolescents under age 18, and pregnant or lactating women.

• Drug hasn't been studied in patients with moderate to severe hepatotoxicity (Child Pugh classes B and C) and isn't recommended in this setting.

• Use cautiously in patients with prolonged QT interval and uncorrected hypokalemia.

• Use cautiously in those with known or suspected CNS disorders or other risk factors that may predispose patients to seizures or lower seizure threshold.

ADVERSE REACTIONS

CNS: dizziness, headache, asthenia, pain, malaise, insomnia, nervousness, anxiety, confusion, somnolence, tremor, vertigo, paresthesia.

CV: *prolongation of QT interval,* chest pain, palpitations, tachycardia, hypertension, peripheral edema.

GI: *pseudomembranous colitis,* nausea, diarrhea, abdominal pain, vomiting, dyspepsia, dry mouth, constipation, oral candidiasis, anorexia, stomatitis, glossitis, flatulence, gastrointestinal disorder, taste perversion.

GU: vaginitis, vaginal candidiasis.

Hematologic: *thrombocytosis, thrombocytopenia, leukopenia,* eosinophilia.

Hepatic: abnormal liver function, cholestatic jaundice.

Musculoskeletal: leg pain, back pain, arthralgia, myalgia, tendon rupture.

Respiratory: dyspnea.

Skin: injection site reaction, rash (maculopapular, purpuric, pustular), pruritus, sweating.

Other: candidiasis, *allergic reaction.*

INTERACTIONS

Drug-drug. *Anticoagulants:* Enhances anticoagulant effects. Monitor PT and INR.

Antipsychotics, erythromycin, tricyclic antidepressants: May have additive effect. Monitor patient and ECG closely; use together with caution.

Class IA (such as procainamide, quinidine) or class III (such as amiodarone, sotalol) antiarrhythmics: May cause risk of arrhythmias. Avoid using together.

NSAIDs: Increases risk of CNS stimulation and seizures. Avoid using together.

Drug-lifestyle. *Sun exposure:* Although photosensitivity hasn't occurred with moxifloxacin, it has been reported with other fluoroquinolones. Advise patient to take precautions.

EFFECTS ON LAB TEST RESULTS

• May increase GGT, amylase, and LDH levels.

• May increase eosinophil count. May decrease PT and WBC count. May increase or decrease platelet count.

ACTION

Inhibits the activity of topoisomerase I and IV in susceptible bacteria. These enzymes are necessary for bacterial DNA replication, transcription, repair, and recombination.

PHARMACOKINETICS

Onset, peak, and duration of drug effect unknown.

Distribution: Widely distributed. About 50% protein bound. Penetrates well into nasal and bronchial secretions, sinus mucosa, and saliva.

Metabolism: To inactive glucuronide and sulfate conjugates.

Excretion: About 20% in urine and 25% in feces. Sulfate metabolite eliminated primarily in feces; glucuronide metabolite renally excreted. Half-life about 12 hours.

CLINICAL CONSIDERATIONS

• Drug is safe to use and effective in elderly patients. Monitor patient for ECG changes.

• Rupture of Achilles' and other tendons has been linked to fluoroquinolones. If pain, inflammation, or tendon rupture occurs, stop drug.

• CNS reactions linked to fluoroquinolones include dizziness, confusion, tremors, hallucinations, depression, and, rarely, suicidal thoughts or acts. These reactions may occur after initial dose. Stop drug and institute appropriate therapy if any of these reactions occur.

• Serious hypersensitivity reactions, including anaphylaxis, have occurred in patients receiving fluoroquinolones. Stop drug and institute supportive measures as indicated.

• Pseudomembranous colitis may occur with moxifloxacin as with other antimicrobials. Consider this diagnosis if diarrhea develops after start of therapy.

• In acute overdose, the patient's stomach should be emptied immediately. Monitor ECG closely because of the risk of QT interval prolongation. Provide adequate hydration and supportive care. It's unknown if drug is dialyzable.

• Switch from I.V. to P.O. therapy when warranted.

PATIENT TEACHING

• Advise patient that the most common adverse reactions include nausea, vomiting, stomach pain, diarrhea, dizziness, and headache. Tell patient to avoid hazardous activities, such as driving an automobile or operating machinery, until effects of drug are known.

• Advise patient to notify health care personnel if he experiences signs of an allergic reaction, heart palpitations, fainting, persistent diarrhea, pain in muscle or tendon.

multivitamins
M.V.I.-12, M.V.I. Pediatric

Pharmacologic class: vitamins and minerals
Therapeutic class: dietary supplement
Pregnancy risk category: NR

INDICATIONS & DOSAGES

➤ **Maintenance of vitamins during parenteral nutrition or in patients who can't take vitamins orally—**
Adults and children age 11 and older: Dosage varies. Maintenance nutrition requires one dose of multivitamin concentrate in I.V. infusion q 24 hours.
Children younger than age 11: 1 vial of M.V.I. Pediatric daily in I.V. infusion.
Neonates weighing 1 to 3 kg (2.2 to 6.6 lb): 65% of M.V.I. Pediatric vial daily in I.V. infusion.
Neonates weighing less than 1 kg: 30% of M.V.I. Pediatric vial daily in I.V. infusion.

ADMINISTRATION

Direct injection: Not recommended.
Intermittent infusion: Infuse diluted solution over ordered amount of time. Add to only one I.V. solution daily.
Continuous infusion: Infuse diluted solution over 24 hours.

PREPARATION & STORAGE

M.V.I.-12 is available in a unit vial container with 5 ml of liquid in vial 1, 5 ml of liquid in vial 2, and 10 ml of lyophilized powder in vial 3. Mix contents of vials 1 and 2 by pressing down to force liquid from upper chamber into lower chamber. Or add 5 ml of sterile water for injection to the 10-ml vial of powder.

M.V.I. Pediatric is available in a 5-ml vial. Reconstitute by adding 5 ml of sterile water for injection, D$_5$W, or normal saline solution. Reconstituted solution is stable for 24 hours if refrigerated.

Dilute all prepared solutions in 500 to 1,000 ml of a compatible solution.

Incompatibilities
Acetazolamide, amino acids (5.5%, 8.5%, or 10%), chlorothiazide sodium, dextrose 5% in Normosol-M, fat emulsions, meropenem, moderately alkaline solutions.

Folic acid: calcium salts.

Some vitamins, particularly thiamine: sodium bisulfite.

CONTRAINDICATIONS & CAUTIONS
● Contraindicated in those hypersensitive to any vitamin and in those with hypervitaminosis.
● Use cautiously in those with hereditary optic nerve atrophy (Leber's disease); cyanocobalamin may cause severe acute optic atrophy.

ADVERSE REACTIONS
CNS: dizziness and faintness with injection of undiluted drug.
Hepatic: *hepatotoxicity (vitamin A toxicity).*
Metabolic: hypercalcemia (vitamin D toxicity).
Other: allergic reactions to thiamine and, rarely, to folic acid; *anaphylaxis;* tissue calcification (vitamin D toxicity).

INTERACTIONS
Drug-drug. *Levodopa:* Decreases effectiveness if given with pyridoxine. Monitor closely; separate administration times if possible.
Methotrexate: May interfere with the body's use of folic acid. Monitor patient closely.

EFFECTS ON LAB TEST RESULTS
● May increase liver enzyme and calcium levels.

ACTION
Vitamin C promotes collagen formation and tissue repair. Vitamin B$_3$ is needed for oxidation-reduction reactions and carbohydrate metabolism; vitamin B$_9$, for nucleoprotein synthesis and erythropoiesis; vitamins B$_5$ and B$_6$ for amino acid metabolism and carbohydrate and lipid metabolism. Vitamin B$_{12}$ plays a vital role in numerous tissues' respiratory systems; vitamin B$_1$, in carbohydrate metabolism; and cyanocobalamin, in nucleoprotein and myelin synthesis, cell reproduction, normal growth, and maintenance of erythropoiesis. Vitamin D helps to regulate calcium level. Although its function is unknown, vitamin E is thought to be an antioxidant. Vitamin A promotes growth, bone development, vision, reproduction, and integrity of mucosal and epithelial surfaces.

PHARMACOKINETICS
Onset, peak, and duration are unknown.
Distribution: Vitamins C, B$_3$, B$_9$, and B$_1$ widely distributed in tissues; vitamin B$_5$ in liver, adrenal glands, heart, and kidneys; vitamin B$_6$ in liver, muscles, and brain; vitamin B$_2$ in GI mucosa, RBCs, and liver; vitamin B$_{12}$ in liver, bone marrow, and other tissues; vitamin A in liver; vitamin D in liver, fat, muscles, skin, and bones; vitamin E in all tissues. All vitamins cross placental barrier.
Metabolism: In liver. Vitamin D also in kidneys.
Excretion: Vitamin A in bile. Vitamins D, E, and B$_{12}$ mainly in feces, with small amounts in urine; all other vitamins in urine.

CLINICAL CONSIDERATIONS
- Osmolality: 4,210 to 4,820 mOsm/kg.
- M.V.I.-12 doesn't provide vitamin K_1; give K_1 separately. M.V.I. Pediatric contains vitamin K_1.
- Folic acid doses exceeding 0.1 mg/day may mask signs of pernicious anemia.
- Fat-soluble vitamins (A, D, E, and K) accumulate in the body. Hypervitaminosis of vitamins A, D, and E can occur.
- Don't use multivitamins in those with severe vitamin deficiency.
- If overdose occurs, provide supportive care and maintain high urine output.

PATIENT TEACHING
- Inform pregnant patient that megadoses of vitamins may be hazardous to the fetus.
- Tell patient not to double a dose if a dose is missed.
- Tell patient to promptly report adverse reactions.

muromonab-CD3
Orthoclone OKT3

Pharmacologic class: murine monoclonal antibody
Therapeutic class: immunosuppressant
Pregnancy risk category: C

INDICATIONS & DOSAGES
➤ **Acute allograft rejection in heart, liver, or kidney transplant—**
Adults: 5 mg daily for 10 to 14 days.
Children weighing 30 kg (66 lb) or less ♦: Initially, 2.5 mg/day I.V. as single bolus over less than 1 minute, for 10 to 14 days. Increase daily dose in 2.5-mg increments to decrease CD3-positive cells.

Children weighing more than 30 kg ♦: Initially, 5 mg/day I.V. as single bolus over less than 1 minute, for 10 to 14 days. Increase daily dose in 2.5-mg increments to decrease CD3-positive cells.

ADMINISTRATION
Direct injection: Give by I.V. push directly into vein over less than 1 minute. Don't give with I.V. fluids.
Intermittent infusion: Not recommended.
Continuous infusion: Not recommended.

PREPARATION & STORAGE
Available in 1-mg/ml ampules. Store in refrigerator unless otherwise specified by the manufacturer. Protect from freezing. Don't shake ampule. Draw solution into syringe through a low-protein-binding 0.2- or 0.22-micrometer filter, then discard filter and attach appropriate needle. Appearance of fine, translucent particles in solution doesn't indicate loss of potency.

Incompatibilities
Other I.V. drugs.

CONTRAINDICATIONS & CAUTIONS
- Contraindicated in those with existing or recent chickenpox or herpes zoster infection and in those with a temperature above 100° F (37.8° C) because of increased risk of severe generalized disease.
- Contraindicated in those with fluid overload, as evidenced by chest X-ray or weight gain greater than 3% within 1 week before treatment because of increased risk of pulmonary edema.
- Use cautiously in those hypersensitive to drug and in those with infection because of risk of severe adverse reactions.
- Use cautiously in breast-feeding patients and in those with a predisposition to or history of seizures.

• Safe use in children hasn't been established.

ADVERSE REACTIONS

CNS: *asthenia,* fatigue, lethargy, malaise, *fever,* **seizures,** dizziness, *headache,* **meningitis,** *tremor,* confusion, depression, nervousness, somnolence.
CV: vasodilation, **arrhythmia,** bradycardia, *hypertension, hypotension,* chest pain, *tachycardia,* vascular occlusion, *edema,* **cardiac arrest, shock, heart failure.**
EENT: photophobia, tinnitus.
GI: anorexia, *diarrhea, nausea,* abdominal pain, GI pain, *vomiting.*
GU: **renal dysfunction.**
Hematologic: anemia, leukocytosis, **leukopenia, thrombocytopenia.**
Musculoskeletal: arthralgia, myalgia.
Respiratory: *dyspnea,* hyperventilation, hypoxia, pneumonia, pulmonary edema, respiratory congestion, wheezing, **adult respiratory distress syndrome.**
Skin: diaphoresis, pruritus, *rash.*
Other: *chills,* pain in trunk area, *cytokine release syndrome, hypersensitivity reactions.*

INTERACTIONS

Drug-drug. *Immunosuppressants:* Increases risk of infection and lymphoproliferative disorders. Monitor patient for infection.
Indomethacin: May cause encephalopathy and other CNS effects. Monitor patient for change in neurological status.
Vaccines with live virus: May potentiate replication of virus, increase adverse effects, and diminish antibody response to vaccine. Postpone immunization, if possible.

EFFECTS ON LAB TEST RESULTS

• May increase BUN and creatinine levels.

ACTION

Reacts in the T-cell membrane with CD3, blocks T-cell functions, and reacts with most T cells in blood and body tissues to block allograft rejection.

PHARMACOKINETICS

Onset, within minutes; duration, 1 week.
Distribution: Widely distributed throughout the body.
Metabolism: Unknown. Drug isn't metabolized but is thought to bind to circulating T cells.
Excretion: Unknown.

CLINICAL CONSIDERATIONS

• Reduce dosage of other immunosuppressants before giving drug.
• Chest X-ray taken 24 hours before treatment begins must be clear.
• To decrease the incidence and severity of cytokine release syndrome, give 8 mg/kg I.V. methylprednisolone sodium succinate 1 to 4 hours before first dose. Give an antipyretic and an antihistamine before therapy to reduce expected pyrexia and chills. Keep cooling blanket available.
• *Alert:* Keep equipment and drugs for advanced life support readily available during first dose.
• First-dose reaction may occur 30 to 60 minutes after initial dose and may last for several hours. Monitor patient closely for 48 hours after initial dose. With each successive dose, both the frequency and severity of symptoms tend to diminish.
• Monitor temperature, CBC, and tests for circulating T cells expressing the CD3 antigen. Monitor renal and hepatic function regularly.
• Aseptic meningitis has been reported in patients treated with drug, although a direct causal relationship hasn't been established.
• Immunosuppressive therapy increases susceptibility to infection and to lym-

phoproliferative disorders. Occurrence of lymphomas seems linked to the intensity and duration of immunosuppression, not to specific drugs, because most patients receive a combination of treatments.

PATIENT TEACHING

• Inform patient of expected adverse effects. Reassure him that adverse effects subside as treatment progresses.

• Instruct patient to avoid immunizations during therapy. Family members should also avoid immunization with oral polio vaccine and any contact with those vaccinated with it.

• Warn patient to avoid exposure to people with bacterial or viral infections.

• Advise any woman of childbearing age to avoid becoming pregnant during therapy.

nafcillin sodium

Pharmacologic class: semi-synthetic penicillinase-resistant penicillin
Therapeutic class: antibiotic
Pregnancy risk category: B
pH: 6 to 8.5

INDICATIONS & DOSAGES
➤ **Severe systemic infections caused by susceptible organisms—**
Adults: 0.5 to 1 g I.V. q 4 hours, depending on severity of infection, for 14 days.
Children older than age 1 month: 50 to 200 mg/kg/day I.V. in equally divided doses q 4 to 6 hours.
Neonates age 7 days and younger, weighing 2 kg (4.4 lb) or less: 25 mg/kg I.V. q 12 hours.
Neonates age 7 days and younger, weighing more than 2 kg: 25 mg/kg I.V. q 8 hours.
Neonates older than age 7 days, weighing 2 kg or less: 25 mg/kg I.V. q 8 hours.
Neonates older than age 7 days, weighing more than 2 kg: 25 mg/kg q I.V. 6 hours.
➤ **Osteomyelitis—**
Adults: 1 to 2 g I.V. q 4 hours for 4 to 8 weeks.
Children older than age 1 month: 100 to 200 mg/kg/day I.V. in equally divided doses q 4 to 6 hours for 4 to 8 weeks.
➤ **Endocarditis—**
Adults: 2 g I.V. q 4 hours for 4 to 6 weeks

Children older than age 1 month: 100 to 200 mg/kg/day I.V. in equally divided doses q 4 to 6 hours for 4 to 8 weeks.
➤ **Meningitis—**
Adults: 100 to 200 mg/kg/day I.V. in equally divided doses q 4 to 6 hours.
Neonates age 7 days and younger, weighing 2 kg or less: 50 mg/kg I.V. q 12 hours.
Neonates age 7 days and younger, weighing more than 2 kg: 50 mg/kg I.V. q 8 hours.
Neonates older than age 7 days, weighing 2 kg or less: 50 mg/kg I.V. q 8 hours.
Neonates older than age 7 days, weighing more than 2 kg: 50 mg/kg q I.V. 6 hours.

ADMINISTRATION
Direct injection: Not recommended.
Intermittent infusion: Infuse dose over at least 30 to 60 minutes.
Continuous infusion: Not recommended.

PREPARATION & STORAGE
Available as 1- and 2-g frozen, premixed dextrose solutions.
Don't force thaw by immersing in hot water bath or by microwave irradiation.
Store at or below -4° F (-20 °C). Thawed solutions are stable for 21 days under refrigeration at 41° F (5° C) or at room temperature of 77° F (25° C).
Don't refreeze solution after being thawed.

Incompatibilities
Aminoglycosides, aminophylline, ascorbic acid, aztreonam, bleomycin,

cytarabine, diltiazem, droperidol, gentamicin, hydrocortisone sodium succinate, insulin (regular), labetalol, meperidine, methylprednisolone sodium succinate, midazolam, nalbuphine, pentazocine lactate, promazine, vancomycin, verapamil hydrochloride, vitamin B complex with C.

CONTRAINDICATIONS & CAUTIONS
• Contraindicated in those hypersensitive to penicillins, cephalosporins, or imipenem.
• Use cautiously in those with a history of an allergy because of predisposition to hypersensitivity reactions.
• Use cautiously in those with hepatic impairment because of increased risk of adverse reactions; in those with eosinophilia or hemolytic anemia because of increased risk of adverse hematologic effects; and in those with GI disorders because of possible pseudomembranous colitis.
• Use cautiously in those with sodium restrictions.

ADVERSE REACTIONS
CNS: fever.
CV: thrombophlebitis.
GI: abdominal pain, diarrhea, dry mouth, *nausea, pseudomembranous colitis,* stomatitis, vomiting.
GU: acute interstitial nephritis, hematuria.
Hematologic: eosinophilia, *neutropenia, thrombocytopenia, agranulocytosis.*
Metabolic: hypokalemia.
Musculoskeletal: arthralgia.
Skin: pruritus, rash, urticaria, pain at injection site.
Other: *anaphylaxis,* bacterial and fungal superinfection, hypersensitivity reactions.

INTERACTIONS
Drug-drug. *Aminoglycosides:* Has synergistic effects and is chemically and physically incompatible. Don't combine in same I.V. solution.
Chloramphenicol, erythromycin, sulfonamides, tetracyclines: Decreases bactericidal activity. Monitor patient closely for clinical effect.
Hormonal contraceptives: May decrease contraceptive effectiveness. Recommend additional form of contraception during penicillin therapy.
Oral anticoagulants: May increase risk of bleeding. Monitor PT and INR closely.
Probenecid: May slow nafcillin excretion. Probenecid may be used for this effect.
Rifampin: Causes dose-dependent antagonism. Monitor patient closely.

EFFECTS ON LAB TEST RESULTS
• May increase AST, ALT, and alkaline phophatase levels. May decrease potassium level.
• May increase eosinophil count. May decrease neutrophil, granulocyte, and platelet counts.
• May falsely elevate turbidimetric urine and serum protein levels in tests using sulfosalicylic acid or trichloroacetic acid. May falsely decrease aminoglycoside level. May alter urinary protein results in tests using biuret or Coomassie brilliant blue method.

ACTION
Acts against gram-positive aerobic bacteria.

PHARMACOKINETICS
Drug level peaks immediately after administration.
Distribution: Readily distributed to most body tissues and fluids; highest level in liver. About 70% to 90% protein bound. Drug crosses the placental barrier and appears in cord blood and amniotic fluid. Slight amounts may appear in breast milk.
Metabolism: In the liver, with about 60% changed to inactive metabolites.

Excretion: Mainly in bile. Small amounts removed in urine by glomerular filtration. Half-life in normal renal function averages 30 to 90 minutes; in renal or hepatic impairment, 1 to 3 hours. Half-life prolonged in neonates.

CLINICAL CONSIDERATIONS

• Osmolality: 300 mOsm/kg.
• Before giving first dose, ask patient about previous allergic reactions to penicillins or cephalosporins. Negative history doesn't rule out future hypersensitivity reaction.
• Obtain specimens for culture and sensitivity tests before giving first dose. Therapy may begin before results are available.
• Change I.V. site every 48 hours to reduce the risk of vein irritation.
• Obtain WBC count and differential before therapy and one to three times weekly during therapy.
• Periodically obtain urinalysis and BUN, AST, and ALT levels.
• Stop drug if patient develops bone marrow toxicity, pseudomembranous colitis, acute interstitial nephritis, eosinophilia, fever, arthralgia, hematuria, or elevated BUN or creatinine levels.
• If diarrhea persists during therapy, collect stool specimens for culture to rule out pseudomembranous colitis.
• Observe patient for fungal and bacterial superinfection with prolonged use.
• Dialysis removes only slight amounts of the drug.

PATIENT TEACHING

• Ask patient to list the drugs he takes and any drug allergies he has.
• Tell patient to notify prescriber if he develops rash, fever, chills, or diarrhea. A rash or diarrhea is the most common allergic reaction.

nalbuphine hydrochloride
Nubain

Pharmacologic class: opioid agonist-antagonist, opioid partial agonist
Therapeutic class: analgesic, adjunct to anesthesia
Pregnancy risk category: B
pH: 3.5 to 3.7

INDICATIONS & DOSAGES

➤ **Moderate to severe pain and preoperative analgesia; supplement to obstetric analgesia—**
Adults: 10 mg (or 0.14 mg/kg) I.V. q 3 to 6 hours, p.r.n. Maximum single dose, 20 mg in nontolerant individuals; maximum daily dose, 160 mg.
➤ **Supplement to balanced anesthesia—**
Adults: 0.3 to 3 mg/kg I.V. over 10 to 15 minutes. Maintenance dosage, 0.25 to 0.5 mg/kg, p.r.n.

ADMINISTRATION

Direct injection: Inject drug directly into vein or into an I.V. line containing a compatible, free-flowing I.V. solution over 2 to 3 minutes or longer. Avoid rapid injection, which can precipitate anaphylaxis, peripheral circulatory collapse, or cardiac arrest.
Intermittent infusion: Not recommended.
Continuous infusion: Not recommended.

PREPARATION & STORAGE

Supplied in 1-ml ampules, 1- and 10-ml vials, and 1-ml disposable syringes in 10- or 20-mg/ml concentration.

Nalbuphine is compatible with D_5W in normal saline, lactated Ringer's, and normal saline solutions.

Reactions may be *common*, uncommon, *life-threatening*, or COMMON AND LIFE-THREATENING.

Protect from freezing, excessive light, and heat. Store at room temperature 59° to 86° F (15° to 30° C).

Incompatibilities
Allopurinol, amphotericin B, cefepime, diazepam, docetaxel, ketorolac, methotrexate sodium, nafcillin, pentobarbital sodium, piperacillin and tazobactam sodium, promethazine, sargramostim, sodium bicarbonate, thiethylperazine.

CONTRAINDICATIONS & CAUTIONS
• Contraindicated in patients hypersensitive to drug and in those with severely altered respiratory function because drug depresses respirations.
• Contraindicated in those with diarrhea caused by pseudomembranous colitis or poisoning because drug may delay removal of toxins from colon, thereby prolonging or worsening diarrhea.
• Use cautiously in those with head injury and increased intracranial pressure because drug can raise CSF pressure.
• Use cautiously in those receiving long-term opioid therapy. High doses of nalbuphine may precipitate withdrawal, but low doses don't suppress the abstinence syndrome.
• Use cautiously in those about to undergo biliary tract surgery and in those with gallbladder disease because drug may induce spasm in the sphincter of Oddi.
• Use cautiously in those with acute abdominal conditions because drug may mask diagnosis; in those with an MI who experience nausea and vomiting because drug may exacerbate these effects; and in those who have recently undergone GI surgery because drug may alter GI motility.
• Use cautiously in those with asthma or chronic respiratory disease because drug may decrease respiratory drive and increase airway resistance.
• Use cautiously in those with a history of seizures because drug's metabolite may induce or exacerbate seizures.
• Use cautiously in those with sensitivity to sulfites because sulfite preservatives in injection may cause allergic reactions.
• Use cautiously in those with prostatic hyperplasia, urinary tract obstruction, urethral stricture, recent urinary tract surgery, or renal dysfunction, because urine retention may worsen.
• Use cautiously in those with hypothyroidism because of increased risk of respiratory and CNS depression, and in those with inflammatory bowel disease because of potential for toxic megacolon.
• Use cautiously in those with hepatic or renal impairment because of slowed drug clearance and increased risk of toxic reaction, and in geriatric patients because of increased sensitivity to drug effects.

ADVERSE REACTIONS
CNS: dizziness, *sedation,* vertigo, headache.
CV: *severe bradycardia or tachycardia, shock.*
GI: dry mouth, nausea, vomiting.
Respiratory: *apnea, respiratory depression, pulmonary edema.*
Skin: sweating, clamminess, injection site reactions.
Other: *anaphylaxis.*

INTERACTIONS
Drug-drug. *Antihypertensives, diuretics:* Potentiates hypotensive effects. Monitor blood pressure closely.
Antimuscarinics: Increases potential for constipation, paralytic ileus, and urine retention. Monitor patient for abdominal pain and distension.
Antiperistaltic antidiarrheals: Increases risk of constipation and CNS depression. Use together cautiously; monitor patient closely.

Buprenorphine: May cause additive respiratory depression. Use together with caution.

CNS depressants, general anesthetics, hypnotics, MAO inhibitors, neuromuscular blockers, phenothiazines and other tranquilizers, sedatives: May deepen CNS and respiratory depression. Use together with caution; monitor patient closely.

Metoclopramide: Decreases effect on GI motility. Monitor patient closely.

Naloxone, naltrexone: Antagonizes analgesic, CNS, and respiratory depressant effects. Use together with caution; monitor patient closely.

Opioid-agonist analgesics: May partially antagonize analgesic effects or precipitate withdrawal symptoms if patient is dependent on opioid-agonist drugs. Use together with caution; monitor patient closely.

Drug-lifestyle. *Alcohol use:* May have additive effects. Discourage use together.

EFFECTS ON LAB TEST RESULTS
• May increase CSF pressure and delay gastric emptying.
• May constrict sphincter of Oddi and increase biliary tract pressure, causing false-positive diagnosis of bile duct obstruction.

ACTION
Binds with opioid receptors at many CNS sites, altering the perception of pain and the emotional response to it.

PHARMACOKINETICS
Onset, 2 to 3 minutes; peak, 30 minutes; duration, 3 to 6 hours.
Distribution: Not well bound to plasma proteins. Placental transfer is high, rapid, and variable. Unknown if drug appears in breast milk.
Metabolism: In the liver.
Excretion: Mostly in feces; less so in urine. Half-life, about 5 hours.

CLINICAL CONSIDERATIONS
• Osmolality: 290 mOsm/kg.
• Give drug with patient in supine position to minimize hypotensive effects.
• Monitor respiratory status for at least 1 hour after administration. Keep resuscitation equipment available. If respirations drop below 8 breaths/minute, rouse patient to stimulate breathing. Notify prescriber, who may order naloxone or respiratory support.
• In long-term use of other opioid agonists, consider giving only 25% of initial nalbuphine dose. Monitor patient for withdrawal symptoms. If needed, give slowly in small increments. If withdrawal symptoms fail to occur, increase dose progressively until reaching desired analgesia level.
• Drug may produce respiratory depression in neonates if drug is used during labor and delivery. Monitor neonate's vital signs.
• Dosage should be reduced when drug is used in elderly patients.
• *Alert:* Drug may contain sulfites.
• Drug's abuse potential equals that of pentazocine but is less than that of codeine or propoxyphene. Monitor patient for habituation and psychological dependence, which may occur with long-term use.
• If overdose occurs, provide airway and respiratory support. Give naloxone, as needed, to reverse respiratory depression. Also, give I.V. fluids and vasopressors to maintain blood pressure.

PATIENT TEACHING
• Tell patient to get up slowly to reduce dizziness and faintness.
• Advise patient to report severe nausea, vomiting, or constipation.

nalmefene hydrochloride
Revex

Pharmacologic class: opioid
antagonist
Therapeutic class: opioid
antagonist
Pregnancy risk category: B
pH: 3.9

INDICATIONS & DOSAGES

➤ **To reverse postoperative opioid effects—**
Adults: Initially, 0.25 mcg/kg I.V., followed by 0.25 mcg/kg I.V. incremental doses at 2- to 5-minute intervals until desired response is obtained. Cumulative total dose above 1 mcg/kg I.V. doesn't provide additional therapeutic effect.

➤ **To manage opioid overdose—**
Adults: Initially, 0.5 mg/70 kg I.V. followed by 1 mg/70 kg I.V. 2 to 5 minutes later, if needed. Cumulative dosages above 1.5 mg/70 kg I.V. aren't likely to have an added effect. If opioid dependence is suspected, give test dose of 0.1 mg/70 kg I.V. If no evidence of withdrawal occurs in 2 minutes after test dose, recommended dose may be given.

Adjust-a-dose: In patients with renal impairment give in incremental doses slowly over 60 seconds, to minimize hypertension and dizziness that may develop after abrupt drug administration.

ADMINISTRATION
Titrate dose to reverse the undesired effects of opioids. After you reverse the opioid effects, stop giving drug.
Direct injection: Give undiluted drug. Drug may be diluted if smaller initial or incremental doses are needed.

Intermittent infusion: Not recommended.
Continuous infusion: Not recommended.

PREPARATION & STORAGE
Supplied in two concentrations: 1-ml ampule (blue label) suitable for postoperative use (concentration, 100 mcg/ml), and 2-ml ampule and syringe (green label) suitable for managing overdose (concentration, 1 mg/ml).

Drug is compatible with D_5W, dextrose 5% in lactated Ringer's, dextrose 5% in half-normal saline, lactated Ringer's, sodium bicarbonate 5%, half-normal saline, and normal saline solutions.

Store at controlled room temperature.

Incompatibilities
Other I.V. drugs.

CONTRAINDICATIONS & CAUTIONS
• Contraindicated in patients hypersensitive to drug.
• Use caution in those with known physical dependence on opioids or after surgery involving high doses of opioids. Abrupt reversal of opioids in postoperative and emergency patients may cause hypertension, hypotension, tachycardia, pulmonary edema, CV instability, ventricular tachycardia, and ventricular fibrillation.
• Use cautiously in patients receiving potentially cardiotoxic drugs and those who are breast-feeding.

ADVERSE REACTIONS
CNS: dizziness, headache, postoperative pain, fever.
CV: hypertension, hypotension, tachycardia, vasodilation.
GI: diarrhea, dry mouth, *nausea,* vomiting.
Other: chills.

INTERACTIONS
Drug-drug. *Flumazenil:* May induce seizures. Use with caution; monitor patient closely.

EFFECTS ON LAB TEST RESULTS
• May increase AST level.

ACTION
Prevents or reverses the effects of opioids, including respiratory depression, sedation, and hypotension.

PHARMACOKINETICS
Onset and peak, immediate; duration, varies. Low dose (1 mcg/kg) may last for 30 to 60 minutes; full reversing doses (1 mg/70 kg) may last for many hours.
Distribution: Rapid; 45% protein bound. Unknown if drug appears in breast milk.
Metabolism: By the liver; primarily by glucuronide conjugation.
Excretion: Less than 5% in urine; 17% in feces.

CLINICAL CONSIDERATIONS
• Isotonic, when mixed with normal saline solution.
• This drug may not completely reverse buprenorphine-induced respiratory depression.
• In postoperative patients at increased risk for CV complications, drug may be diluted 1:1 with saline solution or sterile water for injection using smaller initial and incremental doses.
• Cumulative total doses above 1.5 mg/ 70 kg aren't likely to have an added effect.
• Monitor patient's respiratory depth and rate closely. Duration of opioid's action may exceed that of nalmefene, causing the patient to relapse into respiratory depression. Keep patient under close observation until patient is no longer at risk for recurring respiratory depression.

• *Alert:* Drug may produce acute withdrawal symptoms in patients with known physical dependence on opioids. If opioid dependence is suspected, give test dose of 0.1 mg/70 kg. If no evidence of withdrawal occurs in 2 minutes, recommended dose may be given.
• Before treating a patient with the drug, provide ventilatory assistance, establish circulatory access, and give oxygen.

PATIENT TEACHING
• Explain to patient and family the need for drug and explain how it will be given.
• Reassure family that patient will be monitored closely until narcotic effects are alleviated.

naloxone hydrochloride
Narcan

Pharmacologic class: opioid antagonist
Therapeutic class: opioid antagonist
Pregnancy risk category: B
pH: 3 to 4

INDICATIONS & DOSAGES
➤ **Opioid toxicity—**
Adults: Initially, 0.4 mg to 2 mg I.V., repeated q 2 to 3 minutes, p.r.n.; or 0.4 mg followed by continuous infusion of 0.4 mg/hour, titrated to patient's response.
Children: Initially, 0.01 mg/kg I.V., then 0.1 mg/kg I.V. repeated q 2 to 3 minutes for up to two more doses; or 0.4 mg/hour I.V. by continuous infusion, titrated to patient's response.
Neonates: Initially, 0.01 mg/kg I.V., repeated q 2 to 3 minutes until desired response is obtained.

➤ **Postoperative opioid depression—**
Adults: 0.1 to 0.2 mg I.V. q 2 to 3 minutes until ventilation is adequate; may repeat at 1- or 2-hour intervals. Or, initially, 0.005 mg/kg I.V., repeated in 15 minutes p.r.n. For continuous infusion, 0.0037 mg/kg/hour I.V.
Children: 0.005 to 0.01 mg I.V. q 2 to 3 minutes until ventilation is adequate and child is alert; may be repeated at 1- to 2-hour intervals.

ADMINISTRATION
Direct injection: Inject drug directly into vein or into an established I.V. line containing a free-flowing, compatible solution.
Intermittent infusion: Not recommended.
Continuous infusion: Infuse at rate titrated to patient's needs. Pediatric rate may range from 0.024 to 0.16 mg/kg/hour.

PREPARATION & STORAGE
Available in 0.02-, 0.4-, and 1-mg vials, ampules, and syringes.

For a concentration of 0.004 mg/ml, mix 2 mg of drug in 500 ml of D_5W or normal saline solution. For a concentration of 0.02 mg/ml, dilute 0.5 ml of adult dose (0.4 mg/ml) with 9.5 ml of sterile water or normal saline solution for injection.

Store at 59° to 86° F (15° to 30° C) and protect from light. Avoid freezing. Solution is stable for 24 hours.

Incompatibilities
All other I.V. drugs, especially preparations containing bisulfite, sulfite, long-chain or high–molecular-weight anions, or alkaline solutions.

CONTRAINDICATIONS & CAUTIONS
• Contraindicated in those hypersensitive to drug.
• Use cautiously in those physically dependent on opioids. A sudden reversal of narcotic effect could cause acute abstinence syndrome.
• Use cautiously in postoperative patients with cardiac dysfunction or in those receiving cardiotoxic drugs because cardiac collapse may occur.

ADVERSE REACTIONS
CNS: irritability, pain, *seizures,* tremors.
CV: *arrhythmias,* blood pressure changes, *ventricular tachycardia, ventricular fibrillation.*
GI: nausea, vomiting.
Respiratory: *pulmonary edema.*
Skin: diaphoresis.
Other: withdrawal symptoms including diarrhea, fever, hyperactive reflexes and seizures in neonates, irritability, restlessness, rhinorrhea, sneezing, sweating, tachycardia, tremors, weakness, and yawning.

INTERACTIONS
Drug-drug. *Opioid-agonist analgesics, opioid partial agonists such as butorphanol:* Reverses analgesic effects; may precipitate withdrawal symptoms in patients physically dependent on opioids. Monitor patient closely.

EFFECTS ON LAB TEST RESULTS
None reported.

ACTION
Drug possesses no agonist activity of its own. May antagonize opiate effects by competing for the same CNS receptor sites.

PHARMACOKINETICS
Onset, 2 minutes; peak, 5 to 15 minutes; duration (dose-dependent), about 45 minutes for a 0.4-mg dose.
Distribution: Widely and rapidly to all body fluids and tissues, especially in skeletal muscle, kidneys, liver, brain, lungs, and heart. Drug readily crosses the blood-brain and placental barriers.

Unknown if drug appears in breast milk.
Metabolism: Mainly in the liver, but also in the CNS, kidneys, lungs, and placenta.
Excretion: Principally in urine, with small amounts in feces. Estimated half-life, 60 to 90 minutes; in neonates, about 3 hours.

CLINICAL CONSIDERATIONS
• Osmolality: 289 to 301 mOsm/kg.
• In the detoxified opioid addict, give naloxone challenge test before starting therapy. Give 0.2 mg, then observe for 30 seconds. If patient develops no withdrawal symptoms, give 0.6 mg and continue monitoring for an additional 20 minutes.
• Closely monitor respiratory, cardiac, and hemodynamic status for at least 24 hours. Duration of action of some opioids may be longer than that of naloxone. Also, respiratory rate may suddenly exceed patient's normal rate.
• Because drug's action may be shorter than that of the opioid, continuous infusion may be needed.
• Monitor patient for signs of withdrawal.
• Lack of response indicates condition isn't caused by opioid CNS depressant.
• To reverse effects of opioid agonists used during anesthesia without inhibiting pain control, carefully titrate naloxone dosage.
• *Alert:* Don't confuse naloxone (Narcan) with naltrexone (ReVia, Depade).

PATIENT TEACHING
• Tell patient to report severe pain or tremulousness.
• Inform family of need for drug and explain how it is given.
• Reassure family that patient will be closely monitored until narcotic effects are alleviated.

neostigmine methylsulfate
Prostigmin

Pharmacologic class: anti-cholinesterase
Therapeutic class: muscle stimulant
Pregnancy risk category: C
pH: 5.9

INDICATIONS & DOSAGES
➤ **Symptomatic control of myasthenia gravis—**
Adults: 0.5 to 2.5 mg I.V., p.r.n. Dosage varies widely, depending on patient needs and response.
➤ **Antidote for nondepolarizing neuromuscular blockers—**
Adults: 0.5 to 2.5 mg I.V., repeated p.r.n. to maximum total dose of 5 mg I.V.; give with 0.6 to 1.2 mg atropine I.V. or 0.2 mg glycopyrrolate I.V. for each 1 mg of neostigmine. Give several minutes before neostigmine.
Children: 0.025 to 0.8 mg/kg/dose with 0.01 to 0.03 mg/kg atropine (0.4 mg for each mg of neostigmine) I.V. or 0.004 to 0.015 mg/kg glycopyrrolate (0.2 mg for each mg of neostigmine) I.V.
Infants: 0.025 to 0.1 mg/kg/dose with 0.01 to 0.04 mg/kg atropine (0.4 mg for each mg of neostigmine) I.V. or 0.004 to 0.02 mg/kg glycopyrrolate (0.2 mg for each mg of neostigmine) I.V.

ADMINISTRATION
Direct injection: Inject drug slowly into tubing of patent, free-flowing I.V. line containing D_5W, normal saline, or another compatible I.V. solution.
Intermittent infusion: Not recommended.
Continuous infusion: Not recommended.

Reactions may be *common*, uncommon, *life-threatening*, or COMMON AND LIFE-THREATENING.

PREPARATION & STORAGE
Available in 1-ml ampules of 1:2,000
(0.5 mg/ml) and 1:4,000 (0.25 mg/ml).
Also available in multidose vials of
1:1,000 (1 mg/ml) and 1:2,000
(0.5 mg/ml).

Neostigmine needs no further dilution.

Protect solution from light and avoid
freezing.

Incompatibilities
None reported.

CONTRAINDICATIONS & CAUTIONS
• Contraindicated in those hypersensitive to drug.
• Contraindicated in those with peritonitis or mechanical obstruction of intestinal or urinary tract because drug
increases intestinal and urinary muscle
tone and activity.
• Use cautiously in those with peptic
ulcer disease, epilepsy, or hyperthyroidism.
• Use cautiously in those with asthma,
bradycardia, or arrhythmias, because
drug may worsen these conditions.
• Use cautiously after surgery, because
respiratory difficulty may be aggravated by postoperative pain, sedation, secretions, or atelectasis.

ADVERSE REACTIONS
CNS: confusion, irritability, fatigue,
clumsiness, weakness, *convulsions,*
dizziness, drowsiness, headache.
CV: thrombophlebitis, *severe bradycardia, cardiac arrest,* hypotension.
EENT: blurred vision, pupillary constriction, lacrimation.
GI: *nausea, abdominal cramps, vomiting, diarrhea,* excessive salivation.
GU: urinary frequency and incontinence.
Musculoskeletal: fasciculations, muscle cramps.
Respiratory: aspiration of excessive
oral secretions, dyspnea, *respiratory
paralysis, severe bronchospasm, respi-*
ratory depression, laryngospasm, increased bronchial secretions.
Skin: diaphoresis, rash.
Other: *anaphylaxis,* hypersensitivity
reactions.

INTERACTIONS
Drug-drug. *Aminoglycosides, anticholinergics, atropine, corticosteroids,
local and general anesthetics, magnesium, procainamide, quinidine:* Antagonizes effects of neostigmine. Observe
for lack of drug effect. Stop all other
cholinergics before giving this drug.
Anticholinesterases: May cause additive toxicity. Monitor patient for toxicity.
*Depolarizing neuromuscular blockers,
such as decamethonium and succinylcholine:* Prolongs neuromuscular
blockade. Monitor patient closely.
*Nondepolarizing neuromuscular block-
ers, such as pancuronium and tubocurarine:* Antagonizes muscle relaxant effects. Use with caution; monitor patient
closely.

EFFECTS ON LAB TEST RESULTS
None reported.

ACTION
Blocks effects of acetylcholinesterase,
prolonging increased skeletal muscle
strength and intestinal muscle tone,
bradycardia, ureteral constriction,
bronchial and pupillary constriction,
and salivary and sweat gland secretion.

PHARMACOKINETICS
Onset, within 4 to 8 minutes; peak effect, in 1 to 2 hours; duration, 2 to 4
hours.
Distribution: Throughout most tissues,
highest in liver and heart. Only high
doses cross the blood-brain barrier.
Drug may cross the placental barrier.
Unknown if drug appears in breast
milk.
Metabolism: Cholinesterases hydrolyze
the drug at the neuromuscular junction.

Hepatic microsomal enzymes metabolize it.
Excretion: In urine, by renal tubular secretion. Half-life ranges from 47 to 60 minutes.

CLINICAL CONSIDERATIONS
● Osmolality: 251 mOsm/kg.
● Keep patient on assisted ventilation when drug is used to reverse the effects of nondepolarizing neuromuscular blockers.
● An I.V. dose is much smaller than an oral dose. In critically ill patients, exact dose may be titrated with peripheral nerve stimulators.
● Establish baseline respiratory rate and maintain a patent airway using suctioning, oxygen, and assisted ventilation, as needed.
● Establish baseline heart rate and blood pressure. If heart rate is below 80 beats/minute, give atropine before neostigmine.
● Several minutes before giving adults high doses of neostigmine, give 0.6 to 1.2 mg of atropine I.V. or 0.2 to 0.6 mg glycopyrrolate I.V. for each 1-mg of neostigmine given.
● Measure vital capacity and muscle strength periodically to assess myasthenic patient's response to neostigmine.
● Watch for cholinergic crisis in patients with myasthenia gravis. In cholinergic crisis, muscle weakness is caused by excessive cholinergic stimulation, and usually occurs 1 hour after last dose of neostigmine. It's accompanied by adverse muscarinic effects and fasciculations. Stop drug.
● Monitor and document patient's response after each dose.
● Resistance to neostigmine may develop.
● *Alert:* Don't confuse neostigmine with etomidate (Amidate) vials, which may look alike.
● If overdose occurs, maintain adequate ventilation, stop neostigmine, and give

1 to 4 mg of atropine. Give additional doses of atropine every 5 to 30 minutes, as needed.

PATIENT TEACHING
● Instruct patient to report excessive salivation, muscle weakness, severe abdominal pain, irregular heartbeat, or difficulty breathing.
● Show patient how to observe and record variations in muscle strength.
● Advise patient with myasthenia gravis to wear medical identification bracelet indicating condition.

nesiritide
Natrecor

Pharmacologic class: human B-type natriuretic peptide
Therapeutic class: inotropic vasodilator
Pregnancy risk category: C

INDICATIONS & DOSAGES
➤ **Acutely decompensated heart failure in patients with dyspnea at rest or with minimal activity—**
Adults: 2 mcg/kg by I.V. bolus over 60 seconds followed by continuous infusion of 0.01 mcg/kg/minute.
Adjust-a-dose: If hypotension develops during administration, reduce dosage or stop drug. Monitor patient's blood pressure and give appropriate treatment. Drug may be restarted at a dosage reduced by 30% with no bolus doses once the patient's blood pressure is stabilized.

ADMINISTRATION
Direct injection: Not recommended.
Intermittent infusion: Before giving bolus dose, prime the I.V. tubing with 25 ml of solution before connecting to the patient's I.V. access port. Withdraw the bolus from the infusion bag and

give over 60 seconds through an I.V. port in the tubing. Use this formula to calculate bolus volume (2 mcg/kg): Bolus volume (ml) = 0.33 × patient weight (kg).

Continuous infusion: Immediately after giving bolus, infuse drug at 0.1 ml/kg/ hour to deliver 0.01 mcg/kg/minute. Use this formula to calculate the infusion flow rate (0.01 mcg/kg/minute): Infusion flow rate (ml/hour) = 0.1 ml × patient weight (kg).

PREPARATION & STORAGE

Available as a white to off-white powder contained in a 1.5-mg single-dose vial.

Reconstitute one 1.5-mg vial with 5 ml of diluent (such as D_5W, normal saline solution, dextrose 5% in 0.2% saline solution injection, or dextrose 5% in half-normal saline solution) from a prefilled 250-ml I.V. bag. Gently rock (don't shake) vial until a clear, colorless solution results. Withdraw contents of vial and return solution to the 250-ml I.V. bag to yield 6 mcg/ml. Invert the bag several times to ensure complete mixing.

Use the solution within 24 hours. May store drug at room temperature or refrigerate.

Incompatibilities

Bumetanide, enalaprilat, ethacrynate sodium, furosemide, heparin, hydralazine, insulin, sodium metabisulfite.

CONTRAINDICATIONS & CAUTIONS

• Contraindicated in patients hypersensitive to drug or its components.
• Avoid using drug as primary therapy in patients with cardiogenic shock or patients with systolic blood pressure below 90 mm Hg; low cardiac filling pressures; conditions in which cardiac output is dependent on venous return; or conditions that make vasodilators inappropriate, such as valvular stenosis, restrictive or obstructive cardiomyopa-

thy, constrictive pericarditis, or pericardial tamponade.
• Use cautiously in patients whose baseline systolic blood pressure is less than 100 mm Hg.
• It's unknown whether this drug appears in breast milk or causes fetal harm. Use in pregnant or breast-feeding patients only if the benefit justifies the risk.
• Use cautiously in elderly patients because they might be more sensitive to the drug.

ADVERSE REACTIONS

CNS: fever, headache, confusion, somnolence, insomnia, dizziness, anxiety, paresthesia, tremor.
CV: *hypotension, ventricular tachycardia,* ventricular extrasystoles, angina, *bradycardia,* atrial fibrillation, AV node conduction abnormalities.
EENT: amblyopia
GI: nausea, vomiting, abdominal pain.
Hematologic: anemia.
Musculoskeletal: back pain, leg cramps.
Respiratory: *apnea,* cough, hemoptysis.
Skin: injection site reactions, pain at the site, rash, sweating, pruritus.

INTERACTIONS

Drug-drug. *ACE inhibitors:* Increases hypotension. Monitor blood pressure closely.

EFFECTS ON LAB TEST RESULTS

• May increase creatinine level.
• May decrease hemoglobin and hematocrit.

ACTION

Binds to receptors on vascular smooth muscle and endothelial cells, increasing cGMP level, relaxing smooth muscles, and dilating veins and arteries.

PHARMACOKINETICS

Onset, 15 minutes; peak, 1 hour; duration, 3 hours.
Distribution: Unknown.
Metabolism: Unknown.
Excretion: By lysosomal proteolysis after drug binds to cell surface receptors, proteolytic cleavage by endopeptidases in the vascular lumen, and renal filtration. Half-life, 18 minutes.

CLINICAL CONSIDERATIONS

● *Alert:* Drug binds heparin and could bind the heparin lining of a heparin-coated catheter, decreasing the amount of nesiritide delivered. Don't give nesiritide through a central heparin-coated catheter.
● Don't start at higher-than-recommended dosage because this may increase risk of hypotension and elevated creatinine level.
● Monitor patient's blood pressure closely, particularly if patient also takes an ACE inhibitor.
● Drug may affect renal function in some patients. In patients with severe heart failure whose renal function depends on the renin-angiotensin-aldosterone system, treatment may lead to azotemia. Monitor patient's renal status during drug therapy.
● Be sure to flush the I.V. tubing between each administration of nesiritide and incompatible drugs.
● Monitor patient for any signs or symptoms of drug-induced adverse cardiac events.
● There's limited experience giving this drug for longer than 48 hours.

PATIENT TEACHING

● Tell patient to report discomfort at I.V. site.
● Urge patient to report symptoms of low blood pressure, such as dizziness, light-headedness, blurred vision, or sweating.
● Tell patient to report other adverse effects promptly.

netilmicin sulfate
Netromycin*

Pharmacologic class: semi-synthetic aminoglycoside antibiotic
Therapeutic class: antibiotic
Pregnancy risk category: D
pH: 3.5 to 6

INDICATIONS & DOSAGES

➤ **Severe systemic infections—**
Dosage is based on drug levels. Therapeutic levels are 4 to 12 mcg/ml. Maximum peak levels shouldn't exceed 16 mcg/ml and maximum trough levels shouldn't exceed 4 mcg/ml. Use the following dosages as a guide.
Adults and children older than age 12:
1.3 to 2.2 mg/kg I.V. q 8 hours or 2 to 3.25 mg/kg I.V. q 12 hours for 7 to 14 days.
Children ages 6 weeks to 12 years:
1.83 to 2.67 mg/kg I.V. q 8 hours or 2.75 to 4 mg/kg I.V. q 12 hours for 7 to 14 days.
Neonates younger than age 6 weeks:
2 to 3.25 mg/kg I.V. q 12 hours for 7 to 14 days.
Adjust-a-dose: The dosage for adults with renal impairment depends on drug level. Initially, give a loading dose of 1.3 to 3.25 mg/kg, then 1.3 to 2.2 mg/kg at an hourly interval, calculated by multiplying creatinine level by 8. Supplemental dose of 2 mg/kg is given after each dialysis session.

ADMINISTRATION

Direct injection: Not recommended.
Intermittent infusion: Give diluted solution over 30 minutes to 2 hours into an intermittent infusion device or through tubing containing a free-flowing, compatible solution. After infusion, flush line with normal saline solution or D_5W.

Reactions may be *common,* uncommon, *life-threatening,* or COMMON AND LIFE-THREATENING.

Continuous infusion: Not recommended.

PREPARATION & STORAGE
Available in 1.5-ml vials of 100 mg/ml concentrations in clear, colorless, or pale solutions. Drug may contain sulfites or benzyl alcohol.

Dilute appropriate dose with 50 to 200 ml of any of these compatible solutions: sterile water for injection; normal saline solution ; dextrose 5% in normal saline solution; D₅W or dextrose 10% in water; Ringer's injection; dextrose 5% in lactated Ringer's; lactated Ringer's; Isolyte E, M, or P and dextrose 5%; Plasma-Lyte M, 56, or 148 and dextrose 5%; dextrose 5% and electrolyte #48; Ionosol B or T with dextrose 5%; dextrose 5% with Polysal; 10% invert sugar with Electrolyte #2 or #3; Normosol-R; 10% fructose; or Polysal.

Store vials at room temperature and avoid freezing. Diluted solutions of 2.1 to 3 mg/ml retain potency in glass containers for 72 hours at room temperature or when refrigerated at 39° F (4° C).

Incompatibilities
Allopurinol, amphotericin B, beta-lactam antibiotics, cephalosporins, furosemide, heparin sodium, other I.V. drugs, propofol, vitamin B complex.

CONTRAINDICATIONS & CAUTIONS
• Contraindicated in those hypersensitive to aminoglycosides.
• Use cautiously in those with neuromuscular disease such as myasthenia gravis, parkinsonism, or infant botulism, because drug may cause neuromuscular blockade, thus worsening weakness.
• Use cautiously in those with renal dysfunction or cystic fibrosis because of increased risk of toxic reaction, and in febrile, dehydrated, or severely burned patients because of increased risk of severe dehydration and nephrotoxicity.
• Use cautiously in those with eighth cranial nerve impairment because of possible ototoxicity.

ADVERSE REACTIONS
CNS: paralysis, *seizures, encephalopathy,* damage to cranial nerve VIII resulting in tinnitus and vertigo, peripheral neuropathy, dizziness.
CV: palpitations.
EENT: nystagmus.
GU: hematuria, oliguria, tubular necrosis, proteinuria.
Hematologic: *thrombocytopenia.*
Metabolic: hypomagnesemia, hyperkalemia.
Musculoskeletal: arthralgia, muscle twitching.
Respiratory: *apnea.*
Skin: pruritus, skin tingling.
Other: *anaphylaxis,* bacterial and fungal superinfections, neuromuscular blockade causing *respiratory depression.*

INTERACTIONS
Drug-drug. *Aminoglycosides, amphotericin B, bacitracin, bumetanide, carmustine, cephalosporins, cisplatin, cyclosporine, enflurane, furosemide, methoxyflurane, polymyxin B, streptozocin, vancomycin:* Increases risk of nephrotoxicity or ototoxicity. Monitor renal and auditory function.
Antihistamines, dimenhydrinate, loxapine, phenothiazines, thioxanthenes, trimethobenzamide: May mask signs of ototoxicity. Monitor patient closely; advise him to have regular auditory tests.
Antimyasthenics: May antagonize effects of antimyasthenics. Use with caution; monitor patient closely.
Cephalosporins and penicillins: May inactivate aminoglycosides. Monitor patient for lack of drug effect.
Halogenated hydrocarbon inhalation anesthetics, massive transfusion of citrated blood, neuromuscular blockers:

May potentiate neuromuscular blockade and respiratory failure. Use with caution; monitor patient closely.

I.V. indomethacin: Decreases renal clearance of drug in neonates. Monitor patient closely.

Opioid analgesics: Deepens respiratory depression. Use with caution; monitor respiratory status.

EFFECTS ON LAB TEST RESULTS
• May increase BUN and creatinine, potassium, alkaline phosphatase, ALT, AST, and bilirubin levels. May decrease magnesium level.
• May decrease WBC count.

ACTION
Binds directly to the 30S ribosomal subunit of sensitive microorganisms.

PHARMACOKINETICS
Drug level peaks at end of infusion.
Distribution: Mainly into extracellular fluid. Drug crosses the placental barrier. Small amounts appear in breast milk.
Metabolism: Not metabolized.
Excretion: In urine by glomerular filtration.

CLINICAL CONSIDERATIONS
• Osmolarity: 430 mOsm/kg.
• *Alert:* Drug may contain sulfites and benzyl alcohol.
• Calculate dose in terms of ideal body weight.
• If a cephalosporin or penicillin is ordered concurrently, give at different sites.
• Obtain specimens for culture and sensitivity tests before giving first dose. Therapy may begin before test results are available.
• Monitor respiratory effort, and make sure ventilator is available; neuromuscular blockade may cause respiratory depression. Netilmicin is the most potent neuromuscular blocker of all aminoglycosides.

• Monitor BUN and creatinine levels and urinalysis for signs of nephrotoxicity. Also monitor the function of cranial nerve VIII, and watch for bacterial and fungal superinfection. Keep patient well hydrated to minimize chemical irritation of renal tubules.
• Monitor auditory function in patients receiving prolonged therapy.
• Obtain periodic peak and trough levels. Coordinate collection times with the laboratory. Peak levels are lower in patients with edema, ascites, fever, and severe burns because of altered extracellular fluid volume; peak levels are two to three times higher after rapid infusion.
• Because dialysis may remove drug, dosage may need to be adjusted in those undergoing hemodialysis or peritoneal dialysis.
• Urinalysis may show increased excretion of protein, cells, and casts.

PATIENT TEACHING
• Instruct patient to report ringing in the ears, blood in the urine, or abnormally small amount of urine.
• Instruct patient to complete course of treatment.

nitroglycerin
Nitro-Bid IV, Tridil

Pharmacologic class: nitrate
Therapeutic class: antianginal, vasodilator
Pregnancy risk category: C
pH: 3 to 6.5

INDICATIONS & DOSAGES
➤ **Heart failure and chest pain from MI; acute angina pectoris; blood pressure reduction during surgery—**
Adults: 5 mcg/minute I.V. initially, then increased by 5 mcg/minute I.V. q 3 to 5 minutes until desired response is

achieved. If response is inadequate at 20 mcg/minute, increase dose by 10 to 20 mcg/minute I.V. and give q 3 to 5 minutes if needed. Once partial response is obtained, increases in dosage increments should be reduced and interval between dosage increases should be lengthened. Maximum dose isn't established.

➤ **Acute MI—**
Adults: 12.5 to 25 mcg IV, then 10 to 20 mcg/minute I.V. infusion; increase by 5 to 10 mcg/minute I.V. q 5 to 10 minutes p.r.n. Maximum dose is 200 mcg/minute I.V. Use within 24 to 48 hours of acute MI.

➤ **Hypertensive crisis ♦ —**
Adults: 5 to 100 mcg/minute I.V. infusion.

ADMINISTRATION

Direct injection: Not recommended.
Intermittent infusion: Not recommended.
Continuous infusion: Infuse diluted drug at the rate needed for therapeutic effect. Always use a volume-control device and a microdrip regulator. Closely monitor the patient's response to nitroglycerin.

PREPARATION & STORAGE

Several preparations of nitroglycerin for I.V. injection are available in various concentrations. Each comes with diluent instruction and dosage.

Nitro-Bid IV is supplied in 1-, 5-, and 10-ml vials of 5 mg/ml. Dilute with D_5W or normal saline solution. For a concentration of 50 mcg/ml, mix 1 ml of drug in 100 ml of solution; for 100 mcg/ml, mix 1 ml of drug in 50 ml of solution; for 200 mcg/ml, mix 2 ml of drug in 50 ml of solution.

Tridil is available as a 5-mg/ml concentration in 5- and 10-ml ampules and 5-, 10-, and 20-ml vials and as a 0.5-mg/ml concentration in 10-ml ampules. Mix a 25-mg or 50-mg ampule with 500 ml of D_5W or normal saline solution for 50 or 100 mcg/ml, respectively. Diluting 5 mg of drug in 100 ml of solution yields 50 mcg/ml.

Drug is also available as 100 mcg/ml, 200 mcg/ml, and 400 mcg/ml premixed solution in D_5W.

Store nitroglycerin preparations at room temperature, and protect from light. Avoid freezing. After reconstitution, drug is stable for 48 hours at room temperature and 7 days under refrigeration. Mix and store in glass bottle (bottle and tubing are usually supplied with most products).

The type of infusion set affects the amount of drug delivered. Use only nonabsorbent tubing; polyvinyl chloride tubing may absorb up to 80% of diluted drug from solution. Using polyvinyl chloride extension tubing for the infusion pump may negate advantages of the non–polyvinyl chloride set supplied with the drug.

Incompatibilities
Alteplase, bretylium, hydralazine, other I.V. drugs, phenytoin sodium.

CONTRAINDICATIONS & CAUTIONS
● Contraindicated in patients hypersensitive to drug or to nitrates.
● Contraindicated in those with head trauma or cerebral hemorrhage because drug may increase intracranial pressure, and in those with hypotension or uncorrected hypovolemia because of risk of severe hypotension or shock.
● Contraindicated in those with constrictive pericarditis or pericardial tamponade because drug may further impair coronary circulation, and in those with hypertrophic cardiomyopathy because drug may intensify angina.
● Contraindicated in those with severe anemia or closed-angle glaucoma.
● Use cautiously in those with severe hepatic impairment because drug increases the risk of methemoglobinemia.

• Use cautiously in those with severe renal impairment because of reduced drug excretion.

ADVERSE REACTIONS
CNS: *dizziness, headache,* syncope, weakness, vertigo, anxiety, insomnia.
CV: *reflex tachycardia, orthostatic hypotension, flushing* **palpitations, arrhythmias,** rebound hypertension, atrial fibrillation.
GI: nausea, vomiting, diarrhea, abdominal pain.
GU: dysuria, impotence, urinary frequency.
Musculoskeletal: arthralgia, muscle twitch.
Respiratory: bronchitis, pneumonia, upper respiratory tract infection.
Other: intoxication because of alcohol in diluent, *hypersensitivity reactions.*

INTERACTIONS
Drug-drug. *Antihypertensives, opioid analgesics, other vasodilators, tricyclic antidepressants:* Enhances hypotension. Monitor blood pressure and patient closely.
Ergot alkaloids, sympathomimetics: Reduces antianginal effects. Monitor patient for lack of drug effect.
Heparin: Decreases anticoagulant effectiveness. Monitor PT and INR closely.
Sildenafil: Significantly potentiates nitroglycerin effects. Avoid using together.
Drug-lifestyle. *Alcohol use:* Increases risk of hypotension. Discourage use together.

EFFECTS ON LAB TEST RESULTS
• May increase urine catecholamine and vanillylmandelic acid levels.
• May cause falsely decreased results with cholesterol determination tests using the Zlatkis-Zak color reaction.

ACTION
Relaxes vascular smooth muscle, causing vasodilation and reducing myocardial oxygen requirements and systemic vascular resistance.

PHARMACOKINETICS
Onset, immediate; duration, several minutes.
Distribution: Widely throughout body. Unknown if drug crosses the placental barrier or appears in breast milk.
Metabolism: In the liver, rapidly and nearly completely.
Excretion: In urine. Half-life, 1 to 4 minutes.

CLINICAL CONSIDERATIONS
• Osmolarity: 100 mcg/ml in 5% dextrose is 264 mOsm/L; 200 mcg/ml in 5% dextrose is 277 mOsm/L; 400 mcg/ml in 5% dextrose is 301 mOsm/L.
• Osmolality: 1 mg/ml concentration is 281 mOsm/kg.
• During therapy, monitor blood pressure and heart rate and rhythm continuously; response to drug varies greatly.
• If patient has a pulmonary artery catheter in place, frequently monitor pulmonary artery wedge pressure.
• Help patient sit up and stand until he can tolerate orthostatic hypotension.
• Give an analgesic for headache.
• *Alert:* Don't confuse nitroglycerin with nitroprusside.
• If overdose occurs, elevate patient's legs and reduce infusion rate or temporarily stop infusion. If severe hypotension persists, give phenylephrine I.V., an alpha agonist.

PATIENT TEACHING
• Inform patient that light-headedness, flushing of neck or face, and headache may occur.
• Instruct patient to report chest pain or suffocating pain.
• Tell patient to request assistance with sitting or standing until he can tolerate dizziness upon standing abruptly.

Reactions may be *common,* uncommon, *life-threatening,* or COMMON AND LIFE-THREATENING.

nitroprusside sodium
Nitropress

Pharmacologic class: vasodilator
Therapeutic class: antihypertensive
Pregnancy risk category: C
pH: 3.5 to 6

INDICATIONS & DOSAGES
➤ **Rapid blood pressure reduction in hypertensive emergencies, control of hypertension during anesthesia, reduction of preload and afterload in cardiac pump failure or cardiogenic shock—**
Adults and children who aren't receiving other antihypertensives: 0.3 to 10 mcg/kg/minute I.V.; average dose, 3 mcg/kg/minute I.V. Monitor blood pressure closely and titrate drug to patient's response. Maximum dose, 10 mcg/kg/minute I.V.

ADMINISTRATION
Use nitroprusside only if adequate staff and equipment are available for arterial blood pressure monitoring.
Direct injection: Not recommended.
Intermittent infusion: Not recommended.
Continuous infusion: Using an infusion pump, give diluted solution at a rate that maintains desired hypotensive effect.

PREPARATION & STORAGE
Available as a powder in 50-mg vial.
Reconstitute with 2 to 3 ml of D_5W or sterile water for injection *without* preservatives. Then dilute in 250 to 1,000 ml of D_5W to desired concentration.
Store powder at room temperature, and protect from light, heat, and moisture.
Reconstituted solution is stable for 24 hours. Discard solution if discolored to blue, green, or dark red, which indicates a reaction with another substance. After reconstitution, protect solution from light by covering with aluminum foil or other opaque material; it isn't necessary to cover tubing or drip chamber.

Incompatibilities
Bacteriostatic water for injection, other I.V. drug or preservative.

CONTRAINDICATIONS & CAUTIONS
• Contraindicated in those with inadequate cerebral circulation or coronary artery insufficiency because of reduced tolerance to hypotension.
• Contraindicated in those with compensatory hypertension, as in an AV shunt or coarctation of the aorta, because hypotension may be life-threatening.
• Contraindicated during emergency surgery for patients near death.
• Contraindicated in those with Leber's hereditary optic atrophy or tobacco amblyopia because affected patients lack the enzyme needed to metabolize the drug.
• Contraindicated in those with acute heart failure with reduced peripheral vascular resistance, such as high-output heart failure that may be seen in endotoxic sepsis.
• Use cautiously in those who are poor surgical risks; hypotension may be life-threatening.
• Use cautiously in those with severe renal impairment because of reduced thiocyanate excretion; in those with hepatic insufficiency because of decreased drug metabolism; and in those with hypothyroidism because thiocyanate inhibits iodine uptake and binding.
• Use cautiously in those with pulmonary impairment because drug may aggravate hypovolemia.
• Use cautiously in those with anemia or hypovolemia (correct these before

treatment) because drug decreases tolerance to these conditions, and in those with low vitamin B_{12} levels because drug interferes with vitamin B_{12} metabolism and distribution, worsening the condition.

• Use cautiously in geriatric patients because they are more sensitive to the drug's effects.

ADVERSE REACTIONS
CNS: anxiety, apprehension, *dizziness, headache,* restlessness, loss of consciousness, *increased intracranial pressure.*
CV: *excessive hypotension, bradycardia,* palpitations, reflex tachycardia, ECG changes, flushing.
GI: *abdominal pain, nausea,* vomiting.
Hematologic: *methemoglobinemia.*
Metabolic: lactic acidosis.
Musculoskeletal: *muscle twitching,* retrosternal discomfort.
Skin: *diaphoresis,* rash, irritation at infusion site.
Other: venous streaking; *cyanide toxicity, including absent reflexes, coma, distant heart sounds, extremely shallow breathing, hypotension, imperceptible pulse, pink skin, and widely dilated pupils; thiocyanate intoxication, including anorexia, blurred vision, confusion, delirium, dizziness, dyspnea, fatigue, loss of consciousness, metabolic acidosis, rash, tinnitus, and weakness.*

INTERACTIONS
Drug-drug. *Antihypertensives, ganglionic blockers, general anesthetics such as halothane:* Has additive hypotensive effect. Adjust dosage.
Dobutamine: Increases cardiac output and decreased pulmonary artery wedge pressure. Monitor patient closely.
Estrogens, sympathomimetics: Diminishes hypotensive effect. Monitor patient and blood pressure closely.
Sildenafil: Potentiates hypotensive effects of nitrates. Don't use together.

EFFECTS ON LAB TEST RESULTS
• May increase creatinine and lactate levels.
• May decrease RBC and WBC counts.

ACTION
Dilates vascular smooth muscle, producing peripheral vasodilation and hypotensive action and reducing peripheral vascular resistance and cardiac output.

PHARMACOKINETICS
Onset, immediate; duration, 1 to 10 minutes.
Distribution: Unknown.
Metabolism: Rapidly, in liver.
Excretion: In kidneys. Half-life is 3 days; up to 7 days in patients with renal impairment.

CLINICAL CONSIDERATIONS
• *Alert:* Excessive doses or rapid infusion greater than 10 mcg/kg/minute can cause cyanide toxicity; therefore, if these factors are present, check thiocyanate levels every 72 hours. Levels above 100 mcg/ml are associated with toxic reaction.
• In patients with hepatic impairment, monitor cyanide levels daily after 1 or 2 days.
• In patients with low vitamin B_{12} level, hydroxocobalamin is an antidote for cyanide and may be given before and during nitroprusside administration.
• Adverse reactions seldom occur at recommended dosage in short-term therapy.
• Watch for irritation and infiltration; extravasation can cause tissue damage and necrosis.
• Monitor blood pressure frequently, every 5 minutes at initiation of infusion and every 15 minutes thereafter.
• Slowing infusion rate or temporarily discontinuing drug may alleviate adverse reactions.

Reactions may be *common,* uncommon, *life-threatening,* or COMMON AND LIFE-THREATENING.

- If metabolic acidosis occurs, stop drug and expect to try alternative therapy.
- *Alert:* Don't confuse nitroprusside with nitroglycerin.
- Ask all male patients about the use of sildenafil (Viagra) before using nitrates.
- Hypertensive patients are more sensitive than normotensive patients to nitroprusside. Also, patients taking other antihypertensive drugs are extremely sensitive to nitroprusside. Nitroprusside has been used in patients with acute MI, refractory heart failure, and severe mitral regurgitation.
- The goal of therapy is to reduce the mean arterial pressure by 25% within minutes to 2 hours.
- If overdose occurs, give nitrites to promote methemoglobin formation.
- For a massive overdose, stop nitroprusside and give amyl nitrate by inhalation for 15 to 30 seconds each minute until a 3% sodium nitrite solution can be prepared. Give this solution at a rate of 4 to 6 mg/kg over 2 to 4 minutes. Monitor blood pressure closely. Then give I.V. sodium thiosulfate 150 to 200 mg/kg; a typical dose is 50 ml of the 25% solution. Monitor patient carefully. Half the initial dose may be given after 2 hours. Thiocyanate levels may rise rapidly in patients with renal impairment. Hemodialysis or peritoneal dialysis can remove excess thiocyanate.

PATIENT TEACHING
- Inform patient of the need for frequent blood pressure monitoring and blood tests.
- Tell patient to report adverse reactions promptly.
- Tell patient to inform nurse if discomfort occurs at I.V. site.

norepinephrine bitartrate
Levophed

Pharmacologic class: direct-acting adrenergic
Therapeutic class: vasopressor
Pregnancy risk category: C
pH: 3 to 4.5

INDICATIONS & DOSAGES
➤ **Control of acute hypotensive states and as an adjunct in the treatment of cardiac arrest—**
Adults: Initially, 8 to 12 mcg/minute I.V.; then adjust, usually to 2 to 4 mcg/minute I.V., to maintain desired blood pressure range.
Children: Initially, 2 mcg/minute or 2 mcg/m^2/minute; titrate to maintain blood pressure. For pediatric advanced life support during cardiac resuscitation, give 0.1 mcg/kg/minute initially; then adjust, usually to 2 mcg/minute, to maintain desired blood pressure range.

ADMINISTRATION
Direct injection: Not recommended.
Intermittent injection: Not recommended.
Continuous injection: Insert a plastic I.V. catheter deeply into large vein. Don't use leg veins in geriatric patients or in those with peripheral vascular disease. Use microdrip tubing and an infusion pump to carefully regulate flow rate. Infuse drug at a rate that maintains blood pressure at a low normal, usually 80 to 100 mm Hg systolic or, for previously hypertensive patients, a maximum of 40 mm Hg below previous systolic pressure.

PREPARATION & STORAGE
Available in 4-ml ampules containing 1 mg/ml.
   Store ampules at room temperature. For infusion, mix 1 ampule (4 mg) of

norepinephrine in 1,000 ml of D_5W or dextrose 5% in normal saline solution for a concentration of 4 mcg/ml. Alter concentration, as needed, to reflect patient's drug and fluid volume requirements.

Discard diluted solution after 24 hours. Also discard if solution contains precipitate or if it's brown, pink, or yellow.

Incompatibilities
Aminophylline, amobarbital, chlorothiazide, chlorpheniramine, lidocaine, normal saline solution, pentobarbital sodium, phenobarbital sodium, phenytoin sodium, ranitidine hydrochloride, sodium bicarbonate, streptomycin, thiopental, whole blood.

CONTRAINDICATIONS & CAUTIONS
• Contraindicated in those hypersensitive to norepinephrine, other sympathomimetics, or sulfites.
• Contraindicated in those with hypotension from blood loss because of risk of tissue hypoxia, lactic acidosis, low urine output, and severe vasoconstriction.
• Avoid use in those with mesenteric or peripheral vascular thrombosis or other occlusive vascular disorders—such as arteriosclerosis, Buerger's disease, or diabetes mellitus—because norepinephrine may precipitate or aggravate ischemia.
• Avoid use in those receiving cyclopropane or halothane anesthetics and in those with hypoxia or hypercarbia because norepinephrine produces ventricular tachycardia or fibrillation.
• Use cautiously in geriatric patients and those with hyperthyroidism, hypertension, or severe cardiac disease, because of increased risk of adverse reactions.

ADVERSE REACTIONS
CNS: anxiety, *cerebral hemorrhage, headache,* dizziness, weakness, insomnia, *seizures,* restlessness, tremors.
CV: angina, AV dissociation, bigeminy, *bradycardia,* decreased cardiac output, increased peripheral vascular resistance, junctional rhythm, precordial pain, *severe hypertension, arrhythmias.*
GU: low urine output.
Metabolic: metabolic acidosis, hyperglycemia.
Musculoskeletal: weakness.
Respiratory: asthmatic episodes, *apnea.*
Skin: pallor, tissue necrosis and sloughing with extravasation.
Other: *anaphylaxis.*

INTERACTIONS
Drug-drug. *Antihistamines, atropine, ergot alkaloids, guanadrel, guanethidine, MAO inhibitors, methyldopa, oxytocics, rauwolfia alkaloids, tricyclic antidepressants:* Increases pressor response. Avoid using together.
Antihypertensives: May reduce pressor response. Monitor patient closely for lack of drug effect.
Bretylium, hydrocarbon inhalation anesthetics: Causes ventricular tachycardia or fibrillation. Avoid using together.
CNS stimulants, sympathomimetics: Enhances CNS stimulation and pressor effect. Use together with caution; monitor mental status and vital signs.
Desmopressin, lypressin, vasopressin: Decreases antidiuretic effect. Monitor patient closely.
Diuretics: Decreases arterial responsiveness to pressor effects. Monitor patient closely.

EFFECTS ON LAB TEST RESULTS
• May increase glucose, lactic acid, free fatty acids, and cholesterol levels.

ACTION
Stimulates alpha receptors to produce vasoconstriction and encourages beta receptors to stimulate myocardium and increase cardiac output.

PHARMACOKINETICS
Onset, immediate; duration, 1 to 2 minutes after stopping infusion.
Distribution: Primarily localized to sympathetic nervous tissue. Drug crosses the placental but not the blood-brain barrier. Unknown if drug appears in breast milk.
Metabolism: In the liver and other tissues.
Excretion: In urine.

CLINICAL CONSIDERATIONS
• Osmolality: 319 mOsm/kg.
• Inclusion of heparin at a rate of 100 to 200 units/hour with norepinephrine infusion may reduce the risk of venous thrombosis.
• Correct blood volume depletion before administration. Don't use drug as replacement for blood, plasma, fluids, or electrolytes.
• During infusion, check blood pressure every 2 minutes until stable, then every 5 to 15 minutes, using intra-arterial monitoring.
• Monitor the patient's mental status, skin temperature, and color of extremities, especially earlobes, lips, and nail beds.
• Continuously monitor ECG. Notify prescriber of arrhythmias. Check heart rate every 5 to 15 minutes.
• Insert an indwelling urinary catheter and monitor hourly urine output. If less than 30 ml/hour, notify prescriber.
• Avoid or correct acidosis because it can minimize a patient's response to a vasopressor.
• Watch for irritation and infiltration; extravasation can cause tissue damage and necrosis. Monitor infusion site every 2 minutes until blood pressure stabilizes, then every 5 minutes. If extravasation occurs (infusion site will be blanched and cold) stop infusion immediately and infiltrate area with 5 to 10 mg of phentolamine in 10 to 15 ml of normal saline solution, using a 25G needle. Then remove the I.V. line and protect the area from further trauma. During prolonged infusion, rotate I.V. sites to prevent blanching.
• Avoid prolonged use, when possible, to prevent ischemia of vital organs.
• *Alert:* Drug may contain sulfites.
• Withdraw drug slowly; sudden cessation may cause severe hypotension. Monitor vital signs hourly until stable after stopping infusion. If systolic pressure drops below 70 mm Hg, restart infusion.
• Avoid infusion in lower extremity veins. Infusion into the ankle vein may cause gangrene.
• Early signs and symptoms of overdose include intense sweating, pharyngeal and retrosternal pain, photophobia, and vomiting.

PATIENT TEACHING
• Tell patient to promptly report adverse reactions or any discomfort at I.V. site.

0

octreotide acetate
Sandostatin

Pharmacologic class: synthetic octapeptide
Therapeutic class: somatotropic hormone
Pregnancy risk category: B
pH: 3.9 to 4.5

INDICATIONS & DOSAGES

➤ **Symptomatic treatment of flushing and diarrhea caused by carcinoid tumors—**
Adults: Initially, 100 to 600 mcg I.V. daily in two to four divided doses for first 2 weeks; usual daily dose, 300 mcg I.V. Subsequent dosage based on individual response.

➤ **Symptomatic treatment of watery diarrhea caused by vasoactive intestinal peptide-secreting tumors (VIPomas)—**
Adults: 200 to 300 mcg I.V. daily in two to four divided doses for first 2 weeks of therapy. Subsequent dosage based on individual response, but usually not exceeding 450 mcg daily.

➤ **Acromegaly—**
Adults: Initially, 50 mcg I.V. t.i.d. Subsequent dose based on individual response. Usual dosage, 100 mcg t.i.d. I.V., but some patients require up to 500 mcg t.i.d. I.V. for maximum effectiveness.

➤ **Variceal bleeding ◆ —**
Adults: 25 to 50 mcg/hour I.V. continuous infusion for 18 hours to 5 days.

➤ **Short bowel (ileostomy) syndrome ◆ —**
Adults: 25 mcg/hour I.V.

ADMINISTRATION
Direct injection: Inject directly into vein or compatible I.V. solution over 3 minutes.
Intermittent infusion: Give diluted solution over 15 to 30 minutes.
Continuous infusion: Not recommended.

PREPARATION & STORAGE
Available in 50-, 100-, and 500-mcg/ml ampules and 200- and 1,000-mcg/ml multidose vials.

Dilute in volumes of 50 to 200 ml D_5W or normal saline solution and infuse I.V. or by I.V. push.

Store vials and ampules in refrigerator at 36° to 46° F (2° to 8° C) and protect from light. Stable at room temperature for 14 days if protected from light. Don't warm solution artificially. Solution is stable in sterile isotonic saline solution or D_5W for 24 hours. After initial use, multidose vials should be discarded after 14 days. Discard unused portion of ampules. Don't use if particulates or discoloration, or both, are noted.

Incompatibilities
TPN.

CONTRAINDICATIONS & CAUTIONS
• Contraindicated in those hypersensitive to the drug or its components.
• Use cautiously in the elderly and in those with renal failure because of increased octreotide half-life.
• Use cautiously in pregnant and breast-feeding women.

Reactions may be *common,* uncommon, *life-threatening,* or COMMON AND LIFE-THREATENING.

ADVERSE REACTIONS
CNS: dizziness, fatigue, headache, weakness, depression, anxiety, tremor, *seizures.*
CV: **ARRHYTHMIAS, BRADYCARDIA,** conduction abnormalities, flushing, chest pain, thrombophlebitis, hypertension.
EENT: blurred vision, cold symptoms.
GI: *abdominal pain or discomfort, diarrhea, loose stools, nausea,* constipation, fat malabsorption, flatulence, gallstones or biliary sludge, vomiting, *bleeding, pancreatitis.*
GU: pollakiuria, UTI.
Hematologic: anemia.
Hepatic: *hepatitis,* jaundice.
Metabolic: hyperglycemia, hypoglycemia, hypothyroidism.
Musculoskeletal: joint pain, weakness, backache.
Respiratory: dyspnea, pneumonia, *status asthmaticus.*
Skin: alopecia, edema, pain at injection site, wheals, pruritus, rash, cellulitis.
Other: flulike syndrome, decreased libido.

INTERACTIONS
Drug-drug. *Cyclosporine:* Decreases cyclosporine level. Monitor cyclosporine level.

EFFECTS ON LAB TEST RESULTS
• May increase liver enzyme level. May decrease growth hormone, gastrin, vasoactive intestinal peptide, insulin, glucagon, secretin, motilin, thyroid-stimulating hormone, and pancreatic polypeptide, and vitamin B_{12} levels. May increase or decrease glucose level.
• May alter Schilling test result.

ACTION
Potent inhibitor of growth hormone, glucagon, and insulin. Suppresses luteinizing hormone response to gonadotropin-releasing hormone and inhibits release of serotonin, gastrin, vasoactive intestinal peptide, secretin, motilin, and pancreatic polypeptide.

PHARMACOKINETICS
Onset, rapid after injection; peak, 0.5 hours.
Distribution: To plasma, where it binds to lipoprotein and albumin. Unknown if drug appears in breast milk.
Metabolism: Eliminated from plasma at a slower rate than the naturally occurring hormone. Half-life, $1\frac{1}{2}$ hours.
Excretion: About 35% of drug appears unchanged in urine.

CLINICAL CONSIDERATIONS
• Osmolality: 279 mOsm/kg.
• Half-life of drug may be altered in patients undergoing dialysis for end-stage renal failure. Dosage may need to be adjusted.
• Monitor fluid and electrolyte balance during therapy.
• Perform baseline and periodic testing of thyroid function because drug suppresses thyroid-stimulating hormone secretion.
• Monitor urine 5-hydroxyindoleacetic acid, growth hormone for acromegaly, plasma serotonin, plasma substance P for carcinoid tumors, and vasoactive intestinal peptide (VIP) for VIPomas frequently during therapy.
• Patient may develop mild, transient hypoglycemia or hyperglycemia during therapy. Monitor him closely, and watch for signs and symptoms of both.
• Drug may alter fat absorption and aggravate fat malabsorption. Assess 72-hour fecal fat and carotene levels periodically.
• Monitor vitamin B_{12} levels during long-term therapy because drug may decrease levels.

PATIENT TEACHING
• Instruct patient to notify prescriber if abdominal discomfort occurs because drug may cause gallstones.

• Educate patient regarding signs and symptoms of low and high levels of sugar in the blood, and tell him to notify nurse of unusual symptoms.

ondansetron hydrochloride
Zofran

Pharmacologic class: serotonin type 3 (5-hydroxytryptamine type 3, or 5-HT₃) receptor antagonist
Therapeutic class: antiemetic
Pregnancy risk category: B
pH: 3.3 to 4

INDICATIONS & DOSAGES
➤ **To prevent nausea and vomiting caused by emetogenic chemotherapy—**
Adults and children age 4 and older: Three doses of 0.15 mg/kg I.V. Give first dose 30 minutes before chemotherapy; subsequent doses at 4 and 8 hours after first dose. Or, adults and children ages 12 and older may receive 32-mg infusion over 15 minutes beginning 30 minutes before chemotherapy.
➤ **To prevent postoperative nausea and vomiting—**
Adults: 4 mg I.V., undiluted, over 2 to 5 minutes.
Children ages 2 to 12 who weigh more than 40 kg (88 lb): 4 mg I.V. as a single dose.
Children ages 2 to 12 who weigh 40 kg or less: 0.1 mg/kg I.V. as a single dose.
Adjust-a-dose: In patients with severe hepatic impairment, don't exceed 8 mg daily.

ADMINISTRATION
Direct injection: Give undiluted over 2 to 5 minutes for postoperative nausea and vomiting only.
Intermittent infusion: Dilute drug in 50 ml of compatible solution and infuse over 15 minutes.

Continuous infusion: Not recommended.

PREPARATION & STORAGE
Available for dilution in 2- and 20-ml vials containing 2 mg/ml. Also available as 32 mg/50 ml premixed, preservative-free dextrose solution; don't dilute.

Before administration, dilute drug in 50 ml of compatible solution, such as D₅W injection, normal saline solution injection, dextrose 5% in normal saline solution injection, dextrose 5% in half-normal saline solution injection, and sodium chloride 3% solution injection.

Store at room temperature and protect from light. Inspect solutions for precipitate or discoloration before giving drug.

Drug is stable for up to 48 hours in polyvinyl chloride bags after dilution when refrigerated at 39° F (4° C) or kept at room temperature at 77° F (25° C). When stored in polypropylene syringes, concentrations of 0.25, 0.5, 1, and 2-mg/ml are stable for 3 months at -4 °F (-20° C), 14 days at 39° F (4° C), and 48 hours at 71° to 77° F (22° to 25° C).

Not necessary to protect from light during administration.

Incompatibilities
Acyclovir sodium, allopurinol, aminophylline, amphotericin B, ampicillin sodium, ampicillin sodium and sulbactam sodium, cefepime, cefoperazone, dexamethasone sodium phosphate, droperidol, fluorouracil, furosemide, ganciclovir, lorazepam, meropenem, methylprednisolone sodium succinate, piperacillin sodium, sargramostim, sodium bicarbonate.

CONTRAINDICATIONS & CAUTIONS
• Contraindicated in those hypersensitive to the drug.

• Use cautiously in those with compromised liver function because drug is extensively metabolized by the liver.

ADVERSE REACTIONS
CNS: *headache,* sedation, malaise, fatigue, *dizziness,* fever, anxiety, agitation, cold sensation, paresthesia.
CV: chest pain, hypotension.
GI: *constipation.*
GU: urine retention, dysuria.
Musculoskeletal: *pain.*
Respiratory: bronchospasm.
Skin: rash, pruritus, injection site reaction.

INTERACTIONS
Drug-drug. *Drugs that alter hepatic drug metabolizing enzymes, such as cimetidine or phenobarbital:* May alter drug's pharmacokinetics. Dosage doesn't need to be adjusted.
Drug-herb. *Horehound:* May enhance serotoninergic effects. Discourage use together.

EFFECTS ON LAB TEST RESULTS
• May increase ALT and AST levels.

ACTION
Blocks serotonin type 3 receptors in the CNS to prevent activating the vomiting center. In the peripheral nervous system, it acts at the vagal nerve terminals to prevent abdomen and diaphragm movements that accompany vomiting.

PHARMACOKINETICS
Action: Drug's antiemetic effect varies considerably. Level peaks, 6 to 20 minutes after infusion. Optimum dosage interval about 2 to 8 hours.
Distribution: About 70% to 76% protein bound. Unknown if drug appears in breast milk.
Metabolism: Exclusively in liver; 95% by hydroxylation, glucuronide formation, and *N*-demethylation; about 5% appears in urine as unchanged drug.

Excretion: In urine; 95% excreted as metabolites. Elimination half-life, about 3½ hours; half-life increases to 5½ hours in geriatric patients.

CLINICAL CONSIDERATIONS
• Osmolality: 281 mOsm/kg.
• Osmolarity of premixed solution: 270 mOsm/L.
• Drug controls vomiting better than metoclopramide with fewer adverse effects, such as acute dystonic reactions or akathisia. However, standard course of ondansetron costs about 50% more than similar course of high-dose metoclopramide. Benefits of drug must be weighed against added cost to patient and hospital.
• Dexamethasone combined with ondansetron provides significantly better control of vomiting than ondansetron alone.
• Drug isn't indicated for use in those receiving multiple-day courses of antineoplastic therapy or for prophylaxis of chemotherapy-induced delayed nausea and vomiting.
• Although drug clearance is decreased and half-life is increased in geriatric patients, dosage doesn't need to be adjusted because these changes haven't been linked to reduced safety or efficacy.
• Drug contains methylparaben and propylparaben preservatives.
• Little information is available regarding drug's use in patients with hepatic or renal failure.
• Monitor liver function tests for hepatotoxicity.
• Monitor abdominal surgery patients for ileus or gastric distention.

PATIENT TEACHING
• Instruct patient to alert nurse immediately if breathing difficulty occurs after drug administration.
• Tell patient to immediately report discomfort at I.V. site.

orphenadrine citrate
Banflex, Flexoject, Flexon, Norflex

Pharmacologic class: diphenhydramine analogue
Therapeutic class: skeletal muscle
relaxant
Pregnancy risk category: C
pH: 5 to 6

INDICATIONS & DOSAGES
➤ **Acute pain in musculoskeletal
disorders**—
Adults: 60 mg I.V. q 12 hours.

ADMINISTRATION
Direct injection: Inject drug directly
into a vein or into an I.V. line containing a free-flowing, compatible solution.
Give over 5 to 10 minutes with patient
in supine position.
Intermittent infusion: Not recommended.
Continuous infusion: Not recommended.

PREPARATION & STORAGE
Available in 2-ml ampules and 10-ml
vials with a concentration of 30 mg/ml.
   Store at room temperature; protect
ampules from light. Drug needs no further dilution for injection.

Incompatibilities
None reported.

CONTRAINDICATIONS & CAUTIONS
• Contraindicated in those hypersensitive to the drug.
• Contraindicated in those with glaucoma, myasthenia gravis, stenosing peptic
ulcers, prostatic hyperplasia, bladder-
neck obstruction, duodenal or pyloric
obstruction or cardiospasm because
drug's antimuscarinic action may aggravate these disorders.

• Use cautiously in those hypersensitive
to sulfites since anaphylaxis may occur.
• Use cautiously in patients with CV
disorders (tachycardia, cardiac decompensation, coronary insufficiency, arrhythmias).

ADVERSE REACTIONS
CNS: confusion, dizziness, *drowsiness,*
headache, weakness, hallucinations,
agitation, tremor.
CV: *transient bradycardia,* palpita-
tions, tachycardia.
EENT: visual disturbances.
GI: abdominal cramps, constipation,
dry mouth, nausea, vomiting.
GU: urinary hesitancy or retention.
Hematologic: *aplastic anemia.*
Skin: rash, pruritus.
Other: *anaphylaxis,* hypersensitivity
reactions.

INTERACTIONS
Drug-drug. *Amantadine:* May potentiate orphenadrine's anticholinergic action. Monitor closely; use with caution.
Antimuscarinics: Intensifies antimuscarinic effects. Avoid using together.
CNS depressants: Deepens CNS depression. Avoid using together.
Haloperidol: Decreases haloperidol
levels, causing worsened schizophrenia
and tardive dyskinesia. Monitor patient
closely.
Phenothiazines: Decreases phenothiazine levels. Monitor patient closely.
Propoxyphene: May have additive CNS
effects such as confusion, anxiety, and
tremors. Decrease dose of or stop one
or both drugs.
Drug-lifestyle. *Alcohol use:* Deepens
CNS depression. Discourage use together.

EFFECTS ON LAB TEST RESULTS
• May increase alkaline phosphatase,
ALT, and AST levels.
• May decrease hemoglobin and hemat-
ocrit.

Reactions may be *common,* uncommon, *life-threatening,* or COMMON AND LIFE-THREATENING.

ACTION

Inhibits transmission of spinal cord impulses to skeletal muscle.

PHARMACOKINETICS

Onset, immediate; duration, 12 hours.
Distribution: Probably widespread, especially to the lungs. May cross the placental barrier. Unknown if drug appears in breast milk.
Metabolism: In the liver. Almost totally metabolized to at least eight metabolites.
Excretion: Mainly in urine as metabolites and small amounts of unchanged drug. Small amounts are also excreted in feces. Half-life, about 14 hours.

CLINICAL CONSIDERATIONS

• *Alert:* Drug may contain sulfites.
• *Alert:* Carefully check all doses. Even a slight overdose can cause a toxic reaction.
• Keep patient recumbent for 10 minutes after injection, and then help him sit up slowly.
• Monitor vital signs, input and output.
• During prolonged therapy, monitor liver function and CBC.
• Drug may be used alone or in combination with aspirin as an adjunct to rest, physical therapy, and other comfort measures.
• Replace parenteral therapy with oral therapy as soon as possible.

PATIENT TEACHING

• Advise patient to relieve dry mouth with cool drinks and sugarless gum or candy.
• Instruct patient to inform prescriber if he experiences rash, itching, or urine retention.
• Tell patient to avoid hazardous activities until CNS depressant effects can be determined.

oxacillin sodium

Pharmacologic class: semi-synthetic penicillinase-resistant penicillin
Therapeutic class: antibiotic
Pregnancy risk category: B
pH: 6 to 8.5

INDICATIONS & DOSAGES

➤ **Severe lower respiratory tract infection or disseminated infections caused by susceptible organisms—**
Adults: 1 g I.V. q 4 to 6 hours.
Children age 1 month and older, who weigh less than 40 kg (88 lb): 100 to 200 mg/kg/day I.V. in equally divided doses q 4 to 6 hours.
➤ **Mild to moderate upper respiratory tract infection or skin and skin structure infections caused by susceptible organisms—**
Adults: 250 to 500 mg I.V. q 4 to 6 hours.
Children 1 month and older, who weigh less than 40 kg: 50 mg/kg/day I.V. in equally divided doses q 6 hours.
➤ **Endocarditis caused by susceptible organisms in combination with gentamicin—**
Adults: 2 g I.V. q 4 hours for 4 to 6 weeks.
➤ **Acute or chronic osteomyelitis caused by susceptible organisms—**
Adults: 1.5 to 2 g I.V. q 4 hours for 4 to 8 weeks.
Adjust-a-dose: For adults, if creatinine clearance is less than 10 ml/minute, dosage is 1 g I.V. q 4 to 6 hours.

ADMINISTRATION

Direct injection: Inject drug over 10 minutes through an intermittent infusion device or into an I.V. line containing a free-flowing, compatible solution.
Intermittent infusion: Infuse diluted solution (concentration 0.5 to 40 mg/ml)

through an intermittent infusion device or using an I.V. line containing a free-flowing, compatible solution over the ordered duration.
Continuous infusion: Not recommended.

PREPARATION & STORAGE
Available in powder form in 1- and 2-g vials.

For direct injection, add 10 ml of sterile water injection or normal saline solution to 1-g vial; 20 ml to 2-g vial. Final concentration is 100 mg/ml.

For intermittent infusion, mix 50 to 100 ml of diluent with 1- or 2-g vial.

Compatible solutions include sterile water injection, normal saline solution, D_5W, dextrose 5% in half-normal saline solution, lactated Ringer's, and 10% invert sugar.

Stability depends on concentration of solution, diluent used, and temperature of storing environment. See manufacturer's package insert for stability information.

Incompatibilities
Acidic drugs, aminoglycosides, cytarabine, sodium bicarbonate, verapamil hydrochloride.

CONTRAINDICATIONS & CAUTIONS
• Contraindicated in those hypersensitive to penicillin, cephalosporins, or imipenem.
• Use cautiously in those with interstitial nephritis and in those with a history of GI disease (such as ulcerative colitis, regional enteritis, or antibiotic-associated colitis) because drug may exacerbate these disorders.

ADVERSE REACTIONS
CNS: neurotoxicity, *seizures.*
CV: thrombophlebitis, phlebitis.
GI: diarrhea, nausea, *pseudomembranous colitis,* vomiting.
GU: hematuria, azotemia.

Hematologic: *agranulocytosis,* eosinophilia, *leukopenia, neutropenia, hemolytic anemia.*
Hepatic: *hepatitis,* intrahepatic cholestasis.
Skin: discomfort at injection site.
Other: *anaphylaxis,* bacterial and fungal superinfections.

INTERACTIONS
Drug-drug. *Aminoglycosides:* Produces synergistic bactericidal effects against *Staphylococcus aureus.* This is a therapeutic effect.
Chloramphenicol, erythromycin, sulfonamides, tetracyclines: May reduce bactericidal effect. Monitor patient for clinical effect.
Hormonal contraceptives: May decrease efficacy of hormonal contraceptives. Recommend additional form of contraception during penicillin therapy.
Probenecid: Increases drug level, resulting from inhibited renal tubular secretion. Probenecid may be used for this effect.

EFFECTS ON LAB TEST RESULTS
• May increase creatinine, BUN, ALT, AST, alkaline phosphatase, and LDH levels.
• May increase eosinophil count. May decrease hemoglobin, hematocrit, and platelet, neutrophil, and granulocyte counts.
• May cause falsely elevated turbidimetric urine and serum proteins in tests using sulfosalicylic or trichloroacetic acid. May falsely elevate aminoglycoside level.

ACTION
Adheres to penicillin-binding proteins (PBP-1 and PBP-3), inhibiting bacterial cell-wall synthesis.

PHARMACOKINETICS
Drug level peaks at end of infusion.
Distribution: Into synovial, pleural, pericardial, and ascitic fluids as well as

---

bone, bile, lungs, and sputum. Level in CSF is low but rises with inflamed meninges. Drug crosses the placental barrier and appears in breast milk.
Metabolism: Partially altered to active and inactive metabolites in the liver.
Excretion: Rapidly removed in urine by renal tubular secretion and glomerular filtration. Half-life, 30 minutes to 2 hours.

CLINICAL CONSIDERATIONS

• Osmolality: 1 g in 50 ml D_5W, 326 mOsm/kg; 1 g in 100 ml D_5W, 295 mOsm/kg; 1 g in 50 ml normal saline solution, 353 mOsm/kg; 1 g in 100 ml normal saline solution, 321 mOsm/kg; 2 g in 50 ml D_5W, 379 mOsm/kg; 2 g in 100 ml D_5W, 329 mOsm/kg; 2 g in 50 ml normal saline solution, 406 mOsm/kg; 2 g in 100 ml normal saline solution, 356 mOsm/kg.
• Before giving drug, ask about previous reactions to penicillin or cephalosporins; normal history doesn't rule out future hypersensitivity.
• Obtain specimens for culture and sensitivity tests before giving first dose. Therapy may start immediately.
• Monitor WBC count before therapy and once to three times weekly during therapy.
• Assess renal and hepatic function before therapy and periodically during therapy. Closely monitor neonates for hepatotoxicity and nephrotoxicity.
• Stop drug if signs of hypersensitivity, pseudomembranous colitis, hepatotoxicity, or bacterial or fungal superinfection occur; institute appropriate therapy.
• If diarrhea persists during therapy, obtain stool specimen for culture.
• Hemodialysis removes only minimal amounts of drug.
• Each gram of drug contains 2.5 to 3.1 mEq of sodium.

PATIENT TEACHING

• Instruct patient to notify prescriber if sore throat, fever, ulcers on mucus membranes, rash, or unusual bleeding or bruising occurs.
• Inform patient that discomfort at injection site is a typical reaction.

oxaliplatin
Eloxatin

Pharmacologic class: alkylating drug
Therapeutic class: antineoplastic
Pregnancy risk category: D

INDICATIONS & DOSAGES

➤ **Adjunctive treatment of metastatic colon or rectal cancer that has recurred or progressed during or within 6 months of completion of first-line therapy with 5-fluorouracil (5-FU) and leucovorin and irinotecan—**
Adults: On day 1, give 85 mg/m² oxaliplatin I.V. in 250 to 500 ml D_5W and 200 mg/m² leucovorin I.V. in D_5W simultaneously over 120 minutes, in separate bags using a Y-line, followed by 400 mg/m² 5-FU I.V. bolus over 2 to 4 minutes, followed by 600 mg/m² 5-FU I.V. infusion in 500 ml D_5W over 22 hours.
On day 2, give 200 mg/m² leucovorin I.V. infusion over 120 minutes, followed by 400 mg/m² 5-FU I.V. bolus over 2 to 4 minutes, followed by 600 mg/m² 5-FU I.V. infusion in 500 ml D_5W over 22 hours.
Repeat cycle q 2 weeks.
Adjust-a-dose: In patients with unresolved and persistent grade 2 neurosensory events, reduce oxaliplatin dose to 65 mg/m². In those with persistent grade 3 neurosensory events, consider stopping drug. In patients recovering from grade 3 or 4 GI or hematologic

events, reduce oxaliplatin dose to 65 mg/m^2 and reduce dose of 5-FU by 20%.

ADMINISTRATION
Direct injection: Not recommended.
Intermittent infusion: Give oxaliplatin and leucovorin over 2 hours at the same time in separate bags, using a Y-line. Extend the infusion time to 6 hours to decrease acute toxicities.
Continuous infusion: Not recommended.

PREPARATION & STORAGE
Available in 50- or 100-mg vials.

Reconstitute powder using sterile water injection or D$_5$W. Add 10 ml to a 50-mg vial or 20 ml to a 100-mg vial, for a final concentration of 5 mg/ml. Never reconstitute with sodium chloride solution or other solution containing chloride. Reconstituted solutions must be further diluted in an infusion solution of 250 to 500 ml of D$_5$W.

Visually inspect bag for particulate matter and discoloration before administration and discard if present.

Store unopened vials at room temperature. Reconstituted solutions are stable if refrigerated (36° to 46° F [2° to 8° C]) for up to 24 hours. After final dilution, solutions are stable for 6 hours at room temperature and up to 24 hours under refrigeration.

Incompatibilities
Alkaline solutions or drugs such as 5-FU.

CONTRAINDICATIONS & CAUTIONS
• Contraindicated in patients allergic to drug or other platinum-containing compounds.
• Don't use drug in pregnant women due to risk of fetal harm. Avoid using drug in breast-feeding women.
• Use cautiously in patients with preexisting renal impairment or peripheral sensory neuropathy.

• Use cautiously in elderly patients because it may cause diarrhea, dehydration, hypokalemia, and fatigue.

ADVERSE REACTIONS
CNS: *pain, peripheral neuropathy, fatigue, headache,* dizziness, *insomnia, fever.*
CV: chest pain, ***thromboembolism, edema, flushing, peripheral edema.***
EENT: *rhinitis,* pharyngitis, epistaxis, abnormal lacrimation.
GI: *nausea, vomiting, diarrhea, stomatitis, abdominal pain, anorexia, constipation, dyspepsia, taste perversion,* gastroesophageal reflux, flatulence, mucositis.
GU: dysuria, hematuria.
Hematologic: FEBRILE NEUTROPENIA, *anemia,* LEUKOPENIA, THROMBOCYTOPENIA.
Metabolic: hypokalemia, dehydration.
Musculoskeletal: *back pain, arthralgia.*
Respiratory: *dyspnea, cough, upper respiratory tract infection,* hiccups, ***pulmonary toxicity.***
Skin: *injection site reaction,* rash, alopecia.
Other: ***anaphylaxis,*** *hand-foot syndrome, allergic reaction,* rigors.

INTERACTIONS
Drug-drug. *Nephrotoxic drugs (such as gentamicin):* May decrease elimination of drug and increase level. Monitor patient for signs and symptoms of toxicity.

EFFECTS ON LAB TEST RESULTS
• May increase creatinine, bilirubin, AST, and ALT levels. May decrease potassium level.
• May decrease hemoglobin and neutrophil, WBC, and platelet counts.

ACTION
Exact action is unknown. Probably inhibits cell replication and transcription

---

Reactions may be *common,* uncommon, ***life-threatening,*** or COMMON AND LIFE-THREATENING.

by forming platinum complexes that cross-link with DNA molecules.

PHARMACOKINETICS

Onset, peak, and duration of drug effects unknown.

Absorption: Absorbed I.V.

Distribution: Wide tissue distribution. More than 90% protein bound.

Metabolism: Undergoes nonenzymatic biotransformation. No evidence exists of cytochrome P-450–mediated metabolism.

Excretion: Primarily renal elimination.

CLINICAL CONSIDERATIONS

• Flush infusion line with D_5W before giving any other drugs simultaneously.

• Don't use needles or I.V. administration sets that contain aluminum because they will displace the platinum, causing loss of potency and formation of a black precipitate.

• Follow facility policy to reduce risks because preparation and administration of parenteral form of drug are linked to carcinogenic, mutagenic, and teratogenic risks for staff.

• Drug doesn't require prehydration.

• Premedicate with antiemetics with or without dexamethasone.

• Drug clearance is reduced in patients with renal impairment. Dosage adjustment for patients with renal impairment hasn't been established.

• Monitor CBC, platelet count, and liver and kidney function before each chemotherapy cycle.

• Monitor patient for hypersensitivity reactions, which may occur within minutes of administration.

• Monitor patient for injection site reaction. Watch for irritation and infiltration; extravasation can cause tissue damage and necrosis may occur.

• Monitor patient for neuropathy and pulmonary toxicity. Peripheral neuropathy may be acute or persistent. Acute neuropathy is reversible; it occurs within 2 days of dosing and re-

solves within 14 days. Persistent peripheral neuropathy occurs more than 14 days after dosing and causes paresthesias, dysesthesias, hypoesthesias, and deficits in proprioception that can interfere with daily activities (such as walking or swallowing).

• Avoid ice and cold exposure during infusion of drug because cold temperatures can exacerbate acute neurologic symptoms. Cover patient with a blanket during infusion.

• Avoid using drug in pregnant and breast-feeding women.

• Monitor elderly patients for increase in adverse reactions including diarrhea, dehydration, hypokalemia, and fatigue.

• Signs and symptoms of overdose are thrombocytopenia, myelosuppression, severe nausea, profuse vomiting, and neurotoxicity. Treat with supportive care, including hydration, electrolyte support, and platelet transfusion.

PATIENT TEACHING

• Tell patient to avoid exposure to cold or cold objects (such as cold drinks or ice cubes), which can bring on or worsen acute symptoms of peripheral neuropathy. Advise patient to have warm drinks, wear warm clothing, and cover any exposed skin (hands, face, and head). Have patient warm the air going into his lungs by wearing a scarf or ski cap. Have him wear gloves when touching cold objects (such as foods in the freezer, outside door handles, or mailbox).

• Tell patient to contact prescriber immediately if he has trouble breathing or experiences signs and symptoms of an allergic reaction, such as rash, hives, swelling of lips or tongue, or sudden cough.

• Tell patient to contact prescriber if any of the following occur: fever, signs and symptoms of an infection, persistent vomiting, diarrhea, or signs and symptoms of dehydration (thirst, dry mouth, lightheadedness, and decreased urination).

oxymorphone hydrochloride
Numorphan

Pharmacologic class: opioid
Therapeutic class: analgesic
Pregnancy risk category: C
Controlled substance schedule: II
pH: 2.7 to 4.5

INDICATIONS & DOSAGES
➤ **Moderate to severe pain—**
Adults: Initially, 0.5 mg I.V. May increase dose cautiously in nondebilitated patients.

ADMINISTRATION
Direct injection: Inject dose directly into a vein or into an I.V. line containing a free-flowing, compatible solution. Give over 2 to 3 minutes.
Intermittent infusion: Not recommended.
Continuous infusion: Not recommended.

PREPARATION & STORAGE
Supplied in 1-mg/ml ampules and in 1.5-mg/ml vials.
 No further dilution is needed for direct injection.
 Store between 59° and 86° F (15° and 30° C). Protect from freezing, light, and excessive heat.

Incompatibilities
None reported.

CONTRAINDICATIONS & CAUTIONS
• Contraindicated in those hypersensitive to the drug.
• Contraindicated in those with diarrhea related to pseudomembranous colitis or poisoning because drug may

slow elimination of toxins from GI tract.
• Avoid use in acute respiratory depression because drug may worsen condition.
• Use cautiously in those with altered respiratory function because of possible respiratory depression; and in those with head injury and increased intracranial pressure because drug may mask changes in level of consciousness, impair CNS function, and elevate intracranial pressure.
• Use cautiously in those with hepatic or renal impairment because drug clearance may be slowed.
• Use cautiously in those with prostatic hyperplasia or obstruction, urethral stricture, or recent urinary tract surgery because of increased risk of urine retention.
• Use cautiously in geriatric patients and debilitated patients because of increased sensitivity to drug effects, and in those with inflammatory bowel disease because of increased risk of toxic megacolon.
• Use cautiously in those with history of arrhythmias or seizures because drug may exacerbate symptoms, and in those with hypothyroidism because drug may increase risk of respiratory and CNS depression.
• Use cautiously in those with acute abdominal conditions because drug may mask signs; in those with gallbladder disease because drug may precipitate biliary contractions; and in those who have recently had GI surgery because drug may alter GI motility.
• Use cautiously in those with a history of substance abuse, emotional instability, or suicidal ideation because of possible abuse.

ADVERSE REACTIONS
CNS: confusion, *drowsiness,* faintness, headache, *sedation,* nervousness, severe weakness, *fatigue, euphoria,* depression, hallucinations, paradoxical

---

Reactions may be *common,* uncommon, *life-threatening,* or COMMON AND LIFE-THREATENING.

CNS stimulation, restlessness, trouble sleeping.
CV: *bradycardia,* tachycardia, facial flushing, *hypotension,* palpitations.
EENT: blurred or double vision, pinpoint pupils.
GI: *constipation,* dry mouth, increased gallbladder pain, *nausea, vomiting,* decreased appetite.
GU: urine retention, hesitancy.
Respiratory: *respiratory depression,* atelectasis.
Skin: sweating, itchiness, injection site reaction.
Other: *anaphylaxis,* physical dependence.

INTERACTIONS
Drug-drug. *Anticholinergics, antidiarrheals, antiperistaltics:* Increases risk of severe constipation, urinary retention, and CNS depression. Monitor closely; use with caution.
Antihypertensives, diuretics: Potentiates hypotension. Monitor blood pressure closely.
Antimuscarinics: Causes severe constipation, paralytic ileus, and urine retention. Monitor patient for abdominal pain and distention.
Buprenorphine: Causes withdrawal symptoms in physically dependent patients. Monitor patient for symptoms.
CNS depressants: Has additive CNS depressant effects. Reduce dosage of one or both agents.
Naloxone, naltrexone: Antagonizes effects; causes withdrawal symptoms in physically dependent patients. Use with caution.
Propofol: Increases incidence of bradycardia. Monitor patient closely.
Drug-herb. *St. John's wort:* Increases sedation. Discourage use together.
Drug-lifestyle. *Alcohol use:* Deepens respiratory depression. Discourage use together.

EFFECTS ON LAB TEST RESULTS
• May increase alkaline phosphatase, ALT, AST, bilirubin, LDH levels, amylase, and lipase levels.
• Diagnostic studies may show increased CSF pressure and delayed gastric emptying.

ACTION
Produces analgesia by binding with CNS opiate receptors, altering pain perception and emotional response to it.

PHARMACOKINETICS
Onset, 5 to 10 minutes; peak, 30 to 60 minutes; duration, 3 to 6 hours.
Distribution: Throughout body tissues. Drug crosses the placental and blood-brain barriers. Small amounts appear in breast milk.
Metabolism: In liver.
Excretion: In urine.

CLINICAL CONSIDERATIONS
• To minimize hypotension, keep patient supine when giving drug.
• Don't give drug if respirations are below 12 breaths/minute. Monitor respirations for at least 1 hour after giving dose. Keep resuscitation equipment available. If respirations fall below 8 breaths/minute, awaken patient to stimulate breathing. Notify prescriber, who may order naloxone or respiratory support.
• Assess patient's bowel function, and give a stool softener, if needed.
• For improved analgesia, give before patient has intense pain. Drug isn't intended for mild pain.
• Decreased salivation may contribute to candidiasis, dental caries, and discomfort.
• Dependence can develop with prolonged use.
• If overdose occurs, support airway and respirations. Give naloxone and repeat, as needed, to reverse respiratory

depression. Give I.V. fluids and vasopressors to maintain blood pressure.
• Withdrawal signs and symptoms include abdominal cramps, aching, anorexia, diarrhea, fever, gooseflesh, increased sweating, insomnia, nausea, rhinorrhea, shivering, sneezing, vomiting, and yawning.

PATIENT TEACHING
• Instruct patient to drink frequently, if not contraindicated, and to eat sugar-free candy or gum to relieve dry mouth.
• Advise patient to change positions slowly to avoid dizziness upon standing up quickly.
• Encourage patient to ask for drug before pain becomes intense.

oxytocin, synthetic injection
Pitocin

Pharmacologic class: exogenous hormone
Therapeutic class: oxytocic
Pregnancy risk category: NR
pH: 2.5 to 4.5

INDICATIONS & DOSAGES
➤ **To induce and stimulate labor—**
Adults: Usually, 0.5 to 1 milliunit/minute I.V. Dosage is determined by uterine response. May be increased q 30 to 60 minutes in increments of 1 to 2 milliunits/minute I.V. until contraction pattern simulates that of normal labor. Maximum dosage, 10 milliunits/minute I.V.
➤ **Incomplete or inevitable abortion—**
Adults: 10 to 20 milliunits/minute I.V. Don't exceed 30 units in a 12-hour period because this may cause water intoxication.

➤ **To control postpartum uterine bleeding—**
Adults: 20 to 40 milliunits/minute I.V. to total of 10 units.
➤ **To evaluate fetal distress after 31 weeks' gestation ◆ —**
Adults: Initially, 0.5 milliunit/minute I.V., then increase q 15 to 30 minutes to maximum dosage of 20 milliunits/minute I.V. Stop infusion when three moderate contractions occur within 10 minutes.

ADMINISTRATION
Direct injection: Not recommended.
Intermittent infusion: Not recommended.
Continuous infusion: Use an infusion pump. Start I.V. line with normal saline solution, adding oxytocin-containing solution as a secondary line to port as close to infusion needle as possible. Stop infusion at first sign of uterine hyperactivity or fetal distress. Don't give drug for longer than 8 hours.

PREPARATION & STORAGE
Available in a concentration of 10 units/ ml in 1-ml vials, ampules, disposable syringes.
    For infusion to start labor, add 1 ml of drug to 1,000 ml of normal saline solution or lactated Ringer's. For infusion to control postpartum bleeding, add 1 to 4 ml to 1,000 ml of D_5W or normal saline solution. For use after abortion, thoroughly mix 1 ml of drug with 500 ml of D_5W or normal saline solution. For evaluation of fetal distress, dilute 0.5 to 1 ml in 1,000 ml of D_5W.
    Store between 36° and 46° F (2 and 8° C).

Incompatibilities
Fibrinolysin, norepinephrine bitartrate, Normosol-M with dextrose 5%, prochlorperazine, warfarin sodium.

CONTRAINDICATIONS & CAUTIONS

• Contraindicated in those hypersensitive to drug.
• Contraindicated during labor in those with significant cephalopelvic disproportion, cord presentation or prolapse, total placenta previa, uterine inertia, severe toxemia, hypertonic uterine contractions, and fetal distress when delivery isn't imminent.
• Contraindicated in those for whom adequate uterine activity fails to achieve satisfactory progress and fetal position is unfavorable, so predelivery rotations are needed.
• Avoid use in those for whom vaginal delivery is contraindicated, as in those with cervical cancer, and in those who have had cervical or uterine surgery.
• Except in unusual circumstances, avoid use in those with abruptio placentae, borderline cephalopelvic disproportion, or grand multiparity; in those older than age 35; and in those with history of sepsis, difficult or traumatic delivery, partial placenta previa, unengaged fetal head, or prematurity.
• Use cautiously during abortion that uses hypertonic saline because of increased risk of water intoxication and in those with cardiac disease because of increased risk of fluid overload, arrhythmias, hypotension, and reflex tachycardia.

ADVERSE REACTIONS

CNS: *subarachnoid hemorrhage, seizures, fetal intracranial hemorrhage, coma.*
CV: *arrhythmias, fetal bradycardia,* hypertension, hypotension, increased cardiac output, increased venous return, PVCs, tachycardia.
EENT: fetal retinal hemorrhage.
GI: nausea, vomiting.
GU: *uterine hyperstimulation (resulting in abruptio placentae, amniotic fluid embolism, impaired uterine blood flow, tetanic contractions, and uterine rupture, paradoxical inhibi-*

tion of expulsion of placenta), pelvic hematoma.
Hematologic: *afibrinogenemia, hemorrhage,* increased postpartum bleeding because of drug-induced afibrinogenemia, hypoprothrombinemia, and thrombocytopenia.
Hepatic: neonatal jaundice.
Metabolic: hypochloremia, hyponatremia.
Respiratory: *fetal anoxia or asphyxia.*
Other: *hypersensitivity reactions, low fetal Apgar score,* water intoxification, infection.

INTERACTIONS

Drug-drug. *Caudal block anesthetics with vasoconstrictors:* May cause severe hypertension. Use together cautiously. Monitor blood pressure closely.
Cyclopropane, enflurane, halothane, isoflurane: Alters CV effects, including bradycardia, worsened hypotension, abnormal AV rhythms. Use together cautiously. Monitor ECG closely.
Sympathomimetic pressor amines: Causes severe, persistent hypertension. Monitor blood pressure closely.

EFFECTS ON LAB TEST RESULTS

• May decrease sodium, chloride, fibrinogen, and prothrombin levels.
• May decrease platelet count.

ACTION

Thought to act selectively on uterine and mammary gland smooth muscle, increasing uterine tone and frequency of established contractions. Drug facilitates lactation.

PHARMACOKINETICS

Onset, immediate; duration, 20 to 60 minutes.
Distribution: Throughout extracellular fluid. Drug probably crosses the placental barrier and appears in breast milk.
Metabolism: In the liver and kidneys. Drug is destroyed by oxytocinase.

Excretion: In urine. Half-life, 3 to 5 minutes.

CLINICAL CONSIDERATIONS
● Osmolality: 24 mOsm/kg.
● Oxytocin should be given only by qualified staff in a hospital with intensive care and surgical facilities.
● Don't give drug simultaneously by more than one route.
● Keep 20% solution of magnesium sulfate available to relax myometrium.
● Continuously monitor frequency, duration, and force of uterine contractions; resting uterine tone; fetal heart rate; maternal blood pressure; and intrauterine pressure.
● Stop infusion if contractions occur fewer than 2 minutes apart, exceed 50 mm Hg, or last longer than 90 seconds. Turn patient on her side, and notify prescriber.
● To avoid antidiuretic effects, restrict fluid intake, avoid prolonged infusion of low-sodium fluids and high oxytocin doses, and monitor intake and output.

PATIENT TEACHING
● Instruct patient to inform prescriber promptly if palpitations or other adverse reactions occur.
● Explain to patient and family the use and administration of drug.

paclitaxel
Onxol, Taxol

Pharmacologic class: antimicro-tubule agent
Therapeutic class: antineoplastic
Pregnancy risk category: D
pH: 4.4 to 5.6

INDICATIONS & DOSAGES
Premedicate all patients with 20 mg of dexamethasone P.O., at 12 hours and at 6 hours before therapy (reduce to 10 mg in patient's with AIDS-related Kaposi's sarcoma); 50 mg of diphen-hydramine I.V., 30 to 60 minutes before therapy; and 300 mg of cimetidine I.V., 20 mg famotidine I.V., or 50 mg of ranitidine I.V., 30 to 60 minutes before therapy.
➤ **First-line and subsequent therapy for advanced ovarian cancer**—
Adults (previously untreated):
175 mg/m² I.V. over 3 hours q 3 weeks followed by 75 mg/m² cisplatin I.V.; or 135 mg/m² I.V. over 24 hours in combination with 75 mg/m² cisplatin I.V. q 3 weeks.
Adults (previously treated): 135 or 175 mg/m² I.V. over 3 hours q 3 weeks.
➤ **Breast cancer after failure of combination chemotherapy for metastatic disease or relapse within 6 months of adjuvant chemotherapy (prior therapy should have included an anthracycline unless clinically contraindicated); adjuvant treatment of node-positive breast cancer given sequentially to standard doxorubicin-containing combination chemotherapy**—
Adults: 175 mg/m² I.V. over 3 hours q 3 weeks.
➤ **Initial treatment of advanced non–small-cell lung cancer for patients who aren't candidates for curative surgery or radiation**—
Adults: 135 mg/m² I.V. infusion over 24 hours, followed by 75 mg/m² cisplatin. Repeat cycle q 3 weeks.
Adjust-a-dose: Subsequent courses shouldn't be repeated until neutrophil count is at least 1,500 cells/mm³ and platelet count is at least 100,000 cells/mm³.
➤ **AIDS-related Kaposi's sarcoma**—
Adults: 135 mg/m² I.V. over 3 hours q 3 weeks, or 100 mg/m² I.V. over 3 hours q 2 weeks.
Adjust-a-dose: In patients with HIV, don't give full dose of drug if baseline or subsequent neutrophil counts are less than 1,000 cells/mm³. Reduce subsequent dosages by 20% in HIV patients with neutrophil counts less than 500 cells/mm³ that persist for a week or longer.

ADMINISTRATION
Direct injection: Not recommended.
Intermittent infusion: Infuse over 3 hours through a 0.22-micron in-line filter. Changing the filter every 12 hours may be needed because of clogging. Don't use polyvinyl chloride containers or administration sets.
Continuous infusion: Infuse over 24 hours.

PREPARATION & STORAGE
To avoid mutagenic, teratogenic, and carcinogenic risks, follow institutional guidelines for the safe handling, prepa-

---

ration, administration, and disposal of chemotherapeutic drugs.

Available in a 5-ml single-dose vial and 16.7-, 25-, and 50-ml multidose vials containing 30 mg/5 ml.

To prepare, calculate dose and dilute in normal saline solution, D_5W, dextrose 5% in normal saline solution, or dextrose 5% in lactated Ringer's solution to a final concentration of 0.3 to 1.2 mg/ml. Diluted solutions are physically and chemically stable for up to 27 hours at ambient room temperature 77° F (25° C) and room lighting conditions. Diluted solutions may show haziness attributable to the formulation vehicle.

Vials are stable when stored at room temperature 68° to 77° F (20° to 25° C). Keep product in its original package to protect from light.

Avoid contact of undiluted concentrate with polyvinyl chloride equipment or devices. Store diluted solutions in glass or polypropylene bottles or polypropylene, polyolefin bags and give through polyethylene-lined administration sets.

Incompatibilities

Amphotericin B, chlorpromazine, cisplatin, doxorubicin liposomal, hydroxyzine hydrochloride, methylprednisolone sodium succinate, mitoxantrone.

CONTRAINDICATIONS & CAUTIONS

• Contraindicated in those hypersensitive to the drug or to other drugs formulated in polyoxyethylated castor oil and in those with baseline neutropenia of less than 1,500 cells/mm³.
• Contraindicated in patients with AIDS-related Kaposi's sarcoma with baseline neutrophils less than 1,000 cells/mm³.
• Use cautiously in those with cardiac conduction abnormalities or hepatic dysfunction and in those who were previously treated with other cytotoxic drugs or radiation.

ADVERSE REACTIONS

CNS: headache, *peripheral neuropathy, asthenia,* fatigue, fever.
CV: *bradycardia,* hypotension, *abnormal ECG.*
GI: *diarrhea, mucositis, nausea, vomiting,* taste perversion.
Hematologic: anemia, bleeding, LEUKOPENIA, NEUTROPENIA, THROMBOCYTOPENIA.
Hepatic: *liver dysfunction.*
Musculoskeletal: *arthralgia, myalgia.*
Respiratory: *bronchospasm,* dyspnea.
Skin: generalized urticaria, injection site reaction, *alopecia, cellulitis and phlebitis at injection site.*
Other: hypersensitivity reactions, ***anaphylaxis,*** infection, ***angioedema.***

INTERACTIONS

Drug-drug. *Cisplatin:* Increases myelosuppression. Give paclitaxel before cisplatin.
Doxorubicin: May increase doxorubicin effect. Use together cautiously.
Drugs that inhibit the P-450 isoenzymes CYP 2C8 or CYP 3A4 (cyclosporine, diazepam, doxorubicin, felodipine, ketoconazole, midazolam, retinoic acid): Inhibits paclitaxel metabolism. Use together cautiously and monitor patient for toxicity.
Drugs that induce the P-450 isoenzyme CYP 3A4 (carbamazepine, phenobarbital): May induce metabolism of paclitaxel. Monitor patient closely.

EFFECTS ON LAB TEST RESULTS

• May increase alkaline phosphatase, AST, bilirubin, and triglyceride levels.
• May decrease hemoglobin, hematocrit, and neutrophil, WBC, and platelet counts.

ACTION

Inhibits mitosis. Enhances the assembly of cellular microtubules and prevents their depolymerization. Induces abnormal arrays or bundles of microtubules throughout the cell cycle and multiple esters of microtubules during mitosis.

PHARMACOKINETICS

Onset, peak, and duration of drug effect unknown.

Distribution: Extensive extravascular distribution to the peripheral compartment; 89% to 98% protein-bound.

Metabolism: Probably hepatic.

Excretion: Extensive nonrenal clearance; high levels reported in bile.

CLINICAL CONSIDERATIONS

• Give the drug only under the supervision of a health care provider experienced in use of chemotherapeutic drugs.

• Position needle carefully in vein to avoid extravasation. Watch for irritation and infiltration; extravasation can cause tissue damage and necrosis.

• Monitor hematocrit, hemoglobin, and WBC and platelet counts before and periodically during treatment. Adjust dosage as needed. Monitor vital signs frequently, especially during first hour.

• Monitor patient continuously, particularly during first 30 minutes of infusion. Have epinephrine, oxygen, and other drugs and equipment for treatment of anaphylaxis available during administration.

• Watch patients who develop neutropenia for signs of infection; antibiotics may be needed.

• *Alert:* Severe hypersensitivity reactions, including dyspnea, hypotension, angioedema, and generalized urticaria may occur in patients receiving paclitaxel. Pretreat patients with corticosteroids, antihistamines, and H_2-receptor antagonist.

• Don't use drug again in patients who have experienced severe hypersensitivity reactions to drug.

• Risk and severity of neurotoxicity and hematologic toxicity increase with dose, especially above 190 mg/m^2.

• Use caution during drug preparation and administration; wear gloves. If solution contacts skin, wash immediately

and thoroughly with soap and water. If drug contacts mucous membranes, flush thoroughly with water. Mark all waste materials with CHEMOTHERAPY HAZARD labels.

• *Alert:* Don't confuse Taxol (paclitaxel) with Taxotere (docetaxel).

PATIENT TEACHING

• Tell patient to watch for signs and symptoms of infection, including fever, sore throat, fatigue, and chills, and signs and symptoms of bleeding, such as easy bruising, bleeding gums, or tarry stools. Tell patient to take his temperature daily.

• Inform patient that temporary hair loss may occur.

• Advise woman of childbearing age to avoid becoming pregnant during therapy because of potential harm to fetus.

• Teach patient signs and symptoms of peripheral neuropathy, such as tingling, burning sensation, or numbness in the extremities, and advise him to report them immediately.

pamidronate disodium
Aredia

Pharmacologic class: bisphosphonate, pyrophosphate analogue
Therapeutic class: antihypercalcemic
Pregnancy risk category: D
pH: 6 to 7.4

INDICATIONS & DOSAGES

➤ **Moderate to severe hypercalcemia caused by malignancy (with or without metastases)—**
Dosage depends on severity of hypercalcemia. Calcium levels are corrected for albumin as follows:

$$\text{Corrected calcium (CCa)} = \text{calcium} + 0.8\,(4 - \text{albumin})$$
(in mg/dl)   (in mg/dl)   (in g/dl)

Patients with moderate hypercalcemia (CCa levels of 12 to 13.5 mg/dl) may receive 60 to 90 mg I.V. infusion as a single dose over 2 to 24 hours, depending on dilution. Patients with severe hypercalcemia (CCa levels over 13.5 mg/dl) may receive 90 mg over 2 to 24 hours. Repeat doses shouldn't be given sooner than 7 days to allow for full response to initial dose.

➤ **Osteolytic bone lesions of multiple myeloma—**
Adults: 90 mg I.V. daily over 4 hours once monthly.

➤ **Osteolytic bone lesions of breast cancer—**
Adults: 90 mg I.V. daily over 2 hours every 3 to weeks.

➤ **Paget's disease—**
Adults: 30 mg I.V. daily over 4 hours for 3 consecutive days for a total of 90 mg.

Adjust-a-dose: Patients with renal impairment may require reduced dosage and slower infusion rate of drug.

ADMINISTRATION
Direct injection: Not recommended.
Intermittent infusion: Not recommended.
Continuous infusion: Infuse as directed for specific indication and dosage. Longer infusions (more than 2 hours) may reduce the risk for renal toxicity, particularly in patients with pre-existing renal insufficiency.

PREPARATION & STORAGE
Available as 30- and 90-mg lyophilized powder and as 3 mg/ml, 6 mg/ml, and 90 mg/ml solution in single-dose vials.

To prepare, reconstitute with 10 ml sterile water for injection. Allow drug to dissolve completely. Reconstituted solution is stable for up to 24 hours when refrigerated at 36° to 46° F (2° to 8° C). Once drug is completely dissolved, add to 250 ml (2-hour infusion), 500 ml (4-hour infusion), or 1,000 ml (up to 24-hour infusion) bag of 0.45% or normal saline solution injection or D$_5$W.

Store at 59° to 86° F (15° to 30° C). Don't freeze.

Incompatibilities
Calcium-containing infusion solutions such as Ringer's injection or lactated Ringer's solution.

CONTRAINDICATIONS & CAUTIONS
• Contraindicated in those hypersensitive to bisphosphonates.
• Avoid using drug in pregnant patients.
• Use cautiously in those with cardiac failure or renal impairment.
• Use cautiously in breast-feeding women.

ADVERSE REACTIONS
CNS: *seizures,* somnolence, syncope, fatigue, insomnia, fever, *pain, headache.*
CV: *atrial fibrillation,* hypertension, tachycardia.
EENT: abnormal vision, rhinitis.
GI: *abdominal pain, anorexia, constipation,* **GI hemorrhage,** *nausea, vomiting.*
GU: *UTI,* renal dysfunction, ***renal failure.***
Hematologic: *anemia,* **leukopenia, thrombocytopenia.**
Metabolic: *hypocalcemia, hypokalemia, hypomagnesemia, hypophosphatemia, fluid overload,* hypothyroidism.
Musculoskeletal: *bone pain.*
Respiratory: crackles.
Skin: *infusion site reaction.*

INTERACTIONS
Drug-drug. *Calcium-containing preparations, vitamin D:* May antagonize effects of pamidronate. Monitor patient closely.

EFFECTS ON LAB TEST RESULTS
• May increase creatinine level. May decrease phosphate, potassium, magnesium, and calcium levels.

Reactions may be *common,* uncommon, *life-threatening,* or COMMON AND LIFE-THREATENING.

• May decrease hemoglobin, hematocrit, and WBC and platelet counts.

ACTION
Inhibits resorption of bone but not bone formation or mineralization.

PHARMACOKINETICS
Onset, peak, and duration of drug effect unknown.
Distribution: 50% to 60% rapidly absorbed into bone, preferentially in areas of high turnover.
Metabolism: Not metabolized.
Excretion: 51% excreted unchanged in urine within 72 hours.

CLINICAL CONSIDERATIONS
• Vigorously hydrate patient with saline before use, if not contraindicated. In those with mild to moderate hypercalcemia, hydration alone may be sufficient. Avoid overhydration in those with the potential for cardiac failure.
• For multiple myeloma patients, there is limited information on use in patients with creatinine greater than 3 mg/dl. Also, patients with marked Bence-Jones proteinuria and dehydration should receive adequate hydration before pamidronate infusion. Optimal duration of therapy is unknown; in studies, 21 months demonstrated overall benefits.
• For breast cancer patients, optimal duration of therapy is unknown; in studies, 24 months demonstrated overall benefits.
• A corticosteroid may be helpful for those with hypercalcemia associated with hematologic cancer.
• *Alert:* Due to the risk of renal dysfunction, leading to renal failure, single doses of pamidronate should not exceed 90 mg.
• Patients treated for bone metastases who have renal dysfunction should have the dose withheld until renal function returns to baseline. Treatment of bone metastases in patients with severe

renal impairment is not recommended. In other indications, clinical judgment should determine whether the potential benefit outweighs the potential risk in such patients.
• Drug is excreted intact primarily via the kidney, and the risk of renal adverse reactions may be greater in patients with impaired renal function.
• During therapy, periodically monitor alkaline phosphatase, a disease marker for Paget's disease.
• Monitor electrolyte levels, including calcium, potassium, magnesium, and phosphate. Monitor hemoglobin and creatinine levels, hematocrit, and CBC with differential periodically during therapy.
• Carefully monitor patients with pre-existing anemia, leukopenia, or thrombocytopenia during first 2 weeks after therapy.

PATIENT TEACHING
• Teach patient about foods rich in calcium and vitamin D.
• Tell patient to promptly report adverse reactions.
• Explain use of drug and its administration to patient and family.
• Tell women of childbearing age to avoid pregnancy during therapy.

---

pancuronium bromide*

Pharmacologic class: nondepolarizing neuromuscular blocker
Therapeutic class: skeletal muscle relaxant
Pregnancy risk category: C
pH: 3.8 to 4.2

INDICATIONS & DOSAGES
➤ **Adjunct to anesthesia—**
Adults and children older than age 1 month: 0.04 to 0.1 mg/kg I.V. Addition-

al doses of 0.01 mg/kg I.V. may be given at 25- to 60-minute intervals.
Neonates: Carefully individualized. A test dose of 0.02 mg/kg I.V. should be given to assess responsiveness.
➤ **To facilitate management of mechanically ventilated patients and endotracheal intubation—**
Adults and children older than age 1 month: 0.06 to 0.1 mg/kg I.V.
Neonates: Carefully individualized. A test dose of 0.02 mg/kg I.V. should be given to assess responsiveness.

ADMINISTRATION
Direct injection: Slowly inject into an established I.V. line containing a compatible, free-flowing solution.
Intermittent infusion: Infuse diluted drug at ordered rate.
Continuous infusion: Not recommended.

PREPARATION & STORAGE
Available in 2- and 5-ml ampules, vials, and syringes containing 2 mg/ml, and in 10-ml vials containing 1 mg/ml. Drug may contain benzyl alcohol.
    Store refrigerated at 36° to 46° F (2° to 8° C) for 18 months or expiration date on label. Drug remains potent for 6 months at room temperature. Don't store in plastic containers; however, you may give drug in plastic syringes. For infusion, dilute pancuronium with ordered amount of D_5W, normal saline solution, or lactated Ringer's solution. Drug will remain stable for 48 hours in a compatible solution.

Incompatibilities
Barbiturates, diazepam, other alkaline solution.

CONTRAINDICATIONS & CAUTIONS
• Contraindicated in those hypersensitive to pancuronium or bromides, in those with tachycardia, and in those for whom an increased heart rate is undesirable.

• Use cautiously in those with bronchogenic carcinoma, myasthenia gravis, or Eaton-Lambert syndrome, because of increased neuromuscular blockade risk.
• Use cautiously in those with renal impairment because of possible prolonged neuromuscular blockade, and in those with electrolyte imbalance because of possible altered neuromuscular blocking effects.
• Use cautiously in those with hepatic impairment or hyperthermia because of possible diminished intensity or duration of drug effect.
• Use cautiously in those with pulmonary impairment or respiratory depression because of possible worsened respiratory depression, and in those who are severely obese or have neuromuscular disease because of possible airway or ventilatory problems.
• Use cautiously in breast-feeding women, and in neonates because of increased sensitivity.

ADVERSE REACTIONS
CV: tachycardia, hypertension, phlebitis.
GI: excessive salivation.
Musculoskeletal: prolonged skeletal muscle relaxation.
Respiratory: *prolonged, dose-related respiratory insufficiency or apnea; bronchospasm.*
Skin: transient rash, excessive sweating.
Other: *hypersensitivity reactions.*

INTERACTIONS
Drug-drug. *Aminoglycosides, bacitracin, clindamycin, inhalation anesthetics, lincomycin, magnesium, polymyxin, quinidine, tetracyclines:* Enhances neuromuscular blockade. Use cautiously during surgical and postoperative periods and monitor patient for prolonged recovery.

Reactions may be *common*, uncommon, *life-threatening*, or COMMON AND LIFE-THREATENING.

Azathioprine: Reverses neuromuscular-blocking effect. Monitor patient closely.

Opioid analgesics: Deepens respiratory depression. Use with extreme caution and reduce dose of pancuronium.

Succinylcholine: Increases intensity and duration of neuromuscular blockade. Allow effects of succinylcholine to subside before giving pancuronium.

EFFECTS ON LAB TEST RESULTS

None significant.

ACTION

Produces skeletal muscle relaxation and inhibits neuromuscular transmission.

PHARMACOKINETICS

Onset, 30 to 45 seconds; duration, 35 to 45 minutes. Duration increases in geriatric and debilitated patients, and with prolonged administration.

Distribution: Widely dispersed in extracellular fluid. Small amounts cross the placental barrier, especially in the first trimester. Unknown if drug appears in breast milk.

Metabolism: In the liver.

Excretion: About 80% removed in urine and up to 10% in feces.

CLINICAL CONSIDERATIONS

• Osmolality: 273 to 277 mOsm/kg for 1 mg/ml solution; 338 mOsm/kg for 2 mg/ml solution.

• *Alert:* Large doses may increase the frequency and severity of tachycardia.

• Drug should be given only by staff trained in giving I.V. anesthetics and managing adverse effects.

• Adequate anesthesia is needed when using pancuronium; drug has no effect on consciousness, pain threshold, or cerebration.

• A nerve stimulator and train-of-four monitoring are recommended to assess recovery of muscle strength. Before attempting pharmacologic reversal with

neostigmine, patient should show some signs of spontaneous recovery.

• Be prepared to give mechanical ventilation or airway support because apnea will follow administration. Keep antagonists (such as neostigmine and edrophonium) and resuscitation equipment available.

• Closely monitor vital signs. Also, monitor electrolyte levels and intake and output.

• When moving the patient in bed, protect him from injury. Take special care with his eyes because of absent blink reflex.

PATIENT TEACHING

• Patient should be well sedated, but continue to explain carefully all procedures.

• Reassure patient and family that he'll be closely monitored and that his needs will be anticipated.

pantoprazole sodium
Panto I.V. ◇ , Protonix I.V.

Pharmacologic class: proton pump inhibitor
Therapeutic class: gastric acid suppressant
Pregnancy risk category: B
pH: 9 to 10

INDICATIONS & DOSAGES

➤ **Short-term treatment of GERD from erosive esophagitis—**

Adults: 40 mg I.V. once daily for 7 to 10 days. Switch to oral form as soon as patient is able to take oral medications.

➤ **Short-term treatment of pathological hypersecretion conditions from Zollinger-Ellison syndrome or other neoplastic conditions—**

Adults: Individualize dose. Usual dosage is 80 mg I.V. q 12 hours for no more than 6 days. For those needing a higher dosage, 80 mg I.V. q 8 hours is expected to maintain acid output below 10 mEq/hour. Maximum daily dosage is 240 mg/day I.V.

ADMINISTRATION
Direct injection: Not recommended.
Intermittent infusion: Infuse via a dedicated I.V. line using the provided filter. Infuse diluted solutions I.V. over 15 minutes at a rate not greater than 3 mg/minute (7 ml/minute) for GERD and 6 mg/minute (7 ml/minute) for pathological hypersecretory conditions.
Continuous infusion: Not recommended.

PREPARATION & STORAGE
Available in 40-mg vials. Reconstitute each vial with 10 ml of 0.9% sodium chloride. Compatible diluents for infusion include 5% dextrose, 0.9% sodium chloride, or lactated Ringer's injection.

For GERD, further dilute with 100 ml of diluent to a final concentration of 0.4 mg/ml.

For hypersecretion conditions, combine two reconstituted vials and further dilute with 80 ml of diluent to a total volume of 100 ml, with a final concentration of 0.8 mg/ml.

The reconstituted solution may be stored for up to 2 hours at room temperature, and the diluted solutions may be stored for up to 12 hours at room temperature.

Incompatibilities
None reported.

CONTRAINDICATIONS & CAUTIONS
Contraindicated in patients hypersensitive to any component of the formulation.

ADVERSE REACTIONS
CNS: headache, insomnia.
EENT: rhinitis.
GI: diarrhea, abdominal pain, constipation, dyspepsia, nausea.

Skin: injection site reaction (thrombophlebitis, abscess).

INTERACTIONS
Drug-drug. *Ampicillin esters, iron salts, ketoconazole:* May decrease absorption of these drugs. Monitor patient closely and try to space out the time intervals of administration.
Drug-herb. *St. John's wort:* May increase risk of sunburn. Advise patient to avoid excessive sunlight exposure.

EFFECTS ON LAB TEST RESULTS
None reported.

ACTION
Binds to hydrogen-potassium adenosine triphosphatase to suppress gastric acid secretion.

PHARMACOKINETICS
Onset, 15 to 30 minutes; peak, unknown; duration, 24 hours.
Distribution: In the extracellular fluid.
Metabolism: Extensively, in liver.
Excretion: About 70% in urine, with 18% in feces.

CLINICAL CONSIDERATIONS
• Symptomatic response to therapy does not preclude the presence of gastric malignancy.
• Anaphylaxis, angioedema, severe skin reactions, hepatic damage, pancreatitis, pancytopenia, rhabdomyolysis have occurred with use of I.V. pantoprazole.
• Treatment with I.V. pantoprazole should be stopped when P.O. is warranted.
• *Alert:* Don't confuse with Protonix tablets, Prilosec, Prozac, or Prevacid.
• It is not known if pantoprazole is excreted in breast milk. Use cautiously in nursing women.
• Overdose with 400 to 600 mg was associated with no adverse effects.
• Pantoprazole is not removed by hemodialysis.

Reactions may be *common*, uncommon, **life-threatening**, or COMMON AND LIFE-THREATENING.

PATIENT TEACHING
• Advise patient to report pain at injection site.
• Advise patient to report any adverse reactions.

---

paricalcitol
Zemplar

Pharmacologic class: synthetic vitamin D analogue
Therapeutic class: hyperparathyroidism drug
Pregnancy risk category: C

INDICATIONS & DOSAGES
➤ **To prevent and treat hyperparathyroidism caused by chronic renal failure—**
Adults: 0.04 to 0.1 mcg/kg (2.8 to 7 mcg) I.V. no more frequently than every other day during dialysis. Doses as high as 0.24 mcg/kg (16.8 mcg) have been safely given. If satisfactory response isn't observed, dosage may be increased by 2 to 4 mcg I.V. at 2- to 4-week intervals.

ADMINISTRATION
Direct injection: Given only as an I.V. bolus.
Intermittent infusion: Not recommended.
Continuous infusion: Not recommended.

PREPARATION & STORAGE
Drug is available in 1- and 2-ml ready-to-use vials.
  Inspect drug for particulate matter and discoloration before use.
  Store drug at room temperature (59° to 86° F [15° to 30° C]). Discard unused portion.

Incompatibilities
None reported.

CONTRAINDICATIONS & CAUTIONS
• Contraindicated in those hypersensitive to drug or its ingredients.
• Contraindicated in those with evidence of vitamin D toxicity or hypercalcemia.
• Use cautiously in patients taking digitalis compounds, since patients are at greater risk of digitalis toxicity when they are hypercalcemic.

ADVERSE REACTIONS
CNS: light-headedness, malaise, fever.
CV: palpitations, edema.
GI: dry mouth, GI bleeding, *nausea,* vomiting.
Respiratory: pneumonia.
Other: chills, flulike syndrome, *sepsis.*

INTERACTIONS
Drug-drug. *Digoxin:* Increases risk of digitalis toxicity because of potential for hypercalcemia. Use cautiously.
Phosphate, vitamin D compounds: Increases risk of hypercalcemia. Avoid using together.

EFFECTS ON LAB TEST RESULTS
• May decrease total alkaline phosphatase level.

ACTION
Reduces parathyroid hormone (PTH) levels.

PHARMACOKINETICS
Onset, immediate; peak, unknown; duration, 15 hours.
Distribution: More than 99% protein bound.
Metabolism: Several unknown metabolites detected in urine and feces.
Excretion: Mostly hepatobiliary. Half-life is about 15 hours.

CLINICAL CONSIDERATIONS
• As PTH level is decreased, paricalcitol dose may need to be decreased.
• Monitor patient for symptoms of hypercalcemia. Early signs may include

---

weakness, headache, somnolence, vomiting, dry mouth, constipation, muscle pain, bone pain, and metallic taste. Late signs may include anorexia, weight loss, conjunctivitis, pancreatitis, photophobia, rhinorrhea, pruritus, hyperthermia, decreased libido, elevated BUN, AST and ALT, hypercholesterolemia, ectopic calcification, hypertension, cardiac arrhythmias, and somnolence. Immediately notify prescriber if hypercalcemia is suspected.

• Monitor calcium and phosphorus levels twice weekly when dose is being adjusted, and then monitor monthly. PTH level should be measured every 3 months during therapy.

• Acute overdose of paricalcitol may cause hypercalcemia, which may require emergency attention.

• *Alert:* Treatment of patients with significant hypercalcemia includes immediate reduction in dose or discontinuation of paricalcitol, low-calcium diet, withdrawal of calcium supplements, patient mobilization, monitoring and treatment of fluid and electrolyte imbalances and ECG abnormalities, and hemodialysis or peritoneal dialysis, as needed.

• Monitor patient for ECG abnormalities.

• For patients with chronic renal failure, appropriate types of phosphate-binding compounds may be needed to control phosphorus levels; however, avoid excessive use of compounds that contain aluminum.

PATIENT TEACHING

• Stress importance of adhering to a dietary regimen of calcium supplementation and phosphorus restriction during drug therapy.

• Caution against use of phosphate or vitamin D–related compounds during drug therapy.

• Explain need for frequent laboratory tests.

• Instruct patient with chronic kidney failure to take phosphate-binding compounds as prescribed, but to avoid excessive use of aluminum compounds.

• Alert patient to early signs and symptoms of excessive calcium levels and vitamin D intoxication, such as weakness, headache, sleepiness, nausea, vomiting, dry mouth, constipation, muscle pain, bone pain, and metallic taste.

• Instruct patient to promptly report adverse reactions.

pegaspargase
(peg-L-asparaginase)
Oncaspar

Pharmacologic class: modified version of the enzyme L-asparaginase
Therapeutic class: antineoplastic
Pregnancy risk category: C

INDICATIONS & DOSAGES

➤ **Acute lymphoblastic leukemia in patients who require L-asparaginase but who have developed hypersensitivity to the native forms of L-asparaginase—**
Adults and children with body surface area (BSA) of at least 0.6 m²:
2,500 IU/m² I.V. q 14 days.
Children with BSA less than 0.6 m²:
82.5 IU/kg I.V. q 14 days.

ADMINISTRATION

Direct injection: Not recommended.
Intermittent infusion: Desired dose should be diluted in 100 ml of normal saline solution or dextrose 5%. The diluted solution should be placed into tubing of a free-flowing compatible I.V. solution over 1 to 2 hours.
Continuous infusion: Not recommended.

PREPARATION & STORAGE

Available in a preservative-free, single-use, 5-ml vial containing 750 IU/ml.

Excessive heat should be avoided. Don't shake the vials. Keep vials refrigerated at 36° to 46° F (2° to 8° C). Don't freeze. Don't use if cloudy or if precipitate is present. Drug is stable at room temperature for 48 hours. Discard unused portions.

Incompatibilities

None reported. Shouldn't be mixed with other drugs.

CONTRAINDICATIONS & CAUTIONS

• Contraindicated in those with pancreatitis or history of pancreatitis, and in those who have had significant hemorrhagic reactions to L-asparaginase in the past.

• Contraindicated in those with previous serious allergic reactions, such as generalized urticaria, bronchospasm, laryngeal edema, hypotension, or other unacceptable adverse reactions to pegaspargase.

• Use cautiously in those with liver dysfunction.

• Use in pregnant women only when clearly indicated.

ADVERSE REACTIONS

CNS: *coma,* confusion, disorientation, dizziness, emotional lability, headache, mental status changes, mood changes, paresthesia, parkinsonism, somnolence, *seizures, status epilepticus,* fatigue, malaise.

CV: chest pain, hypertension, hypotension, subacute bacterial endocarditis, tachycardia, edema.

EENT: epistaxis.

GI: abdominal pain, anorexia, constipation, diarrhea, flatulence, indigestion, mouth tenderness, mucositis, nausea, *pancreatitis (sometimes fulminant and fatal),* vomiting.

GU: hematuria, renal dysfunction, *renal failure,* severe hemorrhagic cystitis, urinary frequency, proteinuria.

Hematologic: *agranulocytosis, DIC,* easy bruising and ecchymosis, *hemolytic anemia, hemorrhage, leukopenia, pancytopenia, thrombocytopenia, thrombosis.*

Hepatic: ascites, bilirubinemia, fatty changes in liver, hypoalbuminemia, jaundice, *liver failure.*

Metabolic: hyperglycemia, hyperuricemia, hypoglycemia, hyponatremia, hypoproteinemia, metabolic acidosis, uric acid nephropathy, weight loss.

Musculoskeletal: arthralgia, cramps, joint stiffness, musculoskeletal pain, myalgia, pain in extremities.

Respiratory: cough, *severe bronchospasm,* upper respiratory tract infection, dyspnea.

Skin: alopecia, erythema simplex, fever blisters, fungal changes, hand whiteness, itching, injection site pain or reaction, localized edema, nail whiteness and ridging, petechial rash, purpura, rash, urticaria.

Other: *hypersensitivity reactions, including anaphylaxis,* erythema, pain, fever, and chills; night sweats; infection; *sepsis; septic shock.*

INTERACTIONS

Drug-drug. *Aspirin, dipyridamole, heparin, NSAIDs, warfarin:* May cause coagulation factor imbalances, predisposing patient to bleeding or thrombosis. Use together cautiously and monitor hematologic studies.

Methotrexate: May decrease methotrexate effect. Monitor patient for decreased effectiveness.

Protein-bound drugs: May increase toxic effects of other drugs that bind to proteins and may decrease detoxification of other drugs. Use together cautiously. Monitor patient for toxic reaction.

EFFECTS ON LAB TEST RESULTS

• May increase BUN, creatinine, amylase, lipase, bilirubin, ALT, AST, uric acid, and ammonia levels. May decrease sodium and protein levels. May increase or decrease glucose level.

● May increase PT, INR, PTT, and thromboplastin. May decrease antithrombin III, hemoglobin, hematocrit, and WBC, RBC, platelet, and granulocyte counts.

ACTION
Inactivates the amino acid asparagine, inhibiting synthesis of DNA and RNA.

PHARMACOKINETICS
Onset, peak, and duration of drug effect unknown.
Distribution: Unknown.
Metabolism: Unknown.
Excretion: Unknown.

CLINICAL CONSIDERATIONS
● Drug should be given under supervision of personnel who are qualified to give cancer chemotherapeutic drugs.
● Take preventive measures, including adequate hydration, before starting treatment. Hyperuricemia may result from rapid lysis of leukemic cells. Allopurinol may be ordered.
● Pegaspargase should be used as sole induction drug only when a combined regimen that uses other chemotherapeutic drugs is inappropriate because of toxicity or other patient-specific factors, or when a patient is refractory to other therapy.
● The I.M. route is preferred because it has the lowest risk of hepatotoxicity, coagulopathy, and GI and renal disorders.
● Don't give drug if it has been frozen. Although there may be no change in appearance, the activity of pegaspargase is destroyed by freezing.
● Drug may be a contact irritant; solution must be handled and given with care. Use gloves, avoid inhaling the vapors, and make sure drug doesn't come in contact with skin or mucous membranes, especially the eyes. In case of contact, wash with copious amounts of water for at least 15 minutes.

● Monitor patient closely for hypersensitivity reactions. Hypersensitivity reactions, including anaphylaxis, may occur during therapy, especially in patients known to be hypersensitive to other forms of L-asparaginase. As a routine precaution, keep patient under observation for 1 hour and have readily available resuscitation equipment and other drugs needed to treat anaphylaxis, such as epinephrine, oxygen, and I.V. corticosteroids. Stop the drug if patient develops moderate to life-threatening hypersensitivity reactions.
● As a guide to therapy effects, monitor patient's peripheral blood count and bone marrow. After therapy is initiated, circulating lymphoblast count may decrease and uric acid levels may increase markedly.
● To detect pancreatitis, frequently check amylase levels. To detect hyperglycemia, monitor patient's glucose during therapy.
● Monitor patient for liver dysfunction when drug is used in conjunction with hepatotoxic chemotherapeutic drugs.
● Drug may affect several plasma proteins; therefore, monitor fibrinogen, PT, INR, and PTT.

PATIENT TEACHING
● Inform patient of the possibility of hypersensitivity reactions and the importance of alerting nurse immediately if signs and symptoms occur.
● Instruct patient not to take other drugs (including OTC preparations) unless his prescriber has approved; bleeding risk is higher when drug is given with certain medications such as aspirin. In addition, the drug may increase the toxic effects of other medications.
● Instruct patient to report signs and symptoms of infection, including fever, chills, and malaise; drug may have immunosuppressive effect.
● Advise patient to avoid pregnancy or breast-feeding during therapy.

• Inform patient that hair loss may occur.

penicillin G potassium
Pfizerpen

penicillin G sodium

Pharmacologic class: natural penicillin
Therapeutic class: antibiotic
Pregnancy risk category: B
pH: penicillin G potassium, 5.5 to 8.5; penicillin G sodium, 6 to 7.5

INDICATIONS & DOSAGES
➤ **Anthrax—**
Adults: 5 to 20 million units I.V. daily given in divided doses q 4 to 6 hours for at least 14 days after symptoms abate. The average adult dose is 4 million units q 4 hours; can also be given as 2 million units q 2 hours.
Children: 100,000 to 150,000 units/kg/day I.V. in divided doses q 4 to 6 hours for at least 14 days after symptoms abate.
➤ ***Clostridium* infection—**
Adults and children older than age 12: 20 million units I.V. daily.
➤ ***Erysipelothrix insidiosa* endocarditis—**
Adults and children older than age 12: 2 to 20 million units I.V. daily for 4 to 6 weeks.
➤ ***Fusobacterium* infection of oropharynx, lower respiratory tract, and genital areas—**
Adults and children older than age 12: 5 to 10 million units I.V. daily.
➤ ***Listeria monocytogene* infection—**
Adults and children older than age 12: 15 to 20 million units I.V. daily in equally divided doses for 2 weeks (meningitis) to 4 weeks (endocarditis).
Neonates: 500,000 to 1 million units I.V. daily.

➤ ***Neisseria meningitidis* infection—**
Adults and children older than age 12: 20 to 30 million units I.V. daily by continuous infusion for at least 10 to 14 days.
➤ ***Pasteurella multocida* infection—**
Adults and children older than age 12: 4 to 6 million units I.V. daily for 2 weeks.
➤ **Pulmonary or abdominal actinomycosis—**
Adults and children older than age 12: 10 to 20 million units I.V. daily for 4 to 6 weeks followed by oral penicillin or tetracycline for an additional 6 to 12 months.
➤ **Rat-bite fever—**
Adults and children older than age 12: 12 to 15 million units I.V. daily for 3 to 4 weeks.
➤ **Syphilis—**
Adults and children older than age 12: 3 to 4 million units I.V. q 4 hours for 10 to 14 days; then given I.M. penicillin G benzathine.
➤ **Adjunct to diphtheria antitoxin for diphtheria ◆ —**
Adults: 100,000 to 150,000 units/kg I.V. daily in 4 divided doses for 14 days.
➤ **Infections caused by Enterobacteriaceae (*Escherichia coli, Enterobacter aerogenes, Alcaligenes faecalis, Salmonella, Shigella, Proteus mirabilis*) ◆ —**
Adults: 20 to 80 million units I.V. daily.
➤ **Alternative treatment for Lyme disease ◆ —**
Adults: 18 to 24 million units I.V. daily in 6 divided doses for 14 to 28 days.
Children: 200,000 to 400,000 units I.V. daily in 4 to 6 divided doses for 14 to 28 days. Don't exceed adult dosage.
➤ **Endocarditis from enterococci—**
Adults and children older than age 12: 18 to 30 million units I.V. daily of penicillin G sodium only, in equally divided doses q 4 hours or by continuous infusion for 4 to 6 weeks.

➤ **Endocarditis from *Streptococcus viridans* nonenterococcal group D streptococci—**

Adults and children older than age 12: 12 to 18 million units I.V. daily of penicillin G sodium only, in equally divided doses q 4 hours or by continuous infusion for 2 to 4 weeks.

Adjust-a-dose: In adults with renal or hepatic impairment, dosage reflects degree of impairment, severity of infection, and susceptibility of causative organism. For patients undergoing dialysis, dosage may need to be adjusted.

For patients with renal impairment, receiving penicillin G potassium and penicillin G sodium, refer to the table below. If patient is uremic and creatinine clearance is more than 10 ml/minute, give full loading dose, then give one-half dose q 4 to 5 hours for additional doses.

Creatinine clearance (ml/min)	Dosage (after full loading dose)
10-50	Usual dose q 8-12 hr
< 10	50% of usual dose q 8-10 hr; or usual dose q 12-18 hr

ADMINISTRATION

Direct injection: Not recommended.
Intermittent infusion: Infuse diluted drug over 1 to 2 hours.
Continuous infusion: Infuse diluted solution over 24 hours.

PREPARATION & STORAGE

Available in vials containing 1, 5, or 20 million units of penicillin G potassium and 5 million units of penicillin G sodium. Penicillin G potassium is also available in premixed frozen I.V. bags containing 1, 2, and 3 million units in 50 ml of dextrose solutions.

Reconstitute vials with sterile water for injection, normal saline solution, or D_5W, as manufacturer directs. For intermittent infusion, dilute in 50 to 100 ml of normal saline solution or D_5W. For continuous infusion, dilute daily dose in 1 to 2 L of compatible I.V. solution.

To prepare, first loosen powder in vial, then hold vial horizontally while rotating it and slowly directing stream of diluent against vial wall. Shake vigorously.

Store vials at room temperature. Diluted solution is stable for 24 hours at room temperature and for 7 days at 36° to 46° F (2° to 8° C). Frozen container should be thawed at room temperature. Thawed solution is stable for 24 hours if kept at room temperature, and 14 days if refrigerated.

Incompatibilities

Penicillin G potassium: alcohol 5%, amikacin, aminoglycosides, aminophylline, amphotericin B sodium, chlorpromazine, dextran, dopamine, heparin sodium, hydroxyzine hydrochloride, lincomycin, metoclopramide, pentobarbital sodium, phenytoin sodium, prochlorperazine mesylate, promethazine hydrochloride, sodium bicarbonate, thiopental, vancomycin, vitamin B complex with C.

Penicillin G sodium: aminoglycosides, amphotericin B, bleomycin, chlorpromazine, cytarabine, fat emulsions 10%, heparin sodium, hydroxyzine hydrochloride, invert sugar 10%, lincomycin, methylprednisolone sodium succinate, potassium chloride, prochlorperazine mesylate, promethazine hydrochloride.

CONTRAINDICATIONS & CAUTIONS

• Contraindicated in those hypersensitive to penicillin, cephalosporins, or imipenem.
• Use cautiously in atopic patients because of increased risk of hypersensitivity, and in those with GI disorders because of increased risk of pseudomembranous colitis.

• Use cautiously in those with renal impairment because of reduced drug elimination.

ADVERSE REACTIONS

CNS: *coma, encephalopathy,* confusion, hallucinations, hyperreflexia, lethargy, *seizures,* twitching.
CV: *heart failure,* phlebitis, thrombophlebitis, hypotension.
GI: dysphagia, nausea, vomiting, enterocolitis, *pseudomembranous colitis.*
GU: acute interstitial nephritis.
Hematologic: coagulation disorders, eosinophilia, *hemolytic anemia, leukopenia, neutropenia, thrombocytopenia,* thrombocytopenic purpura, *agranulocytosis.*
Hepatic: *hepatotoxicity.*
Metabolic: asterixis, hyperkalemia, hypernatremia, metabolic alkalosis.
Musculoskeletal: arthralgia, myoclonus.
Skin: pruritus, rash, exfoliative dermatitis.
Other: *anaphylaxis,* bacterial and fungal superinfections, lymphadenopathy.

INTERACTIONS

Drug-drug. *Anticoagulants:* May increase risk of bleeding. Monitor hematologic studies.
Chloramphenicol, erythromycin, sulfonamides, tetracycline: May antagonize penicillin's bactericidal activity. Monitor patient closely for clinical effects.
Hormonal contraceptives: Decreases contraceptive efficacy with breakthrough bleeding. Recommend additional form of birth control while on penicillin therapy.
NSAIDs, salicylates,: Displaces penicillin from binding sites. Avoid using together.
Potassium-sparing diuretics: Increases risk of hyperkalemia with penicillin G potassium. Avoid using together.

Probenecid, sulfinpyrazone: Increases or prolongs penicillin level. Probenecid may be used for this effect.

EFFECTS ON LAB TEST RESULTS

• May increase potassium, sodium, and liver enzyme levels. May falsely decrease aminoglycoside levels.
• May increase eosinophil count. May decrease hemoglobin, hematocrit, and platelet, WBC, and granulocyte counts.
• May cause false-positive CSF protein test result, false-positive urine protein result if biuret reagent is used, and false-positive Coombs' test result. May alter urine glucose testing using cupric sulfate (Benedict's reagent or Clinitest). May cause unreliable phenylketonuria test results in neonates. May cause rise in specific gravity in patient with dehydration or decreased urine output.

ACTION

Active against susceptible gram-positive aerobic bacteria, anaerobic bacteria, enterococci, and some spirochetes.

PHARMACOKINETICS

Drug's onset, peak, and duration are variable.
Distribution: Widely, to most body fluids and bone. Drug crosses the placental barrier, appears in breast milk, and is 45% to 68% protein-bound.
Metabolism: By hydrolysis.
Excretion: In urine. Half-life, 30 minutes to 1 hour. For those with renal impairment, excretion rate doubles or triples.

CLINICAL CONSIDERATIONS

• Osmolality, penicillin G potassium 250,000 units/ml in sterile water for injection, 749 to 776 mOsm/kg; 50,000 units/ml, 402 to 414 mOsm/kg; 100,000 units/ml, 535 to 554 mOsm/kg. Osmolality, penicillin G sodium 250,000 units/ml in sterile water for injection, 795 mOsm/kg.

• Ask patient about penicillin, cephalosporin, or imipenem allergy before giving first dose.
• Obtain specimens for culture and sensitivity tests before giving first dose. Start therapy immediately.
• Give penicillin and aminoglycosides separately at different sites.
• Take special care to prevent infusion near major peripheral nerves or blood vessels; severe or permanent neurovascular damage may occur.
• *Alert:* Patients with poor renal function are at risk for seizures because of high drug levels.
• Penicillin G potassium and sodium differ only in potassium and sodium content: Penicillin G potassium contains 1.7 mEq (66 mg) of potassium and 0.3 mEq (7 mg) of sodium per 1 million units; penicillin G sodium contains 2 mEq (46 mg) of sodium per 1 million units.
• To treat anaphylaxis, stop drug and treat symptoms. Anaphylaxis may occur within 30 minutes of infusion. Give antihistamines, epinephrine, or corticosteroids as needed. Further treatment may include intubation and CPR.
• Monitor vital signs, CBC, PT, INR, PTT, and BUN, AST, electrolyte, and creatinine levels. Monitor intake and output and give fluids.
• Watch for signs of bleeding or hypersensitivity. Monitor patient for bacterial or fungal superinfection, especially when using indwelling I.V. catheters.
• Use Clinistix or glucose enzymatic test strip for urine glucose tests.
• Hemodialysis removes penicillin, but peritoneal dialysis removes only a minimal amount.

PATIENT TEACHING
• Instruct patient regarding the importance of completing full course of therapy.
• Instruct patient to inform prescriber if fever, sore throat, easy bruising, or bleeding occurs.

• Tell patient to promptly report adverse reactions.
• Instruct patient to promptly report discomfort at the I.V. site.

pentamidine isethionate
Pentacarinat, Pentam 300

Pharmacologic class: diamidine derivative
Therapeutic class: antiprotozoal
Pregnancy risk category: C
pH: 4.09 to 5.4

INDICATIONS & DOSAGES
➤ ***Pneumocystis carinii* pneumonia**—
Adults and children older than 4 months: 3 to 4 mg/kg I.V. once daily for 14 to 21 days. Adults and children with AIDS who don't respond in 14 days may receive drug for 7 more days.
➤ **Leishmaniasis (visceral) caused by *Leishmania donovani* ♦** —
Adults and children: 4 mg/kg I.V. three times weekly for 5 to 25 weeks or longer, depending on response; or 2 to 4 mg/kg I.V. once daily to once q 3 days up to a total of 15 doses.
➤ **Trypanosomiasis ♦** —
Adults and children: 3 to 4 mg/kg I.V. once daily or every other day for 7 to 10 doses.
Adjust-a-dose: For adults with a creatinine clearance of less than 10 ml/minute, give usual dose q 48 hours.

ADMINISTRATION
Direct injection: Not recommended.
Intermittent infusion: Infuse diluted drug over 60 to 120 minutes.
Continuous infusion: Not recommended.

PREPARATION & STORAGE
Available as a powder in 300-mg vials. Drug contains no preservatives.

Reactions may be *common*, uncommon, *life-threatening*, or COMMON AND LIFE-THREATENING.

Reconstitute with 3 to 5 ml of sterile water for injection or D$_5$W. For infusion, dilute further in 50 to 250 ml of D$_5$W.

Store vials at 59° to 86° F (15° to 30° C). Protect both dry powder and reconstituted solution from light. Solutions of 1 to 2.5 mg/ml prepared in dextrose 5% remain potent for up to 48 hours at room temperature. Discard unused portion.

Incompatibilities
Aldesleukin, cephalosporins, fluconazole, foscarnet.

CONTRAINDICATIONS & CAUTIONS
• Contraindicated in those with a history of allergy to pentamidine or diamidine compounds.
• Use cautiously in those with anemia or a history of bleeding disorders because of increased risk of blood dyscrasias, and in those with hepatic or renal impairment because of increased risk of toxic reaction.
• Use cautiously in those with cardiac disease because of possible cardiotoxicity, and in those with diabetes mellitus, hypoglycemia, or hypotension because of possible exacerbation of these conditions.

ADVERSE REACTIONS
CNS: anxiety, confusion, dizziness, drowsiness, hallucinations, headache, neuralgia, fatigue, weakness, fever.
CV: *arrhythmias, hypotension,* rapid and irregular pulse, phlebitis.
EENT: blurred vision.
GI: abdominal pain, *acute pancreatitis,* anorexia, diarrhea, nausea, unusual hunger or thirst, vomiting.
GU: *acute renal failure, nephrotoxicity.*
Hematologic: anemia, *leukopenia, thrombocytopenia.*
Metabolic: *hyperkalemia,* hypocalcemia, *hypoglycemia,* hyperglycemia, diabetes mellitus.

Respiratory: *bronchospasm.*
Skin: flushed, red, and dry skin; pruritus; rash; *toxic epidermal necrolysis; Stevens-Johnson syndrome.*
Other: *anaphylaxis,* chills, Jarisch-Herxheimer reaction.

INTERACTIONS
Drug-drug. *Nephrotoxic drugs including aminoglycosides, amphotericin B, capreomycin, cisplatin, colistin, methoxyflurane, polymyxin B, vancomycin:* May worsen nephrotoxicity. Monitor patient closely.

EFFECTS ON LAB TEST RESULTS
• May increase alkaline phosphatase, ALT, AST, BUN, creatinine, and potassium levels. May increase or decrease glucose level.
• May decrease WBC and platelet counts, hemoglobin, and hematocrit.

ACTION
May inhibit synthesis of DNA, RNA, phospholipids, and protein; blocks folate transformation. Drug acts against many protozoa.

PHARMACOKINETICS
Onset, peak, and duration of action vary with dosage and disease state.
Distribution: Probably extensive and highly protein-bound. Unknown if drug crosses the placental barrier or appears in breast milk.
Metabolism: Unknown.
Excretion: In urine. Half-life varies depending on disease state; longer in renal impairment.

CLINICAL CONSIDERATIONS
• Osmolality: 100 mg/ml in sterile water for injection, 160 mOsm/kg; in D$_5$W, 455 mOsm/kg.
• Because of possible severe adverse reactions, give drug only to patients who test positive for susceptible organisms.

• Because drug may cause severe hypotension, keep patient in a supine position during administration and for several hours afterward. Closely monitor blood pressure, and keep resuscitation equipment available.
• Monitor fluid status, especially in AIDS patients who are at risk for dehydration, to ensure adequate hydration and minimize possible nephrotoxicity.
• Before, during, and after therapy, monitor CBC, platelets, and ECG. Also monitor AST, ALT, BUN, and alkaline phosphatase, bilirubin, calcium, creatinine, and glucose levels.
• *Alert:* Up to 10% of patients end up with a glucose level below 25 mg/dl. Have 50% dextrose available for I.V. use. Monitor blood glucose levels carefully.

PATIENT TEACHING
• Instruct patient of importance of recording input and output. Encourage patient to save urine for measuring.
• Teach patient about signs and symptoms of hypoglycemia and hyperglycemia. Instruct patient to inform prescriber if such symptoms occur.

pentazocine lactate
Talwin

Pharmacologic class: narcotic agonist-antagonist, partial opioid agonist
Therapeutic class: analgesic, adjunct to anesthesia
Pregnancy risk category: C
Controlled substance schedule: IV
pH: 4 to 5

INDICATIONS & DOSAGES
➤ **Moderate to severe pain**—
Adults and children older than age 12: Maximum single dose of 30 mg I.V. q

3 to 4 hours, p.r.n. Maximum daily dose, 360 mg.
➤ **Obstetric pain**—
Adults: 20 mg I.V. when contractions become regular, then 20 mg I.V. q 2 to 3 hours, p.r.n., for two or three doses.
Adjust-a-dose: Geriatric patients and patients with hepatic dysfunction may require lower doses.

ADMINISTRATION
Direct injection: Inject drug slowly into I.V. tubing containing a compatible, free-flowing solution. Monitor patient tolerance. Rapid injection may lead to anaphylaxis, peripheral circulatory collapse, or cardiac arrest.
Intermittent infusion: Not recommended.
Continuous infusion: Not recommended.

PREPARATION & STORAGE
Available in concentrations of 30 mg/ml in 1-, 1.5-, and 2-ml ampules; 1-, 1.5-, and 2-ml disposable syringes; and 10-ml multidose vials.
    Store below 104° F (40° C), preferably at room temperature. Protect from freezing. No dilution needed.

Incompatibilities
Aminophylline, amobarbital, glycopyrrolate, heparin sodium, nafcillin sodium, pentobarbital sodium, phenobarbital sodium, sodium bicarbonate.

CONTRAINDICATIONS & CAUTIONS
• Contraindicated in those hypersensitive to the drug.
• Contraindicated in those with diarrhea associated with pseudomembranous colitis or poisoning because of delayed elimination of toxins, and in those with acute respiratory depression because drug may exacerbate the condition.
• Use cautiously in those with sulfite sensitivity.

• Use cautiously in those with chronic respiratory impairment or acute asthma attack because drug decreases respiratory drive and increases airway resistance, and in those with an acute MI because drug increases arterial pressure and systemic vascular resistance.

• Use cautiously in those with head injury, elevated intracranial pressure, or intracranial lesions because deepened respiratory depression raises intracranial pressure, and drug may mask symptoms.

• Use cautiously in those with hypothyroidism because of possible worsened respiratory depression and prolonged CNS depression.

• Use cautiously in those with gallbladder disease because of possible biliary contraction, and in those with obstructive urinary disease, prostatic hyperplasia, or recent urinary tract surgery because of possible urine retention.

• Use cautiously in those with acute abdominal conditions because drug may mask symptoms, and in those with hepatic impairment because drug metabolism may be decreased.

• Use cautiously in those with renal impairment because of possible increased toxic effects, in those who have recently undergone GI surgery because of possible slowing of GI motility, and in those with seizures or arrhythmias because of possible precipitation or exacerbation.

• Use cautiously in those with a history of substance abuse or emotional instability because of increased risk of habituation, in those with inflammatory bowel disease because of increased risk of toxic megacolon, and in those with opioid-agonist dependence because of increased risk of withdrawal symptoms.

ADVERSE REACTIONS

CNS: confusion, disorientation, insomnia, *dizziness,* drowsiness, *euphoria,* unusual dreams, excitement, faintness, hallucinations, headache, irritability, *light-headedness,* paresthesia, *sedation, seizures,* syncope, vertigo.

CV: *shock,* circulatory depression, edema, flushing, hypertension, tachycardia.

EENT: blurred vision, diplopia, miosis, nystagmus, tinnitus.

GI: abdominal pain, altered taste, anorexia, constipation, diarrhea, dry mouth, *nausea, vomiting.*

GU: dysuria.

Hematologic: *leukopenia.*

Musculoskeletal: muscle tremors.

Respiratory: *respiratory depression, apnea.*

Skin: diaphoresis, pruritus, rash, sclerosis at injection site, *toxic epidermal necrolysis.*

Other: *anaphylaxis,* chills.

INTERACTIONS

Drug-drug. *Antihypertensives, diuretics:* Potentiates hypotensive effect. Monitor blood pressure closely.

CNS depressants, opioid agonist analgesics: Increases risk of CNS and respiratory depression and hypotension; may precipitate withdrawal in opioid-dependent patient. Use together cautiously.

Fluoxetine: Causes transient signs and symptoms of diaphoresis, ataxia, flushing, and tremor. Monitor patient closely.

Neuromuscular blockers: Deepens or prolongs respiratory depression. Avoid using together.

Drug-lifestyle. *Alcohol use:* Has additive CNS effects. Discourage patient use.

Smoking: May increase requirements for pentazocine. Monitor drug's effectiveness.

EFFECTS ON LAB TEST RESULTS

• May increase amylase and lipase levels.

• May decrease WBC.

• May elevate CSF pressure; may delay gastric emptying; may delay visualization during hepatic imaging with technetium-99m disofenin.

ACTION
Binds with opiate receptors, altering pain perception. Drug doesn't reverse opioid-induced respiratory depression, but may precipitate withdrawal in opioid-dependent patient.

PHARMACOKINETICS
Onset, 2 to 3 minutes; peak, 15 to 30 minutes; duration, 2 or 3 hours.
Distribution: Widely, to all tissues. About 60% protein bound; drug crosses the placental barrier and appears in breast milk.
Metabolism: In liver.
Excretion: Less than 5% in urine; small amount in feces.

CLINICAL CONSIDERATIONS
• Osmolality: 307 mOsm/kg.
• Dependence can occur with long-term use. Monitor patient for psychological or physical dependency signs.
• Keep patient in a supine position during administration to minimize orthostatic hypotension.
• *Alert:* Drug may contain sulfites.
• During administration, closely monitor respiratory status.
• Reverse severe respiratory depression with naloxone, and then provide supportive treatment.

PATIENT TEACHING
• Instruct patient to ask for drug before pain becomes intense.
• Advise patient to rise slowly to reduce faintness and dizziness.
• Instruct patient to notify prescriber if rash, confusion, or disorientation occurs.

pentobarbital sodium
Nembutal

Pharmacologic class: barbiturate
Therapeutic class: anticonvulsant, sedative-hypnotic
Pregnancy risk category: D
Controlled substance schedule: II
pH: 9.5

INDICATIONS & DOSAGES
➤ **Insomnia, anesthesia (adjunct), and seizures—**
Adults: 100 mg/70 kg patient initially; then smaller doses, p.r.n., at 1-minute intervals, to maximum of 200 to 500 mg. Dose is lower in geriatric patients.
Children: 50 mg initially; then smaller doses at 1-minute intervals until desired effect is reached.

ADMINISTRATION
Direct injection: Inject drug into I.V. tubing of free-flowing, compatible solution at a rate not exceeding 50 mg/minute. Watch for irritation and infiltration; solution is alkaline and extravasation may cause local tissue damage and necrosis. Guard against inadvertent intra-arterial injection, which may cause arterial spasm, severe pain, and possibly gangrene.
Intermittent infusion: Not recommended.
Continuous infusion: Not recommended.

PREPARATION & STORAGE
Available in concentrations of 50 mg/ml in 2-ml ampules and prefilled syringes, and in 20- and 50-ml multidose vials.
   Drug is compatible with most common solutions, such as D_5W and normal saline solution.
   Store at room temperature.

Incompatibilities
Other I.V. drugs or solutions.

CONTRAINDICATIONS & CAUTIONS
• Contraindicated in those hypersensitive to barbiturates and in those with intermittent or variegate porphyria, because drug may aggravate symptoms.
• Use cautiously in those with severe anemia, hyperkinesis, or hyperthyroidism, because drug may aggravate these conditions.
• Use cautiously in those with pain, because drug may cause paradoxical excitement or mask symptoms, and in depressed patients because drug may worsen suicidal tendencies.
• Use cautiously in those with borderline hyperadrenalism because drug diminishes the effects of exogenous hydrocortisone and endogenous cortisol.
• Use cautiously in those with hepatic impairment because of decreased drug metabolism, and in those with renal impairment because of decreased drug excretion.
• Use cautiously in those with a history of substance abuse or emotional instability because of risk of habituation, in those with asthma because of increased risk of hypersensitivity reactions such as bronchospasm, and in those with respiratory dysfunction because of risk of additive respiratory depression.

ADVERSE REACTIONS
CNS: *coma, somnolence,* CNS depression, delirium, depression, *drowsiness,* euphoria, headache, impaired judgment, *lethargy,* vertigo, mood distortion, neuralgia, paradoxical excitement, restlessness, hangover, insomnia, nightmares, fever.
CV: *severe bradycardia,* junctional rhythms, hypotension, thrombophlebitis, vasodilation, syncope.
GI: constipation, nausea, vomiting.
Hematologic: *agranulocytosis, megaloblastic anemia,* thrombocytopenic purpura.

Respiratory: *apnea, bronchospasm,* cough, *laryngospasm, respiratory depression.*
Skin: exfoliative dermatitis, photosensitivity, pain at injection site, rash, urticaria, *Stevens-Johnson syndrome.*
Other: serum sickness, *angioedema,* physical and psychological dependence.

INTERACTIONS
Drug-drug. *Carbamazepine, cardiac glycosides, corticosteroids, doxycycline, estrogens, griseofulvin, hormonal contraceptives, metronidazole, oral anticoagulants, phenytoin, progestins, quinidine, theophylline, tricyclic antidepressants:* May enhance metabolism of these drugs, decreasing their effectiveness. Monitor patient for decreased effect.
CNS depressants, MAO inhibitors: Has additive CNS and respiratory depression. Use together cautiously.
Divalproex sodium, valproic acid: Decreases pentobarbital metabolism and risk of toxic reaction. Avoid using together.
Drug-herb. *Kava:* May cause additive effects. Discourage use together.
Drug-lifestyle. *Alcohol use:* Causes excessive CNS and respiratory depression. Discourage use together.

EFFECTS ON LAB TEST RESULTS
• May decrease bilirubin level.
• May decrease hemoglobin, hematocrit, and granulocyte and platelet counts.
• May falsely elevate sulfobromophthalein level. May cause false-positive phentolamine test result.

ACTION
Depresses the CNS, interfering with transmission of impulses to cortex.

PHARMACOKINETICS
Onset, within 1 minute; duration, 15 minutes.

Distribution: Widely, with highest levels in brain, liver, and kidneys. Drug readily crosses the placental barrier and appears in breast milk.
Metabolism: In liver.
Excretion: In urine.

CLINICAL CONSIDERATIONS

● For seizures, use minimum doses to avoid augmented postseizure CNS and respiratory depression.
● *Alert:* Keep emergency resuscitation equipment available.
● Monitor vital signs, blood pressure, and cardiac function.
● Monitor EEG and blood levels when used for barbiturate coma. Patient will require mechanical ventilation.

PATIENT TEACHING

● Advise patient to change positions and rise slowly to avoid possible loss of equilibrium and hangover effect.
● Caution patient to avoid activities that require alertness or coordination.
● Instruct patient to inform prescriber if he experiences sore throat, fever, easy bruising, or bleeding.

pentostatin
(2'-deoxycoformycin; DCF)
Nipent

Pharmacologic class: antimetabolite (adenosine deaminase inhibitor)
Therapeutic class: antineoplastic
Pregnancy risk category: D
pH: 7 to 8.5

INDICATIONS & DOSAGES

➤ **Alpha-interferon-refractory hairy cell leukemia—**
Adults with creatinine clearance of 60 ml/minute or greater: 4 mg/m^2 every other week by I.V. bolus or diluted in a larger volume and given over 20 to 30 minutes. Treat until complete response is achieved. Hydrate patient with 500 to 1,000 ml of dextrose 5% in half-normal saline solution before treatment and with 500 ml after treatment to minimize risk of adverse renal effects.

ADMINISTRATION

Direct injection: Give by rapid (over 5 minutes) I.V. bolus.
Intermittent infusion: Infuse diluted solution over 20 to 30 minutes.
Continuous infusion: Not recommended.

PREPARATION & STORAGE

To avoid mutagenic, teratogenic, and carcinogenic risks, follow facility guidelines for the safe handling, preparation, administration, and disposal of chemotherapeutic drugs. Use sodium hypochlorite 5% to treat spills and wastes.

Available as 10-mg/vial powder for injection, in single-dose vials. Store refrigerated at 36° to 46° F (2° to 8° C). To prepare, add 5 ml sterile water for injection to vial and mix to obtain complete dissolution. Resultant solution contains 2 mg/ml of pentostatin. Give as I.V. bolus or further dilute using 25 or 50 ml D$_5$W or normal saline solution and infuse. Use reconstituted vials and diluted infusions within 8 hours if stored at room temperature; drug contains no preservatives.

Incompatibilities

Don't mix with other drugs unless specific compatibility data are available.

CONTRAINDICATIONS & CAUTIONS

● Contraindicated in those hypersensitive to the drug and in those with a creatinine clearance of 60 ml/minute or less.
● Use cautiously in those with CV disease, bone marrow depression, or previous cytotoxic drug therapy or radiation.

Reactions may be *common,* uncommon, *life-threatening,* or COMMON AND LIFE-THREATENING.

• Use only under the supervision of a prescriber qualified and experienced in chemotherapeutic drugs. Adverse reactions after drug therapy are common.
• Treat patients with infections only when potential benefit of the treatment justifies potential risk.

ADVERSE REACTIONS
CNS: asthenia, *headache, fatigue, anxiety, confusion, depression, insomnia, nervousness, paresthesia, somnolence, abnormal thinking, pain, fever.*
CV: *abnormal ECGs, thrombophlebitis, **arrhythmias, hemorrhage, heart failure,** chest pain, peripheral edema.*
EENT: *abnormal vision, conjunctivitis, ear and eye pain,* epistaxis, *pharyngitis, rhinitis, sinusitis.*
GI: *abdominal pain, anorexia, constipation, diarrhea, flatulence, nausea, stomatitis, vomiting.*
GU: *hematuria, dysuria.*
Hematologic: ***myelosuppression,*** *anemia,* ***leukopenia, thrombocytopenia.***
Metabolic: *weight loss.*
Musculoskeletal: *arthralgia, myalgia.*
Respiratory: *bronchitis, cough, dyspnea,* ***pulmonary edema,*** *pneumonia, upper respiratory tract infection.*
Skin: *dry skin, pruritus, rash, sweating, eczema, seborrhea, skin discoloration.*
Other: ***anaphylaxis,*** *chills, herpes simplex or zoster, infection,* ***hypersensitivity reactions,*** *lymphadenopathy,* ***sepsis.***

INTERACTIONS
Drug-drug. *Allopurinol:* Increases risk of rash. Monitor patient closely.
Bone marrow depressants: Causes additive bone marrow depression. Monitor hematologic studies.
Fludarabine: Risk of severe or fatal pulmonary toxicity. Avoid using together.
Vidarabine: Increases risk and severity of adverse effects associated with either drug. Avoid using together.

EFFECTS ON LAB TEST RESULTS
• May increase BUN, creatinine, liver enzymes, and uric acid levels.
• May decrease hemoglobin, hematocrit, and platelet, WBC, and granulocyte counts.

ACTION
Inhibits adenosine deaminase (ADA), which blocks DNA synthesis; also inhibits RNA synthesis.

PHARMACOKINETICS
Drug achieves therapeutic response in 3 to 24 months; inhibits the enzyme ADA 1 week after a single dose.
Distribution: Rapid, to all body tissues. Drug crosses the blood-brain barrier.
Metabolism: In liver.
Excretion: In urine.

CLINICAL CONSIDERATIONS
• Stop drug in patients with evidence of CNS toxicity, severe rash, or active infection.
• Temporarily withhold drug if absolute neutrophil count falls below 200 cells/mm^3. No recommendations exist regarding dosage adjustments in patients with anemia, neutropenia, thrombocytopenia, or renal dysfunction.
• Optimal duration of therapy is unknown. Current recommendations suggest two additional courses of therapy after a complete response. If patient hasn't had a partial response after 6 months, stop drug. If patient has had only a partial response, continue drug for another 6 months or for two courses of therapy after a complete response.
• Monitor hematocrit, WBC, platelet count, and creatinine, hemoglobin, and uric acid levels.

PATIENT TEACHING
• Stress importance of watching for adverse reactions and informing prescriber if they occur.
• Advise any woman of childbearing age not to become pregnant while tak-

ing drug and to consult with prescriber before becoming pregnant.

perphenazine
Trilafon

Pharmacologic class: phenothiazine (piperazine derivative)
Therapeutic class: antiemetic
Pregnancy risk category: C
pH: 4.2 to 5.6

INDICATIONS & DOSAGES
➤ **Severe vomiting, intractable hiccups, violent retching during surgery—**
Adults: 1 mg I.V. at no less than 1- to 2-minute intervals for 5 mg total, or maximum dose of 5 mg by infusion.

ADMINISTRATION
Direct injection: Inject into an I.V. line containing a free-flowing, compatible solution at 1- or 2-minute intervals.
Intermittent infusion: Infuse drug slowly into an I.V. line containing a free-flowing, compatible solution.
Continuous infusion: Not recommended.

PREPARATION & STORAGE
Available in 1-ml ampules containing 5 mg/ml.
Dilute to 0.5 mg/ml by adding 1 ml of drug to 9 ml of normal saline solution for direct injection or to an ordered amount for infusion.
Store at 59° to 86° F (15° to 30° C). Slight yellow discoloration won't affect potency or efficacy, but discard if markedly discolored or if a precipitate forms.

Incompatibilities
Cefoperazone, midazolam hydrochloride, pentobarbital sodium, thiethylperazine.

CONTRAINDICATIONS & CAUTIONS
• Contraindicated in those hypersensitive to the drug or related compounds, and in those with severe CNS depression, coma, severe CV disease, bone marrow depression, or blood dyscrasias.
• Use cautiously in those hypersensitive to sulfites.
• Use cautiously in alcoholic patients because drug may enhance CNS depression, and in those with glaucoma, peptic ulcers, or urine retention, because drug may exacerbate these conditions.
• Use cautiously in those with symptomatic prostatic hyperplasia because drug may increase urine retention, and in those with Reye's syndrome, encephalitis, encephalopathy, intestinal obstruction, brain tumor, meningitis, or tetanus, because drug may mask signs.
• Use cautiously in those with seizure disorders because of lowered seizure threshold, and in geriatric or debilitated patients because of increased sensitivity to the drug's antimuscarinic or sedative effects.
• Use cautiously in those with hepatic impairment, because decreased drug metabolism enhances CNS effects.
• Use cautiously in those with history of hepatic encephalopathy secondary to cirrhosis because of increased sensitivity to CNS effects and in those with renal impairment because of decreased drug excretion.
• Use cautiously in those with chronic respiratory disorders or acute respiratory infections because respiratory depression may worsen, and in those with hypocalcemia because dystonic reactions are more likely.

ADVERSE REACTIONS
CNS: dizziness, syncope, drowsiness, *extrapyramidal reactions,* **neuroleptic malignant syndrome, seizures,** tardive dyskinesia.

Reactions may be *common,* uncommon, *life-threatening,* or COMMON AND LIFE-THREATENING.

CV: *cardiac arrest,* hypotension, tachycardia.
EENT: *blurred vision.*
GI: anorexia, *constipation, dry mouth,* diarrhea, dyspepsia, paralytic ileus.
GU: discoloration of urine, *urine retention, menstrual cycle changes, erectile dysfunction.*
Hematologic: *leukopenia, agranulocytosis, hemolytic anemia, thrombocytopenia.*
Metabolic: *weight gain.*
Skin: dermatitis, photosensitivity, erythema, eczema.

INTERACTIONS

Drug-drug. *Antihypertensives, nitrates:* Increases risk of hypotension. Monitor blood pressure.
Appetite suppressants, dopamine, ephedrine, epinephrine, phenylephrine: Reduces response to these drugs. Monitor patient closely.
Atropine, anticholinergics, antiparkinsonians, antihistamines, MAO inhibitors: Potentiates sedation, paralytic ileus, visual changes, and severe constipation. Monitor patient closely.
Barbiturates: Decreases perphenazine level. Barbiturate level also may decrease. Monitor patient for clinical effect.
Bromocriptine: Antagonizes prolactin secretion. Monitor patient closely.
CNS depressants: Causes additive CNS and respiratory depression and hypotension. Monitor vital signs and neurological status if used together.
Lithium: May induce disorientation, unconsciousness, and extrapyramidal symptoms. Stop drug if any of these symptoms occurs.
Meperidine: Causes excessive sedation and hypotension. Monitor patient closely.
Pimozide: Prolongs QT interval. Avoid using together.
SSRIs, tricyclic antidepressants: Inhibits CYP2D6 hepatic enzymes. Monitor patient closely.

Drug-herb. *Yohimbe:* Increases risk of alpha$_2$ adrenergic antagonism. Discourage use together.
Drug-lifestyle. *Alcohol use:* Increases CNS depression. Discourage use together.
Heavy smoking: Decreases therapeutic response to perphenazine. Discourage smoking.
Sun exposure: May cause photosensitivity reactions. Advise patient to take precautions.

EFFECTS ON LAB TEST RESULTS

• May increase liver function test values and eosinophil count. May decrease hemoglobin, hematocrit, and WBC, granulocyte, and platelet counts.
• May cause false-positive results for urinary porphyrins, urobilinogen, amylase, and 5-hydroxyindoleacetic acid because of darkening of urine by metabolites; false-positive results for urine pregnancy tests that use human chorionic gonadotropin; false-positive results for phenylketonuria tests; may change Q- and T-waves in ECG; may blunt response in gonadorelin test; may reduce corticotropin secretion in metyrapone test.

ACTION

Controls severe nausea and vomiting by inhibiting the medullary chemoreceptor trigger zone.

PHARMACOKINETICS

Onset, peak, and duration of drug effect unknown.
Distribution: To most fluids and tissues, with high levels in the brain, lungs, liver, kidneys, and spleen. Highly protein bound; crosses the placental barrier and probably appears in breast milk.
Metabolism: In liver.
Excretion: Primarily in urine, with some in feces.

CLINICAL CONSIDERATIONS
- Osmolality: 263 mOsm/kg.
- *Alert:* Drug may contain sulfites.
- Prevent contact dermatitis by keeping drug away from skin and clothes.
- Keep patient in a supine position during and for 30 to 60 minutes after administration. Monitor blood pressure before and after administration.
- Monitor weekly bilirubin levels during first month.
- For those with severe hypotension requiring a vasopressor, use norepinephrine or phenylephrine. Don't give epinephrine.

PATIENT TEACHING
- Inform patient that drug may cause drowsiness and to avoid activities that require mental alertness or good coordination until CNS effects of the drug are known.
- Inform patient that drug may discolor urine pink to red-brown.

phenobarbital sodium
Luminal

Pharmacologic class: barbiturate
Therapeutic class: anticonvulsant, sedative-hypnotic
Pregnancy risk category: D
Controlled substance schedule: IV
pH: 9.2 to 10.2

INDICATIONS & DOSAGES
➤ **Status epilepticus and acute seizure disorders—**
Adults: 200 to 320 mg I.V., repeat in 6 hours p.r.n. Give until seizures cease or 20 mg/kg have been given.
Children: 15 to 20 mg/kg I.V. over 10 to 15 minutes. Give until seizures cease or 20 mg/kg have been given.

➤ **Seizures—**
Children: 4 to 6 mg/kg/day I.V. for 7 to 10 days to a blood level of 10 to 15 mcg/ml; or 10 to 15 mg/kg/day I.V.
➤ **Sedation—**
Adults: 30 to 120 mg/day I.V. in 2 or 3 divided doses.
➤ **Insomnia—**
Adults: 100 to 320 mg I.V.
➤ **Preoperative sedation—**
Children: 1 to 3 mg/kg I.V., 60 to 90 minutes before surgery.

ADMINISTRATION
Direct injection: Inject dose slowly, not exceeding 60 mg/minute, into vein or I.V. tubing containing a free-flowing, compatible solution. Observe injection site for signs of thrombophlebitis. If patient reports local pain, stop injection and check cannula placement. Watch for irritation and infiltration; extravasation of high-alkaline drug can cause tissue damage and necrosis.
Intermittent infusion: Not recommended.
Continuous infusion: Not recommended.

PREPARATION & STORAGE
Available in single-dose vials, ampules, and prefilled syringes in concentrations of 30, 60, 65, and 130 mg/ml. Discard if solution contains precipitate.
Drug is compatible with commonly used I.V. solutions including half-normal and normal saline solution, dextrose 5%, and lactated Ringer's solution.

Incompatibilities
Amphotericin B, chlorpromazine, dimenhydrinate, diphenhydramine, ephedrine, hydralazine, hydrocortisone sodium succinate, hydromorphone, insulin (regular), kanamycin, levorphanol, meperidine, morphine, norepinephrine, pentazocine lactate, phenytoin, prochlorperazine mesylate, promethazine hydrochloride, ranitidine

Reactions may be *common*, uncommon, *life-threatening*, or COMMON AND LIFE-THREATENING.

hydrochloride, streptomycin, vancomycin.

CONTRAINDICATIONS & CAUTIONS
• Contraindicated in those hypersensitive to barbiturates.
• Contraindicated in those with severe
pulmonary disease, because drug-
induced respiratory depression further
compromises ventilation, and in those
with a history of acute intermittent or
variegate porphyria because drug exacerbates these disorders.
• Use cautiously in those with hepatic
or renal impairment because of slowed
drug metabolism and excretion, and in
those with CV disease or unstable
blood pressure because of increased adverse CV effects or hypotension.
• Use cautiously in those with elevated
ammonia levels because drug impairs
the liver's ability to metabolize ammonia.
• Use cautiously in those with acute or
chronic pain, in geriatric patients, and
in children, because these groups are
more susceptible to paradoxical CNS
excitement.
• Use cautiously in those with diabetes
mellitus, hyperthyroidism, or hypothyroidism because symptoms may wors-
en; and in those with a history of drug
abuse, depression, or suicidal tendencies because of potential for sedative
effects and abuse.

ADVERSE REACTIONS
CNS: somnolence, *drowsiness, hangover, lethargy,* paradoxical excitement,
changes in EEG patterns.
CV: *bradycardia,* hypotension, thrombophlebitis, *shock.*
GI: diarrhea, epigastric pain, vomiting,
nausea.
Hematologic: *agranulocytosis, megaloblastic anemia,* thrombocytopenic
purpura.
Respiratory: *respiratory depression,
apnea with rapid injection, bronchospasm, hypoventilation, laryngospasm.*

Skin: *erythema multiforme, Stevens-
Johnson syndrome,* pain at injection
site, *severe subcutaneous necrosis,*
rash, swelling.
Other: physical and psychological dependence, *angioedema.*

INTERACTIONS
Drug-drug. *Antihypertensives, calcium
channel blockers, guanadrel, guanethidine:* Causes additive hypotension.
Monitor blood pressure closely.
*Carbamazepine, cardiac glycosides,
clonidine, corticosteroids, doxorubicin,
doxycycline, felodipine, hormonal contraceptives, metronidazole, oral anticoagulants, phenytoin, quinidine, theophylline, verapamil:* May enhance
metabolism of these drugs, decreasing
their effectiveness. Monitor patient for
decreased effect.
Chloramphenicol: Inhibits phenobarbital metabolism. Barbiturates may enhance chloramphenicol metabolism.
Use cautiously together.
CNS depressants, MAO inhibitors:
Causes additive CNS depression. Monitor patient closely.
Divalproex sodium, valproic acid: Decreases phenobarbital metabolism and
risk of toxic reaction. Monitor patient
for toxic reaction.
Rifampin: Induces hepatic enzymes
and decreases the effectiveness of barbiturates. Avoid using together.
Drug-herb. *Evening primrose oil:* May
increase anticonvulsant requirements.
Discourage use together.
Drug-lifestyle. *Alcohol use:* Increases
CNS depression. Discourage use together.

EFFECTS ON LAB TEST RESULTS
• May decrease bilirubin level.
• May decrease hemoglobin, hematocrit, and granulocyte and platelet
counts.
• May cause false-positive phentolamine test result.

ACTION
Probably decreases nerve cell excitability in cerebral cortex and reticular formation. Anticonvulsant effect may result from gamma-aminobutyric acid–like activity in the motor cortex.

PHARMACOKINETICS
Onset, 5 minutes; peak, 30 minutes; duration, 4 to 6 hours, but sedative effect may persist for up to 10 hours.
Distribution: Widely, to all tissues. Drug is 20% to 45% protein-bound. Drug crosses the blood-brain and placental barriers and appears in breast milk.
Metabolism: In liver.
Excretion: Primarily in urine. Small amounts are removed in feces. Half-life, 2 to 5 days.

CLINICAL CONSIDERATIONS
• Osmolality: 65 mg/ml is 9,285 to 15,570 mOsm/kg; 200 mg/ml is 10,800 mOsm/kg; 100 mg in 50 ml D_5W or normal saline solution is 296 to 325 mOsm/kg; 100 mg in 100 ml D_5W or normal saline solution is 289 to 317 mOsm/kg.
• Patient may develop tolerance after about 2 weeks of therapy.
• Drug dependence and severe withdrawal symptoms may follow long-term therapy. When discontinuing drug, withdraw single dose over 5 to 6 days to prevent withdrawal symptoms and rebound REM sleep.
• Don't give drug within 24 hours of liver function tests.
• Diazepam is drug of choice for those with status epilepticus. Because of slow onset time, phenobarbital's usefulness in these patients is limited.
• Establish baseline blood pressure, and continuously monitor patient for hypotension.
• Obtain baseline respiratory rate, and continuously monitor. If rate falls below 12 breaths/minute, notify prescriber. If it falls below 8 breaths/minute, rouse patient and encourage him to breathe more deeply to rate of at least 12 breaths/minute. If patient can't be roused, manually ventilate him at 12 to 16 breaths/minute with handheld ventilator. Notify prescriber immediately, and prepare for possible intubation.
• Stop drug immediately if a skin reaction occurs; it may indicate a fatal reaction.
• For full anticonvulsant effect, wait 30 minutes after initial dose before giving additional doses. Maintain drug level at 15 to 40 mcg/ml. Halt injections when seizures stop or when total dose is reached.
• In patients receiving anticoagulants, closely monitor PT; adjust anticoagulant dosage, as needed.
• Signs of overdose include clammy skin, coma, cyanosis, hypotension, and pupillary constriction.
• If overdose occurs, treatment is chiefly supportive. Maintain a patent airway, using oxygen and assisted ventilation, as needed. Keep patient well hydrated with I.V. fluids, and give sodium bicarbonate to alkalize urine and increase drug excretion.
• For severe overdose, peritoneal dialysis and hemodialysis are helpful. Keep resuscitation equipment readily available.

PATIENT TEACHING
• Instruct patient to change positions and to rise slowly because of potential hangover effects and loss of equilibrium.
• Advise patient to avoid activities that require alertness while receiving drug.
• Advise patient to avoid alcohol and other CNS depressants.

Reactions may be *common*, uncommon, *life-threatening*, or COMMON AND LIFE-THREATENING.

phentolamine mesylate
Regitine

Pharmacologic class: alpha blocker
Therapeutic class: antihypertensive for pheochromocytoma, cutaneous vasodilator
Pregnancy risk category: C
pH: 4.5 to 6.5

INDICATIONS & DOSAGES
➤ **Diagnosis of pheochromocytoma—**
Adults: 5 mg I.V.
Children: 1 mg or 0.1 mg/kg or 3 mg/m² I.V.
➤ **Hypertension in pheochromocytoma before surgical removal of tumor—**
Adults: 5 mg I.V. 1 to 2 hours before surgery; repeat, p.r.n.
Children: 1 mg or 0.1 mg/kg or 3 mg/m² I.V. 1 to 2 hours before surgery; repeat, p.r.n.
➤ **Left-sided heart failure secondary to an acute MI ♦ —**
Adults: 0.17 to 0.4 mg/minute by continuous infusion.
➤ **Norepinephrine or dopamine extravasation—**
Adults: 5 to 10 mg I.V. in 10 to 15 ml of normal saline solution into affected tissues within 12 hours of extravasation.
Children: 0.1 to 0.2 mg/kg I.V., to maximum of 10 mg/dose, into affected tissues within 12 hours of extravasation.
➤ **To prevent severe tissue sloughing in norepinephrine infusion—**
Adults: 10 mg added to each 1,000 ml norepinephrine infusion.
➤ **Hypertensive crisis from interaction between MAO inhibitor and sympathomimetic amines ♦ —**
Adults: 5 to 15 mg I.V.

➤ **Cocaine-induced coronary syndrome ♦ —**
Adults: 2.5 to 5 mg I.V.; repeat q 5 to 10 minutes until blood pressure controlled.
Children: 0.05 to 0.1 mg/kg I.V., not to exceed adult dose; repeat q 5 to 10 minutes until blood pressure controlled.

ADMINISTRATION
Direct injection: Delay injection until venipuncture effect subsides, then rapidly inject desired dose.
Intermittent infusion: Not recommended.
Continuous infusion: Infuse at rate ordered for norepinephrine solution; to treat left-sided heart failure, infuse at rate needed to control symptoms, using infusion pump.

PREPARATION & STORAGE
Supplied in 5-mg vials with 1 ml ampule of sterile water for injection as diluent.
Reconstitute with diluent to 5 mg/ml.
Store unreconstituted powder at room temperature. Manufacturer recommends that solution be used immediately after reconstitution. Reconstituted product remains stable for 48 hours at room temperature or for 7 days at 36° to 46° F (2° to 8° C).

Incompatibilities
None reported.

CONTRAINDICATIONS & CAUTIONS
• Contraindicated in those sensitive to phentolamine or related drugs and in those with an acute MI.
• Use cautiously in those with coronary artery disease, angina, or a previous MI because reflex tachycardia may precipitate angina or heart failure.
• Use cautiously in those with gastritis or peptic ulcer disease to avoid exacerbating these disorders.

ADVERSE REACTIONS
CNS: cerebral vascular spasm, *cerebrovascular occlusion*, *dizziness*, *weakness.*
CV: *acute, prolonged, or orthostatic hypotension;* angina; *arrhythmias, MI, flushing,* tachycardia, *shock.*
EENT: *nasal congestion.*
GI: abdominal pain, *diarrhea*, exacerbation of peptic ulcer disease, *nausea, vomiting.*

INTERACTIONS
Drug-drug. *Epinephrine, ephedrine:* Phentolamine antagonizes vasoconstricting and hypertensive effects of these drugs. Avoid using together.

EFFECTS ON LAB TEST RESULTS
None reported.

ACTION
Inhibits adrenergic stimuli. Causes vasodilation and reduces peripheral vascular resistance. In those with heart failure, drug reduces preload and pulmonary artery pressure, increases cardiac output, and exerts a positive inotropic effect.

PHARMACOKINETICS
Onset, 2 minutes; duration, 15 to 30 minutes.
Distribution: Unknown if drug crosses the blood-brain or placental barriers or appears in breast milk.
Metabolism: Unknown.
Excretion: In urine.

CLINICAL CONSIDERATIONS
• Osmolality: 169 mOsm/kg.
• *Alert:* For those with severe hypotension or other signs of shock, treat with norepinephrine and supportive measures. For arrhythmias, give cardiac glycosides. Don't use epinephrine because it may cause "epinephrine reversal," an additional fall in blood pressure.

• Don't give sedatives or opioids in the 24 hours before pheochromocytoma test. Stop rauwolfia alkaloids at least 4 weeks before test.
• Before performing a pheochromocytoma test, make sure that patient's blood pressure has returned to pretreatment level. Give drug rapidly, recording blood pressure immediately after injection, every 30 seconds for 3 minutes, then every 60 seconds for 7 more minutes. Severe hypotension after test dose indicates pheochromocytoma.
• When treating left-sided heart failure, continuously monitor ECG and left ventricular function.

PATIENT TEACHING
• Instruct patient to inform prescriber of new or increased symptoms of suffocating chest pain.
• Explain to patient the use and administration of drug.
• Tell patient to avoid sudden position changes to minimize orthostatic hypotension.

phenylephrine hydrochloride
Neo-Synephrine

Pharmacologic class: adrenergic
Therapeutic class: vasoconstrictor
Pregnancy risk category: C
pH: 3 to 6.5

INDICATIONS & DOSAGES
➤ **Shock or severe hypotension—**
Adults: Initially, 0.1 to 0.18 mg/minute I.V.; then, after blood pressure stabilizes, 0.04 to 0.06 mg/minute I.V.
➤ **Mild to moderate hypotension—**
Adults: 0.1 to 0.5 mg I.V. (usual dose, 0.2 mg). Give subsequent doses at 10- to 15-minute intervals.

➤ **Paroxysmal supraventricular tachycardia—**
Adults: Initially, no more than 0.5 mg I.V. Give subsequent doses in 0.1- to 0.2-mg increments, depending on blood pressure (systolic shouldn't exceed 160 mm Hg) with no single dose exceeding 1 mg.

➤ **Hypotensive emergencies during spinal anesthesia—**
Adults: Initial dose, 0.2 mg I.V. Give later doses in 0.1- to 0.2-mg increments, with no single dose exceeding 0.5 mg.

ADMINISTRATION

Direct injection: Inject dose over 1 minute to treat mild to moderate hypotension or hypotensive emergencies during spinal anesthesia. Inject dose over 20 to 30 seconds for paroxysmal supraventricular tachycardia; rapid injection may cause short paroxysms of ventricular tachycardia, ventricular extrasystoles, or a sensation of fullness in the head.
Intermittent infusion: Not recommended.
Continuous infusion: Infuse diluted drug at rate needed to maintain adequate blood pressure and tissue perfusion. Regulate rate with microdrip tubing and infusion pump. Give through a patent I.V. line into large vein in the antecubital fossa to prevent extravasation. Closely monitor infusion site.

PREPARATION & STORAGE

Available in 1-ml ampules and 1-, and 5-ml vials (10 mg/ml or 1% solution).
For infusion, dilute 10 mg in 500 ml of D_5W or normal saline solution. For injection, prepare a 0.1% solution (1 mg/ml) by diluting 1 ml of 1% solution with 9 ml sterile water for injection. Discard diluted solutions after 48 hours.
Store at room temperature. Discard brown or precipitate-containing solutions.

Incompatibilities

Alkaline solutions, iron salts, other metals, phenytoin sodium, thiopental sodium.

CONTRAINDICATIONS & CAUTIONS

● Contraindicated in those hypersensitive to the drug.
● Contraindicated in those with ventricular tachycardia because of arrhythmogenic effects; in those with severe hypertension because of possible exacerbation; and in those with an MI because of possible increased cardiac workload and ischemia.
● Contraindicated in those with mesenteric or peripheral vascular thrombosis, acute pancreatitis, or hepatitis because drug may precipitate or aggravate ischemia or infarction in affected organ.
● Use cautiously in those hypersensitive to sulfites.
● Use cautiously in those with hyperthyroidism because of increased risk of bradycardia, and in those with myocardial disease because of increased cardiac workload and possible exacerbation of heart failure.
● Use cautiously in those with incomplete heart block because of possible exacerbation, and in those with severe arteriosclerosis because of possible ischemia.
● Use cautiously in geriatric patients because of diminished cerebral and coronary circulation.

ADVERSE REACTIONS

CNS: excitability, headache, restlessness.
CV: hypertension, *severe bradycardia,* ventricular extrasystoles, *ventricular tachycardia.*
GU: decreased renal perfusion.
Respiratory: *asthmatic episodes.*
Skin: necrosis or tissue sloughing with extravasation, pallor, sweating.
Other: *anaphylaxis.*

INTERACTIONS

Drug-drug. *Alpha blockers, phenothiazines:* Decreases pressor effect. Monitor patient for effect.

Antihypertensives, diuretics: Causes mutual antagonism. Avoid using together.

Atropine, doxapram, ergot alkaloids, guanadrel, guanethidine, MAO inhibitors, oxytocin: Potentiates pressor response, increasing risk of severe hypertension and cerebral hemorrhage. Avoid using together.

Bretylium, cardiac glycosides, hydrocarbon inhalation anesthetics, sympathomimetics: Potentiates pressor response, increasing risk of arrhythmias. Use with extreme caution and monitor ECG.

Tricyclic antidepressants: Increases or decreases sensitivity to phenylephrine.

EFFECTS ON LAB TEST RESULTS

None reported.

ACTION

Primarily stimulates alpha receptors, causing vasoconstriction, increasing blood pressure, and slowing the heart rate.

PHARMACOKINETICS

Onset, immediate; duration, 15 to 20 minutes.

Distribution: In plasma. Unknown if drug appears in breast milk.

Metabolism: In liver and intestines.

Excretion: In urine.

CLINICAL CONSIDERATIONS

• Osmolality: 284 mOsm/kg.

• Correct hypovolemia either before or during drug administration; hypovolemic patients are more susceptible to effects of severe vasoconstriction.

• *Alert:* Drug may contain sulfites.

• During infusion, check blood pressure every 2 minutes until stable, then every 5 to 15 minutes via intra-arterial monitoring. Stop slowly to avoid severe hypotension.

• Monitor central venous pressure or left ventricular filling pressure to help detect hypovolemia. Keep in mind that phenylephrine isn't a substitute for blood, plasma, fluid, or electrolytes.

• Continuously monitor ECG. Note heart rate every 5 to 15 minutes. Notify prescriber of arrhythmias.

• Insert indwelling urinary catheter and monitor urine output hourly. Inform prescriber if urine output falls below 30 ml/hour.

• After stopping infusion, monitor vital signs hourly until stable. Watch for severe hypotension. Restart infusion if systolic pressure drops below 70 mm Hg. Maintain blood pressure slightly below patient's usual blood pressure.

• Prevent hypoxia and acidosis, because they will reduce drug's effectiveness.

• Treat hypertension with phentolamine and cardiac arrhythmias with propranolol, as ordered.

• Watch for irritation and infiltration; extravasation can cause tissue damage and necrosis. If extravasation occurs, stop infusion and restart at another site. Infiltrate area with 5 to 10 mg of phentolamine in 10 to 15 ml of normal saline, using syringe with a fine needle. For best results, treat within 12 hours.

PATIENT TEACHING

• Because drug is used only in emergency situations, patient teaching depends on condition and procedures being performed.

• Instruct patient to notify nurse immediately if discomfort occurs at I.V. site.

---

phenytoin sodium
Dilantin

Pharmacologic class: hydantoin derivative
Therapeutic class: anticonvulsant
Pregnancy risk category: D
pH: 12

INDICATIONS & DOSAGES
➤ **Status epilepticus—**
Adults: Initially, 10 to 15 mg/kg by direct injection, then 100 mg q 6 to 8 hours; or 15 to 18 mg/kg, at a rate not to exceed 50 mg/minute. Maximum total daily dose, 1.5 g I.V. In geriatric patients with heart disease, 50 mg I.V. over 2 to 3 minutes.
Children: 15 to 20 mg/kg I.V. at 1 to 3 mg/kg/minute; or 10 to 15 mg/kg I.V. at a rate of 0.5 to 1.5 mg/kg/minute. Maximum total daily dose, 20 mg/kg I.V.
➤ **Ventricular tachycardia, paroxysmal atrial tachycardia, or arrhythmias caused by digitalis toxicity ♦ —**
Adults: 100 mg I.V. at 5-minute intervals, p.r.n., to terminate arrhythmias; not to exceed a total dose of 1 g.

ADMINISTRATION
Direct injection: Avoid injecting drug into dorsal hand veins to prevent extravasation. Inject dose directly into vein using a 0.22-micron in-line filter. Alternatively, inject into I.V. line containing a compatible solution, infusing at a rate of less than 50 mg/minute. In geriatric or debilitated patients, give at rate of 17 to 25 mg/minute. In children give at a rate of 0.5 to 3 mg/kg/minute.
Intermittent infusion: Infuse prescribed dose at ordered rate, after mixing with normal saline solution.
Continuous infusion: Not recommended.

PREPARATION & STORAGE
Available in 100- and 250-mg ampules, syringes, and vials containing 50 mg/ml.
Store at room temperature; avoid freezing. Solution should be clear. If refrigerated, discard if slight yellowing doesn't clear after slow warming.
Drug may be diluted for intermittent infusion with 25 or 50 ml normal saline injection (maximum 100 ml) to 100 mg drug. Prepare immediately before use, always use an in-line filter, and infuse within 1 hour.

Incompatibilities
Amikacin, aminophylline, amphotericin B, bretylium, cephapirin, ciprofloxacin, D_5W, diltiazem, dobutamine, enalaprilat, fat emulsions, hydromorphone, insulin (regular), levorphanol, lidocaine, lincomycin, meperidine, morphine sulfate, nitroglycerin, norepinephrine, other I.V. drugs or infusion solutions, pentobarbital sodium, potassium chloride, procaine, propofol, streptomycin, sufentanil citrate, theophylline, vitamin B complex with C.

CONTRAINDICATIONS & CAUTIONS
• Contraindicated in those hypersensitive to hydantoins.
• Contraindicated in those with sinus bradycardia, SA block, second- or third-degree AV block, or Stokes-Adams syndrome, because phenytoin delays conduction in cardiac muscle.
• Use cautiously in those with myocardial insufficiency and heart failure because drug depresses pacemaker action and force of myocardial contractility, and in those with impaired thyroid function because drug decreases T_4 levels.
• Use cautiously in those with respiratory depression because drug may exacerbate symptoms, and in those with hypoglycemia-induced seizures or hypoglycemia because drug may worsen hypoglycemia.

◆ Off-label use   *May contain benzyl alcohol   ◇ Canada

• Use cautiously in those with hepatic impairment or renal disease because of altered metabolism, in those with blood dyscrasias because of increased risk of serious infection, and in those with hypotension because of possible exacerbation.

• Use cautiously in those with fever lasting for more than 24 hours, because fever reduces phenytoin levels.

• Use cautiously in pregnant and breast-feeding women because safety has not been established.

ADVERSE REACTIONS

CNS: *ataxia,* nervousness, headache, *confusion,* dizziness, **seizures,** severe CNS depression, *slurred speech,* insomnia, fever.
CV: hypotension if injected too rapidly, **CV collapse, ventricular fibrillation.**
EENT: blurred vision, *diplopia, nystagmus, gingival hyperplasia.*
GI: anorexia, constipation, dysphagia, epigastric pain, loss of taste, *nausea, vomiting.*
Hematologic: *thrombocytopenia, agranulocytosis, pancytopenia, leucopenia.*
Hepatic: *toxic hepatitis,* jaundice.
Metabolic: hyperglycemia, weight loss.
Musculoskeletal: osteomalacia, muscle twitching.
Skin: bullous or purpuric dermatitis, exfoliative dermatitis, rash, *hirsutism,* **Stevens-Johnson syndrome, toxic epidermal necrolysis,** injection site pain, inflammation, tissue necrosis or sloughing.
Other: hypertrichosis, lupus erythematosus, lymphadenopathy.

INTERACTIONS

Drug-drug. *Amiodarone, chloramphenicol, chlordiazepoxide, diazepam, cimetidine, disulfiram, estrogen, famotidine, halothane, isoniazid, methylphenidate, nizatidine, phenothiazines, ranitidine, salicylates, succinimides, sulfonamides, tolbutamide, trazodone:* Increases plasma phenytoin levels and risk of toxic reaction. Monitor patient for toxicity.
Antidiabetics: Phenytoin may increase glucose levels. Dosage may need to be adjusted; monitor glucose levels.
Barbiturates, sodium valproate, valproic acid: Causes unpredictable alterations in phenytoin levels. Monitor levels closely.
Bupropion, carbamazepine, clozapine, haloperidol, molindone, reserpine, tricyclic antidepressants: These drugs may lower the seizure threshold, decreasing phenytoin's effectiveness. Monitor patient closely.
Corticosteroids, cardiac glycosides, doxycycline, estrogen, furosemide, hormonal contraceptives, oral anticoagulants, quinidine, rifampin, theophylline, vitamin D: Phenytoin may enhance metabolism of these drugs, decreasing their effectiveness. Monitor patient for clinical effect.
Drug-lifestyle. *Long-term alcohol use:* Decreases phenytoin activity. Inform patient that heavy alcohol use may diminish drug's benefit.

EFFECTS ON LAB TEST RESULTS

• May increase alkaline phosphatase, GGT, and glucose levels. May decrease dexamethasone, metyrapone, and protein-bound iodine levels.
• May increase uptake of resin or RBC T_3. May decrease hemoglobin, hematocrit, and platelet, WBC, RBC, and granulocyte counts.

ACTION

Reduces voltage and spread of electrical stimulation within the motor cortex.

PHARMACOKINETICS

Onset, 3 to 5 minutes; drug level peaks in 1 to 2 hours.
Distribution: Throughout tissues, with highest levels in the liver and adipose

---

tissue. Drug crosses the placental barrier and appears in breast milk.
Metabolism: In liver. With small dose increases, drug levels are substantially higher in healthy patients but lower in those with renal dysfunction. Metabolized faster in children.
Excretion: In urine, with small amounts in feces. Half-life is 14 hours.

CLINICAL CONSIDERATIONS
● Osmolality: 50 mg/ml: 3,035 to 9,740 mOsm/kg; 500 mg in 50 ml normal saline solution: 336 mOsm/kg; 500 mg in 100 ml normal saline solution: 312 mOsm/kg.
● Flush I.V. tubing before and after use with normal saline solution, to remove drug and reduce venous irritation.
● Monitor ECG, blood pressure, and respiratory status.
● Frequently check I.V. site for irritation and infiltration; phenytoin extravasation causes severe tissue damage.
● Closely monitor drug levels.
● Closely monitor patient for seizures. Keep intubation and aspiration equipment as well as padded side rails available.
● If a measles-like rash appears, immediately stop drug.
● Monitor intake and output; hydration affects seizure threshold.
● Each milliliter of phenytoin for injection contains 0.2 mEq of sodium.
● If overdose occurs, immediately stop drug. Therapeutic level is 10 to 20 mcg/ml; toxic level, above 20 mcg/ml; lethal level, 100 mcg/ml. No specific antidote is available.

PATIENT TEACHING
● Inform patient that drug may turn urine pink or red to reddish brown.
● Teach patient about signs and symptoms of high sugar level in the blood, because drug may increase sugar levels.

● Inform patient that drug may decrease effectiveness of hormonal contraceptives.
● Instruct patient to inform prescriber if sore throat, fever, or malaise occur because this may indicate abnormal blood conditions.
● Encourage proper oral hygiene to reduce likelihood of gum problems.
● Encourage patient to obtain and wear medical identification bracelet stating his seizure disorder.

physostigmine salicylate (eserine salicylate)
Antilirium*

Pharmacologic class: anticholinesterase
Therapeutic class: antimuscarinic antidote
Pregnancy risk category: C

INDICATIONS & DOSAGES
➤ **To reverse anticholinergic effects, except those of atropine or scopolamine, or sedative effects of benzodiazepines—**
Adults: 0.5 to 2 mg I.V. initially, then repeated q 20 minutes to desired effect or until adverse cholinergic effects occur. With recurrence of life-threatening signs, such as arrhythmias or coma, give 1 to 4 mg I.V. at 30- to 60-minute intervals, p.r.n.
Children: 0.02 mg/kg I.V. initially, then repeated at 5- to 10-minute intervals to desired effect or until adverse cholinergic effects occur. Maximum total dose, 2 mg I.V. Or, may receive 0.03 mg/kg or 0.9 mg/m² I.V., p.r.n.
➤ **To reverse anticholinergic effects of atropine or scopolamine hydrobromide as preanesthetics—**
Adults: Dose is twice that of anticholinergic, depending on weight. For example, to reverse effects of 0.5 mg of

atropine, give 1 mg I.V. of physostigmine.

➤ **Postoperative intestinal atony to stimulate peristalsis ♦ —**
Adults: 0.5 to 2 mg I.V.

ADMINISTRATION

Direct injection: Slowly inject drug into large vein or into I.V. tubing containing free-flowing, compatible solution. Don't exceed 1 mg/minute for adults or 0.5 mg/minute for children. Rapid injection can cause bradycardia, breathing difficulty, hypersalivation, and seizures.
Intermittent infusion: Not recommended.
Continuous infusion: Not recommended.

PREPARATION & STORAGE

Available in concentration of 1 mg/ml in 2-ml ampules. Preparations may contain benzyl alcohol. Parenteral solution may be tinted red, blue, or brown. Discard solution if discoloration is marked.

Store in light-resistant containers at room temperature. Avoid freezing.

Incompatibilities

None reported.

CONTRAINDICATIONS & CAUTIONS

• Contraindicated in those with asthma, CV disease, diabetes mellitus, or gangrene because drug may aggravate condition; and in those with mechanical obstruction of the intestinal or urinary tract or vagotonia because drug may worsen the obstruction by increasing muscle tone.
• Use drug only in life-threatening situations when diagnosis of anticholinergic overdose is well established and possibility of mixed drug ingestion has been ruled out.
• Use cautiously in those hypersensitive to the drug or to sulfites.

• Use cautiously in those with a history of seizures because of risk of increased seizures, and in those with bradycardia or parkinsonian syndrome because symptoms may worsen.

ADVERSE REACTIONS

CNS: hallucinations, headache, *restlessness,* **seizures,** muscle twitching, weakness.
CV: *arrhythmias, asystole, bradycardia,* hypotension, palpitations.
EENT: lacrimation, miosis.
GI: abdominal cramps, diarrhea, excessive salivation, nausea, vomiting.
GU: urinary urgency.
Respiratory: *bronchospasm,* dyspnea, increased bronchial secretions, *pulmonary edema, respiratory paralysis.*
Skin: sweating.
Other: cholinergic crisis with overdose.

INTERACTIONS

Drug-drug. *Acetylcholine, bethanechol, carbachol, methacholine:* Enhances effects of physostigmine. Use together cautiously.
Succinylcholine: Has additive depolarizing neuromuscular blockade. Use together cautiously.
Drug-herb. *Jaborandi tree, pillbearing spurge:* May have additive effect when used together. Question patient about herbal use.

EFFECTS ON LAB TEST RESULTS

None reported.

ACTION

Blocks cholinesterase destruction of acetylcholine at central and peripheral cholinergic sites of neurotransmission. Accumulated acetylcholine promotes increased receptor stimulation.

PHARMACOKINETICS

Onset, 3 to 5 minutes; peak, 5 minutes; duration, 1 to 2 hours.

Reactions may be *common,* uncommon, *life-threatening,* or COMMON AND LIFE-THREATENING.

Distribution: Throughout the body. Drug easily crosses the blood-brain barrier and probably crosses the placental barrier. Unknown if drug appears in breast milk.
Metabolism: Hydrolyzed.
Excretion: Small quantities in urine. Half-life 15 to 40 minutes.

CLINICAL CONSIDERATIONS
• Draw physostigmine and atropine into separate syringes.
• Always keep suction and cardiopulmonary resuscitation equipment and atropine available.
• Establish baseline heart rate and blood pressure. During administration, continue to monitor patient for tachycardia, bradycardia, arrhythmias, and hypotension. Immediately report significant changes to prescriber.
• Closely monitor patient for changes in level of consciousness. Because drug's action lasts for only 1 to 2 hours, patient may relapse into coma and need additional doses of the drug.
• Watch for signs and symptoms of cholinergic crisis such as excessive salivation, diaphoresis, miosis, nausea, vomiting, diarrhea, bradycardia or tachycardia, hypotension or hypertension, confusion, seizures, coma, severe muscle weakness, and paralysis. Reduce dosage if sweating or nausea occurs. If excessive salivation, vomiting, urination, cramping, or diarrhea occurs, stop drug and notify prescriber.
• Give 2 to 4 mg of atropine by direct injection at 3- to 10-minute intervals. Use 1 mg for children. Counteract ganglionic and skeletal muscle effects with pralidoxime. Institute mechanical ventilation and suction secretions frequently.
• *Alert:* Drug contains sodium bisulfite and benzyl alcohol.

PATIENT TEACHING
• Tell patient to promptly report adverse reactions.

• Explain use of drug and its administration to patient and family.
• Instruct patient to immediately report any discomfort at I.V. site.

phytonadione (vitamin K₁)*

Pharmacologic class: vitamin K derivative
Therapeutic class: nutritional supplement, blood coagulation modifier
Pregnancy risk category: C
pH: 3.5 to 7

INDICATIONS & DOSAGES
➤ **Drug-induced hypoprothrombinemia with existing or imminent bleeding—**
Adults: 2.5 to 10 mg I.V. q 6 to 8 hours, p.r.n., to a maximum dose of 50 mg. Dosage guided by coagulation studies.
➤ **Hypoprothrombinemia caused by factors limiting absorption or synthesis of vitamin K—**
Adults: 2 to 25 mg I.V., repeated p.r.n., to maximum dose of 50 mg.
Children: 5 to 10 mg I.V. Further dosage guided by coagulation studies.
Infants: 1 to 2 mg I.V. Further dosage guided by coagulation studies.

ADMINISTRATION
Direct injection: Using a 21G or 23G needle, inject diluted drug directly into vein or into I.V. tubing containing a free-flowing, compatible solution at a maximum rate of 1 mg/minute.
Intermittent infusion: Infuse diluted drug at a maximum rate of 1 mg/minute. Give over 3 hours. Wrap infusion container with aluminum foil or other dark cover.
Continuous infusion: Not recommended.

PREPARATION & STORAGE

Available in 0.5-ml ampules and 0.5-ml prefilled syringes as a 2-mg/ml concentration and in 2.5- and 5-ml multidose vials containing 10 mg/ml. Drug may contain benzyl alcohol.

Protect drug from light, even after dilution. For direct injection, dilute with 10 ml of preservative-free D_5W, normal saline solution, or dextrose 5% in normal saline solution. For infusion, dilute with 50 to 100 ml of any of these solutions.

Give immediately after dilution. Discard unused drug. May store drug in 1- or 2- ml Tubex cartridges at room temperature for 3 weeks.

Incompatibilities

Dobutamine, phenytoin sodium, ranitidine.

CONTRAINDICATIONS & CAUTIONS

- Contraindicated in those hypersensitive to vitamin K_1 or any component of the preparation.
- Use cautiously in those with hepatic impairment because drug may exacerbate the condition.

ADVERSE REACTIONS

CNS: convulsive movements, dizziness, dulled consciousness.
CV: *cardiac arrest,* chest pain, *circulatory collapse, shock,* transient hypotension, facial flushing.
GI: unusual taste.
Metabolic: cyanosis.
Respiratory: *bronchospasm,* dyspnea, *respiratory arrest.*
Other: *anaphylaxis and anaphylactoid reactions,* hyperhidrosis.

INTERACTIONS

Drug-drug. *Oral anticoagulants:* Decreases effect. Monitor patient and PT and INR closely.

EFFECTS ON LAB TEST RESULTS

- May increase bilirubin level in neonates.
- May decrease PT and INR.

ACTION

Promotes hepatic formation of coagulation factor II, factor VII; factor IX; and factor X.

PHARMACOKINETICS

Onset, 1 to 2 hours; duration, 12 to 14 hours.
Distribution: Briefly in liver, with small amounts in tissues, which are then destroyed. Drug crosses the placental barrier.
Metabolism: Rapidly, in liver.
Excretion: In urine and feces.

CLINICAL CONSIDERATIONS

- Osmolality: 325 mOsm/kg.
- *Alert:* I.V. use can be fatal; use only when other routes of administration aren't feasible.
- *Alert:* Watch for signs of flushing, weakness, tachycardia, and hypotension; may progress to shock.
- Monitor coagulation studies 12 hours after administration and repeat, as needed.
- Even dilution and slow infusion may not prevent severe reactions. To reverse vitamin K effects, give heparin or warfarin.
- Vitamin K_1 is used in hypoprothrombinemia caused by vitamin K deficiency or in moderate to severe bleeding caused by coumadin or indandione derivatives. It won't antagonize the action of heparin.

PATIENT TEACHING

- Explain use of drug to patient.
- Instruct patient to avoid hazardous activities if dizziness occurs.
- If patient will be sent home on oral anticoagulants, instruct him to restrict foods rich in vitamin K.

Reactions may be *common,* uncommon, *life-threatening,* or COMMON AND LIFE-THREATENING.

piperacillin sodium
Pipracil

Pharmacologic class: extended-spectrum bactericidal penicillin
Therapeutic class: antibiotic
Pregnancy risk category: B
pH: 5.5 to 7.5

INDICATIONS & DOSAGES
➤ **Severe systemic infections caused by susceptible organisms—**
Adults: 200 to 300 mg/kg I.V. or 12 to 18 g daily in divided doses q 4 to 6 hours.
Adjust-a-dose: If creatinine clearance is below 20 ml/minute give 4 g q 12 hours; if it's between 20 and 40 ml/minute, give 4 g I.V. q 8 hours.
➤ **Complicated UTIs—**
Adults: 125 to 200 mg/kg I.V. or 8 to 16 g I.V. daily in divided doses q 6 to 8 hours.
Adjust-a-dose: If creatinine clearance is below 20 ml/minute give 3 g I.V. q 12 hours; if it's between 20 and 40 ml/minute, give 3 g I.V. q 8 hours.
➤ **Uncomplicated UTIs—**
Adults: 100 to 125 mg/kg I.V. or 6 to 8 g I.V. daily in divided doses q 6 to 12 hours.
Adjust-a-dose: If creatinine clearance is below 20 ml/minute, give 3 g I.V. q 12 hours.
➤ **Acute *P. aeruginosa* infection in cystic fibrosis, in conjunction with aminoglycosides—**
Adults: 300 to 600 mg/kg I.V. daily.
➤ **Prophylaxis for abdominal surgery—**
Adults: 2 g I.V. before surgery, during surgery, and q 6 hours after surgery for up to 24 hours.
  Maximum daily adult dose for any indication, 24 g.

ADMINISTRATION
Direct injection: Inject reconstituted drug directly into vein over 3 to 5 minutes.
Intermittent infusion: Infuse reconstituted and diluted solution over 20 to 30 minutes.
Continuous infusion: Inject reconstituted 24-hour dose into daily I.V. volume. Infuse at rate necessary for delivery of needed fluid volume.

PREPARATION & STORAGE
Available in powder form in 2-, 3-, and 4-g vials.
  Reconstitute each gram of drug with 5 ml of sterile bacteriostatic water for injection or bacteriostatic sodium chloride injection. Shake vigorously to dissolve. For infusion, dilute reconstituted solution with at least 50 to 100 ml of D_5W, normal saline solution, dextrose 5% in normal saline solution, or lactated Ringer's.
  Store at room temperature. After reconstitution, drug remains stable for 24 hours at room temperature or for 7 days when refrigerated at 36° to 46° F (2° to 8° C), or for 1 month when frozen.

Incompatibilities
Aminoglycosides, amphotericin B, cisatracurium besylate, filgrastim, fluconazole, gemcitabine, ondansetron, sargramostim, vancomycin, vinorelbine.

CONTRAINDICATIONS & CAUTIONS
• Contraindicated in those hypersensitive to penicillins or cephalosporins.
• Contraindicated in children younger than age 12, because safe use hasn't been established.
• Use cautiously in those with hepatic or renal dysfunction because of increased risk of toxic reaction, and in those with ulcerative colitis because of increased risk of exacerbation.

- Use cautiously in patients with bleeding tendencies or decreased potassium levels.
- Use cautiously in those on sodium-restricted diets. Each gram of piperacillin sodium provides 42.5 mg (1.85 mEq) of sodium.
- Use cautiously in breast-feeding patients because drug appears in low levels in breast milk.

ADVERSE REACTIONS
CNS: headache, dizziness, fatigue.
CV: vein irritation.
GI: *pseudomembranous colitis,* diarrhea.
Hematologic: abnormal platelet aggregation, anemia, *leukopenia, neutropenia, thrombocytopenia.*
Metabolic: hypokalemia, hypernatremia.
Skin: phlebitis, *Stevens-Johnson syndrome,* rash; pain, induration, erythema at injection site
Other: *anaphylaxis, hypersensitivity reaction,* overgrowth of nonsusceptible organisms.

INTERACTIONS
Drug-drug. *Aminoglycosides:* Inactivates aminoglycoside. Avoid using together.
Anticoagulants: Enhances bleeding tendency from inhibition of platelet aggregation. Monitor patient, and PT and INR closely.
Hormonal contraceptives: May decrease efficacy of hormonal contraceptives. Recommend additional form of contraception during penicillin therapy.
Sulfinpyrazone, probenecid: Increases penicillin levels and possible toxic reaction from decreased renal excretion. May be used to increase levels; monitor patient closely.
Vecuronium: Prolongs neuromuscular blockade. Avoid using together.

EFFECTS ON LAB TEST RESULTS
- May increase BUN, creatinine, ALT, AST, alkaline phosphatase, bilirubin, LDH, and sodium levels. May decrease potassium level.
- May increase bleeding times and eosinophil count. May decrease hemoglobin, hematocrit, and platelet, WBC, neutrophil, and granulocyte counts.
- May cause false-positive result for urine glucose tests using copper reduction method (such as Clinitest) and for Coombs' test. May falsely decrease aminoglycoside level.

ACTION
Inhibits synthesis of cell-wall mucopeptide, rendering the wall unstable. Inadequate dosage may result in only bacteriostatic action. Active against susceptible gram-positive and gram-negative aerobic bacteria.

PHARMACOKINETICS
Onset, immediate; duration, 3 to 5 hours.
Distribution: Into most tissues. Usually low CSF levels but level increases in meningeal inflammation. Readily crosses the placental barrier and appears in small amounts in breast milk.
Metabolism: Minimal.
Excretion: Mostly in urine; 10% to 20% in feces. Usual half-life, 30 to 90 minutes; may be prolonged in neonates, infants, and patients with renal or hepatic impairment.

CLINICAL CONSIDERATIONS
- Osmolality: 346 to 399 mOsm/kg.
- Drug contains 1.85 mEq (42.5 mg) of sodium per 1 g of drug.
- *Alert:* Before giving drug, ask patient if he's had allergic reactions to penicillin.
- Obtain specimens for culture and sensitivity tests before giving first dose. Therapy may start before test results are available.

Reactions may be *common,* uncommon, *life-threatening,* or **COMMON AND LIFE-THREATENING.**

• To avoid vein irritation, change I.V. site every 48 hours or per facility policy.
• Closely monitor patient for possible hypersensitivity for at least 30 minutes after administration. Treat anaphylaxis symptomatically. Keep emergency equipment available.
• Check CBC frequently and monitor potassium level. Monitor PT and bleeding times.
• Establish baseline renal function, then periodically monitor renal, hepatic, and CV status in patients on prolonged therapy.
• Observe patient for fungal and bacterial superinfection with prolonged use.
• Although hemodialysis removes drug, peritoneal dialysis doesn't.

PATIENT TEACHING
• Instruct patient to inform prescriber if he experiences sore throat, fever, rash, easy bruising or bleeding.
• Tell patient to promptly report adverse reactions.
• Instruct patient to report discomfort at I.V. site immediately.

piperacillin sodium and tazobactam sodium
Tazocin ◊, Zosyn

Pharmacologic class: extended-spectrum penicillin, beta-lactamase inhibitor
Therapeutic class: antibiotic
Pregnancy risk category: B
pH: 4.5 to 6.8

INDICATIONS & DOSAGES
➤ **Appendicitis complicated by rupture or abscess, peritonitis, uncomplicated and complicated skin and skin structure infections, postpartum endometritis, pelvic inflammatory disease, and community-acquired pneumonia caused by piperacillin-resistant organisms—**
Adults: 12 g piperacillin and 1.5 g tazobactam, given as 3.375 g (3 g piperacillin and 0.375 g tazobactam) q 6 hours by I.V. infusion.
Adjust-a-dose: If creatinine clearance is 20 to 40 ml/minute, give 8 g of piperacillin and 1 g of tazobactam daily in divided doses of 2.25 g q 6 hours; if it's below 20 ml/minute, give 6 g of piperacillin and 0.75 g of tazobactam daily in divided doses of 2.25 g q 8 hours.
    In continuous ambulatory peritoneal dialysis (CAPD) patients, give 2.25 g q 12 hours. In hemodialysis patients, give 2.25 g q 12 hours with a supplemental dose of 0.75 g after each dialysis period.
➤ **Moderate to severe nosocomial pneumonia caused by piperacillin-resistant organisms—**
Adults: 4.5 g (4 g piperacillin/0.5 g tazobactam) I.V. q 6 hours in combination with aminoglycoside. Patients with *Pseudomonas aeruginosa* should continue aminoglycoside treatment; if *P. aeruginosa* hasn't been isolated, aminoglycoside treatment may be stopped. Duration of treatment, 7 to 14 days.
Adjust-a-dose: If creatinine clearance is 20 to 40 ml/minute, 3.375 g I.V. q 6 hours; if it's below 20 ml/minute, 2.25 g I.V. q 6 hours. In CAPD patients, 2.25 g I.V. q 8 hours. In hemodialysis patients, 2.25 g I.V. q 8 hours with a supplemental dose of 0.75 g after each dialysis period.

ADMINISTRATION
Direct injection: Not recommended.
Intermittent infusion: Infuse over 30 minutes.
Continuous infusion: Not recommended.

PREPARATION & STORAGE

Available as powder for injection in single-dose vials and as an iso-osmotic frozen solution containing 2 g of piperacillin and 0.25 g of tazobactam, 3 g of piperacillin and 0.375 g of tazobactam, 4 g of piperacillin and 0.5 g of tazobactam.

Reconstitute drug with 5 ml of suitable diluent for each 1 g of piperacillin. Shake well until dissolved. May further dilute to the desired volume of at least 50 to 150 ml. Drug is compatible with normal saline solution, sterile water for injection, dextran 6% in normal saline solution, D_5W, potassium chloride 40 mEq, bacteriostatic saline solution with parabens, bacteriostatic water with parabens, bacteriostatic water with benzyl alcohol, or bacteriostatic saline solution with benzyl alcohol.

Use reconstituted single-dose vials immediately. Discard unused portion after 24 hours if stored at room temperature or 48 hours if refrigerated. Don't freeze vials after reconstituting. After reconstitution, product is stable in I.V. bags for up to 24 hours at room temperature and up to 1 week if refrigerated. Also stable in ambulatory I.V. infusion pump for 12 hours at room temperature. ADD-Vantage system solution is stable for 24 hours at room temperature.

Thaw frozen iso-osmotic solution at room temperature or under refrigeration; don't thaw by warm water bath or microwave radiation. Don't refreeze thawed solutions. After thawing, solution is stable for 24 hours at room temperature or for 14 days under refrigeration.

Incompatibilities

Acyclovir sodium, aminoglycosides, amphotericin B, chlorpromazine, cisatracurium, cisplatin, dacarbazine, daunorubicin, dobutamine, doxorubicin, doxycycline hyclate, droperidol, famotidine, ganciclovir, gemcitabine, haloperidol lactate, hydroxyzine hydrochloride, idarubicin, lactated Ringer's solution, minocycline, mitomycin, mitoxantrone, nalbuphine, prochlorperazine edisylate, promethazine hydrochloride, streptozocin, vancomycin.

CONTRAINDICATIONS & CAUTIONS

● Contraindicated in those hypersensitive to penicillins, cephalosporins, or beta-lactam inhibitors.

● Use cautiously in those who have renal impairment, bleeding tendencies, uremia, or hypokalemia and in those who must restrict their sodium intake.

ADVERSE REACTIONS

CNS: agitation, anxiety, dizziness, pain, headache, *seizures,* insomnia, fever.

CV: hypertension, edema, chest pain.

EENT: rhinitis.

GI: abdominal pain, constipation, *diarrhea,* dyspepsia, nausea, **pseudomembranous colitis,** stool changes, vomiting.

GU: hematuria, proteinuria, pyuria.

Hematologic: eosinophilia, **leukopenia, neutropenia, thrombocytopenia.**

Metabolic: electrolyte abnormalities, hyperglycemia.

Respiratory: dyspnea.

Skin: pruritus, rash, ***Stevens-Johnson syndrome.***

Other: *anaphylaxis,* candidiasis.

INTERACTIONS

Drug-drug. *Aminoglycosides:* Inactivates aminoglycoside. Avoid using together.

Anticoagulants: Prolongs effectiveness. Monitor coagulation studies closely.

Hormonal contraceptives: May decrease efficacy of hormonal contraceptives. Recommend additional form of contraception during penicillin therapy.

Probenecid: Blocks tubular secretion of piperacillin. Probenecid may be used for this purpose.

Reactions may be *common,* uncommon, **life-threatening,** or COMMON AND LIFE-THREATENING.

Vecuronium: Prolongs neuromuscular blockade. Monitor patient closely.

EFFECTS ON LAB TEST RESULTS
• May increase BUN, creatinine, glucose, bilirubin, ALT, AST, alkaline phosphatase, and LDH levels, and urinary protein and blood levels. May decrease albumin level. May alter sodium, potassium, and calcium levels.
• May increase eosinophil and urinary WBC counts. May decrease hemoglobin and hematocrit and WBC, neutrophil, and platelet counts; may prolong PT and PTT.
• May cause false-positive result for urine glucose tests using copper reduction method (such as Clinitest) and for Coombs' test.

ACTION
Piperacillin component inhibits cell-wall synthesis during active bactericidal multiplication; tazobactam component inhibits beta-lactam enzymes, decreasing bacterial resistance to piperacillin.

PHARMACOKINETICS
Drug level peaks at end of infusion.
Distribution: To urine, bile, wound fluid, prostate, heart, gallbladder, fat, and skeletal muscle.
Metabolism: To minor active desethyl metabolite.
Excretion: In urine and bile.

CLINICAL CONSIDERATIONS
• *Alert:* Before giving drug, ask patient about any allergies to penicillin.
• Consider a diagnosis of pseudomembranous colitis in patients with persistent diarrhea.
• Obtain specimen for culture and sensitivity tests before giving first dose. Therapy may begin pending results.
• Monitor CBC, differential blood count, platelet count, and electrolyte level, especially potassium. Observe for occult bleeding.

• Monitor neurologic status; high drug levels may cause seizures when dosage isn't adjusted in those with renal impairment.
• Leukopenia and neutropenia may be reversible and are usually caused by prolonged therapy of more than 21 days.
• Because hemodialysis removes 6% of the piperacillin dose and 21% of the tazobactam dose, patient may need supplemental doses after hemodialysis.
• In patients with cystic fibrosis, there appears to be increased incidences of fever and rash.
• Bacterial and fungal superinfection may occur. Monitor patient carefully.
• Use drug with an aminoglycoside to treat infections caused by *P. aeruginosa.*
• Remember when treating patients requiring restricted sodium intake that drug contains 2.35 mEq (54 mg) of sodium per 1 g of piperacillin in combination product.

PATIENT TEACHING
• Instruct patient to inform prescriber if he experiences sore throat, fever, rash, and easy bruising or bleeding.
• Tell patient to promptly report adverse reactions and discomfort at the I.V. site.

plasma (fresh frozen plasma, liquid plasma)

Pharmacologic class: blood derivative
Therapeutic class: coagulant
Pregnancy risk category: NR

INDICATIONS & DOSAGES
➤ **Coagulation disorders from liver disease, DIC, congenital clotting factor deficiencies, and dilutional coagu-**

lopathy after massive blood replacement—

Adults: Dose reflects disorder and patient's condition.
Children: 15 to 30 ml/kg I.V. for acute hemorrhage and 10 to 15 ml/kg I.V. for clotting factor deficiency. Repeat p.r.n.

ADMINISTRATION

Direct injection: Not recommended.
Intermittent infusion: Give over 1 to 2 hours through a transfusion set containing a 170-micron filter. Begin transfusion slowly, following institutional guidelines. Take vital signs. If patient shows no evidence of a reaction, adjust flow to prescribed rate. Closely monitor patient throughout transfusion.
Continuous infusion: Not recommended.

PREPARATION & STORAGE

Before administration, thaw fresh frozen plasma at 99° F (37° C). Thawing takes 45 to 60 minutes. Then refrigerate at 39° F (4° C) for maximum of 24 hours, pending transfusion.

Liquid plasma may be refrigerated at 39° F for a maximum of 47 days or frozen at 0° F (-18° C) for maximum of 5 years.

Incompatibilities

All I.V. drugs and solutions, except normal saline solution.

CONTRAINDICATIONS & CAUTIONS

• Contraindicated for use as a volume expander because of risk of transmitting blood-borne viral disease, which doesn't occur with crystalloid or colloid solution.
• Contraindicated as a protein source in those with nutritional deficiencies.
• Avoid giving liquid plasma to replace clotting factors V and VIII because these factors degenerate rapidly in a liquid state.

ADVERSE REACTIONS

CV: flushing.
Hepatic: *hepatitis B, non-A and non-B hepatitis.*
Metabolic: volume overload.
Skin: itching, urticaria.
Other: *AIDS, anaphylaxis,* CMV infection.

INTERACTIONS

None reported.

EFFECTS ON LAB TEST RESULTS

None reported.

COMPOSITION

Fresh frozen plasma and liquid plasma each contain 91% water, 2% carbohydrates, and 7% proteins, specifically globulins, antibodies, and clotting factors. Freezing within 6 hours of collection preserves all clotting factors—about 1 unit/ml. Storage in liquid state results in loss of clotting factors V and VIII. One unit of plasma has a volume of 200 to 250 ml.

CLINICAL CONSIDERATIONS

• Follow facility policy for giving blood and blood products.
• Plasma contains virtually no RBCs, making RBC crossmatching unnecessary. Plasma should be ABO compatible with recipient RBCs: Recipient type A is compatible with plasma type A or AB; type B, with B or AB; type AB, with AB; and type O, with O, A, B, or AB.
• Before requesting release of plasma from the blood bank, record vital signs and establish a patent venous catheter.
• To reduce risk of volume overload, use clotting factor concentrates, such as cryoprecipitate, lyophilized factors VIII and IX, if available. If volume overload occurs, stop transfusion and keep vein open with a slow drip of normal saline solution. Place patient's feet in a dependent position, and notify prescriber.

Treat symptomatically and give a diuretic.
• Rh type is insignificant. Patient can receive either Rh-positive or Rh-negative plasma.
• Acute onset of anaphylaxis is accompanied by anxiety, urticaria, and wheezing, progressing to cyanosis, shock, and cardiac arrest. Stop transfusion immediately at the hub of the needle, and keep vein open with normal saline solution. Notify prescriber. Support blood pressure, prepare 0.4 ml of 1:1,000 epinephrine for injection, and treat symptomatically.
• If flushing, itching, or urticaria occurs, slow transfusion until symptoms resolve. Give antihistamines if needed.

PATIENT TEACHING
• Tell patient to immediately report unusual symptoms.
• Explain therapy and related tests to patient.

plasma protein fraction 5%
Plasmanate, Plasma-Plex, Plasmatein, Protenate

Pharmacologic class: blood derivative
Therapeutic class: plasma volume expander
Pregnancy risk category: C
pH: 6.7 to 7.3

INDICATIONS & DOSAGES
➤ **Hypovolemic shock—**
Adults: Initially, 250 to 500 ml I.V. (12.5 to 25 g protein).
Infants and children: Initially, 6.6 to 33 ml/kg I.V. (0.33 to 1.65 g protein). Rate and volume reflect patient's condition and response.
➤ **Hypoproteinemia—**
Adults: 1,000 to 1,500 ml I.V. daily. Larger doses may be needed in severe

hypoproteinemia with continuing loss of plasma proteins.

ADMINISTRATION
Direct injection: Not recommended.
Intermittent infusion: Infuse undiluted or in combination with other parenteral solutions, such as whole blood, plasma, normal saline solution, glucose, or sodium lactate. Don't give near site of infection or trauma. Infusion rate depends on response but shouldn't exceed 10 ml/minute. Faster rates may result in sudden hypotension. As volume approaches normal, reduce rate to 5 to 8 ml/minute. In infants and children, infuse at 5 to 10 ml/minute. Make sure administration set has adequate filter, which the manufacturer provides.
Continuous infusion: Not recommended.

PREPARATION & STORAGE
Plasma protein fraction (PPF) is ready for use. Solution is available in 50-, 250-, and 500-ml vials. Solution varies from nearly colorless to straw color to dark brown.
    Drug is compatible with whole blood, packed red blood cells, and standard I.V. carbohydrate and electrolyte solutions.
    Store at room temperature, not more than 86° F (30° C). Don't use if solution is cloudy, has been frozen, or contains sediment. Give within 4 hours of opening container. Use bottle only once; it contains no preservatives. Discard unused portion.

Incompatibilities
Alcohol-containing solutions, norepinephrine, protein hydrolysates.

CONTRAINDICATIONS & CAUTIONS
• Contraindicated in those with allergic reactions to albumin or other plasma-containing products.
• Contraindicated in those with nutritional deficiencies because of increased

risk of viral infection and in those with cardiac failure because of increased risk of pulmonary edema.
• Contraindicated in those with severe anemia because increased blood volume significantly reduces hemoglobin level and in those having cardiopulmonary bypass surgery because rapid infusion may cause hypotension.
• Contraindicated in first 24 hours after burn injury because of rapid protein loss.
• Use cautiously in those with hepatic or renal failure because of added protein, fluid, and sodium and in those with hypertension, cardiac disease, and severe pulmonary infection because of increased blood volume and blood pressure after infusion.

ADVERSE REACTIONS
CNS: headache, fever.
CV: *hypotension, vascular overload,* flushing, tachycardia.
GI: hypersalivation, nausea, vomiting.
Musculoskeletal: back pain.
Respiratory: *pulmonary edema.*
Skin: erythema, urticaria.
Other: *anaphylaxis,* Creutzfeldt-Jakob disease, chills.

INTERACTIONS
None reported.

EFFECTS ON LAB TEST RESULTS
• May increase alkaline phosphatase level.

COMPOSITION
PPF is a 5% solution of proteins derived from pooled human blood, serum, or plasma containing 83% to 90% albumin and no more than 17% globulin and other proteins. Each milliliter of PPF contains 4.4 g of albumin. Solution is isotonic and equivalent to normal plasma, both osmotically and oncotically. Because blood group isoagglutinins have been removed, PPF may be given without regard to patient's blood group. Its sodium content is 130 to 160 mEq/L.

CLINICAL CONSIDERATIONS
• Although PPF is a pooled human plasma derivative, crossmatching isn't needed.
• PPF isn't normally used for temporary albumin redistribution from major surgery.
• Frequently monitor blood pressure in shock patients; widening pulse pressure correlates with increased stroke volume or cardiac output. Hypotension risk is greater when infusion rates exceed 10 ml/minute.
• Stop infusion if blood pressure suddenly falls. Correct with vasopressors.
• Watch for signs of vascular overload (heart failure, pulmonary edema, widening pulse pressure).
• If allergic reaction occurs, stop drug and give antihistamines.
• Monitor hemoglobin level; increased blood volume may cause significant fall. Transfusion of whole blood or packed RBCs may be needed.
• Monitor albumin levels in patients with hypoproteinemia. Treating the underlying disorder and replacing amino acids and proteins restores albumin levels more effectively than PPF or albumin infusions.
• After PPF infusion, closely observe injured or postoperative patient; elevated blood pressure may cause bleeding from severed blood vessels that may not have bled at lower blood pressure.
• If patient is dehydrated, give additional fluids either P.O. or I.V.
• Each liter contains 130 to 160 mEq of sodium.

PATIENT TEACHING
• Tell patient to immediately report unusual symptoms.
• Explain therapy and related tests to the patient.

platelets (thrombocytes)
Platelet Concentrate

Pharmacologic class: blood derivative
Therapeutic class: clotting factor
Pregnancy risk category: NR

INDICATIONS & DOSAGES
➤ **To treat or prevent hemorrhage in thrombocytopenia or platelet dysfunction—**
Adults: 4 to 10 units I.V., depending on patient's condition.
Children: 1 unit/7 to 10 kg I.V.

ADMINISTRATION
Direct injection: Draw prefiltered platelet concentrate into a syringe, and inject slowly through a 19G to 23G catheter. Direct injection is used primarily in neonatal transfusion.
Intermittent infusion: Infuse through blood component recipient set with a 170-micron filter via a 19G to 21G needle. Begin infusion slowly, according to facility guidelines. Take vital signs. Adjust flow gradually to prescribed rate and closely monitor the patient. Infuse as rapidly as patient can tolerate, within 4 hours or less. Blood bank can reduce volume if circulatory overload is a risk. Avoid passing platelet concentrates through depth-type filters. Also, don't use recipient sets with rubber connections, to which platelets can adhere.
Continuous infusion: Not recommended.

PREPARATION & STORAGE
Random-donor platelets are separated from 1 unit of whole blood within 6 hours of collection. Usually, multiple units are pooled into a single container to provide the needed dose. Single-donor platelets are prepared by platelet pheresis. Store at room temperature in the blood bank for maximum of 5 days. After sterile seal is broken, give within 4 hours.

Incompatibilities
All I.V. drugs and solutions, except normal saline solution.

CONTRAINDICATIONS & CAUTIONS
• Contraindicated in those with bleeding caused by abnormal clotting factors.
• Contraindicated in those with rapid platelet destruction, as in idiopathic thrombocytopenic purpura or untreated DIC.
• Contraindicated in those with thrombocytopenia caused by septicemia or hypersplenism because platelets wouldn't be effective.
• Human leukocyte antigen (HLA)–matched platelets are unnecessary in those for whom HLA antibodies haven't been documented.

ADVERSE REACTIONS
CNS: anxiety, headache.
CV: flushing.
Hepatic: *hepatitis B, hepatitis C.*
Musculoskeletal: myalgia.
Skin: pruritus, urticaria.
Other: *AIDS,* alloimmunization, *anaphylaxis,* chills, Creutzfeldt-Jakob disease, CMV infection, febrile nonhemolytic reactions.

INTERACTIONS
None reported.

EFFECTS ON LAB TEST RESULTS
• May increase platelet count.

COMPOSITION
Platelets are irregularly shaped disks about half the size of RBCs. They migrate and adhere to damaged blood vessels to stop bleeding. Normal platelet count is 150,000 to 400,000/mm^3. Random-donor platelets are derived

from 1 unit of whole blood containing at least 5.5×10^{10} platelets and a variable number of lymphocytes suspended in 50 to 70 ml of plasma. With single-donor platelets, 1 unit contains at least 3×10^{11} platelets, equivalent to 6 random units, and a variable number of lymphocytes suspended in 200 to 400 ml of plasma.

CLINICAL CONSIDERATIONS

● Document thrombocytopenia or platelet dysfunction before giving platelets.

● Because of increased risk of hemorrhage, nonbleeding patients with platelet level below 20,000/mm³ and surgical patients with levels less than 100,000/mm³ may require platelet therapy. Platelets may also be used to treat hemorrhage if platelet count is below 50,000/mm³.

● Because platelets contain few RBCs, RBC crossmatching isn't needed. However, platelet-rich plasma should be ABO compatible with recipient RBCs if volume exceeds 120 ml for adults or 1 to 2 ml/kg for infants and children.

● Alloimmunization occurs in many previously transfused or pregnant patients. It may inhibit platelet survival and cause febrile, nonhemolytic reactions. Giving HLA-matched platelets may prevent premature platelet destruction if anti-HLA antibodies have formed.

● Single-donor platelet transfusion reduces risk of disease transmission and HLA antibody formation.

● Record vital signs and establish a patent venous catheter before requesting the release of platelets from the blood bank. Allow 15 to 30 minutes for blood bank to prepare and label platelets.

● If flushing, itching, or urticaria occurs, slow transfusion until symptoms resolve; prescriber may prescribe antihistamines.

● If patient develops febrile, non-hemolytic reaction, stop transfusion. Keep vein open with normal saline solution, and treat symptomatically. Give an antipyretic. Leukocyte-poor platelets prepared by resedimentation may prevent recurrence.

● Treat anaphylaxis by stopping transfusion at the hub of the needle and by keeping vein open with normal saline solution. Notify prescriber. Provide symptomatic treatment. Prepare 0.4 ml of 1:1,000 epinephrine for injection.

PATIENT TEACHING

● Instruct patient to immediately report unusual symptoms.

● Explain therapy and related tests to patient.

polymyxin B sulfate

Pharmacologic class: polymyxin antibiotic
Therapeutic class: bactericidal antibiotic
Pregnancy risk category: NR
pH: 5 to 7.5

INDICATIONS & DOSAGES

➤ **Acute UTI or septicemia caused by sensitive organisms—**
Adults and children ages 2 and older: 15,000 to 25,000 units/kg I.V. daily divided q 12 hours.
Children younger than age 2: Up to 40,000 units/kg I.V. daily divided q 12 hours.
Adjust-a-dose: If creatinine clearance is above 20 ml/minute, give 75% to 100% of usual daily dose q 12 hours; if clearance is between 5 and 20 ml/minute, give 50% of usual dose divided q 12 hours; and if clearance is below 5 ml/minute, give 15% of usual dose divided q 12 hours.

ADMINISTRATION

Direct injection: Not recommended.
Intermittent infusion: Infuse diluted drug over 60 to 90 minutes.
Continuous infusion: Add daily dose to total fluids scheduled for compatible infusion over 24 hours. Rate depends on volume.

PREPARATION & STORAGE

Available as powder in 500,000-unit vials.
  Dilute in 300 to 500 ml D₅W.
  Protect vials from light and store below 86° F (30° C). Store solution in refrigerator, and use within 72 hours.

Incompatibilities

Alkalies and strong acid solutions, ampicillin sodium, amphotericin B, calcium salts, cefazolin, chloramphenicol sodium succinate, chlorothiazide, heparin sodium, magnesium.

CONTRAINDICATIONS & CAUTIONS

• Use only if less toxic antibiotics are ineffective.
• Contraindicated in patients hypersensitive to the drug.
• Use cautiously in those with renal impairment or nitrogen retention because of possible nephrotoxicity and neurotoxicity.
• Use cautiously in those with myasthenia gravis.

ADVERSE REACTIONS

CNS: ataxia, *coma,* confusion, dizziness, drowsiness, *neurotoxicity with respiratory paralysis,* paresthesia, *seizures,* slurred speech, weakness, fever.
CV: thrombophlebitis, flushing.
EENT: blurred vision, nystagmus.
GU: albuminuria, azotemia, *nephrotoxicity.*
Hematologic: eosinophilia.
Respiratory: *apnea.*
Skin: urticaria.

Other: *anaphylaxis,* bacterial and fungal superinfections.

INTERACTIONS

Drug-drug. *Anesthetics, neuromuscular blockers:* May cause respiratory paralysis because of neuromuscular blockade. Avoid using together.
Nephrotoxic drugs: Has additive nephrotoxicity. Monitor renal function tests.

EFFECTS ON LAB TEST RESULTS

• May increase BUN and creatinine levels.
• May increase eosinophil count.

ACTION

Drug alters permeability of the cell-wall membrane of bacteria, resulting in cell leakage. Active against most aerobic gram-negative bacilli, except for most species of *Proteus* and *Neisseria.*

PHARMACOKINETICS

Drug level peak, unknown.
Distribution: Widely, to tissues. Drug doesn't cross the placental barrier or appear in CSF, even with inflamed meninges, synovial fluid, or aqueous humor. Unknown if drug appears in breast milk.
Metabolism: Unknown.
Excretion: Primarily by glomerular filtration. Half-life, about 4 to 6 hours in adults, 2 to 3 days if creatinine clearance is below 10 ml/minute; 8 hours in infants.

CLINICAL CONSIDERATIONS

• Osmolality: 10 mOsm/kg.
• Give only to hospitalized patients for whom baseline renal function tests have been performed.
• Obtain specimens for culture and sensitivity tests before starting therapy. Therapy may begin pending test results.

• If drug is used with an anesthetic or neuromuscular blocker, keep ventilatory support equipment available.
• During therapy, monitor renal function, intake and output, and drug levels, especially in those with renal impairment. Adjust dosage, as needed.
• If urine output declines, creatinine or BUN level rises, or patient develops respiratory paralysis, stop drug.
• Watch for signs of bacterial or fungal superinfection, and treat appropriately if superinfection occurs.
• Dialysis doesn't remove appreciable amounts of drug.

PATIENT TEACHING
• Instruct patient to notify prescriber if difficulty in breathing or change in voiding pattern occurs.
• Instruct patient to take in plenty of fluids, if not contraindicated, to maintain adequate urine output.

potassium chloride

Pharmacologic class: potassium supplement
Therapeutic class: therapeutic drug for electrolyte balance
Pregnancy risk category: C
pH: 4 to 8

INDICATIONS & DOSAGES
➤ **Hypokalemia**—
Adults and children: Use I.V. potassium chloride when oral replacement isn't feasible. Maximum dose of diluted I.V. potassium chloride is 20 mEq/hour at 40 mEq/L. Further dose based on potassium determinations.

  Further doses are based on potassium levels and blood pH. I.V. potassium replacement should be carried out only with ECG monitoring and frequent potassium determinations.

➤ **Severe hypokalemia**—
Adults and children: Potassium chloride should be diluted in a suitable I.V. solution of less than 80 mEq/L and given at no more than 40 mEq/hour. Further dose based on potassium determinations. Don't exceed 150 mEq I.V. daily in adults, and 3 mEq/kg I.V. daily or 40 mEq/m^2 daily for children. I.V. potassium replacement should be carried out only with ECG monitoring and frequent potassium determinations.
➤ **Acute MI ♦**—
Adults: High dose, 80 mEq/L at 1.5 ml/kg/hour for 24 hours with an I.V. infusion of 25% dextrose and 50 units/L regular insulin. Low dose, 40 mEq/L at 1 ml/kg/hour for 24 hours, with an I.V. infusion of 10% dextrose and 20 units/L regular insulin.

ADMINISTRATION
Direct injection: Not used.
Intermittent infusion: Infuse diluted solution slowly, not to exceed 10 to 20 mEq/hour. Overly rapid infusion can cause fatal hyperkalemia. Infusion rate shouldn't exceed 1 mEq/minute for adults or 0.02 mEq/kg/minute for children.
Continuous infusion: Same as intermittent infusion.

PREPARATION & STORAGE
Supplied as injection for I.V. infusion 0.1 mEq/ml, 0.2 mEq/ml, 0.3 mEq/ml, 0.4 mEq/ml; and injection concentrate 1.5 mEq/ml, 2 mEq/ml.
  Always dilute before use. Dilution varies widely, but potassium concentration usually shouldn't exceed 40 mEq/L. In emergencies, maximum concentration of 80 mEq/L may be temporarily exceeded.
  Store at room temperature.

Incompatibilities
Amikacin, amphotericin B, diazepam, dobutamine, ergotamine, fat emulsion 10%, methylprednisolone sodium suc-

cinate, penicillin G sodium, phenytoin sodium, promethazine hydrochloride.

CONTRAINDICATIONS & CAUTIONS

• Contraindicated in patients with severe renal impairment, untreated Addison's disease, hyperkalemia, acute dehydration, heat cramps, or burns because elevated potassium levels can exacerbate these conditions.
• Use cautiously in those with cardiac disorders because potassium may trigger conduction disturbances and in those with myotonia congenita because potassium may worsen symptoms.
• Use cautiously in those who require a cardiac glycoside and in those with renal impairment because of increased risk of hyperkalemia.
• Use cautiously in breast-feeding patients.

ADVERSE REACTIONS

CNS: anxiety, confusion, paresthesia, fatigue.
CV: *arrhythmias, cardiac arrest, heart block,* ECG changes, hypotension.
Metabolic: *hyperkalemia.*
Musculoskeletal: leg heaviness or weakness.
Respiratory: *respiratory paralysis,* dyspnea.
Skin: *phlebitis and pain at injection site.*

INTERACTIONS

Drug-drug. *ACE inhibitors, potassium-sparing diuretics:* May cause severe hyperkalemia. Use with extreme caution; monitor potassium level closely.
Corticosteroids: May decrease effectiveness of potassium supplements. Monitor patient closely.
Digoxin: Hypokalemia may cause digoxin toxicity. Use cautiously together and monitor potassium and digoxin levels.
Drug-food. *Salt substitutes containing potassium salts:* May cause hyperkalemia. Avoid using together.

EFFECTS ON LAB TEST RESULTS

• May increase potassium level.

ACTION

Essential for enzymatic reactions and nerve impulse transmission in the heart, brain, and skeletal muscle and for maintaining normal renal function, acid-base balance, and cellular metabolic processes.

PHARMACOKINETICS

Onset, immediate; duration, unknown.
Distribution: In extracellular fluid and cells. Drug appears in breast milk.
Metabolism: None.
Excretion: In urine, with small amounts in sweat and feces.

CLINICAL CONSIDERATIONS

• Osmolarity: 3,000 mOsm/L for 1.5 mEq/ml solution; 4,000 mOsm/L for 2 mEq/ml solution.
• Osmolality: 2 mEq/ml is 3,440 to 4,355 mOsm/kg; 7.5% solution is 1,895 mOsm/kg.
• *Alert:* Never give potassium chloride undiluted.
• Potassium chloride is usually the salt of choice in treating hypokalemia; the chloride ion corrects hypochloremia, which commonly accompanies hypokalemia.
• In dehydrated patients, give 1 L of potassium-free fluid before potassium therapy.
• Review renal function tests before giving potassium. Adequate renal function is essential to prevent hyperkalemia.
• Adding concentrated potassium chloride solutions to a hanging flexible plastic container can cause hyperkalemia because of inadequate mixing. When adding potassium solutions, invert the plastic container to avoid pooling of concentrated potassium at its base. Then knead the container to mix contents.

• Don't give potassium chloride post-operatively until urine flow is established.

• Monitor intake and output, ECG, pH, and potassium, BUN, and creatinine levels.

• If patient develops signs of renal dysfunction, especially oliguria and elevated creatinine levels, stop infusion.

• For patients receiving a cardiac glycoside, treat hyperkalemia with caution; rapid reduction of potassium levels may result in a toxic reaction.

• If overdose occurs, stop potassium-containing foods and drugs. Give insulin I.V. in dextrose 10% to 25% solution (10 units insulin/20 g dextrose) at 300 to 500 ml/hour. Also give sodium bicarbonate I.V. to correct acidosis. May use exchange resins, hemodialysis, or peritoneal dialysis.

PATIENT TEACHING

• Instruct patient to inform prescriber of adverse symptoms, including irregular or rapid heartbeats.

• Instruct patient to immediately notify prescriber if discomfort occurs at I.V. site.

potassium phosphate

Pharmacologic class: potassium supplement
Therapeutic class: therapeutic drug for electrolyte balance
Pregnancy risk category: C
pH: 7 to 7.8

INDICATIONS & DOSAGES

➤ **Electrolyte imbalance—**
Adults: Equivalent of 10 to 15 mmol or 310 to 465 mg I.V. of phosphorus per liter of total parenteral nutrition solution.
Children: Equivalent of 1.5 to 2 mmol/kg/day or 46.5 to 62 mg/kg/day I.V. of

phosphorus. Dose must be individualized.

ADMINISTRATION

Direct injection: Not recommended.
Intermittent infusion: Infuse diluted solution slowly over the ordered time to avoid phosphate intoxication and severe hyperkalemia. Rate must be individualized and shouldn't exceed 10 to 20 mEq/hour.
Continuous infusion: Same as intermittent infusion.

PREPARATION & STORAGE

Supplied in 5-, 10-, 15-, and 30-ml vials. Available strength is equivalent to 3 mmol or 93 mg/ml of phosphate and 4.4 mEq/ml of potassium.

For infusion, dilute and thoroughly mix in a larger volume of compatible fluid (D_5W or normal saline solution).

Store at room temperature.

Incompatibilities

Dobutamine and solutions that contain calcium and magnesium, such as lactated Ringer's, Ringer's injection, dextrose 5% and Ringer's injection, dextrose 10% in normal saline solution, and Ionosol D-CM, Ionosol D-CM in D_5W, Ionosol D with invert sugar 10%, and Ionosol D modified with invert sugar 10%.

CONTRAINDICATIONS & CAUTIONS

• Contraindicated in those with hyperkalemia, hyperphosphatemia, infected urolithiasis caused by magnesium ammonium phosphate stones, or severe renal dysfunction because of increased risk of toxic reaction.

• Use cautiously in those with hypoparathyroidism because of increased risk of hyperphosphatemia and in those with osteomalacia, acute pancreatitis, chronic renal disease, or vitamin D deficiency because of increased risk of hypocalcemia.

• Use cautiously in those with cardiac disorders, especially those taking a cardiac glycoside, because elevated potassium levels can cause conduction disturbances.

• Use cautiously in those with Addison's disease, acute dehydration, myotonia congenita, severe renal insufficiency, or extensive tissue necrosis resulting from severe burns because of possible hyperkalemia.

ADVERSE REACTIONS

CNS: confusion, dizziness, headache, paresthesia, *seizures,* fatigue, weakness.
CV: *cardiac depression, arrhythmia.*
GU: oliguria.
Metabolic: hypocalcemic tetany, *hyperkalemia,* hyperphosphatemia.
Musculoskeletal: arm and leg pain, bone and joint pain, heaviness of legs, muscle cramps.
Respiratory: dyspnea.
Skin: phlebitis, pain at injection site.
Other: edema of hands and feet.

INTERACTIONS

Drug-drug. *ACE inhibitors, potassium-containing drugs, potassium-sparing diuretics:* May cause hyperkalemia. Use with caution; monitor potassium level closely.
Cardiac glycosides: Increases risk of arrhythmias if hyperkalemia occurs. Monitor potassium level and ECG closely.

EFFECTS ON LAB TEST RESULTS

• May increase potassium and phosphate levels. May decrease calcium level.

• May decrease bone uptake of technetium-99m in radionuclide bone imaging.

ACTION

Helps to maintain acid-base equilibrium of renal tubular fluids, regulate renal excretion of hydrogen ions, and acidify urine.

PHARMACOKINETICS

Onset, immediate; duration, unknown.
Distribution: Into extracellular fluid and cells.
Metabolism: Unknown.
Excretion: 90% in kidneys; 10% in feces.

CLINICAL CONSIDERATIONS

• Osmolarity: 12 mOsm/ml.
• *Alert:*Never give potassium phosphate undiluted.
• Don't give postoperatively until urine flow is established.
• I.V. infusion of phosphates in high concentrations can cause hypocalcemia.
• Frequently monitor electrolyte levels, including calcium, phosphorus, potassium, and sodium, and renal function, including BUN and creatinine levels. Also monitor ECG for signs of conduction disturbances.

PATIENT TEACHING

• Instruct patient to inform prescriber of irregular or rapid heartbeat.
• Tell patient to promptly report adverse reactions and any discomfort at the I.V. site.

pralidoxime chloride
Protopam Chloride

Pharmacologic class: cholinesterase reactivator
Therapeutic class: antidote
Pregnancy risk category: C
pH: 3.5 to 4.5

INDICATIONS & DOSAGES
➤**Poisoning by organophosphate anticholinesterases—**
Adults: 1 to 2 g I.V. Give atropine at the same time at doses of 2 to 6 mg every 5 to 60 minutes until muscarinic signs and symptoms subside; repeat in 1 hour if signs and symptoms reappear.

Children: 20 to 40 mg/kg I.V. May be repeated in 1 hour if weakness persists.

➤ **Overdose of anticholinesterases (including ambenonium, neostigmine, and pyridostigmine) used in myasthenia gravis—**

Adults: Initially, 1 to 2 g I.V., then 250 mg I.V. q 5 minutes.

➤ **Exposure to nerve agents in chemical warfare—**

Adults, children, and infants: 15 mg/kg I.V. Maximum 1 g I.V.

Elderly: 5 to 10 mg/kg I.V.

Adjust-a-dose: Reduce dosage in patients with renal impairment.

ADMINISTRATION

Direct injection: Inject dose over at least 5 minutes directly into vein or into I.V. tubing containing a free-flowing, compatible solution. Injection rate shouldn't exceed 200 mg/minute.

Intermittent infusion: Dilute with normal saline solution to a volume of 100 ml and infuse diluted drug over 15 to 30 minutes.

Continuous infusion: Not recommended.

PREPARATION & STORAGE

Supplied in a 20-ml vial containing 1 g of drug in white to off-white porous cake.

Reconstitute with 20 ml of sterile water for injection, without preservatives, for a concentration of 50 mg/ml. For I.V. infusion, the calculated dose of reconstituted solution is further diluted to a volume of 100 ml of normal saline solution.

Store vial at room temperature. Use solution within a few hours.

Incompatibilities

None reported.

CONTRAINDICATIONS & CAUTIONS

• Contraindicated in those hypersensitive to any component of the drug.

• Contraindicated in those with carbaryl exposure because pralidoxime may increase carbaryl toxicity.

• Contraindicated in those taking concomitant morphine, aminophylline, theophylline, or succinylcholine.

• Use cautiously in those receiving an anticholinesterase for myasthenia gravis because drug may precipitate myasthenic crisis.

• Always give drug under close medical supervision.

ADVERSE REACTIONS

CNS: dizziness, drowsiness, headache.
CV: hypertension, tachycardia.
EENT: blurred vision, diplopia.
GI: nausea.
Musculoskeletal: muscle weakness.
Respiratory: hyperventilation, laryngospasm.
Skin: maculopapular rash.

INTERACTIONS

Drug-drug. *Anticholinergics:* May cause earlier reactions of flushing, mydriasis, tachycardia, and dry nose and mouth. Use with caution; monitor patient closely.

Barbiturates: Barbiturates are potentiated by anticholinesterase exposure. Use cautiously, especially when treating convulsions.

EFFECTS ON LAB TEST RESULTS

• May increase ALT, AST, and CK levels for 2 weeks after drug administration.

ACTION

Reactivates phosphorylated and carbamylated cholinesterase at neuromuscular junctions and autonomic effector sites and, to a lesser degree, within the CNS. Cholinesterase reactivation reverses anticholinesterase-induced paralysis of respiratory and skeletal muscles.

PHARMACOKINETICS
Onset, 5 to 15 minutes after injection; duration, unknown.
Distribution: Throughout extracellular fluid, with poor protein binding. Drug penetrates the CNS. Unknown if drug appears in breast milk.
Metabolism: May occur in liver.
Excretion: Rapidly, in urine. Half-life, 74 to 77 minutes.

CLINICAL CONSIDERATIONS
• During administration, keep oxygen available as well as equipment for suctioning, emergency tracheotomy, and gastric lavage.
• Give atropine at the same time, to treat poisoning with organophosphate anticholinesterases. Watch closely for signs and symptoms of atropine toxicity, such as blurred vision, delirium, dry mouth, excitement, hallucinations, and tachycardia. Concurrent administration speeds onset of toxic effects.
• Not effective for treating poisoning resulting from phosphorus, inorganic phosphates, or organophosphates with no anticholinesterase activity.
• Monitor vital signs, and intake and output.
• Reduce administration rate or stop drug if patient develops hypertension. Give 5 mg of phentolamine I.V.
• If patient has ingested poison, carefully monitor patient for 48 to 72 hours because of possible delayed intestinal absorption.
• Observe for rapid weakening in myasthenia gravis patients treated for overdose of carbamate anticholinesterases. Patients can pass quickly from cholinergic crisis to myasthenic crisis. Keep edrophonium available to establish differential diagnosis and to help reverse myasthenic crisis.
• If overdose occurs, give artificial respiration and other supportive measures, as needed. It may be difficult to differentiate adverse reactions caused by the drug or the poison.

PATIENT TEACHING
• Instruct patient to inform prescriber immediately of breathing difficulty.
• Tell patient to promptly report other adverse reactions.
• Explain use of drug and its administration to patient and family.

prednisolone sodium phosphate
Hydeltrasol, Key-Pred-SP

Pharmacologic class: synthetic glucocorticoid, mineralocorticoid
Therapeutic class: anti-inflammatory, immunosuppressant
Pregnancy risk category: C
pH: 7 to 8

INDICATIONS & DOSAGES
➤ **Severe inflammation, immunosuppression—**
Adults: 5 to 60 mg I.V. daily
Children: Initially, 0.14 to 2 mg/kg/day I.V. or 4 to 60 mg/m^2/day I.V. in 3 or 4 divided doses.

ADMINISTRATION
Direct injection: Inject undiluted drug over 1 minute.
Intermittent infusion: Infuse ordered dose over prescribed duration.
Continuous infusion: Infuse ordered dose over prescribed duration.

PREPARATION & STORAGE
Available in 2-, 5-, and 10-ml vials containing 20 mg/ml.
   For infusion, dilute with D$_5$W, normal saline solution, or dextrose 5% in normal saline solution.
   Store between 59° and 86° F (15° and 30° C). Protect from freezing and light.

Incompatibilities

Calcium gluconate, dimenhydrinate, methotrexate sodium, polymyxin B, prochlorperazine edisylate, promazine, promethazine hydrochloride.

CONTRAINDICATIONS & CAUTIONS

• Contraindicated in those hypersensitive to corticosteroids or to any component of prednisolone.
• Contraindicated in those with sepsis or septic shock because of anti-inflammatory and immunosuppressive effects.
• Use cautiously in those with systemic fungal infections or uncontrolled viral or bacterial infections, because drug may exacerbate these infections.
• Use cautiously in those with open-angle glaucoma because drug may raise intraocular pressure, and in those with renal impairment or renal calculi because drug may exacerbate fluid retention.
• Use cautiously in those with hyperlipidemia because drug may further increase fatty acid or cholesterol levels, and in those with myasthenia gravis because drug may worsen weakness initially and produce respiratory distress.
• Use cautiously in those with osteoporosis because drug may exacerbate bone loss, and in those with diabetes mellitus and latent or active tuberculosis or a positive skin test for tuberculosis, because drug may exacerbate or activate these disorders.
• Use cautiously in those with AIDS or a predisposition to AIDS because of increased risk of severe, uncontrollable infections and neoplasms.
• Use cautiously in those with hepatic impairment because of increased risk of toxic reaction.
• Use cautiously in those with hypoalbuminemia or a condition predisposing them to this disorder, such as cirrhosis or nephrotic syndrome, because of increased risk of toxic reaction.

• Use cautiously in those with ocular herpes simplex infections because of possible corneal perforation.
• Use cautiously in those with hyperthyroidism because increased metabolism may reduce drug effects, and in those with hypothyroidism because decreased metabolism may enhance drug effects.
• Use cautiously in those with cardiac disease, heart failure, or hypertension, because fluid retention may be hazardous.
• Use cautiously in children and in geriatric patients. Children may develop increased intracranial pressure, causing papilledema, oculomotor or abducens nerve paralysis, vision loss, and headache; geriatric patients may develop hypertension.

ADVERSE REACTIONS

CNS: anxiety, pain, vertigo, headache, paresthesia, depression or other mood changes, hallucinations, restlessness, *seizures, pseudotumor cerebri, euphoria, insomnia.*
CV: *arrhythmias after rapid and high dose infusion, heart failure, thromboembolism,* chest pain, facial flushing, hypertension, hypotension, irregular or bounding heartbeat, edema, thrombophlebitis.
EENT: blurred or decreased vision.
GI: GI upset, increased appetite and thirst, *pancreatitis.*
GU: menstrual irregularities, urinary frequency.
Metabolic: hyperglycemia, sodium and fluid retention, *acute adrenal insufficiency,* cushingoid state, weight gain, hypokalemia, hypercholesterolemia.
Musculoskeletal: muscle weakness, osteoporosis, growth suppression.
Respiratory: dyspnea, wheezing.
Skin: burning, tingling, numbness at injection site, rash, urticaria, hirsutism, delayed wound healing, acne.
Other: *anaphylaxis,* infection.

Reactions may be *common,* uncommon, *life-threatening,* or **COMMON AND LIFE-THREATENING.**

INTERACTIONS

Drug-drug. *Acetaminophen:* Increases risk of hepatotoxicity. Monitor hepatic function.

Anticholinesterases: Causes severe weakness in myasthenia gravis patient. Monitor patient closely.

Anticoagulants: Usually decreases effects; rarely, increases effects. Monitor PT and INR closely.

Barbiturates, phenytoin, rifampin: Enhances prednisolone metabolism. May require increased corticosteroid dose.

Cardiac glycosides: Increases risk of arrhythmias or digitalis toxicity. Monitor ECG, potassium, and digoxin levels closely.

Estrogens, hormonal contraceptives, ketoconazole: Increases half-life and decreases clearance of prednisolone. Monitor patient closely.

Isoniazid, salicylates: Prednisolone enhances the metabolism of these drugs. Monitor patient for clinical response.

Nondepolarizing neuromuscular blockers: Increases or prolongs respiratory depression or paralysis. Avoid using together.

Potassium-wasting drugs: Enhances potassium-wasting effects of prednisolone. Monitor potassium level.

Sodium-containing drugs: Causes risk of edema and elevated blood pressure. Monitor patient and blood pressure closely.

Thyroid hormones: Decreases prednisolone metabolism. Monitor patient for increased adverse reactions.

Toxoids, vaccines: Diminishes response. Postpone immunization, if possible.

Ulcerogenic drugs: Increases risk of GI ulcers. Monitor patient for GI pain and bleeding.

Drug-herb. *Echinacea:* Decreases immunostimulation effects. Discourage use together.

Ginseng: Increases immune-modulatory response. Discourage use together.

EFFECTS ON LAB TEST RESULTS

• May increase glucose and cholesterol levels. May decrease T_3, T_4, potassium, and calcium levels.

• May cause decreased ^{131}I uptake and protein-bound iodine levels in thyroid function tests. May cause false-negative result in the nitroblue tetrazolium test for systemic bacterial infections. May alter reactions to skin tests.

ACTION

Decreases or prevents inflammation. Drug suppresses immune response and pituitary release of corticotropin, stimulates protein catabolism, increases glucose level, enhances lipolysis and mobilization of fatty acids from adipose tissues, decreases bone formation, and increases bone resorption.

PHARMACOKINETICS

Onset, rapid; duration, short but variable. Drug level peaks in 1 to 2 hours.

Distribution: Rapidly, to muscles, liver, skin, intestines, and kidneys. May bind to protein transcortin; only unbound drug is active. Drug crosses the placental barrier and appears in breast milk.

Metabolism: Primarily in the liver; some in other tissues.

Excretion: In urine. Half-life, about 2 to 3½ hours.

CLINICAL CONSIDERATIONS

• Osmolality: 247 mOsm/kg.

• In patients with severe or life-threatening conditions (such as organ transplant rejection, acute nephritis associated with systemic lupus erythematosus, or acute respiratory distress syndrome), single-dose or short-term therapy with exceedingly high doses may be effective.

• In those with acute adrenal insufficiency, expect to begin therapy by direct injection, then continue with slow I.V. infusion or I.M. administration.

• Monitor ECG for arrhythmias, observe for signs of infection, and watch

for depression or psychotic episodes, especially with high-dose therapy.
• In patients with diabetes, monitor urine and glucose levels. May need to increase insulin dose.
• Monitor drug effect. Gradually titrate drug to lowest effective dose and give for shortest possible time. Reduce dose gradually when discontinuing drug.
• After stoppage of short-term, high-dose therapy of up to 5 days, adrenal recovery may take 1 week; after prolonged, high-dose therapy, recovery may take up to 1 year or may never occur.
• *Alert:* Drug may contain sulfites.
• *Alert:* Because of risk of anaphylactoid reactions, keep emergency resuscitation equipment nearby.

PATIENT TEACHING
• Alert patient to the signs and symptoms of high blood sugar and teach him about home blood glucose monitoring, if appropriate.
• Instruct patient to report signs or symptoms of infection, including sore throat, fever, and malaise.
• Inform a woman that she may experience menstrual irregularities.

procainamide hydrochloride
Pronestyl*

Pharmacologic class: procaine derivative
Therapeutic class: ventricular antiarrhythmic, supraventricular antiarrhythmic
Pregnancy risk category: C
pH: 4 to 6

INDICATIONS & DOSAGES
➤ **Symptomatic PVCs; life-threatening ventricular tachycardia—**
Adults: 100 mg q 5 minutes by slow I.V. push, no faster than 25 to 50 mg/

minute, until arrhythmias disappear, adverse effects develop, or 500 mg has been given. Usual effective loading dose is 500 to 600 mg. Or, give a loading dose of 500 to 600 mg I.V. infusion over 25 to 30 minutes. Maximum total dose is 1 g. When arrhythmias disappear, give continuous infusion of 2 to 6 mg/minute. If arrhythmias recur, repeat bolus as above and increase infusion rate.
Children ◆ *:* Although dosage hasn't been established for children, recommendations include 2 to 5 mg/kg I.V. not exceeding 100 mg repeated p.r.n. at 5- to 10-minute intervals, not exceeding 15 mg/kg in 24 hours or 500 mg in a 30-minute period. Or, give15 mg/kg I.V. infused over 30 to 60 minutes, followed by maintenance infusion of 0.02 to 0.08 mg/kg/minute.
➤ **Malignant hyperthermia** ◆ —
Adults: 200 to 900 mg I.V., followed by an infusion.
Adjust-a-dose: For all indications, patients with heart failure or renal impairment may need a reduced dose.

ADMINISTRATION
Direct injection: Inject dose over 2 minutes or longer directly into vein or into I.V. tubing containing a free-flowing, compatible solution.
Intermittent infusion: Give loading infusion at 1 ml/minute for 25 to 30 minutes. Therapeutic effects usually occur after infusion of 100 to 200 mg. If no effect occurs after infusing 500 mg, wait at least 10 minutes to allow for drug distribution, then continue administration.
Continuous infusion: Using an infusion pump, give diluted solution at ordered rate, usually 2 to 6 mg/minute.

PREPARATION & STORAGE
Supplied in 10-ml (100 mg/ml) vials and 2-ml (500 mg/ml) vials and syringes. Drug may contain benzyl alcohol and sulfites.

For injection or loading infusion, dilute 1 g with 50 ml of D_5W to yield 20 mg/ml. For continuous infusion, dilute 1 g with 500 ml of D_5W to yield 2 mg/ml. In patients with fluid restrictions, dilute 1 g with 250 ml of D_5W to yield 4 mg/ml. Note that drug may form a complex with dextrose, causing gradual loss of potency.

Store at room temperature. Protect from light and freezing. Don't use if markedly discolored (light amber color) or if precipitate has formed. Solution is stable for 24 hours at room temperature and 7 days at 35° to 46° F (2° to 8° C).

Incompatibilities
Bretylium, esmolol, ethacrynate, milrinone, phenytoin sodium.

CONTRAINDICATIONS & CAUTIONS
• Contraindicated in patients hypersensitive to procaine or other local anesthetics.
• Contraindicated in those with second- or third-degree or complete AV heart block because of possible additive myocardial depression and in those with atypical ventricular tachycardia because drug may exacerbate these conditions.
• Use cautiously in those with digitalis toxicity, severe first-degree AV block, or bundle-branch heart block because of risk of enhanced myocardial depression with ventricular tachycardia or asystole.
• Use cautiously in those with heart failure or hepatic or renal impairment because of possible drug accumulation and toxic reaction, and in those with bronchial asthma because of possible hypersensitivity.
• Use cautiously in those with myasthenia gravis because drug may worsen weakness, and in those with systemic lupus erythematosus because drug may cause exacerbations.

• Use cautiously in those with sensitivity to sulfites.

ADVERSE REACTIONS
CNS: confusion, depression, dizziness, drowsiness, hallucinations, lightheadedness, *seizures*, fatigue, weakness, fever.
CV: *asystole, severe hypotension*, tachycardia (sympathetic response to hypotension), *ventricular fibrillation, bradycardia, flushing.*
GI: anorexia, diarrhea, nausea, vomiting.
Hematologic: *agranulocytosis*, hemolytic anemia, *thrombocytopenia, neutropenia.*
Musculoskeletal: joint swelling or pain.
Skin: *pruritus, rash, urticaria.*
Other: chills, *systemic lupus erythematosus–like syndrome, angioneurotic edema.*

INTERACTIONS
Drug-drug. *Amiodarone:* May increase procainamide level. Reduce procainamide dosage.
Antiarrhythmics: May have additive or antagonized effects. Avoid using together.
Antidyskinetics, antihistamines, antimuscarinics, especially atropine and related drugs: May intensify atropine-like effects. Monitor patient closely.
Antihypertensives: May cause additive hypotension. Monitor blood pressure closely.
Antimyasthenics: May decrease effects. Monitor patient.
Bethanechol and other cholinergics: Antagonizes cholinergic effects. Avoid using together.
Cimetidine, trimethoprim: Elevates procainamide level. Monitor patient for toxicity.
Neuromuscular blockers: Prolongs or enhances effects. Monitor patient closely.

Drug-herb. *Jimsonweed:* May adversely affect CV function. Discourage use together.

Licorice: May prolong the QT interval and may be additive. Discourage use together.

Drug-lifestyle. *Alcohol use:* Increases metabolism of procainamide. Discourage use together.

EFFECTS ON LAB TEST RESULTS

• May increase ALT, AST, alkaline phosphatase, LDH, and bilirubin levels.
• May decrease hemoglobin, hematocrit, and granulocyte, neutrophil, and platelet counts.
• May alter bentiromide test results and edrophonium test results, and may cause positive antinuclear antibody (ANA) titers, positive direct antiglobulin (Coombs') test results, and ECG changes.

ACTION

Decreases myocardial automaticity, excitability, and conduction velocity.

PHARMACOKINETICS

Drug level peaks immediately after infusion.

Distribution: Rapidly, to liver, spleen, kidneys, lungs, heart, muscles, CSF, and brain. Drug crosses the placental barrier, and both procainamide and N-acetylprocainamide (NAPA), an active metabolite, appear in breast milk.

Metabolism: In liver. About 40% of drug is converted in patients with rapid acetylation or renal impairment.

Excretion: In urine. Half-life of drug, 2½ to 5 hours; half-life of NAPA, about 7 hours. In renal impairment or heart failure, NAPA accumulates to toxic levels; procainamide levels remain normal.

CLINICAL CONSIDERATIONS

• Osmolality: 2,000 mOsm/kg.

• Keep phenylephrine or norepinephrine available to treat severe hypotension.
• During administration, continuously monitor blood pressure and cardiac function including ECG. Place patient in a supine position for blood pressure monitoring. Stop drug if patient develops excessive hypotension, widened QRS complexes of over 50%, prolonged PR or QT intervals, or signs of impending MI.
• In ventricular tachycardia, stop infusion if ventricular rate declines significantly without attaining regular AV conduction.
• Because drug may invalidate results of bentiromide test, stop giving drug at least 3 days before test.
• **Alert:** Drug may contain sulfites.
• Stop drug if signs of systemic lupus erythematosus or hemolytic anemia appear.
• Therapeutic level of procainamide is 3 to 10 mcg/ml; therapeutic levels of NAPA are 10 to 30 mcg/ml.
• Signs and symptoms of overdose include severe hypotension, confusion, dizziness or fainting, drowsiness, nausea, vomiting, oliguria, and unusually rapid or irregular heartbeat.
• If overdose occurs, stop drug immediately. Replace fluids, then give norepinephrine or phenylephrine. Maintain airway patency and ventilate the patient, as needed. Infusion of 1/6 M sodium lactate injection may reverse procainamide's cardiotoxic effects. Hemodialysis reduces half-life of procainamide, removing both procainamide and NAPA.

PATIENT TEACHING

• Instruct patient to inform prescriber of sore throat, fever, malaise, easy bruising or bleeding, or excessive gastrointestinal upset.
• Explain use of drug and its administration to patient and family.

Reactions may be *common*, uncommon, *life-threatening*, or COMMON AND LIFE-THREATENING.

prochlorperazine edisylate
Compazine*

Pharmacologic class: phenothiazine (piperazine derivative)
Therapeutic class: antiemetic
Pregnancy risk category: C
pH: 4.2 to 6.2

INDICATIONS & DOSAGES
➤ **Severe nausea and vomiting—**
Adults: 2.5 mg to 10 mg (0.5 to 2 ml) I.V. Don't exceed 40 mg/day.
➤ **To prevent nausea and vomiting during surgery—**
Adults: 5 mg to 10 mg by direct injection 15 to 30 minutes before induction of anesthesia. Repeat dose once before surgery, p.r.n. Or, give 20 mg/L by infusion 15 to 30 minutes before induction of anesthesia. Maximum dose, 40 mg daily.

ADMINISTRATION
Direct injection: Slowly inject undiluted drug at a rate of 5 mg/minute. Never give as bolus injection.
Intermittent infusion: Not recommended.
Continuous infusion: Infuse diluted drug at ordered rate over prescribed duration.

PREPARATION & STORAGE
Available as a 5-mg/ml concentration in 2-ml ampules, 2- and 10-ml vials, and 2-ml disposable syringes. Drug may contain benzyl alcohol and sulfites.

Dilute for continuous infusion with at least 1 L of a compatible isotonic solution, such as normal saline solution, to yield 20 mg/L.

Store at room temperature and protect from light and freezing. Don't use drug if it's markedly discolored or contains a precipitate.

Incompatibilities
Aldesleukin, allopurinol, amifostine, aminophylline, amphotericin B, ampicillin sodium, aztreonam, calcium gluconate, chloramphenicol sodium succinate, chlorothiazide, dexamethasone sodium phosphate, dimenhydrinate, etoposide, filgrastim, fludarabine, foscarnet, furosemide, gemcitabine, heparin sodium, hydrocortisone sodium succinate, hydromorphone, ketorolac, methylhexital, solutions containing methylparabens, midazolam hydrochloride, morphine, penicillin G potassium, penicillin G sodium, pentobarbital, phenobarbital sodium, phenytoin sodium, piperacillin sodium and tazobactam sodium, solutions containing propylparabens, thiopental, vitamin B complex with C.

CONTRAINDICATIONS & CAUTIONS
• Contraindicated in those hypersensitive to the drug or other phenothiazines.
• Contraindicated in those with severe CNS depression, coma, or severe CV disease because drug may worsen these conditions.
• Avoid use in pregnant patients unless nausea is severe and benefits of drug therapy outweigh the risks.
• Use cautiously in those with seizure disorders because drug may precipitate seizures, in those exposed to extreme heat because drug may disrupt the thermoregulatory mechanism, and in those with glaucoma or a predisposition to glaucoma because drug may potentiate the disorder.
• Use cautiously in debilitated patients because they usually require lowered doses.
• Use cautiously in those with Parkinson's disease because of risk of enhanced extrapyramidal effects.

• Use cautiously in those with myelo-suppression because of increased risk of bone marrow toxicity, and in those with CV disease because of increased risk of transient hypotension.

• Use cautiously in those with symptomatic prostatic hyperplasia because of increased risk of urine retention.

• Use cautiously in those with hepatic impairment because of possible altered drug metabolism, and in alcoholic patients because of possible deepened CNS depression.

• Use cautiously in those with peptic ulcer, chronic respiratory disorders, or urine retention, because of possible exacerbation.

• Use cautiously in those with increased sensitivity to CNS effects.

• Use cautiously in those with increased sensitivity to sulfites.

• Use cautiously in breast-feeding patients.

ADVERSE REACTIONS

CNS: difficulty speaking, dizziness, drowsiness, dystonic reactions, fainting, restlessness, *seizures, neuroleptic malignant syndrome,* fatigue, fever, pseudo-parkinsonism, tardive dyskinesia, *extrapyramidal reactions,* sedation, EEG changes.
CV: *arrhythmias, cardiac arrest, hypotension,* irregular or rapid pulse, ECG changes.
EENT: *visual changes,* nasal congestion.
GI: *constipation, dry mouth,* dysphagia, increased appetite, ileus.
GU: dark urine, menstrual irregularities, *urinary difficulty* or incontinence, inhibited ejaculation.
Hematologic: *agranulocytosis, leukopenia, thrombocytopenia,* hemolytic anemia.
Metabolic: weight gain, hyperglycemia, hypoglycemia.
Musculoskeletal: muscle spasms, shuffling gait, stiffness, trembling of hands and fingers.

Respiratory: *bronchospasm,* dyspnea.
Skin: discolored skin and eyes, increased or decreased sweating, pale skin, rash, exfoliative dermatitis, photosensitivity.
Other: *anaphylaxis,* akathisia, breast pain or swelling, chewing movements, lip smacking, masklike facies, rapid wormlike tongue movements, unusual breast milk secretion.

INTERACTIONS

Drug-drug. *Amantadine, anticholinergics, antidyskinetics, antihistamines, MAO inhibitors, tricyclic antidepressants:* Has additive anticholinergic effects. Use together cautiously.
Anorexiants, guanadrel, guanethidine, levodopa: Decreases effectiveness of these drugs. Avoid using together.
Anticonvulsants: Decreases seizure threshold. Adjust anticonvulsant therapy.
Antihypertensives: Causes additive hypotension. Use together cautiously.
Barbiturates: Decreases phenothiazine levels. Barbiturate levels may also decrease. Use together cautiously.
Beta blockers: Elevates levels of both drugs. Use together cautiously.
Bromocriptine: Inhibits bromocriptine effects. Use together cautiously.
CNS depressants: Worsens CNS depression. Avoid using together.
Epinephrine, norepinephrine: Decreases response to these drugs. Avoid using together.
Lithium: May cause disorientation, unconsciousness, and extrapyramidal symptoms. Monitor patient closely.
Oral anticoagulants: Decreases effectiveness. Monitor PT and INR closely.
Photosensitizing drugs: Causes additive toxicity. Monitor patient closely.
Pimozide: Prolongs QT interval. Avoid using together.
Quinidine: Has additive cardiac effects. Use with caution; monitor patient closely.

Reactions may be *common,* uncommon, *life-threatening*, or COMMON AND LIFE-THREATENING.

EFFECTS ON LAB TEST RESULTS
• May increase or decrease glucose level.
• May decrease WBC and granulocyte counts. May alter liver function test result values.
• May cause false-positive results in tests for phenylketonuria, urine amylase, 5-hydroxyindoleacetic acid, porphobilinogens, urobilinogen, or uroporphyrins. May cause false-negative results in tests for urine bilirubin. May cause false-positive or false-negative results in urine pregnancy tests.

ACTION
Thought to directly affect the medullary chemoreceptor trigger zone, apparently by blocking dopamine receptors.

PHARMACOKINETICS
Onset, almost immediate; duration, varied—up to 12 hours.
Distribution: Widespread, with high levels in the brain, lungs, liver, kidney, and spleen. Drug readily crosses the placental and blood-brain barriers. Small amounts appear in breast milk.
Metabolism: Mostly in the liver.
Excretion: In feces, principally as metabolites, and in urine as metabolites and unchanged drug.

CLINICAL CONSIDERATIONS
• Osmolality: 282 mOsm/kg.
• Because of risk of hypotension, use I.V. route only for closely monitored patients.
• Initially, give low doses to geriatric patients and increase gradually.
• Skin contact with drug can cause contact dermatitis.
• *Alert:* Drug may contain sulfites.
• Antiemetic effect may mask signs of drug toxicity or obscure diagnosis of conditions having nausea as a primary symptom.

• Anticholinergic antiparkinsonians may help to control extrapyramidal reactions.
• Monitor CBC and liver function studies during long-term therapy.

PATIENT TEACHING
• Instruct patient to inform prescriber if he develops a sore throat, fever, or malaise.
• Encourage patient to change positions and to rise slowly to avoid dizziness upon standing up quickly.
• Inform patient that drug may discolor urine from pink to red-brown.
• Warn patient that drug may impair body's temperature regulation. Avoid extreme heat.

promethazine hydrochloride
Phenergan

Pharmacologic class: phenothiazine derivative
Therapeutic class: antiemetic; antivertigo drug; antihistamine (H_1-receptor antagonist); preoperative, postoperative, or obstetric sedative; adjunct to analgesics
Pregnancy risk category: C
pH: 4 to 5.5

INDICATIONS & DOSAGES
➤ **Allergic reactions**—
Adults: 25 mg I.V., repeated in 2 hours, p.r.n.
Children age 2 and older: Don't exceed one-half adult dose.
➤ **Nausea and vomiting**—
Adults: 12.5 to 25 mg I.V. q 4 hours, p.r.n.
Children: 0.25 to 0.5 mg/kg I.V. four to six times daily.
➤ **Obstetric sedation**—
Adults: 50 mg I.V. during early labor stage; then 25 to 75 mg in established labor given with an opioid agonist. If

needed, 25 to 50 mg dose may be repeated once or twice at 4-hour intervals. Maximum dosage, 100 mg in 24 hours.

➤ **Sedation and relief from apprehension, postoperative pain as anesthesia and analgesia adjunct—**
Adults: 25 to 50 mg I.V., p.r.n.; maximum dosage, 150 mg daily.
Children 2 years and older: 12.5 to 25 mg I.V. or 0.5 to 1.1 mg/kg I.V.
Adjust-a-dose: Reduce dosage in dehydrated patients or those with oliguria because diminished urine excretion may potentiate toxic effects.

When giving barbiturates with promethazine, decrease barbiturate dosage by at least 50%. When giving opioids with drug, reduce opioid dosage by 25% to 50%.

ADMINISTRATION
Direct injection: Inject at a rate not exceeding 25 mg/minute into an I.V. line containing a free-flowing, compatible solution. Rapid administration may reduce blood pressure temporarily.

Concentration shouldn't exceed 25 mg/ml. Make sure I.V. line is patent before injection. Watch for irritation and infiltration; extravasation can cause tissue damage and necrosis. Also avoid inadvertent intra-arterial injection because of possible gangrene or severe arteriospasm.
Intermittent infusion: Not recommended.
Continuous infusion: Not recommended.

PREPARATION & STORAGE
Available as 25-mg/ml and 50-mg/ml concentrations in 1-ml ampules.

Store at room temperature and protect from light and freezing. Don't use if solution is discolored or if a precipitate is present.

Incompatibilities
Aldesleukin, allopurinol, aminophylline, amphotericin B, cephalosporins, chloramphenicol sodium succinate, chloroquine phosphate, chlorothiazide, diatrizoate meglumine (34.3%) and diatrizoate sodium (35%), diatrizoate meglumine (52%) and diatrizoate sodium (8%), diatrizoate sodium (75%), dimenhydrinate, doxorubicin liposomal, foscarnet, furosemide, heparin sodium, hydrocortisone sodium succinate, iodipamide meglumine (52%), iothalamate meglumine (60%), iothalamate sodium (80%), ketorolac, methohexital, morphine, nalbuphine, penicillin G potassium and sodium, pentobarbital sodium, phenobarbital sodium, phenytoin sodium, thiopental, vitamin B complex.

CONTRAINDICATIONS & CAUTIONS
• Contraindicated in those hypersensitive to drug and in breast-feeding patients.
• Avoid use in comatose patients because high doses may exacerbate the condition.
• Use cautiously in those hypersensitive to sulfites.
• Use cautiously in patients with bladder neck obstruction, symptomatic prostatic hyperplasia, or predisposition to urine retention because drug may precipitate or aggravate urine retention.
• Use cautiously in those with hypertension or jaundice because drug may worsen these disorders, and in those with epilepsy because drug may intensify seizures.
• Use cautiously in those with acute asthma or respiratory disorders because antimuscarinic drying effects may thicken secretions, impairing expectoration. Drug may also suppress the cough reflex.
• Use cautiously in those who are severely obese and in those who have neuromuscular disease, because of possible airway or ventilation problems.

• Use cautiously in those with hepatic impairment because of decreased drug metabolism, in those with myelosuppression because of increased risk of leukopenia and agranulocytosis, and in those with CV disease because of possible transient hypotension.

• Use cautiously in those with angle-closure glaucoma or predisposition to this condition because increased intraocular pressure may precipitate an acute attack.

• Use cautiously in those with stenosis caused by peptic ulcer and in those with history of peptic ulcer because drug may reduce GI motility and tone, resulting in obstruction and gastric retention.

• Use cautiously in geriatric patients who are more susceptible to dizziness, sedation, confusion, and hypotension.

ADVERSE REACTIONS

CNS: fever, extrapyramidal effects, such as ticlike movements of head and face, decreased alertness, *sedation,* dizziness, *drowsiness,* excitement, irritability, nervousness, restlessness, *seizures,* unsteadiness, nightmares.

CV: hypotension, tachycardia, flushing, hypertension.

EENT: blurred vision; dry nose and throat; sore throat; tinnitus.

GI: GI upset, nausea, vomiting, *dry mouth.*

GU: urine retention.

Hematologic: *agranulocytosis, leukopenia, thrombocytopenia.*

Hepatic: obstructive jaundice.

Metabolic: hyperglycemia.

Musculoskeletal: muscle spasm, especially in neck and back.

Respiratory: *bronchospasm,* dyspnea, laryngospasm.

Skin: rash, photosensitivity.

Other: *anaphylaxis.*

INTERACTIONS

Drug-drug. *Amantadine, anticholinergics, antidyskinetics, antihistamines, MAO inhibitors, tricyclic antidepressants:* Has additive anticholinergic effects. Use together cautiously.

Anorexiants, guanadrel, guanethidine, levodopa: Decreases effectiveness of these drugs. Avoid using together.

Anticonvulsants: Decreases seizure threshold. Adjust anticonvulsant therapy.

Antihypertensives: Causes additive hypotension. Use together cautiously.

Barbiturates: Decreases phenothiazine levels. Barbiturate levels may also decrease. Use together cautiously.

Beta blockers: Elevates levels of both drugs. Use together cautiously.

Bromocriptine: Inhibits bromocriptine effects. Use together cautiously.

CNS depressants: Worsens CNS depression. Avoid using together.

Epinephrine, norepinephrine: Decreases response to these drugs. Avoid using together.

Lithium: May cause disorientation, unconsciousness, and extrapyramidal symptoms. Monitor patient closely.

Oral anticoagulants: May decrease effectiveness. Monitor PT and INR closely.

Photosensitizing drugs: May cause additive drug toxicity. Monitor patient closely.

Quinidine: Causes additive cardiac effects. Use together with caution; monitor patient closely.

Pimozide: Prolongs QT interval. Avoid using together.

Drug-herb. *Kava:* Increases risk or severity of dystonic reactions. Discourage use together.

Yohimbe: Increases risk of toxicity. Discourage use together.

Drug-lifestyle. *Alcohol use:* May increase CNS effects. Discourage use together.

Sun exposure: May cause photosensitivity reactions. Advise patient to avoid excessive sunlight exposure.

EFFECTS ON LAB TEST RESULTS
• May increase glucose level.
• May decrease hemoglobin and WBC, platelet, and granulocyte counts.
• May cause false-negative result in skin test using allergen extracts. May cause false-positive or false-negative result in urine pregnancy tests.

ACTION
Prevents histamine-mediated spasmodic and congestive responses. Drug has antiemetic and antivertigo effects and acts as a sedative-hypnotic.

PHARMACOKINETICS
Onset, 3 to 5 minutes; duration, 6 to 12 hours as antihistamine, 2 to 8 hours as sedative.
Distribution: Widely, in tissues. Drug readily crosses the placental barrier; unknown if drug appears in breast milk.
Metabolism: In liver.
Excretion: Slowly in urine and feces.

CLINICAL CONSIDERATIONS
• Osmolality: 291 mOsm/kg.
• *Alert:* Drug may contain sulfites.
• Antiemetic effects may obscure signs of intestinal obstruction, brain tumor, or promethazine overdose.
• Watch for extrapyramidal reactions, especially in geriatric patients.
• Monitor blood pressure closely.
• Give oxygen and I.V. fluids, as needed, to maintain cardiopulmonary function. Give phenylephrine or norepinephrine to treat hypotension. Don't use epinephrine, which may further lower blood pressure. Also give anticholinergic antiparkinsonians, diphenhydramine, or barbiturates, to treat extrapyramidal symptoms.

PATIENT TEACHING
• Instruct patient to notify prescriber if rash, difficulty breathing, sore throat, fever, or easy bruising or bleeding occurs.

• Instruct patient to avoid activities that require mental alertness.
• Warn patient that drug may impair body's temperature regulation. Tell him to avoid extreme heat.

propofol
Diprivan

Pharmacologic class: phenol derivative
Therapeutic class: anesthetic
Pregnancy risk category: B
pH: 7 to 8.5

INDICATIONS & DOSAGES
➤ **Induce anesthesia—**
Adults: Doses must be individualized according to patient's condition and age. Most patients classified as American Society of Anesthesiologists (ASA) Physical Status category (PS) I or II younger than age 55 require 2 to 2.5 mg/kg I.V. Drug is usually given in 40-mg boluses q 10 seconds until desired response is obtained. Geriatric, debilitated, or hypovolemic patients or those in ASA PS III or IV should receive half of usual induction dose— 20-mg boluses q 10 seconds. For cardiac anesthesia, patients require 20 mg (0.5 to 1.5 mg/kg) I.V. q 10 seconds until desired response is achieved. Neurosurgical patients require 20 mg (1 to 2 mg/kg) I.V. q 10 seconds until desired response is achieved.
Children 3 to 16 years: 2.5 to 3.5 mg/kg I.V. over 20 to 30 seconds.
➤ **Maintenance of anesthesia—**
Adults: May be given as a variable rate infusion, titrated to clinical effect. Most patients may be maintained with 0.1 to 0.2 mg/kg/minute I.V. (6 to 12 mg/kg/hour). Alternatively, increments of 20 to 50 mg intermittent I.V. boluses may be given p.r.n. Geriatric, debilitated, or hypovolemic patients or those in ASA

PS III or IV should receive half of usual maintenance dose (0.05 to 0.1 mg/kg/minute or 3 to 6 mg/kg/hour) I.V. For cardiac anesthesia with secondary opioid, patients require 100 to 150 mcg/kg/minute I.V.; for low dose with primary opioid, patients require 50 to 100 mcg/kg/minute I.V. Neurosurgical patients require 100 to 200 mcg/kg/minute (6 to 12 mg/kg/hour) I.V.
Children 2 months to 16 years: 125 to 300 mcg/kg/minute (7.5 to 18 mg/kg/hour) I.V.

➤**Monitored anesthesia care—**
Adults: Initially, most patients require 100 to 150 mcg/kg/minute (6 to 9 mg/kg/hour) I.V. for 3 to 5 minutes or a slow injection of 0.5 mg/kg over 3 to 5 minutes. For maintenance dose, most patients require an infusion of 25 to 75 mcg/kg/minute (1.5 to 4.5 mg/kg/hour) I.V. or incremental bolus doses of 10 or 20 mg. Geriatric, debilitated, or ASA PS III or IV patients require 80% of usual adult maintenance dose. Rapid bolus shouldn't be used.

➤**Sedation of intubated ICU patients—**
Adults: Initial infusion is 5 mcg/kg/minute (0.3 mg/kg/hour) I.V. for 5 minutes. Increments of 5 to 10 mcg/kg/minute (0.3 to 0.6 mg/kg/hour) I.V. over 5 to 10 minutes may be used until desired sedation is achieved. Maintenance rate is 5 to 50 mcg/kg/minute (0.3 to 3 mg/kg/hour) I.V.

ADMINISTRATION

Direct injection: For induction in adults, give 40 mg every 10 seconds until desired response is obtained. For maintenance of anesthesia in adults, 25 to 50 mg (2.5 to 5 ml) boluses are given, as needed, based on patient's change in vital signs.
Intermittent infusion: Not recommended.
Continuous infusion: For maintenance of anesthesia in adults, give 0.1 to 0.2 mg/kg/minute.

PREPARATION & STORAGE

Supplied in 20-ml ampules containing 10 mg/ml. If drug is to be diluted before infusion, use only D_5W, and don't dilute to a concentration less than 2 mg/ml. After dilution, drug is probably more stable in glass containers than in plastic ones.

When given into a running I.V., propofol emulsion is compatible with D_5W, lactated Ringer's injection, lactated Ringer's and 5% dextrose injection, 5% dextrose and half-normal injection, and 5% dextrose and 0.2% sodium chloride injection. Store unopened ampules above 40° F (4° C) and below 72° F (22° C). Don't refrigerate.

Strict aseptic technique must always be maintained during handling. Propofol injectable emulsion is a single-use parenteral product that contains 0.005% disodium edetate to retard the rate of growth of microorganisms in the event of accidental extrinsic contamination. However, propofol can still support the growth of microorganisms as it isn't an antimicrobially preserved product.

Incompatibilities
Other I.V. drugs.

CONTRAINDICATIONS & CAUTIONS
• Contraindicated in those hypersensitive to the drug or components of the emulsion, including soybean oil, egg lecithin, and glycerol.
• Avoid using for obstetric anesthesia, because safety to fetus hasn't been established.
• Avoid using in those with increased intracranial pressure or impaired cerebral circulation, because hypotension may substantially reduce cerebral perfusion.
• Use cautiously in those with history of epilepsy.
• Use cautiously in those with diabetic hyperlipidemia or a history of lipid metabolism disorders, such as pancreatitis

---

or primary hyperlipoproteinemia, because drug is given as an emulsion.

● Use cautiously in geriatric or debilitated patients and in those with circulatory disorders. Although drug's hemodynamic effects can vary, a major effect in those maintaining spontaneous ventilation is hypotension with little or no change in heart rate and cardiac output. Blood pressures can decrease by as much as 30%. However, incidence and degree of diminished cardiac output increases in those undergoing assisted or controlled positive-pressure ventilation.

● Drug isn't recommended for breast-feeding patients because drug appears in breast milk.

ADVERSE REACTIONS

CNS: dizziness, headache, pain, fever.
CV: *asystole, bradycardia,* hypertension, *hypotension,* flushing.
GI: abdominal cramps, nausea, vomiting.
Musculoskeletal: clonic-myoclonic movements, twitching.
Respiratory: *apnea,* cough, pulmonary edema, hiccups.
Skin: burning, coldness, numbness, stinging at injection site, rash, pruritus.

INTERACTIONS

Drug-drug. *Potent inhalation anesthetics, such as enflurane, halothane, and isoflurane, supplemental anesthetics, such as nitrous oxide and opioids:* May enhance anesthetic and CV actions of propofol. Monitor patient closely.
Premedication with opioids or opioids with sedatives: May enhance reduction of systolic, diastolic, and mean arterial pressure as well as cause a more pronounced decrease in cardiac output. Induction dose requirements also may be decreased. Monitor patient closely.

EFFECTS ON LAB TEST RESULTS

● May increase lipid levels.

ACTION

Produces dose-dependent CNS depression similar to benzodiazepines and barbiturates. Causes hypnosis rapidly with minimal excitation.

PHARMACOKINETICS

Onset, within 40 seconds; duration, 3 to 5 minutes.
Distribution: Rapidly to well-perfused tissues and subsequently redistributes to lean muscle and fat. Cessation of drug effects results partly from this rapid redistribution.
Metabolism: Not fully characterized. Drug is principally conjugated within the liver.
Excretion: Primarily renal; 70% of drug is excreted in urine within 24 hours and 90% within 5 days.

CLINICAL CONSIDERATIONS

● Tonicity: isotonic.
● Drug should be given only by personnel familiar with airway management and administration of I.V. anesthetics.
● Drug's pharmacokinetics aren't altered by hepatic cirrhosis, chronic renal failure, or patient's sex.
● Drug has no vagolytic activity. Premedication with anticholinergics, such as glycopyrrolate or atropine, may help manage potential increases in vagal tone caused by other drugs or surgery.
● Avoid abrupt discontinuation of drug before weaning. This may result in sudden awakening with anxiety, agitation, and resistance to mechanical ventilation.
● Treatment of significant hypotension or bradycardia includes increased rate of fluid administration, pressors, elevation of lower extremities, or atropine. Apnea commonly occurs during induction and may persist for longer than 60 seconds. Ventilatory support may be needed.
● Monitor lipid levels daily.

Reactions may be *common,* uncommon, *life-threatening,* or COMMON AND LIFE-THREATENING.

PATIENT TEACHING
• Inform patient about what to expect with drug administration, including rapid sleep onset.
• Assure patient and family that he will be monitored continuously.

propranolol hydrochloride
Inderal

Pharmacologic class: beta blocker
Therapeutic class: antiarrhythmic
Pregnancy risk category: C
pH: 2.8 to 3.5

INDICATIONS & DOSAGES
➤ **Life-threatening arrhythmias or those occurring under anesthesia**—
Adults: 1 to 3 mg I.V. repeated after 2 minutes and again after 4 hours, p.r.n.
Children ◆ : 0.01 to 0.02 mg/kg I.V. over 10 minutes.
Adjust-a-dose: In geriatric patients base dosage on their response to drug. In patients with hepatic impairment, reduce dose.

ADMINISTRATION
Direct injection: Inject drug at a maximum rate of 1 mg/minute through an I.V. line containing a free-flowing, compatible solution.
Intermittent infusion: In children, infuse over 10 minutes.
Continuous infusion: Not recommended.

PREPARATION & STORAGE
Available in 1-ml ampules and vials containing 1 mg/ml.
   Compatible with normal saline solution and D_5W.
   Store at room temperature and protect from light and freezing.

Incompatibilities
Amphotericin B, diazoxide.

CONTRAINDICATIONS & CAUTIONS
• Contraindicated in those with Raynaud's syndrome or malignant hypertension because of possible peripheral arterial insufficiency, and in those with bronchial asthma because beta blockade may lead to increased airway resistance and bronchospasm.
• Contraindicated in those with sinus bradycardia, heart block greater than first degree, MI with systolic pressure below 100 mm Hg, heart failure unless caused by tachyarrhythmia treatable with propranolol, or cardiogenic shock. Further myocardial depression can occur with these conditions.
• Avoid use in those with myasthenia gravis, because drug may exacerbate symptoms.
• Use cautiously in those with cardiac impairment, because drug may precipitate heart failure, and in those with hyperthyroidism because drug may mask tachycardia.
• Use cautiously in those with diabetes mellitus who are receiving an oral antidiabetic; drug may trigger hyperglycemic reactions or hypoglycemia and may inhibit pancreatic insulin release.
• Use cautiously in those with nonallergic bronchospastic disease because drug may increase airway resistance and bronchospasm.
• Use cautiously in those with depression because of possible exacerbation.
• Use cautiously in those with hepatic or renal failure because of risk of adverse reactions.
• Use cautiously in breast-feeding patients.
• Pediatric safety and efficacy haven't been established.

ADVERSE REACTIONS
CNS: light-headedness, *fatigue, lethargy,* vivid dreams, depression, insomnia, fever.
CV: atrioventricular dissociation, ***bradycardia, cardiac arrest, heart fail-***

ure, fluid retention, *hypotension,* peripheral arterial insufficiency, ***ventricular fibrillation, worsening of AV block,*** intermittent claudication.
EENT: pharyngitis, rhinitis.
GI: constipation, diarrhea, dry mouth, flatulence, nausea, vomiting.
Hematologic: transient eosinophilia, ***agranulocytosis.***
Metabolic: *hyperkalemia,* hyperuricemia.
Respiratory: ***bronchospasm,*** laryngospasm, pulmonary edema, respiratory distress.
Skin: alopecia, rash.
Other: systemic lupus erythematosus-like reaction.

INTERACTIONS
Drug-drug. *Antiarrhythmics:* Enhances cardiac toxicity. Use together cautiously.
Atropine, other antimuscarinics, tricyclic antidepressants: May reverse drug-induced bradycardia. Monitor patient closely.
Cimetidine: Reduces propranolol clearance. Monitor patient for increased beta blocker effect.
Diuretics, other antihypertensives, phenothiazine: Potentiates hypotension. Monitor blood pressure closely.
Haloperidol: May cause cardiac arrest. Avoid using together.
Levodopa, sympathomimetics: Antagonizes effects. Avoid using together.
Neuromuscular blockers: May potentiate effects. Use together with extreme caution.
NSAIDs: Antagonizes hypotensive effects. Monitor patient closely.
Drug-herb. *Betel palm:* Decreases temperature-elevating effects and enhances CNS effects. Discourage use together.
Drug-lifestyle. *Cocaine use:* Increases angina-inducing potential of cocaine. Discourage use together.

EFFECTS ON LAB TEST RESULTS
● May increase BUN, creatinine, potassium, uric acid, alkaline phosphatase, ALT, AST, and LDH levels.
● May increase antinuclear antibody titers and eosinophil count. May decrease intraocular pressure and granulocyte count.

ACTION
Blocks beta receptors in the myocardium; reduces heart rate, conduction velocity, myocardial automaticity, myocardial contractility, and cardiac output and increases systolic ejection time and cardiac volume.

PHARMACOKINETICS
Onset, immediate; duration, 6 to 8 hours.
Distribution: Widely, throughout tissues, including lungs, liver, kidneys, and heart. Drug crosses blood-brain and placental barriers, and small amounts appear in breast milk.
Metabolism: In liver.
Excretion: Primarily in urine, with 1% to 4% in feces; fecal excretion rises in severe renal impairment. Half-life 2 to 6 hours, decreasing in renal impairment.

CLINICAL CONSIDERATIONS
● Osmolality: 12 mOsm/kg.
● *Alert:* Keep in mind that I.V. doses are appreciably smaller than oral ones.
● Carefully monitor ECG, blood pressure, and central venous pressure during administration.
● Correct severe bradycardia with atropine I.V. and, if needed, give isoproterenol. For PVCs, give I.V. lidocaine or phenytoin. For cardiac failure, give oxygen, diuretics, and cardiac glycosides. A transvenous pacemaker may be used if drug therapy is unsuccessful.
● For hypotension, place patient in the Trendelenburg position and give I.V. fluids (unless patient is experiencing pulmonary edema) and an I.V. vaso-

---

Reactions may be *common,* uncommon, ***life-threatening,*** or **COMMON AND LIFE-THREATENING.**

pressor such as epinephrine. If seizures occur, give I.V. diazepam or phenytoin, if needed. For bronchospasm, give isoproterenol or a theophylline derivative. Glucagon may be used to counter CV effects of propranolol overdose.

PATIENT TEACHING
• Inform diabetic patient that normal signs of low blood sugar may be masked.
• Instruct patient to inform prescriber if difficulty breathing, light-headedness, or dizziness occurs.
• Encourage patient to rise slowly to avoid dizziness.

protamine sulfate

Pharmacologic class: antidote
Therapeutic class: heparin antagonist
Pregnancy risk category: C
pH: 6 to 7

INDICATIONS & DOSAGES
➤ **Severe heparin overdose—**
Adults: Dosage reflects heparin dose, route, and time elapsed since administration. Typically, 1 mg of protamine sulfate neutralizes about 90 units of heparin sodium derived from bovine lung tissue, or 115 units of heparin sodium derived from porcine intestinal mucosa.
　　Dosage is 1 to 1.5 mg/100 units heparin when given a few minutes after I.V. heparin injection; 0.5 to 0.75 mg/100 units heparin when given 30 to 60 minutes after I.V. heparin injection; 0.25 to 0.375 mg/100 units heparin when given more than 2 hours after I.V. heparin injection; 25 to 50 mg after continuous infusion of heparin; 1 to 1.5 mg/100 units heparin after deep S.C. heparin injection, or 25 to 50 mg by slow I.V. injection; and the rest of

calculated dose given by continuous I.V. infusion over 8 to 16 hours or expected duration of heparin absorption.
➤ **To neutralize heparin given during extracorporeal circulation in arterial and cardiac surgery or dialysis procedures** ◆ —
Adults and children: Usually, 1.5 mg/100 units heparin I.V.

ADMINISTRATION
Direct injection: Inject reconstituted drug slowly over 1 to 3 minutes. Don't give more than 50 mg in 10 minutes. Overly rapid administration can cause severe hypotension and anaphylactoid reactions.
Intermittent infusion: Not recommended.
Continuous infusion: Not recommended.

PREPARATION & STORAGE
Available in a concentration of 10 mg/ml as liquid in 5- and 25-ml vials or supplied as powder in 50- and 250-mg vials. Store liquid in refrigerator and powder at room temperature. Avoid freezing.
　　Reconstitute powder with sterile water for injection or bacteriostatic water for injection containing 0.9% benzyl alcohol (5 ml for 50 mg vial or 25 ml for 250 mg vial) to yield 10 mg/ml. Shake vigorously. If reconstituted with sterile water, use immediately and discard unused portions. If reconstituted with bacteriostatic water and benzyl alcohol, solution remains stable for 72 hours at room temperature.
　　Reconstituted solutions aren't intended for further dilution, but if desired, may be diluted in D_5W or normal saline solution. Don't store diluted solutions; they contain no preservatives.

Incompatibilities
Cephalosporins, diatrizoate meglumine 52% and diatrizoate sodium 8%, diatrizoate sodium 60%, ioxaglate meglu-

mine 39.3% and ioxaglate sodium 19.6%, penicillins.

CONTRAINDICATIONS & CAUTIONS
● Contraindicated in those hypersensitive to the drug.
● Contraindicated in neonates if drug is reconstituted with bacteriostatic water containing benzyl alcohol.
● Use cautiously in those with allergies to fish, because drug is derived from fish sperm.
● Use cautiously in those with diabetes who receive protamine zinc insulin, and in infertile or vasectomized men because of increased risk of protamine sensitivity.
● Use cautiously in those who have received high doses of drug in the past.

ADVERSE REACTIONS
CNS: malaise, weakness.
CV: *bradycardia,* hypotension, *circulatory collapse,* flushing.
GI: nausea, vomiting.
Respiratory: *pulmonary edema, acute pulmonary hypertension,* coughing, dyspnea, wheezing.
Other: *anaphylaxis, anaphylactoid reactions,* heparin rebound, warm sensation.

INTERACTIONS
None reported.

EFFECTS ON LAB TEST RESULTS
None reported.

ACTION
When given after heparin, drug forms a stable complex with strongly acidic heparin sodium or heparin calcium. This complex possesses no anticoagulant activity. When given without heparin, drug is a weak anticoagulant.

PHARMACOKINETICS
Onset, 30 to 60 seconds; duration, about 2 hours, depending on body temperature.

Distribution: Combines with heparin in the bloodstream. Not known if drug crosses the placental barrier or appears in breast milk.
Metabolism: May be partly metabolized or degraded, thus freeing heparin.
Excretion: Unknown.

CLINICAL CONSIDERATIONS
● Osmolality: 290 mOsm/kg.
● Before giving drug, ensure adequate blood volume. Correct hypovolemia with I.V. fluids or with blood transfusions if patient hemorrhaged from heparin overdose.
● Carefully titrate drug dose, especially if patient received a large heparin dose.
● Don't give more than 100 mg over 2 hours—drug's duration of action—unless coagulation studies indicate need for higher dosage.
● Drug is used to treat severe heparin overdose only. Mild overdose can be corrected by discontinuing heparin.
● Keep epinephrine 1:1,000 available to treat hypersensitivity.
● Monitor patient continuously throughout therapy. Check vital signs frequently.
● Monitor coagulation studies, such as activated clotting time, aPTT, or thrombin time. These should be performed 5 to 15 minutes after therapy and repeated, as needed.
● Closely observe patient who has undergone extracorporeal circulation during arterial and cardiac surgery or hemodialysis. Heparin rebound with bleeding can occur 30 minutes to 18 hours later despite heparin neutralization by protamine sulfate.

PATIENT TEACHING
● Advise patient that he may experience temporary flushing after drug administration.
● Instruct patient to inform nurse immediately if bleeding occurs.

Reactions may be *common,* uncommon, *life-threatening,* or COMMON AND LIFE-THREATENING.

pyridostigmine bromide
Regonol*

Pharmacologic class: anticholinesterase
Therapeutic class: muscle stimulant
Pregnancy risk category: C
pH: 5

INDICATIONS & DOSAGES
➤ **Myasthenia gravis—**
Adults: Dosage varies widely; 2 mg I.V. q 2 to 3 hours or about one-thirtieth of patient's oral maintenance dose.
➤ **Antidote for nondepolarizing neuromuscular blockers, such as gallamine, metocurine, pancuronium, and tubocurarine—**
Adults: 10 to 20 mg I.V. or 0.1 to 0.25 mg/kg I.V., given with or shortly after 0.6 to 1.2 mg of atropine sulfate I.V. or 0.2 to 0.6 mg of glycopyrrolate I.V., about 0.2 mg of glycopyrrolate for each 5 mg of pyridostigmine bromide.

ADMINISTRATION
Direct injection: Inject undiluted drug very slowly into an I.V. line containing a compatible, free-flowing solution. Observe for thrombophlebitis at I.V. site.
Intermittent infusion: Not recommended.
Continuous infusion: Not recommended

PREPARATION & STORAGE
Available in a concentration of 5 mg/ml in 2-ml ampules and 5-ml vials. Products may contain benzyl alcohol.
  Store at room temperature. Protect from light and freezing.

Incompatibilities
Alkaline solutions.

CONTRAINDICATIONS & CAUTIONS
• Contraindicated in those hypersensitive to anticholinesterases or bromides and in breast-feeding patients.
• Contraindicated in those with mechanical obstruction of the intestinal or urinary tract because drug increases smooth-muscle tone and activity.
• Use cautiously in those with asthma, pneumonia, postoperative atelectasis, UTIs, or arrhythmias—especially bradycardia, AV block, or recent coronary occlusion—because drug may exacerbate these conditions.
• Use cautiously after surgery because drug may exacerbate breathing difficulty caused by pain, sedation, secretions, or atelectasis.
• Use cautiously in those with epilepsy, hyperthyroidism, peptic ulcer, or vagotonia because drug may mask their signs and symptoms.

ADVERSE REACTIONS
CNS: agitation, anxiety, clumsiness, confusion, fasciculations, headache, irritability, restlessness, *seizures,* slurred speech.
CV: *cardiac arrest, bradycardia,* hypotension, thrombophlebitis.
EENT: blurred vision, lacrimation, pupillary constriction.
GI: abdominal cramps, severe diarrhea, excessive salivation, nausea, vomiting.
Musculoskeletal: increased weakness, especially in arms, neck, shoulders, and tongue.
Respiratory: *bronchospasm,* bronchoconstriction, increased bronchial secretions, *respiratory paralysis.*
Skin: acne, diaphoresis.

INTERACTIONS
Drug-drug. *Aminoglycosides, capreomycin, guanadrel, guanethidine, hydrocarbon inhalation anesthetics such as halothane, lincomycin, parenteral local anesthetics, polymyxins, procainamide, quinidine, quinine:* Possible

antagonized antimyasthenic effects. Use cautiously together; observe patient closely.

Antimuscarinics especially atropine: Antagonizes muscarinic effects. Use cautiously together; observe patient closely.

Depolarizing neuromuscular blockers such as succinylcholine: Prolongs neuromuscular blockade. Use cautiously together; observe patient closely.

Edrophonium, other anticholinesterases: Has additive effects. Monitor patient closely.

Local ester-derivative anesthetics: Increases risk of toxicity. Monitor patient closely.

Nondepolarizing neuromuscular blockers: Antagonizes effects. Monitor patient closely.

EFFECTS ON LAB TEST RESULTS
None reported.

ACTION
Blocks effects of acetylcholinesterase, resulting in miosis, bradycardia, increased muscle tone, constricted bronchi and ureters, and increased salivary and sweat gland secretion.

PHARMACOKINETICS
Onset, 2 to 5 minutes; duration, 2 to 3 hours.

Distribution: Widespread. Drug crosses the blood-brain barrier only with high doses; also crosses the placental barrier and appears in breast milk.

Metabolism: Hydrolyzed by cholinesterases and metabolized by liver enzymes.

Excretion: In urine. Half-life, about 90 minutes.

CLINICAL CONSIDERATIONS
• Osmolality: 132 mOsm/kg.
• Stop all other cholinergics during pyridostigmine therapy to avoid toxicity.

• Always keep atropine sulfate available in a separate syringe when giving pyridostigmine. Give 0.6 to 1.2 mg of atropine before or with high doses of pyridostigmine.
• If heart rate is below 80 beats/minute, give atropine before pyridostigmine.
• Establish baseline respiratory rate, heart rate, and blood pressure.
• Maintain a patent airway using suctioning, oxygen, and assisted ventilation, as needed.
• When giving drug to reverse effects of nondepolarizing neuromuscular blockers, keep patient on ventilator. Wait 15 to 30 minutes for full effects. Observe closely for possible recurrence of respiratory depression. Delayed recovery is associated with hypokalemia, debilitation, carcinomatosis, aminoglycoside antibiotic therapy, and use of anesthetics, such as ether.
• Severe myasthenia gravis is associated with accelerated pyridostigmine metabolism and excretion. This results in resistance to drug effects.
• Periodically measure vital capacity and muscle strength to assess myasthenic patient's response to drug, especially with increasing doses.
• In myasthenia gravis, muscle groups may respond differently to the same drug. No response and persistent weakness may occur in one muscle group, increased strength in another.
• Signs of drug's muscarinic effects include abdominal cramps, diaphoresis, diarrhea, excessive bronchial and salivary secretions, lacrimation, nausea, and vomiting. If these signs or symptoms occur, promptly stop drug. Give atropine sulfate I.V., 1 to 4 mg, then additional doses every 5 to 30 minutes, as needed. Maintain airway and adequate ventilation.
• Be alert for cholinergic crisis, which can occur with overdose. Stop anticholinesterase therapy. In cholinergic crisis, muscle weakness usually occurs 1 hour after last pyridostigmine dose.

Reactions may be *common*, uncommon, ***life-threatening***, or **COMMON AND LIFE-THREATENING**.

It's accompanied by adverse muscarinic effects and fasciculations. Weakness that occurs 3 or more hours after the last drug dose may indicate myasthenic crisis and need for more drug. An edrophonium chloride (Tensilon) test may also be used to differentiate cholinergic crisis from myasthenic crisis.

PATIENT TEACHING
• Instruct patient to notify prescriber about excessive salivation or sweating, or frequent urination or diarrhea.
• Instruct patient to notify prescriber if difficulty breathing or severe muscle weakness occurs.
• Instruct patient to wear medical identification bracelet indicating he has myasthenia gravis.

pyridoxine hydrochloride (vitamin B₆)

Pharmacologic class: water-soluble vitamin
Therapeutic class: nutritional supplement
Pregnancy risk category: A (C for dosage greater than RDA)
pH: 2 to 3.8

INDICATIONS & DOSAGES
➤ **Pyridoxine dependency syndrome—**
Infants with seizures: 10 to 100 mg I.V. during seizure.
➤ **Isoniazid poisoning—**
Adults: Dose equal to amount of isoniazid ingested, usually 1 to 4 g I.V., followed by 1 g I.M. q 30 minutes until entire dose is given. Usually given with anticonvulsants, p.r.n.
➤ **Hydrazine poisoning—**
Adults: 25 mg/kg; one-third given I.M. and remainder by I.V. over 3 hours.

➤ **Mushroom poisoning (genus *Gyromitra*)—**
Adults: 25 mg/kg I.V. infused over 15 to 30 minutes repeated, p.r.n. Maximum dosage, 15 to 20 g I.V. daily.
Adjust-a-dose: Increase dosage in hemodialysis patients.

ADMINISTRATION
Direct injection: Inject undiluted drug into I.V. line containing a free-flowing, compatible solution.
Intermittent infusion: Infuse diluted drug over prescribed duration.
Continuous infusion: Not used.

PREPARATION & STORAGE
Available in 1 ml vials, containing a concentration of 100 mg/ml.
    For intermittent infusion, dilute with recommended solutions to ordered concentrations.
    Store at room temperature, and protect from light and freezing.

Incompatibilities
Alkaline solutions, erythromycin estolate, iron salts, kanamycin, oxidizers, riboflavin phosphate sodium, streptomycin.

CONTRAINDICATIONS & CAUTIONS
• Contraindicated in those hypersensitive to pyridoxine.

ADVERSE REACTIONS
CNS: drowsiness, headache, paresthesia, weakness, unsteady gait, numbness, somnolence, peripheral neuropathies, *seizures after high I.V. doses.*
GI: nausea.
Other: hypersensitivity reactions.

INTERACTIONS
Drug-drug. *Hydralazine, isoniazid:* These drugs increase daily pyridoxine requirements. May need to adjust dosage.

Levodopa: Increases breakdown of levodopa in the periphery of the body, decreasing effectiveness. Avoid using together.

Phenytoin sodium: Decreases phenytoin blood levels. Avoid using together.

Drug-lifestyle. *Alcohol use:* May cause delirium and lactic acidosis after drinking alcohol. Discourage patient use.

EFFECTS ON LAB TEST RESULTS
● May increase AST level. May decrease folic acid level.
● May cause false-positive results in tests for urine urobilinogen.

ACTION
Active as coenzyme in protein, carbohydrate, and fat metabolism. Also converts tryptophan to niacin or serotonin.

PHARMACOKINETICS
Unknown onset and duration.
Distribution: In liver, muscle, and brain. Drug isn't protein bound. Drug crosses the placental barrier and appears in breast milk.
Metabolism: In RBCs and liver.
Excretion: In urine. Half-life 15 to 20 days.

CLINICAL CONSIDERATIONS
● Osmolality: 852 to 870 mOsm/kg.
● Signs and symptoms of vitamin B_6 deficiency include personality changes, stomatitis, and heightened risk of GU infections.
● Give pyridoxine I.V. when oral route is unsuitable, as in nausea, vomiting, and preoperative and postoperative conditions or impossible, as in malabsorption syndrome or after gastric resection.
● Dosages of 200 mg daily for more than 30 days may cause pyridoxine dependency syndrome.
● In patients receiving high doses for several weeks or months, watch for symptoms of overdose, including ataxia and severe neuropathy.

● High drug doses during pregnancy may cause pyridoxine dependency seizures in neonates.
● Infants with hereditary pyridoxine dependency syndrome require high drug doses in first week of life to prevent seizures and mental retardation. Drug usually stops seizures within 3 minutes.

PATIENT TEACHING
● Instruct patient to maintain good nutrition to prevent recurrence, as appropriate.
● Inform patient of injection site burning with drug administration.
● Explain use of drug and its administration to patient and family.

Reactions may be *common,* uncommon, *life-threatening,* or COMMON AND LIFE-THREATENING.

quinidine gluconate

Pharmacologic class: cinchona alkaloid
Therapeutic class: class IA antiarrhythmic, antimalarial
Pregnancy risk category: C
pH: 5.5 to 7

INDICATIONS & DOSAGES
➤**Arrhythmias, including atrial fibrillation or flutter, paroxysmal atrial or junctional tachycardia, ventricular or atrial premature contractions, and ventricular tachycardia in the absence of heart block—**
Adults: Initially, up to 0.25 mg/kg/minute I.V. infusion, then adjusted to control arrhythmias. Usual dose needed to control arrhythmias is up to 5 mg/kg, but up to 10 mg/kg may be required.
Children ♦ : 30 mg/kg daily or 900 mg/m² daily in five divided doses.
➤**Severe malaria caused by *Plasmodium falciparum* when I.V. quinine dihydrochloride isn't available—**
Adults: Centers for Disease Control and Prevention (CDC) recommends 10 mg/kg diluted in 250 ml of normal saline solution given over 1 to 2 hours, followed by a continuous infusion of 0.02 mg/kg/minute for 72 hours or until parasitemia is reduced to less than 1%. Or, for intermittent infusion, give loading dose of 24 mg/kg in 250 ml normal saline solution over 4 hours, then 4 hours later begin maintenance doses of 12 mg/kg I.V. given over 4 hours q 8 hours for 7 days or until oral therapy is tolerated.

Children ♦ : CDC recommends 10 mg/kg diluted in 250 ml of normal saline solution given over 1 to 2 hours, followed by a continuous infusion of 0.02 mg/kg/minute for 72 hours or until parasitemia is reduced to less than 1%.

ADMINISTRATION
Direct injection: Not recommended.
Intermittent infusion: Infuse solution through I.V. line over prescribed duration.
Continuous infusion: Infuse solution through I.V. line initially at prescribed rate, then adjust rate to control arrhythmias. Rate not to exceed 0.25 mg/kg/minute.

PREPARATION & STORAGE
Available in 10-ml vials (80 mg/ml).
    For intermittent infusion, dilute with D₅W to ordered concentration. For continuous infusion, dilute 800 mg (1 vial) with 40 ml of D₅W to yield 16 mg/ml. Don't use solution if it's brown.
    Store at room temperature and protect from light and freezing. Diluted solutions are stable at room temperature for 24 hours, or refrigerated for 48 hours.

Incompatibilities
Alkalies, amiodarone, atracurium besylate, furosemide, heparin sodium, iodides.

CONTRAINDICATIONS & CAUTIONS
• Contraindicated in those hypersensitive to the drug or cinchona derivatives.
• Contraindicated in those with myasthenia gravis because drug may exacerbate weakness.

• Contraindicated in those with cardiac glycoside-induced AV conduction disorders, complete AV block, severe intraventricular conduction defects caused by a widened QRS complex, or escape junctional or ventricular rhythms because of additive cardiac depression.

• Contraindicated in those with a history of quinidine-linked thrombocytopenia purpura.

• Use cautiously in geriatric patients and in those with hepatic or renal impairment because of decreased drug metabolism and risk of toxic reaction and in those with hypokalemia because of possible reduced drug effect.

• Use cautiously in those with asthma, emphysema, weakness, or febrile infection because symptoms can mask those of quinidine hypersensitivity.

• Use cautiously in those with incomplete AV block because of potential for complete block and in those with heart failure or hypotension because drug may decrease myocardial contractility or blood pressure and aggravate these conditions.

• Use cautiously in those with digitalis toxicity because drug may intensify cardiac depression and inhibit intracardial conduction, and in those with psoriasis or a history of thrombocytopenia because drug may worsen these disorders.

• Safety and efficacy in pediatric patients haven't been established.

ADVERSE REACTIONS

CNS: confusion, *headache, light-headedness, vertigo, fatigue,* ataxia, depression, dementia, fever.
CV: *ECG changes, PVC, ventricular tachycardia, torsades de pointes, ventricular fibrillation, hypotension, complete AV block, tachycardia,* flushing.
EENT: blurred vision and other visual changes, *tinnitus.*
GI: *diarrhea, nausea, vomiting,* abdominal pain.

Hematologic: *agranulocytosis, hemolytic anemia, thrombocytopenia.*
Hepatic: *hepatotoxicity,* jaundice.
Musculoskeletal: arthralgia, myalgia.
Skin: pallor, pruritus, rash, photosensitivity, urticaria.
Other: *anaphylaxis, angioedema,* cinchonism, lupus erythematosus.

INTERACTIONS

Drug-drug. *Amiodarone, cimetidine:* Potentiates quinidine toxicity. Monitor patient closely.
Antiarrhythmics such as lidocaine, procainamide, and propranolol: May cause additive cardiac effects. Monitor patient closely.
Anticholinergics: Potentiates effects of anticholinergics. Monitor patient closely.
Antihypertensives: Causes excessive hypotension. Avoid using together.
Bethanechol, cholinergics: May antagonize cholinergic effects. Monitor patient closely.
Digoxin: Increases digoxin level. Monitor digoxin level, and adjust dose as needed.
Drugs that alkalize urine such as acetazolamide, sodium bicarbonate, some antacids, propranolol, and thiazide diuretics: Increases quinidine level. Dosage may need to be adjusted.
Fosphenytoin, phenobarbital, phenytoin: May decrease quinidine effects. Monitor patient closely.
Rifampin: May increase metabolism of quinidine, reducing drug's therapeutic effects. Monitor therapeutic response. Dosage may need to be adjusted.
Neuromuscular blockers such as cisatracurium, gallamine, metocurine, pancuronium, succinylcholine, tubocurarine: Potentiates effects of neuromuscular blockade. Monitor patient closely.
Nifedipine: May decrease quinidine level and reduce therapeutic response. Monitor patient closely.
Warfarin: Increases bleeding tendency. Monitor INR closely.

Reactions may be *common*, uncommon, *life-threatening*, or COMMON AND LIFE-THREATENING.

Drug-herb. *Jimsonweed:* May adversely affect CV function. Discourage use together.
Licorice: May prolong QT interval and cause additive effects. Discourage use together.
Drug-lifestyle. *Sun exposure:* Increases risk of photosensitivity reactions. Advise patient to avoid excessive sunlight exposure.

EFFECTS ON LAB TEST RESULTS
● May decrease hemoglobin and platelet and granulocyte counts.

ACTION
Exerts direct action on myocardial cell membranes and indirect effects on cardiac tissue. Drug decreases conduction velocity and membrane responsiveness.

PHARMACOKINETICS
Drug level peaks in 1 to 4 hours; 1 or 2 hours in a healthy adult.
Distribution: To all tissues except those of the brain; 80% to 90% protein bound. Highest levels appear in the heart, liver, kidneys, and skeletal muscles. Drug also binds to hemoglobin and crosses the placental barrier.
Metabolism: In the liver.
Excretion: Probably by glomerular filtration, with 10% to 50% excreted unchanged in urine in 24 hours. Excretion increases with acidic urine and decreases in alkaline urine. Normal drug half-life, 6 to 8 hours; range, 3 to 16 hours or longer. Small amounts of drug appear in breast milk.

CLINICAL CONSIDERATIONS
● Osmolality: 80 mg/ml is 220 mOsm/kg.
● Use I.V. administration when a rapid therapeutic effect is needed or patient can't take drug orally.
● During infusion, continuously monitor blood pressure and cardiac function, including ECG. Rapid infusion of as little as 200 mg may reduce blood pressure by 40 to 50 mm Hg.
● Monitor quinidine and potassium levels; quinidine level greater than 8 mcg/ml is toxic.
● *Alert:* Stop quinidine if QRS complex widens to over 25% greater than before infusion, P wave disappears, a rapid heart rate declines to 120 beats/minute, or normal sinus rhythm is restored.
● GI adverse effects, especially diarrhea, are signs of toxic reaction.
● Quinidine toxicity is called cinchonism, an acute anticholinergic syndrome of headache, fever, visual disturbance, mydriasis, tinnitus, nausea, vomiting, coma, and cardiorespiratory arrest.
● Signs and symptoms of overdose include absence of P waves and widening of QRS complex and PR and QT intervals, anuria, apnea, ataxia, extrasystoles, hallucinations, hypotension, irritability, lethargy, respiratory distress, seizures, thrashing, twitching, and ventricular arrhythmias.
● If overdose occurs, promptly discontinue drug and give oxygen and ventilatory support. Assist with cardiac pacing and give hypertensives, urine acidifiers, and I.V. fluids, as needed. Replace fluids, then give metaraminol or norepinephrine, as ordered, to treat hypotension. Infuse 1/6 M sodium lactate to reduce quinidine's cardiotoxic effects. Don't give CNS depressants.

PATIENT TEACHING
● Inform patient that diarrhea commonly occurs early in therapy.
● Instruct patient to immediately report any light-headedness, difficulty breathing, or palpitations. Dosage may need to be reduced.

quinupristin and dalfopristin
Synercid

Pharmacologic class: streptogramin antibacterial
Therapeutic class: antibiotic
Pregnancy risk category: B
pH: 4.4 to 5.1

INDICATIONS & DOSAGES
➤ **Serious or life-threatening infections caused by vancomycin-resistant
Enterococcus faecium bacteremia—**
*Adults and adolescents ages 16 and
older:* 7.5 mg/kg I.V. infusion over 1
hour q 8 hours. Length of treatment depends on site and severity of infection.
➤ **Complicated skin and skin-
structure infections caused by
methicillin-susceptible *Staphylococcus aureus* or *Streptococcus
pyogenes*—**
*Adults and adolescents ages 16 and
older:* 7.5 mg/kg by I.V. infusion over
1 hour q 12 hours for at least 7 days.
Adjust-a-dose: Dosage may need to be
reduced in those with hepatic insufficiency.

ADMINISTRATION
Direct injection: Not recommended.
Intermittent infusion: Give by I.V. infusion over 1 hour. An infusion pump or
device may be used to control rate of
infusion.
Continuous infusion: Not recommended.

PREPARATION & STORAGE
Available as 150 mg quinupristin and
350 mg dalfopristin in 10-ml vials.
    Reconstitute powder for injection by
adding 5 ml of either sterile water for
injection or D_5W. Gently swirl the vial
by manual rotation to ensure dissolution; avoid shaking to limit foaming.

Reconstituted solutions must be further
diluted.
    The appropriate dose of reconstitut-
ed solution, determined by the patient's
weight, should be added to 250 ml of
D_5W to make a final concentration of
no more than 2 mg/ml. Fluid-restricted
patients with a central venous catheter
may receive the dose in 100 ml of D_5W.
This concentration isn't recommended
for peripheral venous administration.
Flush the I.V. line with D_5W before and
after administration.
    Store vials at 36° to 46° F (2° to
8° C). Use reconstituted solution within 30 minutes. The diluted solution is
stable for 5 hours if kept at room temperature or 54 hours if refrigerated at
36° to 46° F (2° to 8° C). Avoid freezing. Drug is compatible at the Y-site
with aztreonam, ciprofloxacin, fluconi-
zole, haloperidol, metoclopramide, and
potassium chloride.

Incompatibilities
Saline and heparin solutions. Do not
mix with other drugs except those listed above.

CONTRAINDICATIONS & CAUTIONS
• Contraindicated in those hypersensitive to the drug or other streptogramin
antibiotics.
• Use cautiously in breast-feeding
women because it's unknown if drug
appears in breast milk.

ADVERSE REACTIONS
CNS: headache, pain.
CV: thrombophlebitis.
GI: nausea, diarrhea, vomiting.
Skin: rash; pruritus; *infusion site reac-
tion; inflammation, pain, and edema at
infusion site.*

INTERACTIONS
Drug-drug. *Cyclosporine:* Reduces
metabolism and may increase cyclosporine level. Monitor level.

Reactions may be *common*, uncommon, ***life-threatening***, or COMMON AND LIFE-THREATENING.

Drugs metabolized by cytochrome P-450 3A4, such as carbamazepine, delavirdine, diazepam, diltiazem, disopyramide, docetaxel, indinavir, lidocaine, lovastatin, methylprednisolone, midazolam, nevirapine, nifedipine, paclitaxel, ritonavir, tacrolimus, verapamil, and vinblastine: Increases levels of these drugs, which could increase their therapeutic effects and adverse reactions. Use together cautiously.

Drugs metabolized by cytochrome P-450 3A4 that may prolong the QTc interval, such as quinidine: Decreases metabolism of these drugs, prolonging the QTc interval. Avoid using together.

EFFECTS ON LAB TEST RESULTS
• May increase AST, ALT, and bilirubin levels.

ACTION
Dalfopristin inhibits the early phase of protein synthesis in the bacterial ribosome, and quinupristin inhibits the late phase. Without the ability to manufacture new proteins, the bacterial cells are inactivated or die.

PHARMACOKINETICS
Onset, unknown; peak, unknown; duration, unknown.
Distribution: Moderately protein bound.
Metabolism: Quinupristin and dalfopristin are converted to several active metabolites by nonenzymatic reactions.
Excretion: About 75% in feces and 15% in urine. Half-lives of quinupristin and dalfopristin are 0.85 and 0.7 hours, respectively.

CLINICAL CONSIDERATIONS
• If moderate to severe peripheral venous irritation occurs, consider increasing infusion volume to 500 or 750 ml, changing injection site, or infusing by a central venous catheter.

• Drug isn't active against *Enterococcus faecalis*. Appropriate blood cultures are needed to avoid misidentifying *E. faecalis* as *E. faecium*.
• Drug may cause mild to life-threatening pseudomembranous colitis, so consider this diagnosis in patients who develop diarrhea during or after therapy with the drug.
• Adverse reactions, such as arthralgia and myalgia, may be reduced by decreasing the dosing interval to every 12 hours.
• Monitor patient closely for signs and symptoms of superinfection because overgrowth of nonsusceptible organisms may occur.
• Monitor liver function test results during therapy.

PATIENT TEACHING
• Advise patient to immediately report irritation at I.V. site, pain in joints or muscles, and diarrhea.
• Tell patient about importance of reporting persistent or worsening signs and symptoms of infection, such as pain and fever.

R

ranitidine hydrochloride
Zantac

Pharmacologic class: H$_2$-receptor antagonist
Therapeutic class: antiulcerative
Pregnancy risk category: B
pH: 6.7 to 7.3

INDICATIONS & DOSAGES
➤ **Active duodenal or gastric ulcer and pathologic hypersecretory conditions, such as Zollinger-Ellison syndrome and multiple endocrine adenomas, in hospitalized patients who can't take drug orally—**
Adults: 50 mg q 6 to 8 hours; continuous infusion at 6.25 mg/hour over 24 hours. Maximum dose, 400 mg daily.
Adjust-a-dose: Adjust dosage in renal impairment. For adults with creatinine clearance less than 50 ml/minute, dosage is 50 mg q 18 to 24 hours, increasing to q 12 hours or more often, if needed. Give dose after hemodialysis.

ADMINISTRATION
Direct injection: Inject diluted drug into a patent I.V. line over at least 5 minutes. Don't exceed 4 ml/minute.
Intermittent infusion: Infuse diluted drug into a patent I.V. line through a piggyback set over 15 to 20 minutes. Don't exceed 5 to 7 ml/minute.
Continuous infusion: Infuse over 24 hours at a rate of 6.25 mg/hour. No loading dose is needed.

PREPARATION & STORAGE
Available in 2- and 6-ml vials containing 25 mg/ml and as 1-mg/ml premixed solution in 50-ml container.

For direct injection, dilute 50 mg with compatible I.V. solution such as normal saline, D$_5$W, dextrose 10% in water, or lactated Ringer's solution to a total volume of 20 ml. For intermittent infusion, dilute 50 mg dose with 100 ml of a compatible I.V. solution. For continuous infusion, dilute 150 mg in 250 ml of D$_5$W.

Store I.V. vial at 39° to 86° F (4° to 30° C). Store premixed containers at 36° to 77° F (2° to 25° C). Protect from light and freezing. Solutions remain stable for 48 hours at room temperature. Don't use if discolored or if a precipitate is present.

Incompatibilities
Amphotericin B, atracurium, cefazolin, cefoxitin, ceftazidime, cefuroxime, chlorpromazine, clindamycin phosphate, diazepam, ethacrynate sodium, hetastarch, hydroxyzine, insulin (regular), methotrimeprazine, midazolam, norepinephrine, pentobarbital sodium, phenobarbital, phytonadione.

CONTRAINDICATIONS & CAUTIONS
● Contraindicated in those hypersensitive to the drug.
● Use cautiously in breast-feeding women; also use cautiously in those with renal or hepatic impairment because drug levels may be increased.

ADVERSE REACTIONS
CNS: agitation, headache, vertigo, malaise.
EENT: blurred vision.

Reactions may be *common*, uncommon, *life-threatening*, or COMMON AND LIFE-THREATENING.

GI: constipation, diarrhea, nausea, vomiting, abdominal pain.
GU: impotence.
Hematologic: eosinophilia, *granulocytopenia, leukopenia, pancytopenia, thrombocytopenia.*
Hepatic: jaundice.
Skin: rash; burning, pain, or itching at I.V. site.
Other: *anaphylaxis,* gynecomastia, decreased libido, *angioneurotic edema, hypersensitivity reactions.*

INTERACTIONS
Drug-drug. *Glipizide:* May increase hypoglycemic effects. Adjust glipizide dosage if needed.
Procainamide: Decreases renal clearance of procainamide. Monitor patient closely for toxicity.
Warfarin: May interfere with warfarin clearance. Monitor PT and INR.
Drug-lifestyle. *Tobacco:* May inhibit ranitidine's ability to suppress nocturnal gastric acid secretion. Discourage use together.

EFFECTS ON LAB TEST RESULTS
• May increase creatinine, AST, ALT, alkaline phosphatase, and bilirubin levels.
• May decrease hemoglobin, hematocrit, and WBC, granulocyte, and platelet counts.
• May cause false-negative skin test results because of inhibited cutaneous histamine response. May cause false-positive results of Multistix test. May reduce response to pentagastrin in gastric acid secretion test.

ACTION
H_2-receptor antagonist that inhibits histamine's action on gastric parietal cells, thus reducing basal and nocturnal gastric acid secretion. It also inhibits stimulation of gastric acid secretion by food, betazole, pentagastrin, insulin, and vagal reflex.

Other effects include increased gastric nitrate–reducing organisms; a small, transient, dose-related increase in prolactin level; and possibly impaired vasopressin release.

PHARMACOKINETICS
Drug level peaks in 15 minutes.
Distribution: Widely distributed, with 10% to 19% protein bound. Drug enters CSF. Unknown if it crosses the placental barrier.
Metabolism: In the liver.
Excretion: Primarily in urine, with about 70% removed unchanged. Half-life, 2 to 2½ hours. Drug appears in breast milk.

CLINICAL CONSIDERATIONS
• Osmolality: 10 mg/ml is 59 mOsm/kg, 1 mg/ml is 260 to 302 mOsm/kg, 2 mg/ml is 257 to 294 mOsm/kg.
• Osmolarity: 180 mOsm/L for premixed 1 mg/ml solution in normal saline solution.
• Malignant GI neoplasm should be ruled out before drug therapy.
• Monitor ALT levels if patient receives 400 mg daily for 5 days or longer. Begin on fifth day of therapy and check daily until discontinuation.
• Patients with hepatic or renal impairment should receive a reduced dose.
• Hemodialysis removes the drug.
• *Alert:* Don't confuse ranitidine (Zantac) with cetirizine (Zyrtec).

PATIENT TEACHING
• Instruct patient to inform prescriber if rash, sore throat, fever, or easy bruising or bleeding occurs.

red blood cells, packed

Pharmacologic class: human blood derivative
Therapeutic class: RBC replacement
Pregnancy risk category: NR
pH: 7.6 at day 1; 6.71 at day 35

INDICATIONS & DOSAGES

➤ **To replace RBCs or restore or maintain adequate oxygenation with minimal expansion of blood volume, especially in severe symptomatic anemia, slow blood loss, or heart failure—**
Adults: Number of units is determined by clinical status.
Children: 10 ml/kg, not to exceed 15 ml/kg.

ADMINISTRATION

Direct injection: Appropriate only for neonatal transfusion. Draw prefiltered RBCs into a 50-ml syringe and inject slowly through a 19G to 21G needle or catheter.
Intermittent infusion: Infuse through a Y-type set with at least a 170-micron filter at a rate of 1 unit over 2 to 3 hours for adults and 2 to 5 ml/kg hourly for children. If infusion will exceed 4 hours, the blood bank can divide units into several bags with small volumes. For optimal flow rate, use at least a 19G needle. In children and adults with small veins, use a 21G or 23G needle, if needed.

Use automatic infusion devices only if they've been tested and approved for transfusion by the manufacturer. Don't inflate manual pressure cuffs above 300 mm Hg.

Begin infusion slowly, and remain at bedside. Monitor vital signs. If patient shows no signs of transfusion reaction, adjust flow to prescribed rate. During rapid, massive infusion, use a microaggregate filter with a 20- to 40-micron pore size. Used with or as replacement for standard blood filters, these filters remove small WBC particulates that aggregate during storage. Aggregates may migrate to the lungs and cause dyspnea.
Continuous infusion: Not used.

PREPARATION & STORAGE

For rapid infusion, dilute with 50 to 100 ml of normal saline solution. Add the normal saline solution via a closed sterile system using a Y-type infusion set connected to the saline container and the packed RBC bag. Invert the bag, and open the roller clamps from the saline to the packed RBCs.

Store packed RBCs at 34° to 43° F (1° to 6° C) in a continuously monitored refrigerator. If temperature goes beyond this range, risk increases for reduced viability, hemolysis, and bacterial proliferation. Maximum storage time is 35 to 42 days, depending on preservative or anticoagulant used. If patient is at risk for circulatory overload, preservatives, such as adenine, saline, and dextrose are removed before transfusion.

Incompatibilities

All I.V. drugs and solutions, except normal saline solution.

CONTRAINDICATIONS & CAUTIONS

• Contraindicated in those with asymptomatic anemia or conditions that may be managed effectively with crystalloid or colloid solutions.
• Give large amounts of packed RBCs cautiously because of risk of hypervolemia.

ADVERSE REACTIONS

CNS: anxiety, headache, fever above 100.4° F (38° C) or an increase of more than 2° F.
CV: volume overload, flushing.

Reactions may be *common,* uncommon, *life-threatening,* or COMMON AND LIFE-THREATENING.

Hematologic: *acute hemolytic reaction, hemosiderosis.*
Hepatic: *hepatitis.*
Musculoskeletal: myalgia.
Skin: pruritus, urticaria.
Other: Creutzfeldt-Jakob disease, *graft-versus-host disease,* transmission of viral infections including *AIDS.*

INTERACTIONS
None reported.

EFFECTS ON LAB TEST RESULTS
None reported.

COMPOSITION
Derived from whole blood after sedimentation or centrifugation, packed RBCs are suspended in about 50 ml of plasma or 100 ml of an additive nutrient solution.

This product and whole blood have equal oxygen-carrying capacities because they contain equal numbers of RBCs, but packed RBCs contain less sodium and potassium than whole blood. The volume of each unit of packed RBCs is 250 to 350 ml; hematocrit is 65% to 80%.

CLINICAL CONSIDERATIONS
• Confirm recipient's identity by comparing name and identification number on blood bag tag with patient identification bracelet. Verify blood compatibility by matching blood group and type on bag to chart or other blood bank record. Have another qualified staff member also check this information.
• RBCs needn't always match patient's group and type, but they must always be compatible. Type O is compatible with RBC type O; type A with A or O; type B with B or O; and type AB with AB, O, A, or B. If recipient's blood is Rh-positive, it's compatible with Rh-positive and Rh-negative RBCs; if it's

Rh-negative, it's compatible with Rh-negative RBCs.
• Don't give any drug through a line used for blood product transfusion.
• Patients having repeat febrile reactions may better tolerate leukocyte-poor blood. Use a leukocyte-depleting filter with the standard blood filter or as a replacement for it.
• Blood warmers may be used during transfusion to prevent arrhythmias caused by rapid infusion of cold blood. Prewarmed blood should also be used in transfusions to patients with cold agglutinin disease. Use coil-tubing or heated-plate warmers designed to allow close temperature monitoring; RBC hemolysis can occur if temperature exceeds 104° F (40° C).
• Allow at least 1 hour for a routine crossmatch. In an emergency, O-negative RBCs may be safely transfused.
• Take vital signs, record results, and establish a patent venous catheter before requesting release of RBCs from the blood bank.
• Monitor vital signs every 15 minutes until 1 hour after transfusion. Record vital signs, product number, starting and ending times, volume, and response to transfusion.
• Monitor patient for chills, fever, hypotension, low back pain, tachycardia, and tachypnea. These may signal an acute hemolytic reaction, especially if they occur during administration of the first 50 ml of RBCs.
• If acute hemolytic reaction occurs, stop transfusion at the needle hub and rapidly infuse normal saline. Notify the prescriber and blood bank, and treat symptomatically to maintain renal blood flow. Also arrange for a serologic evaluation of urine and blood.
• Alloimmunization (the development of antibodies to foreign antigens) occurs in 1% or 2% of previously transfused or pregnant patients, and may be responsible for delayed hemolytic reac-

tions. Subsequent crossmatching is more difficult in these patients.

PATIENT TEACHING
• Instruct patient to immediately inform nurse if unusual symptoms occur.
• Teach patient about need for transfusion, how it's done, and related tests.

red blood cells, washed (leukocyte-poor RBCs, washed packed cells)

Pharmacologic class: human blood derivative
Therapeutic class: RBC replacement
Pregnancy risk category: NR

INDICATIONS & DOSAGES
➤ **To replace RBCs or restore or maintain adequate oxygenation with minimal expansion of blood volume in severe or recurrent febrile nonhemolytic transfusion reactions or urticarial allergic reactions—**
Adults: Number of units is determined by clinical status.

ADMINISTRATION
Direct injection: Not used.
Intermittent infusion: Infuse through a Y-type set with at least a 170-micron filter. Give at a rate of 1 unit over 2 to 3 hours for adults and 2 to 5 ml/kg hourly for children. The blood bank can divide units into several bags containing small volumes if infusion will exceed 4 hours. For optimal rate, use at least a 19G needle or, in children and adults with smaller veins, a 21G or 23G winged infusion set.
  Begin infusion slowly. Take vital signs. If patient shows no evidence of transfusion reaction, adjust flow to the prescribed rate.

Infusion devices are useful for exceedingly slow rates, especially in children and neonates, but packed or washed cells are likely to undergo hemolysis when given through a pressurized infusion pump. Consult pump manufacturer before use.
Continuous infusion: Not used.

PREPARATION & STORAGE
Storage of frozen, thawed RBCs is limited to 24 hours at 34° to 43° F (1° to 6° C) because deglycerolization and resuspension occur in transfer from the original bag for washing.

Incompatibilities
All I.V. drugs and solutions, except normal saline.

CONTRAINDICATIONS & CAUTIONS
• Contraindicated in those with only one previous transfusion reaction.
• Use cautiously if infusing large amounts of washed RBCs because of risk of hypervolemia.

ADVERSE REACTIONS
CNS: malaise, fever.
CV: hypervolemia.
Hematologic: *acute hemolytic anemia.*
Hepatic: jaundice, *hepatitis.*
Other: Creutzfeldt-Jakob disease, transmission of viral infections including *AIDS.*

INTERACTIONS
None reported.

EFFECTS ON LAB TEST RESULTS
None reported.

COMPOSITION
Washed RBCs are derived from whole blood. About 200 to 250 ml of plasma are first removed from a collected pint of blood of about 500 ml. Then the RBC buffy coat, consisting of WBCs and platelets, is removed by saline

washing, inverted centrifugation, or microaggregate blood filters.

The American Association of Blood Banks' standards specify elimination of 70% of WBCs with less than 30% loss of RBCs. After washing, the concentration of RBCs is about 70% to 90%. The volume of each unit of washed RBCs is 250 to 300 ml.

CLINICAL CONSIDERATIONS

• Confirm recipient's identity by comparing name and identification number on blood bag tag with patient identification bracelet. Verify blood compatibility by matching blood group and type on bag with chart or other blood bank record. Have another qualified staff member also perform this check.

• RBCs needn't always match patient's blood group and type, but they must always be compatible. Type O is compatible with RBC type O; type A with A or O; type B with B or O; and type AB with AB, O, A, or B. If recipient's blood is Rh-positive, it's compatible with Rh-positive and Rh-negative RBCs; if it's Rh-negative, it's compatible with Rh-negative cells.

• Don't give any drug through a line used for transfusion.

• Use blood warmers during transfusion to prevent arrhythmias caused by rapid infusion of cold blood. Use prewarmed blood in transfusions to patients with cold agglutinin disease. Use coil-tubing or heated-plate warmers designed to allow close monitoring of temperature; RBC hemolysis can occur if temperature exceeds 104° F (40° C). However, routine blood warming is unnecessary and usually slows infusion rate.

• If patient continues to have reactions even after administration of washed cells, use of frozen thawed deglycerolized RBCs may be effective.

• If patient has had one febrile or allergic transfusion reaction, he usually doesn't have a second. Repeat reactions are more common in women who have had multiple pregnancies and in those who receive frequent transfusions. Repeated transfusion reactions are needed before receiving washed RBCs.

• Alloimmunization occurs in 1% to 2% of previously transfused or pregnant patients and may be responsible for delayed hemolytic transfusion reactions. Subsequent blood crossmatching is more difficult in these patients.

• Washing RBCs removes plasma and WBCs, further reducing risk of allergic reaction to donor plasma.

• Washing RBCs may result in loss of some RBCs. Frequent transfusions may be needed.

• Urticarial reactions are nearly eliminated by using washed RBCs.

• Allow at least 1 hour for a routine blood crossmatch. In an emergency, O-negative RBCs may be safely transfused to all patients.

• Take vital signs, record results, and establish a patent venous catheter before requesting release of RBCs from the blood bank.

• Monitor vital signs every 15 minutes until 1 hour after transfusion. Record vital signs, product number, starting and ending times, volume, and response to transfusion.

• Observe patient for fever, falling hematocrit, jaundice, and malaise, which may indicate a delayed hemolytic reaction.

PATIENT TEACHING

• Instruct patient to immediately inform prescriber if unusual symptoms occur.

• Teach patient about need for transfusion, how it will be given, and related tests.

remifentanil hydrochloride
Ultiva

Pharmacologic class: mu-opioid
agonist
Therapeutic class: analgesic
anesthetic
Pregnancy risk category: C
Controlled substance schedule: II
pH: 2.5 to 3.5

INDICATIONS & DOSAGES
➤ **To induce or maintain general
anesthesia—**
Adults and children age 2 and older:
0.5 to 1 mcg/kg/minute with a hypnotic
or volatile drug; may load with 1 mcg/
kg over 30 to 60 seconds if endotracheal
intubation is to occur in less than 8 minutes after start of remifentanil infusion.
➤ **To maintain anesthesia—**
Adults and children age 2 and older:
0.05 to 2 mcg/kg/minute, depending on
concurrent anesthetic modalities—that
is, nitrous oxide, isoflurane, and propofol. Increase doses by 25% to 100%
and decrease by 25% to 50% q 2 to 5
minutes, p.r.n. If rate exceeds 1 mcg/
kg/minute, consider increases in other
anesthetics. May supplement with
1-mcg/kg boluses over 30 to 60 seconds q 2 to 5 minutes, p.r.n.
➤ **To continue as analgesic immediately postoperatively—**
Adults and children age 2 and older:
0.1 mcg/kg/minute, followed by infusion rate of 0.025 to 0.2 mcg/kg/
minute. Adjust rate by 0.025-mcg/kg/
minute increments q 5 minutes. Rates
above 0.2 mcg/kg/minute are linked to
respiratory depression of fewer than
8 breaths/minute.
➤ **Monitored anesthesia care—**
Adults and children age 2 and older:
As a single I.V. dose, give 0.5 to 1 mcg/
kg over 30 to 60 seconds starting 90
seconds before placement of local or

regional anesthetic. Decrease dose by
50% if given with 2 mg midazolam. As
continuous I.V. infusion, give 0.1 mcg/
kg/minute beginning 5 minutes before
local anesthetic is given; after placement of local anesthetic, adjust rate to
0.05 mcg/kg/minute. Adjust rate by
0.025 mcg/kg/minute q 5 minutes,
p.r.n. Rates exceeding 0.2 mcg/kg/
minute are linked to respiratory depression of fewer than 8 breaths/minute.
Bolus doses given simultaneously with
continuously infusing remifentanil to
spontaneously breathing patients aren't
recommended.
Adjust-a-dose: In patients older than
age 65, decrease dose by 50%. In patients who weigh over 30% more than
their ideal body weight, base the starting dose on ideal body weight.

ADMINISTRATION
Direct injection: Inject directly into a
vein over 30 to 60 seconds.
Intermittent infusion: Not recommended.
Continuous infusion: Give by I.V. infusion device only. Injection site should
be close to the venous cannula and
should be cleared when the infusion is
stopped.

PREPARATION & STORAGE
Available in preservative-free 3-, 5-,
and 10-ml lyophilized powder vials.
    Reconstitute with 1 ml of diluent per
milligram of drug, resulting in a clear,
colorless liquid. Shake well, and dilute
to a final concentration of 25, 50, or
250 mcg/ml. Don't give undiluted.
    Drug may be given in a running I.V.
administration set with lactated
Ringer's or dextrose 5% in lactated
Ringer's solution, but it may not be
mixed with those solutions.
    Store vials at room temperature. Di-
luted final product is stable for 24 hours
at room temperature when diluted with
sterile water, D_5W, dextrose 5% in nor-

mal saline solution, half-normal saline solution, or normal saline solution.

Incompatibilities
Amphotericin B, blood products, cefoperazone, chlorpromazine, dextrose 5% in lactated Ringer's solution, diazepam, lactated Ringer's solution.

CONTRAINDICATIONS & CAUTIONS
• Contraindicated in those hypersensitive to fentanyl analogues.
• Don't give via epidural or intrathecal routes because preparation contains glycine.
• Don't use as a single drug in general anesthesia.
• Use cautiously in morbidly obese patients because of changes in CV or respiratory physiology. Base initial doses on ideal body weight.
• Use cautiously in breast-feeding patients because fentanyl analogues appear in breast milk.

ADVERSE REACTIONS
CNS: dizziness, headache, visual disturbances, sedation, fever, *coma.*
CV: *bradycardia,* hypertension, hypotension, tachycardia, flushing, *circulatory depression, CV arrest.*
EENT: visual disturbances.
GI: nausea, vomiting.
Musculoskeletal: muscle rigidity.
Respiratory: *apnea, hypoxia, respiratory depression or arrest, hypoventilation.*
Skin: pruritus, sweating, pain at injection site.
Other: chills, shivering, warm sensation, postoperative pain, *shock.*

INTERACTIONS
Drug-drug. *Benzodiazepines, hypnotics, inhaled anesthetics:* Causes synergistic response. Monitor patient closely.

EFFECTS ON LAB TEST RESULTS
None reported.

ACTION
Binds to mu-opiate receptors throughout the CNS, resulting in analgesia.

PHARMACOKINETICS
Onset of analgesic effects, 1 to 3 minutes; offset 1 to 3 minutes. Steady-state levels occur within 5 to 10 minutes of changes in infusion rate. Rapid titration occurs when infusion rate or bolus amount changes.
Distribution: Initially, throughout blood and rapidly perfused tissues; then into peripheral tissues. Up to 92% protein bound.
Metabolism: Rapidly metabolized by hydrolysis via blood and tissue enzymes.
Excretion: Excreted by the kidneys with an elimination half-life of about 90 minutes. Clearance of active drug is high, with an elimination half-life of 3 to 10 minutes.

CLINICAL CONSIDERATIONS
• Drug should be used only by personnel trained in monitored anesthetic settings. Make sure that oxygen, an opioid antagonist, and equipment for resuscitation and intubation are available. Monitor oxygen saturation.
• An infusion device must be used with a continuous infusion.
• Give as an I.V. bolus only when maintaining general anesthesia.
• Interruption of infusions will result in rapid offset of effect.
• Establish adequate postoperative analgesia before stopping drug.
• Manage respiratory depression in those breathing spontaneously by decreasing infusion rate by 50% or by temporarily discontinuing infusion.
• Monitor vital signs and oxygenation continually while giving drug.
• Skeletal muscle rigidity may occur and is treated by stopping or decreasing rate of infusion in those breathing spontaneously. If rigidity occurs during

anesthesia, give neuromuscular blockers and concurrent induction drugs.
• Drug-induced bradycardia may be treated with ephedrine, atropine, and glycopyrrolate.
• If hypotension occurs, decrease rate of drug administration and give I.V. fluids or vasopressors.
• Intraoperative awareness in patients younger than age 55 has been reported when drug is given with propofol infusion rates of 75 mcg/kg/minute or less.

PATIENT TEACHING
• Explain anesthetic effect of drug and postoperative care measures to prevent atelectasis.
• Inform patient that another drug will be used to control pain once the effects of remifentanil have worn off.

respiratory syncytial virus immune globulin intravenous, human (RSV-IGIV)
RespiGam

Pharmacologic class: immuno-globulin G
Therapeutic class: prevention of RSV
Pregnancy risk category: C

INDICATIONS & DOSAGES
➤ **To prevent serious lower respiratory tract infections caused by RSV in children with bronchopulmonary dysplasia (BPD) or history of premature birth of 35 weeks' gestation or less—**
Premature infants and children younger than age 2: Single infusion monthly (November through April). Give 1.5 ml/kg/hour for 15 minutes; then, if clinical condition allows a higher rate, increase to 3.6 ml/kg/hour until infusion is complete. Maximum

recommended total dose per monthly infusion, 750 mg/kg.

ADMINISTRATION
Direct injection: Not recommended.
Intermittent infusion: Begin infusion within 6 hours and complete within 12 hours after vial has been entered. Give drug using a constant infusion pump. Don't predilute drug. If possible, give through a separate I.V. line, although it may be piggybacked into a compatible solution. Filters aren't needed, but an in-line filter with a pore size larger than 15 micrometers may be used.
Continuous infusion: Not recommended.

PREPARATION & STORAGE
Available as 20 ml and 50 ml single-use vial containing 40 to 60 mg/ml. Don't shake vial; avoid foaming. Discard after use.
    RespiGam is compatible, with or without normal saline solution, with dextrose 2.5%, 5%, 10%, and 20% in water. Don't dilute drug more than 1:2 with any of these solutions.
    Store between 35.6° and 46.4° F (2° and 8° C). Don't freeze.

Incompatibilities
Other I.V. drugs.

CONTRAINDICATIONS & CAUTIONS
• Contraindicated in those with a history of severe hypersensitivity to the drug or other human immunoglobulin and selective immunoglobulin A (IgA) deficiency, which may lead to allergic reactions.
• Don't use in children with fluid overload.
• Use cautiously in infants with heart disease.

ADVERSE REACTIONS
CNS: anxiety, dizziness, fever.
CV: chest pain, fluid overload, hypertension, palpitations, tachycardia, flushing.

Reactions may be *common,* uncommon, *life-threatening,* or COMMON AND LIFE-THREATENING.

GI: abdominal cramps, diarrhea, gastroenteritis, vomiting.
Musculoskeletal: arthralgia, myalgia.
Respiratory: dyspnea, hypoxia, crackles, *respiratory distress,* tachypnea, wheezing, hypoxemia.
Skin: injection site inflammation, rash, pruritus.
Other: *anaphylaxis.*

INTERACTIONS
Drug-drug. *Vaccines with live virus, such as mumps, rubella, and especially measles:* May interfere with response. If such vaccines are given during or within 10 months after RespiGam, reimmunization is recommended, if appropriate.

EFFECTS ON LAB TEST RESULTS
None reported.

ACTION
Provides passive immunity to RSV.

PHARMACOKINETICS
Antibodies persist for at least 1 month.
Distribution: Unknown.
Metabolism: Unknown.
Excretion: Unknown.

CLINICAL CONSIDERATIONS
• In children with congenital heart disease, especially those with right-to-left shunts, drug may increase the risk of cardiac surgery and severe, life-threatening adverse reactions.
• Give first dose before RSV season begins and subsequent doses monthly during the RSV season to maintain protection. Children with RSV should continue to receive monthly doses for duration of RSV season.
• Adhere to infusion rate guidelines; most adverse reactions may be related to rate used. In especially ill children with BPD, slower rates may be indicated.
• Assess cardiopulmonary status and vital signs before beginning infusion, before each rate increase, and every

30 minutes thereafter until 30 minutes after completion of infusion.
• Monitor patient closely for signs of fluid overload; children with BPD may be at higher risk for this condition. Report increases in heart rate, respiratory rate, retractions, or crackles. Have a loop diuretic, such as furosemide or bumetanide, available.
• If patient develops hypotension, anaphylaxis, or severe allergic reaction, stop infusion and give epinephrine (1:1,000). Patients with selective IgA deficiency can develop antibodies to IgA and have anaphylactic or allergic reactions to subsequent administration of blood products containing IgA, including RSV-IGIV.

PATIENT TEACHING
• Explain to parents the importance of their child receiving drug monthly throughout the RSV season, even if already infected.
• Tell parents how drug is given and which adverse reactions are linked to administration. Instruct parents to promptly report adverse reactions.

---

reteplase, recombinant
Retavase

Pharmacologic class: tissue-plasminogen activator
Therapeutic class: thrombolytic
Pregnancy risk category: C
pH: 6

INDICATIONS & DOSAGES
➤ **To manage acute MI—**
Adults: Double-bolus injection of 10 + 10 units. Give each bolus I.V. over 2 minutes. If complications such as serious bleeding or an anaphylactoid reaction don't occur after first bolus, give second bolus 30 minutes after start of first bolus.

ADMINISTRATION
Direct injection: Give as an I.V. bolus over 2 minutes.
Intermittent infusion: Not recommended.
Continuous infusion: Not recommended.

PREPARATION & STORAGE
Available as a sterile, preservative-free lyophilized powder in 10.8-unit (18.8-mg) vials.

Reconstitute only with materials that the manufacturer has provided. Gently swirl; avoid shaking. Reconstitute with 10 ml of sterile water for injection. Reconstitution results in solution containing 1 unit/ml. Solution should be colorless. If foaming occurs, allow vial to stand for several minutes. Inspect for precipitation.

Solution may be used within 4 hours of reconstitution when stored at 36° to 86° F (2° to 30° C). Protect from light. Don't use if solution develops particulate matter or becomes discolored. Overfill of 0.7 ml will remain in vial.

Incompatibilities
Other I.V. drugs.

CONTRAINDICATIONS & CAUTIONS
● Contraindicated in those with active internal bleeding, known bleeding diathesis, history of CVA, severe uncontrolled hypertension, intracranial neoplasm, arteriovenous malformation, aneurysm, or recent intracranial hemorrhage, intraspinal surgery, or trauma.
● Use cautiously in those who within the past 10 days have had major surgery, obstetric delivery, organ biopsy, or trauma.
● Use cautiously in those with previous puncture of noncompressible vessels; cerebrovascular disease; recent GI or GU bleeding; hypertension with systolic pressure of 180 mm Hg or more or diastolic pressure of 110 mm Hg or more; a condition that may lead to left-sided heart thrombus such as mitral stenosis; acute pericarditis; subacute bacterial endocarditis; a hemostatic defect; diabetic hemorrhagic retinopathy; septic thrombophlebitis; or a condition in which bleeding would be difficult to control.
● Use cautiously in breast-feeding patients and in those age 75 or older.
● Use in pregnancy only if the benefit justifies potential risk to the fetus.

ADVERSE REACTIONS
CNS: *intracranial hemorrhage.*
CV: *arrhythmias, cholesterol emboli.*
GI: *hemorrhage.*
GU: hematuria.
Hematologic: anemia, *hemorrhage.*
Skin: *bleeding at puncture sites.*

INTERACTIONS
Drug-drug. *Heparin; oral anticoagulants; platelet inhibitors such as aspirin, dipyridamole, and abciximab; eptifibatide:* May increase risk of bleeding. Use together cautiously.

EFFECTS ON LAB TEST RESULTS
● May increase PT, PTT, and INR. May decrease hemoglobin.
● May alter coagulation study results.

ACTION
Enhances cleavage of plasminogen to generate plasmin, which leads to fibrinolysis.

PHARMACOKINETICS
Onset 30 minutes for coronary thrombolysis, drug level peaks at 30 to 90 minutes.
Distribution: Unknown.
Metabolism: 32% inactivated in blood.
Excretion: Cleared primarily by the liver and kidney. Half-life, 13 to 16 minutes.

CLINICAL CONSIDERATIONS
● Potency is expressed in terms of units specific for reteplase that aren't comparable to those of other thrombolytics.

Reactions may be *common,* uncommon, *life-threatening,* or COMMON AND LIFE-THREATENING.

- Avoid use of noncompressible pressure sites during therapy. If an arterial puncture is needed, use an upper-extremity vessel that can be compressed manually. Apply pressure for at least 30 minutes; then apply a pressure dressing. Check site frequently.
- Carefully monitor ECG during treatment. Coronary thrombolysis may result in arrhythmias caused by reperfusion. Be prepared to treat bradycardia or ventricular irritability.
- Carefully monitor patient for bleeding. Avoid I.M. injections, invasive procedures, and nonessential handling of patient. Bleeding is the most common adverse reaction and may occur internally or at external puncture sites. If local measures don't control serious bleeding, stop anticoagulation therapy and notify prescriber. Withhold second bolus of reteplase.

PATIENT TEACHING
- Explain to patient and family about use and administration of drug.
- Tell patient to immediately report adverse reactions, including bleeding or pain.

Rh$_0$(D) immune globulin intravenous, human (Rh$_0$[D] IGIV)
WinRho SDF

Pharmacologic class: immune serum
Therapeutic class: anti-Rh$_0$ (D)–positive prophylaxis
Pregnancy risk category: C

INDICATIONS & DOSAGES
➤ **After spontaneous or induced abortion or ectopic pregnancy occurring anytime up to 13 weeks' gestation; amniocentesis after 34 weeks' gestation; other manipulation late in pregnancy after 34 weeks' gestation linked to increased risk of Rh isoimmunization—**
Adults: 120 mcg I.V. Must give within 72 hours after delivery, miscarriage, or manipulation.
➤ **Pregnancy—**
Adults: 300 mcg I.V. at 28 weeks' gestation. If early in pregnancy, give additional doses at 12-week intervals to maintain adequate levels of passively acquired anti-Rh antibodies. Then, within 72 hours of delivery, give 120 mcg. If 72 hours have elapsed, give drug as soon as possible, up to 28 days.
➤ **Transfusion accidents—**
Adults: 600 mcg I.V. q 8 hours until total dose is given. Total dose depends on volume of packed RBCs or whole blood transfused. Give within 72 hours after exposure.
➤ **Immune thrombocytopenic purpura in patients who are Rh$_0$(D) antigen positive—**
Adults and children: Initially, 50 mcg/kg I.V. If hemoglobin is less than 10 g/dl, initial dose is reduced to 25 to 40 mcg/kg. Initial dose may be given as single dose or as two divided doses given on separate days. Then, 25 to 60 mcg/kg may be given, p.r.n., to elevate platelet counts with specific dosage that's determined individually.

ADMINISTRATION
Direct injection: Inject directly into vein or free-flowing compatible I.V. solution over 3 to 5 minutes.
Intermittent infusion: Not recommended.
Continuous infusion: Not recommended.

PREPARATION & STORAGE
Available in kits containing either 120- or 300-mcg single-dose vials of anti-Rh$_0$(D) IGIV, a single-dose vial of 2.5 ml normal saline injection, or 1,000 mcg single-dose vial with 8.5 ml normal saline injection.

Reconstitute drug with accompanying vial of normal saline injection only.

Store at 35° to 46° F (2° to 8° C). Don't freeze or shake vials. If reconstituted product isn't used immediately, store at room temperature for no longer than 12 hours. Don't freeze reconstituted product. Discard unused portion.

Incompatibilities
Other I.V. drugs.

CONTRAINDICATIONS & CAUTIONS
• Contraindicated in those who are Rh$_o$(D)-positive or D^u-positive and in those who have been previously immunized to Rh$_o$(D) blood factor.
• Contraindicated in those with anaphylactic or severe systemic reactions to human globulin.
• Use cautiously in those with immunoglobulin A (IgA) deficiency. These patients may have the potential for developing IgA antibodies and have anaphylactic reactions. Potential benefit of treatment must be weighed against that for hypersensitivity reactions.

ADVERSE REACTIONS
CNS: headache, slight fever.
Skin: discomfort at injection site.
Other: *anaphylaxis,* chills.

INTERACTIONS
Drug-drug. *Vaccines with live virus:* May interfere with response. Postpone immunization, if possible.

EFFECTS ON LAB TEST RESULTS
• May decrease hemoglobin and hematocrit.
• May cause weakly positive direct antiglobulin (Coombs') test results in infants born to women who received drug. May cause detection of anti-A, anti-B, anti-C, and anti-E blood group antibodies in thrombocytopenic purpura patients undergoing direct or indirect antiglobulin (Coombs') test.

ACTION
Suppresses active antibody response and formation of anti-Rh$_o$(D) antibodies in Rh$_o$(D)-negative, D^u-negative patients exposed to Rh-positive blood. Rh$_o$(D) immune globulin I.V. may form complexes with RBCs blocking platelet destruction in adults who are Rh$_o$(D) antigen–positive.

PHARMACOKINETICS
Onset, unknown; peak, within 2 hours of administration; duration, unknown. Half-life, about 24 days.
Distribution: Unknown.
Metabolism: Unknown.
Excretion: Unknown.

CLINICAL CONSIDERATIONS
• This immune serum provides passive immunity to patient exposed to Rh$_o$-positive fetal blood during pregnancy. Drug prevents formation of maternal antibodies (active immunity), which would endanger future Rh$_o$-positive pregnancies.
• Immediately after delivery, send a sample of neonate's cord blood to laboratory for typing and crossmatching. Confirm if mother is Rh$_o$(D)-negative and D^u-negative. Give drug to mother, as needed, only if infant is Rh$_o$(D)-positive or D^u-positive.
• Obtain history of allergies and reaction to immunization. Make sure epinephrine 1:1,000 is available in case of anaphylaxis.
• Reconstitute drug with normal saline solution only.
• Minidose preparations are recommended for every patient undergoing abortion or miscarriage up to 12 weeks' gestation unless she is Rh$_o$(D)-positive or D^u-positive or has Rh antibodies, or unless the father or fetus is Rh-negative.
• In patients treated for immune thrombocytopenic purpura, destruction of Rh-positive RBCs will cause a decrease in hemoglobin level.

Reactions may be *common,* uncommon, *life-threatening,* or COMMON AND LIFE-THREATENING.

PATIENT TEACHING

• Inform patient that vaccinations with live-virus vaccines should be postponed for 3 months after $Rh_0(D)$ immune globulin is given.
• Explain to patient how drug protects future Rh_0-positive fetuses, if used because of pregnancy; or explain other use if indicated.
• Warn patient about adverse reactions caused by drug.

rifampin
Rifadin

Pharmacologic class: semisynthetic rifamycin B derivative (macrocyclic antibiotic)
Therapeutic class: antituberculotic
Pregnancy risk category: C

INDICATIONS & DOSAGES

➤ *Neisseria meningitidis* **carriers—**
Adults: 600 mg b.i.d. for 2 days or 600 mg once daily for 4 days.
Children ages 1 month to 12 years: 10 mg/kg q 12 hours for 2 days or 10 to 20 mg/kg (maximum 600 mg) once daily for 4 days.
Infants younger than age 1 month: 5 mg/kg q 12 hours for 2 days.
➤ **Primary treatment in pulmonary tuberculosis—**
Adults: 10 mg/kg up to 600 mg daily as a single dose.
Children older than age 5: 10 to 20 mg/kg daily as a single dose. Maximum dose, 600 mg daily.

ADMINISTRATION

Direct injection: Not recommended.
Intermittent infusion: Infuse 100 ml over 30 minutes; 500 ml over 3 hours.
Continuous infusion: Not recommended.

PREPARATION & STORAGE

Available as lyophilized powder in a 600-mg vial.
Reconstitute using 10 ml of sterile water to make solution of 60 mg/ml. Immediately before use, withdraw the calculated amount of rifampin and add to 500 ml D_5W or normal saline and infuse over 3 hours; if patient's condition permits, add to 100 ml of D_5W and infuse over 30 minutes.
Store vials at room temperature, protect from light, and avoid excessive heat above 104° F (40° C). Reconstituted solutions are stable at room temperature for 24 hours. Dilutions containing D_5W are stable at room temperature for 4 hours; normal saline is stable at room temperature for 24 hours.

Incompatibilities
Diltiazem, minocycline, other IV solutions.

CONTRAINDICATIONS & CAUTIONS

• Contraindicated in those hypersensitive to rifamycin and in those with active hepatitis.
• Use cautiously in those with hepatic disease and in those receiving other hepatotoxic drugs. Carefully assess benefits and risks.

ADVERSE REACTIONS

CNS: confusion, dizziness, drowsiness, headache, ataxia, fatigue, inability to concentrate, psychoses, fever.
CV: flushing.
GI: anorexia, diarrhea, flatulence, nausea, vomiting, *pseudomembranous colitis.*
GU: menstrual irregularities, interstitial nephritis, acute tubular necrosis.
Hematologic: eosinophilia, *hemolytic anemia, thrombocytopenia, transient leukopenia, DIC.*
Hepatic: *hepatotoxicity,* jaundice.
Metabolic: hyperuricemia.
Musculoskeletal: muscular weakness, pain and numbness in joints.

Respiratory: dyspnea, wheezing.
Skin: pruritus, rash, urticaria.
Other: edema of face and hands, flu-like syndrome, *hypersensitivity reactions, shock.*

INTERACTIONS

Drug-drug. *ACE inhibitors, aminosalicylic acid, antiarrhythmics, anticoagulants, barbiturates, benzodiazepines, beta blockers, chloramphenicol, corticosteroids, cyclosporine, delavirdine, digoxin, doxycycline, estrogens, fluoroquinolones, haloperidol, hormonal contraceptives, losartan, methadone, morphine, nifedipine, ondansetron, phenytoin, progestins, quinidine, sulfonylureas, tacrolimus, theophylline, thyroid hormones, tricyclic antidepressants, verapamil, zidovudine, zolpidem:* Increases metabolism of these drugs, possibly reducing their activity. Monitor patient closely.
Clarithromycin, other macrolides: Decreases metabolism of rifampin and increases metabolism of macrolides. Monitor patient for increased side effects and decreased efficacy of macrolides.
Isoniazid: Increases hepatotoxicity. Monitor liver function test results frequently.
Ketoconazole: Decreases levels of both drugs. Dosages may need to be adjusted.
Protease inhibitors: Decreases metabolism of rifampin and increases metabolism of protease inhibitors. Avoid using together.
Drug-lifestyle. *Alcohol use:* May increase risk of hepatotoxicity. Discourage use together.

EFFECTS ON LAB TEST RESULTS

• May increase ALT, AST, alkaline phosphatase, bilirubin, creatinine, BUN, and uric acid levels.
• May increase eosinophil count. May decrease hemoglobin and platelet and WBC counts.

• May alter standard folate and vitamin B_{12} assay results. May cause temporary retention of sulfobromophthalein in the liver excretion test and interfere with contrast material in gallbladder studies and urinalysis based on spectrophotometry.

ACTION

Inhibits DNA-dependent RNA polymerase, thus impairing RNA synthesis (bactericidal).

PHARMACOKINETICS

Drug level peaks within 30 minutes; duration, 8 to 12 hours.
Distribution: Widely into most body tissues, many organs, and CSF; 84% to 91% protein bound.
Metabolism: In the liver.
Excretion: Biliary; 6% to 30% excreted in urine.

CLINICAL CONSIDERATIONS

• Don't give I.M. or S.C.; injection is I.V. only. Watch for irritation and infiltration; extravasation can cause tissue damage and necrosis.
• Don't use for treatment of meningococcal disease because of rapid resistance.
• Monitor blood counts.
• Drug may cause hyperbilirubinemia shortly after treatment is initiated. Watch closely for signs of hepatic impairment. Monitor AST, ALT, and bilirubin levels.

PATIENT TEACHING

• Inform patient that urine, feces, saliva, sputum, sweat, and tears may turn red or orange during treatment, and soft contact lenses can be permanently stained.
• Inform patient that oral anticoagulants, hormonal contraceptives, and oral antidiabetics may be less effective during treatment with this drug.

• Instruct patient to inform prescriber if sore throat, fever, malaise, easy bruising, or bleeding occurs.

Ringer's injection

Pharmacologic class: isotonic multiple electrolyte solution
Therapeutic class: electrolyte and fluid replenishment
Pregnancy risk category: NR
pH: 6

INDICATIONS & DOSAGES
➤ **To replace extracellular fluid and electrolyte losses—**
Adults and children: Dose highly individualized but usually 1.5 to 3 L daily (2% to 6% of body weight).

ADMINISTRATION
Direct injection: Not used.
Intermittent infusion: Not used.
Continuous infusion: Infuse through central or peripheral I.V. line over ordered duration.

PREPARATION & STORAGE
Available in 500- and 1,000-ml containers.
   Before administration, inspect for precipitates and discoloration. Don't use unless solution is clear and container undamaged.
   Store at room temperature. Avoid excessive heat; however, brief exposure to higher temperatures, up to 104° F (40° C), doesn't adversely affect solution. Protect from freezing.

Incompatibilities
Ampicillin sodium, chlordiazepoxide, diazepam, erythromycin lactobionate, potassium phosphate, sodium bicarbonate, thiopental.

CONTRAINDICATIONS & CAUTIONS
• Contraindicated in those with renal failure, except as an emergency volume expander.
• Don't use as a replacement for blood or a substitute for plasma volume expanders, except in emergencies.
• Use cautiously in those with heart failure, hyperkalemia, hypoproteinemia, severe renal failure, or sodium retention because Ringer's injection may worsen these conditions.
• Use in pregnant patient only if clearly indicated. Unknown if Ringer's injection can harm fetus.

ADVERSE REACTIONS
CNS: fever.
CV: fluid overload, vein thrombosis, phlebitis.
Metabolic: electrolyte imbalance.
Respiratory: pulmonary edema.
Skin: infection at injection site.

INTERACTIONS
Drug-drug. *Corticosteroids, corticotropin:* Increased risk of hypernatremia. Monitor patient closely.
Potassium-sparing diuretics, potassium supplements: Increased risk of hyperkalemia. Use together with caution.

EFFECTS ON LAB TEST RESULTS
• May cause electrolyte imbalances.

COMPOSITION
Contains the principal ionic constituents of normal plasma. Each 100 ml contains 860 mg of sodium chloride, 30 mg of potassium chloride, and 33 mg of calcium chloride dehydrate. A liter of Ringer's injection provides 147 mEq of sodium, 4 mEq of potassium, 4 mEq of calcium, and 155 mEq of chloride.

CLINICAL CONSIDERATIONS
• Osmolarity: 309 to 310 mOsm/L.
• Solution may be given with dextrose, other carbohydrates, or sodium lactate.

• I.V. administration of Ringer's injection can cause fluid or solute overload, resulting in dilution of electrolyte levels, overhydration, or pulmonary edema.
• Monitor for changes in fluid and electrolyte balance during prolonged therapy.
• Electrolyte content is insufficient for treating severe electrolyte deficiencies.
• If an adverse reaction occurs, stop infusion and treat symptomatically. Save remainder of solution for examination, if needed.

PATIENT TEACHING
• Instruct patient to promptly report breathing problems.

Ringer's injection, lactated

Pharmacologic class: electrolyte carbohydrate solution
Therapeutic class: electrolyte and fluid replenishment
Pregnancy risk category: NR
pH: 6.5

INDICATIONS & DOSAGES
➤ **To replace extracellular fluid and electrolyte losses—**
Adults and children: Dose highly individualized, but usually 1.5 to 3 L (2% to 6% of body weight) daily.

ADMINISTRATION
Direct injection: Not used.
Intermittent infusion: Not used.
Continuous infusion: Infuse ordered amount through peripheral or central I.V. line over 18 to 24 hours.

PREPARATION & STORAGE
Available in 250-, 500-, and 1,000-ml containers.
    Store at room temperature. Avoid excessive heat; however, brief exposure

to temperatures up to 104° F (40° C) doesn't adversely affect solution.

Incompatibilities
Amphotericin B, ampicillin sodium, chlordiazepoxide, diazepam, erythromycin lactobionate, methylprednisolone sodium succinate, phenytoin sodium, potassium phosphate, sodium bicarbonate, thiopental, whole blood.

CONTRAINDICATIONS & CAUTIONS
• Contraindicated in those with hyperkalemia, severe renal failure, or potassium retention because of possible worsening of these conditions.
• Contraindicated in those with lactic acidosis.
• Use cautiously in all patients because excess lactate levels may cause metabolic acidosis.
• Use cautiously in those with heart failure, edema, severe renal insufficiency, sodium retention, or metabolic or respiratory alkalosis because lactated Ringer's injection may exacerbate these conditions.
• Use cautiously in those with hepatic insufficiency because of increased level or impaired use of lactate ions.

ADVERSE REACTIONS
CNS: fever.
CV: hypervolemia.
Metabolic: electrolyte imbalance.
Skin: extravasation, infection at injection site.

INTERACTIONS
Drug-drug. *Corticosteroids, corticotropin:* Increases risk of hypernatremia. Monitor patient closely.
Potassium-sparing diuretics, potassium supplements: Increases risk of hyperkalemia. Use together with caution.

EFFECTS ON LAB TEST RESULTS
• May cause electrolyte imbalance.

Reactions may be *common,* uncommon, *life-threatening,* or COMMON AND LIFE-THREATENING.

COMPOSITION

Consists of 130 mEq of sodium, 4 mEq of potassium, 3 mEq of calcium, 109 mEq of chloride, and 28 mEq of lactate per liter. A liter of this isotonic solution contains 9 calories from lactate. Solutions containing D_5W or dextrose 10% in water provide additional calories.

CLINICAL CONSIDERATIONS

- Osmolarity: 273 mOsm/L.
- During long-term therapy, monitor fluid and electrolyte balance.

PATIENT TEACHING

- Instruct patient to report pain or swelling at infusion site.
- Inform patient of reason for infusion and of need to report adverse reactions.

rituximab
Rituxan

Pharmacologic class: murine monoclonal antibody
Therapeutic class: antineoplastic
Pregnancy risk category: C
pH: 6.5

INDICATIONS & DOSAGES

➤ **Relapsed or refractory low-grade or follicular, CD20-positive, B-cell non-Hodgkin's malignant lymphoma—**
Adults: Initially, 375 mg/m^2 I.V. infusion once weekly for four or eight doses, given at rate of 50 mg/hour. If hypersensitivity or infusion-related events don't occur, increase rate by 50-mg/hour increments q 30 minutes, to maximum of 400 mg/hour. Give subsequent infusions at initial rate of 100 mg/hour and increase by 100-mg/hour increments q 30 minutes, to maximum of 400 mg/hour, as tolerated. Retreatment for patients with progressive disease,

375 mg/m^2 I.V. infusion once weekly for four doses.
Adjust-a-dose: If hypersensitivity occurs, temporarily slow or interrupt infusion; after symptoms have resolved, continue infusion at half the previous rate.

ADMINISTRATION

Direct injection: Don't give by I.V. bolus or push.
Intermittent infusion: Not recommended.
Continuous infusion: Give at a rate of 50 mg/hour for initial infusion and 100 mg/hour for subsequent infusions, if tolerated.

PREPARATION & STORAGE

Available as 10 mg/ml in 10- and 50-ml single-use vials.

Dilute to a final concentration of 1 to 4 mg/ml in bag of D_5W or normal saline solution. Gently invert bag to mix the solution. Discard unused portion left in vial.

Protect vials from direct sunlight. Vials and diluted solutions are stable for 24 hours when stored at 36° to 46° F (2° to 8° C). Infusion is stable for 48 hours when stored at room temperature.

Incompatibilities

Other I.V. drugs.

CONTRAINDICATIONS & CAUTIONS

- Contraindicated in those with type I hypersensitivity or anaphylactic reactions to murine proteins or to any component of rituximab.

ADVERSE REACTIONS

CNS: dizziness, *asthenia, headache,* fatigue, paresthesia, malaise, agitation, insomnia, hypesthesia, hypertonia, nervousness, anxiety, general pain, fever.
CV: *hypotension,* **arrhythmias,** hypertension, peripheral edema, chest pain,

tachycardia, orthostatic hypotension, *bradycardia,* flushing.
EENT: sore throat, rhinitis, sinusitis, lacrimation disorder, conjunctivitis.
GI: *nausea,* vomiting, abdominal pain or enlargement, diarrhea, dyspepsia, anorexia, taste perversion.
Hematologic: *leukopenia, thrombocytopenia, neutropenia,* anemia.
Metabolic: hyperglycemia, hypocalcemia.
Musculoskeletal: myalgia, back pain, arthralgia.
Respiratory: *bronchospasm,* dyspnea, increased cough, bronchitis.
Skin: *pruritus, rash,* urticaria, *severe mucocutaneous reactions,* pain at injection site.
Other: *angioedema,* chills, rigors, tumor pain.

INTERACTIONS
None reported.

EFFECTS ON LAB TEST RESULTS
• May increase glucose and LDH levels. May decrease calcium level.
• May decrease hemoglobin, hematocrit, and WBC, platelet, and neutrophil counts.

ACTION
Action is directed against the CD20 antigen found on the surface of normal and malignant B-lymphocytes. Binding to this antigen mediates the lysis of the B cells.

PHARMACOKINETICS
Onset, variable; peak, variable; duration, 6 to 12 months.
Distribution: Unknown.
Metabolism: Unknown.
Excretion: Unknown.

CLINICAL CONSIDERATIONS
• Severe mucocutaneous reactions (including toxic epidermal necrolysis, Stevens-Johnson syndrome, paraneoplastic pemphigus, and lichenoid or vesiculobullous dermatitis) have occurred in patients receiving rituximab. Further infusions should be avoided; treatment of the skin reaction should be started promptly.
• Consider premedicating the patient with acetaminophen and diphenhydramine before each infusion. Infusion reactions generally occur within 30 minutes to 2 hours of beginning the first infusion.
• The risk of infusion-related effects decreases with subsequent infusions.
• Monitor patient closely for signs and symptoms of hypersensitivity reaction. Have drugs such as epinephrine, antihistamine, and corticosteroids available to immediately treat such a reaction.
• Obtain CBCs at regular intervals and more frequently in those who develop cytopenias.
• Monitor patient's blood pressure closely during infusion. If hypotension, bronchospasm, or angioedema occurs, stop infusion and restart at a 50% rate reduction when symptoms resolve.
• Stop infusion if serious or life-threatening arrhythmias occur. Patients who develop significant arrhythmias should undergo cardiac monitoring during and after subsequent infusions of the drug.

PATIENT TEACHING
• Tell patient to report symptoms during and after infusion.
• Tell patient to watch for signs and symptoms of infection, such as fever, sore throat, and fatigue, and signs and symptoms of bleeding, such as easy bruising, nosebleeds, bleeding gums, and melena. Tell patient to take his temperature daily.
• Advise breast-feeding patients to stop breast-feeding until drug levels become undetectable in the blood.

rocuronium bromide
Zemuron

Pharmacologic class: nondepolarizing neuromuscular blocker
Therapeutic class: skeletal muscle
relaxant
Pregnancy risk category: C

INDICATIONS & DOSAGES
➤ **Adjunct to general anesthesia to
facilitate endotracheal intubation or
to provide skeletal muscle relaxation
during surgery or mechanical ventilation—**
*Adults and children older than age 3
months:* Dosage depends on anesthetic
used, individual needs, and response.
Dosages are representative and must be
individualized. Initially, 0.6 mg/kg I.V.
bolus. In most patients, tracheal intubation may be performed within 2 minutes; muscle paralysis lasts about 30
minutes.

A maintenance dose for adults of
0.1 mg/kg provides an additional 12
minutes of muscle relaxation to duration of effect; 0.15 mg/kg, an additional 17 minutes; and 0.2 mg/kg, an additional 24 minutes.

A maintenance dose for children of
0.075 to 0.125 mg/kg provides clinical
relaxation for 7 to 10 minutes. Continuous infusion may be used to maintain
neuromuscular blockade. Infusion for
adults may start at rate of 0.01 to
0.012 mg/kg/minute after early evidence of spontaneous recovery from
intubating dose. Infusion for children
may start at rate of 0.012 mg/kg/minute
after one twitch is present in train-of-
four. Dosages are adjusted to patient's
twitch response.

ADMINISTRATION
Direct injection: Give undiluted drug
by rapid injection.

Intermittent infusion: Not recommended.
Continuous infusion: Give diluted drug
by infusion pump. Infusion rates are
highly individualized but have ranged
from 0.004 to 0.016 mg/kg/minute.

PREPARATION & STORAGE
Available in 5- and 10-ml vials containing 10 mg/ml.

If drug is given by continuous infusion, dilute with D_5W, normal saline injection, dextrose 5% in normal saline
injection, sterile water for injection, or
lactated Ringer's solution.

Store vials refrigerated at 36° to
46° F (2° to 8° C), but don't freeze.
Use vial within 60 days after removal
to room temperature (77° F [25° C]).
Use opened vials within 30 days. Inspect for precipitates before use.

Incompatibilities
Alkaline solutions such as barbiturates;
other drugs.

CONTRAINDICATIONS & CAUTIONS
● Contraindicated in those hypersensitive to bromides or rocuronium.
● Don't use drug during rapid sequence
induction for cesarean delivery.
● Use cautiously in elderly patients and
those with hepatic disease, severe obesity, bronchogenic cancer, electrolyte
disturbances, neuromuscular disease,
altered circulation, or edema.

ADVERSE REACTIONS
CNS: prolonged neuromuscular block-
ade.
CV: abnormal ECG, *arrhythmias,*
tachycardia.
GI: nausea, vomiting.
Respiratory: asthma, *bronchospasm,*
rhonchi, wheezing, hiccups.
Skin: injection site edema, pruritus,
rash.

INTERACTIONS

Drug-drug. *Aminoglycoside antibiotics; clindamycin; general anesthetics, such as enflurane, halothane, and isoflurane; ketamine; lithium; magnesium salts; nitrates; piperacillin; polymyxin antibiotics, including colistin and polymyxin B sulfate; quinidine; thiazide diuretics, verapamil:* Potentiates neuromuscular blockade, leading to increased skeletal muscle relaxation and possible respiratory paralysis. Avoid using together.

Beta blockers, corticosteroids, phenytoin, ranitidine, theophylline: Shortens duration of neuromuscular blockade and resistance to rocuronium's effects. Dosage may need to be adjusted. Monitor patient closely.

EFFECTS ON LAB TEST RESULTS

None reported.

ACTION

Prevents acetylcholine from binding to the receptors on the muscle end-plate, thus blocking depolarization.

PHARMACOKINETICS

Onset, within 1 to 1.5 minutes; effects peak within 2 minutes in most patients; duration, dose-dependent; maximal blockade at about 30 minutes; 25% recovery of muscle-twitch strength occurs within 22 to 67 minutes.

Distribution: About 30% protein bound.

Metabolism: Minimal metabolism.

Excretion: In bile, 33% in urine.

CLINICAL CONSIDERATIONS

● Drug should be given only by personnel experienced in airway management. Have emergency respiratory support materials, including endotracheal equipment, ventilator, oxygen, atropine, edrophonium, epinephrine, and neostigmine, readily available.

● If prescribed, give sedatives or general anesthetics before rocuronium.

● Patients with liver disease may require higher doses of drug to achieve adequate muscle relaxation. Such patients also exhibit prolonged effects from the drug. Monitor patient closely.

● Drug is well tolerated in patients with renal failure because it's metabolized and excreted by the liver.

● Neuromuscular blockers don't alter consciousness or the pain threshold.

● Prior administration of succinylcholine may enhance rocuronium's neuromuscular blocking effect and prolong its duration of action.

● A nerve stimulator and train-of-four monitoring are recommended to confirm antagonism of neuromuscular blockade and recovery of muscle strength. Before attempting pharmacologic reversal, some evidence of spontaneous recovery should be evident. Once spontaneous recovery starts, drug-induced neuromuscular blockade may be reversed with an anticholinesterase, such as neostigmine or edrophonium, which is usually given with an anticholinergic, such as atropine.

● Monitor respirations until patient has fully recovered from neuromuscular blockade, as evidenced by tests of muscle strength. Including hand grip, head lift, and ability to cough.

● If overdose occurs, provide supportive treatment. Keep airway clear and assist ventilation until some spontaneous neuromuscular recovery is apparent.

PATIENT TEACHING

● Teach patient about procedures being performed.

● Explain everything to patient, because he can still hear.

● Reassure patient and family that he'll be closely monitored and his needs anticipated.

Reactions may be *common,* uncommon, ***life-threatening,*** or **COMMON AND LIFE-THREATENING.**

sargramostim (GM-CSF, granulocyte macrophage–colony stimulating factor)
Leukine*

Pharmacologic class: biologic response modifier
Therapeutic class: colony-stimulating factor
Pregnancy risk category: C
pH: 7.1 to 7.7

INDICATIONS & DOSAGES
➤ **To accelerate myeloid reconstitution after autologous bone marrow transplantation in patients with malignant lymphoma, acute lymphoblastic leukemia, or Hodgkin's disease**—
Adults: 250 mcg/m² daily for 21 consecutive days over 2 hours, beginning 2 to 4 hours after transplantation.
➤ **Bone marrow transplantation failure or engraftment delay**—
Adults: 250 mcg/m²/day for 14 days, over 2 hours. May repeat after patient has stopped therapy for 7 days, if engraftment hasn't occurred; may try third course of therapy at 500 mcg/m²/day for 14 days after patient has stopped second course of therapy for 7 days. If patient hasn't improved, further treatment probably won't be beneficial.
➤ **Neutrophil recovery after chemotherapy in acute myelogenous leukemia**—
Adults age 55 and older: 250 mcg/m²/day over 4 hours starting on about day 11 or 4 days after completion of induction chemotherapy, if day-10 bone mar-

row is hypoplastic with fewer than 5% blasts. If second cycle of induction chemotherapy is needed, give about 4 days after completion of chemotherapy if bone marrow is hypoplastic with fewer than 5% blasts. Continue until an absolute neutrophil count (ANC) exceeds 1,500/mm³ for three consecutive days or a maximum of 42 days.
➤ **To mobilize peripheral blood progenitor cells**—
Adults: 250 mcg/m²/day over 24 hours. Dosing should continue at the same dose through the period of peripheral blood progenitor cell collection.
➤ **After infusion of peripheral blood progenitor cells**—
Adults: 250 mcg/m²/day over 24 hours beginning immediately after infusion of progenitor cells and continuing until ANC exceeds 1,500/mm³ for three consecutive days.
➤ **To increase neutrophil count in myelodysplastic syndrome ♦**—
Adults: 15 to 500 mcg/m² once daily over 1 to 2 hours; or 30 to 500 mcg/m² continuous infusion over 24 hours.
➤ **Moderate to severe aplastic anemia ♦**—
Adults: 15 to 480 mcg/m² over 1 to 12 hours; or 120 to 500 mcg/m² continuous infusion over 24 hours.
➤ **Neutropenia caused by HIV infection ♦**—
Adults and adolescents: 250 mcg/m² I.V. infusion once daily for 2 to 4 weeks.
Adjust-a-dose: If ANC exceeds 20,000 cells/mm³ or WBC count exceeds 50,000 cells/mm³, reduce the dose by 50% or stop therapy temporarily.

ADMINISTRATION
Direct injection: Not recommended.
Intermittent infusion: Infuse over 2 to 4 hours by a central line; don't use in-line membrane filter.
Continuous infusion: Give recommended dose over 24 hours.

PREPARATION & STORAGE
Available as a lyophilized powder in 250-mg preservative-free single-dose vials and as a liquid in 500-mcg/ml multidose vials.

Reconstitute powder with 1 ml sterile water, directing stream against side of vial and swirling contents gently to minimize foaming. Dilute in normal saline solution to make a concentration greater than 10 mcg/ml. If final concentration is below 10 mcg/ml, add human albumin at a final concentration of 0.1% to the normal saline solution before adding sargramostim to prevent adsorption. For a final concentration of 0.1% human albumin, add 1 mg human albumin/1 ml normal saline solution.

When reconstituted with sterile water for injection, use within 6 hours and discard unused portion. When reconstituted with bacteriostatic water, drug remains stable for 20 days if stored between 36° and 46° F (2° and 8° C). When diluted with normal saline solution, drug remains stable for 48 hours if kept at room temperature or if refrigerated. Don't reuse single-dose vial.

Liquid-containing multidose vials and reconstituted solutions are stable refrigerated at 36° and 46° F (2° and 8° C). Don't freeze or shake. Liquid-containing multidose vials may be stored refrigerated for up to 20 days once vial has been entered.

Incompatibilities
Other I.V. drugs, unless specific compatibility data are available.

CONTRAINDICATIONS & CAUTIONS
● Contraindicated in those hypersensitive to the drug, its components, or yeast-derived products and in those with excessive leukemic myeloid blasts in bone marrow or peripheral blood.
● Contraindicated with cytotoxic chemotherapy or radiotherapy, or administration 24 hours preceding or after chemotherapy or radiotherapy.
● Use cautiously in those with preexisting cardiac disease or fluid retention, hypoxia, pulmonary infiltrates, heart failure, or impaired renal or hepatic function.
● Safety and efficacy in children haven't been established, but no differences in toxic effects have been found.

ADVERSE REACTIONS
CNS: *anxiety, headache, insomnia, pain, paresthesia,* **CNS hemorrhage,** *asthenia, malaise, fever.*
CV: *chest pain, hypertension, tachycardia, hypotension,* pericardial effusion, *edema, peripheral edema,* **supraventricular arrhythmias.**
EENT: *mucous membrane disorder, eye hemorrhage, pharyngitis, epistaxis, rhinitis.*
GI: *nausea, diarrhea, vomiting, anorexia, abdominal pain, dyspepsia, hematemesis, dysphagia,* constipation, abdominal distention, **GI hemorrhage,** *stomatitis.*
GU: hematuria, *urinary tract disorder,* abnormal renal function.
Hematologic: ***thrombocytopenia, leukopenia, agranulocytosis, hemorrhage,*** stimulation of hematopoiesis.
Hepatic: ***hepatotoxicity,*** hyperbilirubinemia.
Metabolic: *weight loss,* weight gain, *hyperglycemia, hypercholesterolemia, hypomagnesemia,* hypocalcemia.
Musculoskeletal: *bone pain, arthralgia,* myalgia, back pain.
Respiratory: *dyspnea, lung disorder,* pleural effusion.

Reactions may be *common*, uncommon, ***life-threatening***, or COMMON AND LIFE-THREATENING.

Skin: *alopecia, rash, pruritus,* petechiae, sweats.
Other: SEPSIS, *chills, infection.*

INTERACTIONS
Drug-drug. *Corticosteroids, lithium:* May potentiate myeloproliferative effects of sargramostim. Use together cautiously.

EFFECTS ON LAB TEST RESULTS
• May increase BUN, creatinine, glucose, cholesterol, alkaline phosphatase, AST, ALT, and bilirubin levels. May decrease albumin, magnesium, and calcium levels.

ACTION
A glycoprotein that contains 127 amino acids manufactured by recombinant DNA technology in a yeast expression system. Drug differs from natural human GM-CSF because leucine is substituted for arginine at position 23. The carbohydrate moiety may also be different. Drug induces partially committed progenitor cells to divide and differentiate in the granulocyte-macrophage pathways.

PHARMACOKINETICS
Decrease in circulating neutrophils, eosinophils, and monocytes, with drug levels peaking in 30 minutes, and rebounding to baseline or above in 2 hours. Apparent biphasic response: initial leukocyte count plateaus after 3 to 7 days, followed by another increase and another plateau.
Distribution: Drug levels are detected in blood within 12 to 17 minutes of administration; bound to specific receptors on target cells.
Metabolism: Unknown.
Excretion: Renal, less than 0.2%.

CLINICAL CONSIDERATIONS
• Tonicity is isotonic.
• Drug also may be given by S.C. injection, which may be more convenient for self-administration or during prolonged therapy.
• Monitor for first-dose reaction, including hypotension, tachycardia, fever, rigors, chills, diaphoresis, back pain, leg spasms, and dyspnea.
• Closely monitor respiratory symptoms during and immediately after infusion.
• If severe adverse reactions occur, reduce dosage or temporarily stop drug until reactions abate. If blast cells appear or disease progression occurs, stop therapy.
• Transient rash and local injection site reactions may occur; no serious allergic or anaphylactic reactions have been reported.
• Stimulation of marrow precursors may result in rapid rise of WBC count; monitor CBC with differential biweekly, including examination for blast cells.
• If blast cells appear or increase to 10% or more of WBC count or if the underlying disease progresses, stop therapy. Blood counts return to baseline or normal levels 3 to 7 days after treatment is stopped.
• Monitor renal and hepatic function in patients with renal or hepatic dysfunction before starting treatment and at least every other week during therapy. Carefully monitor body weight and hydration status.
• Drug can act as a growth factor for any tumor type, particularly myeloid cancers.
• Drug is effective in accelerating myeloid recovery in patients receiving bone marrow purged from monoclonal antibodies.
• Drug has limited effect in patients who have received extensive radiotherapy to hematopoietic sites for treatment of primary disease in the abdomen or chest or who have been exposed to multiple drugs, including alkylating drugs, anthracycline antibiotics, and

antimetabolites, before autologous bone marrow transplantation.

PATIENT TEACHING

• Tell patient to report adverse reactions.

• Inform patients with tumors (especially myeloid malignancies) that drug may act as a growth factor for the tumor.

• Advise patient that most adverse reactions subside if the dosage is reduced or the infusion stopped.

scopolamine hydrobromide (hyoscine hydrobromide)

Pharmacologic class: anticholinergic
Therapeutic class: antimuscarinic, cycloplegic mydriatic
Pregnancy risk category: C
pH: 3.5 to 6.5

INDICATIONS & DOSAGES

➤ **Premedication to reduce secretions; to treat or prevent nausea—**
Adults: 300 to 600 mcg (0.3 to 0.6 mg) as single dose.
Children: 6 mcg (0.006 mg)/kg or 200 mcg (0.2 mg)/m² as single dose 45 to 60 minutes before procedure.
➤ **Premedication as anesthesia adjunct for amnesia—**
Adults: 320 to 650 mcg (0.32 to 0.65 mg) as single dose.
Children: 6 mcg (0.006 mg)/kg or 200 mcg (0.2 mg)/m² as single dose.
➤ **Premedication as anesthesia adjunct for sedation—**
Adults: 600 mcg (0.6 mg) given 30 minutes before procedure. May repeat three or four times.
Children: 6 mcg (0.006 mg)/kg or 200 mcg (0.2 mg)/m² given 30 minutes before procedure.

ADMINISTRATION

Direct injection: Inject diluted drug at ordered rate through patent I.V. line.
Intermittent infusion: Not recommended.
Continuous infusion: Not recommended.

PREPARATION & STORAGE

Available in 1-ml vials containing 300 mcg/ml, 400 mcg/ml, or 1 mg/ml and in 0.5-ml ampules containing 400 mcg/ml, or 860 mcg/ml.

For direct injection, dilute with sterile water for injection according to manufacturer's instructions.

Store at room temperature. Protect from light and freezing.

Incompatibilities

Alkalies, anticholinergics, methohexital.

CONTRAINDICATIONS & CAUTIONS

• Contraindicated in patients hypersensitive to the drug and in those with myasthenia gravis.

• Contraindicated in those with paralytic ileus because drug further slows gastric emptying and increases risk of obstruction.

• Contraindicated in those with bladder-neck obstruction caused by prostatic hyperplasia because drug may worsen urine retention, in those with pyloric obstruction because drug may aggravate disorder, and in those with angle-closure glaucoma because antimuscarinic action may raise intraocular pressure.

• Contraindicated in those with tachycardia stemming from cardiac insufficiency or thyrotoxicosis because of possible exacerbation.

• Use cautiously in those with fever, which may worsen because of suppressed sweat gland activity.

• Use cautiously in those with reflux esophagitis or hiatal hernia because

---

Reactions may be *common*, uncommon, *life-threatening*, or COMMON AND LIFE-THREATENING.

drug promotes gastric retention and aggravates reflux.

• Use cautiously in those with obstructive GI diseases, such as achalasia and pyloroduodenal stenosis, because drug may decrease GI motility and tone, resulting in obstruction and gastric retention.

• Use cautiously in those with ulcerative colitis because large doses may suppress GI motility and cause paralytic ileus and in those with megacolon because drug may cause or aggravate this condition.

• Use cautiously in children with brain damage because drug may exacerbate CNS effect and in those with hypertension or myasthenia gravis because drug may aggravate these conditions.

• Use cautiously in those with chronic lung disease, especially infants, young children, and debilitated patients, because drug may promote bronchial mucus plug formation.

• Use cautiously in those with nonobstructive prostatic hyperplasia, urine retention, or obstructive uropathy because drug may aggravate or precipitate urine retention and in those with autonomic neuropathy because drug may worsen urine retention and cycloplegia.

• Use cautiously in those with spastic paralysis because of possible enhanced response and in geriatric or debilitated patients with intestinal atony because of possible obstruction.

• Use cautiously in those with Down syndrome because of risk of abnormally increased pupillary dilation and tachycardia.

• Use cautiously in those with cardiac disease, especially arrhythmias, heart failure, coronary heart disease, and mitral stenosis because increased heart rate may be hazardous.

• Use cautiously in those with acute hemorrhage related to unstable CV status because heart rate may rise and in toxemia of pregnancy because hypertension may worsen.

• Use cautiously in those with hepatic or renal impairment because of increased risk of adverse reactions.

• Use cautiously in those with xerostomia because prolonged use may further curtail salivary flow.

• Use cautiously in breast-feeding patients.

ADVERSE REACTIONS

CNS: headache, mental confusion, drowsiness, dizziness, hallucinations, delirium, fever, disorientation, restlessness, irritability.
CV: tachycardia, palpitation, flushing, *paradoxical bradycardia.*
EENT: blurred vision, cycloplegia, mydriasis, photophobia, increased ocular tension.
GI: *constipation, nausea,* vomiting, dry mouth, loss of taste, dysphagia, *epigastric distress.*
GU: urinary hesitancy, urine retention.
Respiratory: bronchial plugging, respiratory depression.
Skin: rash, decreased sweating.

INTERACTIONS

Drug-drug. *Amantadine, anticholinergics, antihistamines, buclizine, cyclizine, cyclobenzaprine, disopyramide, ipratropium, loxapine, MAO inhibitors, maprotiline, methylphenidate, molindone, orphenadrine, phenothiazines, pimozide, procainamide, thioxanthenes, tricyclic antidepressants:* Enhances anticholinergic effects. Monitor patient closely.
CNS depressants: Increases sedation. Avoid using together.
Digoxin: Elevates digoxin level. Monitor level.
Potassium chloride, especially waxmatrix preparations: Increases risk of GI lesions. Use together cautiously.
Drug-herb. *Pill-bearing spurge:* Choline may decrease effect of scopolamine. Discourage use together.

◆ Off-label use   *May contain benzyl alcohol   ◇ Canada

Squaw vine: Tannic acid may decrease metabolic breakdown. Discourage use together.
Drug-lifestyle. *Alcohol use:* CNS depression. Discourage use together.

EFFECTS ON LAB TEST RESULTS
• May interfere with gastric secretion test results.

ACTION
Acts on the iris and ciliary body of the eye and on salivary, bronchial, and sweat glands. Unlike other antimuscarinics, drug also produces CNS depression. As an antiemetic, it reduces excitability of the labyrinthine receptors and depresses conduction in the vestibular cerebellar pathway. It also has antivertigo effects, probably resulting from action on the cerebral cortex or the membranous labyrinth of the vestibular system.

PHARMACOKINETICS
Onset, 10 minutes; duration, 2 hours.
Distribution: Binds minimally to plasma proteins and crosses the placental and blood-brain barriers.
Metabolism: In the liver by enzymatic hydrolysis.
Excretion: In urine, as unchanged drug and metabolites. Half-life, 8 hours. Unknown if drug appears in breast milk.

CLINICAL CONSIDERATIONS
• Osmolality: 303 mOsm/kg.
• To control excitement or delirium, give small doses of a short-acting barbiturate, such as 100 mg of thiopental sodium, or a benzodiazepine, or rectally infuse 2% solution of chloral hydrate. Respiratory depression may require mechanical ventilation. Maintain adequate hydration and provide symptomatic treatment.
• Raise the geriatric patient's bedside rails and take other safety precautions. Confusion, agitation, excitement, and drowsiness may occur even with usual doses. Reorient patient, as needed. Lower doses may be needed.
• Geriatric patients and children are especially susceptible to adverse antimuscarinic effects.
• Monitor bowel sounds, fluid intake and output, blood pressure, and for nausea and vomiting.
• When given for pain without morphine or meperidine, scopolamine can act as a stimulant, producing delirium.
• Parenteral use in pregnant women before onset of labor may cause neonatal CNS depression and hemorrhage.
• With prolonged use, patient may develop tolerance to some adverse effects, and drug's effectiveness may be reduced.
• After drug is stopped, watch for rebound reduction in duration of REM sleep. Signs and symptoms include anxiety, irritability, nightmares, and insomnia. Treatment may be needed.
• Avoid giving drug for 24 hours before gastric acid secretion test.
• If overdose occurs, give physostigmine I.V. slowly, less than 1 mg/minute, to reverse severe antimuscarinic symptoms. In adults, repeat doses of 0.5 to 2 mg, up to total dose of 5 mg, as needed; in children, repeat doses of 0.5 to 1 mg, up to total dose of 2 mg, as needed. Or in adults, give 0.5 to 1 mg of neostigmine methylsulfate I.M., repeated every 2 to 3 hours, or 0.5 to 2 mg I.V., repeated as needed.

PATIENT TEACHING
• Advise patient to report adverse effects.
• Encourage good oral hygiene.
• Notify patient of potential for tolerance to adverse effects with prolonged use.
• Notify patient of childbearing age of risks of taking drug during pregnancy.

sodium bicarbonate
Sodium Bicarbonate

Pharmacologic class: alkalizer
Therapeutic class: systemic and urine alkalizer, systemic hydrogen ion buffer, oral antacid
Pregnancy risk category: C
pH: 7 to 8.5

INDICATIONS & DOSAGES
➤ **Adjunct to advanced CV life support during CPR—**
Adults: Although no longer routinely recommended, inject either 300 to 500 ml of a 5% solution or 200 to 300 mEq of a 7.5% or 8.4% solution as rapidly as possible. Base further doses on subsequent blood gas values. Or, for adults, 1 mEq/kg dose, then repeat 0.5 mEq/kg q 10 minutes.
Children age 2 or younger: 1 mEq/kg I.V. or intraosseous injection of a 4.2 % to 8.4% solution. Give slowly. Don't exceed daily dose of 8 mEq/kg.
➤ **Severe metabolic acidosis—**
Adults: Dose depends on blood carbon dioxide content, pH, and patient's clinical condition. Generally, give 90 to 180 mEq/L I.V. during first hour, then adjust p.r.n.
➤ **Less-urgent metabolic acidosis—**
Adults and adolescents: 2 to 5 mEq/kg as a 4- to 8-hour I.V. infusion.

ADMINISTRATION
Direct injection: For cardiac arrest, flush I.V. line before and after use. In adults, inject rapidly into patent primary I.V. line. In neonates and children younger than age 2, inject ordered dose into patent primary I.V. line over 1 to 2 minutes. Injection flow rate faster than 10 ml/minute can cause hypernatremia, decreased CSF pressure, intracranial hemorrhage, severe alkalosis, hyperirritability, or tetany.

Intermittent infusion: Not recommended.
Continuous infusion: Flush I.V. line before and after use.

PREPARATION & STORAGE
Available as vials, ampules, and syringes in concentrations of 4.2%, 5%, 7.5%, and 8.4%.

To dilute for infusion, follow manufacturer's instructions, using sterile water for injection or other standard electrolyte solutions. In neonates and children younger than age 2, use 4.2% sodium bicarbonate solution or dilute 7.5% or 8.4% sodium bicarbonate solution 1:1 with D_5W.

Store at room temperature, always below 104° F (40° C), and protect from freezing and heat. Stability may be increased by refrigerating sodium bicarbonate injection and syringes before preparation, rinsing syringes twice with refrigerated sterile water for injection, and minimizing contact with air. To do this, expel air from syringes and tape the plungers in place to reduce movement caused by escaping carbon dioxide. The 7.5% solution in polypropylene syringes is stable up to 100 days if refrigerated or up to 45 days at room temperature. Don't use solution if it's cloudy or contains a precipitate.

Incompatibilities
Alcohol 5% in dextrose 5%; allopurinol; amiodarone; amphotericin B; amino acids; ascorbic acid injection; bupivacaine; calcium salts; carboplatin; carmustine; cefotaxime; ciprofloxacin; cisatracurium; cisplatin; corticotropin; dextrose 5% in lactated Ringer's injection; diltiazem; dobutamine; dopamine; doxorubicin liposomal; epinephrine hydrochloride; fat emulsion 10%; glycopyrrolate; hydromorphone; idarubicin; imipenem-cilastatin sodium; Ionosol B, D, or G with invert sugar 10%; isoproterenol; labetalol; lactated Ringer's injection; levorphanol; leucovorin calci-

um; lidocaine; magnesium sulfate; meperidine; meropenem; methylprednisolone sodium succinate; metoclopramide; midazolam; morphine sulfate; nalbuphine; norepinephrine bitartrate; ondansetron; oxacillin; penicillin G potassium; pentazocine lactate; pentobarbital sodium; procaine; Ringer's injection; sargramostim; 1/6 M sodium lactate; streptomycin; succinylcholine; thiopental; ticarcillin disodium and clavulanate potassium; vancomycin; verapamil; vinca alkaloids; vitamin B complex with vitamin C.

CONTRAINDICATIONS & CAUTIONS

• Contraindicated in those with metabolic or respiratory alkalosis because sodium bicarbonate may exacerbate them.
• Contraindicated in those with chloride loss from vomiting or continuous GI suctioning because of increased risk of severe alkalosis; and in those with hypocalcemia because of increased risk of alkalosis resulting in tetany.
• Contraindicated in those at risk for developing diuretic-induced hypochloremic alkalosis.
• Use cautiously in those with hypertension, renal insufficiency, or edematous sodium-retaining conditions, such as cirrhosis of the liver, heart failure, or toxemia of pregnancy because sodium content may cause exacerbation.
• Give to pregnant patients only when clearly needed because it's unknown if drug harms fetus.

ADVERSE REACTIONS

CNS: *intracranial hemorrhage with rapid administration in children younger than age 2,* hyperirritability.
CV: peripheral edema.
Metabolic: *metabolic alkalosis,* hypernatremia.
Musculoskeletal: tetany.
Respiratory: pulmonary edema.
Other: tissue necrosis, sloughing or ulceration with infiltration of I.V. site.

INTERACTIONS

Drug-drug. *Amphetamines, anorexiants, anticholinergics, ephedrine, flecainide, mecamylamine, mexiletine, quinidine:* May cause toxic reaction from inhibited urine excretion. Use together with caution. Monitor patient closely.
Chlorpropamide, lithium, methotrexate, salicylates, tetracyclines: Increases urinary excretion of these drugs. Dosage may need to be adjusted.
Corticosteroids: Increases risk of hypernatremia with frequent or high-dose administration of sodium bicarbonate. Monitor patient closely.

EFFECTS ON LAB TEST RESULTS

• May increase sodium and lactate levels. May decrease potassium level.

ACTION

Increases plasma bicarbonate and buffers excess hydrogen ion concentration.

PHARMACOKINETICS

Onset, immediate; duration, unknown.
Distribution: Throughout extracellular fluid. Drug probably crosses the placental barrier and may appear in breast milk.
Metabolism: Dissociated in water to sodium and bicarbonate ions. Bicarbonate anion is converted to carbonic acid, then to its volatile form, carbon dioxide.
Excretion: In urine, by glomerular filtration as bicarbonate. Usually less than 1% is excreted. Carbon dioxide is excreted by the lungs.

CLINICAL CONSIDERATIONS

• Osmolarity: 1,000 to 2,000 mOsm/L, depending on concentration.
• Osmolality: 815 to 1,815 mOsm/kg, depending on concentration.
• Sodium bicarbonate is commonly overused during cardiac arrest. The American Heart Association no longer

recommends its routine use in initial stages of advanced life support. Instead, initial treatment should include basic life support and defibrillation, hyperventilation, and pharmacologic therapy.

• For patients in cardiac arrest, make sure drug administration is preceded by manual or mechanical hyperventilation to lower partial pressure of carbon dioxide.

• When possible, correct electrolyte imbalances, especially hypokalemia and hypocalcemia, before or during therapy.

• Throughout therapy, monitor pH, arterial blood gas, and bicarbonate levels; renal function, especially in long-term therapy; and urine pH, especially when drug is used for alkalization.

• Don't attempt full correction of bicarbonate deficit during first 24 hours of therapy; this may produce metabolic alkalosis from delayed compensatory mechanisms.

• Give repeated small doses to avoid overdose and resultant metabolic alkalosis. Excessive doses may induce hypokalemia and predispose the patient to arrhythmias.

• If alkalosis develops as a result of overdose, have patient rebreathe expired air from a mask or paper bag. If alkalosis is severe, give calcium gluconate I.V., as ordered.

PATIENT TEACHING

• Advise patient to promptly report adverse reactions.

• Advise patient that adverse reactions can usually be reversed with appropriate treatment of electrolyte imbalances.

• Notify patient of risk of extravasation, and encourage him to report pain at I.V. site immediately.

sodium chloride

Pharmacologic class: electrolyte
Therapeutic class: sodium and chloride replacement
Pregnancy risk category: C
pH: 4.5 to 7

INDICATIONS & DOSAGES

Dosage depends on the disorder and patient's age, weight, and fluid, electrolyte, and acid-base balance. For children, concentration and dosage are based on weight or body surface area.

➤ **Fluid and electrolyte replacement—**
Adults: Usually 1 L daily of normal saline solution or 1 to 2 L daily of half-normal saline solution.

➤ **Fluid and electrolyte replacement in ketoacidosis—**
Children: 0.225% or 0.3% normal saline solution.

➤ **Severe sodium chloride depletion requiring rapid replacement—**
Adults: 100 ml of 3% or 5% sodium chloride solution over 1 hour, then additional doses determined by electrolyte levels.

ADMINISTRATION

Direct injection: Used only as drug diluent.

Intermittent infusion: Used only as drug diluent.

Continuous infusion: Infuse through a peripheral or central vein at ordered rate. Infuse 3% or 5% solutions through a large vein, at a rate not exceeding 100 ml/hour. Watch for irritation and infiltration; extravasation can cause tissue damage and necrosis. Observe infusion site carefully for signs of phlebitis.

PREPARATION & STORAGE

Available in glass or flexible polyvinyl chloride containers. Solutions of half-normal saline solution and normal saline solution are available in various volumes ranging from 2 to 1,000 ml. Solutions of 3% and 5% sodium chloride are available in 500-ml containers. Store solutions at room temperature.

Incompatibilities

Amphotericin B, chlordiazepoxide, diazepam, fat emulsion, mannitol, methylprednisolone sodium succinate, phenytoin sodium.

CONTRAINDICATIONS & CAUTIONS

● Contraindicated in those with conditions in which sodium and chloride administration is hazardous.
● Contraindicated in patients with hypernatremia or fluid retention.
● Use hypertonic solutions only in patients with severe sodium and chloride deficits.
● Use cautiously in those with heart failure, other sodium-retaining conditions, or severe renal disease or insufficiency because of increased risk of fluid retention.
● Use cautiously in geriatric or postoperative patients because fluid retention may worsen.

ADVERSE REACTIONS

CNS: fever.
CV: *heart failure,* venous thrombosis, phlebitis.
Metabolic: metabolic acidosis, fluid and electrolyte overload, hypernatremia, hypokalemia.
Respiratory: pulmonary edema.
Skin: extravasation, infection at injection site.

INTERACTIONS

Drug-drug. *Corticosteroids:* Increases risk of hypernatremia. Monitor sodium levels.

EFFECTS ON LAB TEST RESULTS

● May increase sodium level. May decrease potassium level.
● May cause electrolyte imbalance.

COMPOSITION

These solutions consist of sodium chloride and sterile water with no bacteriostatic or antimicrobials or added buffers.

The half-normal saline solution is hypotonic with 77 mEq/L of sodium and of chloride and an osmolarity of 154 to 155 mOsm/L. The normal saline solution is isotonic, contains 154 mEq/L of sodium and of chloride, and has an osmolarity of 308 to 310 mOsm/L. The 3% concentration is hypertonic and contains 513 mEq/L of sodium and of chloride with an osmolarity of 1,026 to 1,030 mOsm/L. Also hypertonic, 5% sodium chloride contains 855 mEq/L of sodium and of chloride. Its osmolarity is 1,710 to 1,711 mOsm/L.

CLINICAL CONSIDERATIONS

● Osmolarity: 0.9% solution is 308 mOsm/L, 14.6% solution is 4,990 mOsm/L. 23.4% solution is 8,010 mOsm/L.
● Osmolality: 14.6% solution is 4,783 to 5,370 mOsm/kg.
● Monitor electrolyte levels, especially sodium and potassium levels; also check chloride and bicarbonate levels.
● If fluid overload occurs, stop infusion and start corrective measures.

PATIENT TEACHING

● Notify patient of potential adverse effects.
● Advise patient to report adverse effects.
● Advise patient to report pain at I.V. site immediately.

sodium ferric gluconate complex
Ferrlecit*

Pharmacologic class: macro-molecular iron complex
Therapeutic class: hematinic
Pregnancy risk category: B
pH: 7.7 to 9.7

INDICATIONS & DOSAGES
➤ **Iron-deficiency anemia in patients undergoing long-term hemodialysis who are receiving erythropoietin—**
Adults: Test dose of 25 mg elemental iron, followed by 125 mg of elemental iron I.V. over eight sessions at sequential dialysis treatments for a total of 1 g of elemental iron. Once iron stores are adequately replete, iron therapy may continue at the lowest effective dose to maintain adequate iron status.

ADMINISTRATION
Direct injection: Not recommended.
Intermittent infusion: Give over 1 hour.
Continuous infusion: Not recommended.

PREPARATION & STORAGE
Available in 5-ml ampules containing 62.5 mg of elemental iron (12.5 mg/ml).
Dilute test dose of sodium ferric gluconate complex in 50 ml normal saline solution, and give over 1 hour. Dilute therapeutic doses of drug in 100 ml normal saline solution, and give over 1 hour.
Store drug at 68° to 77° F (20° to 25° C). Use immediately after dilution in normal saline solution.

Incompatibilities
Other I.V. drugs.

CONTRAINDICATIONS & CAUTIONS
• Contraindicated in those hypersensitive to sodium ferric gluconate complex or its components, such as benzyl alcohol.
• Contraindicated in those with anemias not caused by iron deficiency. Don't give to patients with iron overload.
• Use cautiously in geriatric patients.

ADVERSE REACTIONS
CNS: asthenia, headache, fatigue, *pain,* malaise, *dizziness,* paresthesia, agitation, insomnia, somnolence, syncope, fever.
CV: *hypotension, hypertension,* tachycardia, **bradycardia,** angina, *chest pain,* edema, flushing, **MI.**
EENT: conjunctivitis, abnormal vision, rhinitis.
GI: *nausea, vomiting, diarrhea,* rectal disorder, dyspepsia, eructation, flatulence, melena, abdominal pain.
GU: UTI.
Hematologic: *abnormal erythrocytes,* anemia.
Metabolic: hyperkalemia, ***hypoglycemia,*** hypokalemia, hypervolemia.
Musculoskeletal: myalgia, arthralgia, back pain, arm pain, *cramps.*
Respiratory: *dyspnea,* coughing, upper respiratory tract infections, pneumonia, pulmonary edema.
Skin: pruritus, increased sweating, rash, injection site reaction.
Other: infection, rigors, chills, flulike syndrome, ***sepsis, carcinoma, hypersensitivity reactions,*** lymphadenopathy.

INTERACTIONS
Drug-drug. *Enalapril:* May potentiate adverse effects of sodium ferric gluconate complex. Use together cautiously.

EFFECTS ON LAB TEST RESULTS
• May increase or decrease potassium level. May decrease glucose level.

• May decrease hemoglobin and hematocrit.

ACTION
Replenishes and maintains total body content of iron.

PHARMACOKINETICS
Onset, peak, and duration of drug effect unknown.
Distribution: Unknown.
Metabolism: Unknown.
Excretion: Unknown.

CLINICAL CONSIDERATIONS
• Don't use drug in those with iron overload, which generally occurs in hemoglobinopathies and other refractory anemias.
• *Alert:* Potentially life-threatening hypersensitivity reactions characterized by CV collapse, cardiac arrest, bronchospasm, oral or pharyngeal edema, dyspnea, angioedema, urticaria, pruritus, and pain and muscle spasm of chest or back may occur during infusion. Have adequate supportive measures readily available. Monitor patient closely during infusion.
• After rapid I.V. iron administration, patient may experience profound hypotension with flushing, lightheadedness, malaise, fatigue, weakness, or severe chest, back, flank, or groin pain. Rapid administration, not hypersensitivity, probably causes these reactions. Don't exceed 2.1 mg/minute, the recommended rate of administration. Monitor patient closely during infusion.
• Monitor hematocrit and hemoglobin, ferritin, and iron saturation levels during therapy.
• Iron levels greater than 300 mcg/dl, with transferrin oversaturation, may indicate iron poisoning.
• Some adverse reactions in hemodialysis patients may be related to dialysis itself or to chronic renal failure.

• Check with patient about other potential sources of iron, such as nonprescription iron preparations and iron-containing multiple vitamins with minerals.
• Signs and symptoms of overdose include abdominal pain, diarrhea, and vomiting that progresses to pallor or cyanosis; lassitude; drowsiness; hyperventilation caused by acidosis; and CV collapse.
• Treat overdose with supportive measures. Dialysis doesn't remove the drug.

PATIENT TEACHING
• Advise patient not to take additional iron supplements.
• Advise patient to immediately report signs and symptoms of possible overdose, such as abdominal pain, diarrhea, vomiting, drowsiness, or rapid breathing.

sodium lactate (1/6 M sodium lactate)

Pharmacologic class: acid salt
Therapeutic class: sodium chloride laxative
Pregnancy risk category: C
pH: 6 to 7.3

INDICATIONS & DOSAGES
➤ **Mild to moderate metabolic acidosis—**
Adults: To calculate suggested dose in milliliters, multiply 0.8 by body weight in pounds. Then multiply this figure by 60 minus the plasma carbon dioxide level. Actual dose depends on severity of acidosis, results of plasma glucose and serum electrolyte level tests, and patient's age, weight, and underlying disorder.

ADMINISTRATION
Direct injection: Not recommended.
Intermittent infusion: Not recommended.
Continuous infusion: Infuse diluted solution through primary I.V. line or piggyback at ordered rate. Don't exceed 300 ml/hour in adults.

PREPARATION & STORAGE
Available in 500-, and 1,000-ml containers of solution having sodium and lactate ions, each in concentrations of 167 mEq/L. Also available in 10-ml flip-top vials containing 5 mEq/ml.

For infusion, dilute sodium lactate in ordered volume of solution if desired concentration isn't commercially available.

Store at 104° F (40° C) or below. Protect from freezing and extreme heat. Discard any unused portions.

Incompatibilities
Sodium bicarbonate.

CONTRAINDICATIONS & CAUTIONS
• Contraindicated in those with lactic acidosis because lactate metabolism is impaired and bicarbonate doesn't form.
• Contraindicated in those with hypernatremia or other conditions in which sodium administration is harmful.
• Use cautiously in those with edema or sodium-retaining conditions, such as heart failure, oliguria, or anuria.
• Use cautiously in those with metabolic or respiratory alkalosis because sodium bicarbonate is an alkalizing drug and can exacerbate these conditions.
• Use cautiously in those with conditions that increase lactate use, such as severe hepatic insufficiency, shock, hypoxia, or beriberi. Additional lactate may worsen these conditions.
• Use cautiously in those with metabolic acidosis associated with circulatory insufficiency, extracorporeal circulation, hypothermia, glycogen storage disease, liver dysfunction, respiratory

alkalosis, shock, cardiac decompensation, or other conditions involving reduced tissue perfusion. Tissue anoxia and impaired lactate metabolism reduce lactate conversion to bicarbonate.

ADVERSE REACTIONS
CNS: fever.
CV: phlebitis.
Metabolic: hypovolemia, hypokalemia, *metabolic alkalosis with overdose,* hypernatremia with or without edema.
Respiratory: pulmonary edema.
Skin: local pain, extravasation.
Other: injection site infection.

INTERACTIONS
None significant.

EFFECTS ON LAB TEST RESULTS
• May increase sodium level.

ACTION
This alkalinizing drug's action depends on conversion to bicarbonate, the principal extracellular buffer, which acts to maintain acid-base balance.

PHARMACOKINETICS
Onset, peak, and duration of drug effect unknown.
Distribution: Unknown.
Metabolism: In the liver.
Excretion: Unknown.

CLINICAL CONSIDERATIONS
• Osmolarity: 330 mOsm/L.
• Osmolality: 10,665 to 11,490 mOsm/kg.
• Carefully monitor glucose level, fluid and electrolyte balance, and acid-base balance throughout therapy.
• Notify prescriber and stop infusion if an adverse reaction occurs. Save remaining solution for examination, if needed.
• One gram of sodium lactate provides 8.9 mEq of sodium and 8.9 mEq of lactate.

PATIENT TEACHING
• Advise patient of potential adverse effects.
• Advise patient to report adverse effects.
• Reassure patient that sodium lactate is generally well tolerated and adverse effects are rare.

---

streptokinase
Streptase

Pharmacologic class: plasminogen activator
Therapeutic class: thrombolytic enzyme
Pregnancy risk category: C
pH: 6 to 8

INDICATIONS & DOSAGES
➤ **Pulmonary embolism, deep vein thrombosis, arterial embolism, or thrombosis—**
Adults: Loading dose 250,000 IU; maintenance dose 100,000 IU/hour.
Children ♦ : Loading dose 1,000 IU/kg; up to 3,000 IU/kg have been used. For maintenance infusion, 1,000 IU/kg/hour for up to 12 hours; up to 1,500 IU/kg/hour for up to 24 hours have been used.
➤ **Acute, obstructing coronary artery thrombi from an evolving acute MI—**
Adults: 1.5 million IU over 60 minutes.
➤ **Arteriovenous cannula occlusion—**
Adults: 250,000 IU in 2 ml of I.V. solution.

ADMINISTRATION
Direct injection: To clear arteriovenous cannula obstruction, use an infusion pump to slowly deliver 250,000 IU of reconstituted drug into each occluded cannula over 25 to 35 minutes. Then clamp off the cannulas for 2 hours.

Closely observe patient for possible adverse reactions. After 2 hours, aspirate contents of the cannulas and flush with normal saline solution. Reconnect cannula.
Intermittent infusion: Not recommended.
Continuous infusion: For loading dose in pulmonary embolism, deep vein thrombosis, or arterial embolism or thrombosis, give diluted drug through a peripheral I.V. line, using an infusion pump to deliver 250,000 IU over 30 minutes. Set rate at 30 ml/hour for 750,000 IU vial or 90 ml/hour for 250,000 IU vial with dilution equaling 45 ml.

For maintenance dose, set infusion pump to deliver 100,000 IU/hour. Continue infusion for 24 hours for pulmonary embolism, 24 to 72 hours for arterial embolism or thrombosis, and 72 hours for deep vein thrombosis.

For coronary artery thrombi, give diluted drug through a peripheral I.V. line, using an infusion pump with rate set at 1.5 million IU/hour for 1 hour. No maintenance dose is needed.

PREPARATION & STORAGE
Available in powder form in 6.5-ml vials containing 250,000, 750,000, or 1.5 million IU.

For arteriovenous cannula clearance, reconstitute using 5 ml of normal saline injection or dextrose 5% injection for each 250,000 IU of streptokinase. Add diluent slowly, directed at the side of the vial rather than onto the powder. Roll and tilt the vial gently; avoid shaking which may cause foaming and an increase in flocculation. Slight flocculation doesn't interfere with safe use; however, solutions containing many particles should be discarded.

For infusion, reconstitute with normal saline injection or dextrose 5% injection. Further dilute, generally to a volume of 45 ml, a loading dose infu-

---

sion, or to a multiple of 45 ml to a maximum of 500 ml for continuous maintenance infusion, with the same solution used for reconstitution. Infusions should be given through a 0.8-micrometer filter or larger. Use volumetric or syringe pumps because reconstituted streptokinase solution may alter drop size, influencing the accuracy of drop-counting infusion devices.

Store unopened vials at room temperature. Store reconstituted solutions at 36° to 39° F (2° to 4° C); discard after 24 hours. Don't add any other drugs to the solution.

Incompatibilities
Dextrans, other I.V. drugs.

CONTRAINDICATIONS & CAUTIONS
• Contraindicated in those with previous severe allergic reaction to drug.
• Contraindicated in those with active internal bleeding, intracranial neoplasm, severe uncontrolled hypertension, or CVA or intracranial or intraspinal surgery within the past 2 months because thrombolytic therapy increases risk of bleeding.
• Contraindicated in those with an increased risk of bleeding, such as those in childbirth; those who have had an invasive procedure, including organ biopsy and puncture of a noncompressible vessel, or surgery within the past 10 days; those who have had severe GI bleeding within the past 10 days; and those who have a dissecting aneurysm, subacute bacterial endocarditis, diabetic hemorrhagic retinopathy, GI lesion or ulcer, moderate hypertension, active tuberculosis with recent-onset cavitation, or either minor or severe recent trauma, including possible internal injury caused by CPR.
• Use cautiously in those with mitral stenosis and atrial fibrillation or other indications of probable left-sided heart thrombus and in those with conditions that increase the risk of cerebral embolism.
• Use cautiously in those with sepsis at or near thrombus site, obstructed intravenous catheter, or occluded arteriovenous cannula because of increased risk of systemic infection.
• Use cautiously in those with recent streptococcal infection and in those receiving drug because elevated streptokinase antibody levels may cause resistance to therapy.

ADVERSE REACTIONS
CV: *arrhythmias,* hypotension.
Hematologic: *hemorrhage.*
Respiratory: pulmonary edema.
Other: *angioedema, delayed hypersensitivity reactions such as vasculitis or interstitial nephritis,* hypersensitivity reactions (fever, shivering, minor breathing difficulty, *bronchospasm,* periorbital edema, *angioneurotic edema,* urticaria, itching, flushing, nausea, headache, musculoskeletal pain, *anaphylaxis).*

INTERACTIONS
Drug-drug. *Antifibrinolytics such as aminocaproic acid:* Reverses streptokinase effects. Avoid using together.
Aspirin, dipyridamole, corticosteroids, heparin, NSAIDs, oral anticoagulants: Increases risk of severe hemorrhage. Use together with caution. Monitor patient closely.
Drug-herb. *Dong quai, feverfew, garlic, ginger, horse chestnut, red clover:* Increases risk of bleeding. Discourage use together.

EFFECTS ON LAB TEST RESULTS
• May increase transaminase levels.
• May increase PT, PTT, and INR. May decrease hematocrit.

ACTION
Promotes thrombolysis by converting residual plasminogen to plasmin (fibrinolysin), which degrades fibrin clots,

fibrinogen, and precoagulant factors V and VII. Also decreases blood and plasma viscosity and reduces erythrocytes' tendency to form aggregates, thereby increasing perfusion of collateral blood vessels. Drug is strongly antigenic; it promotes antibody formation, which diminishes its effects and may cause allergic reactions.

PHARMACOKINETICS

Onset, rapid; duration, a few hours after therapy is stopped.

Distribution: In plasma. Drug crosses the placental barrier minimally. It's unknown if drug appears in breast milk.

Metabolism: None.

Excretion: Rapidly cleared from the circulation by antibodies and the reticuloendothelial system. Initial half-life, about 18 minutes from antibody action against streptokinase; subsequent half-life, about 83 minutes in absence of antibodies.

CLINICAL CONSIDERATIONS

• Only those trained in managing thrombotic disease and working in hospitals equipped to monitor thrombin time and perform other needed laboratory tests should give this drug.

• Before starting therapy, obtain a blood sample to determine thrombin time, aPTT, PT, hematocrit, and platelet count. This is especially important in pretreatment with heparin.

• Monitor vital signs, including blood pressure for infusion-related hypotension, and monitor clotting status.

• To avoid dislodging deep venous thrombi, don't take blood pressure in patient's lower extremities.

• Assess percutaneous puncture sites and cuts for oozing because streptokinase may lyse fibrin deposits at these sites.

• Avoid invasive arterial procedures before and during therapy. If needed, use patient's arm.

• Perform venipunctures carefully and as infrequently as possible.

• Avoid I.M. injections and unnecessary handling of patient.

• Because exposure to streptococci, source of streptokinase, is common, a loading dose is used to neutralize the antibodies present in many patients. To help establish dose, determine patient resistance to streptokinase. Don't give loading dose exceeding 1 million IU.

• Drug may not be effective if given between 5 days and 12 months of earlier administration or streptococcal infections. Ask patient if he has recently had a streptococcal infection, such as streptococcal pharyngitis, acute rheumatic fever, or acute glomerulonephritis secondary to a streptococcal infection before treatment.

• Although heparin isn't recommended during streptokinase therapy, it may be used soon afterward to minimize risk of recurrent thrombosis and pulmonary emboli.

• If hemorrhage develops as a result of overdose, discontinue drug immediately. If needed, give whole blood (preferably fresh blood), packed RBCs, and cryoprecipitate or fresh frozen plasma. Don't use dextrans. Aminocaproic acid may be given in an emergency, although its use as an antidote hasn't been established.

PATIENT TEACHING

• Advise patient to report adverse reactions.

• Advise patient to report bleeding or bruising.

• Inform patient of potential for symptomatic hypotension.

---

streptozocin
Zanosar

Pharmacologic class: nitrosourea
antineoplastic antibiotic (cell
cycle–phase nonspecific)
Therapeutic class: antineoplastic
Pregnancy risk category: C
pH: 3.5 to 4.5

INDICATIONS & DOSAGES
➤ **Metastatic islet cell carcinoma of
pancreas—**
Adults: 500 mg/m^2 daily for five consecutive days q 6 weeks. Alternatively,
1 g/m^2 in a single dose weekly for 2
weeks; then, if needed, up to 1.5 g/m^2
weekly. Dosage depends on renal,
hematologic, and hepatic response and
tolerance to drug.

ADMINISTRATION
Direct injection: Rapidly inject reconstituted drug through port of primary
I.V. line containing a free-flowing,
compatible solution.
Intermittent infusion: Infuse diluted
drug over ordered duration, usually 15
minutes to 6 hours, via I.V. line containing a free-flowing, compatible solution.
Continuous infusion: Infuse diluted
drug over ordered duration. Continuous
5-day I.V. infusions have been given,
but prolonged continuous administration may cause CNS toxicity.

PREPARATION & STORAGE
Supplied in powder form in 1-g vials.
   To avoid mutagenic, teratogenic, and
carcinogenic risks, use a biological
containment cabinet, wear gloves and
mask, and use syringes with luer-lock
fittings to prevent leakage of drug solution. Correctly dispose of needles,
vials, and unused drug, and avoid contaminating work surfaces. If skin or mucous membrane contact occurs, wash
area thoroughly with soap and water.
   Reconstitute with 9.5 ml of dextrose
5% injection or normal saline injection
to yield 100 mg/ml.
   Dilute reconstituted drug with dextrose 5% injection, normal saline solution, or dextrose 5% in normal saline
injection. Usual dilution for intermittent infusion is 100 mg/ml of streptozocin solution added to 10 to 200 ml of
dextrose 5% injection.
   Store vials at 36° to 46° F (2° to
8° C) and protect from light. If kept at
room temperature, reconstituted drug
should be used within 12 hours. Discard if color changes from pale gold to
dark brown, indicating decomposition.

Incompatibilities
Allopurinol, aztreonam, cefepime,
piperacillin sodium and tazobactam
sodium.

CONTRAINDICATIONS & CAUTIONS
• Contraindicated in those with current
or recent chickenpox or herpes zoster
infection because of risk of severe generalized disease.
• Use cautiously in those with bone
marrow depression or infection because of possible hematologic toxicity
and in those with renal and hepatic impairment because of increased risk of
toxicity.
• Use cautiously in those with diabetes
mellitus because drug aggravates the
disorder and in those with previous cytotoxic or radiation therapy because
drug causes further bone marrow depression.

ADVERSE REACTIONS
CNS: confusion, lethargy, and depression with continuous infusion.
GI: *nausea, vomiting,* diarrhea.
GU: NEPHROTOXICITY, azotemia,
anuria, glycosuria, proteinuria, renal
tubular acidosis.

Hematologic: bleeding, anemia, LEU-KOPENIA, THROMBOCYTOPENIA.
Hepatic: *hepatotoxicity.*
Metabolic: hypophosphatemia, glucose intolerance.
Skin: extravasation, burning sensation from injection site up the arm, tenderness, edema, erythema.

INTERACTIONS
Drug-drug. *Bone marrow depressants, radiation therapy:* Enhances bone marrow depression. Use together with caution.
Corticosteroids, corticotropin: Increases hyperglycemic effect of streptozocin. Monitor patient closely.
Doxorubicin: Prolongs half-life. Monitor patient closely and decrease dosage of doxorubicin.
Nephrotoxic drugs: Causes cumulative nephrotoxicity. Avoid using together.
Phenytoin: Decreases therapeutic effects of streptozocin. Monitor patient closely.

EFFECTS ON LAB TEST RESULTS
● May increase AST, ALT, LDH, alkaline phosphatase, bilirubin, BUN, creatinine, and chloride levels. May decrease phosphorus, potassium, and calcium levels.
● May decrease hemoglobin, hematocrit, and WBC and platelet counts.

ACTION
Cytotoxic action probably stems from cross-linking of DNA strands, impairing DNA synthesis. Its action is cell cycle–nonspecific, although it inhibits progression of the G_2 phase of cell division. It's active against gram-positive and gram-negative bacteria, but cytotoxicity limits its use as an antibiotic. Drug also has diabetogenic or hyperglycemic effects, with selective uptake by pancreatic islet beta cells. Irreversible cell damage results in degranulation and stops insulin secretion.

PHARMACOKINETICS
Onset, peak, and duration of drug's effects are unknown.
Distribution: Only small amounts of drug cross the blood-brain barrier, but metabolites readily enter CSF. Drug appears in liver, kidneys, intestine, and pancreas before it appears in plasma. Drug crosses the placental barrier, but it's unknown if it appears in breast milk.
Metabolism: Probably in liver and kidneys.
Excretion: Mostly in urine, with significant amounts in respiration. Less than 1% in feces. Terminal phase half-life is 35 minutes for unchanged drug and 40 hours for metabolites.

CLINICAL CONSIDERATIONS
● Keep I.V. dextrose available, especially with first dose of streptozocin, because of risk of hypoglycemia.
● If extravasation occurs, stop infusion. Apply cold compresses and elevate the arm. Complete administration in another vein.
● To detect nephrotoxicity, monitor BUN, creatinine, electrolyte, and urine creatinine levels and urinalysis before and at least weekly during therapy. After each course, monitor weekly for 4 to 6 weeks. Also, watch for proteinuria, often the first sign of dose-related, cumulative nephrotoxicity.
● Monitor CBC and liver function studies weekly during and after therapy.

PATIENT TEACHING
● Warn patient to watch for signs of infection such as chills, fever, and sore throat, and to report them immediately.
● Encourage patient to drink plenty of fluids to help clear active metabolites.
● Tell patient that because drug has a low therapeutic index, toxicity usually accompanies therapeutic effects.
● Advise breast-feeding patient to discontinue nursing during therapy.

strontium-89 chloride
Metastron

Pharmacologic class: radioisotope
Therapeutic class: radioisotope for metastatic bone pain
Pregnancy risk category: D

INDICATIONS & DOSAGES
➤ **Relief from bone pain with painful skeletal metastases—**
Adults: 4 millicuries (mCi) slowly over 1 to 2 minutes. Alternatively, 40 to 60 microcuries (mcCi)/kg may be used; repeated administration is based on patient response, current symptoms, and hematologic status. Don't repeat dose at intervals of less than 90 days.

ADMINISTRATION
Direct injection: Give slowly, over 1 to 2 minutes.
Intermittent infusion: Not recommended.
Continuous infusion: Not recommended.

PREPARATION & STORAGE
Available in preservative-free 10-ml vials containing 4 mCi strontium-89 (^{89}Sr). Vials are shipped in a container shielded with 3-mm lead walls.
    Store vial and its contents in the container at room temperature (59° to 77° F [15° to 25° C]).

Incompatibilities
Other I.V. drugs.

CONTRAINDICATIONS & CAUTIONS
• Contraindicated in patients with cancer that doesn't involve bone or in those with seriously compromised bone marrow from previous therapy or disease infiltration.

• Use cautiously in patients with platelet counts below 60,000 cells/mm^3 and WBC counts below 2,400 cells/mm^3.
• Use cautiously in patients with renal dysfunction.

ADVERSE REACTIONS
CNS: fever.
Hematologic: *neutropenia, thrombocytopenia.*
Musculoskeletal: transient increase in bone pain.
Other: flushing sensation after rapid injection; chills.

INTERACTIONS
Drug-drug. *Calcium supplements:* Decreases strontium effectiveness. Monitor patient closely.
Other cytotoxic drugs: Additive bone marrow toxicity. Use together with caution.

EFFECTS ON LAB TEST RESULTS
• May decrease WBC and platelet counts.

ACTION
A radioisotope, ^{89}Sr is a true beta emitter, selectively irradiating primary metastatic bone sites. Soluble strontium ions behave like their calcium analogues, clearing rapidly from blood and localizing selectively in bone mineral.

PHARMACOKINETICS
Onset of pain relief, 7 to 20 days after injection.
Distribution: Local, in bone mineral, preferentially in sites of active osteogenesis; retained in metastatic bone lesions longer than in normal bone.
Metabolism: Progressive decay by beta emission (radioisotope).
Excretion: 66% in urine, 33% in feces.

CLINICAL CONSIDERATIONS
• Verify dose and patient identification before giving because ^{89}Sr delivers a relatively high dose of radioactivity.

Handle drug with care and take appropriate safety measures to minimize exposure to radiation.
- [89]Sr should be used only by qualified and trained prescribers who have been approved by a government licensing agency in the safe use and handling of radionuclides.
- Take special precautions with incontinent patients to minimize risk of radioactive contamination of bed, clothing, linen, and patient's room and immediate environment. Consider catheterization.
- Monitor for increased bone pain, which may occur 2 to 3 days after injection.
- Give increased doses of pain drug, as needed, if bone pain is increased.
- Monitor peripheral blood counts.

PATIENT TEACHING
- Advise patient to report adverse effects.
- Advise patient of radioactivity precautions.
- During first week after injection, advise patient to use toilet, not urinal, and flush toilet twice; wipe any spilled urine with a tissue and flush; wash hands thoroughly after using toilet; immediately wash separately and rinse thoroughly any linen and clothes that become stained with blood or urine; and immediately rinse blood if a cut occurs.
- Advise patient to notify all prescribers that he has received strontium-89 chloride.
- Notify patient of potential increase in bone pain beginning 2 or 3 days after the injection. After about 1 to 2 weeks, the pain should begin to diminish and continue to abate for several months.

succinylcholine chloride*
Anectine, Anectine Flo-Pack, Quelicin

Pharmacologic class: depolarizing neuromuscular blocker
Therapeutic class: skeletal muscle relaxant
Pregnancy risk category: C
pH: 3 to 4.5

INDICATIONS & DOSAGES
➤ **Skeletal muscle relaxant for short procedures, such as endotracheal intubation, endoscopy, and orthopedic manipulations—**
Adults: Initially, 0.6 mg/kg, with range of 0.3 to 1.1 mg/kg. Subsequent doses based on response to drug.
Children: Initially, 1 to 2 mg/kg. Subsequent doses based on first dose.
➤ **Skeletal muscle relaxant for prolonged surgical procedures—**
Adults: Average dose of 2.5 to 4.3 mg/minute, with range of 0.5 to 10 mg/minute, by continuous infusion. Or initially, 0.3 to 1.1 mg/kg by intermittent injection; subsequent doses 0.04 to 0.07 mg/kg, p.r.n., to maintain relaxation.

ADMINISTRATION
Direct injection: Inject ordered amount of commercially prepared or diluted drug over 10 to 30 seconds into a primary I.V. line containing a free-flowing, compatible solution.
Intermittent infusion: Not recommended. Administration of repeated intermittent doses may produce tachyphylaxis and prolonged apnea.
Continuous infusion: Infuse diluted drug through an I.V. line containing a free-flowing, compatible solution at 2.5 mg/minute, initially; then adjust to 0.5 to 10 mg/minute, depending on patient response.

To avoid overdose and detect development of nondepolarizing neuromuscular blockade, monitor neuromuscular function with a peripheral nerve stimulator when giving drug by infusion.

PREPARATION & STORAGE

Available in 5-ml syringes and 10-ml vials containing 20 mg/ml, in 10-ml ampules containing 50 mg/ml, and in 5- and 10-ml vials containing 100 mg/ml. Also available in powder form in strengths of 500 mg, and 1 g in 5-ml unit-dose vials.

Reconstitute powder with compatible diluent, such as dextrose 5% injection or normal saline solution, according to manufacturer's instructions.

For continuous infusion, dilute to a concentration of 1 to 2 mg/ml. Add 1 g of powder, 10 ml of solution (100 mg/ml), or 20 ml of solution (50 mg/ml) to 1 L or 500 ml of compatible diluent, such as dextrose 5% injection, dextrose 5% in normal saline solution, normal saline solution, or 1/6 M sodium lactate. Or, add 500 mg of powder, 5 ml of solution (100 mg/ml), or 10 ml of solution (50 mg/ml) to 500 or 250 ml of diluent to yield 1 or 2 mg/ml succinylcholine, respectively.

For direct injection, use prepared solution, if possible; or dilute with compatible solution to yield concentration, volume, and dosage ordered.

Store solutions at 36° to 46° F (2° to 8° C). Multidose vials are stable for 14 days at room temperature. Powders don't need refrigeration. Discard unused solutions within 24 hours.

Incompatibilities

Barbiturates, nafcillin, sodium bicarbonate, solutions with pH above 4.5, thiopental sodium.

CONTRAINDICATIONS & CAUTIONS

• Contraindicated in those with low pseudocholinesterase levels because of risk of apnea or prolonged muscle paralysis and in those with myopathies associated with elevated serum creatine kinase levels because drug may worsen the disorder.

• Contraindicated in those with personal or family history of malignant hyperthermia because drug may induce the disorder and in those with angle-closure glaucoma and penetrating eye injuries because drug may increase intraocular pressure.

• Use cautiously in those who have had recent digoxin therapy or digoxin toxicity, severe burns, degenerative or dystrophic neuromuscular disease, paraplegia, spinal cord injury, or severe trauma because of enhanced risk of arrhythmias or cardiac arrest.

• Use cautiously in those with bronchogenic carcinoma because drug may enhance neuromuscular blocking action; in electrolyte or acid-base imbalance because drug action may be altered; in conditions in which histamine release would be hazardous because drug may cause histamine release; and in hyperkalemia because drug may worsen the disorder.

• Give carefully in anemia; dehydration; exposure to neurotoxic insecticides; severe hepatic disease or cirrhosis; malnutrition; pregnancy; recessive hereditary trait, such as plasma pseudocholinesterase, because of potential for prolonged respiratory depression or apnea; and in pulmonary impairment or respiratory depression because of risk of further respiratory depression.

• Use cautiously in severe obesity or neuromuscular disease because of possible airway or ventilation problems.

• Use drug cautiously in open eye injury, chronic open-angle glaucoma, or during ocular surgery, because of risk of increased intraocular pressure.

• Use cautiously in fractures or muscle spasm because initial muscle fasciculations may result in additional trauma.
• Give carefully in patients with hepatic impairment because decreased pseudocholinesterase activity may result in apnea or respiratory depression; and in renal impairment because of possible slowed drug clearance and prolonged effect.
• In hyperthermia, drug intensity and duration may decrease; in hypothermia, they may increase. Use succinylcholine cautiously.
• Continuous I.V. infusion is considered unsafe in infants and children because of risk of malignant hypertension.

ADVERSE REACTIONS

CV: *cardiac arrest, arrhythmias, bradycardia,* tachycardia, hypotension, hypertension.
EENT: excessive salivation, increased intraocular pressure.
Metabolic: hyperkalemia.
Musculoskeletal: jaw rigidity, muscle fasciculation, postoperative muscle pain, myalgia.
Respiratory: *respiratory depression, apnea.*
Skin: rash.
Other: *malignant hyperthermia.*

INTERACTIONS

Drug-drug. *Amphotericin B, thiazide diuretics:* Increases effects of succinylcholine caused by electrolyte imbalance. Reduce dosage in patients with hypocalcemia and hypokalemia.
Beta-blockers, cimetidine, corticosteroids, cyclophosphamide, chloroquine, furosemide, lidocaine in I.V. doses exceeding 5 mg/kg, lithium, magnesium salts, neostigmine, hormonal contraceptives, oxytocin, pancuronium, phenelzine, phenothiazines, procainamide, promazine, quinidine, thiotepa:

Increases neuromuscular blockade. Use together with caution.
Cardiac glycosides: May increase cardiac effects. Monitor cardiac status closely.
Diazepam: Reduces neuromuscular blockade duration. Monitor patient closely.
Inhalation anesthetics, opioid analgesics: Increases incidence of bradycardia, arrhythmias, sinus arrest, and apnea.
Procaine I.V.: Prolongs neuromuscular blockade. Use together with caution. Monitor patient closely.
Drug-herb. *Melatonin:* Potentiates blocking properties of succinylcholine. Discourage use together.

EFFECTS ON LAB TEST RESULTS

• May increase myoglobin and potassium levels.

ACTION

Paralyzes skeletal muscle by blocking impulse transmission at the neuromuscular junction. It competes with acetylcholine for cholinergic receptors of the motor end plate. Like acetylcholine, succinylcholine binds with these receptors and produces depolarization; however, depolarization is more prolonged.

PHARMACOKINETICS

Onset, 30 to 60 seconds; duration, usually 4 to 10 minutes after a single injection—longer with continuous I.V. infusion.
Distribution: Widely dispersed by plasma. Doesn't cross the blood-brain barrier but crosses the placental barrier in small amounts. Not known if drug appears in breast milk.
Metabolism: Rapidly hydrolyzed by plasma pseudocholinesterase to the active metabolite succinylmonocholine and to choline. Succinylmonocholine is further metabolized, principally by al-

kaline hydrolysis, to inactive succinate acid and choline.

Excretion: In urine as active and inactive metabolites and small amounts, about 10%, of unchanged drug.

CLINICAL CONSIDERATIONS

• Osmolality: 409 mOsm/kg for 50-mg/ml concentration.

• Drug should be given only by staff trained to give anesthetics and manage their adverse reactions.

• *Alert:* Drug may contain benzyl alcohol.

• When giving succinylcholine, keep emergency resuscitation equipment available.

• In prolonged administration, if the depolarizing neuromuscular blockade changes to nondepolarizing blockade, determined by nerve stimulator, give small doses of an anticholinesterase, as ordered. Give atropine with an anticholinesterase to counteract muscarinic adverse effects. Observe patient for at least 1 hour after reversal of nondepolarizing blockade for possible return of muscle relaxation.

• To determine patient's sensitivity and recovery time to drug, a test dose of 0.1 mg/kg (about 10 mg) may be given after induction but while patient is still breathing spontaneously.

• Premedicate with atropine or scopolamine to prevent excessive salivation. Also premedicate with atropine or thiopental sodium to inhibit transient bradycardia accompanied by hypotension, arrhythmias, and temporary sinus arrest resulting from vagal stimulation.

• Succinylcholine fasciculations can cause postoperative myalgia, which may be intense. Some prescribers advocate giving a small dose of succinylcholine to reduce severity of fasciculations.

• Giving a small dose of tubocurarine before succinylcholine may decrease

the incidence of myoglobinuria in children.

• *Alert:* Neuromuscular blockers have no known effect on consciousness or pain threshold. Avoid giving drug until unconsciousness has been induced.

• In a patient who has taken an overdose, use a peripheral nerve stimulator to determine nature and degree of neuromuscular blockade. Overdose may result in prolonged respiratory depression or apnea and CV collapse. Maintain airway and give manual or mechanical ventilation until independent respiration resumes. Give fluids and vasopressors, as needed, to treat shock or severe hypotension.

PATIENT TEACHING

• Advise patient to report adverse effects.

• Advise patient of potential for postoperative myalgia.

• Reassure patient that postoperative myalgia will subside in 24 to 48 hours.

sufentanil citrate
Sufenta

Pharmacologic class: opioid
Therapeutic class: analgesic, adjunct to anesthesia, anesthetic
Pregnancy risk category: C
Controlled substance schedule: II
pH: 3.5 to 6

INDICATIONS & DOSAGES

➤ **Adjunct in anesthesia—**
Adults: Low initial dose, 1 to 2 mcg/kg, with supplemental doses of 10 to 25 mcg, p.r.n., to maintain analgesia or anesthesia; moderate initial dose, 2 to 8 mcg/kg, with supplemental doses of 10 to 50 mcg, p.r.n.

   If used with nitrous oxide and oxygen for procedures lasting 8 hours or longer, total dose is 1 mcg/kg/hour or less.

➤ **Primary anesthesia—**
Adults: Initially, 8 to 30 mcg/kg with 100% oxygen, with supplemental doses of 25 to 50 mcg, p.r.n., to maintain anesthesia. Loading dose followed by continuous infusion is recommended for prolonged procedures.
Children younger than age 12 undergoing CV surgery: Initially, 10 to 25 mcg/kg with 100% oxygen, with supplemental doses of 25 to 50 mcg, p.r.n.—maximum total, 1 to 2 mcg/kg—to maintain anesthesia.

ADMINISTRATION

Only those trained in giving I.V. anesthetics and managing their adverse reactions should give this drug.
Direct injection: Inject slowly, especially with large doses, over 1 to 2 minutes. Use a 1-ml syringe for small doses.
Intermittent infusion: Not recommended.
Continuous infusion: After loading dose, infuse 1 mcg/kg or less over 1 hour.

PREPARATION & STORAGE

Available in preservative-free 1-, 2-, and 5-ml ampules containing 50 mcg/ml.

For continuous infusion, dilute with a compatible solution such as D_5W. Store at room temperature 59° to 77° F (15° to 25° C). Protect from light and freezing.

Incompatibilities

Acidic solutions, diazepam, lorazepam, phenobarbital, phenytoin, thiopental.

CONTRAINDICATIONS & CAUTIONS

• Contraindicated in those with sensitivity to sufentanil or other fentanyl derivatives.
• Use with caution in patients receiving MAO inhibitors within the previous 14 days; sufentanil test dose recommended.
• Use with caution in patients with altered respiratory function because of risk of further respiratory depression and increased airway resistance.
• Use cautiously in patients with head injury and increased intracranial pressure. Sufentanil can obscure changes in level of consciousness and raise intracranial pressure.
• Reduce dose in those with hepatic or renal impairment because of increased risk of toxicity, and in those with hypothyroidism because of risk of respiratory depression and prolonged CNS depression.
• In geriatric and debilitated patients and in neonates, give cautiously because of increased risk of adverse reactions, especially respiratory depression. Lower doses may be needed.
• Give carefully in patients with bradyarrhythmias because drug may worsen the condition, and in patients with poor cardiac reserve because of enhanced risk of severe bradycardia or large decrease in blood pressure.

ADVERSE REACTIONS

CNS: somnolence.
CV: *bradycardia,* hypertension, hypotension, *arrhythmias,* tachycardia.
GI: nausea, vomiting.
Musculoskeletal: chest wall rigidity, intraoperative muscle movement.
Respiratory: *apnea, bronchospasm, postoperative respiratory depression.*
Skin: *pruritus,* erythema.
Other: chills.

INTERACTIONS

Drug-drug. *Anesthetics—spinal or epidural:* Causes additive respiratory depression, bradycardia, or hypotension. Use together cautiously.
Benzodiazepines: Speeds up loss of consciousness. May need to reduce sufentanil dose.

Reactions may be *common*, uncommon, *life-threatening*, or COMMON AND LIFE-THREATENING.

Beta blockers: Reduces severity or frequency of hypertensive response; enhances risk of bradycardia. Monitor cardiac status closely.

CNS depressants, opioid analgesics: Heightens risk of CNS and respiratory depression and hypotension. Avoid using together.

MAO inhibitors: Increases risk of severe hypertension, hypotension, and tachycardia. Avoid using within 14 days of each other.

Nalbuphine, pentazocine: Causes partial antagonism of sufentanil's anesthetic and CNS and respiratory depressant effects. Monitor patient closely.

Naloxone, naltrexone: Antagonizes sufentanil effects. Use together with caution. Monitor patient closely.

Neuromuscular blockers: Causes additive respiratory depression. High doses of sufentanil may allow lower doses of blockers. Assess for dosage adjustment.

Nitrous oxide: Deepens CNS and respiratory depression and increases hypotension; reduces blood pressure, heart rate, and cardiac output. Avoid using together.

EFFECTS ON LAB TEST RESULTS
● May increase plasma amylase, lipase, and prolactin levels.

ACTION
Acts as an agonist at stereospecific opiate receptor sites in the CNS to produce analgesic effect. Alters both the perception of pain and the emotional response to it.

PHARMACOKINETICS
Onset, about 1 to 3 minutes; duration, dose-dependent, ranging from 5 minutes with analgesic doses of less than 8 mcg/kg to about 3 hours with anesthetic doses higher than 8 mcg/kg.

Distribution: Rapidly and extensively dispersed throughout body tissues. Not known if drug crosses the placental barrier. Not known if drug appears in breast milk.

Metabolism: Primarily metabolized in the liver and small intestine.

Excretion: Mainly eliminated in urine, but also in feces. Half-life, about 2.5 hours.

CLINICAL CONSIDERATIONS
● Sufentanil is used to supplement general, regional, or local anesthetics and as a primary drug to maintain anesthesia in certain types of major surgery.

● Dosage depends on which other drugs the patient is receiving, especially if he's receiving an anesthetic; type and expected length of surgery; and patient's age, ideal weight, size, physical condition, underlying disorder, and response to drug.

● Sufentanil is five to seven times more potent than fentanyl.

● *Alert:* Only those experienced in giving parenteral anesthetics to patients under general anesthesia, intubated, and receiving oxygen should give sufentanil.

● During therapy with sufentanil, keep resuscitation equipment available.

● Use of a benzodiazepine or other amnestic is recommended during surgical anesthesia with sufentanil.

● Patients who are tolerant of other opioids may be tolerant of sufentanil.

● High doses may produce muscle rigidity, which can be reversed by giving neuromuscular blockers.

● Give drug with patient in supine position to minimize orthostatic hypotensive effects.

● Monitor patient's breathing for at least 1 hour after dose. If rate drops below 8 breaths/minute, rouse patient to stimulate breathing and notify prescriber.

● Closely monitor for signs of withdrawal when discontinuing sufentanil after prolonged use. Physical dependence is possible.

• If overdose occurs, maintain airway patency and provide respiratory support. Give naloxone, as needed, to reverse respiratory depression. Also give I.V. fluids and vasopressors, as ordered, to maintain blood pressure and neuromuscular blockers to relieve muscle rigidity.

PATIENT TEACHING

• Tell patient to report adverse effects.
• Warn patient to get up slowly after treatment to reduce dizziness and faintness.
• Advise patient of the potential for dependence.

tacrolimus (FK506)
Prograf

Pharmacologic class: bacteria-derived macrolide
Therapeutic class: immunosuppressant
Pregnancy risk category: C

INDICATIONS & DOSAGES
➤ **To prevent organ rejection in allogenic liver or kidney transplants—**
Adults: 0.03 to 0.05 mg/kg/day I.V. as a continuous infusion given no sooner than 6 hours after transplantation. Substitute P.O. therapy as soon as possible, with first oral dose given 8 to 12 hours after stopping I.V. infusion.
Children: Initially, 0.03 to 0.05 mg/kg/day I.V., followed by 0.15 to 0.2 mg/kg/day P.O. on a schedule similar to adults, adjusted p.r.n.
Adjust-a-dose: For patients with renal or hepatic impairment, use lowest recommended dose.

ADMINISTRATION
Direct injection: Not recommended.
Intermittent infusion: Not recommended.
Continuous infusion: Give as a continuous infusion based on weight.

PREPARATION & STORAGE
Available as a 5 mg/ml concentrated solution in a 1-ml ampule.
Dilute drug with 250 to 1,000 ml of normal saline injection or D_5W injection to a concentration between 0.004 mg/ml and 0.02 mg/ml before use.

Store drug from 41° to 77° F (5° to 25° C). Store diluted infusion solution for no more than 24 hours in glass or polyethylene containers. Inspect drug for particulate matter and any discoloration before giving it.

Incompatibilities
Solutions or I.V. drugs with a pH above 9, such as acyclovir and ganciclovir.

CONTRAINDICATIONS & CAUTIONS
• Contraindicated in those hypersensitive to drug or castor oil derivatives.

ADVERSE REACTIONS
CNS: *headache, tremor, insomnia, pain, paresthesia,* delirium, **coma,** *asthenia, dizziness, fever.*
CV: *hypertension, peripheral edema, chest pain, edema.*
GI: *diarrhea, nausea, constipation, anorexia, vomiting, abdominal pain, dyspepsia.*
GU: *abnormal renal function, UTI, oliguria.*
Hematologic: *anemia, leukocytosis,* THROMBOCYTOPENIA, LEUKOPENIA.
Metabolic: *hyperkalemia, hypokalemia, hyperglycemia, hypomagnesemia, diabetes mellitus,* hyperlipidemia, hypophosphatemia.
Musculoskeletal: *back pain, arthralgia.*
Respiratory: *pleural effusion, atelectasis, dyspnea, increased cough.*
Skin: *pruritus, rash,* alopecia.
Other: *ascites, infection,* **anaphylaxis.**

INTERACTIONS
Drug-drug. *Antifungals, bromocriptine, calcium channel blockers, cimetidine, clarithromycin, chloramphenicol, danazol, erythromycin, ethinyl estradiol,*

methylprednisolone, metoclopramide, metronidazole, nefazodone, omeprazole, protease inhibitors, other inhibitors of cytochrome P-450 enzyme system: May increase tacrolimus level. Monitor patient for adverse reactions.

Carbamazepine, fosphenytoin, phenobarbital, phenytoin, rifabutin, rifampin, and other inducers of cytochrome P-450 enzyme system: May decrease tacrolimus levels. Monitor tacrolimus effectiveness.

Immunosuppressants, except adrenal corticosteroids: May oversuppress immune system. Monitor patient closely, especially in stressful times.

Mycophenolate mofetil: Increases mycophenolate mofetil trough levels and increases risk of side effects. Use together cautiously.

Nephrotoxic drugs, such as aminoglycosides, amphotericin B, cisplatin, and cyclosporine: Increases risk of nephrotoxicity. Don't give cyclosporine within 24 hours of drug. Monitor patient closely.

Viral vaccines: May interfere with the immune response to vaccines with live virus. Postpone routine immunizations.

Drug-herb. *St. John's wort:* May decrease tacrolimus level. Monitor patient for effectiveness.

EFFECTS ON LAB TEST RESULTS
● May increase BUN, creatinine, AST, ALT, LDH, alkaline phosphatase, bilirubin, and glucose levels. May decrease magnesium and phosphate levels. May increase or decrease potassium level.
● May decrease hemoglobin and WBC and platelet counts.

ACTION
Precise mechanism unknown. Inhibits T-lymphocyte activation, which results in immunosuppression.

PHARMACOKINETICS
Onset, rapid; peak, 1 to 2 hours; duration, unknown.

Distribution: About 99% protein bound.
Metabolism: Extensive, by mixed-function oxidase, primarily cytochrome P-450 systems (3A4).
Excretion: Half-life, about 34 hours; less than 1% excreted unchanged in the urine.

CLINICAL CONSIDERATIONS
● Because of risk of anaphylaxis, use injection only in patients who can't take the oral form.
● Monitor patient continuously during the first 30 minutes of I.V. administration and frequently thereafter for signs and symptoms of anaphylaxis.
● Keep epinephrine 1:1,000 and oxygen available to treat anaphylaxis.
● Monitor patient for signs and symptoms of electrolyte disturbances and drug-related toxicities.
● Monitor tacrolimus trough concentrations, as ordered.
● Adrenal corticosteroids should be used together with drug.
● Children with normal renal and hepatic function may require higher doses than adults.

PATIENT TEACHING
● Instruct patient to check with prescriber before taking other drugs during therapy.
● Tell patient to promptly report adverse reactions.

---

tenecteplase
TNKase

Pharmacologic class: recombinant tissue plasminogen activator
Therapeutic class: thrombolytic agent
Pregnancy risk category: C
pH: 7.3

INDICATIONS & DOSAGES

➤ **To reduce chance of death from acute MI—**

Adults weighing less than 60 kg (132 lb): 30 mg (6 ml) by I.V. bolus over 5 seconds.

Adults weighing 60 to 69 kg (132 to 152 lb): 35 mg (7 ml) by I.V. bolus over 5 seconds.

Adults weighing 70 to 79 kg (154 to 174 lb): 40 mg (8 ml) by I.V. bolus over 5 seconds.

Adults weighing 80 to 89 kg (176 to 196 lb): 45 mg (9 ml) by I.V. bolus over 5 seconds.

Adults weighing 90 kg (198 lb) or more: 50 mg (10 ml) by I.V. bolus over 5 seconds.

Maximum dose is 50 mg.

ADMINISTRATION

Direct injection: Give reconstituted drug as a single I.V. bolus over 5 seconds.

Intermittent infusion: Not recommended.

Continuous infusion: Not recommended.

PREPARATION & STORAGE

Available as lyophilized powder in 50-mg vials.

Reconstitute with 10 ml sterile water supplied with the drug to yield a concentration of 5 mg/ml. Gently swirl vial to dissolve. Don't shake. Discard unused solution.

Store powder at room temperature below 86° F (30° C) or under refrigeration at 36° to 46° F (2° to 8° C). Reconstituted drug may be refrigerated at 36° to 46° F (2° to 8° C) and used within 8 hours.

Incompatibilities

Solutions containing dextrose.

CONTRAINDICATIONS & CAUTIONS

• Contraindicated in patients with an active internal bleed; history of CVA;

intracranial or intraspinal surgery or trauma within the previous 2 months; intracranial neoplasm, aneurysm, or arteriovenous malformation; severe uncontrolled hypertension; or known bleeding diathesis.

• Use with caution in patients who have had a recent major surgery such as coronary artery bypass graft (CABG), organ biopsy, obstetrical delivery or previous puncture of noncompressible vessels.

• Use cautiously in patients with recent trauma; recent GI or GU bleeding; high risk of left ventricular thrombus; acute pericarditis; hypertension (systolic blood pressure 180 mm Hg or higher or diastolic blood pressure 110 mm Hg or higher); severe hepatic dysfunction; hemostatic defects; subacute bacterial endocarditis; pregnancy; septic thrombophlebitis; diabetic hemorrhagic retinopathy; cerebrovascular disease, and in patients age 75 and older.

ADVERSE REACTIONS

CNS: *intracranial hemorrhage, CVA.*
EENT: pharyngeal bleed, epistaxis.
GI: GI bleeding.
GU: hematuria.
Skin: *hematoma,* bleeding at puncture site.

INTERACTIONS

Drug-drug. *Anticoagulants (heparin, vitamin K antagonists), drugs that alter platelet function (acetylsalicylic acid, dipyridamole, glycoprotein IIb or IIIa inhibitors):* Increases risk of bleeding when used before, during, or after therapy with tenecteplase. Use together cautiously.

EFFECTS ON LAB TEST RESULTS

• May increase PT, PTT, and INR. May decrease hemoglobin.

ACTION

A human tissue plasminogen activator that binds to fibrin and converts plasminogen to plasmin. The specificity to fibrin decreases systemic activation of plasminogen and the resulting breakdown of circulating fibrinogen.

PHARMACOKINETICS
Onset, immediate; peak, immediate; duration, unknown.
Distribution: Related to weight and is an approximation of plasma volume.
Metabolism: Primarily hepatic.
Excretion: Initial half-life is 20 to 24 minutes with terminal half-life of 90 to 130 minutes.

CLINICAL CONSIDERATIONS
• Osmolality: 290 mOsm/kg.
• Begin therapy as soon as possible after onset of MI symptoms.
• Minimize arterial and venous punctures during treatment. Avoid noncompressible arterial punctures and internal jugular and subclavian venous punctures.
• Don't give in the same I.V. line as dextrose. Flush dextrose-containing lines with normal saline solution before administration.
• Give heparin with tenecteplase but not in the same I.V. line.
• Monitor patient for bleeding. If serious bleeding occurs, stop heparin and antiplatelet agents immediately.
• Monitor ECG for reperfusion arrhythmias.
• *Alert:* Cholesterol embolism is rarely linked to thrombolytic use, but may be lethal. Signs and symptoms may include livedo reticularis, "purple toe" syndrome, acute renal failure, gangrenous digits, hypertension, pancreatitis, MI, cerebral infarction, spinal cord infarction, retinal artery occlusion, bowel infarction, and rhabdomyolysis.

PATIENT TEACHING
• Advise patient about proper dental care to avoid excessive gum bleeding.
• Advise patient to report any adverse events or excess bleeding immediately.

• Explain to patient and family about the use of tenecteplase.

teniposide (VM-26)
Vumon*

Pharmacologic class: podophyllotoxin (G_2-phase and late S-phase specific)
Therapeutic class: antineoplastic
Pregnancy risk category: D
pH: 5

INDICATIONS & DOSAGES
➤ **Acute lymphocytic leukemia induction therapy—**
Children: Optimum dose hasn't been established. One protocol reported by manufacturer is 165 mg/m² I.V. teniposide with cytarabine 300 mg/m² I.V. twice weekly for eight or nine doses. Another protocol is 250 mg/m² I.V. teniposide and 1.5 mg/m² I.V. vincristine weekly for 4 to 8 weeks, along with prednisone 40 mg/m² P.O. daily for 28 days.
Adjust-a-dose: Dosage adjustment may be necessary for patients with significant renal and hepatic impairment. In patients with Down syndrome, reduce the first course of teniposide by half. Increase subsequent doses if appropriate.

ADMINISTRATION
Direct injection: Not recommended.
Intermittent infusion: Using a 23G or 25G winged-tip needle, give over at least 30 to 60 minutes to avoid hypotension. Use distal rather than major veins. Choose a new site for each infusion. If extravasation occurs, apply ice to the area. Injection of a corticosteroid and irrigation with copious amounts of normal saline solution may decrease swelling.
Continuous infusion: Not recommended.

PREPARATION & STORAGE

Supplied in ampules of 50 mg/5 ml that must be refrigerated and protected from incandescent light. Use extreme caution when preparing and giving drug to avoid mutagenic, teratogenic, and carcinogenic risks. Use a biological containment cabinet, wear gloves and mask, and use syringes with luer-lock fittings to prevent drug leakage. Avoid contaminating work surfaces, and dispose of needles, syringes, ampules, and unused drug correctly. Avoid inhaling drug particles or solutions or allowing contact with skin or mucosa. If contact occurs, wash the area immediately with soap and water.

For infusion, dilute to a final concentration of 0.1 mg/ml, 0.2 mg/ml, 0.4 mg/ml, or 1 mg/ml with D_5W or normal saline solution. Avoid agitation during mixing and minimize storage time. Teniposide concentrate may soften plastic, causing cracking and leaking. Glass bottles and nonpolyvinyl chloride plastic administration sets are recommended. Solution may appear slightly opalescent from surfactants in the formulation.

Refrigerate ampules and protect from light. Give 1 mg/ml solutions within 4 hours of preparation. Diluted solutions with lower concentrations are stable for 24 hours at room temperature.

Incompatibilities

Heparin, idarubicin.

CONTRAINDICATIONS & CAUTIONS

• Contraindicated in patients who have demonstrated a previous hypersensitivity to teniposide or polyoxyethylated castor oil.
• Use with caution in patients with renal or hepatic dysfunction, and in those with Down syndrome.

ADVERSE REACTIONS

CNS: fever.
CV: hypotension.
GI: *diarrhea, nausea, vomiting, mucositis.*
Hematologic: MYELOSUPPRESSION, NEUTROPENIA, THROMBOCYTOPENIA, LEUKOPENIA, *anemia,* bleeding.
Respiratory: *bronchospasm.*
Skin: rash, alopecia.
Other: *anaphylaxis, infection, hypersensitivity reactions, secondary acute myeloid leukemia.*

INTERACTIONS

Drug-drug. *Methotrexate:* Clearance of methotrexate may be increased. Intracellular levels of methotrexate may also be increased. Avoid using together.
Sodium salicylate, tolbutamide: Enhances toxic effects of teniposide. Avoid using together.

EFFECTS ON LAB TEST RESULTS

• May decrease hemoglobin and WBC, platelet, and neutrophil counts.

ACTION

Stops cell mitosis in metaphase, causing a marked decrease in the mitotic index.

PHARMACOKINETICS

Drug level peaks immediately after infusion.
Distribution: Accumulates in kidneys, small intestine, liver, and adrenals. Minimal amounts cross the blood-brain barrier into the CNS; drug may cross the placental barrier. Drug probably appears in breast milk.
Metabolism: In liver; extensively protein bound.
Excretion: Primarily in feces, with significant amounts in urine.

CLINICAL CONSIDERATIONS

• *Alert:* Keep diphenhydramine, epinephrine, hydrocortisone, and an airway available in case of anaphylaxis.
• *Alert:* Drug may contain benzyl alcohol.

• Monitor blood pressure before, during, and after infusion. If systolic pressure falls below 90 mm Hg, stop infusion and notify prescriber.

• Monitor CBC during and after treatment; leukopenia nadir occurs in 3 to 14 days.

• Monitor Down syndrome patients for myelosuppression and mucositis. Adjust dosage as needed.

• If overdose occurs, provide supportive care. Give blood products and antibiotics, as needed.

PATIENT TEACHING

• Instruct patient to report signs of bleeding or infection.

• Advise patient to report adverse effects.

• Encourage patient to drink plenty of fluids to increase urine output and facilitate uric acid excretion.

• Advise patient that alopecia is temporary.

• Advise any home care patient to avoid exposure to those with infection.

• Explain need for and administration of drug to patient and family and answer questions. Encourage them to express concerns.

terbutaline sulfate
Brethine

Pharmacologic class: adrenergic (beta₂ agonist)
Therapeutic class: tocolytic
Pregnancy risk category: B
pH: 3 to 5

INDICATIONS & DOSAGES

➤**Premature labor after 20 weeks' gestation ♦** —
Adults: Initially, 2.5 to 10 mcg/minute, increased gradually q 10 to 20 minutes until contractions stop or reach maximum rate of 80 mcg/minute. Once contractions have stopped for 30 to 60 minutes, maintain at minimum effective rate for at least 12 hours. Then switch to oral form.

ADMINISTRATION

Direct injection: Not recommended.
Intermittent infusion: Not recommended.
Continuous infusion: Before administration, start a primary I.V. infusion. Hang terbutaline solution as a secondary I.V. line to allow immediate discontinuation if adverse effects occur. Use an infusion pump and continuously monitor cardiac status.

PREPARATION & STORAGE

Available in 2-ml ampules containing 1 mg/ml. Solution is clear and colorless; don't use if discolored.

For infusion, add 10 mg of drug to 250 ml of D₅W, normal or half-normal saline solution to yield 40 mcg/ml.

Store ampules at room temperature and protect from light.

Incompatibilities
Bleomycin.

CONTRAINDICATIONS & CAUTIONS

• Contraindicated in those hypersensitive to sympathomimetics.

• Use cautiously in those with diabetes mellitus, hyperthyroidism, hypertension, cardiac disease, or a history of seizures because drug may exacerbate these conditions.

ADVERSE REACTIONS

CNS: *tremors, nervousness, dizziness, drowsiness, headache,* weakness.
CV: *arrhythmias, palpitations,* tachycardia, flushing.
GI: *nausea, vomiting,* heartburn.
Metabolic: hypokalemia.

Respiratory: dyspnea, chest discomfort, pulmonary edema, *paradoxical bronchospasm with prolonged use.*
Skin: sweating, pain at injection site.

INTERACTIONS
Drug-drug. *Beta-blockers:* Antagonizes effects of terbutaline. Avoid using together.
Cardiac glycosides, levodopa, MAO inhibitors, tricyclic antidepressants: Enhanced CV effects. Monitor cardiac status. Avoid using together.
CNS stimulants, cyclopropane, halogenated inhaled anesthetics, other sympathomimetics, xanthines: May cause additive CNS stimulation. Monitor patient closely.

EFFECTS ON LAB TEST RESULTS
• May decrease potassium level.
• May inhibit allergy test responses. May interfere with results of thyroid hormone tests.

ACTION
Stimulates beta$_2$ receptors and causes uterine relaxation, along with other sympathetic effects.

PHARMACOKINETICS
Onset, within 15 minutes; duration, 1½ to 4 hours.
Distribution: Widespread. Drug crosses the placental and blood-brain barriers.
Metabolism: Partly in liver, mainly to inactive metabolites.
Excretion: About 60% removed unchanged in urine. Drug appears in breast milk at levels 1% less than maternal levels.

CLINICAL CONSIDERATIONS
• Osmolality: 283 mOsm/kg.
• *Alert:* Don't confuse terbutaline with terbinafine or tolbutamide.
• Monitor potassium levels closely during infusion.

• Record intake and output and assess for signs of pulmonary edema. Limit I.V. fluids to 50 ml/hour.
• Monitor fetus continuously for CV effects.
• S.C. therapy followed by oral maintenance therapy may be as effective as I.V. therapy and pose less risk to the patient. Check references for S.C. dosing.

PATIENT TEACHING
• Alert patient to the drug's adverse effects, and advise him to notify his prescriber if he experiences any of these effects.
• Reassure patient that adverse effects are usually transient and don't require treatment.

theophylline

Pharmacologic class: xanthine derivative
Therapeutic class: bronchodilator
Pregnancy risk category: C
pH: 3.5 to 6.5

INDICATIONS & DOSAGES
➤ **Acute bronchial asthma and reversible bronchospasm caused by chronic bronchitis and emphysema—**
Nonsmoking adults not receiving theophylline: Initially, 4.7 mg/kg, followed by maintenance dose of 0.55 mg/kg/hour for 12 hours, then 0.39 mg/kg/hour.
Adult smokers not receiving theophylline: 0.79 mg/kg/hour for 12 hours, then 0.63 mg/kg/hour.
Geriatric patients and those with cor pulmonale not receiving theophylline: 0.47 mg/kg/hour for 12 hours, then 0.24 mg/kg/hour.
Patients with heart failure or liver failure not receiving theophylline:

0.39 mg/kg/hour for 12 hours, then 0.08 to 0.16 mg/kg/hour.
Children ages 6 months to 9 years not receiving theophylline: 0.95 mg/kg/hour for 12 hours, then 0.79 mg/kg/hour.
Children ages 9 to 16 not receiving theophylline: 0.79 mg/kg/hour for 12 hours, then 0.63 mg/kg/hour.
Adults and children receiving theophylline: Dosage form, amount, time, and administration rate of last theophylline dose determine initial dose. Ideally, initial dose is postponed until theophylline level can be determined.

ADMINISTRATION
Direct injection: Not recommended.
Intermittent infusion: Give slowly at a rate not exceeding 20 mg/minute. Give loading doses over 20 to 30 minutes.
Continuous infusion: Adjust infusion rate to deliver prescribed amount each hour.

PREPARATION & STORAGE
Available in containers of premixed drug in D_5W as 0.4 mg/ml in 1,000 ml; 0.8 mg/ml in 500 ml and 1,000 ml; 1.6 mg/ml in 250 ml and 500 ml; 2 mg/ml in 100 ml; 3.2 mg/ml in 250 ml; and 4 mg/ml in 50 and 100 ml. Inspect for precipitates before use.
  Store containers at room temperature and protect from freezing, heat, and light.

Incompatibilities
Ascorbic acid, ceftriaxone, cimetidine, hetastarch, phenytoin.

CONTRAINDICATIONS & CAUTIONS
● Contraindicated in those hypersensitive to theophylline, caffeine, theobromine, or other xanthine compounds.
● Use cautiously in those with severe cardiac disease, severe hypoxemia, hypertension, hyperthyroidism, peptic ulcer, diabetes mellitus, acute MI, or heart failure because drug may exacerbate these conditions.
● Use cautiously in neonates, geriatric patients, and in those with liver disease because of risk of toxic reaction.
● Use cautiously in those with cor pulmonale, prolonged fever, or febrile viral respiratory infections because of theophylline's prolonged half-life.

ADVERSE REACTIONS
CNS: headache, irritability, *restlessness, insomnia, dizziness,* reflex hyperexcitability, muscle twitching, ***seizures.***
CV: *palpitation, tachycardia,* hypotension, extrasystoles, ***circulatory failure, ventricular arrhythmias,*** flushing.
GI: *nausea, vomiting,* epigastric pain, hematemesis, diarrhea.
GU: urinary catecholamines.
Metabolic: hyperglycemia.
Respiratory: tachypnea, ***respiratory arrest.***
Skin: rash, alopecia.
Other: potentiation of diuresis, SIADH.

INTERACTIONS
Drug-drug. *Adenosine:* Decreases antiarrhythmic effectiveness. Higher doses of adenosine may be needed.
Allopurinol, calcium channel blockers, cimetidine, disulfiram, hormonal contraceptives, influenza virus vaccine, interferon, macrolide antibiotics (such as erythromycin), methotrexate, quinolone antibiotics (such as ciprofloxacin): May increase theophylline level. Dosage may need to be adjusted.
Barbiturates, nicotine, phenytoin, rifampin: Enhances metabolism and decreased theophylline level. Dosage may need to be adjusted.
Beta blockers: Causes antagonism, may mutually inhibit therapeutic effects and reduce theophylline clearance; propranolol and nadolol, especially, may cause bronchospasm. Avoid using together.

Reactions may be *common,* uncommon, ***life-threatening,*** or COMMON AND LIFE-THREATENING.

Caffeine and other xanthines, CNS stimulants, ephedrine: Increases potential for toxic effects. Use together with caution.

Carbamazepine, isoniazid, loop diuretics: May increase or decrease theophylline level. Monitor theophylline level.

Lithium: Enhances lithium excretion. Monitor level and therapeutic effect of lithium.

Oral anticoagulants: Increases risk of bleeding. Monitor patient closely.

Drug-herb. *Cacao tree:* May inhibit theophylline metabolism. Discourage use together.

Cayenne: Increases risk of theophylline toxicity. Advise patient to use together cautiously.

Ephedra: May increase risk of adverse reactions. Discourage use together.

Guarana: May cause additive CNS and CV effects. Discourage use together.

Ipriflavone: May increase risk of theophylline toxicity. Discourage use together.

St. John's wort: May decrease levels of theophylline. Discourage use together.

Drug-food. *Caffeine:* Decreases hepatic clearance of theophylline; may increase theophylline level. Monitor patient for evidence of toxicity.

Drug-lifestyle. *Smoking:* May increase elimination of theophylline. Monitor therapeutic response and theophylline level. Dosage may need to be adjusted.

EFFECTS ON LAB TEST RESULTS
● May increase free fatty acid levels.
● May falsely elevate uric acid levels with Bittner or colorimetric methods.

ACTION
May act as an adenosine receptor antagonist or phosphodiesterase—the enzyme that degrades cAMP—inhibitor, altering intracellular calcium levels and relaxing bronchial smooth muscles and pulmonary vessels. Acts as CNS stimulator and has CVS-positive inotropic effect at SA node. Causes coronary vasodilation, diuresis, and cardiac, cerebral, and skeletal muscle stimulation. Also increases medullary sensitivity to carbon dioxide.

PHARMACOKINETICS
Onset, at end of infusion; duration, varies with age, sex, and level of physical activity.

Distribution: Rapidly, throughout extracellular fluids and body tissues. Drug crosses the placental barrier and partially penetrates RBCs.

Metabolism: In liver.

Excretion: Mainly in urine; small amounts unchanged in feces. Also appears in breast milk in levels about 70% of serum levels. Half-life, 3 to 12 hours in nonsmoking asthmatic adults; 1½ to 9½ hours in children.

CLINICAL CONSIDERATIONS
● Base dosage on lean body weight and theophylline level. Optimum therapeutic range is 10 to 20 mcg/ml.
● Expect to reduce dosage in neonates, geriatric patients, and in patients with influenza, COPD, or cardiac, renal, or hepatic dysfunction because these patients show reduced drug clearance.
● Monitor patient's vital signs during infusion.
● Monitor theophylline level.
● If overdose occurs, stop drug immediately and provide supportive care. Avoid sympathomimetics.

PATIENT TEACHING
● Advise patient of potential adverse effects.
● Advise patient to immediately report adverse effects.
● Encourage patient to report to prescriber a history of or current use of tobacco products or marijuana because these products may affect body's response to theophylline.

thiamine hydrochloride (vitamin B₁)
Betaxin ◊ *

Pharmacologic class: water-soluble vitamin
Therapeutic class: nutritional supplement
Pregnancy risk category: A (C if greater than RDA)
pH: 2.5 to 4.5

INDICATIONS & DOSAGES
➤ **Severe thiamine deficiency (beriberi)**—
Adults: 5 to 100 mg t.i.d.
Children: 10 to 25 mg daily.
➤ **Wernicke's encephalopathy**—
Adults: Initially, 100 mg, followed by 50 to 100 mg daily.
➤ **Wet beriberi with heart failure**—
Adults and children: 10 to 30 mg I.V. for emergency treatment.

ADMINISTRATION
Direct injection: Not recommended.
Intermittent infusion: Give ordered amount at a rate not exceeding 20 mg/minute. Use an infusion pump for high doses.
Continuous infusion: Add ordered dose to maintenance fluids and infuse at a rate not to exceed 20 mg/minute.

PREPARATION & STORAGE
Supplied in 1-ml prefilled syringes and 1- and 2-ml vials containing 100 or 200 mg/ml.
    Dilute if needed in normal saline solution, D₅W, or a combination of these solutions.
    Refrigerate drug, don't freeze, and protect from light.

Incompatibilities
Alkali carbonates, barbiturates, citrates, erythromycin estolate, kanamycin, streptomycin, sulfites.

CONTRAINDICATIONS & CAUTIONS
• Contraindicated in those hypersensitive to thiamine.

ADVERSE REACTIONS
CNS: weakness, restlessness, tingling, pain.
CV: *CV collapse,* transient vasodilation, hypotension.
EENT: tightness of throat.
GI: nausea, *hemorrhage.*
Respiratory: respiratory distress, cyanosis, pulmonary edema.
Skin: pruritus, urticaria, sweating.
Other: *hypersensitivity reactions,* feelings of warmth, *angioedema.*

INTERACTIONS
Neuromuscular blockers: Enhances effects of these drugs. Monitor patient closely.

EFFECTS ON LAB TEST RESULTS
• May cause false-positive uric acid results with phosphotungstate method and false-positive urine urobilinogen results with Ehrlich's reagents. May alter theophylline levels with Schack and Waxler spectrophotometric methods.

ACTION
Combines with adenosine triphosphate to form a coenzyme needed for carbohydrate metabolism.

PHARMACOKINETICS
Onset, immediately after administration; duration, unknown.
Distribution: Throughout tissues. Drug probably crosses the placental barrier. Drug may appear in breast milk.
Metabolism: In liver.
Excretion: In urine as metabolites after therapeutic dose and as unchanged thi-

---

Reactions may be *common,* uncommon, *life-threatening,* or COMMON AND LIFE-THREATENING.

amine and metabolites after higher doses, resulting from tissue saturation.

CLINICAL CONSIDERATIONS
• Osmolality: 777 mOsm/kg for 100 mg/ml.
• *Alert:* Drug may contain benzyl alcohol.
• Never give thiamine by direct injection because of risk of anaphylaxis.
• Use I.V. route only if oral or I.M. administration isn't feasible.
• If patient becomes thiamine-deficient during total parenteral nutrition, acute pernicious beriberi may occur. Disorder has mortality rate near 50%.
• Signs and symptoms of mild thiamine deficiency include paresthesia, hyperesthesia, anesthesia, weakness, and possible foot drop and wrist drop. Severe thiamine deficiency may be marked by cardiomegaly, tachycardia, and dependent edema.

PATIENT TEACHING
• Advise patient to report adverse effects.
• Advise patient to report history of sensitivity to thiamine.
• Notify patient that adverse effects usually occur after repeated doses of thiamine.

thiopental sodium
Pentothal

Pharmacologic class: barbiturate
Therapeutic class: anesthetic
Pregnancy risk category: C
Controlled substance schedule: III
pH: 10 to 11

INDICATIONS & DOSAGES
Dosage individualized, based on desired depth of anesthesia, concurrent use of other drugs, and patient's age, weight, sex, and condition.

➤ **Sole anesthesia for brief 15-minute procedures—**
Adults: Initially, 50 to 75 mg q 20 to 40 seconds until anesthesia is established, then 25 to 50 mg, p.r.n.
Children ages 15 and younger: Initially, 3 to 5 mg/kg, then 1 mg/kg, p.r.n.
➤ **Seizure control during or after inhalation or local anesthesia—**
Adults: 75 to 125 mg (3 to 5 ml of 2.5% solution) as soon as possible after start of seizure.
➤ **Increased intracranial pressure in neurosurgery with adequate ventilation—**
Adults: 1.5 to 3.5 mg/kg, repeated p.r.n.
➤ **Increased intracranial pressure caused by trauma—**
Children 3 months to 15 years: 5 to 10 mg/kg I.V. followed by a continuous infusion of 1 to 4 mg/kg/day.
➤ **Narcoanalysis and narcosynthesis in psychiatric patients—**
Adults: 100 mg/minute of 2.5% solution until patient is semidrowsy but can speak and respond.
Adjust-a-dose: In patients with renal or hepatic dysfunction, decrease dosage and rate of administration.

ADMINISTRATION
Direct injection: Inject ordered dose through I.V. tubing containing a free-flowing, compatible solution. Give over 20 to 30 seconds. Repeat, as needed, to maintain anesthesia. Concentration of solution should be 2% to 5% (usually 2% to 2.5%).
Intermittent infusion: Not recommended.
Continuous infusion: Infuse a concentration of 0.2% to 0.4% (200 to 400 mg/100 ml) at a rate not exceeding 50 ml/hour. Monitor drug levels. Prolonged continuous infusion may cause respiratory and circulatory depression.

PREPARATION & STORAGE
Available in 250-, 400-, and 500-mg syringes; in 500- and 1,000-mg vials;

and in 1-, 2.5-, and 5-g containers in kits.

Reconstitute with 10 to 250 ml of sterile water injection, normal saline solution, or D_5W to yield 0.2% to 5% concentration, usually 2.5%.

Compatible solutions include dextrose 2.5% in water, D_5W, half-normal saline solution, dextran 6% in D_5W or normal saline solution, and 1/6 M sodium lactate.

Store thiopental at room temperature before reconstituting. Reconstituted solutions are stable for 24 hours. Drug contains no bacteriostatic agents.

Incompatibilities

Amikacin, ascorbic acid, atracurium, chlorpromazine, cimetidine, cisatracurium, clindamycin, dextrose 10% in water or normal saline solution, diltiazem, dimenhydrinate, diphenhydramine, dobutamine, dopamine, doxapram, droperidol, ephedrine, epinephrine, fentanyl, fructose 10%, furosemide, glycopyrrolate, human fibrinolysin, hydromorphone, insulin (regular), invert sugar 5% and 10% in normal saline solution, isoproterenol, labetalol, lactated Ringer's solution, levorphanol, lidocaine, lorazepam, meperidine, methadone, midazolam, morphine, nicardipine, norepinephrine, Normosol solutions except Normosol-R, pancuronium, penicillin G potassium, pentazocine lactate, phenylephrine, prochlorperazine edisylate, promethazine hydrochloride, Ringer's injection, sodium bicarbonate, succinylcholine, sufentanil, vecuronium.

CONTRAINDICATIONS & CAUTIONS

• Contraindicated in those hypersensitive to barbiturates.
• Contraindicated in those with status asthmaticus because drug provokes histamine release, which could precipitate an asthma attack.

• Contraindicated in those with porphyria because of possible aggravated symptoms.
• Use cautiously in those with severe CV disease, hypotension, or shock because of worsened CV depression.
• Use cautiously in those with severe obesity or neuromuscular disease because of possible airway or ventilation problems.
• Use cautiously in those with conditions that may prolong hypnotic effect. Use cautiously in patients with renal or hepatic dysfunction, intracranial pressure, ophthalmoplegia, asthma, myasthenia gravis, and in those with endocrine disorders.

ADVERSE REACTIONS

CNS: headache, confusion, anxiety, restlessness, retrograde amnesia, prolonged somnolence, dose-dependent alteration in EEG patterns.
CV: thrombophlebitis, hypotension, tachycardia, peripheral vascular collapse, *myocardial depression, arrhythmias.*
GI: nausea, vomiting, abdominal pain, diarrhea, cramping.
Musculoskeletal: muscle twitching.
Respiratory: coughing, sneezing, hiccups, *respiratory depression, apnea, laryngospasm, bronchospasm.*
Skin: pain, swelling, ulceration, necrosis on extravasation (unlikely at levels less than 2.5%), local irritation.
Other: *allergic reactions,* shivering.

INTERACTIONS

Drug-drug. *Antihistamines, benzodiazepines, hypnotics, narcotics, phenothiazines, sedatives:* Increases CNS effect. Monitor patient closely.
Aspirin, meprobamate, sulfisoxazole: Potentiates hypnotic effects. Avoid using together.
Clonidine I.V., metoclopramide before anesthesia: Causes additive anesthetic effects. Thiopental dose may need to be reduced.

Reactions may be *common,* uncommon, *life-threatening,* or COMMON AND LIFE-THREATENING.

Probenecid: Prolongs hypnotic effects. Thiopental dose may need to be reduced.

Drug-lifestyle. *Alcohol use:* Increases CNS depressant effects. Avoid using together.

EFFECTS ON LAB TEST RESULTS
None reported.

ACTION
May facilitate synaptic actions of inhibitory neurotransmitters and block synaptic actions of excitatory neurotransmitters.

PHARMACOKINETICS
Onset, 30 to 60 seconds; duration, 10 to 30 minutes.

Distribution: Rapidly dispersed to CNS, then redistributed first to highly perfused tissues and eventually to fatty tissue. Drug crosses the placental barrier and is 80% protein bound. In large doses, drug appears in small amounts in breast milk.

Metabolism: In liver and kidneys.

Excretion: Minimally, in urine.

CLINICAL CONSIDERATIONS
● Osmolality: 215 mOsm/kg for 25 mg/ml; 942 mOsm/kg for 100 mg/ml. A 3.4% solution in sterile water for injection is isotonic.

● **Alert:** Avoid solutions with concentrations less than 2% prepared with sterile water for injection. Solution is hypotonic and causes hemolysis.

● Only staff specially trained to give anesthetics and to manage their adverse effects should give the drug.

● Patients tolerant of other barbiturates or alcohol may require higher doses.

● Avoid giving drug S.C. or intra-arterially; drug may cause sloughing and necrosis. If inadvertent intra-arterial injection occurs, dilute injected thiopental by removing the tourniquet. Leave needle or I.V. catheter in place

and inject artery with 40 to 80 mg of papaverine or 1% procaine.

● Use warming blankets, chlorpromazine, or methylphenidate, as needed, to treat shivering.

● Closely monitor patient during continuous infusion for respiratory and circulatory depression.

● Monitor drug levels.

PATIENT TEACHING
● Advise patient to report adverse effects.

● After administration, warn patient to avoid alcohol or other CNS depressants.

● Advise patient that psychomotor skills may be impaired for 24 hours and to use caution when operating machinery or driving a car.

thiotepa (TESPA, TSPA)
Thioplex

Pharmacologic class: alkylating drug (cell cycle phase–nonspecific)
Therapeutic class: antineoplastic
Pregnancy risk category: D
pH: 5.5 to 7.5

INDICATIONS & DOSAGES
Dosage reflects response to the drug and appearance or degree of toxic reaction. Maintenance doses are based on hematologic studies.

➤ **Palliative treatment of adeno-carcinomas of breast and ovary, lymphomas—**
Adults and children ages 12 and older: 0.3 to 0.4 mg/kg q 1 to 4 weeks.

ADMINISTRATION
Direct injection: Using a 21G or 23G needle, inject rapidly.

Intermittent infusion: Give diluted drug over ordered duration. Start a primary I.V. line or use the infusion port of an existing primary line.

Continuous infusion: Not recommended.

PREPARATION & STORAGE

Available as a powder in 15-mg vials. Use extreme caution when preparing and giving drug to avoid mutagenic, teratogenic, and carcinogenic risks. Use a biological containment cabinet, wear gloves and mask, and use syringes with luer-lock fittings to prevent leakage. Dispose of needles, vials, and unused drug correctly, and avoid contaminating work surfaces.

Reconstitute with 1.5 ml of sterile water for injection to yield a concentration of 10 mg/ml. For infusion, further dilute drug in sodium chloride injection, dextrose injection, dextrose and sodium chloride injection, Ringer's injection, or lactated Ringer's injection.

Refrigerate powder and reconstituted solution at 36° to 46° F (2° to 8° C), and protect from light. Use reconstituted solution within 8 hours of preparation. Don't use if solution is grossly opaque or contains precipitates, as microbial contamination is possible.

Incompatibilities

Cisplatin, filgrastim, minocycline, vinorelbine.

CONTRAINDICATIONS & CAUTIONS

• Contraindicated in those hypersensitive to the drug and in pregnant patients.
• Contraindicated in those with existing or recent exposure to chickenpox or herpes zoster because of risk of severe generalized disease.
• Use cautiously in those with bone marrow depression, gout, or history of urate renal calculi because of risk of hyperuricemia.
• Use cautiously in those with tumor cell infiltration of bone marrow, previous cytotoxic drug therapy, or radiation therapy because of risk of further myelosuppression and in those with in-

fection because myelosuppression complicates treatment.
• Use cautiously in those with renal or hepatic impairment because of increased risk of toxic reaction.

ADVERSE REACTIONS

CNS: dizziness, headache, fatigue, weakness.
EENT: blurred vision, conjunctivitis.
GI: nausea, vomiting, abdominal pain, anorexia.
GU: dysuria, urine retention, amenorrhea, interference with spermatogenesis.
Hematologic: *leukopenia, thrombocytopenia,* anemia.
Metabolic: hyperuricemia.
Skin: alopecia, dermatitis, pain at injection site.
Other: allergic reaction, *hypersensitivity reactions, anaphylactic shock.*

INTERACTIONS

Drug-drug. *Myelosuppressives, radiation therapy:* Increases myelosuppression. Avoid using together.
Pancuronium: May enhance neuromuscular blockade. Use together cautiously.

EFFECTS ON LAB TEST RESULTS

• May increase uric acid level. May decrease pseudocholinesterase level.
• May decrease hemoglobin and lymphocyte, platelet, WBC, RBC, and neutrophil counts.

ACTION

Interferes with DNA replication and RNA transcription, ultimately disrupting nucleic acid function. Also has some immunosuppressive activity.

PHARMACOKINETICS

Onset and duration of drug effect unknown.
Distribution: 8% to 13% protein bound. Rapidly cleared from plasma and found primarily within cells. Drug

crosses the placental barrier; unknown if drug appears in breast milk.
Metabolism: Partially metabolized to triethylenephosphoramide.
Excretion: In urine; 60% to 85% excreted within 24 to 72 hours.

CLINICAL CONSIDERATIONS

- Osmolality: 269 to 277 mOsm/kg.
- Expect to give lower doses in those with renal, hepatic, or hematopoietic impairment. Monitor patient carefully.
- To prevent hyperuricemia with resulting uric acid nephropathy, allopurinol may be given; keep patient well hydrated.
- Avoid all I.M. injections when platelet count is less than 100,000/mm³. Stop drug if WBC count decreases to less than 3,000/mm³ or if platelet count decreases to less than 150,000/mm³.
- Before and during therapy, monitor WBC and platelet counts, hematocrit, and BUN, AST, ALT, bilirubin, creatinine, LDH, and uric acid levels.
- At the first sign of a sudden large drop in WBC count—particularly granulocytes—or platelet count, stop drug or reduce dosage, as ordered, to prevent irreversible myelosuppression. WBC nadir may occur at 10 to 14 days when given weekly. Resume therapy when counts return to acceptable levels.
- Watch carefully for signs and symptoms of infection in patients with leukopenia. If infection develops, give an antibiotic, as needed.
- Provide adequate oral hydration, which may prevent or delay uric acid nephropathy. Allopurinol administration may also be helpful.
- Drug is highly toxic with a low therapeutic index; many adverse effects are unavoidable. Some effects, such as leukopenia, indicate the drug's effectiveness and aid in dosage adjustment.
- If overdose occurs, give transfusions of whole blood, platelets, or WBCs, as ordered, to relieve hematopoietic toxicity.

PATIENT TEACHING

- Inform patient of drug's adverse effects.
- Advise patient to report signs and symptoms of bleeding, including epistaxis; easy bruising; change in color of urine; and black stools.
- Advise patient to report signs and symptoms of infection, such as fever and chills.
- Stress the importance of adequate fluid intake.
- Advise home care patient to avoid contact with people with infections.
- Advise patient to avoid taking OTC products containing aspirin.
- Advise patient to use effective contraception to prevent pregnancy during treatment.

ticarcillin disodium
Ticar

Pharmacologic class: extended-spectrum penicillin, alpha-carboxypenicillin
Therapeutic class: antibiotic
Pregnancy risk category: B
pH: 6 to 8

INDICATIONS & DOSAGES

➤ **Septicemia; respiratory tract, skin, soft-tissue, intra-abdominal, female pelvic, and genital tract infections—**
Adults and children: 200 to 300 mg/kg/day in divided doses q 4 to 6 hours.
Neonates weighing 2 kg (4.4 lb) or more: 75 mg/kg q 8 hours for first week of life; then 100 mg/kg q 8 hours.
Neonates weighing less than 2 kg (4.4 lb): 75 mg/kg q 12 hours for first week of life; then 75 mg/kg q 8 hours.

➤ **UTI, complicated—**
Adults and children: 150 to 200 mg/kg/day in divided doses q 4 to 6 hours.
➤ **UTI, uncomplicated—**
Adults and children weighing more than 40 kg: 1 g q 6 hours.
Children weighing less than 40 kg: 50 to 100 mg/kg/day in divided doses q 6 to 8 hours.
Adjust-a-dose: In adults with renal impairment, give initial 3 g I.V. loading dose, then base maintenance doses on creatinine clearance as follows: for those with a clearance of 30 to 60 ml/minute, 2 g q 4 hours; for those with a clearance of 10 to 30 ml/minute, 2 g q 8 hours; for those with a clearance of below 10 ml/minute, 2 g q 12 hours; and for those with hepatic impairment and a creatinine clearance of below 10 ml/minute, 2 g q 24 hours. For patients on peritoneal dialysis, give 3 g q 12 hours; for those on hemodialysis, 2 g q 12 hours, then 3 g after each dialysis session.

ADMINISTRATION

Direct injection: Give slowly. Solution concentrations should be 50 mg/ml or less.
Intermittent infusion: Infuse diluted solution directly into vein via an established I.V. line. To minimize vein irritation, use solutions containing 50 mg/ml or less and infuse slowly, over 30 minutes to 2 hours in adults or 10 to 20 minutes in neonates.
Continuous infusion: Add the total daily dose of reconstituted drug to ordered volume of compatible solution. Adjust rate to deliver needed 24-hour volume.

PREPARATION & STORAGE

Supplied as a white to pale yellow powder or lyophilized cake in 1-, 3-, and 6-g vials.
Reconstitute by adding 4 ml of normal saline solution, D_5W, or lactated Ringer's solution for each gram of drug to yield a concentration of 200 mg/ml. For continuous infusion, dilute further with 10 to 100 ml of a compatible I.V. solution. Reconstituted solution is clear and colorless or pale yellow.

Store powder at room temperature. Refrigerate reconstituted solution or use within 30 minutes. Diluted solutions are stable for 72 hours at room temperature with sterile water for injection, D_5W, and normal saline solution at 10 to 100 mg/ml; and for 48 hours at room temperature with Ringer's injection or lactated Ringer's solution at 10 to 100 mg/ml. Solutions with dextrose 5% in 0.225% or half-normal saline solution or with 5% alcohol are stable at room temperature for 72 hours at 10 to 50 mg/ml.

All solutions are stable for 14 days when refrigerated at 39° F (4° C) but shouldn't be used for multiple doses if stored for more than 72 hours. Reconstituted solutions may also be frozen at 0° F (-18° C) and are stable for up to 30 days. Use thawed solution within 24 hours.

Incompatibilities

Aminoglycosides, amphotericin B, ciprofloxacin, doxapram, fluconazole, gentamicin, methylprednisolone sodium succinate, vancomycin.

CONTRAINDICATIONS & CAUTIONS

• Contraindicated in those hypersensitive to penicillin or other beta-lactam antibiotics.
• Use cautiously in those with renal impairment because of increased risk of toxic reaction and in those with sodium restriction. Sodium content is 6.5 mEq/g of drug.
• Use cautiously in those with hypokalemia because condition may be aggravated. Check potassium level frequently.
• Use cautiously in those with history of allergic disorders because of increased risk of hypersensitivity.
• Use cautiously in those with bleeding disorders because drug may cause platelet dysfunction, increasing risk of hemorrhage.

Reactions may be *common*, uncommon, *life-threatening*, or COMMON AND LIFE-THREATENING.

• Use cautiously in those with a history of ulcerative colitis, regional enteritis, or antibiotic-associated colitis because of increased risk of pseudomembranous colitis.

ADVERSE REACTIONS

CNS: *seizures,* neuromuscular excitability.
CV: vein irritation, phlebitis.
GI: nausea, diarrhea, vomiting, *pseudomembranous colitis.*
Hematologic: *leukopenia,* eosinophilia, *neutropenia, thrombocytopenia,* hemolytic anemia.
Metabolic: hypokalemia, hypernatremia.
Skin: pain at injection site.
Other: hypersensitivity reactions (rash, pruritus, urticaria, chills, fever, edema, *anaphylaxis*), overgrowth of nonsusceptible organisms.

INTERACTIONS

Drug-drug. *Aminoglycosides:* Inactivates aminoglycosides in vitro. Avoid using together.
Anticoagulants, NSAIDs, platelet aggregation inhibitors, salicylates, sulfinpyrazone, thrombolytics: May increase risk of hemorrhage. Use together with caution.
Chloramphenicol, erythromycin, sulfonamides, tetracyclines: May interfere with ticarcillin's bactericidal effect. Avoid using together.
Hormonal contraceptives: Decreases efficacy of contraceptive. Advise patient to use another contraceptive method.
Lithium: May affect lithium level. Dosage may need to be adjusted. Monitor lithium level.
Probenecid: Decreases ticarcillin elimination. Monitor patient closely.

EFFECTS ON LAB TEST RESULTS

• May increase PT, INR, ALT, AST, alkaline phosphatase, LDH, and sodium levels. May decrease potassium level.

• May increase eosinophil count. May decrease hemoglobin and platelet, WBC, and granulocyte counts.
• May cause false-positive Coombs', urine protein, acetic acid, biuret reaction, and nitric acid test results. May falsely decrease aminoglycoside levels.

ACTION

Inhibits bacterial septum and cell-wall synthesis by preventing cross-linkage of peptidoglycan chains and inhibits cell division and growth. Active against susceptible gram-positive, gram-negative, and anaerobic bacteria. Rapidly dividing bacteria are most susceptible.

PHARMACOKINETICS

Drug level peaks in 30 to 75 minutes.
Distribution: Readily to pleural and interstitial fluid, skin, kidneys, bone, bile, and sputum. Penetrates CSF with meningeal irritation; 45% to 65% protein bound. Drug appears in breast milk in small amounts and probably crosses the placental barrier.
Metabolism: In liver.
Excretion: Mostly in urine, by renal tubular secretion and glomerular filtration, and partially in feces. Usual half-life, about 1 hour, with 80% to 93% excreted within 24 hours. Half-life is prolonged in renal or hepatic impairment.

CLINICAL CONSIDERATIONS

• Osmolality: 420 to 579 mOsm/kg.
• Before giving drug, ask about allergic reactions to penicillin or other beta-lactam drugs.
• Ticarcillin is almost always used with another antibiotic, such as an aminoglycoside, in life-threatening situations.
• Obtain specimens for culture and sensitivity tests before giving first dose. Therapy may begin before results are complete. Give drug at least 1 hour before bacteriostatic antibiotics.
• Monitor CBC and electrolyte levels, especially potassium, and cardiac status

frequently, because drug's high sodium content may cause electrolyte imbalance and arrhythmias.

• Ticarcillin contains about 5.2 mEq (120 mg) of sodium per gram of drug. Use with caution in patients with sodium restriction.

• Observe patient for fungal and bacterial superinfection with prolonged use.

• With prolonged treatment, monitor patient for renal, hepatic, and hematopoietic dysfunction. Monitor bleeding times closely.

• Monitor neurologic status. High levels may cause seizures.

• If diarrhea persists during treatment, obtain stool culture to rule out pseudomembranous colitis.

PATIENT TEACHING

• Warn patient of potential for allergic reaction.

• Advise patient to report adverse reactions.

• Advise patient to report unusual bleeding or bruising.

ticarcillin disodium and clavulanate potassium
Timentin

Pharmacologic class: extended-spectrum penicillin, beta-lactamase inhibitor
Therapeutic class: antibiotic
Pregnancy risk category: B
pH: 5.5 to 7.5

INDICATIONS & DOSAGES

➤ **Systemic infections and UTI, particularly those caused by beta-lactamase–producing organisms—**
Adults and children age 3 months and older weighing more than 60 kg (132 lb): 3.1 g (3 g ticarcillin and 100 mg clavulanic acid) q 4 to 6 hours.

Adults and children age 3 months and older weighing less than 60 kg: 200 to 300 mg/kg/day given in divided doses q 4 to 6 hours.

Adjust-a-dose: Loading dose for adults with renal failure is 3.1 g (as 3 g ticarcillin with 100 mg clavulanate) and maintenance doses are based on creatinine clearance. If creatinine clearance is below 10 ml/minute, 2 g q 12 hours. If clearance is 10 to 30 ml/minute, give 2 g q 8 hours; if clearance is 30 to 60 ml/minute, give 2 g q 4 hours. If clearance is below 10 ml/minute and patient has liver failure, give 2 g q 24 hours. For patients on hemodialysis, give 2 g q 12 hours, then 3.1 g after treatment; for those on peritoneal dialysis, 3.1 g q 12 hours.

ADMINISTRATION

Direct injection: Not recommended.
Intermittent infusion: Give diluted dose over 30 minutes by infusion through a Y tubing, or use the piggyback method. Temporarily stop giving primary solutions during administration.
Continuous infusion: Not recommended.

PREPARATION & STORAGE

Supplied as a white to pale yellow powder in vials containing 3.1 g as 3 g ticarcillin and 100 mg clavulanic acid, and as a frozen premixed solution in 100 ml water.

Reconstitute by adding 13 ml of sterile water or normal saline solution for a ticarcillin concentration of 200 mg/ml and a clavulanate concentration of 6.7 mg/ml. Before infusion, dilute solution in 50 to 100 ml of normal saline solution, D_5W, or lactated Ringer's solution.

Thaw frozen premixed solutions at room temperature or under refrigeration, not by warm water bath or microwave radiation. Don't refreeze.

Store powder at 70° to 75° F (21° to 24° C). After reconstitution, solutions of 200 mg ticarcillin/ml are potent for 6 hours at room temperature and for up to 72 hours if refrigerated. Lactated Ringer's solution and normal saline solutions of 10 to 100 mg ticarcillin/ml remain potent for 24 hours if kept at room temperature and for 7 days if refrigerated. D₅W solutions remain potent for 24 hours if kept at room temperature and for 3 days if refrigerated. Solutions of 100 mg ticarcillin/ml or less in normal saline or lactated Ringer's solution may be frozen and stored up to 30 days; 7 days for solutions in D₅W. Use thawed solutions within 8 hours.

Incompatibilities
Aminoglycosides, amphotericin B, cisatracurium, other anti-infective drugs, sodium bicarbonate, vancomycin.

CONTRAINDICATIONS & CAUTIONS
• Contraindicated in those hypersensitive to penicillin and other beta-lactam antibiotics.
• Use cautiously in those with renal impairment because of increased risk of toxic reaction and in those with a history of allergic disorders because of increased risk of hypersensitivity.
• Use cautiously in those with ulcerative colitis, regional enteritis, or antibiotic-associated colitis because of increased risk of pseudomembranous colitis.
• Use cautiously in those with electrolyte imbalance because of risk of arrhythmias.
• Use cautiously in those with sodium restriction because the sodium content is about 4.75 mEq/g of ticarcillin.
• Use cautiously in patients with renal or hepatic dysfunction.

ADVERSE REACTIONS
CNS: *seizures,* neuromuscular excitability, headache, giddiness.
CV: thrombophlebitis, vein irritation.
EENT: disturbance of taste and smell.
GI: flatulence, nausea, vomiting, diarrhea, epigastric pain, *pseudomembranous colitis,* stomatitis.
Hematologic: *thrombocytopenia, leukopenia, neutropenia,* eosinophilia, anemia.
Metabolic: hypokalemia, hypernatremia.
Skin: pain at injection site.
Other: hypersensitivity reactions (*anaphylaxis,* fever, chills, rash, pruritus, urticaria, edema), overgrowth of nonsusceptible organisms.

INTERACTIONS
Drug-drug. *Chloramphenicol, erythromycin, sulfonamides, tetracyclines:* May reduce ticarcillin's effects. Dosage may need to be adjusted.
Hormonal contraceptives: Decreases contraceptive effect. Advise patient to use another contraceptive method.
Probenecid: Increases and prolongs ticarcillin level. Dosage may need to be adjusted.

EFFECTS ON LAB TEST RESULTS
• May increase ALT, AST, alkaline phosphatase, LDH, and sodium levels. May decrease potassium level.
• May increase eosinophil count. May decrease hemoglobin, and platelet, WBC, and granulocyte counts.
• May cause false-positive Coombs' test results. May cause false-positive urine protein results with turbidimetric methods using sulfosalicylic acid, trichloroacetic acid, acetic acid, or nitric acid.

ACTION
Inhibits bacterial cell-wall synthesis. Clavulanic acid, a beta-lactamase inhibitor, provides a synergistic bactericidal effect. It binds to certain beta-lactamases that usually inhibit ticarcillin. This results in a broadened spectrum of activity. Active against susceptible gram-positive, gram-negative, and anaerobic bacteria.

PHARMACOKINETICS

Drug level peaks immediately after infusion.

Distribution: Readily into pleural and interstitial fluid, blister fluid, skin, kidneys, bone, lymph tissue, urine, and gallbladder. Clavulanic acid is distributed poorly into respiratory tract. CSF penetration occurs with meningeal irritation; drug is 45% to 65% protein bound. Clavulanic acid and probably ticarcillin cross the placental barrier. Both drugs appear in breast milk in small amounts.

Metabolism: In liver, extensively for clavulanic acid, minimally for ticarcillin.

Excretion: In urine, with 60% to 70% of ticarcillin and 35% to 45% of clavulanic acid excreted unchanged within 6 to 12 hours. Half-life of ticarcillin, about 1 hour; clavulanic acid, about 1 to 1½ hours. Half-lives lengthen in renal dysfunction.

CLINICAL CONSIDERATIONS

● Osmolality: 546 to 562 mOsm/kg.

● Obtain specimens for culture and sensitivity tests before giving first dose. Therapy may begin before results are complete.

● Give drug at least 1 hour before bacteriostatic antibiotics.

● Before giving drug, ask patient about allergic reactions to penicillin. A negative allergy history doesn't rule out future allergic reactions.

● Drug is almost always used with another antibiotic such as an aminoglycoside in life-threatening situations.

● Drug is particularly useful in infections caused by ticarcillin-resistant organisms—for example, peritonitis—and in nosocomial urinary or respiratory tract infections.

● Monitor sodium and potassium levels closely. Drug has a high sodium content (4.75 mEq/g of drug), and clavulanic acid contributes about 0.15 mEq (6 mg) of potassium/100 mg. Frozen preparations (3.1 g/100 ml) have 0.187 mEq of sodium and 0.005 mEq of potassium.

● Monitor renal and hepatic function, CBC, PT, and bleeding times. Watch for bleeding tendencies and stop drug if bleeding occurs.

● If diarrhea persists during therapy, obtain stool culture to rule out pseudomembranous colitis.

● Observe patient for fungal and bacterial superinfection with prolonged use.

● Monitor neurologic status. High levels may cause seizures.

● If patient is receiving dialysis, give drug after session is complete.

PATIENT TEACHING

● Advise patient to report adverse effects.

● Advise penicillin-allergic or allergy-prone patient of potential for hypersensitivity reaction.

● Notify patient on sodium restricted diet of salt content in drug.

● Advise patient to report unusual bleeding or bruising.

---

tirofiban hydrochloride
Aggrastat

Pharmacologic class: glycoprotein (GP) IIb/IIIa receptor blocker
Therapeutic class: antiplatelet drug
Pregnancy risk category: B
pH: 5.5 to 6.5

INDICATIONS & DOSAGES

➤ **Acute coronary syndrome, in combination with heparin, in patients who are to be managed medically and those undergoing percutaneous transluminal coronary angioplasty (PTCA) or atherectomy—**
Adults: I.V. loading dose of 0.4 mcg/kg/minute for 30 minutes followed by a continuous I.V. infusion of 0.1 mcg/kg/minute. Continue infusion through an-

---

giography and for 12 to 24 hours after angioplasty or atherectomy.

Adjust-a-dose: In patients with a creatinine clearance below 30 ml/minute, loading dose is 0.2 mcg/kg/minute for 30 minutes followed by a continuous infusion of 0.05 mcg/kg/minute. Continue infusion through procedure and for 12 to 24 hours after.

ADMINISTRATION

Direct injection: Not recommended.
Intermittent infusion: Not recommended.
Continuous infusion: Give loading dose over 30 minutes, then continue maintenance infusion for 12 to 24 hours after procedure.

PREPARATION & STORAGE

Available as 250 mcg/ml solution in 25- and 50-ml vials or 50 mcg/ml premixed injection in 250- and 500-ml single-dose containers.

Dilute vials 250 mcg/ml to 50 mcg/ml as follows: withdraw and discard 100 ml from a 500-ml bag of sterile normal saline solution or D$_5$W and replace this volume with 100 ml of tirofiban injection from two 50-ml vials or four 25-ml vials; or withdraw 50 ml from a 250-ml bag of sterile normal saline solution or D$_5$W and replace this volume with 50 ml of tirofiban injection, to achieve a concentration of 50 mcg/ml; or add the content of 25-ml vial of tirofiban to 100-ml bag of sterile normal saline solution or D$_5$W.

Inspect solution for particulate matter before administration, and check for leaks by squeezing the inner bag firmly. If visible particles are present or if leaks occur, discard solution. Store drug at room temperature. Protect from light. Discard unused solution 24 hours after the start of infusion.

Incompatibilities

Diazepam.

CONTRAINDICATIONS & CAUTIONS

• Contraindicated in those hypersensitive to the drug or its components and in those who use another parenteral GP IIb/IIIa inhibitor.

• Contraindicated in those with active internal bleeding or history of bleeding diathesis within the previous 30 days and in those with acute pericarditis.

• Contraindicated in those with history of intracranial hemorrhage, intracranial neoplasm, arteriovenous malformation, or aneurysm and in those with history of thrombocytopenia after prior exposure to the drug.

• Contraindicated in those with history of stroke within 30 days of receiving drug or history of hemorrhagic stroke and in those with history, symptoms, or findings suggestive of aortic dissection.

• Contraindicated in those with severe hypertension with systolic blood pressure over 180 mm Hg or diastolic blood pressure over 110 mm Hg and in those who have had a major surgical procedure or severe physical trauma within previous month.

• Use cautiously in those with increased risk of bleeding, including those with hemorrhagic retinopathy or platelet count below 150,000/mm^3.

ADVERSE REACTIONS

CNS: dizziness, fever, headache.
CV: *bradycardia,* coronary artery dissection, vasovagal reaction, edema.
GI: nausea, *occult bleeding.*
Hematologic: *bleeding, thrombocytopenia.*
Musculoskeletal: pelvic pain, leg pain.
Skin: sweating.
Other: bleeding at arterial access site.

INTERACTIONS

Drug-drug. *Anticoagulants such as warfarin, clopidogrel, dipyridamole, heparin, NSAIDs, thrombolytics, ticlopidine:* Increases risk of bleeding. Monitor patient closely.

Levothyroxine, omeprazole: Increases renal clearance of tirofiban. Monitor patient.

Drug-herb. *Dong quai, feverfew, garlic, ginger, horse chestnut, red clover:* May increase risk of bleeding. Discourage use together.

EFFECTS ON LAB TEST RESULTS
• May decrease hemoglobin, hematocrit, and platelet count.

ACTION
Reversibly binds to the GP IIb/IIIa receptor on human platelets and inhibits platelet aggregation.

PHARMACOKINETICS
Onset, immediate; peak, immediate; duration, 4 to 8 hours after end of infusion.
Distribution: Not highly protein bound.
Metabolism: Limited.
Excretion: Elimination half-life is about 2 hours. About 65% is eliminated in urine; 25%, in feces.

CLINICAL CONSIDERATIONS
• Minimize use of arterial and venous punctures, I.M. injections, urinary catheters, nasotracheal intubation, and nasogastric tubes. Avoid noncompressible I.V. access sites, such as subclavian or jugular veins.
• Give drug along with aspirin and heparin.
• If thrombocytopenia occurs, notify the prescriber.
• The most common adverse effect is bleeding at the arterial access site for cardiac catheterization.
• Monitor hemoglobin level, hematocrit, and platelet counts before starting therapy, 6 hours after loading dose, and at least daily during therapy.
• Drug is linked to increases in bleeding rates, particularly at the site of arterial access for femoral sheath placement. Before pulling the sheath, stop heparin for 3 to 4 hours and document

activated clotting time less than 180 seconds or aPTT less than 45 seconds. Sheath hemostasis should be achieved at least 4 hours before hospital discharge.
• *Alert:* Don't confuse Aggrastat (tirofiban) with argatroban.

PATIENT TEACHING
• Explain that drug is a blood thinner that's used to prevent chest pain and heart attacks.
• Explain that risk of serious bleeding is far outweighed by the benefits of the drug.
• Instruct patient to immediately report chest discomfort or other adverse reactions.
• Inform patient that frequent blood sampling may be needed to evaluate therapy.

tobramycin sulfate
Nebcin

Pharmacologic class: aminoglycoside
Therapeutic class: antibiotic
Pregnancy risk category: D
pH: 3 to 6.5

INDICATIONS & DOSAGES
➤ **Serious bacterial infections, including septicemia, lower respiratory tract infection, meningitis, intraabdominal infections, complicated or recurrent UTI, and infections of skin, bone, and skin structure—**
Dosage based on actual pretreatment body weight.
Adults: 3 mg/kg daily in equal doses q 8 hours. May be increased to 5 mg/kg daily in three or four equal doses for life-threatening infections.
Children: 6 to 7.5 mg/kg daily in three or four equal doses.

Neonates younger than age 1 week:
4 mg/kg daily or less in equal doses q
12 hours.

Adjust-a-dose: For adults with renal
impairment, initial dose is same as for
patients with normal renal function.
Subsequent doses and frequency determined by renal function study results
and blood levels. Keep peak drug levels
between 4 and 10 mcg/ml, and trough
drug levels between 1 and 2 mcg/ml.

Hemodialysis removes 50% to 75%
of a dose in 6 hours. In anephric patients maintained by dialysis, 1.5 to
2 mg/kg after each dialysis usually
maintains therapeutic, nontoxic drug
levels. Patients receiving peritoneal
dialysis twice a week should receive a
1.5 to 2 mg/kg loading dose followed
by 1 mg/kg q 3 days; those receiving
dialysis q 2 days should receive a
1.5 mg/kg loading dose after first dialysis and 0.75 mg/kg after each subsequent dialysis.

ADMINISTRATION

Direct injection: Not recommended.
Intermittent infusion: Infuse diluted solution over 30 to 60 minutes.
Continuous infusion: Not recommended.

PREPARATION & STORAGE

Available as a clear, colorless solution
in rubber-stopped vials and syringes
containing in 40 mg/ml, and as pediatric
injection in 2-ml vials containing
10 mg/ml. Also available as a dry powder (1.2 g), which should be reconstituted with 30 ml of sterile water for injection to a 40 mg/ml concentration.

For adults, further dilute the calculated dose in 50 to 100 ml of normal
saline solution or D₅W. For children,
dilution depends on patient needs.

Store vials and syringes at room
temperature. Diluted tobramycin is stable for 24 hours at room temperature
and for 96 hours when refrigerated.

Incompatibilities

Allopurinol; amphotericin B, beta lac-
tam antibiotics, dextrose 5% in Isolyte
E, M, or P; heparin sodium; hetastarch;
indomethacin; I.V. solutions containing
alcohol; other I.V. drugs; propofol; sargramostim.

CONTRAINDICATIONS & CAUTIONS

• Contraindicated in those hypersensitive to the drug or other aminoglycosides.
• Use cautiously in geriatric patients,
neonates, premature infants, and patients with renal impairment or dehydration because of increased risk of
nephrotoxicity.
• Use cautiously in cranial nerve VIII
damage because of increased risk of
ototoxicity.
• Use cautiously in infants with botulism and in those with myasthenia
gravis or Parkinson's disease because
of risk of neuromuscular blockade and
increased skeletal muscle weakness.

ADVERSE REACTIONS

CNS: headache, mental confusion,
seizures, disorientation, lethargy.
EENT: *ototoxicity.*
GI: nausea, vomiting, diarrhea.
GU: *nephrotoxicity.*
Hematologic: anemia, eosinophilia,
*leukopenia, granulocytopenia, throm-
bocytopenia.*
Skin: rash, exfoliative dermatitis, itch-
ing, urticaria, pain at injection site.

INTERACTIONS

Drug-drug. *Antiemetics, antihistamines, antivertigo agents, dimenhydrinate, loxapine, phenothiazines,
thioxanthenes:* May mask signs of ototoxicity. Avoid using together.
Diuretics: May alter tissue tobramycin
levels; may increase risk of ototoxicity.
Monitor patient closely.
*Hydrocarbon inhalation anesthetics,
neuromuscular blockers:* May increase
neuromuscular blockade, resulting in

respiratory depression. Avoid using together.

Nephrotoxic or neurotoxic antibiotics: Increases risk of toxic reaction. Avoid using together.

EFFECTS ON LAB TEST RESULTS
• May increase BUN, creatinine, and nonprotein nitrogen and nitrogenous compound levels. May decrease calcium, magnesium, and potassium levels.
• May increase eosinophil count. May decrease WBC, platelet, and granulocyte counts.

ACTION
Inhibits protein synthesis by binding to the 30S subunit, which results in production of a nonfunctional protein. Drug is bactericidal.

Susceptible gram-negative bacteria include *Acinetobacter, Citrobacter, Enterobacter, Escherichia coli, Klebsiella, Morganella morganii, Proteus, Providencia, Pseudomonas, Salmonella,* and *Serratia.*

Susceptible gram-positive bacteria include most strains of *Staphylococcus aureus* and *S. epidermidis.*

PHARMACOKINETICS
Drug level peaks 30 to 90 minutes after infusion.

Distribution: Widely distributed to tissues and fluids, including sputum and peritoneal, synovial, ascitic, and abscess fluid. Drug readily crosses the placental barrier. CSF penetration varies and is poor even with inflamed meninges. Small amounts appear in breast milk.

Metabolism: Not metabolized.

Excretion: In urine by glomerular filtration, with 84% excreted within 8 hours and nearly all removed within 24 hours.

CLINICAL CONSIDERATIONS
• Osmolality: 10 mg/ml is 133 to 213 mOsm/kg; 1 mg/ml is 254 to 288 mOsm/kg; 2.5 mg/ml is 261 to 283 mOsm/kg; 80 mg/100 ml is 285 to 315 mOsm/kg; 80 mg/50 ml is 289 to 319 mOsm/kg.
• *Alert:* Drug may contain sulfites. Limit treatment to the short term whenever possible. Usual duration of treatment is 7 to 10 days.
• Adjust dosage according to drug levels. A peak drug level of 8 to 10 mcg/ml is needed in patients with pneumonia.
• Obtain specimens for culture and sensitivity tests before giving first dose. Therapy may begin before results are complete.
• Monitor drug levels, especially in neonates, geriatric patients, and those with renal impairment. Therapeutic concentration is 4 to 10 mcg/ml. Avoid prolonged peak levels of 12 mcg/ml; trough levels, 2 mcg/ml. Coordinate blood sampling and drug administration with laboratory. Draw trough levels before next dose and peak levels 30 minutes after the end of the infusion.
• Monitor renal function by obtaining periodic BUN and creatinine levels.
• If possible, obtain serial audiograms for patients at high risk for ototoxicity.
• Observe patient for fungal and bacterial superinfection with prolonged use.
• If overdose occurs, ensure adequate airway, oxygenation, and ventilation. Ensure adequate hydration and urine output. Hemodialysis effectively reduces drug levels (50% of a dose in 6 hours) and may be needed in those with abnormal renal function.

PATIENT TEACHING
• Advise patient to report sulfite sensitivity.
• Tell patient to report tinnitus or hearing loss.
• Advise any woman of childbearing age that drug may harm the fetus if given during pregnancy.

topotecan hydrochloride
Hycamtin

Pharmacologic class: sulfamate-substituted monosaccharide
Therapeutic class: antineoplastic
Pregnancy risk category: D
pH: 2.5 to 3.5

INDICATIONS & DOSAGES
➤ **Metastatic carcinoma of the ovary and small-cell lung cancer after failure of initial or subsequent chemotherapy—**
Adults: 1.5 mg/m² given over 30 minutes daily for 5 consecutive days, starting on day 1 of a 21-day cycle. Minimum of four cycles should be given.
Adjust-a-dose: In those with a creatinine clearance of 20 to 39 ml/minute, decrease dose to 0.75 mg/m². If severe neutropenia occurs, reduce dose by 0.25 mg/m² for subsequent courses. Alternatively, if severe neutropenia occurs, granulocyte colony-stimulating factor (G-CSF) may be given after the subsequent course, before resorting to dosage reduction, starting from day 6 of the course, 24 hours after completing drug administration.

ADMINISTRATION
Direct injection: Not recommended.
Intermittent infusion: Infuse ordered amount over 30 minutes.
Continuous infusion: Not recommended.

PREPARATION & STORAGE
Available in 4-mg single-dose vials. Use caution with preparation and prepare under a vertical laminar flow hood while wearing gloves and protective clothing. If solution touches the skin or mucous membranes, wash thoroughly with soap and water.

Reconstitute drug in each 4-mg vial with 4 ml of sterile water for injection. Further dilute the appropriate volume of the reconstituted solution with 50 to 250 ml of normal saline solution or D₅W before administration.
Use reconstituted product immediately. Store the vials at controlled room temperature (68° to 77° F [20° to 25° C]). Protect from light. Reconstituted vials diluted for infusion are stable at room temperature and ambient lighting conditions for 24 hours. Infusion solutions of 0.025 and 0.05 mg/ml in normal saline solution or D₅W are stable for 28 days at room temperature or refrigerated when protected from light.

Incompatibilities
Dexamethasone, mitomycin.

CONTRAINDICATIONS & CAUTIONS
• Contraindicated in those hypersensitive to the drug or its ingredients.
• Contraindicated in pregnant or breast-feeding patients and in those with severe bone marrow depression.
• Use cautiously in those with hepatic or renal impairment.

ADVERSE REACTIONS
CNS: *headache,* paresthesia, *fatigue,* malaise, *asthenia,* pain, fever.
GI: *nausea, vomiting, diarrhea, constipation, abdominal pain,* intestinal obstruction, stomatitis.
Hematologic: *neutropenia, leukopenia, thrombocytopenia,* anemia.
Respiratory: dyspnea, cough.
Skin: alopecia, rash.
Other: *sepsis.*

INTERACTIONS
Drug-drug. *Cisplatin:* Increases severity of myelosuppression. Avoid using together.
Filgrastim: Prolongs neutropenia. Don't start filgrastim until day 6 of

therapy, 24 hours after topotecan treatment is completed.

EFFECTS ON LAB TEST RESULTS
● May increase ALT, AST, and bilirubin levels.
● May decrease hemoglobin and WBC, platelet, and neutrophil counts.

ACTION
Relieves torsional strain in DNA by inducing reversible single-strand breaks. Binds to the topoisomerase I–DNA complex and prevents religation of these single-strand breaks.

PHARMACOKINETICS
Onset, peak, and duration of drug effect unknown.
Distribution: 35% protein bound. It's unknown if drug appears in breast milk.
Metabolism: In liver to active and inactive metabolites.
Excretion: About 30% in urine. Terminal half-life, 2 to 3 hours.

CLINICAL CONSIDERATIONS
● Bone marrow suppression is the dose-limiting toxicity for topotecan. Nadir occurs in about 11 days. Neutropenia isn't cumulative over time.
● Duration of thrombocytopenia is about 5 days, nadir at 15 days. Blood or platelet transfusions may be needed.
● *Alert:* Before first dose is given, patient must have baseline neutrophil count above 1,500 cells/mm^3 and platelet count above 100,000 cells/mm^3.
● Frequently monitor CBC. Don't treat patient with subsequent courses of drug until neutrophil counts recover to more than 1,000 cells/mm^3, platelet counts recover to more than 100,000 cells/mm^3, and hemoglobin levels recover to more than 9 mg/dl, with transfusion if needed.
● Inadvertent extravasation of topotecan may cause mild local reactions, such as erythema and bruising.

● If drug solution contacts the skin, wash the skin immediately and thoroughly with soap and water. If mucous membranes are affected, flush areas thoroughly with water.

PATIENT TEACHING
● Advise patient to immediately report sore throat, fever, chills, or unusual bleeding or bruising.
● Advise patient of potential adverse reactions and need for frequent monitoring of blood counts.
● Advise any woman of childbearing age to avoid becoming pregnant during treatment.

torsemide
Demadex

Pharmacologic class: loop diuretic
Therapeutic class: diuretic
Pregnancy risk category: B

INDICATIONS & DOSAGES
➤ **Edema resulting from heart failure resistant to furosemide—**
Adults: 10 or 20 mg once daily. If response is inadequate, double the dose until desired diuretic response is obtained. Single doses of more than 200 mg haven't been adequately studied.
➤ **Chronic renal failure—**
Adults: 20 mg once daily. Titrate dosage upward by doubling previous dose until desired diuretic response is obtained. Single doses of more than 200 mg haven't been adequately studied.
➤ **Hepatic cirrhosis—**
Adults: 5 or 10 mg once daily given with an aldosterone antagonist or a potassium-sparing diuretic. Titrate dose upward by doubling previous dose until desired diuretic response is obtained.

Reactions may be *common*, uncommon, *life-threatening*, or COMMON AND LIFE-THREATENING.

Single doses of more than 40 mg haven't been adequately studied.

ADMINISTRATION
Direct injection: Give slowly over 2 minutes.
Intermittent infusion: Not recommended.
Continuous infusion: Not recommended.

PREPARATION & STORAGE
Available in clear ampules containing 2 ml (20 mg) or 5 ml (50 mg) of a 10 mg/ml solution.
   Store at room temperature. Don't freeze.

Incompatibilities
None reported.

CONTRAINDICATIONS & CAUTIONS
• Contraindicated in those hypersensitive to the drug or other sulfonamide derivatives and in those who are anuric.
• Use cautiously in those with anemia, diabetes, gout, hyperlipidemia, ototoxicity, or a history of pancreatitis.
• Use cautiously in those with cirrhosis and ascites because sudden changes in fluid and electrolyte status caused by rapid diuresis may precipitate hepatic coma.

ADVERSE REACTIONS
CNS: headache, dizziness, nervousness, insomnia, asthenia, syncope.
CV: ECG abnormality, chest pain, edema.
EENT: rhinitis, sore throat.
GI: diarrhea, constipation, nausea, dyspepsia, *hemorrhage.*
GU: *excessive urination.*
Metabolic: *dehydration,* electrolyte imbalance.
Musculoskeletal: arthralgia, myalgia.
Respiratory: *cough.*

INTERACTIONS
Drug-drug. *Aminoglycosides and other ototoxic drugs:* Causes auditory toxicity. Monitor patient carefully.
Indomethacin, probenecid: Decreases diuretic activity. Dosage may need to be adjusted.
Lithium: Causes lithium toxicity. Monitor lithium level.
NSAIDs: May decrease diuresis and cause renal dysfunction. Use together cautiously.
Salicylates: May cause salicylate toxicity. Avoid using together.
Drug-herb. *Dandelion:* May interfere with antidiuretic activity. Discourage use together.
Licorice root: May contribute to the potassium depletion caused by thiazides. Discourage use together.

EFFECTS ON LAB TEST RESULTS
• May increase BUN, creatinine, cholesterol, and uric acid levels. May decrease potassium and magnesium levels.

ACTION
Inhibits reabsorption of sodium and chloride at the proximal portion of the ascending loop of Henle.

PHARMACOKINETICS
Onset within 10 minutes; effects peak within 1 hour, half-life, 3 to 6 hours.
Distribution: 97% to 99% protein bound.
Metabolism: In the liver.
Excretion: In the kidney, 69% as metabolites; 21% unchanged in urine.

CLINICAL CONSIDERATIONS
• Flush I.V. line with normal saline solution before and after administration.
• In diuretic potency, 10 to 20 mg of torsemide is about equivalent to 40 mg of furosemide or 1 mg of bumetanide. It has a longer duration of action than furosemide, allowing once-daily dosing.

• Monitor patient for evidence of electrolyte imbalance, hypovolemia, or prerenal azotemia.

• Patients may be switched to and from the I.V. and P.O. forms without dosage change.

• Dosage doesn't need to be adjusted in geriatric patients.

• CV disease (especially in patients receiving cardiac glycosides) and diuretic-induced hypokalemia may be risk factors for the development of arrhythmias.

• *Alert:* The risk of hypokalemia is greatest in patients with hepatic cirrhosis, brisk diuresis, inadequate oral intake of electrolytes, or concurrent therapy with corticosteroids or corticotropin. Perform periodic monitoring of potassium and other electrolytes.

• Excessive diuresis may cause dehydration, blood-volume reduction, and possibly thrombosis and embolism, especially in geriatric patients.

• Monitor fluid intake and output, electrolyte levels, blood pressure, weight, and pulse rate during rapid diuresis and routinely with chronic use. If fluid and electrolyte imbalances occur, stop drug until the imbalances are corrected. Drug may then be restarted at a lower dose.

• *Alert:* Don't confuse torsemide with furosemide (Lasix).

• Monitor patient for signs of ototoxicity.

PATIENT TEACHING

• Advise patient to report adverse effects.

• Advise patient being switched to oral form that tablets may be taken without regard to meals.

• Advise patient of potential drug interactions.

• Instruct patient to report ringing in ears immediately because this may indicate toxicity.

trace elements (chromium, copper, manganese, selenium, zinc)

Pharmacologic class: trace elements
Therapeutic class: nutritional supplements
Pregnancy risk category: C
pH: 2

INDICATIONS & DOSAGES

➤ **As a combination product to prevent trace element deficiencies in long-term TPN—**
Adults: 5 ml/day.

➤ **As a single-element product to prevent trace element deficiencies in long-term TPN—**
chromium
Adults: 10 to 15 mcg daily (20 mcg daily with intestinal fluid loss).
Children: 0.14 to 0.2 mcg/kg daily.
copper
Adults: 0.5 to 1.5 mg daily.
Children: 20 mcg/kg daily.
manganese
Adults: 0.15 to 0.8 mg daily.
Children: 2 to 10 mcg/kg daily.
selenium
Adults: 20 to 40 mcg daily (100 mcg daily for 24 to 31 days with selenium deficiency resulting from long-term TPN).
Children: 3 mcg/kg daily.
zinc
Adults: 2.5 to 4 mg daily. Add 2 mg daily to this dose in those in acute catabolic states; 12.2 mg/L in those with fluid loss from the small intestine; or 17.1 mg/kg in those with stool or ileostomy output.
Children ages 5 and younger: 100 mcg/kg daily.
Premature infants weighing less than 3 kg (6.6 lb): 300 mcg/kg daily.

ADMINISTRATION
Direct injection: Not recommended.
Intermittent infusion: Not recommended.
Continuous infusion: Give diluted solution through a patent I.V. line over the ordered duration.

PREPARATION & STORAGE
Multitrace available in 10-ml vials containing 4 mcg of chromium, 0.4 mg of copper, 0.1 mg of manganese, 20 mcg of selenium, or 1 mg of zinc. Dilute for infusion in the appropriate TPN solution to a minimum dilution of 1:200. Chromium, copper, and manganese are available as single-element products in 5-, 10-, and 30-ml vials. Selenium is available in 10- and 30-ml vials; zinc, in 5-, 10-, 30-, and 50-ml vials. As ordered, dilute for infusion in the appropriate TPN solution.

Store at room temperature and avoid excessive heat. Don't use unless solution is clear and seal is intact. Discard unused portion within 24 hours after opening vial.

Incompatibilities
None reported.

CONTRAINDICATIONS & CAUTIONS
• Use cautiously in those with renal impairment because of increased risk of trace element retention.
• Use cautiously in those with biliary obstruction because copper and manganese are eliminated in bile.
• Dosage may need to be adjusted in those with diabetes mellitus because chromium is important in glucose metabolism. Give cautiously.

ADVERSE REACTIONS
Chromium
CNS: *seizures, coma.*
GI: nausea, vomiting, ulcers.
Hepatic: *hepatotoxicity.*
Copper
CNS: behavior changes.

EENT: photophobia.
GI: diarrhea.
Hepatic: *hepatotoxicity.*
Musculoskeletal: hypotonia.
Other: prostration, marasmus, peripheral edema.
Manganese
CNS: irritability, abnormal gait, headache, apathy, speech disturbance.
GI: anorexia.
GU: impotence.
Selenium
CNS: nervousness, depression.
EENT: metallic taste.
GI: vomiting, GI disorders.
Skin: dermatitis, hair loss, weak nails.
Other: dental defects
Zinc
CNS: decreased consciousness.
CV: tachycardia.
EENT: blurred vision.
Skin: sweating.
Other: hypothermia.

INTERACTIONS
None reported.

EFFECTS ON LAB TEST RESULTS
None reported.

ACTION
Helps maintain trace element levels and prevent deficiency; mechanism of action not well understood.

Chromium maintains normal glucose metabolism and peripheral nerve function and also activates insulin-mediated reactions. Essential in many enzymes, copper maintains normal rates of RBC and WBC formation and is a cofactor for ceruloplasmin. Manganese aids in developing normal skeletal and connective tissue and activates enzymes involved in the synthesis of fatty acids, cholesterol, and mucopolysaccharides; the formation of urea; and the structure and function of mitochondria. An essential component of the enzyme glutathione peroxidase, selenium aids in cell growth, release of energy to cells, development of sperm cells, and liver function. Zinc facilitates wound healing, promotes growth, and plays a role in skin hydration and the senses of taste and smell. It acts as cofactor for numerous enzymes.

PHARMACOKINETICS

Onset and duration of drug effect unknown.
Distribution: Chromium tends to accumulate in skin, muscle, fat, and hair. Copper, found in all tissues, reaches its highest levels in the brain and liver. Manganese appears in small amounts in bone, the pituitary, pancreas, intestinal mucosa, liver, and other tissues. It also crosses the placental barrier. Only small amounts, 12 to 20 mg, are stored in the body. Selenium appears in all tissues except fat, with highest levels in the kidneys, heart, spleen, and liver. Zinc is distributed to all tissues, with about 70% appearing in the skeleton and high amounts in the skin, hair, and testes. Most zinc is protein-bound.
Metabolism: None.
Excretion: Chromium is primarily excreted in urine, with small amounts in feces. Copper and manganese are eliminated primarily in bile. A small amount of manganese is excreted in urine. Selenium's excretion isn't well defined. *Zinc* is eliminated primarily in feces, with small amounts in urine.

CLINICAL CONSIDERATIONS

● Don't give by direct I.V. injection or by I.M. injection because the solution's acidic pH, about 2, may irritate tissues.
● Monitor levels of trace elements. Use results to guide further administration, especially with high maintenance dose.
● Watch for signs and symptoms of toxic reaction.
● Signs and symptoms of chromium deficiency include weight loss, hyperglycemia, abnormal glucose tolerance, and a diabetes-like peripheral neuropathy.

● Signs and symptoms of copper toxicity include nausea, vomiting, intestinal cramps, diarrhea, intravascular hemolysis, and renal impairment. Copper deficiency in adults receiving total parenteral nutrition may cause anemia, leukopenia, and neutropenia. D-penicillamine is the antidote for copper toxicity.
● Manganese toxicity is rare but may cause signs and symptoms resembling Parkinson's disease.
● Signs and symptoms of selenium deficiency include severe muscle pain, thigh tenderness, and cardiomyopathy.
● Signs and symptoms of zinc toxicity include fever, nausea, vomiting, and diarrhea. Calcium supplements may protect against this toxicity.

PATIENT TEACHING

● Alert patient to the signs and symptoms of various deficiencies as well as to those of toxic reaction.
● Advise patient to report adverse effects.

trastuzumab
Herceptin*

Pharmacologic class: humanized monoclonal IgG$_1$ kappa antibody
Therapeutic class: antineoplastic, human epidermal growth factor receptor-2 (HER2) antagonist
Pregnancy risk category: B
pH: 6

INDICATIONS & DOSAGES

➤ **Single-drug treatment of metastatic breast cancer in patients whose tumors overexpress the HER2 protein and who have received one or more chemotherapy regimens for their metastatic disease; combined with paclitaxel for metastatic breast cancer in patients whose tumors**

overexpress the HER2 protein and who haven't received chemotherapy for their metastatic disease—
Adults: Initial loading dose 4 mg/kg I.V. over 90 minutes. Maintenance dose is 2 mg/kg I.V. weekly as a 30-minute I.V. infusion if initial loading dose is well tolerated.

ADMINISTRATION
Direct injection: Don't give as an I.V. push or bolus.
Intermittent infusion: Initial load is given over 90 minutes, and weekly maintenance dose is given over 30 minutes.
Continuous infusion: Not recommended.

PREPARATION & STORAGE
Available as 440 mg lyophilized powder.

Reconstitute drug in each vial with 20 ml of bacteriostatic water for injection, 1.1% benzyl alcohol preserved, as supplied, to yield a multidose solution containing 21 mg/ml. Immediately after reconstitution, label vial for drug expiration 28 days from date of reconstitution.

If patient is hypersensitive to benzyl alcohol, drug may be reconstituted with sterile water for injection; however, drug must be used immediately and unused portion discarded.

Determine dose of drug needed, based on a loading dose of 4 mg/kg or a maintenance dose of 2 mg/kg. Calculate volume of 21 mg/ml solution, withdraw this amount from vial and add it to an infusion bag containing 250 ml of normal saline solution. Gently invert bag to mix solution. Vials of drug are stable at 36° to 46° F (2° to 8° C) before reconstitution. Discard reconstituted solution after 28 days. Don't freeze drug that has been reconstituted. Solution of drug diluted in normal saline injection should be stored at 36° to 46° F (2° to 8° C) before use, and is stable for up to 24 hours.

Incompatibilities
Mixing or diluting drug with other drugs; D$_5$W solution for reconstitution.

CONTRAINDICATIONS & CAUTIONS
• Use only in those with metastatic breast cancer whose tumors have HER2 protein overexpression.
• Use cautiously in those hypersensitive to the drug or its components, in those with preexisting cardiac dysfunction, and in geriatric patients.

ADVERSE REACTIONS
CNS: depression, *dizziness, insomnia,* neuropathy, paresthesia, peripheral neuritis, *asthenia, pain, headache, fever.*
CV: *heart failure, peripheral edema,* tachycardia, cardiomyopathy, decreased ejection fraction.
EENT: *rhinitis, pharyngitis,* sinusitis.
GI: *anorexia, abdominal pain, diarrhea, nausea, vomiting.*
GU: UTI.
Hematologic: *leukopenia,* anemia.
Musculoskeletal: arthralgia, *back pain,* bone pain.
Respiratory: dyspnea, increased cough.
Skin: acne, *rash.*
Other: *allergic reaction,* chills, *flulike syndrome, infection,* herpes simplex.

INTERACTIONS
Drug-drug. *Anthracyclines:* Increases risk of cardiotoxicity. Avoid using together.
Paclitaxel: Increases trastuzumab level. Monitor patient closely.

EFFECTS ON LAB TEST RESULTS
• May decrease hemoglobin, hematocrit, and WBC count.

ACTION
A recombinant DNA-derived monoclonal antibody that selectively binds to HER2, inhibiting the proliferation of human tumor cells that overexpress HER2.

PHARMACOKINETICS

Onset, peak, and duration of drug effect unknown.
Distribution: Unknown.
Metabolism: Unknown.
Excretion: Half-life ranges from 1.7 to 12 days.

CLINICAL CONSIDERATIONS

• Before starting therapy, patient should undergo a thorough baseline cardiac assessment, including history and physical examination and appropriate evaluation methods to identify those at risk for developing cardiotoxicity.
• Monitor patient for first-infusion symptom complex, commonly consisting of chills and fever. Treat with acetaminophen, diphenhydramine, and meperidine, with or without reducing the rate of infusion, as ordered. Other signs or symptoms include nausea, vomiting, pain, rigors, headache, dizziness, dyspnea, hypotension, rash, and asthenia; these occur infrequently with subsequent infusions.
• Monitor patient for dyspnea, increased cough, paroxysmal nocturnal dyspnea, peripheral edema, or S_3 gallop.
• *Alert:* Diluent may contain benzyl alcohol.
• Drug treatment may be stopped in patients who develop a significant decrease in left ventricular function.
• Monitor patient receiving both drug and chemotherapy closely for cardiac dysfunction or failure, anemia, leukopenia, diarrhea, and infection.

PATIENT TEACHING

• Tell patient about risk of first-dose infusion-associated adverse reactions.
• Instruct patient to notify prescriber immediately if signs or symptoms of cardiac dysfunction occur, such as shortness of breath, increased cough, or peripheral edema.
• Instruct patient to report adverse effects to prescriber.   ·

• Advise breast-feeding patient to stop breast-feeding during drug therapy and for 6 months after last dose of drug.

trimetrexate glucuronate
Neutrexin

Pharmacologic class: dihydrofolate reductase inhibitor
Therapeutic class: antimicrobial, antiprotozoal
Pregnancy risk category: D
pH: 3.5 to 5.5

INDICATIONS & DOSAGES

➤ **Alternative treatment of moderate to severe *Pneumocystis carinii* pneumonia in immunocompromised patients intolerant of or refractory to trimethoprim or in whom trimethoprim is contraindicated, given concurrently with leucovorin for 72 hours after the last trimetrexate dose—**
Recommended course of therapy calls for trimetrexate for 21 days and leucovorin for 24 days.
Adults: 45 mg/m² once daily over 60 to 90 minutes. Infuse 20 mg/m² leucovorin over 5 to 10 minutes q 6 hours for total daily dose of 80 mg/m². Leucovorin may be given P.O. throughout the day as four equally divided doses of 20 mg/m², with P.O. dose rounded to the next higher 25-mg increment.
Adjust-a-dose: Modify trimetrexate and leucovorin doses according to hematologic toxicity. For toxicity grade 1, where the neutrophil count is above 1,000/mm³ and platelet count is above 75,000/mm³, give usual dose.
    For toxicity grade 2, where the neutrophil count is 750 to 1,000/mm³ and platelet count is 50,000 to 75,000/mm³, give 45 mg/m² of trimetrexate once daily and 40 mg/m² of leucovorin q 6 hours.

For toxicity grade 3, where the neutrophil count is 500 to 749/mm^3, and platelet count is 25,000 to 49,999/mm^3, give 22 mg/m^2 of trimetrexate once daily and 40 mg/m^2 of leucovorin q 6 hours.

For toxicity grade 4, where the neutrophil count is below 500/mm^3 and platelet count below 25,000, treatment varies with onset of toxicity. If it occurs before day 10 of therapy, stop trimetrexate and give 40 mg/m^2 of leucovorin I.V. q 6 hours for an additional 72 hours. If grade 4 toxicity occurs on or after day 10, hold trimetrexate dose for up to 96 hours to allow blood counts to recover. If recovery doesn't occur within 96 hours, stop trimetrexate therapy. If recovery to grade 3 occurs, resume trimetrexate at 22 mg/m^3 and maintain leucovorin treatment at 40 mg/m^2 q 6 hours. When both counts recover to grade 2 levels, increase trimetrexate dosage to 45 mg/m^2 and keep leucovorin treatment at 40 mg/m^2 for the duration of therapy.

ADMINISTRATION
Direct injection: Not recommended.
Intermittent infusion: Infuse over 60 to 90 minutes, using an infusion pump. Flush line with at least 10 ml D$_5$W before and after infusion. Leucovorin may be given before or after trimetrexate; flush I.V. line thoroughly with at least 10 ml of D$_5$W before and after leucovorin administration. Dilute leucovorin as directed in package insert and give over 5 to 10 minutes every 6 hours.
Continuous infusion: Not recommended.

PREPARATION & STORAGE
Available as a single-dose, 5-ml vial containing 25 mg as a lyophilized powder and a 30 ml vial containing 200 mg.

Reconstitute the 5-ml and 30-ml vials with 2 ml or 16 ml, respectively, of sterile water or D$_5$W to yield a solution of 12.5 mg/ml of trimetrexate. Filter this solution using a 0.22-micron filter before further dilution with D$_5$W to yield a final concentration of 0.25 to 2 mg trimetrexate/ml. Store vials at room temperature (59° to 66° F [15° to 19° C]), and protect from light. Solution should be colorless to a pale greenish yellow and is stable for up to 24 hours whether kept at room temperature or refrigerated; don't freeze. Discard unused portions 2 hours after initial reconstitution.

If drug contacts the skin or mucosa, immediately wash thoroughly with soap and water.

Incompatibilities
Foscarnet, indomethacin, solutions containing chloride ions or leucovorin.

CONTRAINDICATIONS & CAUTIONS
• Contraindicated in those hypersensitive to trimetrexate, leucovorin, or methotrexate.
• Give with leucovorin to avoid potentially serious adverse effects. Leucovorin therapy must extend for 72 hours past the last dose of the drug.
• Use cautiously in those with impaired hematologic, hepatic, or renal function.
• Drug may cause fetal harm if given to a pregnant woman.

ADVERSE REACTIONS
CNS: confusion, fatigue, fever, peripheral neuropathy.
GI: nausea, vomiting, stomatitis.
Hematologic: *neutropenia, thrombocytopenia,* anemia.
Hepatic: *hepatotoxicity.*
Metabolic: hyponatremia, hypocalcemia.
Skin: rash, pruritus.

INTERACTIONS
Drug-drug. *Acetaminophen, cimetidine, clotrimazole, erythromycin, miconazole, fluconazole, ketoconazole, ri-*

fabutin, rifampin: Causes trimetrexate toxicity. Monitor patient closely.
Hepatotoxic, myelosuppressive, nephrotoxic drugs: Enhances toxicity. Use together cautiously.
Rotavirus vaccine: Causes severe infection. Avoid using together.

EFFECTS ON LAB TEST RESULTS
• May increase AST, ALT, alkaline phosphatase, BUN, and creatinine levels. May decrease calcium and sodium levels.
• May decrease hemoglobin, hematocrit, and WBC and platelet counts.

ACTION
A folic acid antagonist that inhibits the enzyme dihydrofolate reductase and disrupts DNA, RNA, and protein synthesis, thereby causing cell death.

PHARMACOKINETICS
Onset, peak, and duration of drug effect unknown.
Distribution: 95% to 98% protein bound. Good distribution to lung tissue, poor distribution to CSF. Half-life is 57 minutes. It's unknown if drug appears in breast milk.
Metabolism: In intestinal mucosa and in liver.
Excretion: In kidney, 10% to 30% unchanged, 10% to 30% as glucuronide metabolite; small amount in feces. Half-life is 15 to 17 hours.

CLINICAL CONSIDERATIONS
• Concurrent diagnoses requiring cyclic or intermittent treatment regimens that may overlap or coincide with the 21-day trimetrexate course of therapy should be documented.
• Other myelosuppressant or nephrotoxic therapy should be interrupted or stopped during trimetrexate therapy.
• Monitor absolute neutrophil and platelet counts and creatinine, BUN, ALT, AST, and alkaline phosphatase

levels at least twice weekly during therapy.
• Check and record patient's temperature at least daily. If temperature goes above 101° F (38° C), antipyretics may be used.
• If extravasation occurs, apply warm compresses to site, insert a new catheter at another site, and restart infusion. Trimetrexate isn't a vesicant.
• If overdose occurs, immediately stop drug and give leucovorin dose of 40 mg/m^2 every 6 hours for 3 days.

PATIENT TEACHING
• Advise patient to report fever.
• Instruct patient to report rash, flulike signs or symptoms, numbness or tingling in the extremities, nausea, vomiting, abdominal pain, mouth sores, increased bruising or bleeding, and black, tarry stools.
• Advise any woman of childbearing age to avoid becoming pregnant during treatment.

tromethamine
Tham

Pharmacologic class: sodium-free organic amine
Therapeutic class: systemic alkalizer
Pregnancy risk category: C
pH: 7.4

INDICATIONS & DOSAGES
➤ **To correct metabolic acidosis caused by cardiopulmonary bypass surgery—**
Adults: Dosage depends on bicarbonate deficit. When using Tham without electrolytes, needed milliliters of 0.3 M tromethamine solution is equivalent to body weight in kilograms multiplied by bicarbonate deficit in mEq/L multiplied by 1.1. Total dose shouldn't exceed

500 mg/kg. Average dose is 9 ml/kg or a single dose of 500 ml (150 mEq). For severe acidosis, up to 1,000 ml of solution may be given.

➤ **To reduce excess acidity in acid citrate-dextrose stored blood before transfusion—**
Adults: 15 to 77 ml solution added to each 500-ml unit of blood.

ADMINISTRATION
Direct injection: Not recommended.
Intermittent infusion: Give over 1 hour, not exceeding 5 ml/minute, through an 18G needle into a central line or an antecubital vein. Use an infusion pump, if possible. In children, infuse over 6 hours.

When infusing peripherally, use largest possible vein to avoid extravasation.
Continuous infusion: Not recommended.

PREPARATION & STORAGE
Supplied in 500-ml (150 mEq) single-dose containers. Use undiluted after cardiac arrest or dilute in needed volume of blood during bypass surgery or for transfusion. Solution concentration shouldn't exceed 0.3 M. Protect from heat and freezing, and discard unused solution within 24 hours.

Incompatibilities
None reported.

CONTRAINDICATIONS & CAUTIONS
• Contraindicated in those with uremia or anuria because of risk of drug accumulation.
• Contraindicated in those with chronic respiratory acidosis because drug may depress respiratory drive and exaggerate hypoxia.
• Don't use drug for more than 1 day, except in life-threatening situations.
• Use cautiously in those with renal dysfunction because of risk of severe hyperkalemia.

ADVERSE REACTIONS
CV: venous thrombosis or phlebitis.
Hepatic: *hepatic necrosis.*
Metabolic: *hyperkalemia,* hypoglycemia, hypervolemia.
Respiratory: *respiratory depression.*
Other: tissue damage and sloughing with extravasation.

INTERACTIONS
Drug-drug. *Other CNS, respiratory depressants:* Increases risk of respiratory depression. Avoid using together.

EFFECTS ON LAB TEST RESULTS
• May increase potassium level. May decrease glucose level.

ACTION
Combines with hydrogen ions from carbonic, lactic, and other metabolic acids, neutralizing acids within intracellular fluid. Increases blood pH and decreases carbon dioxide levels.

PHARMACOKINETICS
Onset, immediately after administration; duration, 8 hours.
Distribution: Widespread. It's unknown if drug crosses the placental barrier or appears in breast milk.
Metabolism: Not appreciably metabolized.
Excretion: By kidneys.

CLINICAL CONSIDERATIONS
• The American Heart Association doesn't recommend use of the drug in patients with cardiac arrest.
• Assess respiratory function during and after therapy, and keep a mechanical ventilator nearby.
• Monitor arterial blood gases and glucose and electrolyte levels before, during, and after therapy.
• In those with renal disease, monitor potassium levels closely and place patient on cardiac telemetry.
• Drug may be used experimentally to treat increased CSF pressure.

PATIENT TEACHING

● Advise patient to report adverse effects.
● Notify patient that adverse reactions occur infrequently.
● Notify patient of potential for serious tissue damage with extravasation, and advise him to report pain at I.V. site.

tubocurarine chloride (curare, d-tubocurarine chloride)*

Pharmacologic class: nondepolarizing neuromuscular blocker
Therapeutic class: skeletal muscle relaxant
Pregnancy risk category: C
pH: 2.5 to 5

INDICATIONS & DOSAGES

➤ **Adjunct to general anesthesia—**
Adults: 6 to 9 mg, then 3 to 4.5 mg in 3 to 5 minutes, if needed. Additional doses may be given during long procedures.
➤ **To aid mechanical ventilation—**
Adults: 0.0165 mg/kg; subsequent dosage determined by response.
➤ **To diagnose myasthenia gravis—**
Adults: 0.004 to 0.033 mg/kg as a single dose.
➤ **To weaken muscle contractions in pharmacologically or electrically induced seizures—**
Adults: Initially, 0.165 mg/kg I.V. As a precaution, 3 mg less than the calculated dose should be given initially.
Adjust-a-dose: Dosage is usually decreased by one-third when given with halogenated anesthetics.

ADMINISTRATION

Only staff trained to give anesthetics and to manage their adverse effects should give this drug.

Direct injection: Give ordered dose over 1 to 1½ minutes. Give subsequent doses, usually 20% to 25% of initial dose, at 40- to 60-minute intervals. Lengthen intervals, as ordered, in geriatric or debilitated patients.
Intermittent infusion: Not recommended.
Continuous infusion: Not recommended.

PREPARATION & STORAGE

Supplied in 10- and 20-ml multidose vials and 5-ml syringes containing 3 mg/ml (20 units of crude curare extract/ml).

Store at room temperature, avoiding excessive heat and freezing. Don't use if solution is discolored.

Incompatibilities

Alkaline solutions, including barbiturates; other drugs with high pH; sodium bicarbonate; trimethaphan.

CONTRAINDICATIONS & CAUTIONS

● Contraindicated in conscious patients and in those hypersensitive to the drug.
● Use cautiously in those with asthma-like respiratory conditions, bronchogenic carcinoma, or myasthenia gravis because of possible enhanced neuromuscular blockade.
● Use cautiously in those with conditions in which histamine release is hazardous.
● Use cautiously in those with hypothermia because of increased drug effects and in those with CV impairment because of potentiated CV effects.
● Use cautiously in those with hepatic failure or hyperthermia because of possible reduced drug effects and in those with renal failure or shock because of possible prolonged drug effects.
● Use cautiously in those with dehydration, endocrine imbalance, or electrolyte imbalance because of possible altered drug action.

Reactions may be *common*, uncommon, **life-threatening,** or **COMMON AND LIFE-THREATENING.**

• Use cautiously in those with hypotension because drug may exacerbate this condition and in those with pulmonary impairment and respiratory depression because drug may deepen respiratory depression.
• Use cautiously in those with severe obesity or neuromuscular disease because of possible airway or ventilation problems.
• Use cautiously in breast-feeding patients.

ADVERSE REACTIONS
CV: tachycardia, hypertension, hypotension, *circulatory collapse, arrhythmias, cardiac arrest, bradycardia,* flushing, edema.
GI: excessive salivation.
Musculoskeletal: profound and prolonged muscle relaxation, idiosyncrasy, residual muscle weakness.
Respiratory: *apnea, bronchospasm, respiratory depression.*
Skin: rash, erythema.
Other: acute porphyria, *hypersensitivity reactions.*

INTERACTIONS
Drug-drug. *Aminoglycosides, amphotericin B, beta blockers, calcium salts, diazepam, halogenated inhalation anesthetics, lidocaine, lithium, magnesium sulfate, MAO inhibitors, methotrimeprazine, quinidine salts, thiazide diuretics:* May prolong neuromuscular effects. Use together with extreme caution.
Antimyasthenics, edrophonium: Antagonizes effects. Monitor patient closely.
Doxapram: May mask tubocurarine's residual effects. Avoid using together.
Opioid analgesics: Causes additive respiratory depression. Avoid using together.

EFFECTS ON LAB TEST RESULTS
None reported.

ACTION
Combines with cholinergic (nicotinic) receptor sites at neuromuscular postjunctional membranes, competitively blocking depolarization of acetylcholine. Flaccid paralysis results from lack of muscle depolarization.

PHARMACOKINETICS
Onset, within 1 minute; peak, 3 to 5 minutes; duration, 20 to 90 minutes.
Distribution: Throughout the body. Drug crosses the placental barrier. About 40% to 50% is protein-bound. It's unknown if drug appears in breast milk.
Metabolism: Minimal; only 1% metabolized by liver. Drug may saturate tissues and be stored for up to 24 hours after last dose.
Excretion: 38% to 75% excreted unchanged in urine within 24 hours; 12% removed unchanged in bile—40% in renal failure. Metabolite also excreted in urine.

CLINICAL CONSIDERATIONS
• Osmolality: 296 mOsm/kg (3 mg/ml).
• When giving tubocurarine, keep patient's airway clear and have resuscitation equipment and anticholinergics, such as neostigmine or pyridostigmine, available.
• Allow succinylcholine's effects to subside before giving tubocurarine.
• Drug doesn't affect consciousness or relieve pain. Assess patient's need for analgesic or sedative.
• *Alert:* Drug may contain sulfites.
• A nerve stimulator and train-of-four monitoring are recommended to assess recovery of muscle strength. Before attempting pharmacologic reversal with neostigmine, some evidence of spontaneous recovery should be apparent.
• In early signs of paralysis, including inability to keep eyelids open and eyes focused, or difficulty swallowing or speaking, notify prescriber immediately. If overdose occurs, give neostigmine

or edrophonium, as ordered, to reverse drug's effects, and provide supportive, symptomatic treatment.
• Check vital signs every 15 minutes, and notify prescriber if changes occur.
• Monitor baseline electrolyte levels; electrolyte imbalance can potentiate neuromuscular effects. Also monitor intake and output because renal dysfunction prolongs duration of action.
• Check for bowel sounds because peristaltic action may be suppressed.

PATIENT TEACHING
• Advise patient to report adverse effects.
• Advise patient that adverse effects are more common in children and with repeated doses.
• Advise patient to report sulfite sensitivity.

urea (carbamide)
Ureaphil

Pharmacologic class: carbonic acid salt
Therapeutic class: osmotic diuretic
Pregnancy risk category: C
pH: 5.5 to 7

INDICATIONS & DOSAGES
➤ **To reduce intracranial or intraocular pressure—**
Adults: 1 to 1.5 g/kg infused over 1 to 2.5 hours. Maximum dosage is 120 g daily.
Children ages 2 and older: 0.5 to 1.5 g/kg infused over 1 to 2.5 hours.
Children younger than age 2: 0.1 g/kg infused over 1 to 2.5 hours.
➤ **To rapidly correct hyponatremia in SIADH secretion ♦ —**
Adults: 80 g infused over 6 hours.
Adjust-a-dose: If BUN level is 75 mg/dl or more, or if diuresis doesn't occur within 1 to 2 hours, dosage may need to be reduced or drug withheld until patient can be reevaluated and renal function reassessed.

ADMINISTRATION
Direct injection: Not recommended.
Intermittent infusion: Infuse diluted dose into a large vein. Don't use leg veins. Geriatric patients have a greater risk of phlebitis and thrombosis of superficial and deep veins. Watch for irritation and infiltration; extravasation can cause tissue damage and necrosis.

Infuse at prescribed rate for adults and children. Don't exceed dosage of 1.5 g/kg or 120 g in 24-hour period, or a rate of 4 ml (30% solution)/minute. Rapid infusion can cause hemolysis and cerebral vasomotor symptoms.

When used preoperatively, start infusion 60 minutes before ocular surgery or at the time of scalp incision for intracranial surgery.
Continuous infusion: Not recommended.

PREPARATION & STORAGE
Supplied as a powder in 40-g vials.

Add 105 ml of D_5W or dextrose 10% in water or 10% invert sugar injection, unless the patient is fructose intolerant, to the 40-g vial for a solution of 30% concentration (300 mg/ml).

Warm diluent to 122° F (50° C) to dissolve urea; cool before administration. Each dose of urea should be freshly prepared.

Store vials at room temperature. Protect from heat and freezing. Use powdered drug only if seal is intact and container is undamaged, and give solution only if it's clear and free from precipitates and discoloration. Discard unused solution 24 hours after reconstitution.

Incompatibilities
None reported.

CONTRAINDICATIONS & CAUTIONS
• Contraindicated in those with severe renal impairment and marked dehydration because of increased risk of circulatory overload and fulminating heart failure, and in those with severe hepatic impairment or elevated ammonia levels.
• Contraindicated in those with intracranial bleeding, except when used preoperatively for surgical control of

hemorrhage, because reduction of brain edema may increase bleeding.
• Contraindicated in those with fructose intolerance if solutions are prepared with invert sugar.
• Avoid use in those with sickle cell disease who have signs of CNS involvement.
• Use cautiously in those with cardiac disease or CV impairment because of the risk of heart failure and pulmonary edema.
• Use cautiously in those with hypovolemia because drug may mask symptoms.
• Use cautiously in patients with impaired renal or hepatic function and in pregnant or breast-feeding women.

ADVERSE REACTIONS

CNS: *headache,* syncope, disorientation, fever.
CV: venous thrombosis, phlebitis.
GI: *nausea, vomiting.*
Hematologic: arterial oozing and bleeding.
Metabolic: hyponatremia, hypokalemia, hypervolemia.
Skin: infection at injection site, extravasation.

INTERACTIONS

Drug-drug. *Diuretics:* May potentiate diuretic effects. Monitor patient closely.
Lithium: Increases excretion of lithium. Observe patient closely and monitor lithium level.

EFFECTS ON LAB TEST RESULTS

• May increase BUN level. May decrease sodium and potassium levels.

ACTION

Produces osmotic diuresis by elevating the glomerular filtrate's osmotic pressure, hindering renal tubular reabsorption of water and solutes. Urea also elevates plasma osmolality, which enhances water flow from tissues, including the brain and eyes.

PHARMACOKINETICS

Onset, 10 minutes after start of infusion; duration, 3 to 10 hours after infusion for diuresis and reduction of increased intracranial pressure, or 5 to 6 hours for reduction of intraocular pressure.
Distribution: Into extracellular and intracellular fluids, including lymph, blood, bile, and CSF. Highest level is in kidneys. Drug crosses the placental barrier and reaches the eye. Drug probably appears in breast milk.
Metabolism: Partially metabolized in GI tract despite I.V. administration by hydrolysis to ammonia and carbon dioxide. Bacterial urease resynthesizes metabolites into urea.
Excretion: By kidneys, with about 50% reabsorption.

CLINICAL CONSIDERATIONS

• Osmolarity: as a 30% solution, 5,253 mOsm/L in D_5W; 5,506 mOsm/L in dextrose 10% in water; 5,555 mOsm/L in 10% invert sugar.
• Monitor blood pressure, intake and output, and electrolyte and BUN levels before and after administration. Also check injection site for phlebitis.
• Maintain adequate hydration.
• Watch for signs and symptoms of hyponatremia or hypokalemia, including muscle weakness and lethargy.
• Rebound elevation of intraocular and intracranial pressure may occur 12 hours after administration.
• If satisfactory diuresis doesn't occur in 6 to 12 hours, drug should be stopped and renal function reevaluated.
• Urea has been used orally on an investigational basis for migraine prophylaxis, acute sickle-cell crisis prevention, and correction of SIADH.

Reactions may be *common*, uncommon, *life-threatening*, or COMMON AND LIFE-THREATENING.

PATIENT TEACHING
● Advise patient to report adverse reactions or bleeding.
● Inform patient of signs and symptoms of hypokalemia or hyponatremia and tell him to report them immediately.
● Notify patient of potential for extravasation, and advise him to immediately report pain at the I.V. site.

urokinase
Abbokinase

Pharmacologic class: thrombolytic enzyme
Therapeutic class: thrombolytic
Pregnancy risk category: B
pH: 6 to 7.5

INDICATIONS & DOSAGES
➤ **Pulmonary embolism—**
Adults: 4,400 IU/kg initially by infusion over 10 minutes, then 4,400 IU/kg/hour for 12 hours by continuous infusion.
➤ **Venous catheter occlusion ◆ —**
Adults: 1 ml of 5,000 IU/ml solution for each clearing procedure.
➤ **Lysis of coronary artery thrombi in patients with acute MI ◆ —**
Adults: 2 to 3 million units over 45 to 90 minutes, with half or all of the dose given as an initial rapid injection over 5 minutes and the remainder, if any, as a continuous infusion.

ADMINISTRATION
Direct injection: To clear a venous catheter occlusion, slowly inject solution into occluded line, wait 5 minutes, then aspirate. Aspirate every 5 minutes for 30 minutes. If not patent after 30 minutes, cap line and let urokinase work for 30 to 60 minutes before aspirating. May require second injection.
Intermittent infusion: Not recommended.

Continuous infusion: Give initial dose of diluted solution over 10 minutes using an infusion pump. Infuse subsequent doses over 12 hours.

PREPARATION & STORAGE
Supplied as lyophilized white powder in vials containing 250,000 IU.
Reconstitute with 5 ml of sterile water for injection, without preservatives, for a solution of 50,000 IU/ml. Don't use bacteriostatic water; it contains preservatives. Dilute solution further with normal saline or D_5W. Total volume given shouldn't exceed 200 ml.
Reconstituted solution should be clear, practically colorless, and without precipitates. To avoid filament formation, roll and tilt vial during reconstitution; avoid shaking. Solution may be filtered through a 0.45-micron or smaller cellulose filter.
Refrigerate vials at 35° to 47° F (2° to 8° C). Because urokinase contains no preservatives, reconstitute immediately before use and discard unused portion. Don't use highly colored solutions, and don't add other drugs to the solution.

Incompatibilities
Other I.V. drugs.

CONTRAINDICATIONS & CAUTIONS
● Contraindicated in those with active internal bleeding and in those who have had a CVA, intracranial neoplasm, or intracranial or intraspinal surgery within the past 2 months; in those who have had major surgery, severe GI bleeding, organ biopsy, obstetric delivery, or puncture of noncompressible vessels within the past 10 days; in those with severe uncontrolled hypertension; and in those with recent serious trauma.
● Contraindicated in those with recent minor trauma (including CPR) and in those at high risk for left-sided heart thrombus, pregnancy, or infectious endocarditis.

• Contraindicated in those with cerebrovascular disease, diabetic hemorrhagic retinopathy, or hemostatic defects, including those linked to severe renal or hepatic disease.

• Use extremely cautiously in those with any condition in which bleeding would be hazardous or especially difficult to manage.

• Use cautiously in those with atrial fibrillation or another condition with risk of cerebral embolism because of risk of bleeding into the infarcted area.

• Safe use in children hasn't been established.

ADVERSE REACTIONS

CNS: fever.
CV: *reperfusion arrhythmias,* tachycardia, transient hypotension or hypertension.
GI: nausea, vomiting.
Hematologic: *bleeding.*
Respiratory: *bronchospasm,* minor breathing difficulties.
Skin: phlebitis at injection site, rash.
Other: *anaphylaxis,* chills.

INTERACTIONS

Drug-drug. *Anticoagulants, corticosteroids, heparin, salicylates, and other drugs affecting platelet function:* Increases risk of hemorrhage. Monitor patient closely.
Antifibrinolytic drugs, such as aminocaproic acid: Inhibits action of urokinase. Monitor patient closely.

EFFECTS ON LAB RESULT TESTS

• May increase PT, PTT, and INR. May decrease hematocrit.

ACTION

Promotes thrombolysis by converting plasminogen to the fibrinolytic enzyme plasmin.

PHARMACOKINETICS

Onset, immediately after administration; duration, 12 to 24 hours.

Distribution: In plasma. Unknown if drug crosses the placental barrier or appears in breast milk.
Metabolism: Rapid, in liver.
Excretion: Small amounts in bile and urine. Half-life is 10 to 20 minutes but may be longer in hepatic dysfunction.

CLINICAL CONSIDERATIONS

• Osmolality: 391 mOsm/kg.

• Monitor for bleeding every 15 minutes for first hour, every 30 minutes for the next 7 hours, and then once each shift.

• Monitor vital signs. Also monitor pulse, color, and sensitivity of arms and legs every hour.

• Maintain alignment of involved arm or leg to prevent bleeding at infusion site.

• Assess percutaneous puncture sites and cuts for oozing, bruising, and hematomas because urokinase may lyse fibrin deposits.

• Have typed and crossmatched RBCs and whole blood available in case of hemorrhage.

• If hemorrhage occurs, stop drug immediately. Give plasma volume expanders other than dextrans to replace volume deficits. For severe blood loss, give packed RBCs rather than whole blood. For rapid reversal of hyperfibrinolysis, consider giving aminocaproic acid; however, efficacy hasn't been established.

• Watch for signs of hypersensitivity and have corticosteroids available to treat allergic reactions.

• *Alert:* Rare reports of orolingual edema, urticaria, cholesterol embolization, and infusion reactions causing hypoxia, cyanosis, acidosis, and back pain have occurred in patients receiving this drug.

• Avoid I.M. injections, unnecessary handling of patient, and arterial invasive procedures. If an arterial puncture is needed, use an arm, apply pressure at site for 30 minutes, and apply a pres-

---

Reactions may be *common,* uncommon, *life-threatening,* or COMMON AND LIFE-THREATENING.

sure dressing. Check site frequently for bleeding. Also avoid venipuncture, or perform as infrequently as possible.

• Follow with heparin, usually within 1 hour after discontinuation of urokinase, to prevent recurrent thrombosis.

• Hematocrit and fibrinogen and plasminogen levels may decrease for 12 to 24 hours after therapy stops. Levels of fibrin split products increase similarly. Monitor these levels.

PATIENT TEACHING

• Advise patient to report adverse effects.

• Instruct patient to report symptoms of bleeding.

• During venous catheter clearing procedure, advise patient to exhale and hold breath while catheter isn't connected to tubing to prevent air from entering the catheter.

vancomycin hydrochloride
Vancocin, Vancoled

Pharmacologic class: glycopeptide
Therapeutic class: antibiotic
Pregnancy risk category: C
pH: 2.5 to 4.5

INDICATIONS & DOSAGES
➤ **Severe systemic infections caused by susceptible organisms when less toxic drugs are ineffective—**
Adults: 500 mg q 6 hours or 1 g q 12 hours.
Children older than age 1 month: 40 mg/kg daily in four divided doses.
Infants 8 days to 1 month: 15 mg/kg initially, then 10 mg/kg q 8 hours.
Neonates age 8 days or younger: 15 mg/kg initially, then 10 mg/kg q 12 hours.
➤ **To prevent bacterial endocarditis in penicillin-allergic patients at moderate or high risk who are undergoing GI, GU, or biliary tract surgery or instrumentation procedures—**
Adults: 1 g I.V. over 1 to 2 hours with the infusion completed 30 minutes before procedure. Give high-risk patients adjunctive 1.5 mg/kg I.V. gentamicin within 30 minutes of the start of the procedure.
Children: 20 mg/kg 30 to 60 minutes before procedure. Give high-risk patients adjunctive 1.5 mg/kg I.V. gentamicin within 30 minutes of the start of the procedure.
➤ **Bacterial endocarditis caused by methicillin-resistant *Staphylococcus aureus* (MRSA) or methicillin-susceptible staphylococci in patients with native cardiac valves—**
Adults: 30 mg/kg daily I.V. in two equally divided doses (maximum 2 g daily unless drug levels are monitored) for 4 to 6 weeks.
➤ **Bacterial endocarditis caused by MRSA or methicillin-susceptible staphylococci in patients with prosthetic valve or other prosthetic material—**
Adults: 30 mg/kg daily I.V. in two to four equally divided doses (maximum 2 g daily unless drug levels are monitored) for 6 weeks or longer in conjunction with oral rifampin and I.M. or I.V. gentamicin.
➤ **Endocarditis caused by viridans streptococci or *Streptococcus bovis*—**
Adults: 30 mg/kg daily I.V. in two equally divided doses (maximum 2 g daily unless drug levels are monitored) for 4 weeks.
➤ **Enterococcal endocarditis—**
Adults: 30 mg/kg daily I.V. in two equally divided doses (maximum 2 g daily unless drug levels are monitored) for 4 to 6 weeks in conjunction with I.M. or I.V. gentamicin for 4 to 6 weeks.
Adjust-a-dose: In renal impairment, recommended initial dose is 15 mg/kg. Subsequent doses should be adjusted, as appropriate. Some prescribers use the following schedule: If creatinine level is less than 1.5 mg/dl, give 1 g q 12 hours. If creatinine level is 1.5 to 5 mg/dl, give 1 g q 3 to 6 days. If creatinine level is greater than 5 mg/dl, give 1 g q 10 to 14 days.
  For anephric patients on dialysis, initial dose is 15 mg/kg, followed by maintenance dose of 1.9 mg/kg/day.

ADMINISTRATION
Direct injection: Not recommended.
Intermittent infusion: Infuse diluted dose over at least 60 minutes to reduce risk of local reactions and red man syndrome.
Continuous infusion: Use only when intermittent infusion isn't feasible. Add ordered dose to compatible solution and give over 24 hours.

PREPARATION & STORAGE
Available as an off-white to buff powder in 500-mg and 1-g vials.

Reconstitute drug in 500-mg vial with 10 ml and in 1-g vial with 20 ml of sterile water for injection for an average concentration of 50 mg/ml. Reconstituted solution is clear and light yellow to light brown. Before administration, dilute 500 mg in at least 100 ml, and 1 g in at least 200 ml of D_5W or normal saline solution. For continuous infusion, dilute 1 to 2 g in the ordered volume for 24 hours. Inspect before administration for precipitates or discoloration.

Before reconstitution, store vials at room temperature. Reconstituted solutions may be refrigerated for 14 days. When diluted, solutions are stable for 24 hours at room temperature and are stable refrigerated for 2 months.

Incompatibilities
Albumin, alkaline solutions, aminophylline, amobarbital, amphotericin B, aztreonam, cephalosporines, chloramphenicol, chlorothiazide, corticosteroids, dexamethasone sodium phosphate, foscarnet, heavy metals, heparin, hydrocortisone, idarubicin, methotrexate, nafcillin, penicillin G potassium, pentobarbital, phenobarbital, phenytoin, piperacillin, piperacillin sodium-tazobactam sodium, sargramostim, sodium bicarbonate, ticarcillin disodium, ticarcillin disodium-clavulanate potassium, vitamin B complex with C, warfarin.

CONTRAINDICATIONS & CAUTIONS
• Contraindicated in those hypersensitive to the drug.
• Use cautiously in geriatric patients because renal function may decline.
• Use cautiously in premature neonates and young infants because of renal immaturity.
• Use cautiously in those with intestinal obstruction because of increased risk of toxic reaction.
• Use cautiously in those with hearing loss because of risk of ototoxicity and in those who are pregnant because of risk of fetal cranial nerve VIII damage.

ADVERSE REACTIONS
CNS: fever.
CV: hypotension, *red man syndrome,* phlebitis.
EENT: ototoxicity, tinnitus.
GI: *pseudomembranous colitis,* nausea.
GU: *nephrotoxicity.*
Hematologic: *neutropenia, leukopenia,* eosinophilia.
Respiratory: wheezing, dyspnea.
Skin: urticaria, pruritus, rash, *Stevens-Johnson syndrome.*
Other: *anaphylaxis,* chills, superinfection.

INTERACTIONS
Drug-drug. *Aminoglycosides, amphotericin B, bacitracin, bumetanide, carmustine, cisplatin, cyclosporine, furosemide:* Enhances ototoxicity and nephrotoxicity. Avoid using together.
Anesthetics: Increases frequency of infusion-related reactions; in children, erythema and flushing. Monitor patient closely.
Antihistamines, buclizine, cyclizine, meclizine, phenothiazines, thioxanthenes, trimethobenzamide: May mask ototoxicity. Avoid using together.
Nondepolarizing muscle relaxants: Enhances neuromuscular blockade. Use cautiously together.

EFFECTS ON LAB TEST RESULTS
• May increase BUN and creatinine levels.
• May increase eosinophil count. May decrease neutrophil and WBC counts.

ACTION
Narrow-spectrum tricyclic glycopeptide antibiotic with bactericidal action. Inhibits cell-wall biosynthesis, selectively inhibits RNA, and alters bacterial cytoplasmic membrane permeability.

PHARMACOKINETICS
Onset, immediate; effect peaks immediately after 1-hour infusion.
Distribution: Extensive, with therapeutic levels in serum, urine, atrial appendage tissue, and in pleural, pericardial, ascitic, and synovial fluids. Low levels appear in bile. Drug is 52% to 60% protein-bound, and with meningeal irritation, has some diffusion into the CSF. Drug crosses the placental barrier and appears in breast milk.
Metabolism: Usually not metabolized; some hepatic metabolism possible.
Excretion: In urine, with small amounts in feces. Half-life in adults, 4 to 11 hours; children, 2 to 3 hours; infants, 4 to 10 hours. Half-life extends to 6 to 10 days in renal impairment.

CLINICAL CONSIDERATIONS
• Osmolality: 50 mg/ml in sterile water is 57 mOsm/kg; 5 mg/ml is 249 to 291 mOsm/kg.
• Drug is used to treat severe infections in patients who can't receive or have failed to respond to penicillins or cephalosporins.
• When used preoperatively, give 60-minute infusion before anesthetic induction to reduce risk of infusion-related reactions.
• Obtain specimens for culture and sensitivity tests before giving first dose. Therapy may begin before results are available unless drug is being used for prophylaxis.

• Watch for superinfection caused by nonsusceptible organisms.
• Monitor vital signs, especially blood pressure. Check blood pressure every 5 to 10 minutes during initial therapy. Change I.V. sites frequently to help avoid extravasation.
• Obtain periodic WBC counts in prolonged therapy or with administration of other drugs that may cause neutropenia.
• Monitor hearing before and during therapy of more than 2 weeks.
• Monitor renal function, including BUN and creatinine levels, creatinine clearance, urinalysis, and output, and auditory function, including audiograms and signs of ototoxicity, especially in high-risk patients.
• Monitor vancomycin level for toxic levels. Adjust dosage or frequency, if needed.
• Coordinate blood sampling and vancomycin administration with the laboratory. Obtain trough samples before next dose; obtain peak samples 1.5 to 2.5 hours after infusion. Therapeutic peak levels are 25 to 40 mcg/ml; trough levels, 5 to 10 mcg/ml.
• If red man syndrome occurs, stop infusion and notify the prescriber. This syndrome is characterized by upper body flushing and a profound drop in blood pressure. Treat symptomatically; syndrome usually resolves within 20 minutes but may continue for several hours.
• Peritoneal dialysis removes less than 30% of the drug; hemodialysis, none of the drug. Patients receiving these treatments require usual dose only once every 5 to 7 days.

PATIENT TEACHING
• Advise patient to report ringing in ears.
• Advise patient to report diarrhea because of risk of pseudomembranous colitis.

• Notify patient of risk of extravasation, and encourage him to promptly report pain at I.V. site.

vasopressin (antidiuretic hormone [ADH])
Pitressin

Pharmacologic class: posterior pituitary hormone
Therapeutic class: hemostatic
Pregnancy risk category: C
pH: 2.5 to 4.5

INDICATIONS & DOSAGES
➤ **GI hemorrhage ♦** —
Adults: 0.2 to 0.4 unit/minute, with increases to 0.9 unit/minute, if needed. Dosage must be individualized according to patient's response and tolerance. After 24 hours, taper according to patient response.
➤ **CPR ♦** —
Adults: 40 units I.V. as a single dose.
➤ **Vasodilatory shock ♦** —
Adults: 0.02 to 0.1 units/minute as a continuous I.V. infusion.

ADMINISTRATION
Direct injection: Not recommended.
Intermittent infusion: Not recommended.
Continuous infusion: Infuse diluted solution through a peripheral vein with a controlled infusion device.

PREPARATION & STORAGE
Available in 1-ml ampules and in 0.5-, 1-, and 10-ml vials with a concentration of 20 unit/ml.
For I.V. infusion, dilute to a concentration of 0.1 to 1 unit/ml with normal saline solution or D$_5$W.
Store at 59° to 86° F (15° to 30° C). Don't freeze.

Incompatibilities
None reported.

CONTRAINDICATIONS & CAUTIONS
• Contraindicated in those with chronic nephritis complicated by nitrogen retention.
• Use cautiously in those with seizure disorders, migraine, asthma, heart failure, vascular disease, angina, coronary thrombosis, renal disease, goiter with cardiac complications, arteriosclerosis, or other disease in which rapid addition to extracellular fluid may be hazardous.
• Use cautiously in children and in geriatric patients because they're particularly sensitive to the drug.

ADVERSE REACTIONS
CNS: tremor, headache, vertigo.
CV: *arrhythmias, cardiac arrest,* hypertension, *bradycardia, vascular collapse,* coronary insufficiency, peripheral vasoconstriction, angina, myocardial ischemia, *MI (with large doses).*
GI: abdominal cramps, flatulence, nausea, vomiting, diarrhea, eructation.
Respiratory: bronchial constriction.
Skin: sweating, gangrene, urticaria.
Other: circumoral pallor, *hypersensitivity reactions, water intoxication.*

INTERACTIONS
Drug-drug. *Carbamazepine, chlorpropamide, clofibrate, fludrocortisone, tricyclic antidepressants, urea:* Increases antidiuretic response. Use together cautiously.
Demeclocycline, epinephrine, heparin, lithium: Decreases antidiuretic activity. Monitor for effect.
Ganglionic blockers: Increases pressor effects. Use together cautiously.
Drug-lifestyle. *Alcohol use:* Decreases antidiuretic activity. Avoid using together.

EFFECTS ON LAB TEST RESULTS
None reported.

ACTION

Decreases portal blood pressure. Acts to increase reabsorption of water by the renal tubules, and urea by the collecting ducts. Directly stimulates contraction of smooth muscle and produces vasoconstriction. In the intestinal tract, vasopressin increases peristaltic activity, especially of the large bowel.

PHARMACOKINETICS

Duration variable, but usually 2 to 8 hours.
Distribution: Throughout extracellular fluid; doesn't bind to protein.
Metabolism: Metabolized largely in the liver.
Excretion: 5% to 15% of dose appears in urine; plasma half-life, 10 to 20 minutes.

CLINICAL CONSIDERATIONS

• Osmolality: 30 mOsm/kg (20 units/ ml).
• *Alert:* Give I.V. only under the supervision of a practitioner familiar with the pharmacologic effects of drug and all accepted treatments for GI bleeding.
• Establish baseline vital signs, intake and output, and daily weight before therapy.
• Observe for signs and symptoms of early water intoxication, including drowsiness, listlessness, headache, confusion, and weight gain.
• *Alert:* Use caution to avoid extravasation because of risk of necrosis and gangrene.
• Because many of the adverse effects of vasopressin are dose-related, use lowest possible effective dose.
• Monitor electrolyte levels and ECG periodically for disturbances.
• Monitor abdominal distention and GI function; a rectal tube facilitates gas expulsion after vasopressin therapy.
• *Alert:* Never inject during first stage of labor; this may cause ruptured uterus.

• If overdose occurs, stop drug and restrict water intake until polyuria occurs. Severe water intoxication may require osmotic diuresis with mannitol, hypertonic dextrose, or urea, either alone or with furosemide.

PATIENT TEACHING

• Advise patient of potential adverse effects.
• Tell patient to call immediately if chest pain, fever, hives, rash, headache, difficulty urinating, weight gain, unusual drowsiness, wheezing, trouble with breathing, or swelling of face, hands, feet, or mouth occurs.
• Encourage patient to drink one to two glasses of water with each dose of vasopressin, as appropriate, to minimize some adverse reactions.
• Remind patient of need to monitor intake and output closely.

vecuronium bromide
Norcuron*

Pharmacologic class: nondepolarizing neuromuscular blocker
Therapeutic class: skeletal muscle relaxant
Pregnancy risk category: C
pH: 4

INDICATIONS & DOSAGES

➤ **Adjunct to general anesthesia, to facilitate endotracheal intubation, and to provide skeletal muscle relaxation during surgery or mechanical ventilation—**
Dose depends on anesthetic used, individual needs, and response. Doses are representative and must be adjusted.
Adults and children age 10 and older: 0.08 to 0.1 mg/kg initially. Maintenance dose, 0.01 to 0.015 mg/kg 20 to 40 minutes after initial dose, then q 12 to 15 minutes, p.r.n., or continuous

infusion started at 1 mcg/kg/minute (0.001 mg/kg/minute).
Children younger than age 10: May require higher initial dose.
Adjust-a-dose: Reduce dosage in patients with renal or hepatic impairment and in geriatric patients.

ADMINISTRATION
Direct injection: Inject dose directly into tubing of an I.V. line containing a free-flowing, compatible solution.
Intermittent infusion: Not recommended.
Continuous infusion: Begin infusion 20 to 40 minutes after initial dose by direct injection. Determine rates by carefully observing neuromuscular blockade with a peripheral nerve stimulator. Infusion rates range from 0.8 to 1.2 mcg/kg/minute (0.0008 to 0.0012 mg/kg/minute) with a 1:10 dilution.

PREPARATION & STORAGE
Supplied as a sterile, nonpyrogenic, freeze-dried buffered cake composed of fine crystalline particles. Available in 10- and 20-mg vials and accompanying bacteriostatic water for injection diluent.

Reconstitute with bacteriostatic water for injection or sterile water for injection. For infusion, dilute further by adding drug to D_5W, normal saline solution, dextrose 5% in normal saline solution, or lactated Ringer's solution.

Before reconstitution, store at room temperature and protect from light. After reconstitution with bacteriostatic water, use within 5 days when stored at room temperature or refrigerated; with sterile water for injection, use within 24 hours when refrigerated.

Incompatibilities
Alkaline solutions, amphotericin B, diazepam, furosemide, thiopental.

CONTRAINDICATIONS & CAUTIONS
• Contraindicated in those hypersensitive to the drug or bromides.
• Use cautiously in those with neuromuscular diseases or bronchogenic carcinoma because of enhanced neuromuscular blockade and in those with electrolyte imbalance or dehydration because of altered neuromuscular blockade.
• Use cautiously in those with hepatic or renal impairment because of prolonged neuromuscular blockade and prolonged recovery time.
• Use cautiously in geriatric or debilitated patients and in those with CV impairment or edema because circulatory impairment may delay drug onset.
• Use cautiously in those with myasthenia gravis because of the profound effect of even small doses.
• Use cautiously in those with pulmonary impairment or respiratory depression because of deepened respiratory depression.
• Use cautiously in those who are severely obese and in those with neuromuscular disease because of possible airway or ventilation problems.

ADVERSE REACTIONS
Musculoskeletal: muscle weakness, prolonged muscle paralysis.
Respiratory: *apnea, respiratory insufficiency.*

INTERACTIONS
Drug-drug. *Aminoglycosides, bacitracin, colistimethate sodium, colistin, halogenated inhalation anesthetics, other neuromuscular blockers, polymyxin B, procainamide, quinidine, tetracyclines:* Prolongs neuromuscular blockade. Monitor patient closely.
Antimyasthenics, edrophonium: Causes mutual antagonism. Use together cautiously during and after surgery.
Calcium salts: Reverses neuromuscular blockade. Use together cautiously.

Doxapram: May mask vecuronium's residual effects. Monitor patient closely.

Opioid analgesics: Causes additive respiratory depression. Use together cautiously during and after surgery.

Drug-lifestyle. *Smoking:* May induce resistance to therapeutic effects of drug. Discourage use together.

EFFECTS ON LAB TEST RESULTS

None reported.

ACTION

Exerts skeletal muscle relaxant action by competing with acetylcholine for cholinergic receptors at the motor end plate, thus blocking depolarization.

PHARMACOKINETICS

Onset, 2½ to 3 minutes; duration, 25 to 40 minutes, depending on anesthetic used, dose, and number of doses given.
Distribution: In extracellular fluid; rapidly reaches its site of action. About 60% to 90% is protein bound. Volume of distribution is decreased in children younger than age 1 and may be decreased in geriatric patients. Drug crosses the placental barrier in small amounts. It's unknown if drug appears in breast milk.
Metabolism: In liver; rapidly and extensively metabolized.
Excretion: Primarily in feces; also in urine.

CLINICAL CONSIDERATIONS

• Osmolality: 292 mOsm/kg (4 mg/ml).
• Drug should be given only by staff trained to give anesthetics and to manage their adverse effects.
• Administration of vecuronium must be accompanied by adequate anesthesia. Drug doesn't relieve pain or affect consciousness.
• Have emergency respiratory support equipment immediately available.
• Onset is too slow for use in emergency intubations.

• Continuously monitor patient throughout infusion. After procedure, monitor vital signs at least every 15 minutes until patient is stable, then every 30 minutes for next 2 hours. Monitor airway and pattern of respirations until patient has recovered from drug effects.
• A nerve stimulator and train-of-four monitoring are recommended to assess recovery of muscle strength. Before attempting pharmacologic reversal with neostigmine, patient should show some signs of spontaneous recovery.
• Evaluate recovery from neuromuscular blockade by checking strength of patient's hand grip and his ability to breathe naturally, take deep breaths and cough, keep eyes open, and lift head keeping mouth closed.
• Infants are especially sensitive to drug effects. Recovery time may be 1½ times that of an adult.
• Signs and symptoms of overdose include prolonged duration of neuromuscular blockade, skeletal muscle weakness, decreased respiratory reserve, low tidal volume, and apnea.
• If overdose occurs, provide mechanical ventilation with endotracheal intubation until reversal of neuromuscular blockade is adequate. Blockade can be reversed with acetylcholinesterase inhibitors, such as neostigmine, pyridostigmine, or edrophonium given with atropine or glycopyrrolate.

PATIENT TEACHING

• Advise patient of adverse effects.
• Reassure patient that he'll be constantly monitored during the surgical procedure.
• Notify patient that the effects of the drug can be reversed, if needed.
• Inform patient that postprocedure monitoring will involve him demonstrating hand grip, breathing, and coughing.

Reactions may be *common,* uncommon, *life-threatening,* or COMMON AND LIFE-THREATENING.

verapamil hydrochloride

Pharmacologic class: calcium
channel blocker
Therapeutic class: antiarrhythmic
Pregnancy risk category: C
pH: 4 to 6.5

INDICATIONS & DOSAGES
➤ **Supraventricular arrhythmias—**
Adults: 0.075 to 0.15 mg/kg (5 to
10 mg) by I.V. push over 2 minutes,
with continuous ECG and blood pressure monitoring. Repeat dose in 30
minutes if no response occurs.
Children ages 1 to 15 ♦ : 0.1 to 0.3 mg/
kg as bolus over 2 minutes, with continuous ECG monitoring. Repeat dose
in 30 minutes if no response occurs.
Children younger than age 1 ♦ : 0.1 to
0.2 mg/kg as bolus over 2 minutes,
with continuous ECG monitoring. Repeat dose in 30 minutes if no response
occurs.
Adjust-a-dose: Reduce dosage in patients with renal or hepatic impairment.

ADMINISTRATION
Direct injection: Give undiluted drug at
a rate of 5 to 10 mg over at least 2 minutes. Inject directly into vein or into an
I.V. line containing a free-flowing,
compatible solution. In geriatric patients, give over at least 3 minutes to
reduce adverse effects.
Intermittent infusion: Not recommended.
Continuous infusion: Not recommended.

PREPARATION & STORAGE
Supplied as a solution of 2.5 mg/ml.
   Drug is stable for 24 hours at 77° F
(25° C) in most common infusion solutions when protected from light. It's
compatible with D_5W, normal saline
solution, and lactated Ringer's solution.

Store at room temperature and protect from light and freezing.

Incompatibilities
Albumin, aminophylline, amphotericin
B, ampicillin sodium, co-trimoxazole,
dobutamine, hydralazine, nafcillin,
oxacillin, propofol, sodium bicarbonate, solutions with a pH greater than 6.

CONTRAINDICATIONS & CAUTIONS
● Contraindicated in those hypersensitive to the drug.
● Contraindicated in those with second-
or third-degree AV block because of
excessive bradycardia.
● Contraindicated in those with severe
hypotension, cardiogenic shock, or pulmonary artery wedge pressure exceeding 20 mm Hg because drug may exacerbate these conditions and in those
with Wolff-Parkinson-White syndrome
because drug may precipitate severe arrhythmias.
● Use with caution in children, especially neonates, because of the risk of
severe CV adverse effects. Some clinical experts no longer recommend its
use in children.
● Use cautiously in those with
Duchenne-type muscular dystrophy because of risk of respiratory paralysis.
● Use cautiously in those with bradycardia or heart failure because of possible reduction of sinus or AV node activity.
● Use cautiously in those with hypertrophic cardiomyopathy, moderate ventricular dysfunction, or sick sinus syndrome because drug may worsen
symptoms and in those with mild to
moderate hypotension because drug
may exacerbate condition.
● Use cautiously in those with renal impairment or liver failure because of increased risk of toxicity.
● Avoid abrupt withdrawal.

ADVERSE REACTIONS

CNS: dizziness, drowsiness, fatigue, headache, asthenia.

CV: *heart failure, symptomatic hypotension,* severe tachycardia, peripheral edema, *bradycardia, AV block, ventricular asystole, ventricular fibrillation.*

GI: *constipation,* nausea.

Respiratory: *pulmonary edema.*

Skin: rash.

INTERACTIONS

Drug-drug. *Antihypertensives, quinidine:* May cause additive effects. Monitor blood pressure.

Beta blockers: Increases risk of heart failure and AV block. Monitor cardiac status closely, and reduce verapamil dose.

Carbamazepine: Increases carbamazepine levels and subsequent toxicity. Use together with caution; watch for signs of toxicity. May need to reduce carbamazepine dosage by 40% to 50%.

Cimetidine, cyclosporine, hydantoins, oral anticoagulants, prazosin, salicylates, sulfonamides, sulfonylureas, valproates: Increases risk of toxic reaction. Monitor patient closely.

Dantrolene I.V.: Decreases potassium level, causes cardiac depression, and may cause CV collapse. Avoid using together.

Digoxin: Increases digoxin level. Reduce digoxin dosage by half, and monitor subsequent drug levels.

Disopyramide: Causes additive effects and possible heart failure. Monitor cardiac status closely. Stop disopyramide 48 hours before starting verapamil therapy, and don't reinstitute until 24 hours after verapamil has been stopped.

Estrogens, NSAIDs, sympathomimetics: May reduce antihypertensive effects of verapamil. Monitor blood pressure. Dosage may need to be adjusted.

Lithium: Decreases lithium level. Monitor for loss of therapeutic effect. Dosage of lithium may need to be adjusted.

Neuromuscular blockers: May prolong neuromuscular blockade. Use together with caution.

Phenobarbital: May increase verapamil clearance. Monitor cardiac status.

Rifampin: May substantially reduce verapamil's oral bioavailability. Monitor therapeutic effect; adjust dosage of verapamil as needed.

Theophylline: Increases theophylline plasma levels. Monitor patient closely; adjust theophylline dosage as needed.

Vitamin D: Therapeutic effect of verapamil may be reduced. Monitor patient closely.

Drug-herb. *Black catechu:* Causes additive effects. Discourage use together.

Yerba maté: May decrease clearance of yerba maté methylxanthines and cause toxic reaction. Advise patient to use together cautiously.

Drug-lifestyle. *Alcohol use:* Drug may enhance effects of alcohol. Discourage use together.

EFFECTS ON LAB TEST RESULTS

● May increase ALT, AST, alkaline phosphatase, and bilirubin levels.

ACTION

Inhibits influx of extracellular calcium ions across the membranes of myocardial and vascular smooth-muscle cells, without changing calcium levels. Reduces afterload and myocardial contractility and also slows SA and AV node conduction.

PHARMACOKINETICS

Onset, 1 to 5 minutes; duration, up to 6 hours.

Distribution: About 90% bound to protein. Drug crosses the placental barrier and is also distributed into CSF, although poorly. Drug also appears in breast milk.

Metabolism: Rapidly metabolized in the liver to demethylated metabolites.

Reactions may be *common,* uncommon, *life-threatening,* or COMMON AND LIFE-THREATENING.

Excretion: In urine and feces; 16% within 5 days. Biphasic half-life: first phase, 4 minutes; second phase, 2 to 8 hours.

CLINICAL CONSIDERATIONS
• Osmolality: 290 mOsm/kg.
• Monitor ECG and blood pressure continuously during drug administration.
• Notify prescriber if patient shows signs of heart failure, such as dependent edema or dyspnea.
• Breast-feeding patients shouldn't breast-feed while receiving drug because of the potential for serious adverse reactions in the infant.
• If overdose occurs, provide supportive care. Beta agonists and I.V. calcium salts may be ordered.

PATIENT TEACHING
• Advise patient to report adverse effects.
• Alert patient to the potential for symptomatic hypotension.
• Instruct patient to report signs of heart failure, such as swelling of hands and feet or shortness of breath.

vinblastine sulfate (VLB)
Velban, Velbe ◊ *

Pharmacologic class: vinca alkaloid (M-phase specific)
Therapeutic class: antineoplastic
Pregnancy risk category: D
pH: 3.5 to 5

INDICATIONS & DOSAGES
➤ **Hodgkin's disease, lymphocytic lymphoma, histiocytic lymphomas; testicular cancer; Kaposi's sarcoma; advanced mycosis fungoides; chorio-carcinoma; Letterer-Siwe disease; bladder cancer ♦ ; melanoma ♦ ; non–small-cell lung cancer ♦ ; in-tracranial germ cell tumors ♦ ; renal cell cancer ♦ —**
Adults: Initially, 3.7 mg/m² weekly. Successive weekly doses increased by increments of 1.8 to 1.9 mg/m², until WBC count falls to 3,000 cells/mm³, tumor size decreases, or maximum dose of 18.5 mg/m², is reached; usual range, 5.5 to 7.4 mg/m². Subsequent maintenance doses, which are one increment smaller than final initial dose q 7 to 14 days, shouldn't be given until WBC count after preceding dose returns to 4,000 cells/mm³.
Children: Initially, 2.5 mg/m² weekly, then successive weekly doses increased in increments of 1.25 mg/m² until WBC count falls to 3,000 cells/mm³, tumor size decreases, or a maximum dose of 12.5 mg/m² is reached. Subsequent maintenance doses, which are one increment smaller than final initial dose q 7 to 14 days, aren't recommended until WBC count after preceding dose returns to 4,000 cells/mm³.

ADMINISTRATION
Direct injection: Inject dose rapidly into side port of a free-flowing patent I.V. line or inject directly into vein over 1 minute. Avoid injecting drug into arm or leg veins with compromised circulation because of enhanced risk of thrombosis. Don't remove the covering until moment of injection.
   If extravasation occurs, stop the injection immediately and inject remaining dose into another vein. Treat the affected area immediately.
Intermittent infusion: Not recommended.
Continuous infusion: Not recommended.

PREPARATION & STORAGE
Supplied as powder for injection in 10- and 25-mg vials. Also available in 10-ml aqueous solution of 10 mg/ml. To avoid mutagenic, teratogenic, and carcinogenic risks when preparing and

giving drug, use a biological containment cabinet, wear disposable gloves and mask, and use syringes with luer-lock fittings to prevent drug leakage. Dispose of needles, syringes, vials, and unused drug properly, and avoid contaminating work surfaces. If spilled, inactivate with sodium hypochlorite 5%.

Avoid drug contact with eyes because severe irritation and possible corneal ulceration may result. If contact occurs, wash the eye with water immediately.

Reconstitute by adding 10 ml of normal saline injection containing phenol or benzyl alcohol as a preservative to yield 1 mg/ml.

Compatible with normal saline solution, D_5W, and lactated Ringer's solution.

Store powder and reconstituted solution at 36° to 46° F (2° to 8° C). Solution is stable at these temperatures for up to 28 days without significant potency loss.

Incompatibilities
Cefepime, furosemide, heparin.

CONTRAINDICATIONS & CAUTIONS
• *Alert:* Intrathecal use of vinblastine sulfate is fatal.
• Contraindicated in those hypersensitive to the drug.
• Contraindicated in those with leukopenia and granulocytopenia (unless the result of disease being treated).
• Contraindicated in those with bacterial infection because of risk of worsening infection.
• Use cautiously in those with previous cytotoxic drug therapy or radiation therapy.
• Use cautiously in those with hepatic impairment because of increased drug levels from reduced metabolism.
• Use cautiously in debilitated or geriatric patients and in those with skin ulcers because of increased susceptibility to leukopenia.

• Use cautiously in those with a history of gout or urate renal calculi because of risk of hyperuricemia.
• Use cautiously in those with pulmonary dysfunction or ischemic CV disease.

ADVERSE REACTIONS
CNS: *paresthesia, loss of deep tendon reflexes, peripheral neuritis, numbness,* mental depression, headache, dizziness, *seizures, CVA,* malaise, weakness.
CV: hypertension, *MI.*
EENT: vesiculation of the mouth, pharyngitis, ototoxicity.
GI: *constipation, nausea, vomiting,* abdominal pain, *ileus,* diarrhea, hemorrhagic enterocolitis, rectal bleeding, ulcer, bleeding, *anorexia, stomatitis.*
Hematologic: *leukopenia,* anemia, *thrombocytopenia.*
Metabolic: hyperuricemia, *weight loss.*
Musculoskeletal: bone pain, jaw pain, *muscle pain and weakness.*
Respiratory: acute shortness of breath, *acute bronchospasm.*
Skin: *alopecia,* skin vesiculation; cellulitis and phlebitis at site with extravasation
Other: pain in tumor-containing tissue.

INTERACTIONS
Drug-drug. *Drugs that inhibit cytochrome P-450:* May decrease metabolism of vinblastine, increasing levels. Use together cautiously.
Erythromycin: May cause vinblastine toxicity. Monitor patient closely for toxicity.
Mitomycin: Shortness of breath or bronchospasm in patients taking mitomycin within 2 weeks of therapy. Avoid using together.
Phenytoin: May reduce phenytoin level. Monitor patient closely.
Vaccines with killed virus: Decreases values. Avoid using together.
Vaccines with live virus: May cause systemic infection and decreased immune response. Avoid using together.

Reactions may be *common,* uncommon, *life-threatening,* or COMMON AND LIFE-THREATENING.

EFFECTS ON LAB TEST RESULTS
• May increase uric acid level.
• May decrease hemoglobin and WBC and platelet counts.

ACTION
Seems to block mitosis by arresting cells in metaphase; may also inhibiting purine synthesis, urea formation, and citric acid cycle. Also has immunosuppressive action and may affect nucleic acids and protein synthesis.

PHARMACOKINETICS
Onset, unknown; duration, unknown.
Distribution: Rapid, throughout tissues and localized in platelets and WBCs. About 75% is protein bound. Poorly penetrates the blood-brain barrier and doesn't appear in CSF in therapeutic levels. It may cross the placental barrier. It's unknown if drug appears in breast milk.
Metabolism: Extensively in the liver.
Excretion: Slowly, primarily in feces, but also in urine. Half-life is triphasic: alpha phase, 4 minutes; beta phase, about 2 hours; and terminal phase, about 25 hours or longer.

CLINICAL CONSIDERATIONS
• Osmolality: 278 mOsm/kg.
• Vinblastine may be used alone or in combination with other drugs in various schedules and regimens. Dosage reflects response to drug and degree of bone marrow depression.
• *Alert:* Severe irritation may occur if needle isn't properly positioned in the vein before injection of drug.
• Give an antiemetic before drug to reduce nausea.
• Monitor hematocrit, platelet and total and differential WBC counts, and AST, ALT, bilirubin, creatinine, LDH, BUN, and uric acid levels. WBC nadir occurs 5 to 10 days after administration; recovery is usually complete within another 7 to 14 days.

• Patients with marked leukopenia, particularly granulocytopenia, or thrombocytopenia should have therapy stopped. Therapy can resume when WBC counts return to satisfactory levels.
• *Alert:* Monitor for life-threatening acute bronchospasm, and notify prescriber immediately if this occurs.
• To prevent uric acid nephropathy, encourage oral fluids. Allopurinol also may be ordered to alkalinize the urine.
• Weekly drug doses are linked to less risk of serious toxic reaction than long-term daily doses. Give drug at intervals of at least 7 days to allow monitoring of each dose's full effect on WBC count.
• Therapy may continue for 4 to 6 weeks or longer. Some patients, especially those with carcinomas, require a trial of at least 12 weeks.
• *Alert:* Don't confuse vinblastine with vincristine, vindesine, or vinorelbine.
• Spilled drug can be inactivated with household bleach.

PATIENT TEACHING
• Advise patient to use a stool softener to avoid constipation when taking drug.
• Advise patient to report fever, sore throat, chills, sore mouth, or unusual bleeding or bruising. Patient also should avoid exposure to people with infections.
• Advise patient to report symptoms of neurotoxicity, such as numbness, tingling, or "pins and needles" sensation.
• Advise any woman of childbearing age to avoid becoming pregnant during treatment.
• Reassure patient that scalp hair may grow back during therapy.
• Encourage adequate fluid intake to increase urine output and facilitate excretion of uric acid.

vincristine sulfate
Oncovin ◇, Vincasar PFS

Pharmacologic class: vinca alkaloid (M-phase specific)
Therapeutic class: antineoplastic
Pregnancy risk category: D
pH: 3.5 to 5.5

INDICATIONS & DOSAGES
➤ **Acute myeloid or lymphoblastic leukemia; Hodgkin's and non-Hodgkin's lymphomas, mainly diffuse histiocytic or lymphocytic; Wilms' tumor; rhabdomyosarcoma; neuroblastoma; multiple myeloma ♦; small cell lung carcinoma ♦; osteogenic and other AIDS-related sarcomas including Kaposi's and Ewing's sarcomas ♦; brain tumors ♦** —
Adults: Depending on protocol, 1.4 mg/m² weekly as single dose. Maximum single dose is 2 mg/m².
Children weighing more than 10 kg (22 lb): 1.5 to 2 mg/m² weekly as single dose.
Children weighing 10 kg or less or have BSA less than 1 mg/m²: 0.05 mg/kg weekly.
Adjust-a-dose: Dosage may need to be adjusted in those with hepatic impairment. Reduce dose by 50% when bilirubin is greater than 3 mg/dl.

ADMINISTRATION
Direct injection: Inject dose over 1 minute directly into vein or into side port of a newly started I.V. line. Use a 23G or 25G winged-tip infusion set. If possible, use distal rather than major veins, which allows for repeated venipuncture, if needed.
  If extravasation occurs, stop the injection immediately and inject the remaining dose into another vein. Apply moderate heat or cold compresses to minimize discomfort and cellulitis.

Intermittent infusion: Not recommended; however, drug has been diluted and given as a slow infusion over 4 to 8 hours.
Continuous infusion: Not recommended.

PREPARATION & STORAGE
Supplied in 1-, 2-, and 5-ml vials containing 1 mg/ml. Use caution when preparing and giving vincristine to avoid mutagenic, teratogenic, and carcinogenic risks. Use a biological containment cabinet, wear disposable gloves and mask, and use syringes with luer-lock fittings to prevent drug leakage. Dispose of needles, syringes, vials, and unused drug properly and avoid contaminating work surfaces.
  Avoid drug contact with eyes because severe irritation and possible corneal ulceration may result. If contact occurs, wash eye immediately with water.
  For infusion, dilute to ordered concentration and volume with a compatible I.V. solution, such as D₅W or normal saline injection. Undiluted drug is best stored at 36° to 46° F (2° to 8° C); however, it's stable at room temperature for 1 week to 1 month depending on manufacturer. Protect from light to prevent degradation.

Incompatibilities
Cefepime, furosemide, idarubicin, sodium bicarbonate.

CONTRAINDICATIONS & CAUTIONS
• *Alert:* Intrathecal use of vincristine sulfate is fatal.
• Contraindicated in those hypersensitive to the drug and in those receiving radiation therapy through ports that include the liver.
• Contraindicated in patients with the demyelinating form of Charcot-Marie-Tooth syndrome.
• Use cautiously in those with hepatic impairment because of decreased drug

---

metabolism and in those with infection because of decreased resistance.

• Use cautiously in patients with hepatic dysfunction, neuromuscular disease, or infection.

• Use cautiously when large fluid intake is needed because of risk of SIADH.

ADVERSE REACTIONS

CNS: *peripheral neuropathy,* sensory loss, *loss of deep tendon reflexes, paresthesia, wristdrop and footdrop, seizures, coma,* headache, ataxia, cranial nerve palsies, hoarseness, vocal cord paralysis, fever.
CV: hypotension, hypertension.
EENT: diplopia, optic and extraocular neuropathy, ptosis, photophobia, transient cortical blindness, optical atrophy.
GI: diarrhea, *constipation, cramps,* ileus that mimics surgical abdomen, paralytic ileus, *nausea, vomiting,* anorexia, dysphagia, ***intestinal necrosis,*** *stomatitis.*
GU: urine retention, SIADH, dysuria, acute uric acid neuropathy, polyuria.
Hematologic: anemia, ***leukopenia, thrombocytopenia.***
Metabolic: *hyperuricemia,* hyponatremia, weight loss.
Musculoskeletal: *jaw pain, muscle weakness and cramps.*
Respiratory: ***acute bronchospasm,*** dyspnea.
Skin: *reversible alopecia,* severe local reaction with extravasation; *phlebitis,* cellulitis at injection site.

INTERACTIONS

Drug-drug. *Allopurinol, colchicine, probenecid, sulfinpyrazone:* Decreases antigout effectiveness. Monitor patient closely.
Asparaginase: Decreases hepatic clearance of vincristine. Adjust vincristine dosage.
Calcium channel blockers: Enhances vincristine accumulation in cells. Monitor patient closely; adjust vincristine dosage.
Digoxin: Decreases digoxin level. Monitor level.
Methotrexate: Increases therapeutic effect of methotrexate. May require a lower dosage of methotrexate.
Mitomycin: May increase frequency of bronchospasm and acute pulmonary reactions. Avoid using together.
Neurotoxic drugs: Increases neurotoxicity. Monitor patient closely; adjust vincristine dosage as needed.
Phenytoin: May decrease phenytoin level. Monitor phenytoin level.

EFFECTS ON LAB TEST RESULTS

• May decrease sodium level.
• May decrease hemoglobin and WBC and platelet counts.

ACTION

May arrest mitosis in metaphase, prohibiting cell division; may interfere with amino acid metabolism; and may impair nucleic acid and protein synthesis; also acts as immunosuppressive.

PHARMACOKINETICS

Drug level peaks immediately after administration.
Distribution: Rapidly dispersed throughout the body, with peak biliary level 2 to 4 hours after administration. Extensively tissue-bound and protein-bound; penetrates the blood-brain barrier poorly and usually doesn't appear in CSF in cytotoxic levels. It's unknown if drug appears in breast milk.
Metabolism: Probably in liver, but also appears to undergo decomposition within the body.
Excretion: About 67% removed in feces; the rest excreted in urine. Half-life is triphasic: alpha phase, about 1 hour; beta phase, about 2 hours; gamma phase, 85 hours.

CLINICAL CONSIDERATIONS

- Osmolality: 610 mOsm/kg.
- When vincristine is used with other drugs, risk and severity of adverse reactions may be altered.
- Because vincristine is a vesicant, assemble needed supplies for managing extravasation before administration. Also ensure a patent I.V. line.
- Assess patient for numbness, tingling, and altered walking pattern before administration. If hypotension develops after administration, notify the prescriber.
- Monitor hematocrit, platelet, and total and differential WBC counts, and ALT, AST, bilirubin, creatinine, LDH, BUN, and uric acid levels. Leukopenia usually reaches nadir within 4 days.
- Start a prophylactic bowel regimen before treatment and continue throughout treatment to prevent severe constipation and paralytic ileus. A stool softener may prevent upper colon impaction.
- Hematologic toxicity with vincristine is less than that with other antineoplastics. Mild leukopenia, anemia, and thrombocytopenia are rare at usual doses. However, drug is highly toxic with a narrow therapeutic index.
- To prevent or minimize development of uric acid nephropathy, encourage oral fluids. Allopurinol also may be ordered to alkalinize the urine.
- If signs of hyponatremia or inappropriate ADH secretion appear, notify prescriber.
- Because of potential for neurotoxicity, don't give drug more than once weekly. Children are more resistant to neurotoxicity than adults. Neurotoxicity is dose-related and usually reversible.
- *Alert:* Don't confuse vincristine with vinblastine, vinorelbine, or vindesine.
- *Alert:* Monitor patient for life-threatening bronchospasm reaction. It's most likely to occur in patients also receiving mitomycin.
- Inactivate drug with household bleach if it spills or leaks.

PATIENT TEACHING

- Advise patient to report adverse effects.
- Notify patient that sensorimotor dysfunction may worsen with treatment; these symptoms usually disappear by 6 weeks after stopping therapy but may continue for prolonged periods.
- Reassure patient that scalp hair may regrow during therapy.
- Advise women of childbearing age to avoid becoming pregnant during treatment.
- Encourage adequate fluid intake to increase urine output and facilitate excretion of uric acid.
- Tell patient to call regarding use of laxatives if constipation or stomach pain occurs.

vinorelbine tartrate
Navelbine

Pharmacologic class: vinca alkaloid (M-phase specific)
Therapeutic class: antineoplastic
Pregnancy risk category: D
pH: 3.5

INDICATIONS & DOSAGES

➤ **Alone or as adjunct therapy with cisplatin for first-line treatment of ambulatory patients with nonresectable advanced non–small-cell lung cancer (NSCLC); alone or with cisplatin in stage IV of NSCLC; with cisplatin in stage III of NSCLC—**
Adults: 30 mg/m² weekly. In combination therapy, 30 mg/m² with 120 mg/m² of cisplatin, given on days 1 and 29, then q 6 weeks.
Adjust-a dose: Adjust dosage for hematologic toxicity. If granulocyte count is 1,000 to 1,499 cells/mm³, give

15 mg/m²; if it's below 1,000 cells/mm³, don't give drug, and repeat granulocyte count in 1 week. If three consecutive weekly doses are held because granulocyte count is less than 1,000 cells/mm³, stop drug. If granulocytopenia and patient experiences fever or sepsis, or if two consecutive weekly doses were held due to granulocytopenia, if granulocytes are 1,500 cells/mm³ or more, dosage is 22.5 mg/m²; if 1,000 to 1,499 cells/mm³, give 11.25 mg/m².

If total bilirubin is 2.1 to 3 mg/dl, give 15 mg/m²; if more than 3 mg/dl, give 7.5 mg/m².

➤ **Advanced metastatic breast cancer, alone or with first-line and salvage drug ♦** —
Adults: 30 mg/m² weekly over 6 to 10 minutes, or 20 to 30 mg/m² weekly over 20 to 60 minutes.

ADMINISTRATION
Direct injection: Give over 6 to 10 minutes into the side port of a free-flowing I.V. line closest to the I.V. bag, followed by flushing with at least 75 to 125 ml of one of the solutions.
Intermittent infusion: Give diluted solution over 6 to 10 minutes as above.
Continuous infusion: Not recommended.

PREPARATION & STORAGE
Supplied as preservative-free 1-ml and 5-ml single-use vials at a concentration of 10 mg/ml. Use caution when handling and preparing the solution. Gloves are recommended. Skin reactions may occur with accidental exposure. If the solution contacts the skin or mucosa, immediately wash with soap and water. If contact with the eyes occurs, flush with water thoroughly and immediately to prevent severe irritation.

For direct injection, dilute calculated dose to a concentration between 1.5 and 3 mg/ml with D₅W or normal saline injection. For infusion, the calculated dose should be diluted to a concentration between 0.5 and 2 mg/ml with D₅W, normal saline solution, half-normal saline solution, dextrose 5% in half-normal saline solution, Ringer's solution, or lactated Ringer's solution.

Store the vials under refrigeration at 36° to 46° F (2° to 8° C). Vials can be stored at 77° F (25° C) for up to 72 hours. Protect from light. Avoid freezing. Diluted drug may be used for up to 24 hours under normal room light when stored in polypropylene syringes or polyvinyl chloride bags at 41° to 86° F (5° to 30° C).

Incompatibilities
Acyclovir, allopurinol, aminophylline, amphotericin B, ampicillin sodium, cefazolin, cefoperazone, cefotetan, ceftriaxone, cefuroxime, fluorouracil, furosemide, ganciclovir, methylprednisolone, mitomycin, piperacillin, sodium bicarbonate, thiotepa, trimethoprimsulfamethoxazole.

CONTRAINDICATIONS & CAUTIONS
• *Alert:* Intrathecal use may be fatal.
• Contraindicated in those with pretreatment granulocyte counts below 1,000 cells/mm³.
• Use cautiously in those whose bone marrow reserve may have been compromised by previous radiation or chemotherapy or whose bone marrow function is recovering from the effects of previous chemotherapy.
• Use cautiously in those with hepatic, renal, or pulmonary impairment or coronary artery disease.

ADVERSE REACTIONS
CNS: *fatigue, peripheral neuropathy, asthenia.*
CV: chest pain.
GI: *nausea, vomiting, anorexia, diarrhea, constipation, stomatitis.*
Hematologic: ***bone marrow suppression (agranulocytosis,* LEUKOPENIA, *thrombocytopenia,* anemia).**

Hepatic: *abnormal liver function tests, bilirubinemia.*
Musculoskeletal: jaw pain, myalgia, arthralgia.
Respiratory: dyspnea.
Skin: *alopecia,* rash, *injection pain or reaction.*
Other: SIADH.

INTERACTIONS

Drug-drug. *Cisplatin:* Increases risk of bone marrow suppression. Monitor hematologic status closely.
Mitomycin: Acute pulmonary reactions. Monitor respiratory status closely.

EFFECTS ON LAB TEST RESULTS

● May increase bilirubin level.
● May decrease hemoglobin, liver function test values, and granulocyte, WBC, and platelet counts.

ACTION

A vinca alkaloid that exerts its antineoplastic effect by disrupting microtubule assembly, which, in turn, disrupts spindle formation and prevents mitosis.

PHARMACOKINETICS

Onset, peak, and duration of drug effect unknown.
Distribution: Highly bound to platelets and lymphocytes; 79% to 91% protein bound. It's unknown if drug appears in breast milk.
Metabolism: In the liver.
Excretion: Primarily in the feces, but also in the urine. Terminal half-life averages 28 to 44 hours.

CLINICAL CONSIDERATIONS

● *Alert:* Avoid extravasation because of risk of severe tissue irritation, necrosis, and thrombophlebitis. If extravasation occurs, stop drug immediately and use different vein for remaining infusion.
● *Alert:* Don't confuse vinorelbine with vinblastine, vincristine, or vindesine.

● Monitor I.V. site closely.
● Check granulocyte count before administration; it should be 1,000 cells/mm^3 or more for drug to be given.
● Adjust dosage, as needed, according to granulocyte counts. If three consecutive doses are missed because of low granulocyte counts, further treatment with drug should be avoided.
● Monitor blood count throughout therapy. Patients with hepatic impairment should have liver function monitored.
● Monitor deep tendon reflexes; loss may be the result of toxic reaction.
● Monitor patient for hypersensitivity reactions.

PATIENT TEACHING

● Notify patient of potential adverse effects.
● Advise patient to immediately report fever, sore throat, or chills.
● Advise patient to report bleeding or bruising.
● Notify patient to report pain at I.V. site immediately because of potential for tissue damage with extravasation.
● Advise any woman of childbearing age to avoid becoming pregnant during treatment.

voriconazole
Vfend

Pharmacologic class: synthetic triazole
Therapeutic class: antifungal
Pregnancy risk category: D

INDICATIONS & DOSAGES

➤ **Invasive aspergillosis; serious infections caused by *Fusarium* species and *Scedosporium apiospermum* in patients intolerant of or refractory to other therapy—**
Adults: Initially, 6 mg/kg I.V. q 12 hours for two doses, then 4 mg/kg I.V.

q 12 hours. If maintenance dose can't be tolerated, decrease dose to 3 mg/kg q 12 hours. Switch to P.O. form as tolerated.

Adjust-a-dose: In patients with mild to moderate cirrhosis, decrease the maintenance dosage by 50%.

ADMINISTRATION
Direct injection: Not recommended.
Intermittent infusion: Infuse over 1 to 2 hours, at a concentration of 5 mg/ml or less and a maximum hourly rate of 3 mg/kg.
Continuous infusion: Not recommended.

PREPARATION & STORAGE
Available as 200 mg lyophilized powder in a single-use vial. Reconstitute the powder with 19 ml of sterile water for injection to obtain a volume of 20 ml of clear concentrate containing 10 mg/ml of voriconazole. Discard the vial if a vacuum doesn't pull the diluent into the vial. Shake the vial until all the powder is dissolved.

Further dilute the 10-mg/ml solution to a concentration of 5 mg/ml or less. Follow the manufacturer's instructions for diluting.

Store unreconstituted vials at controlled room temperature (59° to 86°F [15° to 30°C]). The reconstituted solution should be used immediately, or it can be stored up to 24 hours at 35° to 46°F (2° to 8°C).

Incompatibilities
Blood products, electrolyte supplements, 4.2% sodium bicarbonate infusion.

CONTRAINDICATIONS & CAUTIONS
• Contraindicated in patients hypersensitive to voriconazole or its components and in those with rare hereditary problems of galactose intolerance, Lapp lactase deficiency, or glucose-galactose malabsorption.

• Contraindicated in patients taking rifampin, carbamazepine, long-acting barbiturates, sirolimus, rifabutin, ergot alkaloids, pimozide, and quinidine.

• Use cautiously in patients hypersensitive to other azoles. Use I.V. form cautiously in patients with moderate to severe renal dysfunction (creatinine clearance less than 50 ml/minute).

ADVERSE REACTIONS
CNS: fever, headache, hallucinations, dizziness.
CV: tachycardia, hypertension, hypotension, vasodilatation, peripheral edema.
EENT: *abnormal vision,* photophobia, chromatopsia.
GI: abdominal pain, nausea, vomiting, diarrhea, dry mouth.
Hepatic: cholestatic jaundice.
Metabolic: hypokalemia, hypomagnesemia.
Skin: rash, pruritus.
Other: chills.

INTERACTIONS
Drug-drug. *Benzodiazepines, calcium channel blockers, lovastatin, omeprazole, sulfonylureas, vinca alkaloids:* Increases levels of these drugs. May need to adjust dosages of these drugs; monitor patient for adverse effects.
Carbamazepine, long-acting barbiturates, rifampin, rifabutin: Decreases voriconazole level. Avoid using together.
Cyclosporine, tacrolimus: Increases levels of these drugs. Monitor levels of these drugs and reduce their dosages both during and after therapy with voriconazole.
Ergot alkaloids (such as ergotamine), sirolimus: Increases levels of these drugs. Avoid using together.
HIV protease inhibitors (amprenavir, nelfinavir, saquinavir), nonnucleoside reverse transcriptase inhibitors (delavirdine, efavirenz): May increase levels of both drugs. Monitor patient for adverse effects.

Phenytoin: Decreases voriconazole level and increases phenytoin level. Increase voriconazole maintenance dose, and monitor phenytoin level.

Pimozide, quinidine: Increases levels of these drugs, possibly leading to prolonged QT interval and torsades de pointes. Avoid using together.

Warfarin: Significantly increases PT. Monitor PT or other appropriate anticoagulant test results.

Drug-lifestyle. *Sun exposure:* May increase risk of photosensitivity reactions. Advise patient to avoid excessive sunlight exposure.

EFFECTS ON LAB TEST RESULTS
• May increase AST, ALT, bilirubin, alkaline phosphatase, and creatinine levels. May decrease potassium and magnesium levels.
• May decrease hemoglobin, hematocrit, and platelet, WBC, and RBC counts.

ACTION
Antifungal action is achieved by inhibiting fungal cytochrome P-450–mediated 14-alpha-lanosterol demethylation, an essential step in fungal ergosterol biosynthesis.

PHARMACOKINETICS
Onset, immediate; peak, 1 to 2 hours; duration, 12 hours.
Distribution: Extensive, into tissue; 58% protein bound.
Metabolism: By cytochrome P-450 enzymes 2C19, 2C9, and 3A4.
Excretion: Less than 2% excreted unchanged in the urine.

CLINICAL CONSIDERATIONS
• Use P.O. form in patients with moderate to severe renal impairment, unless the benefits of I.V. use outweigh its risks.
• Infusion reactions, including flushing, fever, sweating, tachycardia, chest tightness, dyspnea, faintness, nausea, pruritus, and rash, may occur as soon

as infusion is started. Notify prescriber if reaction occurs. Infusion may need to be stopped.
• Monitor liver function test results at the start of and during therapy. Patients who develop abnormal liver function test results should be monitored for more severe hepatic injury. Stop drug if patient develops signs and symptoms of liver disease that may be caused by voriconazole use.
• Monitor visual acuity, visual fields, and color perception if treatment lasts more than 28 days.
• Monitor creatinine level in patients with creatinine clearance less than 50 ml/minute. If creatinine level increases, consider changing to P.O. form of drug.
• Drug may harm fetus. If drug is used during pregnancy or if the patient becomes pregnant while taking the drug, the patient should be informed of the potential hazard to the fetus.

PATIENT TEACHING
• Advise patient to avoid driving or operating machinery while taking drug, especially at night, because vision changes, including blurring and photophobia, may occur.
• Tell patient to avoid strong, direct sunlight during therapy.
• Tell woman of childbearing age to use effective contraception during treatment.

warfarin sodium
Coumadin

Pharmacologic class: coumarin derivative
Therapeutic class: anticoagulant
Pregnancy risk category: X
pH: 8.1 to 8.3

INDICATIONS & DOSAGES
➤ **Venous thrombosis, pulmonary embolism, atrial fibrillation, cardiac valve replacement, thromboembolism, recurrent MI, heart disease, and embolism—**
Adults: 2 to 5 mg daily; adjust dosage based on INR and PT. Maintenance dosage, also based on INR and PT, ranges from 2 to 10 mg daily.

Dosage requirements vary greatly among patients, and dosage must be individualized based on clinical and laboratory findings.

ADMINISTRATION
Direct injection: Inject diluted solution over 1 to 2 minutes in a peripheral vein.
Intermittent infusion: Not recommended.
Continuous infusion: Not recommended.

PREPARATION & STORAGE
Available as 5-mg single-use vials.
For infusion, reconstitute with 2.7 ml of sterile water for injection to yield a concentration of 2 mg/ml. Store vials at controlled room temperature and protect from light. Store reconstituted solution at controlled room temperature and use within 4 hours. Don't refrigerate. Discard unused portion.

Incompatibilities
Aminophylline, ammonium chloride, ceftazidime, cimetidine, ciprofloxacin, dobutamine, esmolol, gentamicin, heparin, labetalol, metronidazole, Ringer's injection, vancomycin.

CONTRAINDICATIONS & CAUTIONS
• Contraindicated in pregnant patients and in those with hemorrhagic tendencies or blood dyscrasias.
• Contraindicated in those who have had recent surgery of the CNS or eye or traumatic surgery resulting in large open surfaces.
• Contraindicated in those with cerebrovascular hemorrhage, aneurysms, pericarditis and pericardial effusions, bacterial endocarditis, or ulcerations of the GI, GU, or respiratory tract.
• Contraindicated in those with threatened abortion, eclampsia, or preeclampsia; unsupervised patients with senility, alcoholism, or psychosis; and uncooperative patients.
• Contraindicated in diagnostic or therapeutic procedures with potential for uncontrolled bleeding, such as spinal puncture, in major regional lumbar block anesthesia, and malignant hypertension.
• Use cautiously in those with hepatic or renal insufficiency, an infectious disease, disturbance of intestinal flora, trauma that may result in internal bleeding, or severe to moderate hypertension.
• Use cautiously in those with indwelling catheters, known or suspected deficiency in protein C–mediated anti-

coagulant response, polycythemia vera, vasculitis, or severe diabetes.

ADVERSE REACTIONS

CNS: *fever.*
GI: anorexia, nausea, vomiting, cramps, *diarrhea,* mouth ulcerations, sore mouth.
GU: hematuria.
Hematologic: *hemorrhage* (with excessive dosage).
Hepatic: *hepatitis,* jaundice.
Skin: dermatitis, urticaria, necrosis, gangrene, alopecia, *rash.*
Other: enhanced uric acid excretion.

INTERACTIONS

Drug-drug. *Acetaminophen:* May increase bleeding with use of acetaminophen longer than 2 weeks and doses higher than 2 g/day. Monitor patient closely.
Allopurinol, amiodarone, anabolic steroids, azithromycin, capecitabine, cephalosporins, chloramphenicol, cimetidine, clofibrate, co-trimoxazole, danazol, diazoxide, disulfiram, erythromycin, fenofibrate, fluoroquinolones, flutamide, glucagon, heparin, influenza virus vaccine, isoniazid, itraconazole, lovastatin, meclofenamate, metronidazole, methimazole, miconazole, neomycin (oral), NSAIDs, omeprazole, pentoxifylline, propafenone, propoxyphene, propylthiouracil, quinidine, quinine, salicylates, simvastatin, SSRIs, streptokinase, sulfonamides, tamoxifen, tetracyclines, thiazides, thyroid drugs, tramadol, tricyclic antidepressants, urokinase, vitamin E, zafirlukast, zileuton: Increases PT. Monitor patient closely for bleeding. May need to reduce warfarin dose.
Aminoglutethimide, atorvastatin, carbamazepine, corticosteroids, ethchlorvynol, glutethimide, griseofulvin, hormonal contraceptives, mercaptopurine, nafcillin, rifampin, spironolactone, trazodone, sucralfate, vitamin K: Decreas-

es anticoagulant effect. Avoid using together.
Anticonvulsants: Increases levels of phenytoin and phenobarbital. Monitor patient closely.
Barbiturates: May inhibit anticoagulant effect for several weeks after barbiturate withdrawal, and fatal hemorrhage can occur after cessation of barbiturate effect. Monitor patient closely. If barbiturates are withdrawn, reduce anticoagulant dose.
Chloral hydrate: May increase or decrease anticoagulant effect of warfarin. Avoid using together.
Ethacrynic acid, indomethacin, mefenamic acid, sulfinpyrazone: Increases anticoagulant effect of warfarin and cause severe GI irritation (may be ulcerogenic). Avoid using together.
Drug-herb. *Angelica root, anise, arnica flower, asafetida, bromelain, celery, chamomile, clove, danshen, devil's claw, dong quai, fenugreek, feverfew, garlic, ginger, ginkgo biloba, horse chestnut, licorice, meadowsweet, motherwort, onion, papain, parsley, passion flower, quassia, reishi mushroom, rue, sweet clover, turmeric:* May increase risk of bleeding. Discourage use together.
Angelica sinensis: May significantly prolong PT. Discourage use together.
Ginseng, St. John's wort, ubiquinone: May decrease anticoagulant effect. Discourage use together.
Green tea: Decreases anticoagulant effect. Advise patient to limit green tea and other foods or nutritional supplements containing vitamin K.
Drug-food. *Foods or enteral supplements containing vitamin K:* May impair anticoagulation. Advise patient to maintain a consistent daily intake of leafy green vegetables.
Drug-lifestyle. *Alcohol use:* May enhance anticoagulant effects. Discourage use together.

Reactions may be *common*, uncommon, ***life-threatening***, or COMMON AND LIFE-THREATENING.

EFFECTS ON LAB TEST RESULTS
• May increase ALT and AST levels.
• May increase INR, PT, and PTT.
• May falsely decrease theophylline levels.

ACTION
Inhibits vitamin K–dependent activation of clotting factors II, VII, IX, and X in the liver.

PHARMACOKINETICS
Onset within 1 hour; drug level peaks within 1 to 12 hours; anticoagulant action 24 to 72 hours; antithrombotic 6 days into therapy; duration of action 4 to 5 days.
Distribution: Distributed to liver, lungs, spleen, and kidneys. About 99% protein bound; crosses the placental barrier but doesn't appear in breast milk.
Metabolism: Metabolized in the liver to inactive metabolites.
Excretion: Excreted in bile, metabolites are reabsorbed and excreted in the urine, and to a lesser extent in bile. Half-life, about 1 to 3 days.

CLINICAL CONSIDERATIONS
• *Alert:* Use of a large loading dose may increase the risk of hemorrhage or other complications and doesn't offer faster protection against thrombi formation.
• Because of potential drug interactions, carefully observe patients for changes in prescribed drug regimens that may cause significant interactions.
• Monitor PT, PTT, and INR. Adjust dosage based on findings.
• Monitor for signs of bleeding.

PATIENT TEACHING
• Advise patient that strict adherence to dosage regimen is needed.
• Warn patient against taking OTC or prescription drugs or herbal medicines without prescriber's advice.

• Advise patient to avoid alcohol consumption during treatment.
• Advise any woman of childbearing age to avoid becoming pregnant during therapy.
• Reinforce importance of monitoring blood counts during therapy.
• Teach patient about appropriate diet, which maintains a consistent amount of vitamin K. Patient should avoid drastic changes in diet.
• Advise patient to report illness—such as diarrhea, infection, or fever—and any signs or symptoms of bleeding.
• Caution patient that the anticoagulant effects of the drug may last for 2 to 5 days after discontinuing.
• Tell patient to promptly report any unusual bruising or bleeding.
• Instruct patient to inform all prescribers (including dentists) about use of warfarin.

white blood cells (granulocyte concentrates, leukocytes)

Pharmacologic class: human whole blood derivative
Therapeutic class: antibacterial, antifungal
Pregnancy risk category: NR

INDICATIONS & DOSAGES
➤ **Life-threatening acquired neutropenia or congenital white cell dysfunction with bacterial and fungal infections unresponsive to antibiotics or other modes of therapy—**
For effective therapy, patient must receive 1 unit of granulocytes each day for at least 4 days or until infection is cured.
Adults: 1 unit q day until improvement or resolution of infection.
Children: 10 ml/kg q day based on 200-ml volume of unit.

ADMINISTRATION

Direct injection: Not recommended.
Intermittent infusion: Infuse through an 18G to 22G I.V. catheter through a Y-type blood set with at least a 170-micron filter. Always use normal saline with granulocyte transfusion. Don't use a small-pore or depth-type filter, which can trap white cells.

Slowly infuse 1 unit of granulocytes over 2 to 4 hours.
Continuous infusion: Not recommended.

PREPARATION & STORAGE

Hemapheresis is used to collect the granulocytes for infusion. Once collection has been completed, the granulocytes should be infused as soon as possible because their survival is less than 24 hours. They should be stored without agitation, for no longer than 24 hours at 68° to 75° F (20° to 24° C).

Incompatibilities

D_5W.

CONTRAINDICATIONS & CAUTIONS

• Contraindicated in those whose bone marrow isn't expected to recover.
• Contraindicated to prevent infection.
• Drug isn't indicated for those with infections that are responsive to antibiotics.

ADVERSE REACTIONS

CNS: disorientation, hallucinations.
CV: hypertension.
Respiratory: coughing, shortness of breath, dyspnea, wheezing, pulmonary infiltrates.
Other: febrile nonhemolytic reactions, shaking chills.

INTERACTIONS

Drug-drug. *Amphotericin B:* May cause pulmonary insufficiency. Don't give amphotericin B within 4 hours of transfusion.

EFFECTS ON LAB TEST RESULTS

None reported.

ACTION

Infusion provides granulocytes that defend the body by engulfing the infection and destroying it. This happens when the granulocytes enter the blood system and attach to the blood vessel wall. The vessel wall becomes porous, allowing the phagocytes to enter the affected tissue. The granulocytes then migrate toward, phagocytize, and kill the bacteria or fungi.

COMPOSITION

WBCs are the body's major resource of inflammatory and immune responses. They're separated into two groups, granulocytes and agranulocytes. Granulocytes derive their name from the granules found in the cytoplasm. They're made up of neutrophils and eosinophils, which act as phagocytes, destroying foreign substances in the body; and basophils, which have an active role in hypersensitivity reactions.

Agranulocytes don't have granules and are made up of monocytes, which are phagocytes and lymphocytes, some of which are responsible for antibody production.

Normal range for WBCs in a nonpregnant adult is 4,500 to 10,800/mm³. Neutrophils account for 50% to 70% of this value.

Granulocytes, collected by pheresis, are given to patients requiring transfusions of WBCs. A unit of granulocyte concentrate contains a minimum of 1×1^{10} granulocytes, a variable amount of lymphocytes—usually less than 10%—6,010 units of platelets, 30 to 50 ml of red cells, and 210 ml of plasma.

CLINICAL CONSIDERATIONS

• Because each unit of granulocytes contains 20% of RBCs and plasma, pa-

tients must be typed and crossmatched to ensure ABO compatibility.
• Rh-negative components may be transfused to Rh-positive patients.
• Ensure a patent venous catheter before calling the blood bank.
• Check blood compatibility by matching patient's name and blood bag number with patient's armband. Have another nurse perform similar check and document according to institutional procedures.
• Flush I.V. site with normal saline solution before and after giving WBCs.
• Use tubing with standard blood filter.
• Premedicate patient with an antihistamine, acetaminophen, a corticosteroid, or meperidine, as needed, to prevent reactions.
• Most reactions can be avoided or lessened by slow infusion and the use of meperidine.
• Take patient's vital signs before, during, and after blood transfusion.
• Observe infusion site for redness, swelling, or tenderness. If site becomes infiltrated, stop infusion and start new line.
• Closely observe patient for signs of reaction during administration.
• If anaphylaxis occurs, stop transfusion at the hub of the needle and keep vein open with normal saline. Notify prescriber and provide symptomatic treatment.
• Return blood product to blood bank for proper storage if there is a delay in administration.
• Continue to monitor patient after transfusion for delayed reactions.

PATIENT TEACHING
• Explain transfusion procedure to patient.
• Make sure patient understands reason for premedication.
• Inform patient of signs and symptoms of transfusion reactions, such as fever, chills, itchiness, and difficulty breathing.

• Instruct patient to notify prescriber if he's uncomfortable or experiences signs or symptoms of reaction.
• If patient is neutropenic, explain neutropenic precautions to patient and family members.

whole blood

Pharmacologic class: human whole blood
Therapeutic class: blood replacement
Pregnancy risk category: NR
pH: 6.8 to 7.2

INDICATIONS & DOSAGES
➤ **Acute, massive blood loss of more than 25% of total blood volume requiring oxygen-carrying properties of RBCs as well as volume expansion of plasma—**
Adults: Number of units depends on patient's condition.
Children: 20 ml/kg initially, followed by volume needed for stabilization.

ADMINISTRATION
Direct injection: Appropriate for neonates only. Draw prefiltered blood into a syringe and inject slowly through a 19G to 21G needle or catheter.
Intermittent infusion: Give through a Y-type or straight infusion set with a minimum 170-micron filter at a rate rapid enough to stabilize hemodynamic status. Use normal saline to prime and clear tubing. Also keep solution available for possible adverse reactions. Use automatic infusion devices only if they have been tested and approved for transfusion by the manufacturer. Don't inflate manual pressure cuffs above 300 mm Hg.
   Begin infusing blood slowly while remaining at the bedside. Take vital signs. If patient shows no evidence of a

transfusion reaction, adjust flow to the prescribed rate.

If rapid, massive transfusion is needed, you may use microaggregate filter (20- to 40-micron) to remove WBC particulates. Microaggregates may migrate to the lungs and cause dyspnea. *Continuous infusion:* Not recommended.

PREPARATION & STORAGE

Available in a sterile pack containing 475 ml of blood and 63 ml of an anticoagulant and preservative, such as citrate phosphate dextrose adenine, which prevents clotting and provides nutrients for long-term cell survival.

Store at 34° to 43° F (1° to 6° C) in a continuously monitored refrigerator; temperatures above or below this range may cause decreased viability, hemolysis, and bacterial proliferation. After removing whole blood from refrigerator and breaking sterile seal, infuse within 4 hours.

Incompatibilities

All drugs and solutions except normal saline solution.

CONTRAINDICATIONS & CAUTIONS

• Because of risk of disease transmission and adverse reactions, don't transfuse homologous blood if crystalloid or colloid solutions can treat the condition sufficiently. Acute loss of up to one-third of total blood volume, 3 to 4 units, can usually be treated effectively without blood transfusion.

ADVERSE REACTIONS

Metabolic: volume overload.
Skin: skin reactions.
Other: acute hemolytic reaction, graft-versus-host disease (GVHD), alloimmunization, febrile nonhemolytic reactions.

INTERACTIONS

None reported.

EFFECTS ON LAB TEST RESULTS

None reported.

COMPOSITION

One unit (513 ml) of whole blood contains about 180 to 240 ml of RBCs, 235 to 295 ml of plasma, and 63 ml of an anticoagulant and preservative. Whole blood may be homologous (collected from a random donor and tested for hepatitis and HIV) or autologous (collected from patient and saved for future use or salvaged during surgery or after trauma). Because autologous blood eliminates risk of alloimmunization and transmission of blood-borne diseases it's used, whenever possible, instead of homologous blood.

CLINICAL CONSIDERATIONS

• Confirm recipient's identity by comparing name and identification number on blood bag tag with that on patient's bracelet.
• Verify blood compatibility by comparing blood group and type on bag to chart or other blood bank record. Have another authorized staff member perform this check also. Accurate identification of recipient before drawing the crossmatch sample and beginning infusion can help prevent acute hemolytic reactions.
• The ABO type of whole blood must be identical to that of the recipient, but Rh-negative blood, lacking the D antigen, may be given to an Rh-positive patient.
• Warm blood to body temperature with an approved blood-warming device to prevent arrhythmias linked to rapid, massive infusions of cold blood.
• Take vital signs, record results, and establish a patent venous catheter before requesting release of blood from the blood bank.
• Monitor vital signs every 15 minutes, which may vary according to hospital protocol, until 1 hour after transfusion. Record vital signs, product number,

starting and ending times, volume infused, and response to transfusion.

• Watch for signs of volume overload, including cough, dyspnea, crackles at lung bases, and distended neck veins. If these occur, stop transfusion, keep the vein open with a slow infusion of normal saline, and contact prescriber. Diuretics and other measures to reduce fluid volume may be ordered. Whenever possible, prevent volume overload by giving concentrated blood components.

• If an acute hemolytic reaction occurs, stop transfusion at the needle hub and rapidly infuse normal saline. Contact the prescriber and blood bank and begin symptomatic treatment to maintain renal blood flow. Arrange a serologic evaluation of blood and urine.

• If a febrile nonhemolytic reaction occurs, stop the transfusion and keep the vein open with normal saline. Confirm recipient's identity and contact the prescriber and blood bank. Arrange a serologic evaluation of blood and urine, and start symptomatic treatment. If ordered, give antipyretics.

• Whole blood stored for more than 24 hours contains insignificant amounts of platelets and labile clotting factors V and VIII. Treat specific clotting deficiencies with component therapy.

PATIENT TEACHING

• Notify patient of potential adverse effects.

• Advise patient to immediately report adverse reactions.

• Tell the patient to report signs and symptoms of GVHD—such as fever, rash, and hepatitis—which may appear 2 to 3 weeks after transfusion. No effective therapy exists, but GVHD can be prevented by exposing blood to ionizing radiation (1,500 rad) before transfusion.

Z

zidovudine
Retrovir I.V. Infusion

Pharmacologic class: thymidine analogue; nucleoside reverse transcriptase inhibitor
Therapeutic class: antiviral
Pregnancy risk category: C
pH: 5.5

INDICATIONS & DOSAGES
➤ **HIV in patients who can't take oral zidovudine—**
Adults: 1 mg/kg I.V. over 1 hour, q 4 hours around-the-clock until oral therapy can be given.
➤ **To reduce risk of transmission of HIV from infected mother to fetus—**
Adults: 100 mg P.O., given between 14 and 34 weeks' gestation and continued throughout pregnancy. During labor, give loading dose of 2 mg/kg I.V. over 1 hour, followed by continuous infusion of 1 mg/kg/hour I.V. until delivery.
Neonates: 1.5 mg/kg I.V. over 30 minutes q 6 hours.
Adjust-a-dose: For those with creatinine clearance less than 15 ml/minute who are receiving dialysis, give 1 mg/ kg I.V. q 6 to 8 hours. For hemoglobin less than 7.5 g/dl, or more than 25% below baseline, or granulocyte count of less than 750 cells/mm^3, or more than 50% below baseline, stop therapy until bone marrow recovers.

In patients with mild to moderate hepatic dysfunction or liver cirrhosis, a reduction in the daily dose may be necessary.

ADMINISTRATION
Direct injection: Not recommended.
Intermittent infusion: Infuse over 1 hour. Dilute in D$_5$W to no more than 4 mg/ml.
Continuous infusion: After loading dose, use during labor and delivery until umbilical cord is clamped.

PREPARATION & STORAGE
Available as 200 mg in 20-ml vials.

To prepare, dilute zidovudine to a concentration not exceeding 4 mg/ml using D$_5$W, normal saline solution, dextrose 5% in normal saline solution, lactated Ringer's solution, or dextrose 5% in lactated Ringer's solution.

Store vials at 59° to 77° F (15° to 25° C) and protect from light. After dilution, resultant solution is stable for 24 hours at room temperature (77° F [25° C]) and 48 hours if refrigerated (36° to 46° F [2° to 8° C]). Give within 8 hours if stored at room temperature; within 24 hours if refrigerated.

Incompatibilities
Biological or colloidal solutions, such as blood products or protein-containing solutions; meropenem.

CONTRAINDICATIONS & CAUTIONS
• Contraindicated in those with known hypersensitivity to the drug.
• Use with caution in those with compromised bone marrow function because significant anemia may occur after 2 to 6 weeks of therapy. Dosage may need to be adjusted, drug may need to be discontinued, or patient may need to receive a transfusion.
• Use cautiously in those with impaired hepatic function; drug is metabolized

in the liver and may result in increased toxic reaction.

• Use cautiously in those with severe impairment of renal function.

ADVERSE REACTIONS

CNS: *headache,* dizziness, paresthesia, insomnia, mania, somnolence, asthenia, *malaise, seizures, fever.*

GI: diarrhea, dyspepsia, GI pain, *nausea, vomiting,* constipation, taste perversion, *anorexia.*

Hematologic: *severe bone marrow suppression resulting in anemia, agranulocytosis, thrombocytopenia.*

Musculoskeletal: myalgia, myopathy, myositis.

Respiratory: dyspnea.

Skin: *rash,* diffuse macular lesions, diaphoresis.

INTERACTIONS

Drug-drug. *Atovaquone, fluconazole, methadone, probenecid, valproic acid:* Increases bioavailability of zidovudine. May need to alter dosage.

Doxorubicin, ribavirin, stavudine: May cause antagonistic effects. Avoid using together.

Ganciclovir, interferon-alpha, and other bone marrow suppressive or cytotoxic agents: May increase hematologic toxicity of zidovudine. Use together cautiously, as with other reverse transcriptase inhibitors.

Nelfinavir, rifampin, ritonavir: Decreases bioavailability of zidovudine. No need to adjust dosage.

Phenytoin: Alters phenytoin level and decreases zidovudine clearance by 30%. Monitor patient closely.

EFFECTS ON LAB TEST RESULTS

• May increase ALT, AST, alkaline phosphatase, and LDH levels.

• May decrease hemoglobin and granulocyte and platelet counts.

ACTION

Converted intracellularly to an active compound that inhibits replication of HIV.

PHARMACOKINETICS

Distribution: Crosses the blood-brain and placental barriers; also appears in semen of HIV-infected patients; 34% to 38% protein bound.

Metabolism: Hepatic; rapidly metabolized to inactive metabolites.

Excretion: Renal, 14% to 18% by glomerular filtration and active tubular secretion in urine; 60% to 74% of inactive metabolite recovered in urine. Half-life, about 1 hour.

CLINICAL CONSIDERATIONS

• Osmolality: 10 mg/ml is 34 mOsm/kg.

• *Alert:* Lactic acidosis and severe hepatomegaly with steatosis has occurred. If unexplained dyspnea, tachypnea, or decreased bicarbonate levels occur, discontinue drug immediately and evaluate patient.

• Monitor CBC and platelet count at least every 2 weeks. Dosage may be reduced or discontinued if hematologic toxicity occurs.

• Significant anemia usually occurs after 4 to 6 weeks of therapy. This usually improves when drug is discontinued or dosage is reduced. Patient may still require blood transfusions even with lower doses.

• Observe patient for signs and symptoms of opportunistic infections.

• *Alert:* Combivir and Trizivir are combination products that contain zidovudine. Don't give with Retrovir IV.

PATIENT TEACHING

• Advise patient that drug won't cure the disease and illnesses linked to HIV infection, such as opportunistic infections, may continue to occur.

• Advise patient to report significant changes in health.

• Notify patient that adverse hematologic effects are more common in those with advanced disease.
• Reinforce importance of monitoring blood counts to prevent toxic reaction.
• Advise patient of potential drug interactions.
• Instruct patient to report muscle weakness, shortness of breath, or symptoms of hepatitis or pancreatitis.
• Advise patient that drug doesn't reduce the ability to transmit HIV.

zoledronic acid
Zometa

Pharmacologic class: bisphosphonate
Therapeutic class: antihypercalcemic
Pregnancy risk category: D
pH: 2

INDICATIONS & DOSAGES
➤ **Hypercalcemia related to malignancy—**
Adults: 4 mg by I.V. infusion over at least 15 minutes. If albumin-corrected calcium level doesn't return to normal, consider retreatment with 4 mg. Allow at least 7 days to pass before retreatment to allow a full response to the initial dose.
➤ **Multiple myeloma and bone metastases of solid tumors in conjunction with standard antineoplastic therapy; prostate cancer that has progressed after at least one course of hormonal therapy—**
Adults: 4 mg I.V. infused over 15 minutes q 3 or 4 weeks. Duration of treatment in the clinical studies was 15 months for prostate cancer, 12 months for breast cancer and multiple myeloma, and 9 months for other solid tumors.

Adjust-a-dose: The following guidelines are for patients who received zoledronic acid, have reduced renal function after the initial dose, and must be retreated with the drug: If the patient had a normal creatinine level before treatment and has an increase in creatinine level of 0.5 mg/dl within 2 weeks of the next dose, drug should be withheld until creatinine level is within 10% of baseline value. Likewise, if patient had an abnormal creatinine level before treatment and has an increase of 1 mg/dl within 2 weeks of the next dose, drug should be withheld until level is within 10% of baseline value.

ADMINISTRATION
Direct injection: Not recommended.
Intermittent infusion: Infuse over 15 minutes or longer.
Continuous infusion: Not recommended.

PREPARATION & STORAGE
Available as a white crystalline powder contained in a 4-mg vial.
  Reconstitute by adding 5 ml of sterile water to each vial. Inspect the solution to rule out particulate matter and discoloration before giving it. Make sure that the drug is completely dissolved. Withdraw 4 mg of drug and further dilute it in 100 ml of normal saline solution or D_5W.
  If not used immediately after reconstitution, the solution must be refrigerated at 36° to 46° F (2° to 8° C). Drug must be given within 24 hours after reconstitution.

Incompatibilities
Other I.V. drugs; solutions that contain calcium, such as lactated Ringer's solution.

CONTRAINDICATIONS & CAUTIONS
• Contraindicated in patients hypersensitive to drug or its components or other bisphosphonates.

Reactions may be *common*, uncommon, *life-threatening*, or COMMON AND LIFE-THREATENING.

• Contraindicated in patients with hypercalcemia of malignancy with creatinine level greater than 4.5 mg/dl or in patients with bone metastases with creatinine level greater than 3 mg/dl.

• Contraindicated in breast-feeding women because it's unknown if drug appears in breast milk.

• Use cautiously in patients with aspirin-sensitive asthma because other bisphosphonates have been linked to bronchoconstriction in aspirin-sensitive patients with asthma.

• Use cautiously in patients with renal impairment because the drug is excreted primarily via the kidneys. Drug should be used in patients with severe renal impairment only if benefits outweigh risks.

• Use cautiously in elderly patients because of the greater likelihood of disease, additional drug therapy, and decreased hepatic, renal, or cardiac function.

ADVERSE REACTIONS

For hypercalcemia trials
CNS: headache, somnolence, *anxiety, confusion, agitation, insomnia, fever.*
CV: *hypotension.*
GI: *nausea, constipation, diarrhea, abdominal pain, vomiting,* anorexia, dysphagia.
GU: *decreased creatinine level, urinary infection, candidiasis.*
Hematologic: anemia, **granulocytopenia, thrombocytopenia, pancytopenia.**
Metabolic: dehydration.
Musculoskeletal: *skeletal pain,* arthralgia.
Respiratory: *dyspnea, cough,* pleural effusion.
Other: PROGRESSION OF CANCER, infection.
For bone metastases trials
CNS: *headache,* anxiety, *insomnia, depression, paresthesia, hypoesthesia, fatigue, weakness, dizziness, fever.*
CV: *hypotension,* leg edema.

GI: *nausea, constipation, diarrhea, abdominal pain, vomiting, anorexia, increased appetite.*
GU: *decreased creatinine level, urinary infection.*
Hematologic: *anemia,* **neutropenia.**
Metabolic: *dehydration, weight loss.*
Musculoskeletal: *skeletal pain, arthralgia, myalgia, back pain.*
Respiratory: dyspnea, cough.
Skin: alopecia, dermatitis.
Other: PROGRESSION OF CANCER, rigors, infection.

INTERACTIONS

Drug-drug. *Aminoglycosides, loop diuretics:* Causes additive effects, which lower calcium level and increase risk of hypocalcemia. Use together cautiously, and monitor calcium level.
Thalidomide: May increase risk of renal dysfunction in multiple myeloma patients. Use together cautiously.

EFFECTS ON LAB TEST RESULTS

• May increase creatinine levels. May decrease calcium, phosphorus, magnesium, and potassium levels.

• May decrease hemoglobin, hematocrit, and RBC, WBC, and platelet counts.

ACTION

Inhibits bone resorption and inhibits calcium release induced by the stimulatory factors produced by tumors.

PHARMACOKINETICS

Duration, 7 to 28 days.
Distribution: About 22% protein bound. The rest is presumed to be bound to bone.
Metabolism: Doesn't inhibit P-450 enzymes or undergo biotransformation in vivo.
Excretion: Mostly in the kidneys; less than 3% in the feces. Half-life, 167 hours.

CLINICAL CONSIDERATIONS

• Make sure patient is adequately hydrated before giving drug; urine output should be about 2 L daily.

• Loop diuretics shouldn't be used until the patient is adequately rehydrated and then only with caution because of the increased risk of hypocalcemia.

• Faster infusion rates and higher-than-recommended doses may increase the risk of renal toxicity

• Monitor renal function and calcium, phosphate, magnesium, and creatinine levels during treatment.

• Monitor respiratory function closely in patients with asthma and aspirin sensitivity.

• Patients should also be given an oral calcium supplement of 500 mg and a multiple vitamin containing 400 IU of vitamin D daily.

• Overdose may cause clinically significant hypocalcemia, hypophosphatemia, and hypomagnesemia. Reductions in calcium, phosphorus, and magnesium levels should be corrected by I.V. administration of calcium gluconate, potassium and sodium phosphate, and magnesium sulfate, respectively.

PATIENT TEACHING

• Review the use and administration of drug with patient and family.

• Instruct patient to immediately report adverse reactions.

• Explain the importance of scheduled laboratory tests to monitor therapy and kidney function.

• Advise patient to alert prescriber if she is pregnant.

Nursing
I.V.
DRUG
HANDBOOK

MAJOR ELECTROLYTE COMPONENTS OF I.V. SOLUTIONS

SOLUTION	Sodium (mEq/L)	Potassium (mEq/L)	Osmolarity (mOsm/L)	
Aminosyn 3.5% M	47	13	477	
Aminosyn 7% with electrolytes	70	66	1,013	
Aminosyn 8.5% with electrolytes	70	66	1,160	
Dextrose 2.5% in half-strength lactated Ringer's injection	~65.5	2	265	
Dextrose 5% in electrolyte no. 48	25	20	348	
Dextrose 5% in electrolyte no. 75	40	35	402	
Dextrose 5% in sodium chloride 0.11%	19	-	290	
Dextrose 5% in sodium chloride 0.2%	34 or 38.5	-	320-330	
Dextrose 5% in sodium chloride 0.33%	51 or 56	-	355-365	
Dextrose 5% in sodium chloride 0.45%	77	-	~405	
Dextrose 5% in sodium chloride 0.9%	154	-	~560	
Dextrose 50% with electrolyte pattern A	84	40	2,800	
Dextrose 50% with electrolyte pattern N	90	80	2,875	
Dextrose 50% with electrolyte no. 1	110	80	2,917	
5% Travert and electrolyte no. 2	56	25	449	
FreAmine III 3% with electrolytes	35	24.5	405	
Ionosol B in dextrose 5% in water	57	25	426	
Ionosol MB in dextrose 5% in water	25	20	352	
Ionosol T in dextrose 5% in water	40	35	432	
Isolyte E	140	10	310	
Isolyte G with dextrose 5%	65	17	555	
Lactated Ringer's injection	130	4	~273	
Normosol-M in dextrose 5%	40	13	363	
Plasma-Lyte A	140	5	294	

Tonicity	Calcium (mEq/L)	Magnesium (mEq/L)	Chloride (mEq/L)	Acetate (mEq/L)	Phosphate (millimoles)	Other (mEq/L)
hypertonic	-	3	40	58	3.5	amino acids 3.5%
hypertonic	-	10	96	124	30	amino acids 7%
hypertonic	-	10	98	142	30	amino acids 8.5%
isotonic	1.4-1.5	~55	-	-	lactate 14	
isotonic	-	3	24	-	3	lactate 23
hypertonic	-	-	48	-	15	lactate 20
isotonic	-	-	19	-	-	-
isotonic	-	-	34 or 38.5	-	-	-
isotonic	-	-	51 or 56	-	-	-
hypertonic	-	-	77	-	-	-
hypertonic	-	-	154	-	-	-
hypertonic	10	16	115	-	-	gluconate 13 sulfate 16
hypertonic	-	16	150	-	28	sulfate 16
hypertonic	-	16	140	36	24	-
hypertonic	-	6	56	-	12.5	lactate 25
hypertonic	-	5	41	44	3.5	amino acids 3%
hypertonic	-	5	49	-	7	lactate 25
hypotonic	-	3	22	-	3	lactate 23
hypertonic	-	-	40	-	15	lactate 20
isotonic	5	3	103	49	-	citrate 8
hypertonic	-	-	149	-	-	ammonium 70
isotonic	2.7-3	-	~109	-	-	lactate 28
hypertonic	-	3	40	16	-	-
isotonic	-	3	98	27	-	gluconate 23

(continued)

SOLUTION	Sodium (mEq/L)	Potassium (mEq/L)	Osmolarity (mOsm/L)	
Plasma-Lyte R	140	10	312	
ProcalAmine	35	24	735	
Ringer's injection	147 or 147.5	4	310	
Sodium bicarbonate 5%	595	-	1,190-1,203	
Sodium chloride 0.45%	77	-	154	
Sodium chloride 0.9%	154	-	308	
Sodium chloride 3%	513	-	1,030	
Sodium chloride 5%	855	-	1,710	
Sodium lactate 1/6 M	167	-	330	
Travasol 3.5% with electrolytes	25	15	450	
Travasol 5.5% with electrolytes	70	60	850	
Travasol 8.5% with electrolytes	70	60	1,160	
Fat emulsion 10%, 20%, 30%	-	-	258-310	

Tonicity	Calcium (mEq/L)	Magnesium (mEq/L)	Chloride (mEq/L)	Acetate (mEq/L)	Phosphate (millimoles)	Other (mEq/L)
isotonic	5	3	103	47	-	lactate 8
hypertonic	3	5	41	47	3.5	amino acids 3% glycerin 3%
isotonic	4 or 4.5	-	155 or 156	-	-	-
hypertonic	-	-	-	-	-	HCO$_3$ 595
hypotonic	-	-	77	-	-	-
isotonic	-	-	154	-	-	-
hypertonic	-	-	513	-	-	-
hypertonic	-	-	855	-	-	-
isotonic	-	-	-	-	-	lactate 167
hypertonic	-	5	25	52	7.5	-
hypertonic	-	10	70	102	30	-
hypertonic	-	10	70	141	30	-
isotonic	-	-	-	-	-	egg yolk phospholipids 1.2%

PREVENTING AND TREATING EXTRAVASATION

Extravasation—the inadvertent administration of a vesicant solution or drug into surrounding tissue—can result from a punctured vein or from leakage around a venipuncture site. Vesicants can cause blisters and severe local tissue damage. This may cause prolonged healing, infection, cosmetic disfigurement, and loss of function and may necessitate multiple debridements or amputation.

Preventing extravasation

To avoid extravasation when giving vesicants, adhere to proper administration techniques and follow these guidelines:

• Don't use an existing I.V. line unless you're sure it's patent. Perform a new venipuncture to ensure correct needle placement and vein patency.

• Select the site carefully. Use a distal vein that allows successive proximal venipunctures. To avoid tendon and nerve damage from extravasation, don't use the back of the hand. Also avoid the wrist and fingers (they're hard to immobilize), previously damaged areas, and areas with poor circulation.

• Start the infusion with D_5W or normal saline solution.

• Use a transparent film dressing to allow inspection.

• Check for extravasation before starting the infusion. Check for blood return. Flush the needle to ensure patency. Palpate the vein and surrounding area while flushing. If swelling occurs at the I.V. site, the solution is infiltrating.

• Give vesicants after the I.V. line is tested with normal saline solution and before multiple manipulations that may dislodge the needle.

• Don't use an infusion pump to give vesicants. A pump will continue the infusion if infiltration occurs.

• Give the drug by slow I.V. push through a free-flowing I.V. line or by small-volume infusion (50 to 100 ml).

• When giving the drug, check the infusion site for erythema or infiltration. Tell the patient to report burning, stinging, pruritus, or temperature changes.

• After giving the drug, instill several milliliters of normal saline solution to flush the drug from the vein and avoid drug leakage when the needle is removed.

Treating extravasation

Extravasation of vesicants requires emergency treatment. Follow your facility's protocol. Essential steps include:

• Stop the I.V. flow, aspirate the remaining drug in the catheter, and remove the I.V. line, unless you need the needle to infiltrate the antidote.

• Estimate the amount of extravasated solution, and notify the prescriber.

• Instill the appropriate antidote, according to facility protocol.

• Have the patient elevate the affected arm or leg, and avoid excessive pressure on the site.

• Record the extravasation site, the patient's symptoms, the estimated amount of infiltrated solution, and the treatment. Include the prescriber's name and the time you notified him. Continue documenting the site's appearance and patient's symptoms.

• Apply either ice packs or warm compresses to the affected area. Apply ice to most extravasated areas for 15 to 20 minutes every 4 to 6 hours for about

3 days. However, for etoposide and vinca alkaloids, apply heat.

• Patient should continue to rest and elevate the site for 48 hours before re-
suming normal activity.

• If skin breakdown occurs, apply silver
sulfadiazine cream and gauze dressings
or wet-to-dry povidone-iodine dressings.

• If severe extravasation occurs, de-
bridement, plastic surgery, and physical
therapy may be needed.

Those who prepare and handle chemotherapeutic drugs face a significant risk. Although the extent of risk hasn't been fully determined, antineoplastics increase the handler's chances of reproductive abnormalities and may cause hematologic problems. Continuous exposure to these drugs may damage the liver and skin. These drugs also pose certain environmental dangers. Therefore, use caution whenever handling chemotherapeutic drugs.

The Occupational Safety and Health Administration (OSHA) has set guidelines to help ensure the safety of both the handler and the environment. These guidelines include two basic requirements:
• All health care workers who handle chemotherapeutic drugs should be specifically trained, with an emphasis on reducing exposure while handling these drugs.
• The drugs must be prepared within a class II or III biological safety cabinet.

Safety equipment

To protect yourself and the environment, wear a face shield or goggles, a long-sleeved gown, surgical gloves made from latex (or nitrile, if you're allergic to latex), with cuffs long enough to tuck over the cuffs of the gown. Wear disposable gowns made of lint-free, low-permeability fabric with a closed front, long sleeves, and elastic or knot closed cuffs if you're preparing or giving drugs. Make sure you have eyewash, a plastic absorbent pad, alcohol wipes, sterile gauze pads, shoe covers, and an impervious container with the label "Caution: Biohazard" for the disposal of any unused drug or equipment.

Also, keep a chemotherapeutic spill kit handy. To create a kit, you need a water-resistant, nonpermeable, long-sleeved gown with cuffs and back closure; shoe covers; two pairs of high-grade, extra-thick latex gloves (for double-gloving); goggles; a mask; a disposable dustpan and a plastic scraper (for collecting broken glass); plastic-lined or absorbent towels; a container of desiccant powder or granules (to absorb wet contents); two disposable sponges; a puncture- and leak-proof container labeled "Biohazard Waste"; and detergent for cleaning the spill area.

Precautions for drug preparation

Prepare the prescribed chemotherapeutic drugs according to product instructions, with special attention to compatibility, stability, and reconstitution technique.
• Wash your hands before and after drug preparation and administration. Prepare the drugs in a class II or III biological safety cabinet. Wear protective garments, including gloves, as required by the facility's policy. Don't wear these garments outside the preparation area. Never eat, drink, smoke, or apply cosmetics in the drug preparation area.
• Before and after preparing the drug, clean the inside of the cabinet according to the drug manufacturer's instructions. When finished, discard cleaning products in a leakproof chemical or biohazard waste container, according to facility policy. Then cover the work surface with a clean, plastic absorbent pad to minimize contamination by droplets or spills. Change the pad at the end of each shift and after any spill.
• All drug preparation equipment and any unused drug are hazardous waste. Dispose of them according to facility policy. Place all chemotherapeutic

waste products in leakproof, sealable, plastic bags or another suitable container, and make sure the container is appropriately labeled.

Special considerations

Reduce exposure to chemotherapeutic drugs by following these guidelines:

• Remember that systemic absorption can occur if contaminated materials are ingested or inhaled or if they come in contact with the skin. You can accidentally inhale a drug while opening a vial, clipping a needle, expelling air from a syringe, or discarding excess drug that splashes. Drug absorption also can result from handling contaminated feces or body fluids.

• Prime I.V. bags containing chemotherapeutic drugs in an approved class II or III biological safety cabinet. Leave the blower on 24 hours a day, 7 days a week.

• If the safety cabinet doesn't have a hood, prepare drugs in a quiet, well-ventilated work space, away from heating or cooling vents and other personnel. Wear a respirator with a high-efficiency filter.

• If you must prime the drug at the administration site, prime the I.V. line with a fluid that doesn't contain the drug or use a backflow-closed system. Discard used supplies with other chemotherapy waste.

• Have the biological safety cabinet examined every 6 months and whenever it's moved by a company that specializes in certifying such equipment.

• Vent vials with a hydrophobic filter, or use negative-pressure techniques. Use a needle with a hydrophobic filter to remove the solution from vials. Break ampules by wrapping a sterile gauze pad or alcohol wipe around the ampule's neck to decrease the chances of droplet contamination.

• Use only syringes and I.V. sets with luer-lock fittings.

• Mark all chemotherapeutic drugs with "Chemotherapy Hazard" labels.

• Don't clip needles, break syringes, or remove needles from syringes used in drug preparation. Use a gauze pad when removing syringes and needles from I.V. bags of chemotherapeutic drugs.

• Place used syringes, needles, and other sharp or breakable items in a puncture-proof container.

• Change gloves every 30 minutes and whenever you spill a drug solution or puncture or tear a glove. Wash your hands before putting on and after removing gloves.

• If the drug touches your skin, wash the area thoroughly with soap (not a germicidal agent) and water. If drug contacts your eye, hold your eyelid open and flood the eye with water or isotonic eyewash for at least 5 minutes. Obtain a medical evaluation as soon as possible after accidental exposure.

• Use a chemotherapeutic spill kit to clean up a major spill.

• Discard disposable gowns and gloves in an appropriately marked, waterproof receptacle whenever they become contaminated or whenever you leave the work area.

• Never place food or drinks in a refrigerator that contains chemotherapeutic drugs.

• Understand individual drug excretion patterns because they vary significantly. Take appropriate precautions when handling a chemotherapy patient's body fluids, especially if he's receiving a drug that's excreted in an active state.

• Wear disposable latex or nitrile gloves when handling body fluids or soiled linens of patients who have received chemotherapeutic drugs in the past 48 hours. Give men a urinal with a tight-fitting lid. Before flushing the toilet, place a waterproof pad over the toilet bowl to prevent splashing. Place soiled linens in designated isolation linen bags.

• Remember that women who are pregnant, trying to conceive, or breast-feeding should be extremely careful when handling chemotherapeutic drugs.

• Document each exposure incident according to facility policy.

Home care considerations

Remember these guidelines when giving chemotherapy to a patient at home:

• If chemotherapeutic drugs aren't provided by the home care agency pharmacy, contact the patient to confirm that he obtained them from a hospital pharmacy or a specialized retail pharmacy. Drug should be packaged in a sealed plastic bag.

• Determine that the home care agency has received precertification or authorization from the patient's insurance company for home administration of these drugs. If the patient's chemotherapy treatment requires a 24-hour continuous infusion, it's typically given through a portable infusion pump. Make sure all infusion equipment is available and ready for use, or bring it with you.

• Teach patient or caregiver to wear two pairs of latex or nitrile gloves whenever he handles chemotherapy equipment, contaminated linens or bedclothes, or body fluids.

• Instruct patient or caregiver to place soiled linens in a separate washable pillowcase and to launder the pillowcase twice, with the soiled linen inside, separate from other household items.

• Teach patient or caregiver how to manage a chemotherapy spill. Provide spill kit or help assemble needed supplies. Give him a phone number with 24-hour availability, and instruct him to contact his prescriber if he has questions or concerns or if a chemotherapy spill occurs.

• Advise patient or caregiver to arrange for pickup and proper disposal of contaminated waste, and help make these arrangements.

• Instruct patient or caregiver to place all treatment equipment in a leakproof container before disposal.

• Advise patient or caregiver to dispose of waste products in the toilet, emptying the container close to the water to minimize splashing. Advise him to close the lid and flush two or three times.

SELECTED DRUGS FOR CONSCIOUS SEDATION IN ADULTS

Defined as the induction of a minimally depressed level of consciousness (LOC), conscious sedation is used during certain short medical procedures to relieve pain and anxiety, produce a hypnotic state, cause short-term amnesia, or achieve a combination of these effects. Conscious sedation has gained widespread popularity and is now performed in gastroenterology, radiology, pulmonology, and cardiac catheterization suites as well as in critical care settings.

Required safeguards
Conscious sedation must occur in a controlled environment with emergency resuscitative equipment readily available. During the procedure, the patient must be able to maintain a patent airway independently and respond appropriately to physical or verbal commands. To avoid deep sedation and cardiopulmonary depression, the sedative dose is titrated to decrease the patient's LOC only to the point of slurred speech and nystagmus.

Drug options
Drugs used for conscious sedation include analgesics, hypnotics, and amnestic drugs. This table gives general dosing guidelines and key nursing considerations for the drugs most commonly used to produce conscious sedation in adults. Given alone or in combination, these drugs produce varying levels of sedation and commonly have potent synergistic effects.

Drug	Dosage	Key considerations
diazepam (Valium) Benzodiazepine with anxiolytic, amnestic, anticonvulsant, skeletal muscle relaxant, and sedative-hypnotic properties	*Adults:* Give up to 10 mg I.V. slowly, immediately before the procedure. If drug is given without opiates, up to 20 mg I.V. may be required. Or, give 5-10 mg I.M. 30 min before the procedure.	●Individualize doses and titrate to achieve desired effect. ●Drug is a potent respiratory depressant, particularly when given with opioids. ●Hypotension and bradycardia may occur in patients premedicated with an opioid. ●Inject directly into large vein at no more than 5 mg/min. Don't inject intra-arterially. ●For reversal of sedative effects, give flumazenil (Romazicon). Individualize dosage; generally, 0.2 mg I.V. over 30 sec. If needed, may follow with 0.3 mg over 30 sec, then 0.5 mg q min, up to a maximum dose of 3 mg.
fentanyl citrate (Sublimaze) Opioid agonist that's 100 times more potent than morphine sulfate; its analgesic activity of 100 mcg is equivalent to 10 mg morphine or 75 mg meperidine	*Adults:* 0.5-1 mcg/kg I.V. titrated in 25-mcg increments over several minutes. *Elderly or debilitated patients with renal or hepatic disease:* Individualize and reduce dosage.	●Watch for bradycardia, hypotension, apnea, respiratory depression, and chest wall rigidity. ●Drug may cause nausea and vomiting. ●Contraindicated in patients with elevated intracranial pressure or head trauma.

(continued)

Drug	Dosage	Key considerations
fentanyl citrate (Sublimaze) *(continued)*		• If overdose occurs, maintain patent airway and provide respiratory and CV support. • Use naloxone (Narcan), to reverse respiratory and CV-depressant effects. Low doses (1-4 mcg/kg) have been used to reverse respiratory depression caused by conscious sedation procedures. Patient may need additional doses (0.1-0.2 mg) based on total dosage and time elapsed since last opioid dose.
lorazepam (Ativan) Benzodiazepine with sedative-hypnotic and anxiolytic properties	*Adults:* 2 mg or 0.044 mg/kg I.V., whichever is less, 15-20 min before the procedure. For greater amnestic effect, give up to 4 mg I.V. *Elderly patients:* Use reduced dosage and wait several minutes to evaluate drug effect before giving additional sedative doses. Don't exceed 2 mg I.V. total in patients older than age 50.	• Individualize doses and titrate to achieve desired effect. • Before I.V. administration, dilute drug with an equal volume of compatible solution and inject directly into the vein or into the tubing of an existing I.V. infusion at a rate not exceeding 2 mg/min. • Have emergency resuscitation equipment available when giving drug I.V. • For reversal of sedative effects, administer flumazenil (Romazicon). Individualize dosage; generally, 0.2 mg I.V. over 15 sec. May repeat p.r.n. Don't exceed 3 mg in any 1-hr period.
midazolam (Versed) Ultrashort-acting, water-soluble benzodiazepine with amnestic, anxiolytic, sedative, muscle relaxant, and anticonvulsant properties	*Healthy adults:* 0.5 mg I.V. over 2 min. For initial dose, don't exceed 2.5 mg. Some patients may respond to as little as 0.5-1 mg. *Adults age 60 and older or debilitated patients with decreased pulmonary reserve:* Incremental doses of 0.25-0.5 mg I.V. over 2 min. Wait several minutes to evaluate drug effect before giving additional sedative doses.	• Individualize doses and titrate to achieve desired effect. • Bolus administration isn't recommended for conscious sedation procedures. • Drug is potent respiratory depressant, particularly when given with opioids. • Hypotension and bradycardia may occur in patients premedicated with an opioid. • Excessive doses or hypoxia may lead to agitation, involuntary movement, hyperactivity, and combativeness. • For reversal of sedative effects, give flumazenil (Romazicon). Reversal dosage is individualized; usually, 0.2 mg is given I.V. over 15 sec. May repeat dose to achieve desired effect. Don't exceed 3 mg in any 1-hr period.
meperidine (Demerol) Opioid analgesic that's also used as an adjunct to anesthesia	*Adults:* 50-100 mg I.M. or S.C. 30-90 min before anesthesia.	• Watch for bradycardia, hypotension, respiratory depression, and apnea. • Drug may cause nausea and vomiting. • If I.V. administration is necessary, decrease dosage and give slowly, preferably as a diluted solution. • Use naloxone (Narcan) to reverse respiratory and CV depressant effects.

INFUSION RATES

The infusion rates are based on the concentrations shown at the top of each table. Be sure to check the label on the drug you're infusing to verify the correct infusion rate.

Epinephrine infusion rates
Mix 1 mg in 250 ml (4 mcg/ml).

Dose (mcg/min)	Infusion rate (ml/hr)
1	15
2	30
3	45
4	60
5	75
6	90
7	105
8	120
9	135
10	150
15	225
20	300
25	375
30	450
35	525
40	600

Isoproterenol infusion rates
Mix 1 mg in 250 ml (4 mcg/ml).

Dose (mcg/min)	Infusion rate (ml/hr)
0.5	8
1	15
2	30
3	45
4	60
5	75
6	90
7	105
8	120
9	135
10	150
15	225
20	300
25	375
30	450

Nitroglycerin infusion rates
Determine the infusion rate in milliliters per hour using the ordered dose and the concentration of the drug solution.

Dose (mcg/min)	25 mg/250 ml (100 mcg/ml)	50 mg/250 ml (200 mcg/ml)	100 mg/250 ml (400 mcg/ml)
5	3	2	1
10	6	3	2
20	12	6	3
30	18	9	5
40	24	12	6
50	30	15	8
60	36	18	9
70	42	21	10
80	48	24	12
90	54	27	14
100	60	30	15
150	90	45	23
200	120	60	30

(continued)

Dobutamine infusion rates

Mix 250 mg in 250 ml of D$_5$W (1,000 mcg/ml). Determine the infusion rate in milliliters per hour using the ordered dose and the patient's weight in pounds or kilograms.

Dose (mcg/kg/ min)	lb 88	99	110	121	132	143	154	165	176	187	198	209	220	231	242
	kg 40	45	50	55	60	65	70	75	80	85	90	95	100	105	110
2.5	6	7	8	8	9	10	11	11	12	13	14	14	15	16	17
5	12	14	15	17	18	20	21	23	24	26	27	29	30	32	33
7.5	18	20	23	25	27	29	32	34	36	38	41	43	45	47	50
10	24	27	30	33	36	39	42	45	48	51	54	57	60	63	66
12.5	30	34	38	41	45	49	53	56	60	64	68	71	75	79	83
15	36	41	45	50	54	59	63	68	72	77	81	86	90	95	99
20	48	54	60	66	72	78	84	90	96	102	108	114	120	126	132
25	60	68	75	83	90	98	105	113	120	128	135	143	150	158	165
30	72	81	90	99	108	117	126	135	144	153	162	171	180	189	198
35	84	95	105	116	126	137	147	158	168	179	189	200	210	221	231
40	96	108	120	132	144	156	168	180	192	204	216	228	240	252	264

Dopamine infusion rates

Mix 400 mg in 250 ml of D$_5$W (1,600 mcg/ml). Determine the infusion rate in milliliters per hour using the ordered dose and the patient's weight in pounds or kilograms.

Dose (mcg/kg/ min)	lb 88	99	110	121	132	143	154	165	176	187	198	209	220	231
	kg 40	45	50	55	60	65	70	75	80	85	90	95	100	105
2.5	4	4	5	5	6	6	7	7	8	8	8	9	9	10
5	8	8	9	10	11	12	13	14	15	16	17	18	19	20
7.5	11	13	14	15	17	18	20	21	23	24	25	27	28	30
10	15	17	19	21	23	24	26	28	30	32	34	36	38	39
12.5	19	21	23	26	28	30	33	35	38	40	42	45	47	49
15	23	25	28	31	34	37	39	42	45	48	51	53	56	59
20	30	34	38	41	45	49	53	56	60	64	68	71	75	79
25	38	42	47	52	56	61	66	70	75	80	84	89	94	98
30	45	51	56	62	67	73	79	84	90	96	101	107	113	118
35	53	59	66	72	79	85	92	98	105	112	118	125	131	138
40	60	68	75	83	90	98	105	113	120	128	135	143	150	158
45	68	76	84	93	101	110	118	127	135	143	152	160	169	177
50	75	84	94	103	113	122	131	141	150	159	169	178	188	197

Nitroprusside infusion rates

Mix 50 mg in 250 ml of D₅W (200 mcg/ml). Determine the infusion rate in milliliters per hour using the ordered dose and the patient's weight in pounds or kilograms.

Dose (mcg/kg/ min)	lb 88	99	110	121	132	143	154	165	176	187	198	209	220	231	242
	kg 40	45	50	55	60	65	70	75	80	85	90	95	100	105	110
0.3	4	4	5	5	5	6	6	7	7	8	8	9	9	9	10
0.5	6	7	8	8	9	10	11	11	12	13	14	14	15	16	17
1	12	14	15	17	18	20	21	23	24	26	27	29	30	32	33
1.5	18	20	23	25	27	29	32	34	36	38	41	43	45	47	50
2	24	27	30	33	36	39	42	45	48	51	54	57	60	63	66
3	36	41	45	50	54	59	63	68	72	77	81	86	90	95	99
4	48	54	60	66	72	78	84	90	96	102	108	114	120	126	132
5	60	68	75	83	90	98	105	113	120	128	135	143	150	158	165
6	72	81	90	99	108	117	126	135	144	153	162	171	180	189	198
7	84	95	105	116	126	137	147	158	168	179	189	200	210	221	231
8	96	108	120	132	144	156	168	180	192	204	216	228	240	252	264
9	108	122	135	149	162	176	189	203	216	230	243	257	270	284	297
10	120	135	150	165	180	195	210	225	240	255	270	285	300	315	330

CANCER CHEMOTHERAPY: ACRONYMS AND PROTOCOLS

This table lists commonly used chemotherapy acronyms and protocols, including standard dosages for specific cancers.

Indication & acronym	Generic drug name	Trade drug name	Dosage
Adenocarcinoma FAM	fluorouracil (5-FU)	Adrucil	600 mg/m^2 I.V., days 1, 8, 29, and 36
	doxorubicin	Adriamycin	30 mg/m^2 I.V., days 1 and 29
	mitomycin	Mutamycin	10 mg/m^2 I.V., day 1 *Repeat cycle q 8 wk.*
Bladder cancer CISCA	cisplatin	Platinol	100 mg/m^2 I.V., day 2
	cyclophosphamide	Cytoxan	650 mg/m^2 I.V., day 1
	doxorubicin	Adriamycin	50 mg/m^2 I.V., day 1 *Repeat cycle q 21-28 days.*
GC	gemcitabine	Gemzar	1 g/m^2 I.V. over 30-60 min, days 1, 8, and 15
	cisplatin	Platinol	70 mg/m^2 I.V., day 2 *Repeat cycle q 28 days.*
MVAC	methotrexate		30 mg/m^2 I.V., days 1, 15, and 22
	vinblastine	Velban	3 mg/m^2 I.V., days 2, 15, and 22
	doxorubicin	Adriamycin	30 mg/m^2 I.V., day 2
	cisplatin	Platinol	70 mg/m^2 I.V., day 2 *Repeat cycle q 28 days.*
Bony sarcoma AC	doxorubicin	Adriamycin	75-90 mg/m^2 (total dose) by 96-hr continuous I.V. infusion
	cisplatin	Platinol	90-120 mg/m^2 intra-arterial or I.V., day 6 *Repeat cycle q 28 days.*
HDMTX (high-dose methotrexate)	methotrexate		8-12 g/m^2 I.V. weekly for 2-12 wk
	leucovorin calcium		15-25 mg/m^2 I.V. or P.O. q 6 hr for 10 doses, beginning 24 hr after methotrexate dose (monitor methotrexate levels) *Repeat cycle q 7 days for 2-4 wk.*
Brain tumors PCV	procarbazine	Matulane	60 mg/m^2 P.O., days 8-21
	lomustine (CCNU)	CeeNu	110 mg/m^2 P.O., day 1
	vincristine	Oncovin	1.4 mg/m^2 (2 mg maximum) I.V., days 8 and 29 *Repeat cycle q 6-8 wk.*

Indication & acronym	Generic drug name	Trade drug name	Dosage
Breast cancer			
AC	doxorubicin	Adriamycin	60 mg/m^2 I.V., day 1
	cyclophosphamide	Cytoxan	600 mg/m^2 I.V., day 1 *Repeat cycle q 21 days.*
CAF	cyclophosphamide	Cytoxan	100 mg/m^2 P.O., days 1-14
	doxorubicin	Adriamycin	30 mg/m^2 I.V., days 1 and 8
	fluorouracil (5-FU)	Adrucil	500 mg/m^2 I.V., days 1 and 8 *Repeat cycle q 28 days.*
	or		
	cyclophosphamide	Cytoxan	500 mg/m^2 I.V., day 1
	doxorubicin	Adriamycin	50 mg/m^2 I.V., day 1
	fluorouracil (5-FU)	Adrucil	500 mg/m^2 I.V., day 1 *Repeat cycle q 21 days.*
CEF	cyclophosphamide	Cytoxan	75 mg/m^2 P.O., days 1-14
	epirubicin	Ellence	60 mg/m^2 I.V., days 1 and 8
	fluorouracil (5-FU)	Adrucil	500 mg/m^2 I.V., days 1 and 8
	co-trimoxazole	Bactrim	2 tablets (single-strength) P.O. twice daily, days 1-28 *Repeat cycle q 28 days.*
CMF	cyclophosphamide	Cytoxan	100 mg/m^2 P.O., days 1-14; or 400-600 mg/m^2 I.V., day 1
	methotrexate		40 mg/m^2 I.V., days 1 and 8
	fluorouracil (5-FU)	Adrucil	400-600 mg/m^2 I.V., days 1 and 8 *Repeat cycle q 28 days.*
Dox-CMF, Sequential	doxorubicin	Adriamycin	75 mg/m^2 I.V., day 1 for 4 cycles, followed by CMF regimen for 8 cycles *Repeat cycle q 21 days.*
FAC (CAF)	fluorouracil (5-FU)	Adrucil	500 mg/m^2 I.V., day 1
	doxorubicin	Adriamycin	50 mg/m^2 I.V., day 1
	cyclophosphamide	Cytoxan	500 mg/m^2 I.V., day 1 *Repeat cycle q 21 days.*
FEC	fluorouracil (5-FU)	Adrucil	500 mg/m^2 I.V., day 1
	epirubicin	Ellence	100 mg/m^2 I.V., day 1
	cyclophosphamide	Cytoxan	500 mg/m^2 I.V., day 1 *Repeat cycle q 21 days.*
Trastuzumab-paclitaxel	trastuzumab	Herceptin	4 mg/kg I.V. over 90 min as loading dose, day 1; then 2 mg/kg I.V. over 30 min weekly, days 1, 8, and 15, except for day 1 of first cycle
	paclitaxel	Taxol	175 mg/m^2 I.V. over 3 hr, day 1 *Repeat cycle q 21 days.*

(continued)

Indication & acronym	Generic drug name	Trade drug name	Dosage
Colorectal cancer F-CL (FU/LV)	fluorouracil (5-FU)	Adrucil	370-425 mg/m² I.V., days 1-5, after starting leucovorin
	leucovorin calcium		20 mg/m² I.V., days 1-5 *Repeat cycle q 28-56 days.*
	or		
	fluorouracil (5-FU)	Adrucil	600 mg/m² I.V., 1 hr after starting leucovorin infusion, weekly for 6 wk; then 2-wk rest period
	leucovorin calcium		500 mg/m² over 2 hr weekly for 6 wk; then 2-wk rest period *Repeat cycle q 28-56 days.*
FU/LV/CPT-11	irinotecan	Camptosar	125 mg/m² I.V. over 90 min, days 1, 8, 15, and 22
	fluorouracil (5-FU)	Adrucil	500 mg/m² I.V., days 1, 8, 15, and 22
	leucovorin calcium		20 mg/m² I.V., days 1, 8, 15, and 22 *Repeat cycle q 42 days.*
Endometrial cancer AP	doxorubicin	Adriamycin	50-60 mg/m² I.V., day 1
	cisplatin	Platinol	50-60 mg/m² I.V., day 1 *Repeat q 21-28 days.*
Gastric cancer FAM	fluorouracil (5-FU)	Adrucil	600 mg/m² I.V., days 1, 8, 29, and 36
	doxorubicin	Adriamycin	30 mg/m² I.V., days 1 and 29
	mitomycin	Mutamycin	10 mg/m² I.V., day 1 *Repeat cycle q 8 wk.*
Head and neck cancer CF	cisplatin	Platinol	100 mg/m² I.V., day 1
	fluorouracil (5-FU)	Adrucil	1,000 mg/m² daily by continuous I.V. infusion, days 1-5 *Repeat cycle q 21-28 days.*
	or		
	carboplatin	Paraplatin	300 mg/m² I.V., day 1
	fluorouracil (5-FU)	Adrucil	1,000 mg/m² daily by continuous I.V. infusion, days 1-5 *Repeat cycle q 21-28 days.*
Hodgkin's disease ABVD	doxorubicin	Adriamycin	25 mg/m² I.V., days 1 and 15
	bleomycin	Blenoxane	10 units/m² I.V., days 1 and 15
	vinblastine	Velban	6 mg/m² I.V., days 1 and 15
	dacarbazine	DTIC-Dome	350-375 mg/m² I.V., days 1 and 15 *Repeat cycle q 28 days.*

Indication & acronym	Generic drug name	Trade drug name	Dosage
Hodgkin's disease *(continued)*			
MOPP	mechlorethamine (nitrogen mustard)	Mustargen	6 mg/m² I.V., days 1 and 8
	vincristine	Oncovin	1.4 mg/m² (2 mg maximum) I.V., days 1 and 8
	procarbazine	Matulane	100 mg/m² P.O., days 1-14
	prednisone	Deltasone	40 mg/m² P.O., days 1-14 *Repeat cycle q 28 days.*
MVPP	mechlorethamine (nitrogen mustard)	Mustargen	6 mg/m² I.V., days 1 and 8
	vinblastine	Velban	4 mg/m² I.V., days 1 and 8
	procarbazine	Matulane	100 mg/m² P.O., days 1-14
	prednisone	Deltasone	40 mg/m² P.O., days 1-14 *Repeat cycle q 4-6 wk.*
Stanford V	mechlorethamine (nitrogen mustard)	Mustargen	6 mg/m² I.V., day 1
	doxorubicin	Adriamycin	25 mg/m² I.V., days 1 and 15
	vinblastine	Velban	6 mg/m² I.V., days 1 and 15
	vincristine	Oncovin	1.4 mg/m² (2 mg maximum) I.V., days 8 and 22
	bleomycin	Blenoxane	5 units/m² I.V., days 8 and 22
	etoposide	VePesid	60 mg/m² I.V., days 15 and 16
	prednisone	Deltasone	40 mg/m² P.O., every other day for 10 wk; then taper off by 10 mg every other day for next 14 days *Repeat cycle q 28 days.*
Leukemia – ALL, adult induction			
Hyper-CVAD	cyclophosphamide	Cytoxan	300 mg/m² I.V. over 3 hr q 12 hr, days 1-3
	mesna	Mesnex	600 mg/m² continuous I.V. infusion, days 1-3
	vincristine	Oncovin	2 mg I.V., days 4 and 11
	doxorubicin	Adriamycin	50 mg/m² I.V., day 4
	dexamethasone	Decadron	40 mg P.O. daily, days 1-4 and 11-14
	filgrastim	Neupogen	5 mcg/kg S.C. b.i.d., day 5, until ANC recovery *Alternate cycles with HD MTX-Ara-C regimen q 3-4 wk.*
HD MTX-Ara-C	methotrexate		200 mg/m² I.V. over 2 hr, day 1, followed by 800 mg/m² over 24 hr, day 1
	cytarabine (ara-C)	Cytosar-U	3 g/m² I.V. over 2 hr q 12 hr, days 2 and 3
	methylprednisolone	Solu-Medrol	50 mg I.V. b.i.d., days 1-3
	filgrastim	Neupogen	5 mcg/kg S.C. b.i.d., day 4, until ANC recovery
	leucovorin calcium		15 mg P.O. q 6 hr for eight doses, starting 24 hr after completion of methotrexate infusion *Alternate cycles with Hyper-CVAD regimen for a total of 8 cycles.*

(continued)

Indication & acronym	Generic drug name	Trade drug name	Dosage
Leukemia – AML, induction			
5 + 2	cytarabine (ara-C)	Cytosar-U	100-200 mg/m^2 by continuous I.V. infusion, days 1-5
	daunorubicin	Cerubidine	45 mg/m^2 I.V., days 1 and 2 *Repeat cycle q 7 days.*
	or		
	cytarabine (ara-C)	Cytosar-U	100-200 mg/m^2 by continuous I.V. infusion, days 1-5
	mitoxantrone	Novantrone	12 mg/m^2 I.V. daily, days 1 and 2 *Repeat cycle q 7 days.*
7 + 3 (with mitoxantrone)	mitoxantrone	Novantrone	12 mg/m^2 I.V. daily, days 1-3
	cytarabine (ara-C)	Cytosar-U	100-200 mg/m^2 daily by continuous I.V. infusion, days 1-7 *Give 1 cycle only.*
7 + 3 (with daunorubicin)	cytarabine (ara-C)	Cytosar-U	100-200 mg/m^2 daily by continuous I.V. infusion, days 1-7
	daunorubicin	Cerubidine	30 or 45 mg/m^2 I.V., days 1-3 *Give 1 cycle only.*
Leukemia – CLL			
CVP	cyclophosphamide	Cytoxan	300-400 mg/m^2 P.O., days 1-5
	vincristine	Oncovin	1.4 mg/m^2 (2 mg maximum) I.V., day 1
	prednisone	Deltasone	100 mg/m^2 P.O., days 1-5 *Repeat cycle q 21 days.*
Melanoma			
DTIC/Tamoxifen	dacarbazine	DTIC–Dome	250 mg/m^2 I.V., days 1-5
	tamoxifen	Nolvadex	20 mg/m^2 P.O., days 1-5 *Repeat cycle q 21 days.*
VDP	vinblastine	Velban	5 mg/m^2 I.V., days 1 and 2
	dacarbazine	DTIC–Dome	150 mg/m^2 I.V., days 1-5
	cisplatin	Platinol	75 mg/m^2 I.V., day 5 *Repeat cycle q 21-28 days.*
Multiple myeloma			
MP	melphalan (L-phenylalanine mustard)	Alkeran	8 mg/m^2 P.O., days 1-4
	prednisone	Deltasone	60 mg/m^2 P.O., days 1-4 *Repeat cycle q 21-28 days.*
VAD	vincristine	Oncovin	0.4 mg by continuous I.V. infusion, days 1-4
	doxorubicin	Adriamycin	9 mg/m^2 by continuous I.V. infusion, days 1-4
	dexamethasone	Decadron	40 mg P.O. on days 1-4, 9-12, and 17-20 *Repeat cycle q 4-5 wk.*

Indication & acronym	Generic drug name	Trade drug name	Dosage
Non-Hodgkin's lymphoma			
CHOP	cyclophosphamide	Cytoxan	750 mg/m^2 I.V., day 1
	doxorubicin	Adriamycin	50 mg/m^2 I.V., day 1
	vincristine	Oncovin	1.4 mg/m^2 (2 mg maximum) I.V., day 1
	prednisone	Deltasone	100 mg P.O., days 1-5 *Repeat cycle q 21-28 days.*
CHOP-BLEO	bleomycin	Blenoxane	15 units/day I.V., days 1-5 Add to CHOP regimen. *Repeat cycle q 21-28 days.*
CHOP-rituximab	rituximab	Rituxan	375 mg/m^2 I.V., day 1 Add to CHOP regimen. *Repeat cycle q 21 days.*
CNOP	cyclophosphamide	Cytoxan	750 mg/m^2 I.V., day 1
	mitoxantrone	Novantrone	12 mg/m^2 I.V., day 1
	vincristine	Oncovin	1.4 mg/m^2 (2 mg maximum) I.V., day 1
	prednisone	Deltasone	50 mg/m^2/day P.O., days 1-5 *Repeat cycle q 21-28 days.*
COPP	cyclophosphamide	Cytoxan	450-600 mg/m^2 I.V., days 1 and 8
	vincristine	Oncovin	1.4 mg/m^2 (2 mg maximum) I.V., days 1 and 8
	procarbazine	Matulane	100 mg/m^2 P.O., days 1-14
	prednisone	Deltasone	40 mg/m^2 P.O., days 1-14 *Repeat cycle q 28 days.*
CVP	cyclophosphamide	Cytoxan	300-400 mg/m^2 P.O., days 1-5
	vincristine	Oncovin	1.4 mg/m^2 (2 mg maximum) I.V., day 1
	prednisone	Deltasone	100 mg/m^2 P.O., days 1-5 *Repeat cycle q 21 days.*
ESHAP	etoposide	VePesid	40-60 mg/m^2/day I.V., days 1-4
	methylprednisolone	Solu-Medrol	250-500 mg I.V., days 1-4 or 1-5
	cisplatin	Platinol	25 mg/m^2 by continuous I.V. infusion, days 1-4
	cytarabine	Cytosar-U	2 g/m^2 I.V., day 5 *Repeat cycle q 21-28 days.*
MACOP-B	methotrexate		400 mg/m^2 I.V., wk 2, 6, and 10
	leucovorin calcium		15 mg/m^2 P.O. q 6 hr for six doses, beginning 24 hr after methotrexate dose
	doxorubicin	Adriamycin	50 mg/m^2 I.V., wk 1, 3, 5, 7, 9, and 11
	cyclophosphamide	Cytoxan	350 mg/m^2 I.V., wk 1, 3, 5, 7, 9, and 11
	vincristine	Oncovin	1.4 mg/m^2 (2 mg maximum) I.V., wk 2, 4, 6, 8, 10, and 12
	bleomycin	Blenoxane	10 units/m^2 I.V. weekly, wk 4, 8, and 12
	prednisone	Deltasone	75 mg P.O., daily for 12 wk; taper dose over last 2 wk *Give only 1 cycle.*

(continued)

Indication & acronym	Generic drug name	Trade drug name	Dosage
Non-Hodgkin's lymphoma *(continued)*			
ProMACE	prednisone	Deltasone	60 mg/m² P.O., days 1-14
	methotrexate		750 mg/m² I.V., day 14
	leucovorin calcium		50 mg/m² I.V. q 6 hr for five to six doses, beginning 24 hr after methotrexate dose
	doxorubicin	Adriamycin	25 mg/m² I.V., days 1 and 8
	cyclophosphamide	Cytoxan	650 mg/m² I.V., days 1 and 8
	etoposide (VP-16)	VePesid	120 mg/m² I.V., days 1 and 8 *Repeat cycle q 28 days.*
ProMACE/cytaBOM	cyclophosphamide	Cytoxan	650 mg/m² I.V., day 1
	doxorubicin	Adriamycin	25 mg/m² I.V., day 1
	etoposide (VP-16)	VePesid	120 mg/m² I.V., day 1
	prednisone	Deltasone	60 mg/m² P.O., days 1-14
	cytarabine (ara-C)	Cytosar-U	300 mg/m² I.V., day 8
	bleomycin	Blenoxane	5 units/m² I.V., day 8
	vincristine	Oncovin	1.4 mg/m² (2 mg maximum) I.V., day 8
	methotrexate		120 mg/m² I.V., day 8
	leucovorin calcium		25 mg/m² P.O. q 6 hr for six doses, beginning 24 hr after methotrexate dose
	co-trimoxazole	Bactrim DS	2 tablets (double-strength) P.O. b.i.d., days 1-28 *Repeat cycle q 21-28 days.*
Non–small cell lung cancer			
CP	carboplatin	Paraplatin	Area under the curve 6 I.V., day 1
	paclitaxel	Taxol	225 mg/m² I.V. over 3 hr, day 1 *Repeat cycle q 21 days.*
CG	cisplatin	Platinol	100 mg/m² I.V. over 30-120 min, day 1
	gemcitabine	Gemzar	1-1.2 g/m² I.V. over 30-60 min, days 1, 8, and 15 *Repeat cycle q 28 days.*
EP	cisplatin	Platinol	80-100 mg/m² I.V., day 1
	etoposide (VP-16)	VePesid	80-120 mg/m² I.V., days 1-3 *Repeat cycle q 21-28 days.*
VC	vinorelbine	Navelbine	30 mg/m² I.V., days 1, 8, 15, and 22
	cisplatin	Platinol	120 mg/m² I.V., days 1 and 29; then give one dose q 6 wk *Repeat cycle q 28 days.*
Ovarian cancer			
Carbo-Tax	paclitaxel	Taxol	175 mg/m² I.V. over 3 hr, day 1
	carboplatin	Paraplatin	Area under the curve 7.5 targeted by Calvert equation, day 1 (after paclitaxel) *Repeat cycle q 21 days.*
CC	carboplatin	Paraplatin	300-350 mg/m² I.V., day 1
	cyclophosphamide	Cytoxan	600 mg/m² I.V., day 1 *Repeat cycle q 28 days.*

Indication & acronym	Generic drug name	Trade drug name	Dosage
Ovarian cancer *(continued)*			
CP	cyclophosphamide	Cytoxan	600-1,000 mg/m^2 I.V., day 1
	cisplatin	Platinol	60-80 mg/m^2 I.V., day 1 *Repeat cycle q 21-28 days.*
Prostate cancer			
FL	flutamide	Eulexin	250 mg P.O. t.i.d.
	leuprolide acetate	Lupron	1 mg S.C. daily
	flutamide	Eulexin	250 mg P.O. t.i.d.
	or		
	leuprolide acetate	Lupron Depot	75 mg I.M. q 28 days or 22.5 mg I.M. q 3 mo
FZ	flutamide	Eulexin	250 P.O. q 8 hr
	goserelin acetate	Zoladex	3.6 mg implant S.C. q 28 days or 10.8 mg implant S.C. q 12 wk
MP	mitoxantrone	Novantrone	12 mg/m^2 by short I.V. infusion q 3 wk
	prednisone	Deltasone	5 mg P.O. b.i.d.
Small-cell lung cancer			
ACE (CAE)	doxorubicin	Adriamycin	45 mg/m^2 I.V., day 1
	cyclophosphamide	Cytoxan	1 g/m^2 I.V., day 1
	etoposide (VP-16)	VePesid	50 mg/m^2 I.V., days 1-5 *Repeat cycle q 21 days.*
CAV	cyclophosphamide	Cytoxan	1 g/m^2 I.V., day 1
	doxorubicin	Adriamycin	40-50 mg/m^2 I.V., day 1
	vincristine	Oncovin	1-1.4 mg/m^2 (2 mg maximum) I.V., day 1 *Repeat cycle q 21 days.*
EP	cisplatin	Platinol	75-100 mg/m^2 I.V., day 1
	etoposide (VP-16)	VePesid	75-100 mg/m^2 I.V., days 1-3 *Repeat cycle q 21-28 days.*
Soft-tissue sarcoma			
AD	doxorubicin	Adriamycin	45-60 mg/m^2 I.V., day 1
	dacarbazine	DTIC-Dome	200-250 mg/m^2 I.V., days 1-5 *Repeat cycle q 21 days.*
CYVADIC	cyclophosphamide	Cytoxan	500 mg/m^2 I.V., day 1
	vincristine	Oncovin	1 mg/m^2 (2 mg maximum) I.V., days 1 and 5
	doxorubicin	Adriamycin	50 mg/m^2 I.V., day 1
	dacarbazine	DTIC-Dome	250 mg/m^2 I.V., days 1-5 *Repeat cycle q 21 days.*

(continued)

Indication & acronym	Generic drug name	Trade drug name	Dosage
Soft-tissue sarcoma *(continued)*			
MAID	mesna	Mesnex	2.5 g/m^2 by continuous I.V. infusion, days 1-4
	doxorubicin	Adriamycin	15 mg/m^2 by continuous I.V. infusion, days 1-4
	ifosfamide	Ifex	2 g/m^2 by continuous I.V. infusion, days 1 to 3
	dacarbazine	DTIC-Dome	250 mg/m^2 by continuous I.V. infusion, days 1-4 *Repeat cycle q 21 days.*
Testicular cancer			
BEP	bleomycin	Blenoxane	30 units I.V., days 2, 9, and 16
	etoposide (VP-16)	VePesid	100 mg/m^2, days 1-5
	cisplatin	Platinol	20 mg/m^2 I.V., days 1-5 *Repeat cycle q 21 days.*
VelP	vinblastine	Velban	0.11 mg/kg I.V., days 1 and 2
	ifosfamide	Ifex	1.2 g/m^2/day by continuous I.V. infusion, days 1-5
	cisplatin	Platinol	20 mg/m^2 I.V. over 1 hr, days 1-5
	mesna	Mesnex	400 mg I.V. 15 min before ifosfamide, day 1; then 1.2 g daily by continuous I.V. infusion, days 1 to 5 *Repeat cycle q 21 days.*
VIP	etoposide (VP-16)	VePesid	75 mg/m^2 I.V., days 1-5
	ifosfamide	Ifex	1.2 g/m^2 by continuous I.V. infusion, days 1-5
	cisplatin	Platinol	20 mg/m^2 I.V., days 1-5
	mesna	Mesnex	400 mg I.V. 15 min before ifosfamide, day 1; then 1.2 g daily by continuous I.V. infusion, days 1-5 *Repeat cycle q 21 days.*

LOOK-ALIKE AND SOUND-ALIKE DRUG NAMES

Watch out for the following drug names that resemble other drug names either in the way they're spelled or the way they sound.

abciximab and infliximab

acetazolamide and acetohexamide

Aggrastat and argatroban

albuterol and atenolol or Albutein

Aldomet and Aldoril or Anzemet

Amicar and Amikin

amiloride and amiodarone

aminophylline and amitriptyline or ampicillin

Aminosyn and amikacin

amiodarone and amiloride

amitriptyline and nortriptyline or aminophylline

Anafranil and enalapril, nafarelin, or alfentanil

anakinra and amikacin

Anzemet and Aldomet

atenolol and timolol or albuterol

Avinza and Invanz

azathioprine and azidothymidine, Azulfidine, or azatadine

bacitracin or baclofen and Bactroban

Benadryl and Bentyl, Aventyl, or Benylin

benztropine and bromocriptine or brimonidine

Bumex and Buprenex

calcifediol and calcitriol

carboplatin and cisplatin

Cardene and Cardura, Coumadin, K-Dur, Cordarone, Cordran, Lodine, or codeine

Cerebyx and Cerezyme, Celexa, or Celebrex

Chloromycetin and chlorambucil

Ciloxan and Cytoxan or cinoxacin

cimetidine and simethicone

clonidine and quinidine, clomiphene, or clomipramine

clotrimazole and co-trimoxazole

Copaxone and Compazine

corticotropin and cosyntropin

cyclosporine and cycloserine

dacarbazine and Dicarbosil or procarbazine

Dantrium and Daraprim

Demerol and Demulen, Dymelor, or Temaril

desmopressin and vasopressin

Desoxyn and digoxin or doxepin

dexamethasone and desoximetasone

Dexedrine and dextran or Excedrin

diazepam and diazoxide

diazoxide and Dyazide

diclofenac and Diflucan or Duphalac

dicyclomine and dyclonine or doxycycline

Dilantin and Dilaudid

dimenhydrinate and diphenhydramine

Diprivan and Ditropan or diazepam

disopyramide and desipramine or dipyridamole

dobutamine and dopamine

doxepin and doxazosin, digoxin, doxapram, doxorubicin, or Doxidan

penicillamine and penicillin

dronabinol and droperidol

enalapril and Anafranil or Eldepryl

epinephrine and ephedrine or norepinephrine

Epogen and Neupogen

Ethmozine and Erythrocin

etidronate and etomidate

fentanyl and alfentanil or sufentanil

floxuridine and fludarabine, fluorouracil, or flucytosine

fluticasone and fluconazole

folic acid and folinic acid

furosemide and torsemide

glucagon and Glaucon

Haldol and Halcion or Halog

hydralazine and hydroxyzine or hydroxyurea

hydrocortisone and hydroxychloroquine

hydromorphone and morphine

Hyperstat and Nitrostat

idarubicin and daunorubicin

ifosfamide and cyclophosphamide

Inderal and Inderide, Isordil, Adderall, Imuran, or Isuprel

Isoptin and Intropin

levothyroxine and liothyronine or liotrix

Lodine and iodine or codeine

lorazepam and alprazolam

Luvox and Lasix

magnesium sulfate and manganese sulfate

melphalan and Mephyton

Mestinon and Mesantoin or Metatensin

metaproterenol and metoprolol, metolazone, or metipranolol

methocarbamol and mephobarbital

methyltestosterone and medroxyprogesterone or methylprednisolone

Mevacor and Mivacron

Minocin and niacin or Mithracin

naloxone and naltrexone

Navane and Nubain or Norvasc

nifedipine and nimodipine or nicardipine

nitroglycerin and nitroprusside

oxymorphone and oxymetholone

Paxil and Doxil, paclitaxel, paroxetine, or Taxol

penicillin and Polycillin or penicillamine

pentobarbital and phenobarbital

pentostatin and pentosan

Persantine and Periactin

phentermine and phentolamine

phenytoin and mephenytoin

Pitocin and Pitressin

pralidoxime and pramoxine or pyridoxine

Pravachol and Prevacid or propranolol

prednisolone and prednisone

Premarin and Primaxin

ProAmatine and protamine

procainamide and probenecid

propranolol and Pravachol

protamine and Protopam or Protropin

pyridoxine and pralidoxime or Pyridium

quinidine and quinine or clonidine

ranitidine and rimantadine

Reminyl and Robinul

Restoril and Vistaril

rifabutin and rifampin or rifapentine

Rifater and Rifadin or Rifamate

Ritalin and Rifadin

Sandimmune and Sandoglobulin or Sandostatin

selegiline and Stelazine

Serentil and Serevent or Aventyl

Solu-Cortef and Solu-Medrol

sotalol and Stadol

streptozocin and streptomycin

sulfasalazine and sulfisoxazole, salsalate, or sulfadiazine

Survanta and Sufenta

Tegretol and Toradol or Foradil

terbutaline and tolbutamide or terbinafine

thiamine and thioridazine or Thorazine

Ticlid and Tequin

Tigan and Ticar

Trandate and Trental

Versed and VePesid

vidarabine and cytarabine

vinblastine and vincristine, vindesine, or vinorelbine

Xanax and Zantac or Tenex

Zofran and Zosyn, Zantac, or Zoloft

MOST COMMON DRUG ERRORS

Drug orders

Prescribing and filling drug orders must be done carefully to avoid potential problems.

Drug name confusion

Error: The approval of Zyvox (linezolid) raises concerns that this drug will be confused with Zovirax (acyclovir sodium). This mix-up could happen easily with either a verbal or a written order.

Best practice or prevention: Be aware of the medications your patient takes regularly, and question any deviations from his regular routine. And, as with any medication, take your time and read the label carefully.

Dangerous abbreviations

Error: Abbreviating drug names is risky. A cancer patient with anemia may receive epoetin alfa, commonly abbreviated EPO, to stimulate RBC production. In one case, when a cancer patient was admitted to a hospital, the prescriber wrote, "May take own supply of EPO." But the patient wasn't anemic. Sensing that something was wrong, the pharmacist interviewed the patient, who confirmed that he was taking "EPO"—evening primrose oil—to lower his cholesterol level.

Best practice or prevention: Ask all prescribers to spell out drug names.

Unclear orders

Error: A patient was supposed to receive doxorubicin 30 mg/m^2 continuous I.V. infusion every day on days 1 to 3 of his chemotherapy cycle. The prescriber's orders read "30 mg/m^2 I.V. continuous infusion days 1 to 3." This was misinterpreted as giving the dose divided over the 3 days, instead of giving the dose every day for 3 days. The

pharmacist caught the error and confirmed it with the prescriber before the dose was given. If this error hadn't been caught, the patient would have received much less than the intended dose.

Best practice or prevention: If you're unfamiliar with a drug, check a drug reference before giving it and clarify the order with the prescriber. When documenting orders, note how much drug was given that day.

Misinterpreted orders

Error: Several reports to the Institute for Safe Medication Practices (ISMP) involved errors related to insulin orders. In one case, an order was written as "add 10U of regular insulin to each TPN bag," and the pharmacist preparing the solution misinterpreted the dose as 100 units. In another case, a pharmacy technician entering orders misinterpreted a sliding scale when the insulin order used "U" for units, an error that could have caused a 10-fold overdose if a nurse hadn't caught it. Yet another report involved a nurse who received a verbal order to resume an insulin drip but wrote "resume heparin drip." Fortunately, the pharmacist caught the error.

Best practice or prevention: Before giving drugs such as insulin or heparin, which are ordered in units, always check the prescriber's written order against the provided dose. Never abbreviate "units." If you must accept a verbal order, have another nurse listen in; then write that order directly onto an order form and repeat it to ensure that you've written it correctly.

Lipid-based drugs

Error: Confusion between certain lipid-based (liposomal) drugs and their conventional counterparts can cause serious drug errors, some fatal. The drugs involved include:

- Lipid-based amphotericin B (Abelcet, Amphotec, AmBisome) and conventional amphotericin B for injection (available generically and as Fungizone)
- The pegylated liposomal form of doxorubicin (Doxil) and its conventional form, doxorubicin hydrochloride (Adriamycin, Rubex)
- A liposomal form of daunorubicin (DaunoXome, daunorubicin citrate liposomal) and conventional daunorubicin hydrochloride (Cerubidine).

Best practice or prevention: Lipid-based products have different dosages than their conventional counterparts. Check the original order and labels carefully to avoid mix-ups.

Misread orders

Error: A report from the ISMP detailed a problem concerning a new insulin protocol instituted at a hospital. The new protocol described the insulin dose in units per hour, while the old protocol described the dose in milliliters per hour. Staff members unfamiliar with the new protocol inevitably gave the insulin infusion as milliliters per hour, not units per hour. In one case, the patient received just 20% of the intended dose.

Best practice or prevention: Protocols can be effective tools only if they are being followed correctly. Staff members must be taught the new protocols to make them aware of confusing points, such as in this example. Always know the concentration of the drug and make sure that you set the pump correctly. Also, be aware of the infusion rates of each drug and check a reference book if you are unfamiliar with the drug.

Drug preparation

When preparing a drug for administration, be alert for potential problems.

Inattentiveness

Error: When a hospital pharmacy received an order for Fludara (fludarabine), a pharmacy technician asked the pharmacist if Navelbine (vinorelbine) was the same as Fludara (both are antineoplastics). The preoccupied pharmacist said "yes." The technician prepared the Navelbine, but labeled it as Fludara. The pharmacist checked the preparation but didn't notice the error, and the patient received the wrong drug.

Best practice or prevention: To prevent errors of this type, the hospital posted tables of antineoplastics and their dosing guidelines in the pharmacy. As an added safeguard, the pharmacy now sends the empty drug vial or box top with the prepared solution for the nurse to double-check before infusing the drug.

Injectable solution color changes

Error: In two cases, alert nurses noticed that antineoplastics prepared in the pharmacy didn't look the way they should.

The first error involved a 6-year-old child who was to receive 12 mg of methotrexate intrathecally. In the pharmacy, a 1-g vial was mistakenly selected instead of a 20-mg vial, and the drug was reconstituted with 10 ml of normal saline solution. The vial containing 100 mg/ml was incorrectly labeled as containing 2 mg/ml, and 6 ml of the solution was drawn into a syringe. Although the syringe label indicated 12 mg of drug, the syringe actually contained 600 mg of drug.

When the nurse received the syringe and noted that the drug's color didn't appear right, she returned it to the pharmacy for verification. The pharmacist retrieved the vial used to prepare the dose and drew the remaining solution into another syringe. The solutions in both syringes matched, and no one noticed the vial's 1-g label. The pharmacist concluded that a manufacturing change caused the color difference.

The child received the 600-mg dose and experienced seizures 45 minutes later. A pharmacist responding to the emergency detected the error. The child received an antidote and recovered.

A similar case involved a 20-year-old patient with leukemia who received mitomycin instead of mitoxantrone. The nurse had questioned the drug's unusual bluish tint, but the pharmacist assured her that the color difference was caused by a change in manufacturer. Fortunately, the patient didn't suffer any harm.

Best practice or prevention: If a familiar drug seems to have an unfamiliar appearance, investigate the cause. If the pharmacist cites a manufacturing change, ask him to double-check whether he has received verification from the manufacturer. Document the appearance discrepancy, your actions, and the pharmacist's response in the patient record.

Diluent mistakes

Error: Just because a drug comes prepackaged with a diluent doesn't mean that it's always the diluent to use. An example of this is the drug chlordiazepoxide (Librium) used to treat acute alcohol withdrawal. When preparing an I.M. injection, the nurse uses the diluent provided. When preparing an I.V. injection, she uses saline solution or sterile water injection. She shouldn't use the prepackaged diluent for the I.V. injection because air bubbles will form on the surface of the solution.

The ISMP has documented several reports regarding errors in the reconstitution of docetaxel (Taxotere) caused by overfill in the drug vial and the enclosed diluent vial. Docetaxel 20 mg and 80 mg vials actually contain 23.6 mg and 94.4 mg of docetaxel, respectively, because of the overfill vol-

umes. The diluent vials also contain overfill. Docetaxel requires two dilutions before administration. First, the entire vial of diluent must be added to the docetaxel for injection concentrate, yielding 10 mg/ml. Next, the docetaxel solution must be further diluted in an infusion bag. The final strength could be miscalculated if the total volume contained in the drug vials is injected into the infusion bag, rather than figuring out what the dose is using milligrams per milliliter and removing that volume from the drug vials and injecting it into the infusion bag.

Best practice or prevention: Review the technique of preparing solutions that you aren't used to handling. Institute readily available guidelines about drugs that are more complicated or confusing to prepare.

Drug administration

When giving a drug, be careful to avoid the following problems.

Calculation errors

Error: A physician assistant wrote the following order for a woman being admitted to the hospital for neck surgery: "methylprednisolone 10.6 g (30 mg/kg) over 1 hour IVPB before surgery" to minimize inflammation. The patient weighed 70 kg (154 lb), so the dose should have been 2.1 g, not 10.6 g. But neither the pharmacist nor the nurse independently checked the calculation, and the patient received an overdose. She developed significant hyperglycemia and hypokalemia but recovered without injury.

Best practice or prevention: Writing the mg/kg or mg/m^2 dose and the calculated dose provides a safeguard against calculation errors. Whenever a prescriber provides the calculation, double-check it and document that the dose was verified.

Dosage equations

Error: A 13-month study at Albany (N.Y.) Medical Center examined 200 prescribing errors arising from the use of dosage equations. Almost 70% involved pediatric patients, for whom dosage equations are commonly used. Mistakes in decimal point placement, mathematical calculation, or expression of the regimen accounted for over 50% of the errors. Examples include prescribing the entire day's drug as a single dose instead of at intervals or using an entire day's dose at each interval. Use of dosage equations invites drug errors.

Best practice or prevention: Alternatives to dosage equations include using preestablished ranges or tables, incorporating a calculator into a computer order-entry system, and requiring both the calculated dose and dosage equation on orders to facilitate independent checks.

After you calculate a drug dosage, always have another nurse calculate it independently to double-check your results. If doubts or questions remain or if the calculations don't match, ask a pharmacist to calculate the dose before giving the drug.

Air bubbles in pump tubing

Error: After starting an I.V. drip to give insulin, 2 units/hour, to a 9-year-old patient, a nurse noted air bubbles in the tubing and pump chamber. To remove them and promote proper flow, she disconnected the tubing and increased the pump rate to 200 ml/hour. When the bubbles were cleared, she reconnected the tubing and restarted the infusion without resetting the rate. The child received about 50 units of insulin before the error was detected. Fortunately, the child wasn't harmed.

Best practice or prevention: To clear bubbles from I.V. tubing, never increase the pump's flow rate to flush the line. Instead, remove the tubing from

the pump, disconnect it from the patient, and use the flow-control clamp to establish gravity flow. When the bubbles have been removed, return the tubing to the pump, restart the infusion, and recheck the flow rate.

Misplaced decimals

Error: A patient in the intensive care unit was to receive the opioid fentanyl, 12.5 to 25 mcg I.V. every 4 to 6 hours, as needed, for pain. Unit stock consisted of 5-ml ampules of fentanyl 0.05 mg/ml, so each ampule contained 0.25 mg (250 mcg). A nurse preparing the dose confused the volume needed when she converted from milligrams to micrograms and gave 5 ml, thinking it contained 25 micrograms. The patient suffered respiratory arrest but was resuscitated.

Best practice or prevention: Numerous serious fentanyl errors have been reported, and a misplaced decimal point caused many of them. A safer alternative for intermittent dosing is I.V. morphine. Fentanyl doses are best prepared in the pharmacy rather than on the unit. If a fentanyl dose must be prepared, refer to dosing charts, follow the facility's protocols, and ask another nurse to check your calculations.

Stress

Error: A nurse-anesthetist gave the sedative midazolam (Versed) to the wrong patient. When she discovered the error, she grabbed what she thought was a vial of the antidote flumazenil (Romazicon), withdrew 2.5 ml, and gave it to the patient. When the patient didn't respond, she realized she'd grabbed a vial of ondansetron (Zofran), an antiemetic, instead. Another practitioner assisted with proper I.V. administration of flumazenil, and the patient recovered without harm.

Best practice or prevention: Committing a serious error can cause enormous stress and cloud your judgment. If you're involved in a drug error, ask another professional to give the antidote.

Giving an I.V. drug too quickly

Error: A report from the ISMP detailed a scenario where the patient experiencing a hypertensive crisis was prescribed labetalol 20 mg I.V. push. The dose was given over a matter of seconds while the patient was en route to the radiology department. The patient immediately suffered a cardiac arrest and couldn't be resuscitated. Later, staff discovered several other cases in which rapid I.V. push of labetalol may have contributed to patient harm.

There have also been reports of furosemide, pancuronium bromide, potassium chloride, vancomycin (causing red-neck syndrome), and verapamil given too quickly.

Best practice or prevention: Practitioners should avoid the terminology "I.V. push" with drugs that need to be given over a minute or longer. When giving orders for drugs, the time frame of injection should be noted. Readily available resources are needed at the point of care to teach prescribers about the drug's maximum rate of administration (as an alert on the medication itself, on automated dispensing cabinet screens, or on the computer).

Drugs with similar names

Error: The ISMP has found many reports of confusion between methylprednisolone acetate (Depo-Medrol) and methylprednisolone sodium succinate (Solu-Medrol). One case described a 3-year-old child who was prescribed Solu-Medrol 40 mg I.V. The nurse accidentally selected methylprednisolone acetate 40 mg, which was the first form and strength of the generic methylprednisolone that appeared on the automated dispensing cabinet screen. Shortly thereafter, the pharmacist who entered the order for Solu-Medrol into the computer noticed that

Depo-Medrol had been removed from the cabinet, and he called the unit to alert the nurse to the error. Fortunately, the nurse had already noticed that she had selected the wrong product and the child received the correct form of the drug.

Best practice or prevention: Teach staff about the differences in the I.V. and I.M. formulations, noting that "depo" or "depot" indicates a long-acting I.M. injection.

Be aware of other look-alike brand and generic name drugs. If possible, create an alert on automated dispensing cabinet screens to remind practitioners by which route the drug can be given. List both brand and generic names of methylprednisolone products in order-entry computer systems to reduce the risk of mix-ups. Even though the I.M. formulation has a small warning on the label saying "Not for I.V. use," affix a warning label, "I.M. use only," to help prevent these errors from occurring. Another idea is to have the pharmacy dispense these products or ensure that a pharmacist has reviewed the order before using products that are stocked on the unit. This way, a double-check system is put into effect.

THERAPEUTIC MONITORING GUIDELINES FOR I.V. DRUGS

Drug	Laboratory test monitored	Therapeutic ranges of test
aminoglycoside anti-biotics (amikacin, gentamicin, tobramycin)	Amikacin peak trough Gentamicin/tobramycin peak trough Creatinine	20-30 mcg/ml 1-8 mcg/ml 4-8 mcg/ml 2 mcg/ml 0.6-1.3 mg/dl
amphotericin B	Creatinine BUN Electrolytes (especially potassium and magnesium) Liver function CBC with differential and platelets	0.6-1.3 mg/dl 5-20 mg/dl Potassium: 3.5-5 mEq/L Magnesium: 1.5-2.5 mEq/L Sodium: 135-145 mEq/L Chloride: 98-106 mEq/L * *****
antibiotics	WBC with differential Cultures and sensitivities	*****
digoxin	Digoxin Electrolytes (especially potassium, magnesium, and calcium) Creatinine	0.8-2 ng/ml Potassium: 3.5-5 mEq/L Magnesium: 1.7-2.1 mEq/L Sodium: 135-145 mEq/L Chloride: 98-106 mEq/L Calcium: 8.6-10 mg/dl 0.6-1.3 mg/dl
diuretics	Electrolytes Creatinine BUN Uric acid Fasting glucose	Potassium: 3.5-5 mEq/L Magnesium: 1.7-2.1 mEq/L Sodium: 135-145 mEq/L Chloride: 98-106 mEq/L Calcium: 8.6-10 mg/dl 0.6-1.3 mg/dl 5-20 mg/dl 2-7 mg/dl 70-110 mg/dl
erythropoietin	Hematocrit Ferritin Transferrin saturation	Women: 36%-48% Men: 42%-52% 10-383 mg/ml 220-400 mg/dl
heparin	aPTT	1.5-2.5 times control

Note: ***** For those areas marked with asterisks, the following values can be used:

Hemoglobin: Women: 12-16 g/dl
  Men: 14-18 g/dl
Hematocrit: Women: 37%-48%
  Men: 42%-52%
RBCs: 4-5.5 x 10⁶/mm³
WBCs: 5-10 x 10³/mm³

Differential: Neutrophils: 45%-74%
  Bands: 0%-8%
  Lymphocytes: 16%-45%
  Monocytes: 4%-10%
  Eosinophils: 0%-7%
  Basophils: 0%-2%

Monitoring guidelines

Wait until you give the third dose to check drug level. Obtain blood for peak level 30 min after I.V. infusion ends or 60 min after I.M. administration. For trough level, draw blood just before next dose. Dosage may need to be adjusted accordingly. Recheck after three doses. Monitor creatinine and BUN levels and urine output for signs of decreasing renal function. Monitor urine for increased proteins, cells, and casts.

Monitor creatinine, BUN, and electrolyte levels at least weekly during therapy. Also, regularly monitor blood counts and liver function test results during therapy.

Specimen cultures and sensitivities will determine the cause of the infection and the best treatment. Monitor WBC with differential weekly during therapy.

Check digoxin level just before the next dose or ≥ 6-8 hr after the last dose. To monitor maintenance therapy, check drug level at least 1-2 wk after starting or changing therapy. Make any adjustments in therapy based on entire clinical picture, not solely on drug level. Also, check electrolyte levels and renal function periodically during therapy.

To monitor fluid and electrolyte balance, obtain baseline and periodic determinations of electrolyte, calcium, BUN, uric acid, and glucose levels.

After starting or changing therapy, monitor the hematocrit twice weekly for 2-6 wk until stabilized in the target range and a maintenance dose determined. Monitor hematocrit regularly thereafter.

When drug is given by continuous I.V. infusion, check aPTT q 4 hr in the early stages of therapy, and daily thereafter. When drug is given by deep S.C. injection, check aPTT 4-6 hr after injection, and daily thereafter.

(continued)

* For those areas marked with one asterisk, the following values can be used:

ALT: 7-56 units/L
AST: 5-40 units/L
Alkaline phosphatase: 17-142 units/L
LDH: 60-220 units/L
GGT: < 40 units/L
Total bilirubin: 0.2-1 mg/dl

Drug	Laboratory test monitored	Therapeutic ranges of test
insulin	Fasting glucose	70-110 mg/dl
	Glycosylated hemoglobin	5.5%-8.5% of total hemoglobin
linezolid	CBC with differential and platelets	*****
	Cultures and sensitivities	
	Platelet count	150-450 $\times$ 10³/mm³
	Liver function	*
	Amylase	35-118 IU/L
	Lipase	10-150 units/L
methotrexate	Methotrexate	Normal elimination:
		~ 10 micromol 24 hours postdose
		~ 1 micromol 48 hours postdose
		< 0.2 micromol 72 hours postdose
	CBC with differential	*****
	Platelet count	150-450 $\times$ 10³/mm³
	Liver function	*
	Creatinine	0.6-1.3 mg/dl
phenytoin	Phenytoin	10-20 mcg/ml
	CBC	*****
potassium chloride	Potassium	3.5-5 mEq/L
procainamide	Procainamide	3-10 mcg/ml (procainamide)
	N-acetylprocainamide (NAPA)	10-30 mcg/ml (combined procainamide and NAPA)
	CBC	*****
quinidine	Quinidine	2-6 mcg/ml
	CBC	*****
	Liver function	*
	Creatinine	0.6-1.3 mg/dl
	Electrolytes (especially potassium)	Potassium: 3.5-5 mEq/L
		Magnesium: 1.7-2.1 mEq/L
		Sodium: 135-145 mEq/L
		Chloride: 98-106 mEq/L
theophylline	Theophylline	10-20 mcg/ml

Note: ***** For those areas marked with asterisks, the following values can be used:

Hemoglobin: Women: 12-16 g/dl
  Men: 14-18 g/dl
Hematocrit: Women: 37%-48%
  Men: 42%-52%
RBCs: 4-5.5 x 10⁶/mm³
WBCs: 5-10 x 10³/mm³

Differential: Neutrophils: 45%-74%
  Bands: 0%-8%
  Lymphocytes: 16%-45%
  Monocytes: 4%-10%
  Eosinophils: 0%-7%
  Basophils: 0%-2%

Monitoring guidelines

Monitor response to therapy by evaluating glucose and glycosylated hemoglobin levels. Glycosylated hemoglobin level is a good measure of long-term control. Patient should monitor glucose levels at home to help measure compliance and response.

Obtain baseline CBC with differential and platelet count. Repeat weekly, especially if > 2 wk of therapy are received. Monitor liver function test results and amylase and lipase levels during therapy.

Monitor methotrexate level according to dosing protocol. Monitor CBC with differential, platelet count, and liver and renal function test results more frequently when therapy is started or changed and when methotrexate level may be elevated, such as when the patient is dehydrated.

Monitor phenytoin level immediately before next dose and 7-10 days after starting or changing therapy. Obtain a baseline CBC, and repeat monthly early in therapy. Watch for toxic effects at therapeutic level. Adjust the measured dose for hypoalbuminemia or renal impairment, which can increase free drug level.

Check level weekly after P.O. replacement therapy is started until stable and q 3-6 mo thereafter.

Measure procainamide level 6-12 hr after a continuous infusion is started or immediately before the next P.O. dose. Combined procainamide and NAPA levels can be used as an index of toxicity when renal impairment exists. Obtain CBC periodically during longer-term therapy.

Obtain drug level immediately before next P.O. dose and 30-35 hr after starting or changing therapy. Periodically obtain blood counts, liver and kidney function test results, and electrolyte level. With more specific assays, therapeutic level is < 1 mcg/1 ml.

Obtain theophylline level immediately before next dose of sustained-release P.O. product and at least 2 days after starting or changing therapy.

(continued)

---

* For those areas marked with one asterisk, the following values can be used:

ALT: 7-56 units/L
AST: 5-40 units/L
Alkaline phosphatase: 17-142 units/L
LDH: 60-220 units/L
GGT: < 40 units/L
Total bilirubin: 0.2-1 mg/dl

Drug	Laboratory test monitored	Therapeutic ranges of test
valproate sodium	Valproic acid	50-100 mcg/ml
	Liver function	*
	Ammonia	15-45 mcg/dl
	Fibrinogen	150-360 mg/dl
	BUN	5-20 mg/dl
	Creatinine	0.6-1.3 mg/dl
	CBC with differential	*****
	Platelet count	150-450 x 10³/mm³
vancomycin	Vancomycin	20-40 mcg/ml (peak)
		5-15 mcg/ml (trough)
	Creatinine	0.6-1.3 mg/dl
warfarin	INR	For an acute MI, atrial fibrillation, treatment of pulmonary embolism, prevention of systemic embolism, tissue heart valves, valvular heart disease, or prophylaxis or treatment of venous thrombosis: 2-3
		For mechanical prosthetic valves or recurrent systemic embolism: 2.5-3.5

Note: ***** For those areas marked with asterisks, the following values can be used:

Hemoglobin: Women: 12-16 g/dl
   Men: 14-18 g/dl
Hematocrit: Women: 37%-48%
   Men: 42%-52%
RBCs: 4-5.5 x 10⁶/mm³
WBCs: 5-10 x 10³/mm³

Differential: Neutrophils: 45%-74%
   Bands: 0%-8%
   Lymphocytes: 16%-45%
   Monocytes: 4%-10%
   Eosinophils: 0%-7%
   Basophils: 0%-2%

Monitoring guidelines

Monitor liver function test results, ammonia level, coagulation test results, renal function test results, CBC, and platelet count at baseline and periodically during therapy. Monitor liver function test results closely during the first 6 mo.

Check vancomycin level when you give the third dose, at the earliest. Draw peak level 1.5-2.5 hr after a 1-hr infusion or I.V. infusion is complete. Draw trough level within 1 hr of the next dose. Renal function can be used to adjust dosing and intervals.

Check INR daily, beginning 3 days after therapy is started. Continue checking INR until therapeutic goal is achieved, and monitor it periodically thereafter. Also, check drug level 7 days after any change in warfarin dose or concomitant, potentially interacting therapy.

---

* For those areas marked with one asterisk, the following values can be used:

ALT: 7-56 units/L
AST: 5-40 units/L
Alkaline phosphatase: 17-142 units/L
LDH: 60-220 units/L
GGT: < 40 units/L
Total bilirubin: 0.2-1 mg/dl

DIALYZABLE DRUGS

The amount of a drug removed by dialysis differs among patients and depends on several factors, including the patient's condition, the drug's properties, length of dialysis and dialysate used, rate of blood flow or dwell time, and purpose of dialysis. This table indicates the effect of hemodialysis on selected drugs.

Drug	Level reduced by hemodialysis	Drug	Level reduced by hemodialysis
acetazolamide	No	ciprofloxacin	Yes
acyclovir	Yes	cisplatin	No
allopurinol	Yes	clindamycin	No
amikacin	Yes	codeine	No
amiodarone	No	colchicine	No
amoxicillin	Yes	co-trimoxazole	Yes
amoxicillin and clavulanatepotassium	Yes	cyclophosphamide	Yes
amphotericin B	No	diazepam	No
ampicillin	Yes	diazoxide	No
ampicillin and sulbactam sodium	Yes	digoxin	No
atenolol	Yes	diltiazem	No
azathioprine	Yes	diphenhydramine	No
aztreonam	Yes	dipyridamole	No
bivalirudin	Yes	doxorubicin	No
carbenicillin	Yes	doxycycline	No
carmustine	No	enalaprilat	Yes
caspofungin	No	ertapenem	Yes
cefazolin	Yes	erythromycin	Yes
cefepime	Yes	ethacrynic acid	No
cefoperazone	Yes	famotidine	No
cefotaxime	Yes	fluconazole	Yes
cefotetan	Yes	fluorouracil	Yes
cefoxitin	Yes	foscarnet	Yes
ceftazidime	Yes	furosemide	No
ceftizoxime	Yes	ganciclovir	Yes
ceftriaxone	No	gatifloxacin	No
cefuroxime	Yes	gemtuzumab	No
chloramphenicol	Yes	gentamicin	Yes
chlordiazepoxide	No	haloperidol	No
chlorpromazine	No	heparin	No
cimetidine	Yes	hydralazine	No
		imipenem and cilastatin	Yes

Drug	Level reduced by hemodialysis
indomethacin	No
insulin	No
iron dextran	No
kanamycin	Yes
ketorolac	No
labetalol	No
levofloxacin	No
lidocaine	No
linezolid	Yes
lorazepam	No
mechlorethamine	No
meperidine	No
meropenem	Yes
methotrexate	Yes
methyldopa	Yes
methylprednisolone	No
metoclopramide	No
metoprolol	No
metronidazole	Yes
midazolam	No
minocycline	No
morphine	No
nafcillin	No
nitroglycerin	No
nitroprusside	Yes
oxacillin	No
pantoprazole	No
penicillin G	Yes
pentamidine	No
pentazocine	Yes
phenobarbital	Yes
phenytoin	No
piperacillin	Yes
piperacillin and tazobactam	Yes
procainamide	Yes
promethazine	No
propranolol	No
pyridoxine	Yes
quinidine	Yes

Drug	Level reduced by hemodialysis
ranitidine	Yes
rifampin	No
theophylline	Yes
ticarcillin	Yes
ticarcillin and clavulanate	Yes
tobramycin	Yes
valproic sodium	No
vancomycin	No
verapamil	No
voriconazole	Yes
warfarin	No

UNDERSTANDING CONTROLLED SUBSTANCE SCHEDULES

Drugs regulated under the jurisdiction of the Controlled Substances Act of 1970 are divided into the following groups, or schedules:

• Schedule I (C-I): High abuse potential and no accepted medical use. Examples include heroin, marijuana, and LSD.

• Schedule II (C-II): High abuse potential with severe dependence liability. Examples include narcotics, amphetamines, and some barbiturates.

• Schedule III (C-III): Less abuse potential than schedule II drugs and moderate dependence liability. Examples include nonbarbiturate sedatives, nonamphetamine stimulants, anabolic steroids, and limited amounts of certain narcotics.

• Schedule IV (C-IV): Less abuse potential than schedule III drugs and limited dependence liability. Examples include some sedatives, anxiolytics, and nonnarcotic analgesics.

• Schedule V (C-V): Limited abuse potential. This category includes mainly small amounts of narcotics, such as codeine, used as antitussives or antidiarrheals. Under federal law, limited quantities of certain C-V drugs may be purchased without a prescription directly from a pharmacist if allowed under specific state statutes. The purchaser must be at least age 18 and must furnish suitable identification. All such transactions must be recorded by the dispensing pharmacist.

RATING PREGNANCY RISK

The Food and Drug Administration (FDA) has established five pregnancy risk categories (A, B, C, D, and X) that reflect a drug's potential for causing birth defects. Although drugs are best avoided during pregnancy, this rating system permits rapid assessment of the risk-benefit ratio, should drug administration to a pregnant woman become necessary.

The FDA defines pregnancy risk categories as follows:

- **A:** Controlled studies show no risk. Adequate studies in pregnant women have failed to demonstrate risk to the fetus.
- **B:** No evidence of risk exists. Either animal findings show risk and human findings don't; or if human studies are lacking, animal findings show no risk.
- **C:** Risk can't be ruled out. Human studies are lacking, and animal findings show risk or are also lacking. However, potential benefits may justify the potential risk.
- **D:** Positive evidence of fetal risk exists. Nevertheless, potential benefits may outweigh potential risks.
- **X:** Contraindicated in pregnancy. Animal or human findings show fetal abnormalities and risk that clearly outweighs any benefits.
- **NR:** Not rated.

OSMOLALITY, OSMOLARITY, AND pH

Osmolality, osmolarity, and pH can be used to identify potential infusion problems, such as phlebitis or fluid shift.

Osmolality
Osmolality is the measure of a solute concentration in terms of kilograms of water and expresses the solution's osmotic pressure. It's measured in milliosmols/kilogram (mOsm/kg).

Osmolarity
Osmolarity is the measure of a solute concentration in terms of liters of solution. It's measured in milliosmols/liter (mOsm/L). The osmolarity of plasma is 290 mOsm/L; of hypotonic solutions, less than 240 mOsm/L; of isotonic solutions, 240 to 340 mOsm/L; and of hypertonic solutions, more than 340 mOsm/L. Hypotonic and hypertonic solutions cause vessel irritation or chemical phlebitis. Hypotonic solutions cause a vascular-to-cellular fluid shift; hypertonic solutions, cellular-to-vascular fluid shift.

pH
The pH is the degree of acidity or alkalinity of a solution. Normal range is 7.35 to 7.45. The pH of an acid is less than 7.35; the pH of a base, more than 7.45. Solutions that are mildly acidic or alkaline usually present no infusion risk, but when values fall outside the normal range, the patient is at risk for vein irritation, chemical phlebitis, or fluid shift.

INDEX

A

Abbokinase, 719
Abbreviations, ix-x
abciximab, 50-51
Abdominal surgery patients, piperacillin for, 589
Abelcet, 96
Abortion
ertapenem for, 321
methylergonovine maleate for, 480
oxytocin, synthetic injection, for, 548
$Rh_o(D)$ immune globulin intravenous, human, for, 643
Abruptio placentae, aminocaproic acid for, 81
acebutolol, 19, 20
acetazolamide sodium, 52-53
Acidosis. *See also* Ketoacidosis
sodium bicarbonate for, 659
sodium lactate for, 664
tromethamine for, 712
Acromegaly, octreotide for, 536
ACT, 231-233
actinomycin D, 231-233
Actinomycosis, penicillin G for, 563
Acute coronary syndrome
eptifibatide for, 319
tirofiban for, 698
Acute lymphocytic leukemia
asparaginase for, 119
chemotherapy protocols for, 771t
cytarabine for, 223
daunorubicin for, 239
doxorubicin for, 286
pegaspargase for, 560
sargramostim for, 653

Acute lymphocytic leukemia *(continued)*
teniposide for, 682
vincristine for, 734
Acute myeloid leukemia
chemotherapy protocols for, 772t
cytarabine for, 223
daunorubicin for, 239
doxorubicin for, 286
gemtuzumab ozogamicin for, 370
idarubicin for, 399
sargramostim for, 653
vincristine for, 734
Acute promyelocytic leukemia, arsenic trioxide for, 115-116
acycloguanosine, 54-55
acyclovir sodium, 54-55
Adenocarcinoma, chemotherapy protocols for, 768t
Adenocard, 56
adenosine, 56-57
ADH, 725-726
Adrenal function testing, cosyntropin for, 214
Adrenalin Chloride, 310
Adrenal insufficiency
adrenocorticoids for, 5
hydrocortisone for, 388
Adrenal stimulation, cosyntropin for, 214
Adrenergics, 1-2
adrenocorticoids, 3-6
Adriamycin PFS, 285
Adriamycin RDF, 285
Adrucil, 352
Advanced cardiac life support
atropine for, 126
calcium salts for, 154
inamrinone for, 410
sodium bicarbonate for, 659
Afterload reduction, nitroprusside for, 531

Agammaglobulinemia, immune globulin for, 407
Aggrastat, 698
Agitation, amobarbital for, 89
AHF, 105-106
A-Hydrocort, 388
Akineton, 138
albumin, 57-59
Albuminar 5% and 25%, 57
Albutein 5% and 25%, 57
albuterol sulfate, 1
Alcohol withdrawal, chlordiazepoxide for, 189
aldesleukin, 59-62
Aldomet, 477
alefacept, 62-64
alemtuzumab, 64-66
Alfenta, 66
alfentanil hydrochloride, 36, 37, 66-68
Alkeran, 462
Allergic reactions
antihistamines for, 14
diphenhydramine for, 271
phenothiazines for, 44
promethazine for, 613
red blood cells, washed, for, 636
allopurinol sodium, 68-69
Aloprim, 68
Alpha-adrenergic blockers, 6-7
$Alpha_1$-antitrypsin deficiency, $alpha_1$-proteinase inhibitor (human) for, 69-70
AlphaNine SD, 336
$alpha_1$-proteinase inhibitor (human), 69-70
alprazolam, 17
alprostadil, 71-72
alteplase, 47, 48, 72-75
Ambenonium overdose, pralidoxime for, 604
AmBisome, 98

t refers to a table.

COMMON CALCULATIONS

$$\text{body surface area in m}^2 = \sqrt{\frac{\text{height in cm} \times \text{weight in kg}}{3{,}600}}$$

$$\text{mcg/ml} = \text{mg/ml} \times 1{,}000$$

$$\text{ml/minute} = \frac{\text{ml/hour}}{60}$$

$$\text{gtt/minute} = \frac{\text{volume in ml to be infused}}{\text{time in minutes}} \times \text{drip factor in gtt/ml}$$

$$\text{mg/minute} = \frac{\text{mg in bag}}{\text{ml in bag}} \times \text{flow rate} \div 60$$

$$\text{mcg/minute} = \frac{\text{mg in bag}}{\text{ml in bag}} \div 0.06 \times \text{flow rate}$$

$$\text{mcg/kg/minute} = \frac{\text{mcg/ml} \times \text{ml/minute}}{\text{weight in kilograms}}$$